Abrams Angiography

Vascular and Interventional Radiology

Abrams Angiography

Vascular and Interventional Radiology

THIRD EDITION

HERBERT L. ABRAMS, M.D.
Editor

Philip H. Cook Professor of Radiology, Harvard Medical School;
Chairman of Radiology, Brigham and Women's Hospital and
Sidney Farber Cancer Institute, Boston

Volume II

Little, Brown and Company   Boston

TO MARILYN

Contents

Volume I

Volume II

IV. The Abdomen and Pelvis
SECTION 1. LUMBAR AORTOGRAPHY

Volume III

V. The Extremities
SECTION 1. ANGIOGRAPHY OF THE
EXTREMITIES

VI. Interventional Techniques
SECTION 1. ANGIOPLASTY

SECTION 2. OCCLUSIVE AND
INFUSION TECHNIQUES

Notice

The indications and dosages of all drugs in this book have been recommended in the medical literature and conform to the practices of the general medical community. The medications described do not necessarily have specific approval by the Food and Drug Administration for use in the diseases and dosages for which they are recommended. The package insert for each drug should be consulted for use and dosage as approved by the FDA. Because standards for usage change, it is advisable to keep abreast of revised recommendations, particularly those concerning new drugs.

IV

The Abdomen
and Pelvis

1. Lumbar Aortography

The Normal Abdominal Aorta

ELLIOT O. LIPCHIK
STANLEY M. ROGOFF

Because most patients studied by lumbar aortography are in the age group in which arteriosclerosis is common, the normal lumbar aortogram has rarely been seen in our radiology department.

Figures 45-1 and 45-2 are diagrammatic representations of the normal aorta, based, in part, on the original aortographic experiences of Muller and Figley [11]. The diagrams express the maximum pattern of vascular identification that reasonably can be expected from aortography. The reader must recognize that two-dimensional roentgenograms exposed under varying clinical and technical conditions cannot result in confident identification of all diagrammed vessels. The so-called typical textbook patterns are seen in a very slight majority of cases. Major and minor variations and aberrations should be expected. The details of anatomical structure beyond those given here may be obtained from Michels' text [10] and from other sources [12, 13].

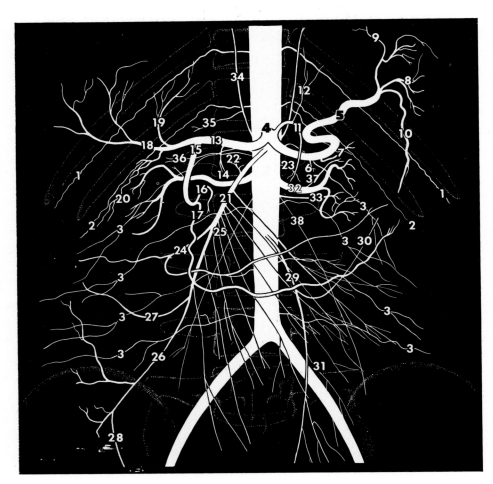

Figure 45-1. Radiographic anatomy of the abdominal aorta. Arteries: *1*, intercostals; *2*, subcostals; *3*, lumbar; *4*, celiac; *5*, splenic; *6*, dorsal pancreatic; *7*, pancreatica magna; *8*, terminal branches to spleen; *9*, short gastric; *10*, left gastroepiploic; *11*, left gastric; *12*, esophageal; *13*, common hepatic; *14*, right gastric; *15*, gastroduodenal; *16*, anterosuperior pancreaticoduodenal; *17*, right gastroepiploic; *18*, right hepatic; *19*, left hepatic; *20*, cystic; *21*, superior mesenteric; *22*, inferior pancreaticoduodenal; *23*, inferior pancreatic; *24*, middle colic; *25*, intestinal; *26*, ileocolic; *27*, right colic; *28*, appendiceal; *29*, inferior mesenteric; *30*, left colic; *31*, sigmoid; *32*, renal; *33*, accessory renal; *34*, inferior phrenic; *35*, superior suprarenal; *36*, middle suprarenal; *37*, inferior suprarenal; *38*, internal spermatic or ovarian. (From Muller and Figley [11]. Reproduced by permission from *AJR*.)

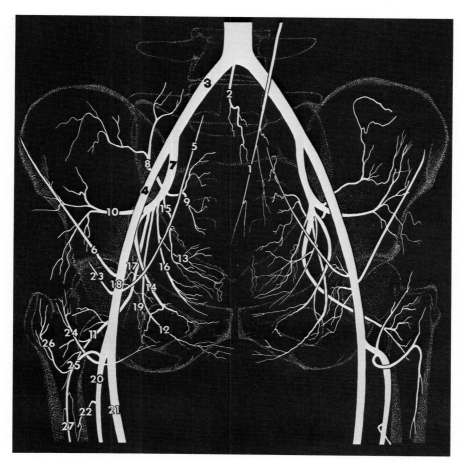

Figure 45-2. Radiographic anatomy of the arteries of the pelvis. Arteries: *1,* superior hemorrhoidal; *2,* middle sacral; *3,* common iliac; *4,* external iliac; *5,* inferior epigastric; *6,* deep circumflex; *7,* internal iliac; *8,* iliolumbar; *9,* lateral sacral; *10,* superior gluteal; *11,* inferior gluteal; *12,* internal pudendal; *13,* middle hemorrhoidal; *14,* obturator; *15,* uterine; *16,* vesical; *17,* superficial epigastric; *18,* common femoral; *19,* external pudendal; *20,* deep femoral (profunda femoris); *21,* superficial femoral; *22,* perforator; *23,* superficial circumflex iliac; *24,* medial femoral circumflex; *25,* lateral femoral circumflex; *26,* lateral femoral circumflex, ascending; *27,* lateral femoral circumflex, descending. (From Muller and Figley [11]. Reproduced by permission from *AJR.*)

Radiographic Anatomy of the Abdominal Aorta

The abdominal aorta begins as it emerges through the diaphragm and ends at its bifurcation into the common iliac arteries. It usually lies either directly on the anterior aspect of the vertebral column or slightly to the left. In severe kyphosis, the aorta follows a normal course, closely associated with the spine, until it reaches the area of deformity, where it bridges the apex of the kyphosis [15]. In this condition and in other vertebral body maldevelopments, the aorta may be shorter than normal.

In thin individuals, the anterior wall of the aorta is surprisingly near the abdominal wall and so may be mistaken for an aneurysm by the neophyte examiner. Too heavy pressure on the stethoscope may also induce "murmurs."

Values for the size of the lumen of the aorta in normal adult patients have been suggested [7, 8]. The internal diameter at the xiphoid level should be about 25 mm and it should decrease to approximately 15 mm at the bifurcation. While the limits of normal are quite broad, any *increase* in the size of the distal lumen is abnormal (see Chap. 48). The diameter should not exceed 30 mm.

At the bifurcation of the normal human aorta into the iliac arteries, there is a mean *decrease* in the size of the vascular bed by a factor of 0.77, which is counter to the *increase* in cross-sectional area that is seen at bifurcations elsewhere in the body [1].

Character and Course of Vessels

Normal main-stem vessels generally have smooth walls and either a straight or a smoothly curving course. Their caliber should be regular and subtly diminishing (Figs. 45-3, 45-4). Any deviations from this norm, such as notching or nicks in the wall of the vessel, are usually an indication of atheromatous change. Beading or slight saccular dilatations are evidence of arteriosclerosis, as is a serpentine course in the main-stem artery (see Chap. 48).

Minor variations in the opacity of a main-stem vessel can be a sign that atheromatous plaques compromise its anteroposterior diameter. This condition is difficult to diagnose unless the contrast is of generally high quality.

Figure 45-3. Normal retrograde femoral aortoarteriogram in a 37-year-old woman. Note the gradually diminishing caliber of the main-stem vessels, the smooth contours of the major vessels, and the gentle curves of the femoral arteries. The slight narrowing of the right common femoral artery is due to vessel spasm about the catheter at the puncture site.

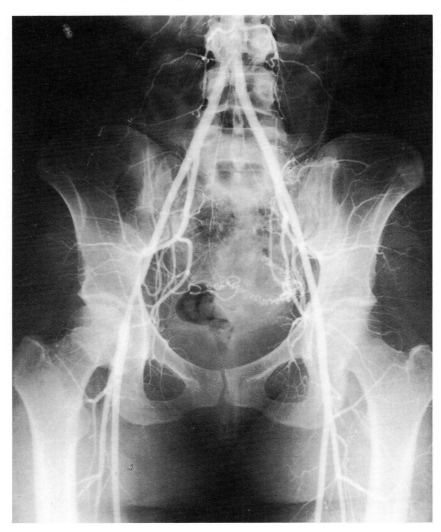

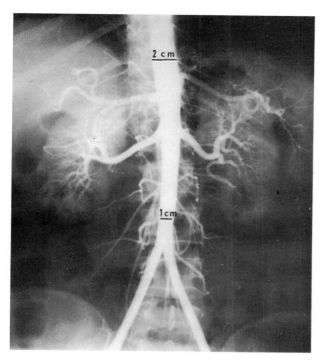

Figure 45-4. Normal abdominal aortoarteriogram in a 40-year-old woman. The diameter of the aorta above the level of the renal and visceral arteries is significantly wider than it is below these vessels. The celiac artery and the first portion of the superior mesenteric artery are obscured by the contrast-filled aorta.

The visceral and parietal branches of the main-stem vessels need not appear smooth walled or smoothly curving in order to be considered normal. They are frequently serpentine and kinked in the normal course of their distributions. They should, however, show a regular diminution in caliber toward their peripheries to be considered normal.

As an aid in the identification of any visceral or parietal branch, it is useful to search the radiograph in the general region of the known parenchymal or organic distributions and then to work back from that point toward the origin. Topographic anatomy has become more important with the increasing use of ultrasonography and computed tomography.

In the rest of the chapter, the numbers in parentheses that follow the names of the arteries refer to numbers in either Figure 45-1 or 45-2, whichever one is appropriate for the area under discussion.

CELIAC ARTERY

The first major branch of the abdominal aorta is the celiac artery, which branches on the ventral surface of the aorta at the superior level of the first lumbar vertebra (Fig. 45-5). Classically, but by no means in all cases, this large trunk divides close to its origin into three major subdivisions: splenic (5), common hepatic (13), and left gastric (11). The inferior phrenic artery (34) often arises from the celiac artery.

The splenic artery provides the dorsal pancreatic artery (6), near its origin, the pancreatica magna in its distal third (7), and then the left gastroepiploic (10) and, frequently, the numerous short gastric arteries (9) before ending in terminal branches to the spleen (8). An inferior pancreatic branch may arise from the dorsal pancreatic artery. The splenic artery is one of the first arteries in the body to show arteriosclerotic changes. The splenic artery lies on the craniodor-

Figure 45-5. Normal retrograde abdominal aortogram, lateral projection, in a 62-year-old woman. Note the ventral origin of the celiac and superior mesenteric arteries and the anterolateral origin of the renal arteries (*), which appear foreshortened and posteriorly arched in this projection. The paired lumbar arteries are also opacified.

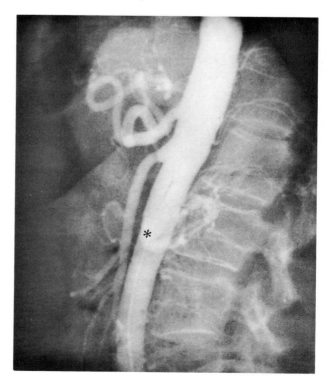

sal surface of the body and tail of the pancreas. The splenic vein is just caudal to the artery.

The common hepatic artery distributes the small right gastric (14) and larger gastroduodenal (15) arteries, which arise, usually in that order, at nearly right angles from the parent vessel, although their origins may be reversed. The position of the stomach influences the direction of the right gastric artery. Near its origin, the gastroduodenal artery, which courses ventral to the head of the pancreas, contributes to the posterosuperior pancreaticoduodenal artery and then descends to terminate in the small anterosuperior pancreaticoduodenal artery (16) and the larger right gastroepiploic artery (17). The latter is directed inferiorly and to the left along the greater curvature of the stomach to join the left gastroepiploic branch of the splenic artery. The hepatic artery teminates by dividing into the right (18) and left (19) hepatic arteries, the former of which usually provides the cystic artery (20). The main hepatic artery lies ventral to the portal vein.

The left gastric artery is frequently obscured by the contrast-filled aorta and by changes in its position due to the position of the stomach. Often it gives rise to small esophageal branches (12), and occasionally it contributes to the left hepatic circulation.

SUPERIOR MESENTERIC ARTERY

The superior mesenteric artery (21) arises 1 or 2 cm below the celiac artery on the ventral aspect of the aorta at the level of the first lumbar vertebra (Fig. 45-5). The origin of the superior mesenteric artery lies posterior to the body of the pancreas. Its first branch is usually the obscure inferior pancreaticoduodenal artery [22]. The right hepatic artery, or the common hepatic or gastroduodenal arteries, may also arise early in the course of the superior mesenteric artery. From this point on, the wide range of arterial movement that follows that of the mesenteric fan makes even major branches difficult to identify when their position varies with the location of the gut from moment to moment in a living person. This is true in the case of the first major branch of the superior mesenteric artery and the middle colic artery (24), as well as of a widely ranging spray of 12 to 20 intestinal arteries (25). But more distally, the main stem of the superior mesenteric artery points inferiorly and to the

right as it branches into the right colic (27), the ileocolic (26), and the appendiceal (29) arteries.

RENAL ARTERIES

The renal arteries (32) arise approximately opposite each other at the level of the lower first lumbar or the upper second lumbar vertebra about 2 cm below the superior mesenteric artery from the lateral (often anterolateral) aspect of the aorta. The right renal artery courses posteriorly to the inferior vena cava.

In about 20 percent of people, multiple renal arteries occur, more often on the left. Most frequently they arise from the aorta below the main artery although their origin may also be above the main renal artery or even aberrantly from the iliac arteries [2]. They usually enter the kidney parenchyma at its nearest point instead of accompanying the main artery into the hilum.

Excessively straight, rigid, and somewhat caudad-directed arteries probably indicate arteriosclerotic changes even if no narrowing is apparent. A mild right posterior oblique position of the supine patient may be most helpful in depicting the origins of the renal arteries during aortography in a hypertensive patient [6]. Perhaps this is so partly because of the rotation of the abdominal aorta in such a patient.

Immediately below the renal artery origins, the aorta abruptly becomes significantly narrower (see Figs. 45-1–45-4). This is a normal occurrence following the origin of the large visceral branches, and it must not be overinterpreted as a sign of atherosclerosis or thrombosis.

INFERIOR MESENTERIC ARTERY

The inferior mesenteric artery (29), which originates at the second to third lumbar vertebra level of the aorta on its ventral aspect, is much smaller than the superior mesenteric artery. Its course is usually downward and almost parallel to the aorta on its left. It soon gives rise to the main left colic artery (30), which bifurcates into *prominent* ascending and descending divisions. These are, therefore, inaccurately displayed in the schematic diagram. It also contributes sigmoid branches (31) before terminating in the pelvis as the superior hemorrhoidal artery (1) (see Fig. 45-2). Neither the arcade among the sigmoid and left colic branches nor the arcade between the middle

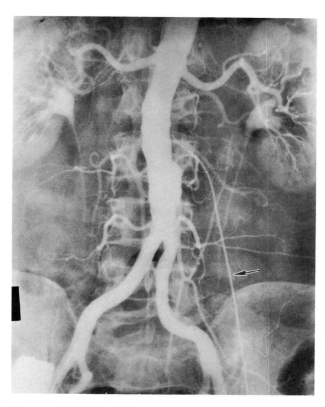

Figure 45-6. The left spermatic artery (*arrow*) is well opacified in this aortogram of a 64-year-old man examined for a thoracic aortic aneurysm. The small aneurysm of the abdominal aorta was unsuspected.

and left colic is depicted in Figures 45-1 and 45-2.

PAIRED LATERAL BRANCHES

The inferior phrenic arteries (*34*) usually arise high on the abdominal aorta just above or lateral to the celiac artery, and they course sharply upward along the diaphragmatic crura. They often spring from a common trunk from the aorta or the celiac axis [9]. The suprarenal or adrenal circulation is contributed by the superior suprarenal arteries (*35*) (branches of the inferior phrenic arteries), the middle suprarenal arteries (*36*) (usually arising from the aorta), and, the largest and most important vessels, the inferior suprarenal arteries (*37*) (originating from the renal arteries) [5].

Originating just below the renal arteries or, occasionally, from the renal arteries themselves are the internal spermatic (testicular) or ovarian arteries (*38*). The long, curved descent of these delicate vessels is accentuated by their lack of branches and their direct course. They are only infrequently opacified (Fig. 45-6).

SEGMENTAL BRANCHES

The segmental branches include the paired intercostal (*1*) and the subcostal arteries (*2*); they also include the four pairs of lumbar arteries (*3*), whose pattern is established on an aortogram by their characteristic association with the lateral margins of the upper four lumbar vertebral segments. The fifth lumbar arteries arise from the middle sacral artery.

MAJOR ANTERIOR RADICULAR ARTERY TO THE SPINAL CORD

This vessel (the artery of Adamkiewicz) may arise from spinal branches from the eighth intercostal to the second lumbar artery, most frequently on the left [4]. It can be clearly identified by selective angiography but rarely by aortography. This important vessel may be perfused heavily during aortography, which could account for many of the earlier neurologic complications of aortography that occurred when more toxic substances were used [14]. Other cervical and thoracic vessels also supply the anterior spinal cord [4].

Radiographic Anatomy of the Arteries of the Pelvis

RIGHT AND LEFT COMMON ILIAC ARTERIES

The abdominal aorta usually terminates at the level of the fourth lumbar vertebra, bifurcating into the right and the left common iliac arteries (*3*). In Figure 45-2, the middle sacral artery (*2*)—the last aortic branch—can be seen at the bifurcation; the fifth lumbar arteries may arise from this vessel. The superior hemorrhoidal artery (*1*), the termination of the inferior mesenteric artery, is also depicted in its descent to the rectum.

The common iliac arteries have only obscure peritoneal, psoas, ureteric, and areolar branches as a rule. However, they may give rise to displaced renal arteries or to the iliolumbar artery, which normally arises from the internal iliac (hypogastric) artery. Because of radiographic distortion, the common iliac arteries appear to branch after a varying distance of 2 to 6 cm at a level from the fifth lumbar to the low first sacral vertebra. The main-stem vessel on each side continues as the larger external iliac artery (4) from the point at which the smaller internal iliac trunk (7) originates.

EXTERNAL ILIAC ARTERY

The external iliac artery curves smoothly down across the lateral sacrum and sacroiliac joint and near the iliopectineal line of the pelvic inlet. Its course is quite ventral as well as inferior and slightly lateral. Because the radiographic beam may not cross it at right angles, it can appear shorter than its true length on the radiograph.

Just above the level of the inguinal ligament, usually from a point projected in the highest level of the hip joint space, the external iliac artery gives rise to (1) the deep circumflex iliac artery (6), which ascends in a fairly straight oblique line, superiorly and laterally, and (2) the inferior epigastric artery (5), which shows a smooth, curved ascent superiorly and medially. In a normal person, these branches are prominent. At this point, the main-stem vessel continues for a distance of 2 to 5 cm below the inguinal ligament as the common femoral artery (18).

COMMON FEMORAL ARTERY

The common femoral artery gives rise laterally to a sometimes obscure superficial circumflex iliac vessel (23) and medially to the equally obscure superficial epigastric artery (17) and deep and superficial external pudendal branches (19).

The main-stem artery becomes the femoral artery (21) at a point where it gives rise to the deep femoral (profunda femoris) branch (20). This point may be appreciably higher than depicted in the diagram. In practice, the femoral artery is often referred to as the *superficial* femoral artery, to distinguish it from the *deep* femoral artery. The femoral artery descends along the medial thigh in a shallow, smooth curve, sending out only small muscular branches until it reaches the level just above the adductor canal. At this point, it gives rise medially to the highest genicular artery before continuing as the popliteal artery.

DEEP FEMORAL ARTERY

The deep femoral artery originates from the common femoral artery as a large branch of the main-stem vessel at the level of the bony landmark of the femoral head. Its exact origin is frequently obscured on the radiograph because it overlaps with the shadow of the main femoral channel. In patients with iliac artery thrombosis, its higher branches are important effluent collateral vessels, from vessels in the abdomen and pelvis (see Chap. 48). Its lower branches are indispensable as affluent collateral vessels around occlusions of the femoral or popliteal system.

The deep femoral artery descends laterally and inferiorly. Near its origin it provides the small medial femoral circumflex artery (24), which branches laterally and superiorly along the trochanteric line of the femoral neck and medially and superiorly toward the obturator foramen. The larger lateral circumflex branch (25) of the deep femoral artery has important ascending (26) and descending (27) components.

INTERNAL ILIAC ARTERY

The branches of the internal iliac (hypogastric) artery (7) are quite variable [3]. On a lateral or an oblique roentgenogram, its main anterior and posterior divisions might be seen, but this spatial relationship is not obvious on the usual frontal projection. The posterior trunk early in its course gives rise to one or two lateral sacral arteries (9), which, in turn, furnish the segmental branches to the sacral foramina, which can be seen (unlabeled) in Figure 45-2. Next, the posterior division furnishes the iliolumbar branch (8) with its iliac and lumbar ramifications. The posterior trunk continues in a transverse or horizontal course through the greater sciatic notch as the superior gluteal artery (10).

The anterior trunk of the internal iliac artery contributes the remaining pelvic arteries. The obturator artery (14) may be identified by tracing back from its terminal branches encircling the obturator foramen. This vessel frequently arises from the inferior epigastric, the deep circumflex iliac, or the external iliac artery. The internal pudendal artery (12) usually crosses the obturator foramen inferior to the obturator artery and terminates with fine branches in the scrotum or labia. The inferior gluteal artery (11) originates with either the superior gluteal or the internal pudendal artery. Its laterally descending course parallels the axis of the femoral neck, and it is often projected over the bone or, as shown in Figure 45-2, just medial to it.

The middle hemorrhoidal (*13*) and vesical (*16*) arteries are quite obscure and inconstant in position. The uterine artery (*15*) comes off high on the anterior trunk and may be identified by its coiled terminal azygos branches in the uterus and vagina. (See Chap. 73 for additional details of pelvic arterial anatomy.)

ACKNOWLEDGMENTS

We appreciate the clinical material and advice of Charles Rob, M.D., and James DeWeese, M.D., of the Departments of Surgery at the East Carolina University School of Medicine, North Carolina, and the University of Rochester, New York, respectively. Frank E. Maddison, M.D., of the Medical College of Wisconsin, also was most kind in supplying case material. We appreciate also the assistance of Mrs. Lois Wahlers in the preparation of this chapter and Chapters 46, 48, and 49.

References

1. Beales, J. S. M., and Steiner, R. E.   Radiological assessment of arterial branching coefficients. *Cardiovasc. Res.* 6:181, 1972.
2. Boijsen, E.   Angiographic studies of the anatomy of single and multiple renal arteries. *Acta Radiol. [Suppl.]* (Stockh.) 183:1, 1959.
3. Braithwaite, J. L.   Variations in origins of parietal branches of internal iliac artery. *J. Anat.* 86:423, 1952.
4. DiChiro, G., Doppman, J., and Ommaya, A. K.   Selective arteriography of arteriovenous aneurysms of spinal cord. *Radiology* 88:1065, 1967.
5. Edsman, G.   Angionephrography and suprarenal angiography. *Acta Radiol. [Suppl.]* (Stockh.) 155:1, 1957.
6. Gerlock, A. J., Goncharenko, V., and Sloan, O. M.   Right posterior oblique: The projection of choice in aortography of hypertensive patients. *Radiology* 127:45, 1978.
7. Goldberg, B. B., and Lehman, J. S.   Aortosonography: Ultrasound measurement of the abdominal and thoracic aorta. *Arch. Surg.* 100:652, 1970.
8. Goldberg, B. B., Ostrum, B. J., and Isard, H. J.   Ultrasonic aortography. *J.A.M.A.* 198:353, 1966.
9. Merklin, R. J. and Michels, N. A.   The variant renal and suprarenal blood supply with data on the inferior phrenic, ureteral and gonadal arteries. *J. Int. Coll. Surg.* 29:41, 1958.
10. Michels, N. A.   *Blood Supply and Anatomy of the Upper Abdominal Organs with a Descriptive Atlas.* Philadelphia: Lippincott, 1955.
11. Muller, R. F., and Figley, M. M.   The arteries of the abdomen, pelvis, and thigh. *AJR* 77:296, 1957.
12. Nebesar, R. A., Kornblith, P. L., Pollard, J. J., and Michels, N. A.   *Celiac and Superior Mesenteric Arteries: A Correlation of Angiograms and Dissections.* Boston: Little, Brown, 1969.
13. Reuter, S. R., and Redman, H. C.   *Gastrointestinal Angiography.* Philadelphia: Saunders, 1972.
14. Tarazi, A. K., Margolis, G., and Grimson, K. S.   Spinal cord lesions produced by aortography in dogs. *Arch. Surg.* 72:38, 1956.
15. Watt, I., and Park, W. M.   Abdominal aorta in spina bifida cystica. *Clin. Radiol.* 29:63, 1978.

Abdominal Aortography: Translumbar, Femoral, and Axillary Artery Catheterization Techniques

ELLIOT O. LIPCHIK
STANLEY M. ROGOFF

Translumbar aortography is a relatively fast, safe, and easy procedure for contrast visualization of the aorta and its lower branches. The angiographer should be well versed in both catheter placement and translumbar techniques; the patient and his problem are paramount, and the best (and safest) technique should be used. In most instances percutaneous catheterization is applicable, whether it is done through the femoral or the axillary arteries. With the availability of the J-shaped catheter [6] and curved-tip and floppy guidewires [44], most arterial tortuosities, plaques, and partial obstructions can be easily negotiated. If the femoral arteries are obstructed and if catheter placement there is impossible, we believe that left axillary artery percutaneous catheterization is the next method of choice [23, 40, 43]. However, there still remain a group of patients who have diffuse arterial occlusive disease or severe atherosclerotic changes and tortuosity that may prevent catheterization. In this group of patients we prefer translumbar aortography rather than intravenous aortography or the more complicated catheter techniques via subclavian [3] or brachial arteriotomy.

The most frequent use of aortography is in the study of atherosclerosis and arteriosclerosis of the aorta and the iliofemoral arteries. It almost always precedes vascular surgery. Many cardiac surgeons request an anatomic roadmap of the aortoiliac system before the possible insertion of an intraaortic balloon assist pump. Other diagnostic indications for aortography preliminary to selective visceral and renal angiography will be discussed in other chapters. Aneurysms will be discussed in Chapter 49.

In the following discussion, translumbar aortography is discussed first. Many of the details of patient preparation and aftercare, equipment, and filming are applicable to femoral and axillary artery catheterizations also and so, therefore, will not be repeated in the sections discussing these techniques.

Translumbar Aortography

Translumbar aortography was first described by the brilliant Portuguese surgeon Reynaldo dos Santos in 1929 [16, 17]. While dos Santos was experimenting with lumbar ganglionic blockade, on several occasions he accidentally punctured a human aorta. Noting the generally benign and uncomplicated nature of these invasions, dos

Santos undertook deliberate aortic puncture, apparently with the intention of using this daring route for parenteral drug therapy.

By 1937 dos Santos had performed 1,000 translumbar aortograms. With the development of the translumbar technique, a major psychologic barrier to the performance of aortography had been cleared. The lack of a suitably benign, easily injectable, and densely opaque contrast substance, however, was a major factor in the failure of this diagnostic procedure to receive unqualified approval during the 20 years following its initial appearance.

In 1936, the surgeons Henline and Moore performed experiments on 21 dogs in anticipation of using aortography in human beings [27]. By the percutaneous translumbar approach and also under direct vision, they injected relatively large volumes of sodium iodide, Skiodan, Uroselectan B, Thorotrast, and Iopax into the aorta above the renal arteries in 19 animals. After percutaneous puncture the animals were rolled onto their backs with the needle in place and they were x-rayed. The authors' description of the dogs' uncontrollable bleeding, renal damage, clonic spasm of the hindquarters, and high mortality was succinct but spectacular.

The work of Henline and Moore, as well as disparaging remarks from other quarters about the technique [5], discouraged the performance of human lumbar aortography in the United States until 1942, when Nelson reported 73 relatively successful lumbar aortograms [39]. Soon thereafter, Doss, a urologic surgeon, and his coworkers described their experience with 70 percent Diodrast for renal arteriography [14]. It then became clear that lumbar aortography was applicable to all diseases and abnormalities involving the renal arteries and kidneys. World War II interrupted this work, but interest was quickly revived in 1946 by Wagner [49] and by Melick and Vitt [35].

In 1947, fortune provided a particularly sweet and final justification for Reynaldo dos Santos' tenacious faith in the clinical value of aortography. His own son, J. Cid dos Santos, reported the first successful thromboendarterectomy before the Académie de Chirurgie on June 4 [15]. Nine months later, Luis Bazy independently described the same operation in the belief that he was its originator. A new horizon unfolded for patients whose comfort and existence were threatened by arteriosclerosis and other diseases

of the large and small vessels, and experience with the method burgeoned.

CONTRAINDICATIONS TO TRANSLUMBAR AORTOGRAPHY

Contraindications to translumbar aortography are:

1. Hemorrhagic diathesis or anticoagulation therapy leading to prothrombin levels below 30 percent of control values.
2. Urticaria and other benign allergic manifestations to contrast material. This is a relatively minor contraindication. Premedication with steroids before the procedure may be of help in patients with a previous history of an anaphylactic response to contrast medium [1, 52].
3. Local infection at the puncture site.
4. Presence of a definable aneurysm at or near the projected site of puncture. However, all workers have (at times) inadvertently punctured aneurysms without untoward sequelae. Heavy calcification in the aorta is not an absolute contraindication for translumbar aortic puncture. In our experience heavy calcification has not been associated with a higher risk of complication.
5. Advanced cardiorenal disease. In general, translumbar aortography should not be performed in patients whose poor physical status precludes surgical exploration. Patients with recent myocardial infarctions or renal disease may fall into this category. The severely ill and dehydrated patient is a poor risk for angiography by any route. (Other contraindications to angiographic procedures are given in Chap. 2.)

PRECAUTIONS

Certain simple precautions, such as proper hydration and avoidance of too large doses of contrast medium, should always be taken. There is special risk to the dehydrated patient with diabetes mellitus, azotemia, or multiple myeloma [1]. An intravenous infusion of low-molecular-weight dextran or mannitol might be started just prior to and/or after the study *in selected cases,* such as the diabetic patient who also has renal dysfunction. Precautions to take in other pathologic conditions, such as multiple myeloma and gout, are discussed in Chapter 2.

TECHNIQUE OF TRANSLUMBAR AORTOGRAPHY

The translumbar approach is technically simple, easy to teach, and diagnostically reliable, and throughout the years it has been comparatively free of complications [13, 24]. It belongs in the armamentarium of vascular radiologists.

Preparation of the Patient

The following points should be considered in preparation of the patient for translumbar aortography:

1. The importance of a careful history and physical examination is so obvious that no further comment is needed.
2. Informed consent is now universal in the United States. In our hospital, a radiologist, preferably the one who is to do the procedure, obtains the consent. There is a growing consensus that the anxieties and fears of the patient contribute significantly to contrast-media reactions and that improperly obtained informed consents may heighten this anxiety state [13, 30].
3. Dehydration is to *be avoided*. Bowel preparation is not required unless barium remains in the gut. Solid foods should not be eaten at least 6 hours before the examination; a clear liquid diet is suggested instead.
4. The angiography room should be equipped with all the apparatus and medications needed for emergency treatment of untoward reactions. The medication tray should be checked daily, and all equipment should be tested periodically. Oxygen and suction apparatus should be within easy reach. An electrocardiograph and defibrillator are probably mandatory standby equipment in all special procedure areas. An intravenous infusion is recommended to provide an immediately available route for emergency supportive measures.
5. Premedications may vary, depending on the patient and the experience and training of the physicians. Ordinarily, 5 to 10 mg of Valium administered intramuscularly or intravenously just before or during the examination suffices. Demerol and morphine are to be avoided be-

cause they may induce hypotension and pre dispose to vasovagal reactions. General anes thesia is very rarely needed; proper loca analgesia and psychologic support for the pa tient offered in the most pleasant and gentl but firm way possible are more than adequat for most patients [30, 41]. Atropine is a ver valuable drug to have at hand.

6. Use of a test dose of contrast material ad ministered intravenously or intradermally ha no scientific basis and is not recommended There is no evidence that such a test has valu in predicting major allergic or idiosyncrati reactions [22].
7. Preliminary radiographs of the abdomen (wit the patient prone) often help estimate th presence and level of an unsuspected an eurysm and demonstrate possible difficultie in approaching the aorta. These films com plement the aortographic examination, per mitting a more accurate definition of the are as well as defining the technical quality of th study.

Positioning of the Patient

The patient lies prone. A small pad is place under the dorsa of the feet to raise the toe comfortably off the table. Conveniently, the toe point inward and the relaxed heels rotate out ward, resulting in an internal oblique projectio of the calf and knee (Fig. 46-1). This produces

Figure 46-1. Internal rotation of the feet and lowe legs with the patient prone during long-film translum bar aortoarteriography projects the popliteal arter trifurcation within the interosseous space. A small pa under the dorsa of the feet raises the toes comfortabl off the table.

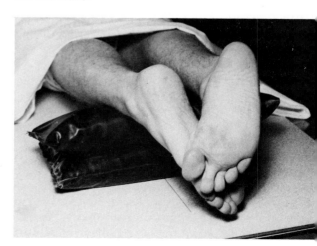

lear picture of the interosseous space and has proved helpful in showing greater detail in the three major arteries of the calf.

Needle, Tubing, and Syringes

An 18-gauge Teflon needle catheter approximately 18 to 24 cm (8–10 inches) in length is preferred [2, 9, 47] because its flexibility prevents damage to the aortic wall if the patient moves. The catheter can be used with a pressure injector. The tip of the catheter's Teflon sleeve should be safely positioned upstream or downstream to prevent intimal disruption or plaque dislodgment [2, 38]. Because the Teflon sleeve bends easily, replacement of the inner metal sharp guidewire is hazardous after the sleeve is in position. We perform all our translumbar studies with this type of needle and flexible guidewire.

Flexible transparent tubing is connected to the needle. The tubing should be as short as possible; the force necessary to accomplish injection will increase in proportion to the length of tubing in the system following an immutable law of hydrodynamics. Luer-Lok fittings are used on all syringes, tubing, and needles to prevent the joints from opening during injection.

Needle Approach to the Aorta

With the use of a flexible Teflon needle, it is no longer necessary to use different puncture sites for *high* (suprarenal) and *low* (infrarenal) injections. With the patient lying prone and the operator standing to the patient's left, the twelfth left thoracic rib is located by palpation or fluoroscopy. The skin is entered 2 cm below the inferior margin of this rib, 8 to 12 cm to the left of the midline (spinous processes). After local anesthesia is administered and a small stab is made in the skin with a #11 blade, the needle with its stylet is advanced ventrally through the muscular mass so that it points at the vental margin of the second to third lumbar vertebral body (Fig. 46-2).

When it is reasonably certain that the anterolateral margin of the body has been struck by the needle point, the position of the needle must be changed slightly. This is done carefully by withdrawal and minimal redirection of the shaft so that the point is directed slightly more ventrad. The aorta is in close approximation to the anterior and lateral aspect of the vertebral body.

As the point of the needle begins to touch the adventitial wall of the aorta, the aorta's pulsation

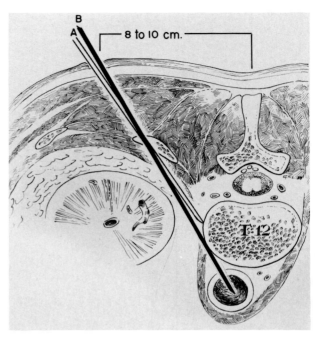

Figure 46-2. Transverse section of prone patient during left lumbar approach to abdominal aorta. The white needle (*A*) indicates the course the needle takes to meet the vertebral body. The black needle (*B*) shows repositioning of the needle to have it slide along the margin into the aorta. It is often necessary to begin 10 to 12 cm to the left of the midline. T12 is illustrated but see text for proper needle approach.

may occasionally be felt. The aortic wall should then be penetrated with a short, controlled stab of the needle for about 1 cm. With experience it is possible to puncture the aorta *without* first engaging the vertebral body. The object is to enter the vessel at the level of the second to third lumbar vertebral body in order to opacify the inferior mesenteric artery but to avoid deliberate injection of the renal, superior mesenteric, or anterior radicular spinal arteries [31]. Slight cephalad or caudad angulation of needle is needed to place the Teflon sheath for, respectively, retrograde and antegrade injections of contrast medium.

Puncture

As the needle pierces the wall of the aorta, a snap, a click, or a release of tension can be felt. The wall can be disconcertingly thick and resistant due to arteriosclerosis or thrombosis. On the needle's accurate entrance into the lumen, a pulsatile flow of blood emerges from the hilt of the needle. In general, the flow at the hilt of the needle is not exceptionally dramatic or ejaculatory; rather it is often only a hurried drip.

Under fluoroscopic control, a curved-tip guidewire is advanced cephalad or caudad through the catheter and into the aorta. The sheath is then guided into the lumen of the aorta over the guidewire.

The flexible transparent tubing is now firmly attached to the needle and connected to the saline drip infusion. With this liquid system in place, it will become apparent quickly whether the aorta has been punctured successfully because blood will invariably pump into the tubing in puffs or spurts no matter how weak the stream from the naked needle hilt seemed to be. The patency of the needle and the accuracy of its position should always be tested with small injections of contrast medium under film or fluoroscopic guidance.

With the flexible Teflon sheath in place, the patient can then be moved easily and without risk into oblique or lateral positions.

Opaque Substance

Any of the newer contrast agents may be safely used. The higher iodine concentrations provide the best density but are significantly more viscous than the iodine compounds of lower concentrations, and so they cause more pain. The intraarterial injection of lidocaine either before or mixed with the contrast medium (1–2 mg/cc of contrast medium) provides significant relief of pain in most patients [26, 27, 49]. Unfortunately, a small percentage of patients still experience severe pain during aortofemoral angiography. Lidocaine should be used only in the lower aorta and in peripheral arteriography. Because lidocaine floats on the contrast material, the injector should be upright or the lidocaine should be mixed thoroughly with the contrast medium. (See Chap. 2 for further discussion of contrast material.)

Filming

In most adult patients, the 14-×-17-inch film can provide detail from the level of the second lumbar body to the common femoral bifurcation.

Serial examinations are always an advantage in dynamic studies of flow and collateral circulation. Homemade film tunnels permitting "slow serialization" are still useful because arterial flow is usually sluggish in atherooclusive disease. Arteries distal to blocked segments maintain their contrast density over many seconds because of the relatively slow flow through collateral systems. Patients with an aneurysm or with so-called polyaneurysmal dystrophy have very slow transit times.

The film timing sequence is *not* crucial if the concepts of blood flow physiology just described are understood. Huge amounts of contrast medium are not needed to opacify the aorta. Twenty-five to 30 cc injected at a rate of 8 to 12 cc per second gives excellent opacification of the lumbar area and allows the use of small-diameter catheters. Somewhat more contrast medium would be needed for good visualization of the origins of the visceral arteries.

If femoral arteriography with visualization of peripheral runoff is the goal, 50 to 75 cc at 8 to 10 cc per second is more than adequate for the contrast medium to replace the blood in a *slow-flowing* system. If the injection lasts 5 to 7 seconds, and the appearance time at the popliteal artery trifurcation is 5 to 7 seconds from the start of the injection, there is a leeway of at least 5 seconds between film exposures.

An all too common misjudgment, particularly of inexperienced angiographers, involves injecting a large contrast bolus very rapidly and then missing the peak concentration of the bolus as it progresses distally. Studies performed in younger patients with little arteriosclerosis, and studies in which postreactive hyperemia is induced, are indications for faster filming since blood flow is relatively faster, often by a factor of two [28] in such cases. Conversely, serial exposures prolonged for 15 to 20 seconds may be necessary in severely atherosclerotic-diseased patients to detect popliteal branches, and up to 40 seconds may be required to see the vessels of the ankle and foot (see Chap. 48).

Predetermination of the circulation time by any means may help to establish the optimum time for exposure of the radiographs although it is not necessary. The abdominal aorta and iliac vessels are usually fully opacified by the first exposure in 2 to 5 seconds after the beginning of the injection.

RADIOGRAPHIC EQUIPMENT

There are numerous types of commercial film changers, some specifically designed for long-film aortoarteriography. It does not serve to enumerate them; all the major x-ray manufacturing and supply companies have the necessary information.

Modern rotating anode tubes and x-ray generators capable of providing sufficient milliamperage to allow 70 to 85 kV and short exposure times during rapid-sequence filming are requirements for angiographic studies. An oscillating or reciprocating grid of any description is adequate to the task of slow serial filming, but in any case the modern fine-line stationary grid is perfectly suitable. Variable programming from rapid sequences of two films per second to one film every 2 to 5 seconds is highly desirable and often necessary.

If the method chosen involves centering over a 36-inch cassette, the tube stand must permit approximately a 52-inch or longer target-to-film distance to cover the film.

Numerous technical manipulations must be employed to obtain uniform density of long radiographs in one exposure from the abdomen to the lower leg. The anode of the tube should be toward the feet to take advantage of the so-called heel effect. Either multiwedged filters [45] or filters of another geometry [12] should be constructed to compensate for the gradations of thickness of the average patient (Fig. 46-3). If the tabletop or x-ray tube can be moved at a preprogrammed speed, automatic changes of the kilovoltage may be possible. Further enhancement of the quality of the radiographs may be achieved by experimentation with intensifying screens of different speeds and even by experimentation with films of different sensitivities under various body parts [45].

COMPLICATIONS

A more detailed overview of complications following arteriography is to be found in Chapter 47. The translumbar approach has remained, through the years, remarkably free of major complications. Paraaortic hemorrhage is a constant finding, but it rarely has any major clinical

Figure 46-3. Variable-thickness aluminum filters used to compensate for the gradation of thickness (abdomen to lower leg) of most patients and so to achieve homogeneous density along the entire length of the film. (A) Side view of the three filters. The top filter is the standard one used for most patients. The patient's lower extremities correspond with the thicker part and the abdomen and pelvis to the thinner part of the filter. (B) Full-face view to show the brass diaphragm that holds the filters and restricts the x-ray beam to a 14-×-36-inch field at a 52-inch target-to-film distance.

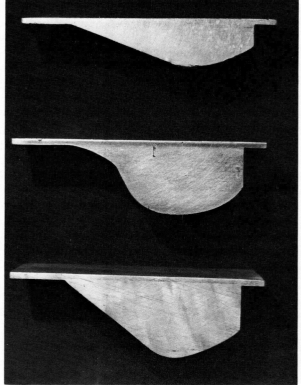

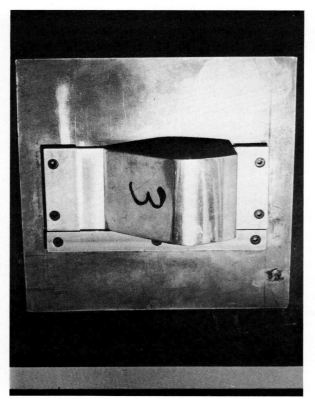

A   *B*

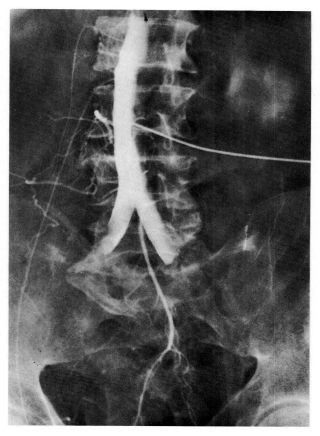

Figure 46-4. Intramural deposition of contrast medium during a translumbar aortogram attempt. The markedly increased density of the contrast medium, the sharply defined proximal and distal edges, and the prolonged holdup in that region are characteristic. There were no clinical sequelae.

sequelae [7, 10]. Figure 46-4 illustrates an intramural deposition, or intravasation, of contrast material.

The total complication rate of translumbar aortography is equal to or perhaps even somewhat less than that of transfemoral aortography [24, 33, 34, 48]. Isolated case reports of such complications as osteomyelitis, dissections, hemothoraces and pneumothoraces, paraplegia, intestinal infarctions, and fatalities are to be found in the literature [21, 32, 34, 38, 51], but these complications rarely occur today, particularly when the Teflon needle/sheath technique is used [24].

AFTERCARE OF PATIENT

Continued hydration is recommended, but induced diuresis is usually not necessary, particularly if only one bolus of contrast material was injected. An excretory urogram is always done after the aortogram as a simple screening test of renal function and anatomy. Most patients show obliteration of the normal psoas muscle margin on the left due to some hemorrhage from the aorta at the puncture site. The patient should be instructed to remain on bed rest for at least 6 to 8 hours and preferably until the next morning. If bleeding is suspected, the usual precautions and checks by both nurses and doctors should be instituted.

Transfemoral Catheterization

As outlined earlier in the chapter, abdominal angiography has had an interesting genesis and history. Angiography as we know and practice it today is a direct extension of the ingenious modification by Seldinger [46] of earlier, more basic techniques. For instance, the first *operative* passage of a catheter (urethral) into the aorta was performed by Fariñas in 1951 [20]. The first person to describe the percutaneous passage of a catheter for angiography was Peirce [42], who punctured the femoral artery with a large-bore needle and threaded a catheter through the needle into the aorta.

TECHNIQUE OF TRANSFEMORAL CATHETERIZATION

Patient preparation, premedication, and precautions are discussed on pages 1030 to 1031. Angiography is to be avoided whenever possible in patients with homocystinuria [37] or homozygous sickle cell disease [1]. The more common contraindications have already been discussed.

Nothing is as conducive to success as experience. Impeccable technique, however, hastens the acquisition of experience; therefore, the emphasis in this chapter is on proper techniques.

The common femoral artery is the safest and most accessible artery for the percutaneous approach. After sterile preparation and draping, the artery is entered below the inguinal ligament, in or near the inguinal crease. The inguinal crease does *not* demarcate the course of the ligament (Fig. 46-5).

Anesthesia is accomplished with the injection of 1 percent lidocaine down to and alongside the vessel wall in the same trajectory that the needle and catheter will follow. The patient will be more comfortable if the subcutaneous layers are infiltrated with lidocaine (via a 25-gauge needle

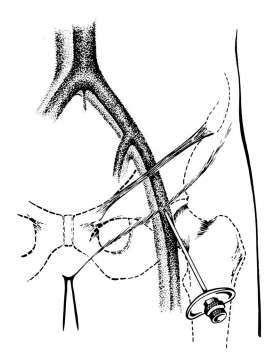

Figure 46-5. Relationship of the femoral arteries, inguinal crease, inguinal ligament, and positioning of the percutaneous needle into the femoral artery.

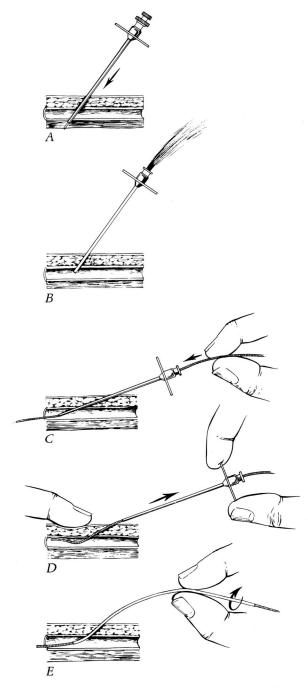

Figure 46-6. Technique for percutaneous catheterization (see text).

fore the intracutaneous wheal is raised. Patients often dread the initial painful intracutaneous needling, but it is hardly noticeable if it is preceded by subcutaneous analgesia. *All aspects of the percutaneous catheterization procedure, except the initial needle puncture, should be pain free.*

A small skin stab with a #11 scalpel blade, followed by spread of the subcutaneous tissues by a small hemostat, allows easier catheter passage. The needle, which need not be larger than an 18 gauge, is directed along the course of the femoral artery at a 45-to-60-degree angle. Arterial pulsations are usually transmitted through the needle. Straddling and fixation of the femoral artery by the index and middle fingers may be necessary in younger patients with mobile vessels, in arteries with very weak pulsations, and occasionally in extremely obese people. With experience, one wall of the common femoral artery can be punctured in most cases, but it is not essential for an uncomplicated procedure (Fig. 46-6A).

The obturator is removed and the needle or Teflon sheath slowly withdrawn while the skin is tamped down by the fingers of the other hand. After the blood spurts from the needle, the needle is lowered to lie more parallel to the skin for the gentle introduction of the guidewire. Lowering the needle while both walls of the vessels are transfixed may damage the posterior wall since the distant part of the needle travels farther than the closer part (Fig. 46-6B, C). Some angiographers advocate advancing the needle into the vessel before insertion of the guidewire. This maneuver may, however, lead to damage of the intima and raising of an intimal flap.

With the guidewire placed intraluminally in the aorta, the needle is removed while hemostasis is maintained with the third, fourth, and fifth fingers and while the thumb and index finger of the same hand hold the guidewire. The catheter is fed over the guidewire into the vessel with minimal rotation (Fig. 46-6C, D, E). The guidewire is most thrombogenic and so should remain in the catheter a minimum of time. If reinsertions of the guidewire are necessary, its surface should be cleaned of all traces of blood.

A curved-tip catheter should be inserted with the curve opened, i.e., with its tip pointed upward, since in this position the compressing finger can help straighten the catheter into the vessel. If the catheter is curved dorsally, the compression may, on the contrary, contribute to further curving and buckling. A short, smaller, and stiffer dilating catheter frequently allows easier passage of the catheter into the vessel, especially through scarred tissue. Figure 46-7 shows and provides a description of a catheter that is most useful in abdominal aortography.

Blood is aspirated from the catheter after the guidewire is removed. A closed-system drip flush is connected with 500 to 1,000 units of heparin per 500 cc of solution. All catheters are also flushed through with this heparinized solution prior to their insertion. Some workers prefer to have the guidewires and catheters "wet" rather than dry since if the guidewire is wiped clean before threading the catheter, the sponge may leave cotton fibers and other debris on the guidewire that can be carried into the vessel by the catheter.

The needle need not be larger than 18 gauge and the guidewires not more than 0.038 inch; the catheters are rarely larger than 7 French. Stiff Teflon catheters are no longer necessary; thin-wall catheters allow a high-enough injection rate for all kinds of study. Larger catheters cause more bleeding and thrombotic complications, and it is our unconfirmed impression that Teflon catheters also are the cause of more frequent femoral artery bleeding.

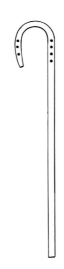

Figure 46-7. Catheter used for most routine abdominal aortograms. *Laterally* placed side holes through one wall at opposing levels in each arm of the catheter give high local bolus concentration of contrast material. (There are more side holes than appear in the illustration.) When the side holes are adjacent to the renal artery origins, excellent opacification can be achieved without overlapping of superior mesenteric artery branches. The catheter can also be withdrawn to straddle the aortic bifurcation for long-film arteriography of the lower extremities. If each arm is situated in each common iliac artery, it is possible to obtain good opacification of these vessels while avoiding repeat contrast flooding of the aorta and its attendant patient discomfort. (Courtesy of Angiograf, Inc. Leeds, Alabama.)

At the close of the procedure, the catheter is withdrawn and compression is maintained on and above the puncture site for 10 minutes. The distal pulse should be controlled and palpable throughout the procedure and during most of the compression time.

"Fishing" (i.e., vigorous aspiration with a syringe by an assistant as the catheter is slowly withdrawn) sometimes results in dramatic "catches." It is not known whether these catches are (1) fibrin elements or clot that is formed on the outside of the catheter while it is in the vessel and that is stripped during removal but sucked into the syringe, (2) formed elements loosened from the vessel wall, or (3) merely fragments of subcutaneous tissues.

Pressure dressings are generally not needed; they may be necessary if a hematoma has formed, for hypertensive patients, and for patients who cannot be relied on to stay on bed rest for the prescribed amount of time. The patient should remain in bed for at least 6 to 8 hours and preferably until the next morning.

Catheter angiography by direct puncture through aortofemoral bypass grafts has been claimed to be safe [19]. However, it is not recommended in the immediate postoperative stages. Because it is technically difficult to pass a catheter through scar tissue and tough graft material, we suggest that in such cases an axillary or translumbar approach be attempted first.

Transaxillary Catheterization

Transaxillary catheterization is another very useful approach. In our hands, the complication rate has been as relatively low as that of the transfemoral approach [unpublished data], but several articles in the literature do indicate a significantly higher rate [3, 18, 36]. Thus, extra care is indicated, and the following discussion is warranted.

The axillary approach may be necessary in patients with severe arteriosclerotic blockage in the aortoiliofemoral system since severe tortuosity may prevent passage of catheters. Recent aortofemoral grafts may also preclude the transfemoral approach. Patients receiving anticoagulants should not undergo *translumbar* aortography, but catheter techniques may be possible since bleeding can be readily controlled by direct manual pressure.

The superficial position of the axillary artery permits easy catheterization and hemostasis. The left side is used for all lower aortic studies. It is surprisingly easy to enter visceral arteries superselectively from this antegrade direction. The actual artery punctured is the high or proximal *brachial artery,* i.e., that part of the artery lying on the humerus, just beyond the axillary fold.

The left arm should be abducted with the hand under the patient's head (Fig. 46-8). Careful lidocaine infiltration is advised to avoid the brachial plexus. The patient will immediately exclaim about an "electric shock" or pain down the arm into the hand if the brachial plexus is touched by the needle. A different brachial artery site should be chosen if the brachial plexus surrounds the artery at the site originally selected.

SUGGESTIONS AND PRECAUTIONS FOR TRANSAXILLARY CATHETERIZATION

We recommend a perpendicular needle approach to the vessel, with the needle about 45 degrees

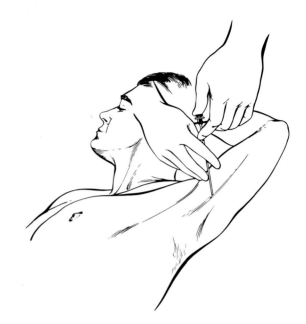

Figure 46-8. Position of patient for percutaneous axillary catheterization.

up from the horizontal. The axillary/brachial artery can be quite mobile, and it needs to be firmly transfixed by two fingers. It does not transmit pulsations through the needle, as does the femoral artery. A useful technique is to have an assistant continuously monitor the radial pulse to indicate when the pulse fades as the needle approaches and compresses the artery. *Single-wall* punctures then are feasible much of the time.

With older patients, it is more difficult to pass the catheter down the descending aorta. The universal catheter that we employ for transfemoral aortography is also useful in helping direct the guidewire *down* the aorta (see Fig. 46-7). A catheter deflector may occasionally be needed. The curved tip of the catheter should be directed posterolaterally to the left (Fig. 46-9). An unsuccessful examination should indeed be a rarity. In those rare instances when all else fails, a flow-directed, gas-filled balloon catheter technique may succeed [8, 29]. All other standard catheter techniques for a safe examination are to be followed and need no further elucidation. We no longer use stiff Teflon catheters for any procedure and never catheters that exceed a 7 French diameter.

Hemostasis is extremely important in the transaxillary approach. Hemorrhage into the brachial plexus sheath is to be avoided. Compression (not obliteration) at, and proximal to, the puncture site for 15 minutes instead of the usual 10 minutes is advised. The radial artery pulse is

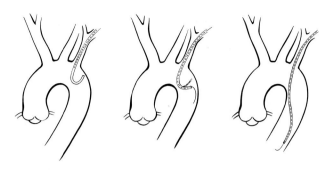

Figure 46-9. Axillary artery catheterization. The curved tip of the catheter is directed posterolaterally to the left for easier access to the descending aorta.

easier to monitor and more reliably present than its counterpart in the foot. The perpendicular needle approach tells exactly where the arterial puncture is located. It may be difficult to obtain hemostasis within the axilla itself since there is no firm or bony floor to compress the artery against. If delayed bleeding occurs within the axillary neurovascular sheath, early surgical axillary sheath decompression may be necessary [18].

References

1. American College of Radiology. *Prevention and Management of Adverse Reactions to Intravascular Contrast Media.* Chicago: American College of Radiology, Committee on Drugs, Bulletin, 1977. P. 2.
2. Amplatz, K.   Translumbar catheterization of the abdominal aorta. *Radiology* 81:927, 1963.
3. Amplatz, K., and Harner, R.   A new subclavian artery catheterization technique: Preliminary report. *Radiology* 78:963, 1962.
4. Antonovic, R., Rösch, J., and Dotter, C. T. Complications of percutaneous transaxillary catheterization for arteriography and selective chemotherapy. *AJR* 126:386, 1976.
5. Balestra, G.   L'esplorazione radiologica dell' aorta abdominale. *Minerva Med.* 2:276, 1932.
6. Baum, S., and Abrams, H. L.   A J-shaped catheter for retrograde catheterization of tortuous vessels. *Radiology* 83:436, 1964.
7. Bergman, A. B., and Neiman, H. L.   Computed tomography in the detection of retroperitoneal hemorrhage after translumbar aortography. *AJR* 131:831, 1978.
8. Buonocore, E., and Lynch, T. P. Flow-directed balloon catheterization for aortofemoral arteriography using the axillary artery approach. *AJR* 131:823, 1978.
9. Carlin, R. A., and Amplatz, K.   Downstream aortography. *AJR* 109:536, 1970.
10. Chuang, V. P., Fried, A. M., and Chen, C-Q.
Computed tomographic evaluation of para-aortic hematoma following translumbar aortography. *Radiology* 130:711, 1979.
11. Dean, R. E., Andrew, J. H., and Read, R. C.   The red cell factor in renal damage from angiographic media; perfusion studies of the in situ canine kidney with cellular and acellular perfusates. *J.A.M.A.* 187:27, 1964.
12. DiLella, D., and Henry, A.   Variable thickness filters for use with 14 × 36 inch film. *Radiol. Technol.* 36:1, 1964.
13. Dorph, S., and Folke, K.   Complications in translumbar aortography. *Acta Radiol.* [*Diagn.*] (Stockh.) 12:750, 1972.
14. Doss, A. K., Thomas, H. C., and Bond, T. B. Renal arteriography: Its clinical value. *Texas Med.* 38:277, 1942.
15. dos Santos, J. C.   Sur la désobstruction des thromboses artérielles anciennes. *Acad. Chir. Bull. Mem.* 73:409, 1947.
16. dos Santos, R., Lamas, A., and Pereira-Caldas, J. Arteriografia da aorta e dos vasos abdominais. *Med. Contemp.* 47:93, 1929.
17. dos Santos, R., Lamas, A., and Pereira-Caldas, J. L'artériographie des membres de l'aorte et de ses branches abdominales. *Soc. Nat. Chir. Bull. Mem.* 55:587, 1929.
18. Dudrick, S., Masland, W., and Mishkin, M. Brachial plexus injury following axillary artery puncture. *Radiology* 88:271, 1967.
19. Eisenberg, R. L., Mani, R. L., and McDonald, E. J., Jr.   The complication rate of catheter angiography by direct puncture through aorto-femoral bypass grafts. *AJR* 126:814, 1976.
20. Fariñas, P. L.   A new technique for the arteriographic examination of the abdominal aorta and its branches. *AJR* 46:641, 1941.
21. Finberg, C., Schechter, D. C., and Barrick, C. W. Gangrene of large intestine and ovaries after translumbar aortography: Report of a case. *J.A.M.A.* 167:1232, 1958.
22. Fischer, H. W., and Doust, V. L.   An evaluation of pre testing in the problem of serious and fatal reactions to excretory urography. *Radiology* 103:497, 1972.
23. Gordon, I. J., and Westcott, J. L.   Intra-arterial lidocaine: An effective analgesic for peripheral angiography. *Radiology* 124:43, 1977.
24. Guthaner, D. F., Silverman, J. F., Hayden, W. G., and Wexler, L.   Intraarterial analgesia in peripheral arteriography. *AJR* 128:737, 1977.
25. Hanafee, W.   Axillary artery approach to carotid, vertebral, abdominal aorta, and coronary angiography. *Radiology* 81:559, 1963.
26. Haut, G., and Amplatz, K.   Complication rates of transfemoral and transaortic catheterization. *Surgery* 63:594 1968.
27. Henline, R. B., and Moore, S. W.   Renal arteriography: Preliminary report of experimental study. *Am. J. Surg.* 32:222, 1936.

28. Kahn, P. C., Boyer, D. N., Moran, J. M., and Callow, A. D.   Reactive hyperemia in lower extremity arteriography: An evaluation. *Radiology* 90:975, 1968.

29. Klatte, E. C., Sloan, O. M., and Yune, H. Y. Balloon-tip guide for selective and subselective arteriography. *Radiology* 103:707, 1972.

30. Lalli, A. F.   Contrast media reactions: Data analysis and hypothesis. *Radiology* 134:1, 1980.

31. Laufman, H., Berggren, R. E., Finley, T., and Anson, B. J.   Anatomical studies of the lumbar arteries: With reference to the safety of translumbar aortography. *Ann. Surg.* 152:621, 1960.

32. Lonni, Y. G. W., Matsumoto, K. K., and Lecky, J. W.   Postaortographic cholesterol (atheromatous) embolization. *Radiology* 93:63, 1969.

33. Maluf, N. S. R., and McCoy, C. B.   Translumbar aortography as a diagnostic procedure in urology, with notes on caval phlebography. *AJR* 73:533, 1955.

34. McAfee, J. G.   A survey of complications of abdominal aortography. *Radiology* 68:825, 1957.

35. Melick, W. F., and Vitt, A. E.   The present status of aortography. *J. Urol.* 60:321, 1948.

36. Molnar, W., and Paul, D. J.   Complications of axillary arteriotomies: Analysis of 1762 consecutive studies. *Radiology* 104:269, 1972.

37. Morreels, C. L., Jr., Fletcher, B. D., Weilbaecher, R. G., and Dorst, J. P.   Roentgenographic features of homocystinuria. *Radiology* 90:1150, 1968.

38. Nebesar, R. A., and Pollard, J. J.   Catheter recoil and whipping in aortography: A potentially serious hazard. *Radiology* 89:845, 1967.

39. Nelson, O. A.   Arteriography of abdominal organs by aortic injection: A preliminary report. *Surg. Gynecol. Obstet.* 74:655, 1942.

40. Newton, T. H.   Axillary artery approach to arteriography of aorta and its branches. *AJR* 89:275, 1963.

41. Osler, W. E.   *Aequanimitas with Other Addresses to Medical Students, Nurses, and Practitioners of Medicine* (3rd ed.). Philadelphia: Blakiston, 1932. P. 1.

42. Peirce, E. C., II.   Percutaneous femoral artery catheterization in man with special reference to aortography. *Surg. Gynecol. Obstet.* 93:56, 1951.

43. Riley, J. M., Hanafee, W., and Weidner, W.   Left axillary approach to abdominal aorta. *Radiology* 84:96, 1965.

44. Rossi, P., and Verdu, C. C.   The floppy wire as an aid in arterial catheterization. *AJR* 97:511, 1966.

45. Roy, P., Jutras, A., and Longtin, M.   Extra large field angiography: Technique and results. *J. Can. Assoc. Radiol.* 12:21, 1961.

46. Seldinger, S. I.   Catheter replacement of the needle in percutaneous arteriography. *Acta Radiol.* 39:368, 1953.

47. Stocks, L. O., Halpern, M., and Turner, A. F. Complete translumbar aortography: The Teflon sleeve technique. *AJR* 107:835, 1969.

48. Szilagyi, D. E., Smith, R. F., Elliot, J. P., Jr., and Hageman, J. H.   Translumbar aortography: A study of its safety and usefulness. *Arch. Surg.* 112:399, 1977.

49. Wagner, F. B., Jr.   Arteriography in renal diagnosis: Preliminary report and critical evaluation. *J. Urol.* 56:625, 1946.

50. Widrich, W. C., Robbins, A. H., Goldstein, S. A., and Singer, R. J.   Adjuvant intra-arterial lidocaine in aortofemoral arteriography: Some further observations. *Radiology* 129:371, 1978.

51. Wohns, R., Glickman, M., and Kerstein, M. D. Osteomyelitis following translumbar aortography. *Angiology* 28:487, 1977.

52. Zweiman, B., Mishkin, M. M., and Hildreth, E. A.   An approach to the performance of contrast studies in contrast media–reactive persons. *Ann. Intern. Med.* 83:159, 1975.

Complications of Angiography and Other Catheter Procedures

SAMUEL J. HESSEL

The percutaneous approach to the vascular system has come a long way in a relatively short period of time. As recently as 1957, renowned surgeons in the United States were making statements like the following:

In the great majority of cases of aneurysms of the abdominal aorta, for example, there is little or no need to perform aortography for these purposes. Similarly, in complete occlusive disease of the aorta, aortography has been found unnecessary for these purposes. Its usefulness lies primarily in patients with incomplete aortic occlusion and in the few patients in whom the diagnosis remains doubtful. . . . The necessity for aortography may be eliminated in the majority of patients with aneurysms and occlusive disease of the abdominal aorta, approximately two-thirds of the cases, with commensurate reduction in the occurrence of complication [35].

The greatest gain has been in the application of the Seldinger technique [110], particularly with reference to catheterization via the femoral and axillary arteries. Advances in percutaneous catheterization have not been met by unbridled enthusiasm, however. In large part, this response has resulted from complications that occurred in temporal relationship to catheterization. Thus in 1963, McGraw wrote, "Except for visualization of the renal arteries, or due to inability to needle the small aorta in children, retrograde abdominal aortography offers no advantages over the translumbar method, and there are definite practical disadvantages" [86]. The actual morbidity and mortality associated with the procedure, coupled with this skeptical view of the advantages of modern angiographic techniques, led to both qualitative and quantitative analyses of the complications occurring with the different approaches to the vascular system. A series of studies, several of them surveys, pinpointed the problem areas and offered suggestions for increasing patient safety [1, 8, 54, 56, 57, 73, 76, 77, 83, 87, 91, 108, 109].

Over the last decade, angiography has become a stable diagnostic modality performed in virtually all hospitals of substantial size. Thus, to assess complications, it is clearly necessary to evaluate a large cross-section of institutions using a large number of different techniques. The results of such a survey form the basis for much of the following discussion. (See Chap. 14, p. 349.)

Angiography

Four major companies that sell catheters provided the names of hospitals that bought catheters (other than coronary and cerebral catheters) from 1974 to 1975. Detailed questionnaires concerning complications of angiography for the year July, 1974, through June, 1975, were sent to 2,066 hospitals. A cover letter asked that the radiologists report only complications that (1) required therapy, (2) complicated the care of the patient, or (3) prolonged the patient's hospital stay. Thus, we hoped to eliminate the reporting of trivial complications.

Five hundred and fourteen (25%) of the hospitals contacted responded, reporting a total of 118,591 angiographic examinations. These hospitals had 159,460 beds, 10.5 percent of the total acute hospital bed capacity in the United States. Each year, 21,944,000 radiologic examinations were performed in these hospitals by a total of 2,227 radiologists, of whom 1,087 performed angiography.

OVERALL COMPLICATION RATES

Table 47-1 shows a significant difference in the overall complication rates of the three angiographic approaches surveyed—transfemoral, transaxillary, and translumbar. These differences were significant (X^2, $p < 0.005$). Femoral arteriography had the lowest overall complication rate, followed by the translumbar approach and the axillary approach, in that order. The complication rate for femoral aortography was slightly less than half of the 3.6 percent reported by Lang [76]. Similarly, the death rate (0.03%), was half of the 0.06 percent reported in Lang's study. By contrast, the complication rate for axillary ar-

Table 47-2. Classification of Causes of Death

Cause of Death	Number of Deaths	Percent of Deaths
Aortic dissection and aneurysm rupture	8	27
Cardiac	5	17
Exsanguinated from gastrointestinal hemorrhage	3	10
Drug reaction	2	7
Neurologic	2	7
Renal failure	2	7
Bowel infarction	1	3
Distal aortic occlusion	1	3
Pulmonary embolism	1	3
Not specified	5	17

teriography was higher than the 2.1 percent reported by Molnar [90]. The total complication rates (including the death rate) for the translumbar approach were significantly less than those reported by Lang [76]. But the complication rate when the death rate was excluded was significantly higher than that in a more recent report by Schreiber [108].

Of the 30 deaths, 8 (27%) were caused by aortic dissection or aneurysm rupture (Table 47-2). At least three of the patients had these lesions prior to angiography. Five patients died of cardiac causes not otherwise specified. Only 2 (7%) of the 30 deaths were attributed to drug reactions.

OTHER SYSTEMIC COMPLICATIONS

The highest incidence of neurologic problems and seizures occurred with the axillary approach. The femoral approach showed a somewhat higher

Table 47-1. Overall Complication Rates in Angiography

	Approach			Statistically Significant Differences Among Approaches (X^2)
	Femoral	Axillary	Translumbar	
Number of cases	83,068	4,590	4,118	
Number of complications	1,441	151	119	
Complications	1.73%	3.29%	2.89%	$p < 0.005$
Number of deaths	24	4	2	
Deaths	0.03%	0.09%	0.05%	$p < 0.05$

Table 47-3. Classification of Systemic Complications

Complication	Percent Complications			Statistically Significant Differences Among Approaches (X^2)
	Femoral Approach	Axillary Approach	Translumbar Approach	
Cardiac	0.29	0.26	0.36	NS
Cardiovascular collapse	0.03	0.04	0.07	NS
Neurologic	0.17	0.46	0.02	$p<0.05$
Seizures	0.06	0.15	0.00	$p<0.01$

NS = not significant.

incidence of neurologic complications than did the translumbar approach (Table 47-3).

The breakdown of cardiac complications associated with the femoral approach (Table 47-4) showed a large number of so-called vasovagal hypotension incidents. The cumulative incidence (0.07%) of other cardiac complications of the femoral approach indicates their relative rarity. Yet they are of sufficient importance that all radiologists should be aware of how to handle these potentially lethal complications. Routine electrocardiographic monitoring and close observation by a member of the catheterization team or a nurse should be part of any catheterization procedure. At no time should a patient be left unattended during the course of an arteriographic examination.

The neurologic complications associated with the femoral approach show a predominance of transient episodes in contrast to more permanent deficits (Table 47-5). Other workers [41, 69, 112] have also reported transient neurologic

problems that have either completely or partiall• cleared over a short period of time. Patients wit• preexisting spinal cord lesions may be at greate• risk for developing particular autonomic nervou• system complications at angiography [43]. Im• mediate lumbar puncture with cerebrospinal flui• removal in 10-cc increments to reduce the ele• vated spinal fluid iodine concentration, followe• by maintenance of the patient in the head-up po• sition, has been recommended for postangio• graphic paraplegia and tetraplegia [89]. A rela• tively higher incidence of severe neurologi• reactions, particularly hemiplegia or death, ha• been associated with the use of older contras• agents (70% Urokon or Diodrast) [1, 70, 83].

In sharp contrast to the studies of Abrams an• McAfee [1, 83], in which 70 percent Diodras• and Urokon were particularly nephrotoxic, rela• tively few cases of renal failure were seen. How• ever, modern diatrizoate contrast media are no• entirely safe and still carry a risk of azotemia [5• 24, 74], particularly in patients with long-standin•

Table 47-4. Classification of Femoral Cardiac Complications

Complication	Number of Episodes	Percent of Cardiac Complications	Approximate Percent of Examinations*
Vasovagal hypotension	111	54	0.16
Arrhythmia	45	22	0.06
Heart failure	15	7	0.02
Myocardial infarction	13	6	0.02
Angina	11	5	0.02
Hypertension	6	3	0.01
Endocarditis	2	1	0.003
Cardiac arrest—resuscitated	1	0.5	0.001

*Calculation assumes that the cardiac complications not classified on the follow-up questionnaire were distributed in the same proportions a• those classified.

Table 47-5. Classification of Femoral Neurologic Complications

Complication	Duration	Number of Episodes	Percent of Neurologic Complications	Approximate Percent of Examinations*
Motor	Transient	20	13	0.03
	Permanent	9	6	0.01
Transient ischemic attack		15	10	0.02
Aphasia	Transient	11	7	0.02
	Permanent	6	4	0.01
Blindness	Transient	14	9	0.02
	Permanent	2	1	0.01
Seizures		53	34	0.07
Other		24	16	0.04

*Calculation assumes that the neurologic complications not classified on the follow-up questionnaire were distributed in the same proportions as those classified.

diabetes who suffer from diabetic complications [68]. Other predisposing factors include acute, severe systemic illness, advanced age, preexisting renal impairment [119], and dehydration [68]. Since evidence of decreased renal function, elevated creatinine levels, oliguria, or persistent nephrogram [95] is usually evident at 24 hours, careful postangiographic monitoring of high-risk patients is recommended so that early, appropriate management may be substituted if needed [123]. Most cases do not require dialysis, and they resolve with conservative treatment. Adequate pre- and postprocedure hydration and careful titration of the dose of contrast medium in patients at risk are important in preventing progressive azotemia.

Other systemic complications occur infrequently (Table 47-6). Postangiographic fevers and chills are, in our experience, most often nonspecific pyrogen reactions rather than evidence of bacteria infection. Shawker and his colleagues [111] showed positive bacterial cultures from catheters and guidewires in 23 of 100 procedures. Four patients had transient bacteremia but none developed local infections, prolonged

Table 47-6. Other Systemic Complications of Arteriography

Complication	Number of Episodes	Percent of Total Arteriographic Cases
Renal failure	13	0.01
Fever, chills	4	0.004
Miscellaneous	8	0.01

bacteremia, or sepsis. They concluded that postprocedural temperature elevations noted had not been proved to be related to catheter-induced infection.

Clearly, excellent sterile technique is very important, particularly in dealing with the increasing numbers of patients taking immunosuppressive drugs. When catheters are reused, the importance of rigid, thorough cleaning techniques before sterilization needs to be emphasized. In our institution, there was an increase in pyrogenic reactions when our scrub room technician went on vacation. Once the association was made, strict, uniform guidelines were established for cleaning catheters, with good results.

ALLERGIC REACTIONS TO CONTRAST AGENTS

Many so-called allergic reactions may actually be autonomic vagal nerve–mediated responses, ameliorated by intravenous atropine [7]. Some workers have suggested that certain systemic symptoms (nausea and vomiting) may be, in part, psychogenic [75]. The incidence of laryngeal edema, as a specific endpoint in evaluating allergic reactions to contrast media, was 0.03 percent for femoral arteriography, 0.07 percent for axillary arteriography, and zero percent for translumbar aortography. These figures should be compared with the 0.08 percent incidence reported by Sigstedt in a much smaller series [114]. The rates did not differ among the three angiographic approaches (X^2, $p > 0.05$). There is controversy concerning the pathogenesis of these reactions. Recent data suggest an allergic im-

Table 47-7. Puncture Site Complications

Complication	Percent Complications			Statistically Significant Differences Among Approaches (X^2)
	Femoral Approach	Axillary Approach	Translumbar Approach	
Hemorrhage	0.26	0.68	0.53	$p < 0.001$
Arterial obstruction	0.14	0.76	0	$p < 0.001$
Pseudoaneurysm	0.05	0.22	0.05	$p < 0.01$
Arteriovenous fistula	0.01	0.02	0.00	NS
Limb amputation	0.01	0.02	0.00	NS
Total	0.47	1.7	0.58	

NS = not significant.

munologic mechanism for some severe contrast media reactions [25]. Pretesting with small doses of contrast media before the administration of large boluses did not identify the patients who were likely to have a serious or fatal reaction. A comparison of death rates of pretested patients and those not pretested showed no significant difference [42].

PUNCTURE SITE COMPLICATIONS

The axillary route had, overall, the highest complication rate (Table 47-7). This was most evident in the incidence of arterial obstruction, hemorrhage, and pseudoaneurysm. Similarly, Molnar [90] reported that 33 (89%) of 37 axillary complications involved one of these three complications. The axillary artery is prone to local complications, most likely because of its small size and its location, which makes hemostasis difficult. Axillary artery hemorrhage can lead to brachial

plexus injuries in a significant number of patients [26, 37, 90, 117]. The proximity of the axillary artery to the cerebral circulation can result in serious problems, including embolization of mural thrombi, causing cerebral ischemia [59] and inadvertent perfusion of cerebrally toxic volumes of drugs such as lidocaine used in peripheral arteriography [31].

Arterial obstruction or embolization (Table 47-8) has received considerable attention. Fogarty [45] postulated that an intimal flap at the puncture site was a nidus for thrombus that resulted in late arterial occlusions. Siegelman [113] demonstrated convincingly, with pullout arteriograms, that there was a high incidence of thrombi on catheters at the completion of femoral arteriograms. He further defined several parameters, including thick catheters and long catheterization times, associated with a high incidence of catheter clots. Scanning electron microscopy studies showed that polyurethane

Table 47-8. Guidewire and Catheter Complications

Complication	Percent Complications			Statistically Significant Differences Among Approaches (X^2)
	Femoral Approach	Axillary Approach	Translumbar Approach	
Perforation or extraluminal contrast injection	0.44	0.37	1.75	$p < 0.001$
Embolism	0.10	0.07	0.00	NS
Breakage	0.10	0.02	0.02	NS
Total	0.64	0.46	1.77	

NS = not significant.

catheters were not as smooth as polyethylene ones [93]. In experimental animals, polyethylene catheters were significantly more thrombogenic than Silastic ones [127]. Formanek [47] showed that polyethylene and siliconized polyurethane catheters were less thrombogenic than Teflon end-occluded catheters. Glancy [52] and Eldh [39] showed that heparinization was effective in reducing thrombus formation on catheters. Jacobsson and Schlossman [66] demonstrated that catheter length, thickness, and material were all significant factors in thromboembolism. McCarty [84] and Ovitt [96] indicated that Teflon-coated wires were more rapidly thrombogenic than stainless steel ones, and they suggested coating all wires with a benzalkonium chloride–heparin solution. Although some authors [71] emphasized that vessel size was an important parameter in the pathogenesis of thrombosis, others [65] tended to minimize the importance of such patient variables.

Intermittent and frequent catheter flushing with heparinized saline or contrast medium [58] is important in preventing intracatheter thrombus formation. Some centers use a closed, constant flushing system under pressure to prevent catheter thrombosis. Other approaches to decreasing thromboses have also been suggested. Jacobsson [64, 65] advocated infusion of 10 cc per kilogram of 6 percent dextran for 2 to 4 hours prior to angiography. In 85 patients so treated, none developed thromboemboli, while 6 of 77 patients in the control group had thromboembolism demonstrated after angiography. Other workers have pointed to their experience in coronary angiography [2, 82, 88, 124] to suggest that systemic heparinization be used routinely in visceral studies [125]. A prospective study of 400 patients in total, 200 of whom received 45 units per kilogram of heparin injected into the abdominal aorta at the beginning of the study and 200 of whom received only a small amount of heparin in the catheter-flushing solution, showed fibrinous sheaths around the catheters in 12 control patients and 8 of the heparinized group. Nonocclusive thrombi at the entry site were found in 13 control patients and 4 of the systemically heparinized patients. This difference was statistically significant (X^2, $p <$ 0.05). There were two patients with femoral artery occlusions; both patients were in the control group. Thus, there appears to be some benefit to heparinization. That benefit has to be balanced against the higher incidence of delayed bleeding, which may be avoided by the use of protamine sulfate at the completion of the angiographic procedure. Systemic heparinization is used rather widely in the cardiac catheterization laboratory, but it has not been as widely used in other angiographic procedures. It may well be that the more critical nature of thromboembolic events in the coronary arteries as compared to the visceral and peripheral circulations makes physicians doing cardiac catheterization more sensitive to these complications.

While intravenous heparin therapy has occasionally been successful with fresh emboli [85], the consensus is that proximal lesions, such as those in the femoral artery, should be removed expeditiously [23, 102]. Fogarty catheters [44] have greatly facilitated this approach. In the case of more peripheral emboli, there are those who advocate conservative management, particularly when the emboli are below the knee [13].

In some hospitals, pressure dressings and/or sandbags are placed on the groin after femoral arteriography. Christenson [29] reported that the use of pressure dressings, especially in hypertensive patients, significantly reduced delayed bleeding requiring medical attention. By contrast, Eisenberg [38] found no significant advantage in either normotensive or hypertensive patients in using pressure dressings after angiography. In addition, he felt that the dressings prevented visual inspection of the groin for hematomas. He, therefore, recommended supine bed rest for 8 hours with the punctured extremity extended. Our standard approach has been to use a sandbag on the groin for a few hours after catheterization. This permits easy visual inspection by the nurse and at the same time, is a reminder to the patient to remain supine, with the leg extended, and not to move about.

Computed tomography has increased our sensitivity in detecting hematomas. Thus, in five of seven patients scanned immediately after translumbar aortography, discrete soft tissue densities consistent with retroperitoneal bleeding were found [17]. While the detection of small hematomas may not be significant, severe periaortic hemorrhage can be detected early and followed with computed tomography.

Pseudoaneurysms occur with the greatest frequency in the axillary artery, where difficulty in compression seems to be an important factor. Hypertension has also been mentioned as an antecedent finding [98]. Arteriovenous fistulas are the least common puncture site complication.

These fistulas can arise not only at the site of percutaneous arterial puncture [34] but also in association with venous punctures [40]. Surgical approaches to both pseudoaneurysms and arteriovenous fistulas are recommended [16, 102].

GUIDEWIRE AND CATHETER COMPLICATIONS

The most significant complications are perforation and extraluminal contrast injection, which can lead to vascular dissection [55]. Gaylis and Laws [50] showed diagrammatically how faulty positioning of an aortography needle can result in intramural injection and aortic dissection. This can progress to occlusion of small aortic branches or the entire aorta. Wolfman and Boblitt [128] found a 10.9 percent incidence of intramural injection, with four deaths, two of which were directly attributable to a dissecting aneurysm. They described the roentgen signs of contrast dissection of the aortic wall [21] and suggested several technical modifications, including the filming of a 5-cc test injection to define precisely the location of the aortography needle. The use of a vascular sheath and a fluoroscopically monitored small test injection minimizes the incidence of intramural contrast injection and dissection. With transfemoral and transaxillary catheters, there may be a different pathophysiology of intramural contrast injection, involving cardiovascular trauma from the angiographic jet originating at the catheter tip [51]. Realization of the importance of these jets led to the development of a mathematical model, validated in experimental animals, that enables the angiographer to calculate the safe operating range of any catheter [81]. In the past, tip-occluded catheters, which preclude subintimal injection but not subintimal hematoma, have been recommended. Subsequently, coiled-tip pigtail catheters were developed to reduce significantly aortic trauma. While such catheters are effective, their flow characteristics can lead to thrombus formation between the last side hole and the end hole [100]. The clot is then expelled with a particularly forceful power injection. A constant, relatively high-pressure catheter-flushing system may prevent this complication. Recent data suggest that the incidence of subintimal contrast injection increases as the catheter position becomes more selective. Injury to the celiac or hepatic arteries is relatively benign, while injuries to the superior mesenteric or renal arteries may have serious consequences [67].

Catheter knotting, though an unusual complication, can be troublesome [80]. It should be standard practice to advance and manipulate catheters only under fluoroscopic control [131]. Multiple techniques have been suggested for reducing arterial catheter knots. The use of a tip deflector [62, 121] has been described.

Overall, of the two selective approaches, the femoral technique is the safer and easier one for selective and superselective angiography. Although the right groin is usually punctured (because most radiologists are right-handed and because of the setup of angiographic suites), there are no intrinsic anatomic reasons why the left groin should not be immediately approached when there is difficulty using the right groin [60]. When technical factors, such as vessel occlusion or tortuosity, prevent use of either femoral artery, the axillary approach should be tried. Recently the translumbar technique provoked debate [11] when it was once more suggested as a safe, simple alternative when selective vascular opacification is not required [101].

COMPLICATIONS VERSUS CASE LOAD

There was a strong inverse relationship between complications and case load (Fig. 47-1). When the hospitals were divided into nonteaching and teaching institutions, this relationship was seen most strikingly in nonteaching hospitals. In

Figure 47-1. Relationship between the yearly number of angiography cases and the complication rates at hospitals with radiology residents (teaching hospitals) and those without residents (nonteaching hospitals).

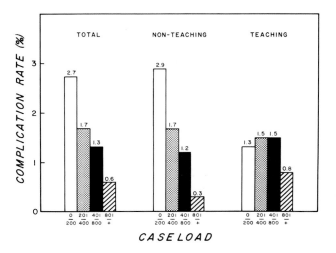

Table 47-9. Relationship Between Percent of Complications and Case Load

| Case Load | Complication | | | | |
	Death	Cardiac	Neurologic	Puncture Site	Guidewire and Catheter
0–200	0.04	0.48	0.32	0.78	1.00
201–400	0.03	0.26	0.22	0.49	0.53
401–800	0.03	0.19	0.21	0.27	0.57
800+	0.03	0.11	0.01	0.18	0.22

teaching hospitals, only when 801 or more cases were handled per year was there a reduction in the complication rates in comparison with smaller numbers of cases. This relationship is similar to that found in studies of coronary angiography [2, 3]. We found no relationship between the complication rates and the number of beds, radiologists, or angiographers or the total number of radiologic procedures. If we divide the complications into the major groups discussed earlier, all the complications except death showed a significant inverse relationship to the number of cases (Table 47-9).

ADRENAL VENOGRAPHY

There were 604 adrenal venograms reported. There was an 8.1 percent incidence of extravasation. Two of these patients (0.4% of the population) had adrenal insufficiency. In both cases, the extravasation was bilateral. The incidence of other, unspecified complications was 0.7 percent.

PHEOCHROMOCYTOMA

There were 228 patients studied for pheochromocytoma. Of these, 7.9 percent had blood pressure elevations during the study that were called *hypertensive crises*. One patient (0.4% of the group studied) died during a study. This is in contrast to translumbar aortography studies using older contrast agents (Urokon or Diodrast), in which 3 of 18 patients died and 5 others (28%) had severe hypertensive crises [106]. As part of a follow-up questionnaire, we ascertained that 66 (35.7%) of 185 patients were premedicated. A total of 10 of these 185 patients had hypertensive episodes, and 5 of the 10 patients had been premedicated. Rossi [106] reported that premedication with phenoxybenzamine, an alpha-adrenergic blocking agent, reduced the severity and frequency of hypertensive crises. In our lim-

ited population, we could not document such an effect. This difference may be related to the reporting radiologists' use of varying definitions of hypertensive episode (we did not ask for the precise level of blood pressure elevation).

PERIPHERAL VENOGRAPHY

Of the 18,342 patients examined, 128 (0.7%) had postvenogram thrombophlebitis. Twenty-seven patients had other complications (Table 47-10) [116]. Albrechtsson and Olsson [4] reported on 61 patients with normal phlebograms; two of these patients had deep venous thrombosis following the phlebogram and two others had scintigraphic evidence of pulmonary embolism. Bettmann and Paulin [19] reported that 24 percent of patients had symptoms after the venogram that were suggestive of thrombophlebitis. In a smaller study, 3 of 23 patients had deep venous thrombosis and 3 others had superficial venous thrombosis after an initially negative venogram using 60 percent sodium methylglucamine diatrizoate [20]. Arndt [10] reported a 4.4 percent incidence of postvenog-

Table 47-10. Complications of Peripheral Venography

Complication	Number of Incidents	Percent of Venographic Complications	Percent of Venograms
Postvenogram thrombophlebitis	128	83	0.7
Skin slough	9	6	0.05
Contrast "allergy"	4	3	0.02
Infection	3	2	0.02
Congestive heart failure	2	1	0.01
Miscellaneous	6	4	0.03
Unspecified	3	2	0.02

Table 47-11. Complications of Pedal Lymphography

Complication	Number of Incidents	Percent of Lymphographic Complications	Percent of Lymphograms
Pulmonary	31	47	0.4
Local infection	13	20	0.17
Evans blue reactions (allergic or overdose)	7	11	0.09
Fever	3	5	0.04
Lymphocele	2	3	0.03
Skin ulceration	2	3	0.03
Thrombophlebitis	2	3	0.03
Contributory to death (pulmonary)	1	2	0.01
Amputation			
Ischemia	1	2	0.01
Osteomyelitis	1	2	0.01
Unspecified	3	5	0.04

raphy thrombophlebitis before a heparin flush was used and a 2 percent incidence after a routine heparin flush was used. In neither of the latter two studies were follow-up venograms performed. The authors of these two studies took as positive evidence of "thrombophlebitis" pain, erythema, and swelling after venography. While contrast agents in experimental settings cause endothelial damage, particularly in association with venostasis [104], there may be some differences in degree between the development de novo of clinical thrombophlebitis and the process that occurs after venography. Regardless, one cannot argue with efforts to minimize the development of symptoms and signs of thrombophlebitis. Thus, dilute ionic contrast media [19, 20] and nonionic contrast media [5], as well as a flush solution of saline or heparin to prevent contrast stasis in the lower extremity veins, may be useful. In 142 leg venograms performed supine with power injections (95 cc of 76% meglumine diatrizoate, 1–2 cc/sec in each limb), only three patients had delayed pain [33]. The authors suggest that shorter endothelial contact time with supine phlebography in contrast to the standard semierect technique [99] accounts for the lower incidence of pain.

PEDAL LYMPHOGRAPHY

In 7,641 examinations reported, 31 of the patients examined (0.4%) had pulmonary complications resulting from a reduction in the diffusion capacity secondary to embolization of oily contrast material. In one case, the pulmonary com-

plications were felt to contribute to the patient's death. Thirty-five patients (0.5%) had other complications (Table 47-11). At least 14 of these complications were related to infection at the site of the cutdown for contrast infusion. This points up the need for sterile, careful technique in doing that procedure.

WEDGE HEPATIC VENOGRAPHY

Wedge hepatic venography to evaluate portal hypertension can result in hemorrhagic hepatic infarction if the contrast medium is injected too rapidly [207]. Subsequent hepatic angiography may show an area of apparent "tumor blush" at the site of the previous wedge injection.

TRANSHEPATIC CATHETERIZATION

Of 26 patients having percutaneous transhepatic catheterization of the biliary or portal venous system using a polyethylene catheter (1.3-mm diameter), 26 percent had arteriovenous fistulas when studied by hepatic arteriography within 1 month of the procedure. Five patients seen 6 months to 3 years after catheterization had no evidence of splenomegaly or esophageal varices. However, angiography was repeated in only one patient, who did not demonstrate a fistula [94].

ARTERIOGRAPHY IN CHILDREN

The effect on limb length of arterial catheterization of young children is controversial. Bassett [14] reported that the catheterized limb was more than 0.3 cm shorter than the contralateral limb, a degree of shortening roughly parallel to the severity of circulatory impairment as judged by oscillometry and diminished pulses. Other workers [105, 115, 120] failed to find chronic impairment of flow to the lower extremity or evidence of shortening after catheterization. In a study of 50 children who had repeat catheterizations, primarily for cardiac lesions, 37 were normal. Six had complete arterial occlusion, three had incomplete occlusions, and four had mural abnormalities. There was a strong correlation between the age at initial catheterization and the subsequent presence of vascular abnormalities. The authors suggest that thrombotic complications in catheterized arteries are secondary to mechanical intimal injuries [92]. Heparin has been recommended for patients 10 years of age or younger who undergo catheterization because of the potential for thrombosis in their small vessels [48]. Aspirin, however, did not seem to have any beneficial effects [49]. Because of the extreme sensitivity of the infant femoral artery to spasm at catheterization, thin-walled needles and catheters and limitation to a single puncture are recommended [18]. In addition, a percutaneous rather than an open arteriotomy [49] is associated with a lower incidence of arterial thrombosis. In adults, transient but definite decreases in limb blood flow and venous capacitance were found after, respectively, femoral arterial and venous catheterizations [122].

REPEATED ARTERIAL AND VENOUS CATHETERIZATION

Seventeen normal volunteers were subjected to one to seven arterial and venous cannulations. Two developed venospasm and thrombophlebitis after an initial catheterization. Two other subjects developed severe arterial spasm. Four subjects had arterial embolization after four or more repeated brachial artery catheterizations. The authors concluded that catheterization of the arm veins in young, healthy individuals is attended by a significant incidence of localized venous occlusion without serious sequelae. Repeated arterial catheterization leads to an increased incidence of thrombus formation and peripheral embolization [79]. From 2 to 8 months after catheterization one patient had persistent arterial symptoms, whereas four had evidence of venous disease.

Pseudocomplications

Simply because a complication, particularly a systemic one, occurs after angiography does not, with absolute certainty, establish a cause-and-effect relationship. It is entirely conceivable that ill patients requiring angiography may be stricken by one or another condition simply because of their deteriorating health rather than as a result of catheterization. Baum [15] evaluated 1,600 consecutive vascular catheterization procedures and found a striking similarity in the incidence and character of untoward reactions occurring 48 hours prior to angiography and those occurring within 48 hours afterward. Hildner [61] evaluated the incidence of pseudocomplications, which he defined as complications occurring in the 48 hours before or the 24 hours after scheduled but unperformed cardiac catheterization. He found a 2.3 percent incidence of pseudocomplications, including a 1.2 percent mortality. In the group that was catheterized, there was a 2.6 percent catheter-related incidence of complications, including a 0.6 percent mortality. Similar types of complications were noted in both groups. The authors concluded that the incidence of complications would have doubled and the mortality tripled if the procedures had been performed on schedule or up to 48 hours earlier in the patients who had the pseudocomplications. They feel that the incidence of complications after cardiac catheterization is materially influenced by unexpected events resulting from severe cardiac disease. These studies make less certain the association between complications (particularly those that do not involve the puncture site or the distal vasculature) and angiographic procedures.

Angiographic Interventional Therapy

As catheter therapy becomes more common, it is likely that a whole new class of complications arising from the use of this modality will be seen. Superior mesenteric artery thrombosis, left gastric artery thrombosis, small bowel gangrene, and false aneurysm have been reported after vasopressin infusion of gastrointestinal bleeding sites [72]. In one instance, angiographic attempts to demonstrate a pancreatic neoplasm resulted in the provocation of massive gastrointestinal hemorrhage [29]. Balsys [12] recently reported multiple aneurysms developing in embolization sites after treatment of an arteriovenous malformation of the scalp. A patient with chronic renal failure who was undergoing bilateral renal infarction for hypertension had reflux of Gelfoam into the aorta from a renal artery, with consequent peripheral embolization [129]. A modified injection technique has been suggested to avoid spill of emboli into the aorta with subsequent deposition in untargeted vessels [78]. Methods to recover other arterial emboli, such as the use of Gianturco coils [30], have been reported.

The use of indwelling arterial catheters is not immune to problems. Infection [118] and thromboembolism [36] occur with some regularity. Clouse [32] reported on 127 transbrachial hepatic artery catheters used in 75 patients for prolonged hepatic chemotherapy infusion. Partial or complete arterial thrombosis was seen in 30 patients. Bleeding and pseudoaneurysm at the arteriotomy site were found in nine patients. Minor complications, including catheter displacement from the hepatic artery, cracks or leaks in the catheter at the arteriotomy site, and clotted catheters, occurred in 77 (61%) of the 127 catheter procedures. Seven (9%) of the 75 patients had a loss of their radial pulses. Because of this high incidence of complications, the authors suggest that a thin-walled 5 French catheter be used and that it be cared for meticulously by the clinical team.

Intravenous Catheters

Indwelling intravenous catheters, for either central venous pressure monitoring or total parenteral nutrition, may cause serious complications, including phlebitis, venous thrombosis, embolism, and sepsis [126]. Hoshal [63] reported the formation of fibrin sleeves around catheters left in place 24 hours or longer. He suggested using graphite–benzalkonium chloride–heparin–bonded catheters to inhibit fibrin formation. Ryan [107] reported superior vena caval thrombosis, pulmonary embolism, and sepsis from catheters used for total parenteral nutrition. He showed that strict aseptic technique significantly reduced the rate of sepsis. In a study of 234 saphenous venous cutdowns, 34 complications, including 10 minor wound infections and 10 episodes of phlebitis, were found. The inci-

dence of phlebitis was directly related to how long the catheter remained in place [22].

Complications of central venous pressure monitoring by flow-directed balloon-tip catheters (Swan-Ganz catheters) have become more common with increasing use of these catheters. Massive pulmonary arterial thrombosis [130], fatal pulmonary hemorrhage [53, 97], and pulmonary embolism [46] have been reported.

INTRAVENOUS CATHETER EMBOLI

A review of 202 intravenous catheter emboli showed that 126 (62.3%) had been removed, 74 at surgery and 52 by a catheter snare [103]. Of those that had not been removed, 42 (55%) of 76 were not associated with complications. However, 16 (21%) of 76 patients had major nonfatal complications, including endocarditis, thrombosis, ventricular perforation, and arrhythmias. Eighteen (24%) of the 76 died. The causes of death included perforation, arrhythmias, endocarditis, and pulmonary thrombosis. Thus, it is important that such catheter fragments be removed. As we become more experienced, the approaches to removal will become more numerous. At present, the choice is of various methods of snaring or grabbing the catheter fragment. The approach we prefer is to use a thin guidewire doubled on itself and inserted into the venous system through a Desilets-Hoffman sheath. This approach facilitates withdrawal of the catheter fragment without injuring the vein at the puncture site.

References

1. Abrams, H. L. Radiologic aspects of operable heart disease: III. The hazards of retrograde thoracic aortography: A survey. *Radiology* 68: 812, 1957.
2. Adams, D. F., and Abrams, H. L. Complications of coronary arteriography: A follow-up report. *Cardiovasc. Radiol.* 2:89, 1979.
3. Adams, D. F., Fraser, D. B., and Abrams, H. L. The complications of coronary arteriography. *Circulation* 48:609, 1973.
4. Albrechtsson, U., and Olsson, C. G. Thrombotic side-effects of lower-limb phlebography. *Lancet* 1:723, 1976.
5. Albrechtsson, U., and Olsson, C. G. Thrombosis following phlebography with ionic and

non-ionic contrast media. *Acta Radiol. [Diagn.]* (Stockh.) 20:46, 1979.

6. Alexander, R. D., Berkes, S. L., and Abuelo, J. G. Contrast media-induced oliguric renal failure. *Arch. Intern. Med.* 138:381, 1978.

7. Andrews, E. J., Jr. The vagus reaction as a possible cause of severe complications of radiological procedures. *Radiology* 121:1, 1976.

8. Ansell, G. A national survey of radiological complications: Interim report. *Clin. Radiol.* 19:175, 1968.

9. Antonovic, R., Rösch, J., and Dotter, C. T. The value of systemic arterial heparinization in transfemoral angiography: A prospective study. *AJR* 127:223, 1976.

10. Arndt, R. D., Grollman, J. H., Jr., Gomes, A. S., and Bos, C. J. The heparin flush: An aid in preventing post-venography thrombophlebitis. *Radiology* 130:249, 1979.

11. Athanasoulis, C. A. On the inadequacies of translumbar aortography. *AJR* 132:500, 1979.

12. Balsys, R., and Cross, R. Multiple aneurysm formation as a complication of interventive angiography. *Radiology* 126:91, 1978.

13. Barnes, R. W., Petersen, J. L., Krugmire, R. B., Jr., and Strandness, D. E., Jr. Complications of percutaneous femoral arterial catheterization: Prospective evaluation with the Doppler ultrasonic velocity detector. *Am. J. Cardiol.* 33:259, 1974.

14. Bassett, F. H., III, Lincoln, C. R., King, T. D., and Canent, R. V., Jr. Inequality in the size of the lower extremity following cardiac catheterization. *South. Med. J.* 61:1013, 1968.

15. Baum, S., Stein, G. N., and Kuroda, K. K. Complications of "no arteriography." *Radiology* 86:835, 1966.

16. Bergentz, S.-E., Hansson, L. O., and Norback, B. Surgical management of complications to arterial puncture. *Ann. Surg.* 164:1021, 1966.

17. Bergman, A. B., and Neiman, H. L. Computed tomography in the detection of retroperitoneal hemorrhage after translumbar aortography. *AJR* 131:831, 1978.

18. Bergström, K., and Jorulf, H. Reaction of femoral and common carotid arteries in infants after puncture or percutaneous catheterization. *Acta Radiol. [Diagn.]* (Stockh.) 17:577, 1976.

19. Bettmann, M. A., and Paulin, S. Leg phlebography: The incidence, nature, and modification of undesirable side effects. *Radiology* 122:101, 1977.

20. Bettmann, M. A., Salzman, E. W., Rosenthal, D., Clagett, P., Davies, G., Nebesar, R., Rabinov, K., Ploetz, J., and Skillman, J. Reduction of venous thrombosis complicating phlebography. *AJR* 134:1169, 1980.

21. Boblitt, D. E., Figley, M. M., and Wolfman, E. F., Jr. Roentgen signs of contrast material dissection of aortic wall in direct aortography. *AJR* 81:826, 1959.

22. Bogen, J. E. Local complications in 167 patients with indwelling venous catheters. *Surg. Gynecol. Obstet.* 110:112, 1960.

23. Bolasny, B. L., and Killen, D. A. Surgical management of arterial injuries secondary to angiography. *Ann. Surg.* 174:962, 1971.

24. Borra, S., Hawkins, D., Duguid, W., and Kaye, M. Acute renal failure and nephrotic syndrome after angiocardiography with meglumine diatrizoate. *N. Engl. J. Med.* 284:592, 1971.

25. Brasch, R. C., and Caldwell, J. L. The allergic theory of radiocontrast agent toxicity: Demonstration of antibody activity in sera of patients suffering major radiocontrast agent reactions. 1976 Memorial award paper. *Invest. Radiol.* 11:347, 1976.

26. Carroll, S. E., and Wilkins, W. W. Two cases of brachial plexus injury following percutaneous arteriograms. *Can. Med. Assoc. J.* 102:861, 1970.

27. Castaneda-Zuniga, W. R., Jauregui, H., Rysavy, J. A., Formanek, A., and Amplatz, K. Complications of wedge hepatic venography. *Radiology* 126:53, 1978.

28. Chait, A., and Dann, R. H. G-I bleed after angiography (letter). *N. Engl. J. Med.* 286:1418, 1972.

29. Christenson, R., Staab, E. V., Burko, H., and Foster, J. Pressure dressings and postarteriographic care of the femoral puncture site. *Radiology* 119:97, 1976.

30. Chuang, V. P. Nonoperative retrieval of Gianturco coils from abdominal aorta. *AJR* 132:996, 1979.

31. Chuang, V. P., and Widrich, W. C. Complications from intraarterial lidocaine in upper extremity arteriography. *AJR* 131:906, 1978.

32. Clouse, M. E., Ahmed, R., Ryan, R. B., Oberfield, R. A., and McCaffrey, J. A. Complications of long term transbrachial hepatic arterial infusion chemotherapy. *AJR* 129:799, 1977.

33. Coel, M. N., and Dodge, W. Complication rate with supine phlebography. *AJR* 131:821, 1978.

34. Cooper, P. W., and Gladstone, R. M. Arteriovenous fistula following brachial arterial puncture for cerebral angiography. *J. Can. Assoc. Radiol.* 25:140, 1974.

35. Crawford, E. S., Beall, A. C., Moyer, J. H., and DeBakey, M. E. Complications of aortography. *Surg. Gynecol. Obstet.* 104:129, 1957.

36. Downs, J. B., Chapman, R. L., and Hawkins, I. F., Jr. Prolonged radial-artery catheterization: An evaluation of heparinized catheters and continuous irrigation. *Arch. Surg.* 108:671, 1974.

37. Dudrick, S., Masland, W., and Mishkin, M.

Brachial plexus injury following axillary artery puncture: Further comments on management. *Radiology* 88:271, 1967.

38. Eisenberg, R. L., and Mani, R. L. Pressure dressings and postangiographic care of the femoral puncture site. *Radiology* 122:677, 1977.

39. Eldh, P., and Jacobsson, B. Heparinized vascular catheters: A clinical trial. *Radiology* 111:289, 1974.

40. Farhat, K., Nakhjavan, F. K., Cope, C., Yazdanfar, S., Fernandez, J., Gooch, A., and Goldberg, H. Iatrogenic arteriovenous fistula: A complication of percutaneous subclavian vein puncture. *Chest* 67:480, 1975.

41. Feigelson, H. H., and Ravin, H. A. Transverse myelitis following selective bronchial arteriography. *Radiology* 85:663, 1965.

42. Fischer, H. W., and Doust, V. L. An evaluation of pretesting in the problem of serious and fatal reactions to excretory urography. *Radiology* 103:497, 1972.

43. Fleischman, S., and Shah, P. Autonomic dysreflexia: An unusual radiologic complication. *Radiology* 124:695, 1977.

44. Fogarty, T. J., Cranley, J. J., Krause, R. J., Strasser, E. S., and Hafner, C. D. A method for extraction of arterial emboli and thrombi. *Surg. Gynecol. Obstet.* 116:241, 1963.

45. Fogarty, T. J., and Krippaehne, W. W. Vascular occlusion following arterial catheterization. *Surg. Gynecol. Obstet.* 121:1295, 1965.

46. Foote, G. A., Schabel, S. I., and Hodges, M. Pulmonary complications of the flow-directed balloon-tipped catheter. *N Engl. J. Med.* 290:927, 1974.

47. Formanek, G., Frech, R. S., and Amplatz, K. Arterial thrombus formation during clinical percutaneous catheterization. *Circulation* 41:833, 1970.

48. Freed, M. D., Keane, J. F., and Rosenthal, A. The use of heparinization to prevent arterial thrombosis after percutaneous cardiac catheterization in children. *Circulation* 50:565, 1974.

49. Freed, M. D., Rosenthal, A., and Fyler, D. Attempts to reduce arterial thrombosis after cardiac catheterization in children: Use of percutaneous technique and aspirin. *Am. Heart J.* 87:283, 1974.

50. Gaylis, H., and Laws, J. W. Dissection of aorta as a complication of translumbar aortography. *Br. Med. J.* 2:1141, 1956.

51. Gilbert, G. J., and Melnick, G. S. Pathophysiology of subintimal hematoma formation during retrograde arteriography. *Radiology* 85:306, 1965.

52. Glancy, J. J., Fishbone, G., and Heinz, E. R. Nonthrombogenic arterial catheters. *AJR* 108:716, 1970.

53. Golden, M. S., Pinder, T., Anderson, W. T., and Cheitlin, M. D. Fatal pulmonary hemorrhage complicating use of a flow-directed balloon-tipped catheter in a patient receiving anticoagulant therapy. *Am. J. Cardiol.* 32:865, 1973.

54. Grainger, R. G. Complications of cardiovascular radiological investigations. *Br. J. Radiol.* 38:201, 1965.

55. Gudbjerg, C. E., and Christensen, J. Dissection of the aortic wall in retrograde lumbar aortography. *Acta Radiol.* 55:364, 1961.

56. Halpern, M. Percutaneous transfemoral arteriography: An analysis of the complications in 1,000 consecutive cases. *AJR* 92:918, 1964.

57. Haut, G., and Amplatz, K. Complication rates of transfemoral and transaortic catheterization. *Surgery* 63:594, 1968.

58. Hawkins, I. F., Jr., and Herbert, L. Contrast material used as a catheter flushing agent: A method to reduce clot formation during angiography. *Radiology* 110:351, 1974.

59. Head, R. M., and Robboy, S. J. Embolic strike from mural thrombi, a fatal complication of axillary artery catheterization. *Radiology* 102:307, 1972.

60. Hessel, S. J., and Sequeira, J. C. Femoral artery catheterization and vessel tortuosity. *Cardiovasc. Intervent. Radiol.* 4:80, 1981.

61. Hildner, F. J., Javier, R. P., Ramaswamy, K., and Samet, P. Pseudo complications of cardiac catheterization. *Chest* 63:15, 1973.

62. Holder, J. C., and Cherry, J. F. The use of a tip deflecting guide in untying a knotted arterial catheter. *Radiology* 128:808, 1978.

63. Hoshal, V. L., Ause, R. G., and Hoskins, P. A. Fibrin sleeve formation on indwelling subclavian central venous catheters. *Arch. Surg.* 102:353, 1971.

64. Jacobsson, B. Use of dextran in prophylaxis against thromboembolic complications in arterial catheterisation. *Acta Chir. Scand. [Suppl.]* 387:103, 1968.

65. Jacobsson, B. Effect of pretreatment with dextran 70 on platelet adhesiveness and thromboembolic complications following percutaneous arterial catheterisation. *Acta Radiol. [Diagn.]* (Stockh.) 8:289, 1969.

66. Jacobsson, B., and Schlossman, D. Thromboembolism of leg following percutaneous catheterisation of femoral artery for angiography: Predisposing factors. *Acta Radiol. [Diagn.]* (Stockh.) 8:109, 1969.

67. Jonsson, K., Lunderquist, A., Pettersson, H., and Sigstedt, B. Subintimal injection of contrast medium as a complication of selective abdominal angiography. *Acta Radiol. [Diagn.]* (Stockh.) 18:55, 1977.

68. Kamdar, A., Weidmann, P., Makoff, D. L., and

Massry, S. G.   Acute renal failure following intravenous use of radiographic contrast dyes in patients with diabetes mellitus. *Diabetes* 26:643, 1977.

69. Kardjiev, V., Symeonov, A., and Chankov, I. Etiology, pathogenesis, and prevention of spinal cord lesions in selective angiography of the bronchial and intercostal arteries. *Radiology* 112:81, 1974.

70. Killen, D. A., and Foster, J. H.   Spinal cord injury as a complication of aortography. *Ann. Surg.* 152:211, 1960.

71. Kloster, F. E., Bristow, J. D., and Griswold, H. E.   Femoral artery occlusion following percutaneous catheterization. *Am. Heart J.* 79:175, 1970.

72. Komaki, S.   Angiographic complications caused by vasopressin infusion of gastrointestinal bleeders. *Nippon Acta Radiol.* 37:657, 1977.

73. Kottke, B. A., Fairbairn, J. F., II, and Davis, G. D.   Complications of aortography. *Circulation* 30:843, 1964.

74. Krumlovsky, F. A., Simon, N., Santhanam, S., del Greco, F., Roxe, D., and Pomarane, M. M. Acute renal failure: Association with administration of radiographic contrast material. *J.A.M.A.* 239:125, 1978.

75. Lalli, A. F.   Urographic contrast media reactions and anxiety. *Radiology* 112:267, 1974.

76. Lang, E. K.   A survey of the complications of percutaneous retrograde arteriography: Seldinger technic. *Radiology* 81:257, 1963.

77. Lang, E. K.   Prevention and treatment of complications following arteriography. *Radiology* 88:950, 1967.

78. Levin, D. C., Beckmann, C. F., and Hillman, B. Experimental determination of flow patterns of Gelfoam emboli: Safety implications. *AJR* 134:525, 1980.

79. Levin, H. S., Messer, J. V., and Pines, J.   Repeated venous and arterial catheterization in man: An analysis of complications. *Am. Heart J.* 73:475, 1967.

80. Lipp, H., O'Donoghue, K., and Resnekov, L. Intracardiac knotting of a flow-directed balloon catheter. *N. Engl. J. Med.* 284:220, 1971.

81. Lipton, M. J., Abbott, J. A., Kosek, J. C., Hayashi, T., Lee, F. C. S., and Bishop, E.   Cardiovascular trauma from angiographic jets—validation of a theoretic concept in dogs. *Radiology* 129:363, 1978.

82. Luepker, R. V., Bouchard, R. J., Burns, R., and Warbasse, J. R.   Systemic heparinization during percutaneous coronary angiography: Evaluation of effectiveness in decreasing thrombotic and embolic catheter complications. *Cathet. Cardiovasc. Diagn.* 1:35, 1975.

83. McAfee, J. G.   A survey of complications of abdominal aortography. *Radiology* 68:825, 1957.

84. McCarty, R. J., and Glasser, S. P.   Throm-bogenicity of guide wires. *Am. J. Cardiol.* 32:943, 1973.

85. McConnell, R. W., Fore, W. W., and Taylor, A. Embolic occlusion of the renal artery following arteriography: Successful management. *Radiology* 107:273, 1973.

86. McGraw, J. Y.   Arteriography of peripheral vessels: A review with report of complications. *Angiology* 14:306, 1963.

87. Meaney, T. F.   Complications of percutaneous femoral angiography. *Geriatrics* 29:61, 1974.

88. Miller, H. C., and Miller, G. A. H.   Experience with systemic heparinization during cardiac catheterization by brachial arteriotomy. *Br. Heart J.* 36:1122, 1974.

89. Mishkin, M. M., Baum, S., and Di Chiro, G. Emergency treatment of angiography-induced paraplegia and tetraplegia (letter). *N. Engl. J. Med.* 288:1184, 1973.

90. Molnar, W., and Paul, D. J.   Complications of axillary arteriotomies: An analysis of 1,762 consecutive studies. *Radiology* 104:269, 1972.

91. Moore, C. H., Wolma, F. J., Brown, R. W., and Derrick, J. R.   Complications of cardiovascular radiology: A review of 1,204 cases. *Am. J. Surg.* 120:591, 1970.

92. Mortensson, W.   Angiography of the femoral artery following percutaneous catheterization in infants and children. *Acta Radiol.* [*Diagn.*] (Stockh.) 17:581, 1976.

93. Nachnani, G. H., Lessin, L. S., Motomiya, T., and Jensen, W. N.   Scanning electron microscopy of thrombogenesis on vascular catheter surfaces. *N. Engl. J. Med.* 286:139, 1972.

94. Okuda, K., Musha, H., Nakajima, Y., Takayasu, K., Suzuki, Y., Morita, M., and Yamasaki, T. Frequency of intrahepatic arteriovenous fistula as a sequela to percutaneous needle puncture of the liver. *Gastroenterology* 74:1204, 1978.

95. Older, R.   Contrast-induced renal failure: A radiological problem and a radiological diagnosis. *Radiology* 131:553, 1979.

96. Ovitt, T. W., Durst, S., Moore, R., and Amplatz, K.   Guide wire thrombogenicity and its reduction. *Radiology* 111:43, 1974.

97. Page, D. W., Teres, D., and Hartshorn, J. W. Fatal hemorrhage from Swan-Ganz catheter (letter). *N. Engl. J. Med.* 291:260, 1974.

98. Perl, S., Wener, L., and Lyons, W. S.   Pseudoaneurysm after angiography. *Med. Ann. D. C.* 42:173, 1973.

99. Rabinov, K., and Paulin, S.   Roentgen diagnosis of venous thrombosis in the leg. *Arch. Surg.* 104:134, 1972.

100. Rashid, A., Hildner, F. J., Fester, A., Javier, R. P., and Samet, P.   Thromboembolism associated with pigtail catheters. *Cathet. Cardiovasc. Diagn.* 1:183, 1975.

101. Reuter, S. R.   On behalf of translumbar aortography (editorial). *AJR* 131:733, 1978.

102. Rich, N. M., Hobson, R. W., II, and Fedde, C. W. Vascular trauma secondary to diagnostic and therapeutic procedures. *Am. J. Surg.* 128:715, 1974.

103. Richardson, J. D., Grover, F. L., and Trinkle, J. K. Intravenous catheter emboli: Experience with twenty cases and collective review. *Am. J. Surg.* 128:722, 1974.

104. Ritchie, W. G. M., Lynch, P. R., and Stewart, G. J. The effect of contrast media on normal and inflamed canine veins: A scanning and transmission electron microscopic study. *Invest. Radiol.* 9:444, 1974.

105. Rosenthal, A., Anderson, M., Thomson, S. J., Pappas, A. M., and Fyler, D. C. Superficial femoral artery catheterization: Effect on extremity length. *Am. J. Dis. Child.* 124:240, 1972.

106. Rossi, P., Young, I. S., and Panke, W. F. Techniques, usefulness, and hazards of arteriography of pheochromocytoma: Review of 99 cases. *J.A.M.A.* 205:547, 1968.

107. Ryan, J. A., Jr., Abel, R. M., Abbott, W. M., Hopkins, C. C., Chesney, T. McC., Colley, R., Phillips, K., and Fischer, J. E. Catheter complications in total parenteral nutrition: A prospective study of 200 consecutive patients. *N. Engl. J. Med.* 290:757, 1974.

108. Schreiber, M. H. Complications of angiography: Incidence and prevention. *Tex. Med.* 67:68, 1971.

109. Seidenberg, B., and Hurwitt, E. S. Retrograde femoral (Seldinger) aortography: Surgical complications in 26 cases. *Ann. Surg.* 163:221, 1966.

110. Seldinger, S. I. Catheter replacement of the needle in percutaneous arteriography. A new technique. *Acta Radiol.* 39:368, 1953.

111. Shawker, T. H., Kluge, R. M., and Ayella, R. J. Bacteremia associated with angiography. *J.A.M.A.* 229:1090, 1974.

112. Shuttleworth, E. C., and Wise, G. R. Transient global amnesia due to arterial embolism. *Arch. Neurol.* 29:340, 1973.

113. Siegelman, S. S., Caplan, L. H., and Annes, G. P. Complications of catheter angiography: Study with oscillometry and "pullout" angiograms. *Radiology* 91:251, 1968.

114. Sigstedt, B., and Lunderquist, A. Complications of angiographic examinations. *AJR* 130:455, 1978.

115. Skovranek, J., and Samanek, M. Chronic impairment of leg muscle blood flow following cardiac catheterisation in childhood. *AJR* 132:71, 1979.

116. Spigos, D. G., Thane, T. T., and Capek, V. Skin necrosis following extravasation during peripheral phlebography. *Radiology* 123:605, 1977.

117. Staal, A., van Voorthuisen, A. E., and van Dijk, L. M. Neurological complications following arterial catheterisation by the axillary approach. *Br. J. Radiol.* 39:115, 1966.

118. Stamm, W. E., Colella, J. J., Anderson, R. L., and Dixon, R. E. Indwelling arterial catheters as a source of nosocomial bacteremia: An outbreak caused by flavobacterium species. *N. Engl. J. Med.* 292:1099, 1975.

119. Stark, F. R., and Coburn, J. W. Renal failure following methylglucamine diatrizoate (Renografin) aortography: Report of a case with unilateral renal artery stenosis. *J. Urol.* 96:848, 1966.

120. Takahashi, O., Zakheim, R., Park, M. K., Mattioli, L., and Diehl, A. M. The effects of transfemoral cardiac catheterization on limb blood flow in children. *Chest* 71:159, 1977.

121. Thomas, H. A., and Sievers, R. E. Nonsurgical reduction of arterial catheter knots. *AJR* 132:1018, 1979.

122. Vyden, J. K., Nagasawa, K., Graettinger, W., Marcus, H. S., Groseth-Dittrich, M., and Swan, H. J. C. The effects of transfemoral catheterization on blood flow in the extremities. *Circulation* 50:741, 1974.

123. Wagoner, R. D. Acute renal failure associated with contrast agents. *Arch. Intern. Med.* 138:353, 1978.

124. Walker, W. J., Mundall, S. L., Broderick, H. G., Prasad, B., Kim, J., and Ravi, J. M. Systemic heparinization for femoral percutaneous coronary arteriography. *N. Engl. J Med.* 288:826, 1973.

125. Wallace, S., Medellin, H., De Jongh, D., and Gianturco, C. Systemic heparinization for angiography. *AJR* 116:204, 1972.

126. Walters, M. B., Stanger, H. A. D., and Rotem, C. E. Complications with percutaneous central venous catheters. *J.A.M.A.* 220:1455, 1972.

127. Welch, G. W., McKeel, D. W., Jr., Silverstein, P., and Walker, H. L. The role of catheter composition in the development of thrombophlebitis. *Surg. Gynecol. Obstet.* 138:421, 1974.

128. Wolfman, E. F., Jr., and Boblitt, D. E. Intramural aortic dissection as a complication of translumbar aortography. *Arch. Surg.* 78:629, 1959.

129. Woodside, J., Schwarz, H., and Bergreen, P. Peripheral embolization complicating bilateral renal infarction with Gelfoam. *AJR* 126:1033, 1976.

130. Yorra, F. H., Oblath, R., Jaffe, H., Simmons, D. H., and Levy, S. E. Massive thrombosis associated with use of the Swan-Ganz catheter. *Chest* 65:682, 1974.

131. Young, D. A., and Maurer, R. M. Successful manipulation of a knotted intravascular catheter allowing nonsurgical removal. *Radiology* 94:155, 1970.

The Abnormal Abdominal Aorta: Arteriosclerosis and Other Diseases

ELLIOT O. LIPCHIK
STANLEY M. ROGOFF

The most common, virtually universal, disease of blood vessels is arteriosclerosis. Arteriosclerosis begins as an intimal change and becomes a palpable, visible hardening and thickening of an arterial wall [67]. Its cause, site of involvement, and microscopic and histopathologic-chemical characteristics may vary greatly from patient to patient. For example, Monckeberg's calcification in the elastic fiber and ground substance of the media of muscular arteries is very similar to calcinosis infantium (i.e., arteriosclerosis in the newborn) [67]. A more precise definition of the disease is thus impossible because of its diverse characteristics.

Arterial disease is not solely associated with old age. The arteries begin to change somewhat in everyone at an early age, and a significant number of patients under 40 years of age have severe occlusive arterial disease of the lower extremities [19]. Almost all people beyond middle age have some signs of atherosclerosis although they often remain asymptomatic—most likely because the width of the aortic lumen remains adequate.

The abdominal aorta below the renal arteries is the commonest site of atherosclerosis. The symptoms of localized aortoiliac disease are often typical, and the diagnosis is easy to substantiate clinically and to measure [18]. Most patients with aortoiliac occlusive disease also have associated femoral and distal arterial occlusions. In diffuse disease, extensions develop fairly rapidly, symptoms worsen, and surgery is required sooner than with localized processes [42]. The progression of the arteriosclerotic process is also faster in diabetic patients [39]. Gastrointestinal bleeding secondary to rupture of a small aneurysm in a sclerotic artery or arteriole and thromboses of visceral arteries with their attendant intestinal changes are part of the arteriosclerotic symptom complex. These associated lesions are more difficult to diagnose and correct.

Reconstruction of the aorta and the iliac arteries by thromboendarterectomy, shunts, or dilatations has proved to be extremely satisfactory therapy for disabling arteriosclerosis obliterans of the aortoiliac system. There are therapeutic procedures available for even poor-risk patients who suffer from significant cardiopulmonary disease as well as disabling ischemic symptoms of the lower extremities [6, 8, 23, 38]. Failure of aortoiliac endarterectomy or any other procedure may be due to unrecognized persistent disease located distally [18]. It must be remembered that arteriosclerosis is a diffuse disease as well as a malignant one, and the long-term survival rate of these patients is dismal, even with treatment. For example, in patients who underwent femoropopliteal bypass reconstruction, DeWeese and Rob [21] showed a 5-year mortality of 48 percent and a 10-year mortality of 73 percent, with most deaths due to vital organ failure secondary to arteriosclerotic disease.

Angiography is the most effective diagnostic approach for the demonstration of aortoiliac obstruction sites, distal runoff vessels or collateral vessels, and associated stenoses or occlusions of the major visceral arteries. Estimation by angiography of hemodynamic changes caused by vessel narrowing is feasible when the stenosis is severe or mild [56]. In moderately severe stenoses (50–75% stenosis), the arteriogram may not accurately indicate the hemodynamic significance [10, 76].

Angiographic Appearance

Disease of the aorta and iliac vessels can produce a variety of roentgenographic signs that reflect the gross morphologic changes. These signs are (1) diffuse narrowing of the vessels; (2) generally irregular vascular contours and diameters; (3) nicks, filling defects, and calcifications along the vessel walls; (4) spotty or ragged density of the opaque column; (5) vessels that are generally large or tortuous or both; (6) saccular dilatations; and (7) aneurysms. Frank occlusion of a vessel is a relatively late sequela, and it is almost always due to obliterative arteriosclerosis.

The surgeon almost invariably finds a greater degree of luminal compromise, intimal atherosclerosis, mural thrombus formation, and palpable hardening of the vessel wall than is shown by the angiograms [25, 77].

DIFFUSE VASCULAR NARROWING

An appearance of smooth, general narrowing of the large vessels is one of the surprising manifestations of arteriosclerosis. The very smoothness of the margins of the opaque column can be deceptive, suggesting vessel spasm more than atherosclerotic disease. At points along the course of the artery, however, there are short constrictions, irregular margins, or even seg-

Figure 48-1. Probable congenital hypoplasia of the femoral arteries. (A) The common femoral arteries are diffusely narrowed on both sides in this 13-year-old girl. Hypertension has been present at least since early childhood, with increasing claudication of the lower extremities. (B) Above the adductor canal, the femoral arteries terminate medially into an anomalous vessel above the knee. There was no evidence of a popliteal artery or normal trifurcation, and there were no dorsal pedal or posterior tibial pulsations. (Courtesy of James Manning, M.D.)

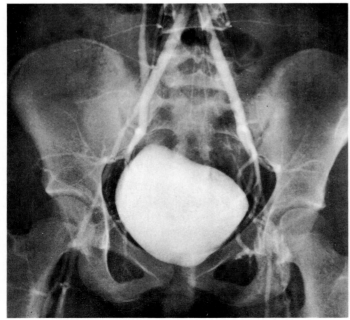

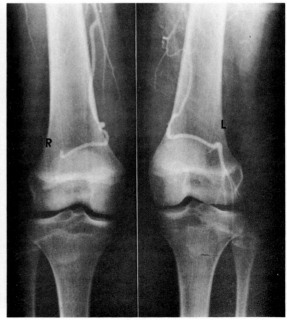

A

B

Figure 48-2. Retroperitoneal fibrosis causing a localized, smooth narrowing of the first portion of the left common iliac artery. This 56-year-old man had typical symptoms of arterial obstruction. The fibrotic process extended up the retroperitoneal space on the left, and it also involved the left ureter. There are also typical atherosclerotic irregularities and notches of the abdominal aorta. (From Neistadt et al., Vascular system involvement by idiopathic retroperitoneal fibrosis. *Surgery* 59:950, 1966. Reproduced with permission.)

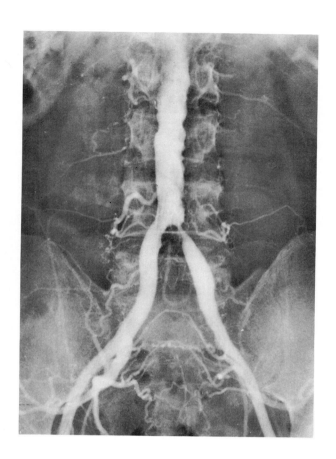

mental occlusions to aid the diagnosis. The pattern becomes clear when a long radiograph is available for study. Diffuse narrowing of the lumen of a vessel, including the aorta, may also be due to a dissecting aneurysm, a thrombus within an aneurysm, aortitis [34], periaortic fibrosis [1], postradiotherapy sequelae [15, 62], congenital hypoplasia (Fig. 48-1), coarctation, or hypercalcemia [45, 55, 63]. Arterial fibrodysplasia can occur in many regions of the vascular tree. Its actual incidence is unknown. There has even been a report of "fibromuscular dysplasia" of the abdominal aorta [41], as well as several reports of involvement of the external iliac arteries [60, 61, 75]. Figure 48-2 is an example of nonarteriosclerotic, smooth narrowing. (Figure 46-4 illustrates narrowing of an ex-

Figure 48-3. Diffuse narrowing and occlusion of the abdominal aorta below the renal arteries in a 60-year-old diabetic woman who had acute paralysis of both legs 2 weeks prior to this examination. The narrowing was due to a thrombus extending up from the iliac arteries and that was secondary to severe arteriosclerotic disease.

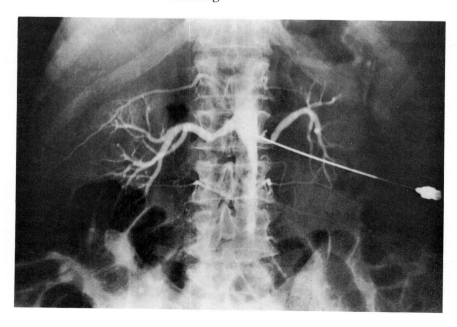

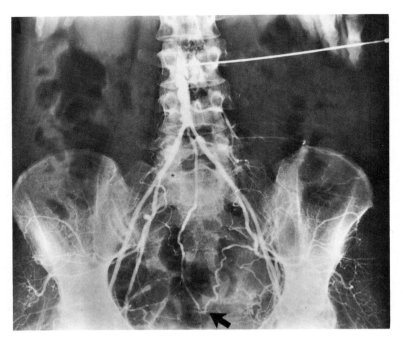

Figure 48-4. Note the slender, smooth, common iliac and common femoral vessels. The ragged aortic column and the narrowed common iliac origins, however, are signs of diffuse atherosclerosis. The prominence of the middle sacral artery and its inosculation (*arrow*) with the left lateral sacral artery is a clue to collateralization around a significant stenosis of the left common iliac origin. The patient is a 57-year-old woman who had diabetes and who, for several years, had claudication about the left hip, both thighs, and the left calf. She had no pulses in either lower extremity.

traluminal contrast material column in the aortic wall after faulty placement of a translumbar needle.) This should not be mistaken for narrowing of the true lumen of the aorta. Figure 48-3 shows diffuse narrowing and occlusion of the aorta caused by extensive thrombosis. Figure 48-4 shows an example of smoother atherosclerotic narrowing following thrombosis.

Takayasu's disease and other nonspecific arteritis may involve all vessels, including the abdominal aorta [34]. (The geographic variations and ethnic distributions of Takayasu's disease are quite intriguing [20].) The angiographic search for involved major vessels should be comprehensive [47, 65].

GENERALLY IRREGULAR VASCULAR DIAMETERS

Because normal main-stem vessels should show a gradual, smoothly tapered diminution in diameter (see Chap. 45), any inconsistency in this geometric pattern is suggestive of arteriosclerosis. Figure 48-5 illustrates an unusual exception to this rule [71]. Most of the aorto-

grams illustrated in this chapter show some degree of wall irregularity.

NICKS, FILLING DEFECTS, OR CALCIFICATIONS ALONG THE VESSEL MARGINS

These are signs of intimal atheromas, mural thrombi, and degenerative calcification (Figs. 48-6, 48-7). They are the classic stigmata of intimal atherosclerosis. Monckeberg's medial calcifications can occur in the aorta although there they are not as clearly divorced from intimal calcifications as in the peripheral vessels [2, 50]. Calcification does not establish that a vessel is thrombosed, and, conversely, 40 percent of deWolfe's patients with chronic aortoiliac thromboses did not have obvious calcification of their large vessels on roentgenograms [22]. Calcification in smaller vessels may have considerably more clinical significance in terms of obstruction than it does in larger vessels. The metastatic calcification of the smaller vessels in patients with chronic renal failure is probably indicative of sec-

Figure 48-5. Stationary arterial waves. A fortuitous finding in an asymptomatic 28-year-old man. These diffuse, symmetric, and regularly spaced narrowings were constant and present during slow manual injections of small amounts of contrast material. The original purpose of the angiogram was to discover the cause of the patient's hematuria.

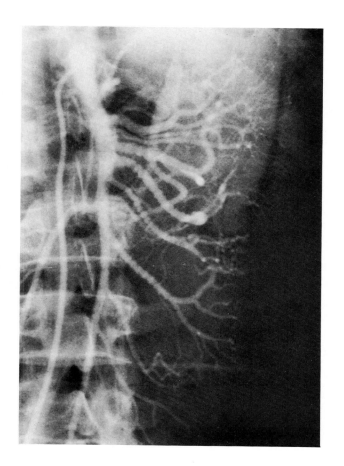

ondary hyperparathyroidism and may even be seen without osteodystrophy [33].

SPOTTY OR RAGGED DENSITY OF THE OPAQUE COLUMN

Atherosclerotic lesions are ofen eccentrically located in the arterial wall. A variation in the density of the contrast column is a clue to the presence of plaques and mural thrombi on the anterior and/or posterior wall of the vessel. Wylie and McGuinness [78] stressed the importance of this subtle finding. Severe anteroposterior narrowing, which can be present even if the vessel's lateral diameter seems adequate on the frontal angiograms, would not be detected without a lateral projection unless one searched for this sign. Oblique and biplane projections should be *routinely* employed in arteriography [69, 72]. However, significantly different projections of the branches of the aorta may be impossible. The three-dimensional character of vessels must be kept in mind constantly. Careful scrutiny of many

Figure 48-6. (A) Heavy linear calcification of the lower abdominal aorta and both iliofemoral systems *(arrows)*. (B) Translumbar aortography shows an occlusion of the right external iliac artery and moderate-to-severe atherosclerotic involvement on the left. Note the areas of decreased density in the contrast column of the left external iliac artery. On later films, the femoral artery was reconstituted via collateral vessels from the right internal iliac system. The obturator artery is quite dilated *(arrow)*.

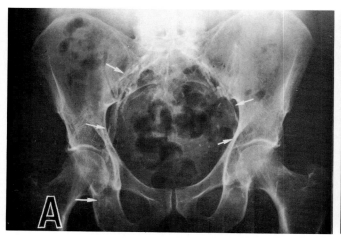
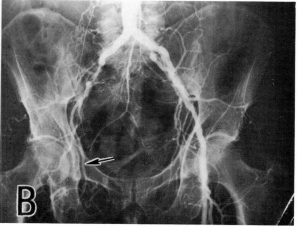

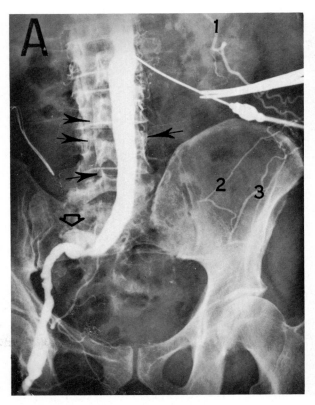
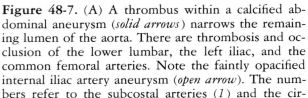
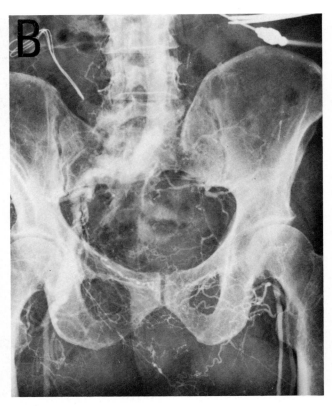

Figure 48-7. (A) A thrombus within a calcified abdominal aneurysm (*solid arrows*) narrows the remaining lumen of the aorta. There are thrombosis and occlusion of the lower lumbar, the left iliac, and the common femoral arteries. Note the faintly opacified internal iliac artery aneurysm (*open arrow*). The numbers refer to the subcostal arteries (*1*) and the cir-

cumflex iliac branches (*2, 3*), which provide collateral supply to the left leg. (B) A film several seconds later revealed opacification of the left superficial and deep femoral arteries from the collateral vessels seen in (A) and probably from the pudendal and inferior hemorrhoidal vessels.

---

of the illustrations in this chapter will reveal areas of irregularly decreased density in the aorta and large vessels.

There are, therefore, limitations to the angiographic identification of even major stenosing atheromas of which all angiographers ought to be aware. In one postmortem series, more than one-fourth of the patients had large plaques on the anterior or posterior walls of the renal arteries that were inconspicuous on the anteroposterior angiograms [3]. So-called intimal flaps secondary to lap-seatbelt injury of the abdominal aorta may also be difficult to visualize on one projection [9]. Not all filling defects projecting into the lumen are arteriosclerotic in origin; for example, Figure 48-8 illustrates the angiographic features of heparin-induced thromboembolism [51]. Such nonatherosclerotic lesions, while not necessarily unique in appearance,

are distinctive, and the diagnosis may be suggested angiographically, especially in the appropriate clinical context.

GENERALLY LARGE AND/OR
TORTUOUS VESSELS

Some arteriosclerotic patients demonstrate a remarkable general dilatation and/or a serpentine course of the aorta and the iliac arteries (Fig. 48-9). Lesser degrees of tortuosity are more common, of course. Despite the disease process, these vessels frequently are widely patent, and some are quite soft to palpation. Diffuse tortuosity and lengthening of the arteries may (very rarely) be seen in very young people, even young children [5, 27]. Histologically, the common denominator in these rare conditions seems to be fragmentation of the internal elastic membrane

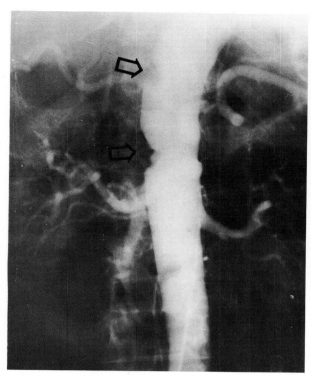

Figure 48-8. Heparin-induced thromboembolism. Abdominal aortogram demonstrating contour deformities and mural filling defects (*arrows*) of adherent mural thrombi composed mostly of platelets and fibrin (white thrombi). (From Lindsey et al. [51]. Reproduced with permission from *Radiology*.)

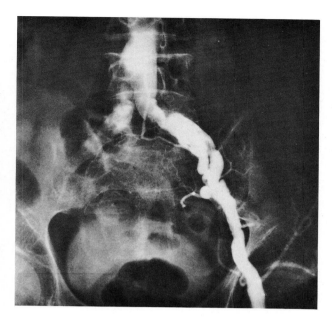

Figure 48-9. Despite the marked tortuosity and irregular aneurysmal dilatations of the left iliac and femoral arteries, a femoral catheter was successfully used to demonstrate the aortoiliac region on both sides.

and hyperplasia and distortion of the elastic fibers. (See Chapter 49 for a discussion of arteriomegaly.)

SACCULAR DILATATIONS

Occasionally there may be small, saccular dilatations or frank aneurysms along the vessel's course (Fig. 48-10). These are often multiple, as in the syndrome of polyaneurysmal dystrophy, described by Fontaine et al. [30].

ANEURYSMS

Aneurysms of the aorta and its pelvic branches are discussed in Chapter 49.

OCCLUSIONS OF THE AORTOILIAC SYSTEM

Although patients frequently present a clinical picture of relatively acute thrombosis of a large vessel, in many cases it is clear from the history that it is simply the terminal event in slowly progressive arteriosclerotic stenosis [4, 53, 78]. The final episode of complete occlusion may in many patients be tolerated without medical attention, and the history of this event may be elicited only on questioning when the patient finally consults his physician because of chronic claudication or other symptoms. Symptoms of arterial ischemia may not appear until arteriosclerotic obliteration is almost complete [25, 78]. The blood flow through a vessel can remain relatively adequate until the vessel's diameter is reduced about 70 percent [46], and in the aortoiliac system the blood flow is not reduced by one-half until the luminal area is decreased 82 percent or more [54].

According to May et al. [56], different vessels have different critical degrees of stenosis (e.g., the carotid arteries, with their slower blood flow, may tolerate a greater degree of stenosis before a pressure drop is seen). It is certainly crucial, therefore, that patients with claudication about the hip, gluteal muscles, or thigh; chronic pain in the lower back or low abdomen; weakness in walking; or difficulty in maintaining an erection [49] be recognized as possibly having chronic aortoiliac thrombosis. If one waits for the symp-

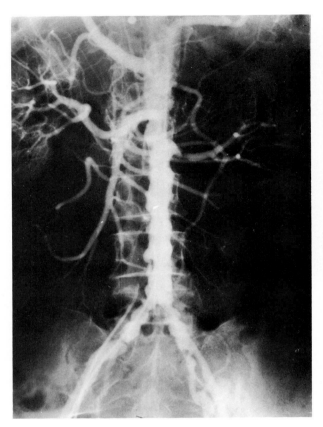

Figure 48-10. Diffuse, severe, multiple saccular dilatations and plaques of the abdominal aorta and iliofemoral arteries. This atheromatous disease process also involved the lower thoracic aorta but spared the superficial femoral and popliteal arteries. Note the severe narrowing of the first portion of the left renal artery. This 62-year-old man with a long history of smoking and hypertension, and diabetes of recent onset, had a cyanotic, painful, great toe. Decreased bilateral kidney function and small kidneys were present. There was no follow-up. (Courtesy of Frank E. Maddison, M.D.)

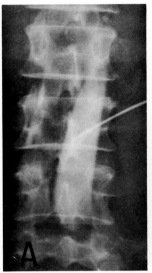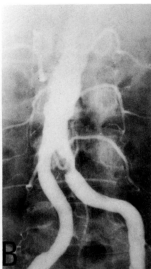

Figure 48-11. (A) A test injection through a translumbar needle revealed an inferior vena cava on the left side. (B) The aortoiliac system is further to the right, as demonstrated a day later by catheter technique. The aorta shows the ragged outlines of atherosclerosis, and the iliac arteries show the moderate tortuosity of arteriosclerosis. There is a localized narrowing in the common iliac on the left which may be hemodynamically significant because the left lumbar arteries are quite dilated. This 59-year-old man suffered from claudication but had no other associated cardiovascular anomalies.

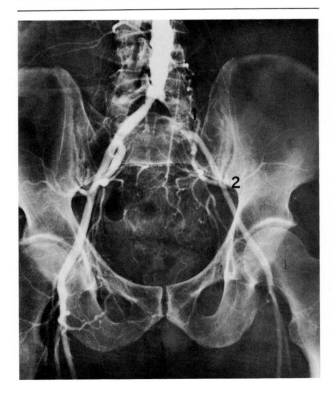

toms of calf claudication or for obvious nutritional disturbances in the legs, many cases will be missed [22]. Conversely, calf claudication may develop first (Figs. 48-11–48-13; see also Figs. 48-9, 48-10).

Acute embolization occurs frequently as a result of mural cardiac thrombi in arteriosclerotic heart disease, often secondary to myocardial infarction. Rheumatic heart disease with thrombus formation in the left atrium is another prominent cause of embolization (Fig. 48-14), and thrombosed prosthetic heart valves as a source of emboli are also well known [7]. In some instances, emboli can arise from atherosclerotic plaques

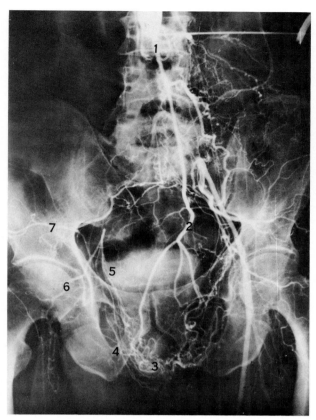

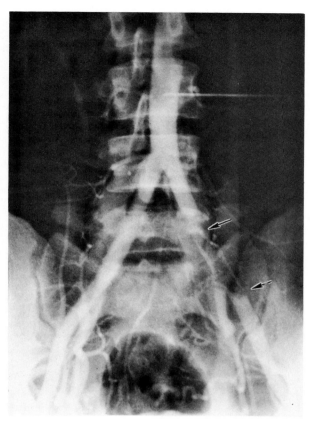

Figure 48-13. Chronic aortoiliac obstruction below the inferior mesenteric artery. The principal affluent collateral vessel is the inferior mesenteric artery (*1*) with its superior hemorrhoidal branch (*2*). Through rich rectal and perirectal anastomoses, the inferior hemorrhoidal (*3*), internal pudendal (*4*), middle hemorrhoidal (*5*), inferior gluteal (*6*), and superior gluteal (*7*) branches of the internal iliac artery are refilled bilaterally. The patient was a 62-year-old man whose only complaint was bilateral calf claudication, worse on the right, of one year's duration.

Figure 48-14. Thrombus in the left common iliac artery extending for a short distance into the external iliac artery (*arrows*). This was an acute occurrence in a patient with long-standing rheumatic heart disease. The aorta and other vessels have normal, smooth, parallel walls. Decreased density in the midportion of the right common iliac artery suggests anteroposterior narrowing or thrombus.

higher in the aorta as well as from aneurysms [29]. So-called cholesterol emboli most commonly involve the kidney and the gastrointestinal system, including the pancreas [44, 57]. It is quite conceivable that rough manipulation of a catheter along an atherosclerotic aortic wall may cause such embolization.

Dramatic symptoms of embolization occur in the absence of a well-developed collateral system. The patient with gradual arteriosclerotic obliteration is more likely to have developed a collateral reserve during the slowly progressive phase of his disease.

In Wylie's complete series of 500 patients with symptoms of occlusion at the abdominopelvic and/or leg level, long-film aortography demonstrated a multiplicity and diffuseness of lesions [77]. The routine depiction of thigh and leg ves-

◀ **Figure 48-12.** Chronic localized iliac thrombosis in a 60-year-old man with claudication of the left hip and gluteal regions. Note the decreased density of the entire left iliofemoral system, indicating a slower or decreased flow of blood. The important collateral vessels arise from the left lumbar, iliolumbar (*1*), and superior gluteal (*2*) arteries.

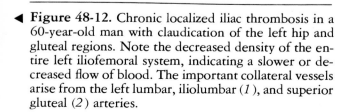

sels during aortography is an important contribution to presurgical evaluation. Those relatively few patients with localized aortoiliac obstruction are likely to be younger, to have a low prevalence of diabetes, and to have a high prevalence of hypercholesterolemia [18]. Approximately one-half of the female patients will have had an artificial menopause [32].

Chronic Aortoiliac Thrombosis

As originally described by Leriche [49], the syndrome of complete obliteration of the aortic bifurcation occurred predominantly in young adult males and included (1) the inability to

Figure 48-15. A translumbar aortogram demonstrating obstruction of the abdominal aorta just distal to the inferior mesenteric artery. Note the aberrant left renal artery to the lower pole. The lower lumbar arteries and the inferior mesenteric artery serve as large affluent collateral vessels. Both femoral arteries were seen to be reconstituted on a lateral film. This 56-year-old laborer had mild hypertension; he complained only of severe, crampy leg pain after walking about 300 feet. An aortofemoral bypass graft was inserted successfully.

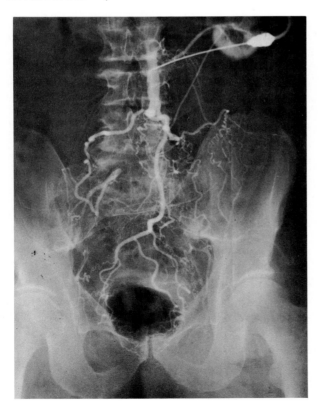

maintain an erection; (2) weakness of the lower extremities without claudication; (3) soft-tissue (so-called global) atrophy of both lower extremities; (4) no trophic changes of the skin or nails; (5) slow wound healing; (6) pallor of the legs and feet, even when standing; and (7) absent pulses over the aorta and iliac arteries and in the thighs and legs. Cases that fit this pattern precisely are quite rare, however, and most authors now use the term *Leriche syndrome* to describe a variable spectrum of clinical symptoms traceable either to complete obstruction (Fig. 48-15; see also Figs. 48-12, 48-13) or to partial obstruction at the aortic bifurcation [4, 22, 35, 77]. The clinical symptoms vary with the adequacy of the collateral circulation, the degree of occlusion, and the coexistence of more peripheral atherosclerotic lesions.

Complete Occlusion of the Aorta

Complete occlusion of the aorta, a somewhat unusual diagnosis, rarely extends upward to occlude the renal arteries totally [48], but the renal and other visceral arteries are frequently found at surgery to be at least partially involved [43]. Total occlusion *above* the renal and visceral arteries is very rare [52, 68]. In such a case, the visceral arteries and the lower aorta have to be supplied by large vessels coursing through the thoracic and abdominal walls (Figs. 48-16, 48-17). Syphilis [37] and aortic coarctation [45, 55] have been reported to cause occlusion near or just below the renal arteries.

In Muller and Figley's report of 19 complete aortic occlusions [59], about half began above the origin of the inferior mesenteric artery and about half began below. All extended down to involve at least the origins of the common iliac arteries, except a single case of a high, short obstruction in which the aortic occlusion terminated above the inferior mesenteric origin (see Fig. 48-15).

Leriche originally postulated that complete thrombosis of the terminal aorta and common iliac arteries originated in the iliac arteries and extended upward [48]. The general incidence of symmetrical atherosclerosis in the iliac arteries and the adjacent aorta corroborates this theory in our experience and that of others [4, 35, 59]. It is logical that the smaller iliac vessels would thrombose before the aorta, but this is by no means

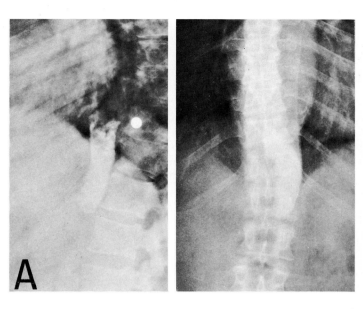

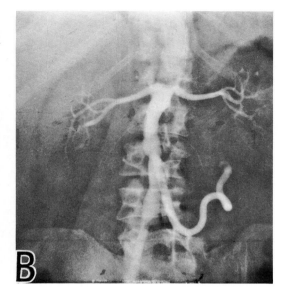

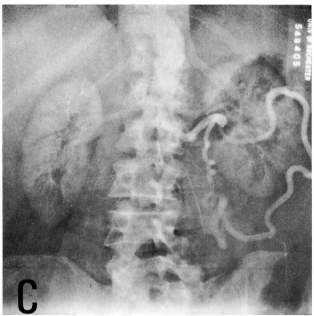

Figure 48-16. Calcified thrombosis with occlusion of the abdominal aorta localized to a segment above the origins of the renal arteries. (A) Anteroposterior and lateral roentgenograms show smoothly marginated, dense calcification within the lumen of the aorta from the eleventh thoracic vertebra to the first lumbar vertebra. (B) A retrograde aortogram (there were good femoral artery pulsations) showing abrupt, convex obstruction to the contrast material corresponding exactly to the inferior limit of the calcified thrombus. (C) A huge branch of the inferior mesenteric artery courses to the left and joins with and fills the proximal portion of the middle colic branch of the superior mesenteric artery. Later films showed opacification of the main trunk of the superior mesenteric artery and its intestinal branches. This 45-year-old man had been severely hypertensive for about 2 years before the study, and aortic calcification had been noted about 4 years before the angiograms. (From Lipchik et al. [52]. Reproduced with permission from *Radiology*.)

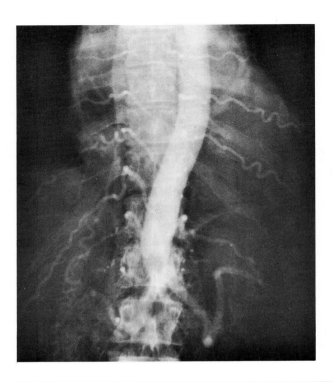

Figure 48-17. Dilated, tortuous intercostal arteries that serve as important collateral vessels in overcoming obstruction of the abdominal aorta in a 57-year-old woman. Rib notching was not yet apparent on plain radiographs of the chest.

invariable. In many cases it is impossible to determine pathologically whether a mass of thrombotic material in a vessel is a thrombus formed at the site or an embolus [66]. Figure 48-18 illustrates occlusion of the abdominal aorta just below the renal arteries due to thrombosis of a large aneurysm.

In one relatively large series of 28 patients with total occlusion of the abdominal aorta, the average age was 54 years, with claudication as the prime symptom in all and heavy tobacco use in most [74]. Surprisingly this group had a low incidence of diabetes and coronary artery disease.

Figure 48-18. Aortic occlusion due to thrombosis of a large aneurysm (10 × 15 × 8 cm). Antegrade injection of contrast material into the upper abdominal aorta through a catheter inserted percutaneously into the left axillary artery. (A) Both renal arteries and the superior mesenteric artery are patent. (B) The superior mesenteric artery supplies the distal inferior mesenteric artery via branches of the middle colic artery (*arrow*). There was later faint opacification of distal femoral vessels. This 68-year-old man had a typical Leriche syndrome; his most troublesome complaint was pain and "tiredness" of both legs and feet. Shortly after surgery, he died of thrombotic occlusion of the superior mesenteric artery with ischemic necrosis of the bowel.

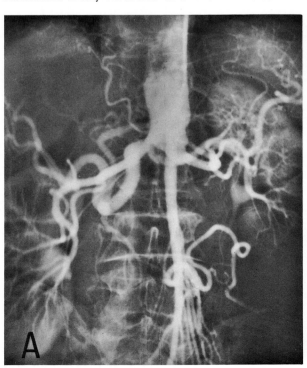

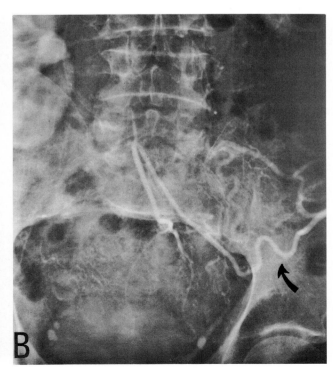

Collateral Pathways

Even incompletely obstructing lesions in mainstem vessels may cause unusual opacification and enlargement of certain branch arteries that are known to serve as collateral vessels. Thus, such collateral prominence can be used as an important angiographic sign in corroborating or raising the suspicion that subtle defects or irregularities in the opaque column in a main artery are truly significant signs of obstruction. To avoid missing important collateral demonstration, the interpreter must be careful to note whether the radiograph has been exposed at a moment when collateral vessels might be expected to be filled.

The arteriographic technique should guarantee the depiction of both the beginning of the mainstem block and its distal reconstitution. Major collateral pathways should all be demonstrated. Because intercostal and epigastric arteries may serve as collateral pathways in obstruction of the abdominal aorta, it would be theoretically desirable to inject contrast material into the ascending aorta (Fig. 48-19). Figure 48-20 is a schematic diagram of the major parietal pathways of collateral circulation.

In discussing collateral circulation, the terminology employed by Edwards and LeMay [24] is helpful. An *affluent* vessel is a collateral branch arising from the patent main vessel above the block or narrowing or from a patent contralateral mate. An *effluent* vessel is a branch below the block that receives blood from the affluent vessel and permits it to flow retrogradely to refill the blocked artery. The affluent vessel may pass blood into the effluent vessel in a bold, continuous line (a phenomenon called *inosculation*), or the affluent vessel may connect with the effluent vessel by a fine network of smaller vessels to form a *retiform anastomosis*. Intermediate anastomoses may also be needed to lead between the affluent vessel and its definitive effluent vessel.

Figure 48-19. Blood supply to the lower extremities via the epigastric arteries. (A) An upper abdominal aortogram shows a complete block of the lower aorta and both common iliac arteries and extensive collateral vessels to the internal iliac systems. The femoral arteries were not opacified at any time after this injection. (B) The second injection of contrast material into the ascending aorta shows good opacification of dilated epigastric arteries (*upper arrow*) reconstituting the femoral arteries (*lower arrow*). This 57-year-old man had bilateral calf claudication, no femoral pulses, yet warm lower limbs and feet. (Courtesy of Frank Maddison, M.D.)

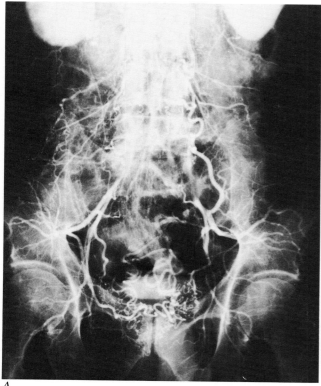

A

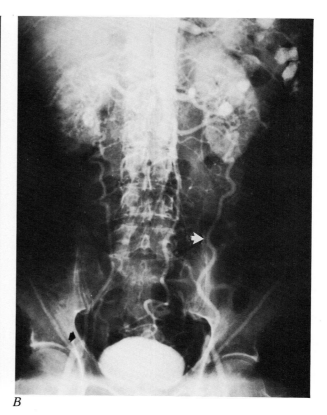

B

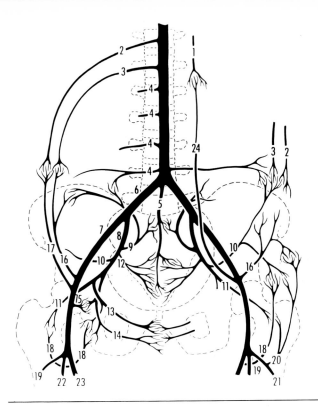

Figure 48-20. Schematic diagram of the major potential parietal pathways of collateral circulation demonstrated in aortoiliofemoral occlusive disease. Arteries: superior epigastric (*1*); intercostal (*2*); subcostal (*3*); lumbar (*4*); middle sacral (*5*); common iliac (*6*); external iliac (*7*); internal iliac (*8*); iliolumbar (*9*); superior gluteal (*10*); inferior gluteal (*11*); lateral sacral (*12*); obturator (*13*); internal pudendal (*14*); external pudendal (*15*); deep iliac circumflex (*16*); superficial iliac circumflex (*17*); medial femoral circumflex (*18*); lateral femoral circumflex (*19*); lateral ascending branch (*20*); lateral descending branch (*21*); profunda femoris (*22*); superficial femoral (*23*); inferior epigastric (*24*). (From Muller and Figley [59]. Reproduced with permission from *AJR*.)

Figure 48-21. Extensive visceral and parietal collateral vessels circumventing occluded left common iliac and right femoral arteries. (A) Note the large affluent last left lumbar artery (*1*) anastomosing with the iliolumbar artery. A large subcostal artery (*2*) sends branches to the left superior gluteal (*3*) and deep circumflex iliac (*4*) arteries. The superior hemorrhoidal branch (*5*) of the inferior mesenteric artery anastomoses with the inferior hemorrhoidal artery and then into a large right obturator artery (*6*) with a strong inosculation with the right medial femoral circumflex artery (*7*). (B) Opacification of the left iliofemoral arteries (*8*) via superior gluteal, internal iliac, and obturator artery anastomoses. This 41-year-old alcoholic man was admitted to the hospital with acute pneumonitis and complaints of severe pain in both legs. (Courtesy of T. VanZandt, M.D.)

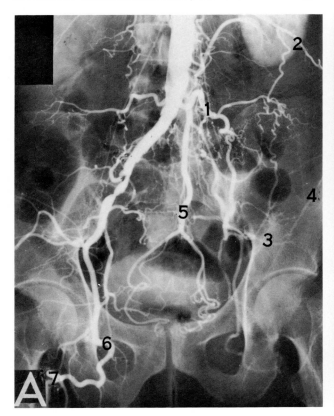

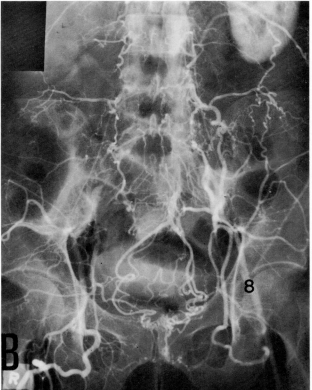

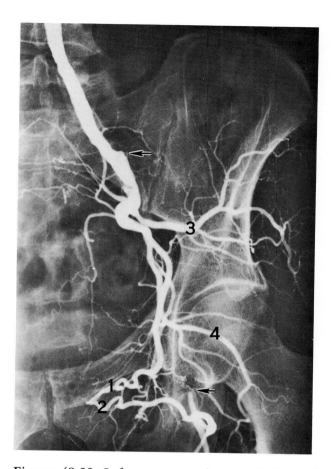

Figure 48-22. Left common and external iliac and superficial femoral artery obstruction (*between arrows*) with refilling of the deep femoral artery (*lower arrow*) via internal iliac affluent vessels. Note the large direct connection (inosculation) between the obturator (*1*) and medial femoral circumflex (*2*) arteries. The superior gluteal artery (*3*) is dilated, but its eventual anastomosis is not yet visible in this phase of the arteriogram. (It usually anastomoses with the lateral femoral circumflex artery via its ascending branch.) The inferior gluteal artery (*4*) is also quite dilated and helps supply the deep femoral artery. These parietal collateral vessels are unusually dilated because the inferior mesenteric and iliolumbar arteries were blocked.

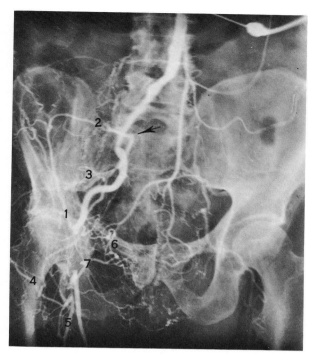

Figure 48-23. Internal iliac artery obstruction on the right. There are also obstructions involving a segment of the right common femoral artery and the iliofemoral system on the left. A large deep circumflex iliac artery (*1*) arises from the external iliac artery and refills the iliac branch of the iliolumbar artery (*2*) back to its common origin (*arrow*) with the superior gluteal and inferior gluteal (*3*) arteries (poorly opacified.) The common femoral artery obstruction is reconstituted by an anastomosis between the refilled gluteal vessels and the lateral femoral circumflex branches (*4*) back into the deep femoral artery (*5*). The inosculation from the obturator artery (*6*) to the medial femoral circumflex artery (*7*) is evident.

Inosculation maintains a good heavy head of pressure and leads to rapid refilling of the main vessel distal to the block, whereas there are inevitably a drop in pressure and a decrease in flow and opacification when collateral blood passes through a retiform connection. Common examples of inosculation are seen between the lumbar and iliolumbar arteries (Fig. 48-21; see also Figs. 48-12, 48-18), between the obturator and medial femoral circumflex arteries (Figs. 48-22, 48-23; see also Fig. 48-21), between the iliolumbar and deep circumflex iliac arteries (see Figs. 48-20, 48-23), between the superior gluteal and deep circumflex iliac arteries (Fig. 48-24; see also Figs. 48-21, 48-23), and between the superior gluteal artery and the ascending branch of the lateral femoral circumflex artery (see Figs. 48-20, 48-23, 48-24). Often the retiform anastomosis is not obvious on the radiograph although one may be certain that it is present because of the obvious proximity of the affluent and effluent vessels.

The following discussion of collateral pathways provides only an orientation for the reader. Different cases are discussed to show various types of collateral development. The presence or absence of specific vessels in any given angiogram depends on many factors other than logic, not the least of which is the diffuseness of the atheroscle-

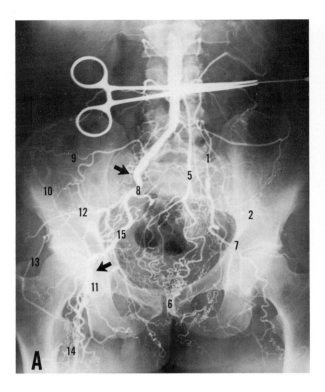

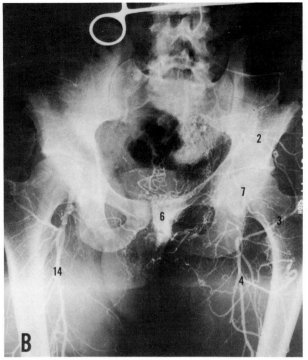

Figure 48-24. Chronic aortoiliofemoral obstruction. Note the importance of serial radiographs. This 44-year-old patient was successfully rehabilitated for work for over a year by insertion of a long aortopopliteal homograft. (A) On the patient's left there is a complete block of the iliofemoral system above the inguinal region. There are three main affluent channels to the left side: the left lumbar branches anatomose both with the left iliolumbar artery's lumbar branch (*1*) and with the left superior gluteal (*2*) and inferior gluteal (*7*, A) arteries, which in turn feed the lateral femoral circumflex (*3*, B) and thereby help to refill the left femoral artery (*4*, B). The superior hemorrhoidal arteries (*5*) inosculate with middle and inferior hemorrhoidal arteries about the rectum (*6*) which act as intermediates across the effluent branches of the left deep femoral artery (*4*, B). The sacral arteries also help to transmit blood to the deep femoral artery via anastomoses with the lumbar and again into the left inferior gluteal branch (*7*, B). On the right side there is an occlusion of the external iliac artery (*upper arrow*). However, inosculating collaterals between the iliac branch (*9*) of the iliolumbar and the deep circumflex iliac arteries (*10*) refill the right common femoral artery (*11*). (B) The later arterial phase shows that the superior gluteal artery (*12*, A) and the lateral femoral circumflex artery (*13*, A; *3*, B) also fill the deep femoral arteries (*14*). The hypogastric artery (*15*) communicates directly with the common femoral artery (*lower arrow*, A). In subsequent films, both distal superficial femoral and popliteal arteries were fully patent.

---

rotic disease process. Technical and flow artifacts may obscure certain channels.

Collateral Circulation in Aortoiliac Occlusion

The regions of the thorax, abdomen, pelvis, and lower extremities are potentially linked by a large network of both parietal and visceral vessels. These vessels may effectively bypass any segment of the aortoiliac system by collateral channel formation. Interconnections between the parietal and visceral systems are frequent. Figure 48-20 is a schematic diagram of the major parietal pathways of collateral circulation.

OCCLUSION OF THE AORTA

Visceral Collateral Network
The superior and inferior mesenteric arteries are the chief sources of visceral collateral circulation to the pelvis (see Figs. 48-15, 48-16, 48-18). When the aorta is occluded above the inferior mesenteric artery, the superior mesenteric artery acts as a main affluent vessel by carrying blood

through the left branch of the middle colic artery and into the intermediate left colic branch of the inferior mesenteric artery [24, 58, 59]. Figure 48-18 demonstrates refilling of distal vessels by this route.

The so-called *meandering mesenteric artery* or *central anastomotic artery* of the colon represents this direct continuation of the left branch of the middle colic into the left colic artery [58] (see Fig. 48-16).

When the distal aorta is thrombosed below the inferior mesenteric artery, the superior hemorrhoidal branch acts as an intermediate pathway to carry blood down to the perirectal area. Rich anastomoses with the middle and inferior hemorrhoidal vessels lead to intermediate pathways into all branches of the internal iliac artery except the iliolumbar [24] and from the internal iliac artery back into the external iliac artery if it is patent.

When the external iliac and common femoral arteries are also occluded, the same internal iliac branches can act as intermediate pathways down to the deep femoral branches. These femoral branches serve as the final retrograde effluent vessels channeling blood back into the common femoral artery.

The inferior mesenteric artery is a prime source of anastomoses to the leg when the aortic obstruction is low enough to leave it patent (see Figs. 48-13, 48-15). Unfortunately, its origin has appeared to be narrow or blocked in a significant percentage of the patients with aortoiliac arteriosclerosis whom we have examined. Its superior hemorrhoidal branch can anastomose richly around the rectum with most of the hypogastric branches deep in the pelvis. In the pelvis, visceral arteries from the vesical, middle, and inferior hemorrhoidal arteries may at some time be involved in forming collateral vessels even to refill the external iliac artery. If the external iliac artery is blocked, the visceral channels may refill the deep femoral artery and then fill the leg arteries.

Parietal Collateral Network

The most important parietal collateral vessels (Fig. 48-25; see also Figs. 48-17, 48-19–48-22), which usually develop on the side ipsilateral to the occlusions they bypass, arise from the intercostal, subcostal, lumbar, and middle sacral branches of the aorta; the iliolumbar, lateral sacral, superior gluteal, and obturator branches of the internal iliac arteries; and the deep iliac circumflex and

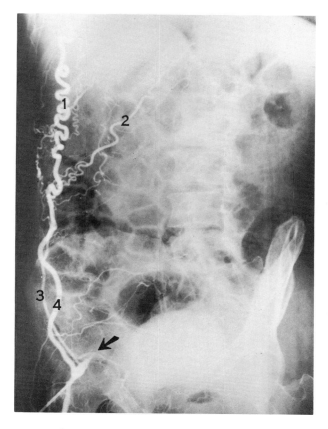

Figure 48-25. Obstruction of the right common iliac artery in a 52-year-old man who had had a distal aorta–bilateral common iliac graft 7 years earlier. A manual injection of contrast material was made through a percutaneous needle into the right common femoral artery with the patient in the right posterior oblique position. The common femoral artery is occluded down to the needle site (*arrow*). Collateral anastomoses between the intercostal (*1*), subcostal (*2*), deep iliac circumflex (*3*), and superficial iliac circumflex (*4*) arteries are demonstrated. (From Friedenberg and Perez [31]. Reproduced by permission from *AJR*.)

the medial and lateral circumflex branches of the external iliac and deep femoral arteries.

When the injection is high enough, the intercostal arteries may be visualized as important affluent vessels to the effluent deep iliac circumflex and lumbar vessels. Both these effluent vessels can supply the common femoral artery. The lumbar vessels may anastomose with the effluent iliolumbar artery (frequently by inosculation). From the iliolumbar artery, blood flows to the superior gluteal artery and, finally, by way of the internal iliac, to the external iliac artery [11, 26, 31, 59]. Rib notching may occur along the lower rib cage in occlusive disease of the upper abdominal aorta [31].

Winslow's Pathway
The epigastric arteries may also form important collateral vessels. Winslow's pathway (i.e., from the intercostal and internal mammary arteries to the external iliac arteries via the epigastric arteries) has been described by Gottlob [36] and Chait [12]. At the point of origin of the inferior epigastric artery, any opacified blood within the external iliac artery may contain a filling defect as the nonopaque blood from the collateral chain enters the main-stem vessels [59]. This pathway is an indication for injection of contrast material into the ascending aorta, or even the subclavian vessels if distal reconstitution is not seen with the usual angiographic technique (see Fig. 48-19).

Lumbar Arteries
Even a high obstruction of the aorta immediately below the renal arteries may leave the first or second lumbar arteries patent to act as prime affluent vessels into the effluent iliolumbar and superior gluteal branches of the internal iliac ar-

tery (Fig. 48-26; see also Figs. 48-21, 48-24). The internal iliac artery may then refill the external iliac artery. There are also communications between the lumbar arteries posteriorly that help to form the so-called subperitoneal parietal plexus of Turner [64]. These communications include the connections anteriorly below the superior and inferior epigastric and deep femoral arteries, which thus join the torso to the legs by a parietal network of collateral vessels within the abdominal wall and posteriorly along the spine.

In an interesting case of a blocked aorta and inferior mesenteric artery described by Chiappa [14], the third lumbar artery carried blood to the iliolumbar artery on one side, then to the lateral sacral artery and into the internal pudendal artery through hemorrhoidal anastomoses, and then back into the inferior mesenteric artery, to be distributed into its left colic branch. This is a striking example of how the distal colon can be supplied when the inferior mesenteric artery is blocked without obvious anastomosis between the superior and inferior mesenteric arteries. The leg in this same patient was presumably nourished by anastomoses originating in the lumbar artery.

Figure 48-26. Left aortoiliofemoral occlusion in a 50-year-old man complaining of claudication of the left lower extremity. A translumbar aortogram shows transpelvic lateral sacral collateral vessels (2) from the right side opacifying the superior (3) and the inferior (4) gluteal arteries of the left internal iliac artery. The large right-sided gluteal arteries are also an expression of the severity of the stenosis of the origin of the right common iliac artery. Note the anastomoses of the iliolumbar artery (1) with the fourth lumbar artery on the right.

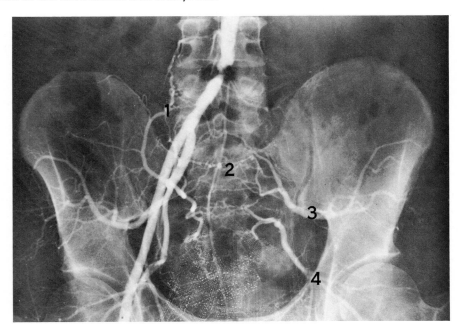

OCCLUSION OF THE COMMON ILIAC ARTERY

With occlusion of the common iliac artery (Fig. 48-27; see also Figs. 48-7, 48-12, 48-14, 48-25), the major possibilities for affluent circulation are the lumbar arteries, and, less often, the superior hemorrhoidal branch of the inferior mesenteric artery, which connects to various internal iliac effluent vessels that refill the external iliac artery. If that main-stem vessel is blocked, the femoral artery can be refilled by internal iliac intermediate vessels or by the lumbar artery to the deep circumflex iliac channels discussed above (see Fig. 48-22). Edwards and LeMay have ob-

Figure 48-27. Occlusion of the common iliac artery on the right. Translumbar aortogram with placement of the needle into a small lower abdominal aortic aneurysm. The internal iliac artery on the right is filled mainly via collateral vessels from the left lateral sacral (*1*) and left internal pudendal (*2*) arteries. There is faint opacification of the right common femoral artery (*arrow*). This 54-year-old woman, a cashier, could walk only one-half block before she had severe pain in both legs; it was much more severe in the right leg. Additional serial films showed patent femoral and popliteal arteries. An aortic-to-femoral bypass graft was successfully inserted.

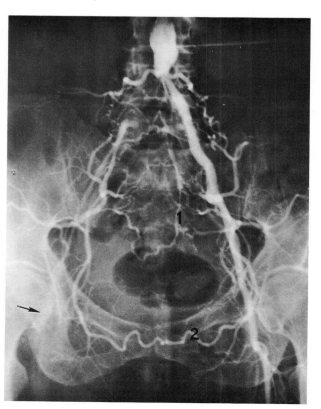

served that the rectal or hemorrhoidal network is not as strikingly filled in these patients as it is in patients with aortic block [24]. Indeed, in our patients with isolated common iliac artery obstruction, the inferior mesenteric artery has often been obscure.

There may also be rich crossover anastomoses with a prominent sacral network from the contralateral internal iliac branches to the involved side. In long occlusions of the iliac artery, the superior hemorrhoidal branch of the inferior mesenteric artery may make important anastomoses with the pudendal arteries, eventually leading to the leg (see Figs. 48-21, 48-24).

OCCLUSION OF THE EXTERNAL ILIAC ARTERY

In occlusion of the external iliac artery, the main collateral pathway may be via the parietal branches, such as a superior gluteal–lateral femoral circumflex connection, as well as the obturator and medial femoral circumflex, as demonstrated in Figures 48-13, 48-23, and 48-26. The internal pudendal artery may also connect with the medial femoral circumflex branch. The importance of the internal iliac branches is clear in such cases. Even when the main internal iliac trunk is blocked, its branches may be refilled to serve as effluent vessels and, in turn, to help refill the external iliac arteries (Fig. 48-28). In rare cases, continuation of the inferior gluteal artery may be via a persistent primitive sciatic artery instead of the usual external iliac continuation [17, 70].

OCCLUSION OF THE COMMON FEMORAL ARTERY

With occlusion of the common femoral artery (see Figs. 48-22, 48-23, 48-24), the so-called cruciate anastomosis is frequently mentioned [59]; the term probably refers to a commonly observed combination of pathways leading from the superior and inferior gluteal and lateral femoral circumflex affluent vessels to refilling of the deep femoral artery. Figure 48-22 represents a case of common femoral artery block and demonstrates those channels that compose part of the cruciate anastomosis. Figures 48-23 and 48-28 illustrate interesting variations on the use of internal iliac branches when the internal iliac main trunk is blocked.

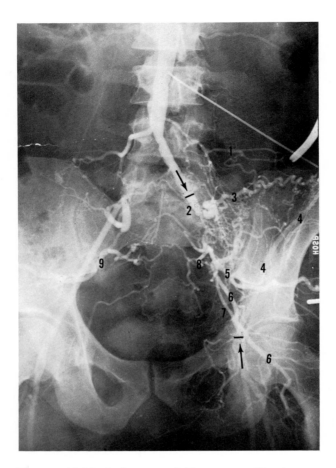

Figure 48-28. Left external iliac artery (*2*) obstruction between arrows as well as occlusion of the proximal main trunk of the internal iliac artery. The right common iliac artery is also occluded. The left fourth lumbar artery (*1*) is anastomosing with other retroperitoneal vessels in the sacral region and with the deep circumflex iliac artery (*4*). The coiled iliac portion (*3*) of the iliolumbar artery helps supply the superior gluteal artery (*5*), which in turn supplies the inferior gluteal (*6*), internal pudendal (*7*), and lateral sacral (*8*) arteries. The lateral sacral artery enables the sacral network to nourish the opposite superior gluteal artery via the lateral sacral artery (*9*) below the right common iliac block.

When there is occlusion of the internal iliac (hypogastric) artery at its origin, various branches are usually patent owing to anastomoses from their contralateral analogues or from the parietal and visceral branches of the aorta above. After ligation or acute block of both internal iliac arteries, these extensive collaterals provide an immediate blood supply to the pelvic organs [13]. Figure 48-23 illustrates an interesting refilling of certain of the internal iliac branches from the external iliac artery.

In conclusion, we would like to impress on the reader that an enormously varied pattern of collateralization is possible. Connections between the parietal and visceral pathways are commonplace, and long distances can be spanned— one report even describes the testicular artery as the major provider of the femoral artery circumventing an obstructed iliac artery [16]. However, most patterns of collateral flow are seen repeatedly because arteriosclerotic occlusions are so commonplace and occur in predilected areas.

AORTIC AND ILIAC GRAFTS

An exact diagnosis of aortic graft–intestinal fistulas may be difficult to make [28]. The most frequent site of fistula formation involves the proximal anastomosis and the third part of the duodenum [42]. Infection at the suture line may be the cause of most graft failures [40]. Rupture occurs on the anterior surface of the anastomosis; thus, prone lateral aortography may be more helpful [73].

References

1. Barnard, W. G.   Diffuse and nodular fibrosis of adventitia of aorta (rheumatic periaortitis). *J. Pathol. Bacteriol.* 32:95, 1929.
2. Barnum, E. N.   The roentgenographic differentiation of peripheral arteriosclerosis. *AJR* 68:619, 1952.
3. Bauer, F. W., and Robbins, S. L.   A postmortem study comparing renal angiograms and renal artery casts in 58 patients. *Arch. Pathol.* 83:307, 1967.
4. Beckwith, R., Huffman, E. R., Eiseman, B., and Blount, S. G., Jr.   Chronic aortoiliac thrombosis: A review of 65 cases. *N. Engl. J. Med.* 258:721, 1958.
5. Beuren, A. J., Hort, W., Kalbfleisch, H., Müller, H., and Stoermer, J.   Dysplasia of the systemic and pulmonary arterial system with tortuosity and lengthening of the arteries. *Circulation* 39:109, 1969.
6. Blaisdell, F. W., and Hall, A. D.   Axillary-femoral artery bypass for lower extremity ischemia. *Surgery* 54:563, 1963.
7. Braunwald, N. S.   Embolus following valve replacement. *Heart Bull.* 19:1, 1970.
8. Bron, K. M.   Thrombotic occlusion of the abdominal aorta: Associated visceral artery lesions and collateral circulation. *AJR* 96:887, 1966.
9. Campbell, D. K., and Austin, R. F.   Seat-belt injury: Injury of the abdominal aorta. *Radiology* 92:123, 1969.

10. Casteneda-Zuniga, W., Knight, L., Formanek, A., Moore, R., D'Souza, V., and Amplatz, K. Hemodynamic assessment of obstructive aortoiliac disease. *AJR* 127:559, 1976.

11. Cevese, P. G., and deMarchi, R. L'anastomosi di Winslow nella ostruzione estesa dell'aorta; studio aorto-seriografico di un caso. *Rass. Ital. Chir. Med.* 5:219, 1956.

12. Chait, A. The internal mammary artery: An overlooked collateral pathway to the leg. *Radiology* 121:621, 1976.

13. Chait, A., Moltz, A., and Nelson, J. H. The collateral arterial circulation in the pelvis: An angiographic study. *AJR* 102:392, 1968.

14. Chiappa, S. Occlusion of the abdominal aorta. *AJR* 80:297, 1958.

15. Colquhoun, J. Hypoplasia of the abdominal aorta following therapeutic irradiation in infancy. *Radiology* 86:454, 1966.

16. Conroy, R. M., and Vander Molen, R. L. Scrotal arteriocele from iliac artery occlusion. *AJR* 127:670, 1976.

17. Cowie, T. N., McKellar, N. J., MacLean, N., and Smith, G. Unilateral congenital absence of the external iliac and femoral arteries. *Br. J. Radiol.* 33:520, 1960.

18. Darling, R. C. Peripheral arterial surgery. *N. Engl. J. Med.* 280:84, 1969.

19. DeBakey, M. E., Crawford, E. S., Garrett, H. E., Cooley, D. A., Morris, G. C., Jr., and Abbott, J. P. Occlusive disease of the lower extremities in patients 16 to 37 years of age. *Ann. Surg.* 159:873, 1964.

20. Deutsch, V., Wexler, L., and Deutsch, H. Takayasu's arteritis, an angiographic study with remarks on ethnic distribution in Israel. *AJR* 122:13, 1974.

21. DeWeese, J. A., and Rob, C. Autogenous venous grafts ten years later. *Surgery* 82:775, 1977.

22. deWolfe, V. G., LeFevre, F. A., Humphries, A. W., Shaw, M. B., and Phalen, G. S. Intermittent claudication of the hip and the syndrome of chronic aortoiliac thrombosis. *Circulation* 9:1, 1954.

23. Dotter, C. T., and Judkins, M. P. Percutaneous transluminal treatment of arteriosclerotic obstruction. *Radiology* 84:631, 1965.

24. Edwards, E. A., and LeMay, M. Occlusion patterns and collaterals in arteriosclerosis of the lower aorta and iliac arteries. *Surgery* 38:950, 1955.

25. Eiseman, B., and Waggener, H. U. Role and interpretation of arteriograms in atherosclerosis and atherosclerotic aneurysms. *Arch. Surg.* 74:934, 1957.

26. Elliott, R. V., and Peck, M. E. Thrombotic occlusion of aorta as demonstrated by translumbar aortograms. *J.A.M.A.* 148:426, 1952.

27. Ertugrul, A. Diffuse tortuosity and lengthening of the arteries. *Circulation* 36:400, 1967.

28. Ferris, E. J., Koltay, M. R. S., Koltay, O. P., and Sciammas, F. D. Abdominal aortic and iliac graft fistulae: Unusual roentgenographic findings. *AJR* 94:416, 1965.

29. Flory, C. M. Arterial occlusions produced by emboli from eroded aortic atheromatous plaques. *Am. J. Pathol.* 21:549, 1945.

30. Fontaine, R., Dany, A., and Müller, J. N. À propos de 2 nouvelles observations de dystrophie polyanéurysmale. *Rev. Chir.* 87:193, 1949.

31. Friedenberg, M. J., and Perez, C. A. Collateral circulation in aorto-ilio-femoral occlusive disease: As demonstrated by a unilateral percutaneous common femoral artery needle injection. *AJR* 94:145, 1965.

32. Friedman, S. A., Holling, H. E., and Roberts, B. Etiologic factors in aortoiliac and femoropopliteal vascular disease: Leriche syndrome. *N. Engl. J. Med.* 27:1382, 1964.

33. Friedman, S. A., Novack, S., and Thomson, G. E. Arterial calcification and gangrene in uremia. *N. Engl. J. Med.* 280:1392, 1969.

34. Gotsman, M. S., Beck, W., and Schrire, V. Selective angiography in arteritis of the aorta and its major branches. *Radiology* 88:232, 1967.

35. Gottlob, R. Über Thrombosen der Aorta und der Iliacalarterien. *Arch. Klin. Chir.* 272:408, 1952.

36. Gottlob, R. Über die "ascendierende Arteriographie," zugleich ein Beitrag zur Auswertung aortographischer Bilder. *Arch. Klin. Chir.* 277:483, 1954.

37. Greenfield, I. Thrombosis and embolism of the abdominal aorta. *Ann. Intern. Med.* 19:656, 1943.

38. Grüntzig, A., and Hopff, H. Percutane Rekanalisation chronischer arterieller Verschlüsse mit einem neuen Dilatationskatheter: Modifikation der Dotter-Technike. *Dtsch. Med. Wochenschr.* 99:2502, 1974.

39. Haimovici, H. Patterns of arteriosclerotic lesions of the lower extremity. *Arch. Surg.* 95:918, 1967.

40. Harrison, J. H. Influence of infection on homografts and synthetic (Teflon) grafts: A comparative study in experimental animals. *Arch. Surg.* 76:67, 1958.

41. Hata, J., and Hosoda, Y. Tubular stenosis of the aorta with aortic fibromuscular dysplasia. *Arch. Pathol. Lab. Med.* 100:652, 1976.

42. Humphries, A. W., Young, J. R., deWolfe, U. G., and Lefevre, F. A. Complications of abdominal aortic surgery: I: Aortoenteric fistula. *Arch. Surg.* 86:43, 1963.

43. Julian, O. Chronic occlusion of aorta and iliac arteries. *Surg. Clin. North Am.* 40:139, 1960.

44. Kassirer, J. P. Atheroembolic renal disease. *N. Engl. J. Med.* 280:812, 1969.

45. Kittrege, R. D., and Anderson, J. W. Coarctation of the lower thoracic and abdominal aorta. *Radiology* 79:799, 1962.

46. Kunkel, P., and Stead, E. A., Jr. Blood flow and vasomotor reactions in the foot in health, in arteriosclerosis, and in thromboangiitis obliterans. *J. Clin. Invest.* 17:715, 1938.

47. Lande, A., and Gross, A. Total aortography in the diagnosis of Takayasu's arteritis. *AJR* 116:165, 1972.

48. Leriche, R. De la résection du carrefour aortoiliaque avec double sympathectomie lombaire pour thrombose artéritique de l'aorte; le syndrome de l'oblitération termino-aortique par arterite. *Presse Med.* 48:601, 1940.

49. Leriche, R., Kunlin, J., and Boely, C. Lesions artéritiques des iliaques et de l'aorte d'après 90 aortographies. *Lyon Chir.* 45:5, 1950.

50. Lindbom, Å. Arteriosclerosis and arterial thrombosis in the lower limb. *Acta Radiol. [Suppl.]* (Stockh.) 80:1, 1950.

51. Lindsey, S. M., Maddison, F. F., and Towne, J. B. Heparin-induced thromboembolism: Angiographic features. *Radiology* 131:771, 1979.

52. Lipchik, E. O., Rob, C. G., and Schwartzberg, S. Obstruction of the abdominal aorta above the level of the renal arteries. *Radiology* 82:443, 1964.

53. Lowenberg, E. L. Changing concepts of the pathology and management of acute arterial occlusion of the lower extremities. *South. Med. J.* 51:35, 1958.

54. Mann, F. C., Herrick, J. F., Essex, H. E., and Baldes, E. J. The effect on the blood flow of decreasing the lumen of a blood vessel. *Surgery* 4:249, 1938.

55. Martin, J. F., and Yount, E. H. Coarctation of the abdominal aorta: Report of a case illustrating the value of aortography as a diagnostic aid. *AJR* 76:782, 1956.

56. May, A. G., DeBerg, L. V., DeWeese, J. A., and Rob, C. G. Critical arterial stenosis. *Surgery* 54:250, 1963.

57. Moldveen, G. M., and Merriam, J. C., Jr. Cholesterol embolization: From pathologic curiosity to clinical entity. *Circulation* 35:946, 1967.

58. Moskowitz, M., Zimmerman, H., and Felson, B. The meandering mesenteric artery of the colon. *AJR* 92:1088, 1964.

59. Muller, R. F., and Figley, M. M. The arteries of the abdomen, pelvis and thigh. *AJR* 77:296, 1957.

60. Najafi, H. Fibromuscular hyperplasia of the external iliac arteries. An unusual case of intermittent claudication. *Arch. Surg.* 92:394, 1966.

61. Palubinskas, A. J., and Ripley, H. R. Fibromuscular hyperplasia in extrarenal arteries. *Radiology* 82:451, 1964.

62. Poulias, G. E., Giannopoulos, G. D., and Fran-gagis, E. Selective constriction of the profunda femoris as a post radiotherapy sequel. *Radiology* 89:127, 1967.

63. Pyörälä, K., Heinonen, O., Koskelo, P., and Heikel, P. Coarctation of the abdominal aorta: Review of 27 cases. *Am. J. Cardiol.* 6:650, 1960.

64. Rian, R. L., and Eyler, W. R. Aortic, iliac and visceral arterial lesions. *Radiol. Clin. North Am.* 5:409, 1967.

65. Sano, K., Aiba, T., and Saito, I. Angiography in pulseless disease. *Radiology* 94:69. 1970.

66. Schenk, E. A. Pathology of occlusive disease of the lower extremities. *Cardiovasc. Clin.* 5:287, 1973.

67. Schettler, F. G., and Boyd, G. S. *Atherosclerosis: Pathology, Physiology, Aetiology, Diagnosis and Clinical Management.* Amsterdam/New York: Elsevier, 1968.

68. Sequeira, J. C., Beckman, C. F., and Levin, D. C. Suprarenal aortic occlusion. *AJR* 132:773, 1979.

69. Sethi, G. K., Scott, S. M., and Takaro, T. Value of oblique projections in translumbar aortography. *AJR* 116:187, 1973.

70. Taylor, D. A., and Fiore, A. S. Arteriography of a persistent primitive left sciatic artery with aneurysm: A case report. *Radiology* 87:714, 1966.

71. Theander, G. Arteriographic demonstration of stationary arterial waves. *Acta Radiol.* (Stockh.) 53:417, 1960.

72. Thomas, M. L., and Andress, M. R. Value of oblique projections in translumbar aortography. *AJR* 116:187, 1972.

73. Thompson, W. M., Jackson, D. C., and Johnsrude, I. S. Aortoenteric and paraprosthetic-enteric fistulas: Radiologic findings. *AJR* 127:235, 1976.

74. Traverso, L. W., Baker, J. D., Dainko, E. A., and Machleder, H. I. Infrarenal aortic occlusion. *Ann. Surg.* 187:397, 1978.

75. Twigg, H. L., and Palmisano, P. J. Fibromuscular hyperplasia of the iliac artery. *AJR* 95:418, 1965.

76. Udoff, E. J., Barth, K. H., Harrington, D. P., Kaufman, S. L., and White, R. I. Hemodynamic significance of iliac artery stenosis: Pressure measurements during angiography. *Radiology* 132:289, 1979.

77. Wylie, E. J., and Goldman, L. The role of aortography in the determination of operability in arteriosclerosis of the lower extremities. *Ann. Surg.* 148:325, 1958.

78. Wylie, E. J., and McGuinness, J. S. The recognition and treatment of arteriosclerotic stenosis of major arteries. *Surg. Gynecol. Obstet.* 97:425, 1953.

Aneurysms of the Abdominal Aorta

ELLIOT O. LIPCHIK
STANLEY M. ROGOFF

Abdominal aortic aneurysm is a lethal disease with a poor, short-term prognosis, especially if it is symptomatic. One-third [20], one-half [7, 30], or two-thirds [26] of the patients can be expected to die of ruptured aneurysms within a short time after diagnosis. In Estes' series of 102 cases [26], 30 percent did not have symptoms at the time of the diagnosis and one-third of the total were dead within a year. Of the patients of Gliedman et al. who were suffering symptoms when diagnosed, 80 percent died within a year [30]. Because surgery and cure may be possible, accurate diagnosis is important in this increasingly common disease.

The clinical diagnosis of the abdominal aneurysm is relatively simple; that is, it is often possible to palpate the aneurysm and to localize it correctly [40, 72]. Despite the feasibility and ease of clinical diagnosis in experienced hands, the mortality in cases of ruptured aortic aneurysm in Western countries appears to be on the rise [41, 49]. Since elective-surgery mortality is relatively low (less than 1%), as compared to the mortality of *over* 50 percent in acute operations for rupture [19, 66], the importance of the detection of abdominal aortic aneurysm in its asymptomatic stage cannot be overemphasized.

The detection of the asymptomatic aneurysm, the rapid noninvasive documentation of the symptomatic aneurysm, and the proper diagnosis in the small but definite number of patients who have misleading symptoms can now be achieved in the majority of cases by ultrasound. Computed tomography has obvious limitations of cost and radiation dose, but with it the aorta can also be reliably identified [4].

In a small number of patients, misleading symptoms [7, 21, 67] are responsible for the failure to make the proper diagnosis (Figs. 49-1, 49-2). Ectatic, tortuous, arteriosclerotic arteries, particularly in elderly, thin individuals, may be mistaken for aneurysms. A review of aneurysms and their immensely varied clinical presentation can be found in Shafer's article [60]. In one series of 200 cases of abdominal aortic aneurysm, 15 cases were misdiagnosed [51]; in three patients who died of ruptured aneurysms the diagnosis was not made until postmortem examination. In an excellent review and history Sondheimer and Steinberg discuss all the gastrointestinal manifestations of abdominal aortic aneurysms [62]. The urologic manifestations of abdominal aortic aneurysm include simulation of ureteral colic, ureteral obstruction, infection, and hematuria

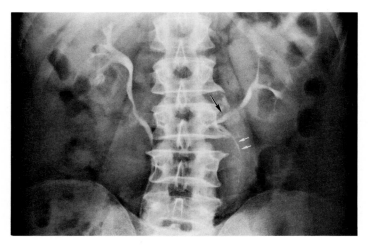

Figure 49-1. Marked displacement without obstruction of the left ureter (*black arrow*) by an aneurysm 5 cm in diameter (*white arrows*). This 59-year-old man complained of dull, aching pains in the left buttock, radiating to the thigh during the previous 3 months. There were no postoperative urograms.

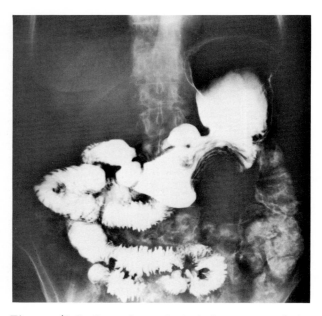

Figure 49-2. Smooth extrinsic indentation and displacement of the greater curvature of the stomach by a large aortic aneurysm. This 84-year-old woman had a 4-day history of progressive weakness and nausea and a 2-day history of hematemesis. She refused surgery.

[25, 43, 67]. In another series, 20 percent of the patients presented only with intermittent claudication; some of them had nonpalpable aneurysms [73].

Pathology

Most of the aneurysms seen today are due to arteriosclerosis and nearly always involve the aorta distal to the origin of the renal arteries. The aneurysms are most common in patients after the fourth decade. In one-half of the cases the aneurysms appear to the left of the lumbar spine, and three-quarters are fusiform [7, 11, 14, 49].

An aneurysm may be defined as a focal saccular or fusiform dilatation of a segment between two normal areas in a blood vessel due to partial destruction of the wall (Fig. 49-3) [34, 49]. *Arteriomegaly* [65], *arteria magna et dolicho* [63], and *arteria magna* [55] are all terms describing the same entity: a profound loss of elastic tissue in the media with resultant extreme vessel dilatation, tortuosity, and elongation—probably a more advanced form of arteriosclerosis.

Dissecting aneurysm is a different disease entity and morphologic problem. Dissection from the thoracic aorta, extending downward to involve the abdominal aorta secondarily, is the most frequent form of abdominal dissection. Dissection beginning in the abdominal aorta without antecedent trauma is rare, with a reported incidence of from 4.0 to 0.28 percent, the latter figure more

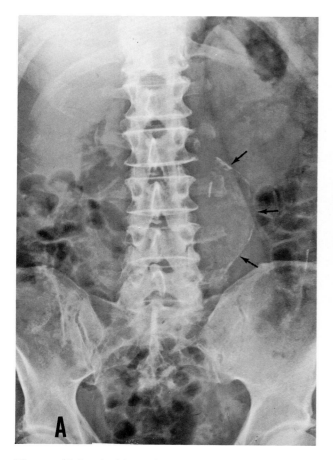

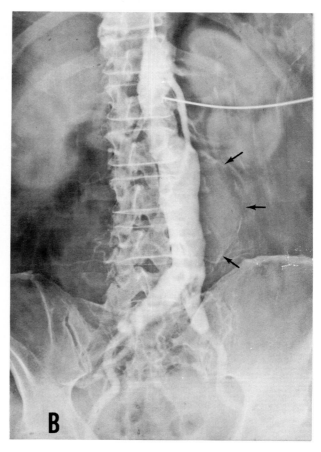

Figure 49-3. (A) Typical curvilinear calcification in a large lower abdominal aortic aneurysm (*arrows*). (B) Translumbar aortogram outlining the large amount of thrombus in the aneurysm. The aneurysmal disease extends into the common iliac arteries. This patient also had a popliteal artery aneurysm.

probably correct [16, 36, 37, 48]. Cystic medial necrosis is the primary etiology.

Arteriovenous fistula does not belong in the category of true aneurysms. An aortocaval fistula may, however, result from a ruptured arteriosclerotic aneurysm [15, 24]. Traumatic rupture of the aorta also is not necessarily predicated on antecedent aneurysm disease [47].

A *mycotic aneurysm* (Fig. 49-4; see also Fig. 49-11) results from an infectious process of the arterial wall. Approximately 2.5 percent of all aneurysms are mycotic in origin [53]. These are usually saccular and quite round and may cause few local symptoms when the aorta is involved [70]. Grossly, they may be tiny or measure several centimeters in diameter, rarely larger. There are no pathognomonic roentgenographic features, only sudden appearance, rapid progression in size, meaningful clinical history, and lack of arteriosclerotic changes in the vicinity (if in a young patient). Such aneurysms have a dangerous propensity for early rupture and recurrence after resection. Angiography and/or ultrasound is necessary for their delineation and follow-up, although mycotic aneurysms may be evidenced on plain films by retroperitoneal gas surrounding the infected aneurysmal mass [68].

A small percentage of other aneurysms may be caused by trauma [9], syphilis, or aortitis [32]. Aneurysms and other vascular abnormalities due to aortitis, while seen most frequently in the Orient and Africa, are also represented in Western countries.

Poststenotic dilatation resembling aneurysm may also occur in coarctation of the abdominal aorta [30]. Other causes of aneurysms are too rare or incompletely documented to be discussed; there are even reports of aneurysms in young children [1, 29, 35, 46].

Pseudoaneurysms communicate with and are

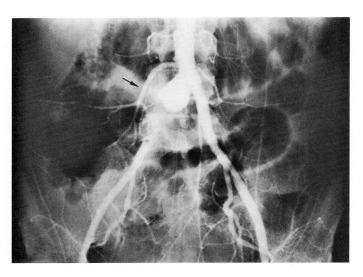

Figure 49-4. Mycotic saccular aneurysm of the right common iliac artery due to a *Salmonella* infection. This 60-year-old man had an acute history of night sweats, shaking chills, and low back pain radiating to the groin and extending to the right lower abdominal quadrant. The initial diagnosis was perforating appendicitis. Two years after surgery (Dacron graft) the patient was free of infection. The right fourth lumbar artery (*arrow*) is dilated, an angiographic indication of poor flow of blood through the right iliac system.

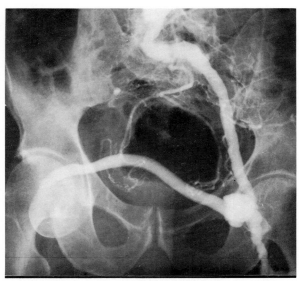

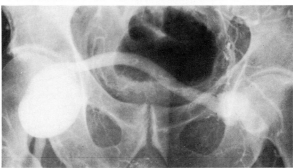

Figure 49-5. Two large pseudoaneurysms developed several years after the insertion of a woven Dacron graft at the site of anastomosis to the femoral arteries. The graft was inserted to overcome a right iliofemoral occlusion. At corrective surgery the silk sutures were fragmented and the graft was separated from the femoral artery on the right side. (Courtesy of James A. DeWeese, M.D.)

confined by the tissues surrounding the aorta or the blood vessel. They are uncommon and can occur as a complication of any type of direct arterial trauma, such as catheterization, graft site infection, leak at the graft site, or the use of silk suture material [54] (Fig. 49-5). A case of lumbar vertebral erosion caused by an aortic pseudoaneurysm has been described [69].

Methods of Diagnosis

Routine radiographs of the lumbar spine in both anteroposterior and lateral projections showed evidence of the aneurysm in 55 to 83 percent of the cases in several large series [20, 26, 58]. The diagnosis is made on the basis of mural calcification, often curvilinear, and of displacement of adjacent organs of the gastrointestinal and genitourinary systems (see Figs. 49-1, 49-2). Unless both walls of the calcified aorta are visualized on the plain films, a tortuous calcified

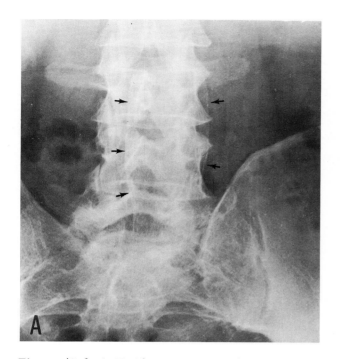
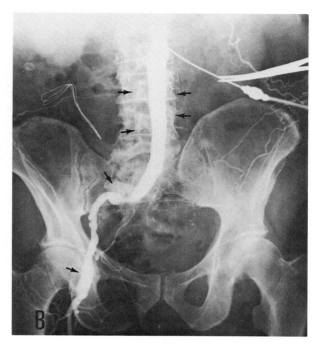

Figure 49-6. (A) Fusiform aneurysm of the abdominal aorta outlined by curvilinear calcification (*arrows*). (B) Aortogram revealing a central channel narrowed to "normal" caliber by laminated thrombus. The left iliac system is blocked. Aneurysms of the right internal iliac and right common femoral arteries (*lower two arrows*) are also present.

aorta may also be mistaken for an aneurysm. The lack of parallelism of the calcification is essential for establishing a correct diagnosis (Fig. 49-6; see also Fig. 49-3).

The principal modern method for diagnosis of abdominal aortic aneurysm is ultrasonography. This type of imaging provides a noninvasive, safe, reliable, and, above all, highly accurate representation of the aneurysm in all dimensions [24]. Aortography is not to be recommended for diagnosis in the routine workup.

The accuracy of ultrasound may be better than 98 percent [27]. Valuable information as to presence of clot or dissection may also be obtained. Certainly ultrasound is the method of choice for serially evaluating the abdominal aorta or the size of the aneurysm. Angiography may be indicated (there is controversy in the literature) if the sonogram is inadequate, if extension of the aneurysm either above the renal arteries or into the iliac arteries is suggested, if organ vascular bed compromise is suspected (such as mesenteric ischemia), or if a map of the vascular anatomy is deemed necessary for surgical planning [13, 31, 42, 57]. It is not clear that visceral infarction (which occurs in 1–2% of cases) would be universally prevented through the additional infor-mation provided by angiography [39, 52], especially with the modern techniques of repair, but if concomitant correction of other aneurysms or vascular disorders is in order, angiography might indeed play a vital role. Furthermore, recent reports of the inability of ultrasonography to detect some clots and its tendency to misdiagnose patency of aneurysms in the presence of total occlusion [2] indicate that caution must still be maintained in totally relying on ultrasound. In the near future, digital videoangiography may replace the need for invasive aortography (see Chap. 7).

Aortographic Techniques and Roentgenographic Findings

While there is some reluctance among radiologists to pass catheters through aneurysms from below via the femoral arteries (Fig. 49-7) because aneurysms predispose to large amounts of thrombus and may have thin walls, the presence of an aneurysm is not a contraindication to a transfemoral approach, although caution is warranted. Percutaneous left axillary retrograde

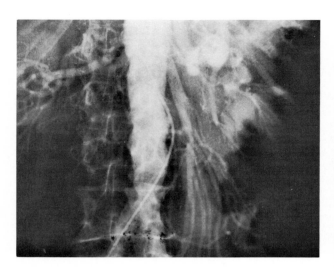

Figure 49-7. Unsuspected small abdominal aortic aneurysm with part of the catheter seemingly extending outside the lumen through thrombus lining the wall. No complications were caused by the procedure.

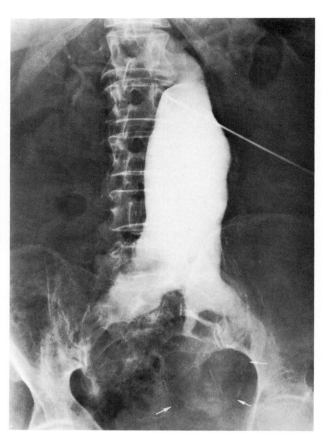

Figure 49-8. Large fusiform aneurysm of the abdominal aorta beginning *above* the translumbar needle insertion but below the renal arteries. Calcification delineating a large left iliac artery aneurysm is outlined by arrows.

catheterization is often the method of choice, although transfemoral catheter passage is generally safe and simple. It is important, when studying an aneurysm from below, to employ a J-shaped or flexible-tip guidewire. Occasionally translumbar aortography with the puncture site above the abnormality may be employed (Fig. 49-8; see also Fig. 49-12). Intravenous angiography has been used, but with this method opacification of the visceral arteries, particularly the renal arteries, may be very poor. Furthermore, blood flow in the aorta is usually extremely slow when severe ectasia, atherosclerosis, or aneurysm is present (Fig. 49-9), resulting in dilution of the contrast material and poor opacification of the aneurysm and the distal vessels [17, 55]. Increased amounts of contrast material and marked prolongation of film sequences may be necessary.

Measurement of the aneurysmal mass has prognostic value. It is generally accepted that a diameter greater than 7 cm represents imminent danger to the patient and makes surgery imperative [27, 59, 61]. It is also important to realize that aneurysms less than 4.5 cm in diameter are usually not palpable [61].

Small aneurysms (less than 4 cm) grow slowly and remain stable for long periods of time, but there is discussion in the literature as to whether small aneurysms are acutely dangerous or whether they can be observed. Most workers believe that aneurysms under 4.5 cm probably do not acutely rupture [6, 10, 71], but there are dis-

senting opinions [22]. Since frequent serial follow-ups with ultrasound are feasible, a more conservative approach for the small aneurysm may be in order for selected patients.

Other classifications do exist that may also be important in the clinical management of the patient [61, 64]. In one angiographic series [64], the average diameter of the normal abdominal aorta did not exceed 30 mm. Therefore, any localized dilatation above this figure may be significant. An extremely important factor in patient survival in this group is the presence or absence of associated severe cardiovascular disease [28, 50, 59].

Most aneurysms are *fusiform* (i.e., concentrically dilated) as compared to *saccular* (i.e., only one of the vessel walls is ballooned out) (Figs. 49-10, 49-11). In either form, filling with contrast medium may be incomplete because of mural thrombosis of the sac. The thickness of the unopacified portion of the aneurysm measured to the curvilinear calcification laterally may be sub-

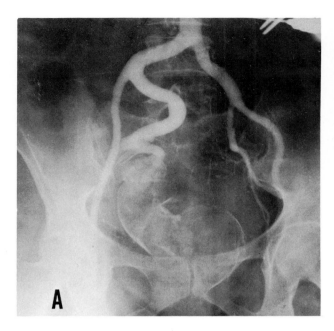

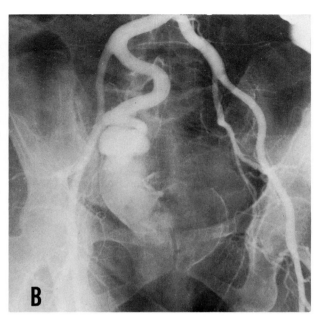

Figure 49-9. Slow circulation in a calcified aneurysm of the right internal iliac artery. (A) First film in a serial aortogram showing normal progression of opaque material into the normal channels on either side. (B) Second exposure showing progressive but still incomplete filling of the aneurysm. The aneurysm remained opacified long after the contrast had washed out of the normal vessels. (Courtesy of John G. McAfee, M.D.)

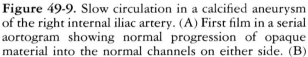

Figure 49-10. Bleeding saccular aneurysm. (A) Plain radiograph of a 54-year-old man with low back pain and vomiting. A large mass obliterates the right psoas muscle shadow and bulges the flank. This proved to be a retroperitoneal hematoma. (B) Aortogram some months later showing the saccular aneurysm along the right wall of the aorta immediately below the renal artery. In addition, there is a fusiform aneurysm of the more distal aorta.

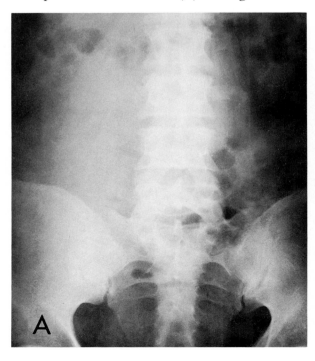

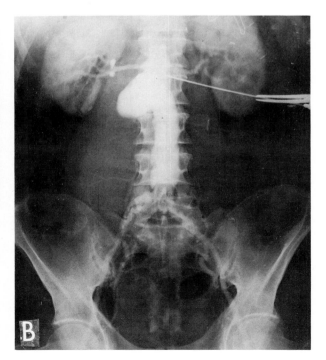

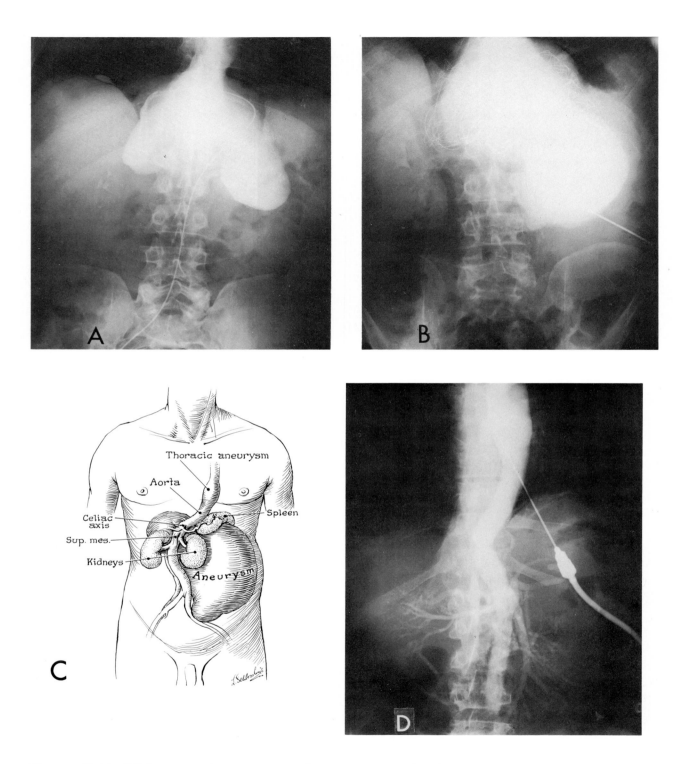

Figure 49-11. Bilobate saccular aneurysm of the upper abdominal aorta in a 45-year-old man who had a positive serologic test for syphilis. (A) Initial aortogram by retrograde femoral catheterization. Below the aneurysm the lower abdominal aorta was normal. (B) Eight months later, after wiring, aneurysm is shown to be increased in all diameters. The soft tissue mass below the translumbar needle and toward the left pelvis proved to be a clot within the aneurysm sac. (C) Sketch of operative findings. A separate fusiform aneurysm of the descending thoracic aorta was also found. (D) Aortogram 1 month after amputation of the saccular aneurysm and tailoring of the remaining aorta. (Reproduced with permission of the author and publisher from *Surgery, Gynecology and Obstetrics* [5].)

stantially wider than that of the opacified lumen. If the lumen is compromised by the thrombus but the wall is not markedly thickened, a dissection has to be considered. Some of the mass density associated with the lesion may also be due to retroperitoneal bleeding. Nonopacification of lumbar arteries and the inferior mesenteric artery during angiography does not necessarily indicate dissection.

Demonstration of thrombus has minor direct importance; most surgeons expect to find thrombus lining the walls of an aneurysm. Thrombus probably does not buttress the aneurysm against rupture. It may, however, prevent angiographic opacification of parietal vessels.

There is frequently kinking at the junction between the elongated, dilated aneurysm and the more normal vessel from which it arises. Any long curvature in the abdominal aorta tends to be to the left and anteriorly because this is the path of least resistance to aortic expansion at the lumbar level. Erosion of the lumbar vertebral bodies is an unusual occurrence in arteriosclerotic aneurysms of the abdominal aorta because these lesions are usually limited to the portion of the aorta that is relatively free and unrestricted. Vertebral erosion may be noted in aneurysms *above* the renal arteries; such aneurysms are often syphilitic.

Ruptured or rupturing aneurysms (see Fig. 49-10) represent an emergency situation and potential catastrophe for the patient. There are no pathognomonic roentgen signs of aortic rupture, but increasing displacement of adjacent organs, an acute change in size of the aneurysm, and increasing soft tissue shadows adjacent to the aorta may provide good clues to the diagnosis [18]. This is especially the case when correlated with the clinical picture and physical examination [38]. The aorta may rupture intraperitoneally or retroperitoneally as well as into the gut, inferior vena cava, and/or ureter—all presenting potential problems in the differential diagnosis [8, 12]. The most common site of rupture is into the retroperitoneum from the posterior aortic wall about 1 to 2 cm distal to the renal arteries [33] (Fig. 49-12).

In the frontal projection an aneurysm may ap-

Figure 49-12. (A) Large fusiform aneurysm of the abdominal aorta below the renal arteries. The translumbar needle was inserted into the aneurysm without complications. At the tip of the needle there is a small intramural accumulation of contrast material. (B) Wire packing of the aneurysm, done because resection was judged not feasible [56]. Six weeks following surgery the patient died after the aneurysm ruptured into the duodenum.

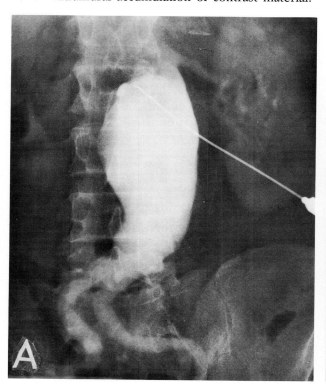

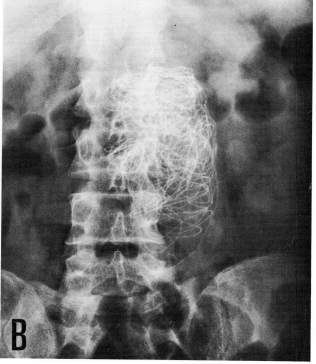

pear to encompass the renal artery origins. However, a lateral projection will usually show the overlay of the dilatation anteriorly, projecting above the level of the normal aorta from which the renal arteries arise. The incidence of renal artery involvement with abdominal aortic aneurysm is less than 5 percent while the iliac arteries are much more frequently involved [44].

References

1. Abrahams, D. G., and Cockshott, W. P. Multiple non-luetic aneurysms in young Nigerians. *Br. Heart J.* 24:83, 1962.
2. Anderson, J. C., Baltaxe, H. A., and Wolf, G. L. Inability to show clot: One limitation of ultrasound of the abdominal aorta. *Radiology* 132:693, 1979.
3. Aurig, G., and Radke, H. Die Bedeutung der Aortographie für die Diagnostik der abdominalen Aortenaneurysmen. *ROEFO* 84:661, 1956.
4. Axelbaum, S. P., Schellinger, D., Gomes, M. N., Ferris, R. A., and Hakkal, H. G. Computed tomographic evaluation of aortic aneurysms. *AJR* 127:75, 1976.
5. Bahnson, H. T. Definitive treatment of saccular aneurysms of the aorta with excision of sac and aortic suture. *Surg. Gynecol. Obstet.* 96:383, 1953.
6. Baker, W. H., and Munns, J. R. Aneurysmectomy in the aged. *Arch. Surg.* 110:513, 1975.
7. Barratt-Boyes, B. F. Symptomatology and prognosis of abdominal aortic aneurysms. *Lancet* 2:716, 1957.
8. Beall, A. C., Cooley, D. A., Morris, G. C., and DeBakey, M. Perforation of arteriosclerotic aneurysms into the inferior vena cava. *Arch. Surg.* 86:809, 1963.
9. Bennett, D. E., and Cherry, J. K. The natural history of traumatic aneurysms of the aorta. *Surgery* 61:516, 1967.
10. Bernstein, E. F. *Controversy in Surgery.* Philadelphia: Saunders, 1976. P. 267.
11. Blakemore, A. H., and Voorhees, A. R., Jr. Aneurysm of the aorta: A review of 365 cases. *Angiology* 5:209, 1954.
12. Blum, L. Ruptured aneurysm of abdominal aorta. *N.Y. State J. Med.* 68:2061, 1968.
13. Brewster, D. C., Retana, A., Waltman, A. C., and Darling, R. C. Angiography in the management of aneurysms of the abdominal aorta, its value and safety. *N. Engl. J. Med.* 292:822, 1975.
14. Brindley, P., and Stembridge, V. A. Aneurysms of the aorta: A clinicopathologic study of 369 necropsy cases. *Am. J. Pathol.* 32:67, 1956.
15. Bulgrin, J. G., and Jacobson, G. Aortographic demonstration of an aortocaval fistula. *Radiology* 71:409, 1958.
16. Burch, G. E., and DePasquale, N. Study of incidence of abdominal aortic aneurysm in New Orleans. *J.A.M.A.* 151:374, 1953.
17. Carlson, D. H., Gryska, P., Seletz, J., and Armstrong, S. Arteriomegaly. *AJR* 125:553, 1975.
18. Chisolm, A. J., and Sprayregen, S. Angiographic manifestations of ruptured abdominal aortic aneurysm. *AJR* 127:769, 1976.
19. Christenson, J., Eklöf, B., and Gustafson, I. Abdominal aortic aneurysms: Should all be resected? *Br. J. Surg.* 64:767, 1977.
20. Crane, C. Arteriosclerotic aneurysm of the abdominal aorta. *N. Engl. J. Med.* 253:954, 1955.
21. Culp, O. S., and Bernatz, P. E. Urologic aspects of lesions in the abdominal aorta. *J. Urol.* 86:189, 1961.
22. Darling, R. C. Ruptured abdominal aortic aneurysm. *Am. J. Surg.* 119:397, 1970.
23. Davis, J. H. Complications of surgery of the abdominal aorta. *Am. J. Surg.* 130:523, 1975.
24. Eiseman, B., and Hughes, R. H. Repair of an abdominal aortic vena cava fistula caused by rupture of an atherosclerotic aneurysm. *Surgery* 39:498, 1956.
25. Enselberg, C. D. The clinical picture of aneurysm of the abdominal aorta. *Ann. Intern. Med.* 44:1163, 1956.
26. Estes, J. E., Jr. Abdominal aortic aneurysm: A study of 102 cases. *Circulation* 2:258, 1950.
27. Filly, R. A., and Goldberg, B. B. Normal Vessels. In B. B. Goldberg (ed.), *Abdominal Grayscale Ultrasonography.* New York: Wiley, 1977.
28. Friedman, S. A., Hufnagel, C. A., Conrad, P. W., Simmons, E. M., and Weintraub, A. Abdominal aortic aneurysms: Clinical status and results of surgery in 100 consecutive cases. *J.A.M.A.* 200:1147, 1967.
29. Gelfand, M. Giant cell arteritis with aneurysmal formation in an infant. *Br. Heart J.* 17:264, 1955.
30. Gliedman, M. L., Ayers, W. B., and Vestal, B. L. Aneurysms of the abdominal aorta and its branches: A study of untreated patients. *Ann. Surg.* 146:207, 1957.
31. Gordon, D. H., Martin, E. C., Schneider, M., Staiano, S. J., and Noyes, M. B. Complementary role of sonography and arteriography in the evaluation of the atheromatous abdominal aorta. *Cardiovasc. Radiol.* 1:165, 1978.
32. Gotsman, M. S., Beck, W., and Schrire, V. Selective angiography in arteritis of the aorta and its major branches. *Radiology* 88:232, 1967.
33. Haimovici, H. Abdominal aortic aneurysm. *N.Y. State J. Med.* 67:691, 1967.
34. Hall, E. M. Blood and Lymphatic Vessels. In W. A. D. Anderson (ed.), *Pathology* (4th ed.). St. Louis: Mosby, 1961.
35. Hills, E. A. Behçet's syndrome with aortic aneurysms. *Br. Med. J.* 4:152, 1967.
36. Hirst, A. E., Jr., Johns, V. J., Jr., and Kime, S. W., Jr. Dissecting aneurysm of the aorta: A review of 505 cases. *Medicine* (Baltimore) 37:217, 1958.

37. Hume, D. M., and Porter, R. R. Acute dissecting aortic aneurysms. *Surgery* 53:122, 1963.
38. Janower, M. L. Ruptured arteriosclerotic aneurysms of the abdominal aorta: Roentgenographic findings on plain films. *N. Engl. J. Med.* 265:12, 1961.
39. Johnson, W. C., and Nabseth, D. C. Visceral infarction following aortic surgery. *Ann. Surg.* 180:312, 1974.
40. Kampmeier, R. H. Aneurysm of abdominal aorta: Study of 73 cases. *Am. J. Med. Sci.* 192:97, 1936.
41. Karp, W., and Eklöf, B. Ultrasonography and angiography in the diagnosis of abdominal aortic aneurysm. *Acta Radiol. [Diagn.]* (Stockh.) 19:955, 1978.
42. Kwaan, J. H. M., Connolly, J. E., Molen, R. V., and Conroy, R. Value of arteriography before abdominal aneurysmectomy. *Am. J. Surg.* 134:108, 1977.
43. Labardini, M. M., and Ratliff, R. K. The abdominal aortic aneurysm and the ureter. *J. Urol.* 98:590, 1967.
44. Lee, K. R., Walls, W. J., Martin, N. L., and Templeton, A. W. A practical approach to the diagnosis of abdominal aortic aneurysm. *Surgery* 78:195, 1975.
45. Leopold, G. R., Goldberger, L. E., and Bernstein, E. F. Ultrasonic detection and evaluation of abdominal aortic aneurysms. *Surgery* 72:939, 1972.
46. Lepow, H. Chu, F., and Muren, O. Multiple aneurysmal formation—an elastic tissue defect. *Am. J. Med.* 24:631, 1958.
47. Lipchik, E. O., and Robinson, K. E. Acute traumatic rupture of the thoracic aorta. *AJR* 104:408, 1968.
48. Lodwick, G. S. Dissecting aneurysms of the thoracic and abdominal aorta: Report of six cases with a discussion of roentgenologic findings and pathologic changes. *AJR* 69:907, 1953.
49. Maniglia, R., and Gregory, J. E. Increasing incidence of arteriosclerotic aortic aneurysms; analysis of 6,000 autopsies. *Arch. Pathol.* 54:298, 1952.
50. May, A. G., DeWeese, J. A., Frank, I., Mahoney, E. B., and Rob, C. G. Surgical treatment of abdominal aortic aneurysms. *Surgery* 63:711, 1968.
51. Moore, W. S., Preger, L., Hall, A., and Maddison, F. E. Abdominal aortic aneurysms: Unusual clinical manifestations. *Calif. Med.* 108:345, 1968.
52. Ottinger, L. W., Darling, R. C., Nathan, M. J., and Linton, R. R. Left colon ischemia complicating aortoiliac reconstruction: Causes, diagnosis, management and prevention. *Arch. Surg.* 105:841, 1972.
53. Parkhurst, G. F., and Decker, J. P. Bacterial aortitis and mycotic aneurysm of aorta: A report of twelve cases. *Am. J. Pathol.* 31:821, 1955.
54. Postlethwait, R. W. Long-term comparative study of nonabsorbable sutures. *Ann. Surg.* 171:892, 1970.
55. Randall, P. A., Omar, M. M., Rohner, R., Hedgcock, M., and Brenner, R. J. Arteria magna revisited. *Radiology* 132:295, 1979.
56. Rob, C. G., and DeWeese, J. A. Treatment of Arterial Aneurysms. In C. G. Rob (ed.), *Operative Surgery* (2nd ed.). Philadelphia: Lippincott, 1968.
57. Rösch, J., Keller, F. S., Porter, J. M., and Baur, G. M. Value of angiography in the management of abdominal aortic aneurysm. *Cardiovasc. Radiol.* 1:83, 1978.
58. Ryan, E. A., Spittell, J. A., Jr., and Kincaid, O. W. Roentgenographic manifestations of abdominal aortic aneurysms. *Postgrad. Med.* 36:A77, Dec. 1964.
59. Schatz, I. J., Fairbairn, J. F., and Juergens, J. L. Abdominal aortic aneurysms—a reappraisal. *Circulation* 26:200, 1962.
60. Shafer, N. Abdominal aortic aneurysms. *N.Y. State J. Med.* 78:1727, 1978.
61. Sommerville, R. L., Allen, E. V., and Edwards, J. E. Bland and infected arteriosclerotic abdominal aortic aneurysms: A clinicopathological study. *Medicine* (Baltimore) 38:207, 1959.
62. Sondheimer, F. K., and Steinberg, I. Gastrointestinal manifestations of abdominal aortic aneurysms. *AJR* 92:1110, 1964.
63. Staple, T. W., Friedenberg, M. J., Anderson, M. S., and Butcher, H. R., Jr. Arteria magna et dolicho of Leriche. *Acta Radiol. [Diagn.]* (Stockh.) 4:293, 1966.
64. Steinberg, I., and Stein, H. L. Visualization of abdominal aortic aneurysms. *AJR* 95:684, 1965.
65. Thomas, M. L. Arteriomegaly. *Br. J. Surg.* 58:690, 1971.
66. Thompson, J. E., Hollier, L. H., Patman, R. D., and Persson, A. V. Surgical management of abdominal aortic aneurysms: Factors influencing mortality and morbidity, a twenty-year experience. *Ann. Surg.* 181:654, 1975.
67. Uhle, C. A. W. The significance of aneurysm of the abdominal aorta masquerading as primary urologic disease: Case reports. *J. Urol.* 45:13, 1941.
68. Upson, J. F., and Culver, G. J. X-ray diagnosis of a mycotic aneurysm: Case report. *Radiology* 86:932, 1966.
69. Usselman, J. A., Vint, V. C., and Kleiman, S. A. CT diagnosis of aortic pseudoaneurysm causing vertebral erosion. *AJR* 133:1177, 1979.
70. Weintraub, R. A., and Abrams. H. L. Mycotic aneurysms. *AJR* 102:354, 1968.
71. Wolffe, J. B., and Colcher, R. E. Diagnosis and conservative management of atherosclerotic aneurysms of the abdominal aorta. *Vasc. Dis.* 3:49, 1966.
72. Wright, I. S., Urdaneta, E., and Wright, B. S. Re-opening the case of the abdominal aortic aneurysm. *Circulation* 13:754, 1956.
73. Yashar, J. J., Indeglia, R. A., and Yashar, J. Surgery for abdominal aortic aneurysms. Factors affecting survival and long-term results. *Am. J. Surg.* 123:398, 1972.

2. Renal Angiography

Techniques and Hazards

ERIK BOIJSEN

Intravenous bolus technique combined with digital subtraction radiography may soon remove those few indications for catheter renal angiography that remain after the recent introduction of computed tomography and ultrasonography. This change is, of course, welcome, because the renal angiographic procedure is not, and can never be, completely free from risks for the patient. Many of the complications can, however, be reduced with proper technique, since it is quite clear that most complications occur because of lack of experience and improper handling of the material. Since renal angiography will continue to be with us in the future, perhaps mainly for therapeutic reasons, there is reason to analyze and discuss what is meant by proper technique and how complications can be avoided.

There are various techniques of renal angiography, but the overwhelmingly important one is the percutaneous femoral catheterization technique introduced by Seldinger [32, 110], which will be the only one discussed in this chapter.

Preparation

The patient should be well informed about what is going to happen. He should know why and how the procedure is performed, and he should also know what discomfort he may experience. There is no reason to frighten the patient by talking about all the complications that can occur, but he should know that there are certain but very small risks with the method and that these must be accepted for proper treatment.

It should be clear that the radiologist has full responsibility for the examination. He should refuse to perform angiography if there is any indication that the patient will not tolerate it or if he feels that the reason for the examination is not good enough. Thus, the case history and the previous clinical and radiologic examinations should be carefully reviewed before a decision is made to perform angiography.

The bowel should be cleansed in a routine way. During the day of examination the patient should be allowed light meals and a free intake of fluids (to prevent dehydration). His groin should be shaved before he is sent to the angiography suite.

It is important that the patient is relaxed during the examination. Therefore, a sedative should be given if he is tense. To the sedative should be added 0.5 mg of atropine to prevent any vasovagal reflex that can occur in predisposed patients. Before the procedure is started, the blood pressure should be recorded and the pulsations of the dorsal pedic artery should be checked.

Guidewires, Catheters, and Catheterization Technique

After local anesthesia, the femoral artery is punctured well below the inguinal ligament. It is important to do so in order to have full control of the puncture site during and after the examination. The puncture needle should allow a 0.9-mm guidewire to pass.

The guidewire has at its tip a flexible core that, preferably, is J shaped in order to avoid dissection [69]. The guidewire should never be allowed to pass into the artery against resistance. When the tip of the guidewire is in the lumbar aorta, the needle is extracted, slight pressure is applied over the entrance, and the catheter (previously selected) is introduced over the guidewire. There are various types of guidewires, all of which are thrombogenic [45, 83, 97, 104]. The Teflon-coated guidewire in particular shows high thrombogenicity; the flat, polished steel guidewire seems to be the least thrombogenic. Heparin coating of the guidewire reduces thrombus deposition.

The *catheter* used for renal angiography depends on the indication for the examination. Two main types of catheters are used, one for aortic injection and one for selective renal angiography. Originally the catheter introduced for aortic injection was of polyethylene with an end hole. The tip was positioned at the level of origin of the renal arteries. The drawback of this type of catheter was that a large part of the bolus of contrast medium reached the splanchnic arteries with consequent reduction of information regarding the renal vasculature. In order to reduce the jet effect, side holes were introduced and the tapered tip occluded [94] (see Fig. 55-11).

Other variations of the catheter design for semiselective aortography (*Etagen-Aortographie*) were developed. A loop catheter [82, 96] (a catheter with no end hole but two side holes, introduced via a Teflon sheath [57]) and a catheter with a long, tapered tip [13] (later called a *pigtail catheter* [68]) were developed. Another type of catheter had two side holes close to the top hole; the top of the catheter was placed in

one renal artery and the two side holes were positioned in the aorta close to the opposite renal artery [41, 124]. With the high injection rate required for renal aortography (20 cc per sec), the risk of subintimal deposit of contrast medium in the catheterized renal artery is obvious. Renal artery dissection was also observed with this technique, and so the use of this catheter was abandoned [124]. The radiopaque catheter most commonly used today for renal angiography has a 6 or 7 French outer diameter, which means it can deliver contrast medium at a rate of about 20 cc per second when it is placed in the lumbar aorta.

It is generally agreed that in renal angiography an aortic injection of contrast medium should precede selective angiography and the selective method should be performed only if the expected information is not obtained by the survey angiogram. In my opinion, there is rarely a need for selective angiography if the quality of the aortic study is good. A good aortic study can be obtained in most cases if *semiselective renal angiography* is performed. The catheter used for this purpose is a thin-walled radiopaque catheter (OD/ID = 2.2/1.45 mm) with a 3-cm tapered part (OD/ID = 1.4/1.0 mm). The catheter has six side holes just proximal to the tapered part (Figs. 50-1, 50-2). The tip of the catheter is positioned

Figure 50-1. Catheter design for selective and semiselective renal angiography.

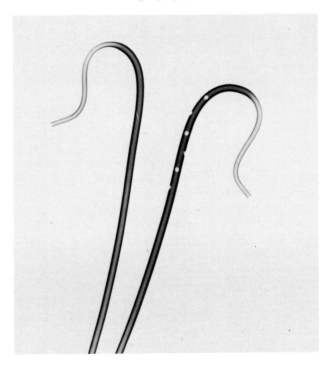

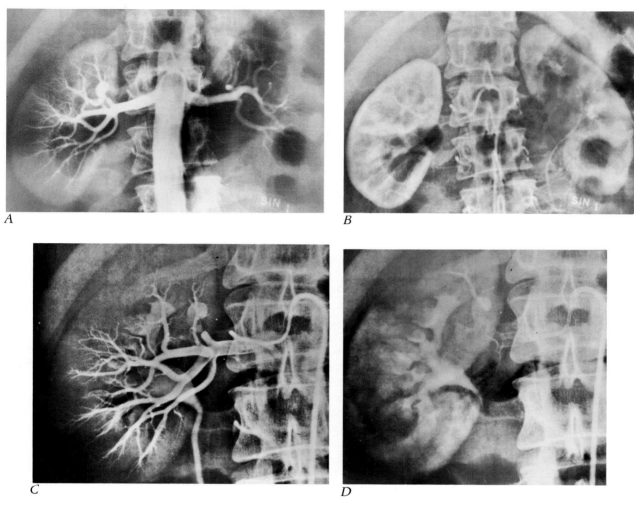

A

B

C

D

Figure 50-2. Renovascular hypertension due to short stenosis in cranial branch of ventral artery with a jet aneurysm. (A and B) Semiselective right renal angiography, arterial and capillary phases. Note the delayed circulation in the branch supplying the anterior part of the upper pole. The catheter is shaped according to the course of the renal artery. (C and D) Selective angiography with a tapered catheter without side holes. Two micrograms of angiotensin was given before the contrast medium injection. Note the marked delay in the perfusion of the ischemic segment. A 1-mm-long stenosis and a jet aneurysm are well demonstrated.

in one of the main renal arteries. When contrast medium is delivered at a rate of 20 cc per second, approximately the same amount passes through the top hole as through each side hole. When the usual total amount of 30 cc is injected, about 5 cc passes through the top hole over a period of 1.5 seconds, and 25 cc is deposited in the aorta, close to the opposite main renal artery (Fig. 50-3C; see also Figs. 50-2A and B, 51-1, 51-2, 51-12, 55-2). Thus at the same time selective and nonselective renal angiography is achieved. If necessary, the tip of the catheter then can be positioned in the contralateral renal artery to gain more detailed information about that kidney. The tapered tip of

the catheter should be formed so that it follows as closely as possible the course of the renal artery. Therefore, a slight bend on the most distal part is appropriate (see Figs. 50-1, 50-2). The rather slow rate of injection into the catheterized renal artery guarantees an atraumatic injection of contrast medium. We have found this technique quite advantageous in, for example, renal hypertension, particularly when marked stenosis is present, because the thin catheter tip can pass such a stenosis without interfering with the blood flow.

The pigtail catheter has been used for nonselective renal angiography with great advantage

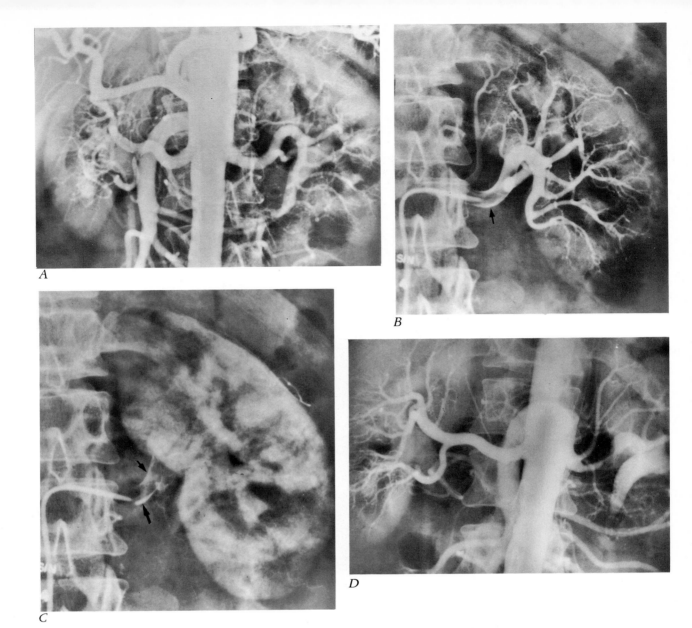

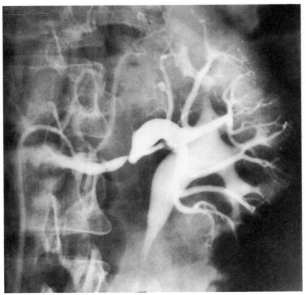

Figure 50-3. A man, 37-years-old, examined because of hematuria. (A) Nonselective renal angiography and (B and C) selective left renal angiography, arterial and nephrographic phases. No abnormality is observed. The sleevelike subintimal deposit of contrast medium (*arrows*) at the tip of the catheter was not recorded. The patient returned 2 years later with severe hypertension. (D) Semiselective right renal angiography and (E) selective left renal angiography reveal marked narrowing of the left main stem extending into the dorsal artery.

E

compared with many other varieties. But a serious complication has been reported with this catheter: the tip of the catheter has entered an intercostal artery during contrast medium injection with consequent spinal cord damage [19]. The reason for this problem seems to be that the tapered part, which is curved, straightens as a result of the jet effect. The straightening does not occur with a semiselective catheter because the main bend is in the more rigid part.

Selective renal angiography requires an exchange of catheters. For this purpose, the same type of catheter as for semiselective angiography, but without side holes, may be used (see Figs. 50-1, 50-2C and D, 50-3E). The catheter has a tapered distal part, with an outer diameter of 1.4 mm. Consequently, the distal part of the catheter does not have a very sharp and rigid tip, as is true of most catheters used selectively.

Subintimal dissection of the renal artery is rarely reported, but when it occurs it has very serious consequences for the patient [11, 29, 40, 46, 48, 53, 103, 124] (Fig. 50-4; see also Fig. 50-3). It may cause instant, severe hypertension, which must be treated with arterial repair or nephrectomy. If the occlusion is not complete, watchful

Figure 50-4. Hematuria and massive proteinuria were the main indications for renal angiography in this 20-year-old woman. At selective test injection into the right renal artery, a subintimal deposit of contrast medium occurred. The catheter was removed, and a nonselective aortogram was performed a few minutes later. (A) A nonselective renal angiogram and (B) a subtraction film of the same show that the contrast medium in the almost normal appearing renal artery on the right is in fact subintimally located and that there is complete occlusion of flow through the right kidney. (C) A urogram made 10 minutes later shows that the nephrographic effect is still present on the right as a consequence of the subintimal dissection.

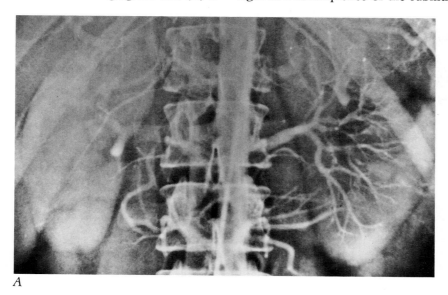

A

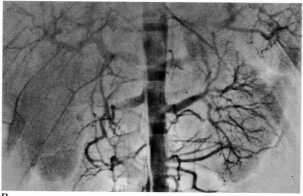

B

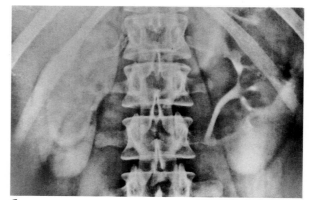

C

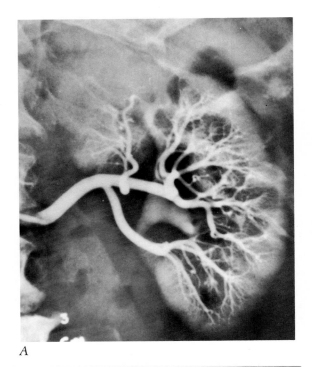

A

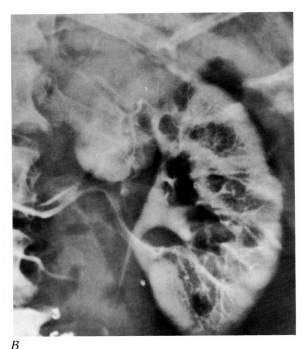

B

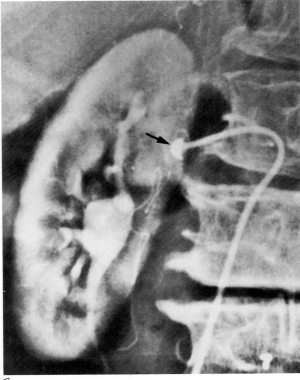

C

Figure 50-5. A subintimal injection of contrast medium into the left and right renal arteries. (A and B) An arterial and a late arterial left renal angiogram reveals a sleevelike deposit of contrast medium at the tip of the catheter not recognized at the time of examination. (C) A nephrographic phase of selective right renal angiography in the right posterior oblique position shows a small deposit of contrast medium at the tip of the catheter (*arrow*). The complications had no deleterious consequences.

waiting and anticoagulant therapy and repeated scintigraphic checks may be the best treatment [115, 124]. It is said that the lesion occurs more often in patients with atherosclerosis or fibromuscular dysplasia with hypertension, but it may occur in any age group. It is of interest that all subintimal renal artery lesions reported in the literature have occurred during the last decade. Certainly, subintimal dissection occurs much more often than reported, a fact that becomes obvious in a well-controlled prospective study [67, 115]. Many of the cases are not reported because they are not recognized at the time of examination (Fig. 50-5; see also Fig. 50-3), particularly when there is only a thin, sleevelike contrast deposit subintimally.

The advantage of using a catheter with a 2- to 3-cm-long tapered part is thus obvious. It is mandatory that no side holes be present on the catheter used for selective angiography; if side holes are present, a small artery may constrict around the tip and yet free flow be present. Injection of contrast medium into an ischemic kidney is bound to cause renal damage [43, 91, 116].

During injection, not only may the contrast medium pass subintimally at the tip of the catheter but also the renal artery may be perforated by the jet effect of the contrast medium [92]. The tip of the catheter may also recoil into a small adrenal or capsular artery originating from the first part of the renal artery, with consequent extravasation (Fig. 50-6).

THROMBOEMBOLIC CONSEQUENCES

Like the guidewires, the catheters are thrombogenic. Scanning electron microscopy and other methods have shown that fibrin deposition on the catheter is a rule. Catheters made of polyurethane and having a very rugged surface are the most thrombogenic; the smoother polyethylene catheters are less thrombogenic [45, 64, 90, 92, 104, 108]. The catheters cause an activation of the coagulation system, which is observed as an increased platelet adhesiveness and a consumption of fibrinogen. The length and diameter of the catheter (i.e., the amount of catheter surface exposed to blood) is related to the amount of fibrin deposited [66, 135]. Consequently, the frequency of complications due to thromboembolism is related to the type of catheter used, an observation that explains the wide range in the incidence of thromboembolic complications reported in the literature.

Figure 50-6. Rupture of a capsular artery. (A and B) Selective right renal angiography in the right posterior oblique position, arterial and capillary phases. During the contrast medium injection, the tip of the catheter recoiled into a small capsular artery (*arrow*, A), with resultant extravasation. The patient had severe pain, followed by marked hypotension, which was difficult to treat.

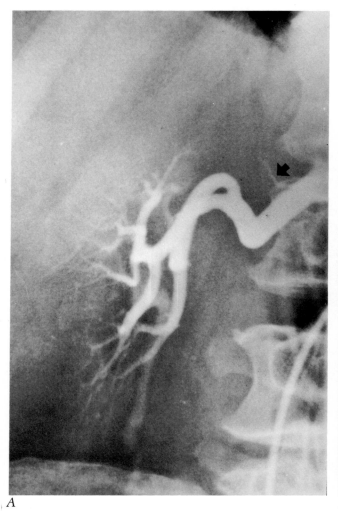

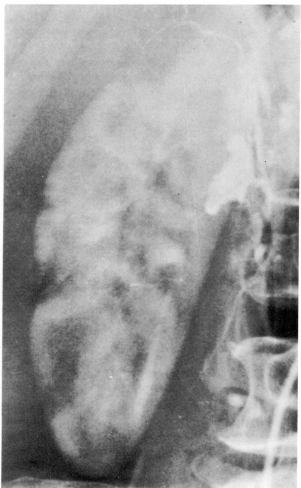

A

B

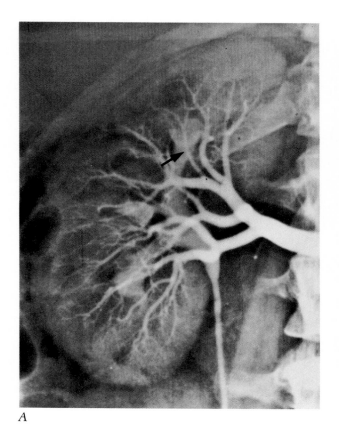

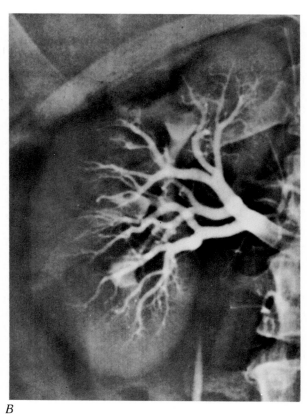

A

B

Figure 50-7. Selective right renal angiogram before (A) and after (B) an occlusion of the interlobar artery (*arrow*) which supplies mainly the third anterior lobe. An embolus was released from the catheter during a prolonged investigation.

These complications are mainly of two types. The most frequently recorded complication occurs when the catheter is withdrawn and the deposits on it are whipped off. This phenomenon occurs in practically every instance, but it seldom gives rise to ischemic symptoms. Occlusion at the puncture site or more distally in the leg resulting in loss of pulse or symptoms occurs in 0.1 to 1.2 percent of cases [10, 44, 52, 56, 78, 85, 107]. Pullout arteriography and oscillometry result in higher rates of this complication [26, 65, 113].

The second most common type of thromboembolic complication occurs when a clot within the catheter is released and causes embolism (Fig. 50-7) [33, 55, 88]. It occurs particularly when the guidewire has to be reintroduced for catheter exchange. With modern interventional embolization techniques, it has become obvious that renal embolism is not as serious a complication as previously thought. Furthermore, both immediate heparinization and transcatheter embolectomy have proved successful in treating this complication [20, 84].

Thromboembolism can be prevented by heparinization of the patient [5, 6, 99, 129]. The recommended dose is 45 units of heparin per kilogram body weight to a maximum of about 3,000 units given through the catheter at the start of the procedure [31, 129]. At the completion of the examination, protamine sulfate can be given [31, 100]. Other workers have recommended the infusion of low-molecular-weight dextran as an effective method of preventing coagulation [79]. Heparin coating of the catheters is still another method [25], but it has the drawback of prolonging the necessary compression time after catheter removal [37].

It is quite clear that clot formation can be reduced dramatically with the technique mentioned above. In modern renal angiography, however, there is rarely any complication of this kind in the adult patient, and so there is no need for the more expensive heparin-coated catheters [115]. Systemic heparinization is, on the other hand, a precaution that should be routinely employed in every catheterization procedure.

OTHER COMPLICATIONS DUE TO GUIDEWIRES AND CATHETERS

Fatal complications are extremely rare but they do occur, even with modern techniques and contrast media [26, 78, 107, 115]. Thromboembolic occlusion requiring surgery in debilitated patients is one potentially fatal complication; another is retroperitoneal hemorrhage due to catheter or guidewire perforation of the iliac arteries or lumbar aorta. Today, acutely and severely ill patients are undergoing renal angiography more often than previously. No doubt, preexisting severe disease is the main factor in fatal outcomes [10]. An increase in the number of deaths that show a time relationship to the procedure is therefore to be expected [56].

Complications at the puncture site can be serious. One such complication is the *subintimal passage* of the guidewire or catheter, or perforation of the artery, a lesion that may cause thrombosis, false aneurysm, or arteriovenous fistula [12, 44, 52 115]. Guidewire breakage is another complication, a rare one [24, 44, 52, 107].

Hematoma formation occurs frequently, and a large hematoma may require surgery [44, 52, 107, 115]. Particularly in patients with hypertension, the hematoma may be a problem; it may occur later, when the patient has been sent back to the ward. In a prospective series, serious delayed bleeding occurred in 0.5 percent of the patients examined by various types of abdominal angiography [115].

Thrombosis of the femoral vein as a consequence of abdominal angiography is rarely reported [44, 131]. It is rather surprising that this complication does not occur more often, considering the fact that the patients in question are old, are bedridden and have poor perfusion of the legs, and have a hematoma that compresses the vein. In a prospective search for this complication in a highly selected group of 20 patients, we found only one patient with a thrombosis secondary to a large hematoma [131].

Subintimal injection of contrast medium into the renal artery was mentioned previously; it may also occur in the abdominal aorta or the iliac arteries. Previously it was regarded as a frequent complication [28, 44, 47, 51]. With the technique recommended above, this complication has diminished markedly.

Embolization due to clot formation has also been mentioned previously. In advanced atherosclerosis, plaque may be dislodged and embolized to various vascular beds [54, 81, 109, 114]. This complication occurs more often than reported, but obviously it is not recognized because the emboli are too small to be observed or to cause symptoms.

Foreign materials, such as surgical glove powder and cotton fiber, were previously reported in the kidneys after selective renal angiography [2, 44, 72, 137]. This complication occurred usually because foreign material fell into the open bowls that had been used in flushing the catheters; the complication was eliminated after closed reservoir-tubing systems were introduced. More recently, glass particles and other material have been found to contaminate contrast media [18, 133], and particulate contamination of all kinds of fluid administration sets and cannulas has been observed [132]. The thrombogenicity of catheters and guidewires has been mentioned above; in addition the rough surfaces of the equipment contribute to the release of particles [5]. At experimental selective renal angiography, the particles have caused renal infarction [134].

Contrast Medium

TECHNIQUES

The delivery rates and the amounts of contrast medium are generally adjusted to the renal blood flow rate, the size of the patient, and the size of the lumbar aorta. In semiselective or nonselective renal angiography, 30 to 40 cc of a 76 percent sodium meglumine salt (diatrizoate or metrizoate) is injected at a rate of 20 cc per second. In selective renal angiography of a normal functioning kidney, 8 to 10 cc of a 60 percent meglumine salt (diatrizoate, iothalamate, or metrizoate) is injected at a rate of 10 cc per second. In renal disease with reduced blood flow, the amount of contrast medium and the injection rate should be reduced. Thus, in severe renal disease, 3 to 4 cc injected at a rate of 2 to 3 cc per second may be sufficient. On the other hand, 30 to 40 cc may be delivered at a rate of 15 cc per second in a kidney that has a richly vascularized carcinoma, when the main purpose is to find out whether the renal vein has been invaded by tumor.

In selected patients, *vasoconstrictors* may be used to obtain additional information [1, 16, 35, 36] (see Fig. 50-2). The most reliable information is obtained with a dose of 0.5 to 2.0 μg of angiotensin injected 10 to 15 seconds before the contrast medium injection.

TOXICITY

Contrast media may cause acute renal failure when administered intravenously, particularly when given intraarterially. In a recent review, Byrd and Sherman [21] found an incidence of 0.15 percent acute renal failure over a 12-month period in patients examined with contrast medium administered intravenously; the frequency in their angiographic studies was 0.53 percent. In fact, an even higher incidence (10–12%) of acute renal failure has been reported for angiography [93, 121]. It is therefore interesting to note that in communications about the general complications of angiography, no or very few cases of renal failure have been mentioned [20, 44, 78, 105]. The main reason for this remarkable discrepancy is that renal failure may be observed only as a slight or moderate azotemia and short-term oliguria, and it passes undetected if it is not particularly looked for. Acute renal failure is almost always reversible. The oliguria usually lasts for no longer than 72 hours [4]. It may, however, be fatal for a patient at risk. An increasing number of cases of acute renal failure following angiography have been reported [17, 21, 75, 76, 101, 119, 121, 130]. The increase may have some relationship to the increasing amounts of contrast media used in angiography.

There are certain factors that increase the risk of renal failure after the delivery of contrast medium [21, 122]. Advanced age, a past or current reduction in renal function, dehydration, hyperuricemia, diabetes, and proteinuria are important risk factors that should be considered before renal angiography is done.

Toxicity is related to the concentration, osmolality, and volume of the contrast medium and to the contact time and the number of injections [63, 89]. The least concentrated contrast medium adequate to the diagnostic task should be used [95]. It is true that large doses of contrast media accidentally injected into the renal artery have not caused significant damage to the kidney [80, 98, 112]. Not even highly concentrated media (the 76% solutions) have proved to be more toxic than the commonly used solutions (the 50–60% solutions) [74, 126]. There is clinical and experimental evidence, however, that there is a short period of decreased renal function and signs of reversible renal damage. Transient enzyme excretion suggests that there is tubular damage [49, 125], and signs of cell injury and regeneration are observed [42]. The isotope nephrogram is often abnormal [71], and the extraction of PAH is reduced for a short period after the intraarterial injection [27, 117]. In humans, an "osmotic nephrosis" has been observed in biopsies performed within a week of arteriography [86]; and in infants, tubular changes, and even medullary necrosis, have been observed [50].

Urinary albumin excretion levels up to five times higher than preinjection levels have been observed in humans [127, 128]. Experimental and clinical tests show that maximum albuminuria is found some 45 minutes after injection and also that metrizamide (Amipaque), which is three times less osmotic, causes similar effects. The cause of the albuminuria is believed to be leakage through the glomeruli rather than tubular damage [58–60, 62]. The most recently developed nonionic contrast media (Iohexol; Nyegaard) does not cause massive proteinuria [61].

The exact mechanism of the nephrotoxic effects of the contrast medium is not definitely known. Hypertonicity certainly plays a role, but it is not the only cause. Most of the effects can be related to the response of the vascular bed. Probably, the increased stiffness of the red cells is an important factor in addition to hyperosmolality and viscosity [8]. Abnormal rigidity of red cells is also caused by the metrizamide; it is observed to a much lesser extent with iohexol [9]. It is hoped, therefore, that the new contrast material may reduce nephrotoxicity.

The renal vascular bed does not respond to contrast medium injection in the same way that other vascular beds do. There is no unanimous description of the changes in renal blood flow, but in all cases described there was a decreased flow [7, 22, 23, 70, 87, 111, 123]. In most reports, the increased resistance is observed at 10 to 15 seconds after injection and it lasts for 1 to 15 minutes. During the first few seconds the kidney volume is reduced, and then a prolonged period of renal distention follows [30].

The pathophysiology of acute renal failure is thus complex. It can be explained by reversible damage of the vascular endothelium causing protein to leak from the glomeruli and into the tubular ducts. Plugging of the ducts, in combination with the osmotic effects of the contrast medium in the ducts and extracellular fluid, explains the increased renal size. The intrarenal pressure rises because the high resistance of the renal capsule causes an increased resistance to flow. The increased contact time of the contrast medium with the tubular cells and a certain

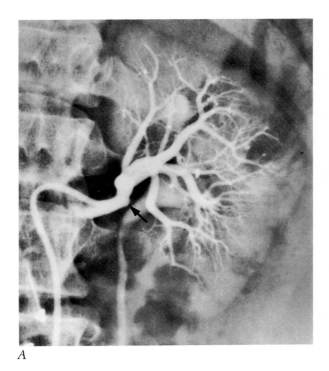
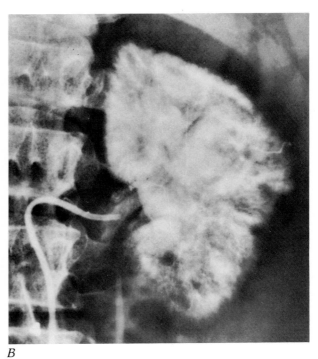

A

B

Figure 50-8. Cortical arterial spasm due to malpositioning of the catheter in the renal artery. (A and B) Selective left renal angiography, early and late arterial phases. Observe that the tip of the catheter causes bulging of the arterial wall (*arrow*, A), with secondary spasm of the cortical arteries and irregular perfusion, which was not demonstrated at nonselective renal angiography.

anoxia can explain the tubular damage. Thus, the decreased flow does not necessarily mean that vasoconstriction is present, but there is evidence that the renin-angiotensin system is activated during selective renal angiography [22, 136].

Vasoconstriction may be observed at renal angiography either as a localized, short, concentric ring at the tip of the catheter or as a long segment of fusiform narrowing. A third type of vasoconstriction comprises multiple small cortical perfusion defects [3, 34, 118] (Fig. 50-8). Because the most common cause is a malpositioning of the catheter in the renal artery, these defects disappear when a vasodilating drug is given or when the catheter's position is corrected.

Spasm of the cortical arteries is also observed if the renal artery is clamped or if intraarterial vasoconstrictors are given before the contrast medium injection [38, 39]. Similar perfusion defects are observed when angiography is performed during hypotension or shock due to hemorrhage [77]. It should be recognized that the use of vasoconstrictors in combination with contrast media increases the risk of renal damage [73, 102].

Radiographic Technique

The radiographic technique varies with the actual situation and the indications for renal angiography. It should always begin with proper positioning of the catheter to obtain as much information as possible about the lumbar aorta and the renal arteries. As mentioned, the most precise information is obtained with a semiselective technique. After a test injection of 10 cc of contrast medium (to check the position of the catheter), the patient is positioned over a film changer. Ordinary radiographic techniques are used (1) to prevent unnecessary scattered irradiation (by compression of the abdomen and careful collimation) and (2) to arrive at the best possible geometry (the patient should be positioned as close as possible to the film changer). The generator should be capable of giving exposures below 0.10 second at 70 to 75 kV.

NONSELECTIVE OR SEMISELECTIVE RENAL ANGIOGRAPHY

During the arterial phase, two frames per second gives enough information in most cases. Since the injection time is about 1.5 seconds, usually six frames over 3 seconds covers the arterial phase. In order to cover the nephrographic and venous phases (see Chap. 51), one frame every other second (i.e., six frames over 12 seconds) is sufficient. Particularly in hypertension, it is important to visualize the origin of the renal arteries from the aorta. Since the arteries often arise from the anterolateral aspect of the aorta, oblique films may be necessary. If the semiselective technique is used, the catheter tip is positioned in the left renal artery in the right posterior oblique projection and in the right renal artery in the left posterior oblique projection.

Selective renal angiography is performed only when the expected information has not been obtained or when a special technique can be expected to give more information. Thus, selective angiography is done when vasoactive drugs are used or when large doses of contrast medium are required for venous demonstration.

The injection time for a normal selective renal angiogram is about 1 second. Usually, four frames over 2 seconds covers the arterial phase, and four frames over 8 seconds covers the nephrographic and venous phases. If vasoconstrictors are injected before the contrast medium, a slower injection rate and longer intervals between the exposures are recommended. Also, when large doses of contrast medium are injected for tumor analysis, one exposure every other second suffices for arterial and venous information.

When possible, a selective angiogram should be performed with 3× magnification (see Figs. 51-1, 51-12). In order to lower the radiation dose to the skin, the number of exposures can be decreased to cover only the later arterial and early nephrographic phases [14, 15, 106, 120].

References

1. Abrams, H. L. The response of neoplastic renal vessels to epinephrine in man. *Radiology* 82:217, 1964.
2. Adams, D. F., Olin, T. B., and Kosek, J. Cotton fiber embolization during angiography. A clinical and experimental study. *Radiology* 84:678, 1965.
3. Albrechtsson, U., and Tylén, U. Spasm of cortical arteries as a complication to selective nephroangiography. *Acta Radiol. [Diagn.]* (Stockh.) 19:785, 1978.
4. Alexander, R. D., Berkes, S. L., and Abuelo, J. G. Contrast media induced oliguric renal failure. *Arch. Intern. Med.* 138:381, 1978.
5. Anderson, J. H., Gianturco, C., Wallace, S., Dodd, G. D., and DeJongh, D. Anticoagulation techniques for angiography: An experimental study. *Radiology* 111:573, 1974.
6. Antonovic, R., Rösch, J., and Dotter, C. T. The value of systemic arterial heparinization in transfemoral angiography: A prospective study. *AJR* 127:223, 1976.
7. Aperia, A., Broberger, O., and Ekengren, K. Renal hemodynamics during selective renal angiography. *Invest. Radiol.* 3:389, 1968.
8. Aspelin, P. Effect of ionic and non-iogenic contrast media on red blood cell morphology and rheology. University of Lund (Malmö) Thesis, 1976.
9. Aspelin, P. Personal communication, 1980.
10. Baum, S., Stein, G. N., and Kuroda, K. K. Complications of "No arteriography." *Radiology* 86:835, 1966.
11. Bergentz, S.-E., Faarup, P., Hegedüs, V., Lindholm, T., and Lindstedt, E. Diagnosis of hypertension due to occlusion of a supplemental renal artery; its localization, treatment by removal from the body, microsurgical repair and reimplantation. A case report. *Ann. Surg.* 178:643, 1973.
12. Bergentz, S.-E., Hansson, L. O., and Norbäck, B. Komplikationer till artärpunktioner. Diagnostik och behandling (in Swedish). *Läkartidningen* 63:2419, 1966.
13. Boijsen, E., and Judkins, M. P. A hook-tail "closed-end" catheter for percutaneous selective cardioangiography. *Radiology* 87:872, 1966.
14. Boijsen, E., and Maly, P. Vergrösserungstechnik in der abdominellen Angiographie. *Radiologe* 18:167, 1978.
15. Bookstein, J. J., Davidson, A. J., Hill, G. S., Hollenberg, N., and Sherwood, T. The Small Renal Vessels. In S. K. Hilal (ed.), *Small Vessel Angiography*. St. Louis: Mosby, 1973.
16. Bookstein, J. J., and Ernst, C. B. Vasodilatory and vasoconstrictive pharmacoangiographic manipulation of renal collateral flow. *Radiology* 108:55, 1973.
17. Borra, S., Hawkins, D., Duguid, W., and Kaye, M. Acute renal failure and nephrotic syndrome after angiocardiography with meglumine diatrizoate. *N. Engl. J. Med.* 284:592, 1971.
18. Brekkan, A., Lexow, P. E., and Woxholt, G.

Glass fragments and other particles contaminating contrast media. *Acta Radiol. [Diagn.]* (Stockh.) 16:600, 1975.

19. Brodey, P. A., Doppman, J. L., and Bisaccia, L. J.   An unusual complication of aortography with the pig-tail catheter. *Radiology* 110:711, 1974.

20. Buxton, D. R., Jr., and Mueller, C. F.   Removal of iatrogenic clot by transcatheter embolectomy. *Radiology* 111:39, 1974.

21. Byrd, L., and Sherman, R. L.   Radiocontrast-induced acute renal failure: A clinical and pathophysiologic review. *Medicine* 58:270, 1979.

22. Caldicott, W. J., Hollenberg, N. K., and Abrams, H. L.   Characteristics of response of renal vascular bed to contrast media: Evidence of vasoconstriction induced by renin-angiotensin system. *Invest. Radiol.* 5:539, 1970.

23. Chou, C. C., Hook, J. B., Hsieh, C. P., et al. Effect of radiopaque dyes on renal vascular resistance. *J. Lab. Clin. Med.* 78:705, 1971.

24. Cope, C.   Intravascular breakage of Seldinger spring guide wires. *J.A.M.A.* 180:1061, 1962.

25. Cramer, A., Frech, R. S., and Amplatz, K.   A preliminary human study with a simple non-thrombogenic catheter. *Radiology* 100:421, 1971.

26. Cramer, R., Morre, R., and Amplatz, K.   Reduction of the surgical complication rate by the use of a hypothrombogenic catheter coating. *Radiology* 109:585, 1973.

27. Danford, R. O., Talner, L. B., and Davidson, A. J.   Effect of graded osmolalities of saline solution and contrast media on renal extraction of PAH in the dog. *Invest. Radiol.* 4:301, 1969.

28. Davidsen, H. G., Gudbjerg, C. E., and Thomsen, G.   Complications of selective angiocardiography and percutaneous transarterial aortography. *Acta Chir. Scand. [Suppl.]* 283:161, 1961.

29. Delin, A., Fernström, I., and Swedenborg, J. Intimal dissection of the renal artery following selective angiography. Report of two cases and review of the literature. *Vasa* 8:78, 1979.

30. Dorph, S.   Changes in renal size following intraarterial administration of water-soluble contrast medium. *Invest. Radiol.* 9:487, 1974.

31. Dotter, C. T., Keller, F. S., Rösch, J., and Buschman, R. W.   The value of protamine following heparin-covered angiography: Double-blind placebo-controlled study. *Radiology* 135:229, 1980.

32. Edholm, P., and Seldinger, S. I.   Percutaneous catheterization of the renal artery. *Acta Radiol.* (Stockh.) 45:15, 1956.

33. Edling, N. P. G., and Ovenfors, C. O.   Risks in selective renal catheterization and arteriography. An experimental study in dogs. *Acta Radiol.* [Diagn.] (Stockh.) 2:241, 1964.

34. Edsman, G.   Angionephrography and suprarenal angiography. *Acta Radiol. [Suppl.]* (Stockh.) 155:1957.

35. Ekelund, L.   Pharmako-Angiographie der Niere. *Radiologe* 13:279, 1973.

36. Ekelund, L., Göthlin, J., and Lunderquist, A.   Diagnostic improvement with angiotensin in renal angiography. *Radiology* 105:33, 1972.

37. Eldh, P., and Jacobsson, B.   Heparinized vascular catheters: A clinical trial. *Radiology* 111:289, 1974.

38. Elkin, M., and Meng, C. H.   Angiographic study of the effect of vasopressors—epinephrine and levarterenol—on renal vascularity. *AJR* 93:904, 1965.

39. Elkin, M., and Meng, C. H.   The effects of angiotensin on renal vascularity in dogs. *AJR* 98:927, 1966.

40. Engberg, A., Eriksson, U., Killander, A., Persson, R., and Wicklund, H.   An unusual complication of selective renal angiography: A case presentation. *Aust. Radiol.* 18:304, 1974.

41. Eriksson, U.   On the technique of selective renal arteriography. *Aust. Radiol.* 17:316, 1973.

42. Evensen, A., and Skalpe, J. A.   Cell injury and cell regeneration in selective renal arteriography in rabbits: A preliminary report. *Invest. Radiol.* 6:299, 1971.

43. Farry, P. J., Beale, L. R., and Macbeth, W. A. A. G.   Intrarenal extravasation complicating selective vessel angiography. *N.Z. Med. J.* 72:17, 1970.

44. Folin, J.   Complications of percutaneous femoral catheterization for renal angiography. *Radiologe* 8:190, 1968.

45. Formanek, G., Frech, R. S., and Amplatz, K.   Arterial thrombus formation during clinical percutaneous catheterization. *Circulation* 41:833, 1970.

46. Gewertz, B. L., Stanley, J. C., and Fry, W. J.   Renal artery dissections. *Arch. Surg.* 112:409, 1977.

47. Gilbert, G. J., and Melnick, G. S.   Pathophysiology of subintimal hematoma formation during retrograde arteriography. *Radiology* 85:306, 1965.

48. Gill, W. B., Cole, A. T., and Wong, R. J.   Renovascular hypertension developing as a complication of selective renal arteriography. *J. Urol.* 107:922, 1972.

49. Goldstein, E. J., Feinfeld, D. A., Fleischner, G. M., and Elkin, M.   Enzymatic evidence of renal tubular damage following renal angiography. *Radiology* 121:617, 1976.

50. Gruskin, A. B., Detliker, O. H., Wolfish, N. M., et al.   Effects of angiography on renal function and histology in infants and piglets. *J. Pediatr.* 76:41, 1970.

51. Gudbjerg, C. E., and Christensen, J.   Dissection

of the aortic wall in retrograde lumbar aortography. *Acta Radiol.* (Stockh.) 55:364, 1961.

52. Halpern, M.   Percutaneous transfemoral arteriography. An analysis of the complications in 1,000 consecutive cases. *AJR* 92:918, 1964.

53. Hare, W. S. C., and Kincaid-Smith, P.   Dissecting aneurysm of the renal artery. *Radiology* 97:255, 1970.

54. Harrington, J. T., Sommers, S. C., and Kassirer, J. P.   Atheromatous emboli with progressive renal failure. Renal arteriography as the probable inciting factor. *Ann. Intern. Med.* 68:152, 1968.

55. Hartmann, H. R., Newcomb, A. W., Barnes, A., and Lowman, R. M.   Renal infarction following selective renal angiography. *Radiology* 86:52, 1966.

56. Herlinger, H.   Aortography and Peripheral Arteriography. In G. Ansell (ed.), *Complications in Diagnostic Radiology.* Oxford: Blackwell, 1976.

57. Hettler, M.   Angiographische Probleme und Möglichkeiten: II. Der perkutane Arterienkateterismus mit an der Spitze verschlossenem Katheter als Grundlage der Etagen-Aortographie. *ROEFO* 92:198, 1960.

58. Holtås, S.   Proteinuria following nephroangiography. University of Lund (Malmö) Thesis, 1978.

59. Holtås, S., Almén, T., Hellsten, S., and Tejler, L.   Proteinuria following nephroangiography: VI. Comparison between metrizoate and metrizamide in man. *Acta Radiol.* [*Diagn.*] (Stockh.) 21:491, 1980.

60. Holtås, S., Almén, T., and Tejler, L.   Proteinuria following nephroangiography: III. Role of osmolality and concentration of contrast medium in renal arteries in dogs. *Acta Radiol.* [*Diagn.*] (Stockh.) 19:401, 1978.

61. Holtås, S., Golman, K., and Törnquist, C.   Proteinuria following nephroangiography: VIII. Comparison between diatrizoate and iohexol in rats. *Acta Radiol.* [*Suppl.*] (Stockh.) 362:53, 1980.

62. Holtås, S., and Tejler, L.   Proteinuria following nephroangiography: IV. Comparison in dogs between ionic and non-ionic contrast media. *Acta Radiol.* [*Diagn.*] (Stockh.) 20:13, 1979.

63. Idbohrn, H., and Berg, N.   On the tolerance of the rabbit's kidney to contrast media in renal angiography: A roentgenologic and histologic investigation. *Acta Radiol.* (Stockh.) 42:121, 1954.

64. Jacobsson, B., Bergentz, S.-E., and Ljungqvist, U.   Platelet adhesion and thrombus formation on vascular catheters in dogs. *Acta Radiol.* [*Diagn.*] (Stockh.) 8:221, 1969.

65. Jacobsson, B., Paulin, S., and Schlossman, D.   Thromboembolism of leg following percutaneous catheterisation of the femoral artery for angiography. Symptoms and signs. *Acta Radiol.* [*Diagn.*] (Stockh.) 8:97, 1969.

66. Jacobsson, B., and Schlossman, D.   Thromboembolism of leg following percutaneous catheterisation of femoral artery for angiography. Predisposing factors. *Acta Radiol.* [*Diagn.*] (Stockh.) 8:109, 1969.

67. Jonsson, K., Lunderquist, A., Pettersson, H., and Sigstedt, B.   Subintimal injection of contrast medium as a complication of selective abdominal angiography. *Acta Radiol.* [*Diagn.*] (Stockh.) 18:55, 1977.

68. Judkins, M. P.   Percutaneous transfemoral selective coronary angiography. *Radiol. Clin. North Am.* 6:467, 1968.

69. Judkins, M. P., Kidd, H. J., Frische, L. H., and Dotter, C. T.   Lumen-following safety J-guide for catheterization of tortuous vessels. *Radiology* 88:1127, 1967.

70. Katzberg, R. W., Morris, T. W., Burgener, F. A., Kamm, D. E., and Fischer, H. W.   Renal renin and hemodynamic responses to selective renal artery catheterization and angiography. *Invest. Radiol.* 12:381, 1977.

71. Kaude, J., and Nordenfelt, I.   Influence of nephroangiography on ^{131}I-hippuran nephrography. *Acta Radiol.* [*Diagn.*] (Stockh.) 14:69, 1973.

72. Kay, J. M., and Wilkins, R. A.   Cotton fibre embolism during angiography. *Clin. Radiol.* 20:410, 1969.

73. Knapp, R., Hollenberg, N. K., Busch, G. J., and Abrams, H. L.   Prolonged unilateral acute renal failure induced by intra-arterial nor-epinephrine infusion in the dog. *Invest. Radiol.* 7:164, 1972.

74. Knox, F. G., Bunnell, J. L., Elwood, C. M., and Sigman, E. N.   The effect of selective renal angiography on glomerular filtration rate and renal plasma flow in man. *Physiologist* 8:210, 1965.

75. Kovnat, P. J., Lin, K. Y., and Popky, G.   Azotemia and nephrogenic diabetes insipidus after arteriography. *Radiology* 108:541, 1973.

76. Krumlovsky, F. A., Simon, N., Santhanam, S., et al.   Acute renal failure—association with administration of radiographic contrast material. *J.A.M.A.* 239:128, 1978.

77. Kupic, E. A., and Abrams, H. L.   Renal vascular alterations induced by hemorrhagic hypotension: Preliminary observations. *Invest. Radiol.* 3:345, 1968.

78. Lang, E. K.   A survey of the complications of percutaneous retrograde arteriography: Seldinger technique. *Radiology* 81:257, 1963.

79. Langsjoen, P. H., and Best, E. B.   Studies in the prevention of complications of angiography. *AJR* 106:425, 1969.

80. Laubscher, W. M. L., and Raper, F. P.   A report of a case of the injection of a massive dose of Urografin into the renal artery. *Br. J. Urol.* 32:160, 1960.

81. Lonni, Y. G. W., Matsumoto, K. K., and Lecky,

J. W.   Postaortographic cholesterol (atheromatous) embolization. *Radiology* 93:63, 1969.

82. Mannila, T. O., and Wiljasalo, M.   Semiselective renal arteriography. *Invest. Radiol.* 2:176, 1967.

83. McCarty, R. J., and Glasser, S. P.   Thrombogenicity of guide wires. *Am. J. Cardiol.* 32:943, 1973.

84. McConnel, R. W., Fore, W. W., and Taylor, A.   Embolic occlusion of the renal artery following arteriography: Successful management. *Radiology* 107:273, 1973.

85. Moore, C. H., Wolma, F. J., Brown, R. W., and Derrick, J. R.   Complications of cardiovascular radiology: A review of 1204 cases. *Am. J. Surg.* 120:591, 1970.

86. Moreau, J. F., Droz, D., Sabto, J., Jungers, P., Kleinknecht, D., Hinglais, N., and Michel, J.-R.   Osmotic nephrosis induced by water-soluble triiodinated contrast media in man: A retrospective study of 47 cases. *Radiology* 115:329, 1975.

87. Morris, T. W., Katzberg, R. W., and Fischer, H. W.   A comparison of the hemodynamic responses to metrizamide and meglumine/sodium diatrizoate in canine renal angiography. *Invest. Radiol.* 13:74, 1978.

88. Morrow, J., and Amplatz, K.   Embolic occlusion of the renal artery during aortography. *Radiology* 86:57, 1966.

89. Mudge, G. H.   Some questions on nephrotoxicity. *Invest. Radiol.* 5:407, 1970.

90. Nachnani, G. H., Lessin, L. S., Motomiya, T., and Jensen, W. N.   Scanning electron microscopy of thrombogenesis on vascular catheter surfaces. *N. Engl. J. Med.* 286:139, 1972.

91. Obrez, I., and Abrams, H. L.   Temporary occlusion of the renal artery: Effects and significance. *Radiology* 104:545, 1972.

92. Olbert, F., Denck, H., and Wicke, L.   Komplikationen bei Katheterangiographien. Ursachen und deren Behandlung. *Wien. Med. Wochenschr.* 123:293, 1973.

93. Older, R. A., Miller, J. P., Jackson, D. C., Johnsrude, J. S., and Thompson, W. M.   Angiographically induced renal failure and its radiographic detection. *AJR* 126:1039, 1976.

94. Olin, T.   Studies in angiographic technique. University of Lund (Malmö) Thesis, 1963.

95. Olsson, O.   Technique and Hazards of Renal Angiography. In H. L. Abrams (ed.), *Angiography* (2nd ed.). Boston: Little, Brown, 1971.

96. Ovitt, T. W., and Amplatz, K.   Semiselective renal angiography. *AJR* 119:767, 1973.

97. Ovitt, T. W., Durst, S., Moore, R., and Amplatz, K.   Guide wire thrombogenicity and its reduction. *Radiology* 111:43, 1974.

98. Pepper, H. W., Korobkin, M. T., and Palubinskas, A. J.   Massive injection of contrast medium into a renal artery segment: A case report. *Radiology* 112:273, 1974.

99. Porstmann, W., and Geisser, W.   Die retrograde Kateterisierung des linken Ventrikels in der A. femoralis und der A. carotis communis dextra. Zwei sich ergänzende Methoden, ihre Indikationen und Ergebnisse. *ROEFO* 91:14, 1959.

100. Porstmann, W., Wierny, L., Warnke, H., et al.   Catheter closure of patent ductus arteriosus. 62 cases treated without thoracotomy. *Radiol. Clin. North Am.* 9:203, 1971.

101. Port, F. K., Wagoner, R. D., and Fulton, R. E.   Acute renal failure after angiography. *AJR* 121:544, 1974.

102. Redman, H. C., Olin, T. B., Saldeen, T., and Reuter, S. R.   Nephrotoxicity of some vasoactive drugs following selective intra-arterial injection. *Invest. Radiol.* 1:458, 1966.

103. Reiss, M. D., Bookstein, J. J., and Bleifer, K. H.   Radiologic aspects of renovascular hypertension: IV. Arteriographic complications. *J.A.M.A.* 221:374, 1972.

104. Roberts, G. M., Roberts, E. E., Davies, R. L., and Lawrie, B. W.   Thrombogenicity of arterial catheters and guidewires. *Br. J. Radiol.* 50:415, 1977.

105. Robertson, P. W., Dyson, M. L., and Sutton, P. D.   Renal angiography. A review of 1750 cases. *Clin. Radiol.* 20:401, 1969.

106. Sakuma, S., Ikeda, H., Ayakawa, Y., Tanaka, Y., and Takahashi, S.   Angiography with direct fourfold magnification. *Invest. Radiol.* 4:310, 1969.

107. Saur, H. T.   Komplikationen bei der indirekten (perkutanen Katheter-) Methode der Aortographie. Folgerungen in Bezug auf ihre Anwendung. *Roentgenblaetter* 19:305, 1966.

108. Schlossman, D.   Thrombogenicity of vascular catheters. University of Gothenburg (Sweden) Thesis, 1972.

109. Schwartz, S., and Waters, L.   Cholesterol embolization. *Radiology* 106:37, 1973.

110. Seldinger, S. I.   Catheter replacement of the needle in percutaneous arteriography. A new technique. *Acta Radiol.* (Stockh.) 39:368, 1953.

111. Sherwood, T., and Lavender, J. P.   Does renal blood flow rise or fall in response to diatrizoate? *Invest. Radiol.* 4:327, 1969.

112. Sidd, J. J., and Decter, A.   Unilateral renal damage due to massive contrast dye injection with recovery. *J. Urol.* 97:30, 1967.

113. Siegelman, S. S., Caplan, L. H., and Annes, G. P.   Complications of catheter angiography. Study with oscillometry and "pull out" angiograms. *Radiology* 91:251, 1968.

114. Sieniewicz, D. J., Moore, S., Moir, F. O., and McDade, D. F.   Atheromatous emboli to the kidneys. *Radiology* 92:1231, 1969.

115. Sigstedt, B., and Lunderquist, A. Complications of angiographic examinations. *AJR* 130:455, 1978.

116. Smiddy, F. G., and Andersson, G. K. Tolerance of the kidneys to the contrast medium Urografin. *Br. J. Urol.* 32:156, 1960.

117. Sorby, W. A., and Hoy, R. J. Renal arteriography and renal function. *Aust. Radiol.* 12:252, 1968.

118. Spriggs, D. W., and Brantley, R. E. Recognition of renal artery spasm during renal angiography. *Radiology* 127:363, 1978.

119. Stark, F. R., and Coburn, J. W. Renal failure following methylglucamine diatrizoate (Renografin) aortography: Report of a case with unilateral renal artery stenosis. *J. Urol.* 96:848, 1966.

120. Stein, H. L. Direct serial magnification. Renal arteriography: A clinical study. *J. Urol.* 109:967, 1973.

121. Swartz, R. D., Rubin, J. E., Leeming, B. W., and Silva, P. Renal failure following major angiography. *Am. J. Med.* 65:31, 1978.

122. Talner, L. B. Renal Complications of Angiography. In G. Ansell (ed.), *Complications in Diagnostic Radiology.* Oxford: Blackwell, 1976.

123. Talner, L. B., and Davidson, A. J. Renal hemodynamic effects of contrast media. *Invest. Radiol.* 3:310, 1968.

124. Talner, L. B., McLaughlin, A. P., and Bookstein, J. J. Renal artery dissection: A complication of catheter arteriography. *Radiology* 117:291, 1975.

125. Talner, L. B., Rushmer, H. N., and Coel, M. N. The effect of renal artery injection of contrast material on urinary enzyme excretion. *Invest. Radiol.* 7:311, 1972.

126. Talner, L. B., and Saltzstein, S. Renal arteriography: The choice of contrast material. *Invest. Radiol.* 10:91, 1975.

127. Tejler, L., Almen, T., and Holtås, S. Proteinuria following nephroangiography: I. Clinical experience. *Acta Radiol.* [*Diagn.*] (Stockh.) 18:634, 1977.

128. Tejler, L., Ekberg, M., Almén, T., et al. Proteinuria following renal arteriography. *Acta Med. Scand.* 202:131, 1977.

129. Wallace, S., Medellin, H., DeJongh, D., and Gianturco, C. Systemic heparinization for angiography. *AJR* 116:204, 1972.

130. Weinrauch, J. A., Healy, R. W., Leland, O. S., et al. Coronary angiography and acute renal failure in diabetic azotemic nephropathy. *Ann. Intern. Med.* 86:56, 1977.

131. Widestadt, B.-M., Bergentz, S.-E., and Boijsen, E. Catheter angiography and venous thrombosis. *Acta Radiol.* [*Diagn.*] (Stockh.) 17:773, 1976.

132. Williams, A., and Barnett, M. J. Particulate contamination in intravenous fluids, administration sets and cannulae. *Pharmacol. J.* 211:190, 1973.

133. Winding, O. Intrinsic particles in angiographic contrast media. *Radiology* 134:317, 1980.

134. Winding, O., Grønwall, J., Faarup, P., and Hegedüs, V. Sequelae of intrinsic foreign-body contamination during selective renal angiography in rabbits. *Radiology* 134:321, 1980.

135. Yellin, A. E., and Shore, E. H. Surgical management of arterial occlusion following percutaneous femoral angiography. *Surgery* 73:772, 1973.

136. Young, D. B., and Rostorfer, H. H. Renin release responses to acute alterations in renal arterial osmolality. *Am. J. Physiol.* 225:1003, 1973.

137. Yunis, E. J., and Landes, R. R. Hazards of glove powder in renal angiography. *J.A.M.A.* 193:304, 1965.

Anatomic and Physiologic Considerations

ERIK BOIJSEN

Renal angiography gives essential information about the morphology of the renal vasculature, the renal cortex, and any abnormal states in the kidney and its vicinity. It also gives information about renal hemodynamics and vascular physiology. With the development of noninvasive radiologic methods, the indications for renal angiography have diminished markedly. Renal angiography is necessary, however, to determine an adequate approach in vascular disease states of various forms as well as before surgery or interventional radiologic procedures. It is therefore just as important today as it was a few years ago to have detailed knowledge about the renal angiogram in order not to misinterpret the many normal variations as renal pathology.

The renal angiogram is composed of the arterial, nephrographic, and venous phases. When contrast medium is injected into the lumbar aorta or into the renal artery, serial filming is performed in order to cover these phases.

Arterial Phase

An aortic injection should precede selective renal angiography. The many variations in origin, number, and size of the renal arteries are thereby defined. An injection of contrast medium well above the renal arteries also gives information about the difference in flow to the kidneys, which, with modern videodensitometric technique, quickly gives reliable information about the renal blood flow [49, 50, 52, 67]. An aortic injection at the level of the renal arteries or as a semiselective study (Fig. 51-1; see also Chap. 50) as a rule gives the information required for therapeutic considerations. If, however, there is a need for more precise information, selective angiography, with magnification if available, should follow. To perform only selective injection would be more comfortable for the patient, but the many variations in the renal blood supply would cause unpredictable problems and would give false information about the renal vessels and parenchyma [46].

ORIGIN

The renal artery or, if multiple arteries are present, the main renal artery arises from the lumbar aorta at the level of L1 and L2. The right renal artery usually arises somewhat higher than the

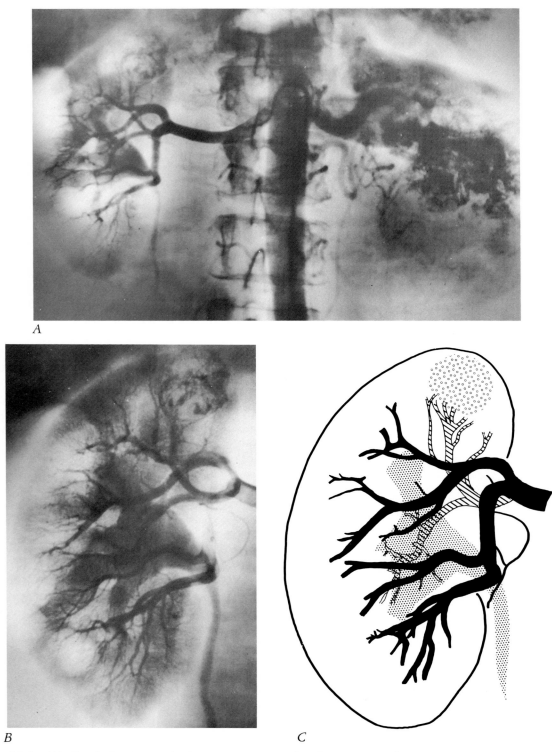

A

B

C

Figure 51-1. (A) Semiselective and (B) 2 × magnification selective right renal angiography in a patient with renal carcinoma on the left and a small metastasis in the right upper renal pole. (C) A typical distribution of the ramifications of the dorsal artery (*hatching*). The dorsal artery supplies the entire superior pole, including the metastasis and the posterior intermediate part. A small middle capsular artery is observed.

left renal artery, and both usually take their origin from the anterolateral part of the aorta [6, 27]. An origin of the renal artery at the level of T11 is extremely rare [22].

COURSE

Because of its rather constant origin, the renal artery has a quite varying course, depending on the site of the kidney. Thus, in ptosis the renal artery has a steep caudolateral course to the renal hilus. In cranial ectopia, the renal artery takes a steep cranial course [56]. Multiple arteries are common; they are discussed in Chapter 55.

CALIBER

The caliber of the single renal artery varies within rather wide limits. In the adult patient, the diameter varies between about 5 mm and 10 mm, as measured on the renal angiogram, with values for the female in the lower part of the range [24, 72]. The diameter or cross-sectional area of the renal artery reflects the function of the renal parenchyma and thus the renal blood flow [44, 45, 55, 71]. Vasoactive substances changing renal blood flow also change the caliber of the renal artery. With an increased blood flow there is dilatation [31, 32, 63], and with decreased blood flow there is a reduced width [1, 61]. The main renal artery has mainly elastic tissue in its wall and may therefore increase in width with increased blood pressure and peripheral resistance [48]. This increase may be observed in malignant hypertension, or the artery may be of normal width despite reduced parenchyma (Fig. 51-2).

As a consequence of aging and arteriosclerosis, various changes occur in the main stem. The width is usually reduced owing to senile involution of the parenchyma, but increased width and tortuosity are often encountered. Increased tortuosity may be regarded as a progression of the changes present in the cortical vessels and arcuate arteries in old age, when the normal tapering disappears. Tortuosity starts in the interlobar arteries [20, 53]. Tortuosity of the extrahilar parts of the renal artery and its branches is in fact more common than usually observed in renal angiography [38]. This is due to the fact that the posterolateral course of the renal artery from the aorta to the renal hilus cannot be fully appreciated in the anteroposterior projection. The normal movements of the kidney from the supine to the erect position require, of course, a certain adaptability of the renal pedicle.

BRANCHES OF THE RENAL ARTERY AND THE SEGMENTAL SUPPLY

The renal artery branches into two, three, or more arteries before it enters the renal hilus. In the normal renal angiogram, the pattern of arborization is smooth and regular (Fig. 51-3). The vessels taper toward the periphery. The branches pass anteriorly and posteriorly to the renal pelvis in the renal sinus. Branches are also observed to the upper pole, the suprarenal gland, and the renal capsule without crossing the renal pelvis. A separate branch to the lower pole is even more common, but this artery crosses the renal pelvis usually on the anterior side. Within the renal sinus, the vessels, whether anterior or posterior, rebranch and give rise to a variable number of interlobar arteries that spread out around the minor calices. Each interlobar artery gives off arcuate arteries, which, in the distal part, run parallel to the renal surface. The arcuate arteries give off the interlobular arteries, which course peripherally in the cortex (Fig. 51-4). They give rise to numerous afferent arterioles to the glomeruli. Selective renal angiography can give information about the renal arterial tree up to this point; the efferent arteriolae and the vasa recta cannot be distinguished.

Many attempts have been made to define a segmental supply of the primary branches of the renal artery by both anatomic dissections and angiography [9, 27, 36–38, 65, 68]. There are various opinions regarding this segmental distribution. In order to understand the ramification and distribution of the renal artery branches, a few facts must be understood. One is that the renal artery branches are end arteries; that is, they have their definite field of supply. Another is that the large variations that exist depend entirely on the macroarchitecture of the kidney. Seven anterior and seven posterior pyramids with the surrounding cortex form seven pairs of lobes [54]. Since the kidney during its fetal stage has to accommodate to surrounding structures, the pyramids undergo fusions and deviations that give the final shape to the kidney. It is therefore the distal branches in the sinus of the kidney, the *interlobar arteries* that run close to the septa of Bertin, that represent the true segmental lobar supply and from which six to eight arcuate arteries arise and enter the kidney tissue at the in-

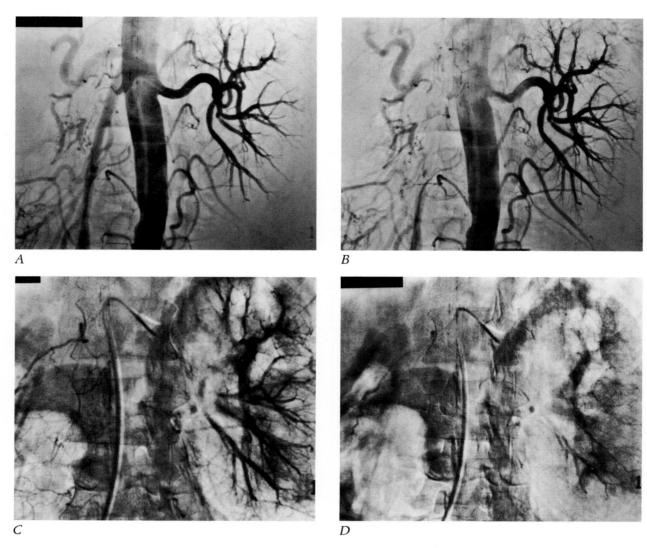

Figure 51-2. Semiselective left renal angiography in a patient with severe malignant hypertension and occlusion of the right renal artery. After the end of the injection of 30 cc of contrast medium, the subtraction films presented were exposed in the following order: (A) 0.1 second, (B) 0.6 second, (C) 3 seconds, and (D) 6.2 seconds. The left renal artery is of normal width despite a marked reduction in renal functioning and an increased resistance to flow. The interlobar and arcuate arteries are still observed 6.2 seconds after the end of the injection. The nephrographic phase is poor, and there is no demarcation of the cortex.

terphase between the cortex and the medulla [42] (Fig. 51-4). Each lobe is supplied by at least two interlobar arteries that can be traced backward to the renal hilus, where they join to form segmental vessels, which thus supply more than one lobe.

In an attempt to systematize the segmental supply of the renal artery, I have suggested that there are four main segments made up of two polar and two intermediate segments [9] (Fig. 51-5). Since each interlobar artery supplies two adjacent lobes, the segmental distribution is not limited to the exact border of the lobes. Nevertheless, it is of practical value to have this segmental orientation in order to understand the variations of the normal anatomy. The intermediate segments are made up of three anterior and three posterior lobes, and the upper and lower polar segments are made up of two pairs of lobes each. The main value of this suggestion is that it can be used to identify a dorsal artery supplying the intermediate posterior segment and a ventral artery going to the corresponding anterior segment. The interlobar arteries are thus

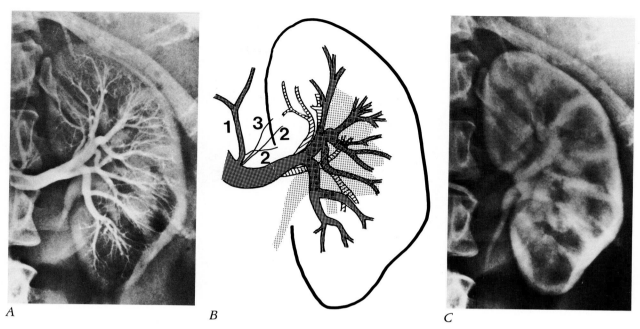

Figure 51-3. Normal selective left renal angiography. (A and B) arterial phase. (C) Late cortical nephrogram and early venous phase. A common trunk for the inferior phrenic (*1*), superior capsular (*2*), and adrenal arteries (*3*) arises early from the renal artery. The dorsal artery (*hatching,* B) arises as the first renal branch and supplies the posterior lobes in the upper and intermediate parts of the kidney. The cortex is thin, and the columns of Bertin are prominent.

Figure 51-4. Diagrammatic presentation of the blood supply of the renal parenchyma. Interlobar arteries (*1*); arcuate arteries (*2*); interlobular arteries (*3*); afferent arteries (*4*); peritubular plexus (*5*); arteriolae rectae (*6, 7*); perforating arteries (*8*); and spiral arteries (*9*). (Adapted from Davidson [18], Hodson [42], and Meiisel and Apitzsch [58]. Reproduced by permission from Saunders, University of California Press, and Springer-Verlag, respectively.)

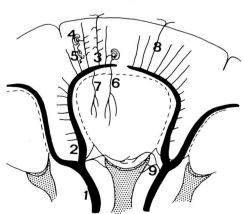

Figure 51-5. The four renal segments as they are projected on the renal surface according to Boijsen [9]. (Reproduced by permission from *Acta Radiol.*)

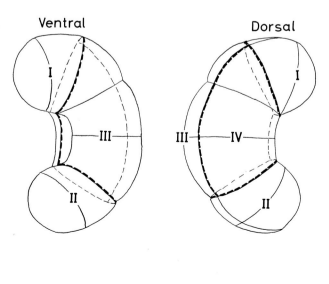

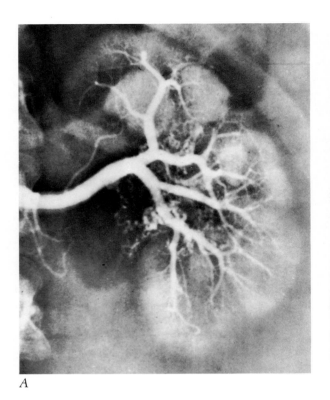

A

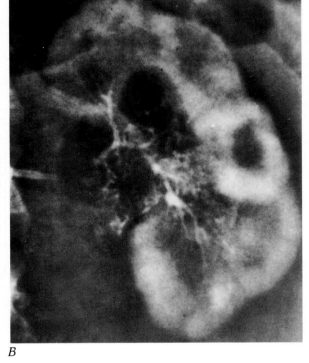

B

Figure 51-6. Dorsal renal artery ligated at pyelolithotomy. (A) At selective renal angiography, only ventral artery branches are filled in addition to numerous wide pelvic arteries that serve as collateral vessels to the dorsal artery. In the renal sinus, the ventral branches do not cross each other. (B) In the nephrographic phase, the distribution of the dorsal artery branches is well observed. Note the lobulation, mainly the result of the reduced volume of the dorsal parenchyma.

subsegmental arteries. Because of the position of the kidney in the body, the ventral artery in the anteroposterior projection always supplies the lateral border, and the dorsal artery always supplies the medial border of the intermediate part of the kidney (see Figs. 51-1, 51-3). From there on, the vessels can be traced back to their origin from the renal artery, where certain characteristics appear. One characteristic is that the branches of the ventral artery do not, as a rule, cross each other; nor do the branches of the dorsal artery in the renal sinus. Another characteristic is that the dorsal artery is usually smaller in caliber and appears as a branch of the renal artery, while the ventral artery appears more as a direct continuation of the renal artery. Furthermore, the dorsal artery appears as the first branch of the renal artery in some 50 percent of kidneys. These are simple observations, but they are easily overlooked in, for example, a kidney whose dorsal artery has been ligated [3, 41] (Fig. 51-6). Because of the ligation, the dorsal lobes are reduced

in size, and the ventral lobes are hyperplastic. The kidney may still be of normal size.

The variations of the supply of the upper and lower poles are many (Figs. 51-7, 51-8). There may be only two branches, one dorsal artery supplying the posterior lobes and one ventral artery supplying the anterior lobes; but this phenomenon occurs only in some 15 percent of kidneys. Most often, the ventral artery supplies the entire lower pole as well as the anterior intermediate part, a phenomenon that occurs in some 60 percent of kidneys. The dorsal artery supplies the entire upper pole and the posterior intermediate segment in about 20 percent of kidneys, but it rarely supplies the anterior part of the lower pole.

COURSE IN THE RENAL SINUS

The dorsal and ventral arteries are very close when they enter the upper part of the renal hilus. They often appear to squeeze the ramus of the

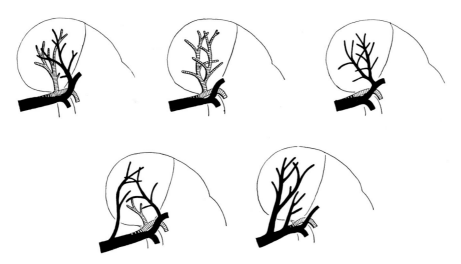

Figure 51-7. The left upper renal pole showing common variations of arterial supply. (From Boijsen [9]. Reproduced by permission from *Acta Radiol.*)

Figure 51-8. Left lower pole showing common variations in origin, course, and field of supply of the lower polar artery. (From Boijsen [9]. Reproduced by permission from *Acta Radiol.*)

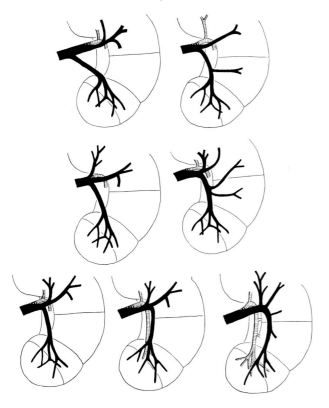

renal pelvis to the upper pole (Fig. 51-9). At this point, a vascular impression is often observed in the renal pelvis [8, 9, 29, 33, 34, 47, 66]. A combination of dilatation and papillary destruction of the upper pole and a vascular impression of the upper ramus has been falsely regarded as an obstruction to flow that causes pain [29, 30]. Surgery has been performed on the crossing artery because of this combination. Vascular impressions causing obstruction to flow from the upper pole probably can occur only when a large aneurysm is present or when a mass displaces the artery [12]. Aneurysms usually cause deformation of the upper part of the renal pelvis, which may cause differential diagnostic problems [25].

The dorsal artery usually follows the posterior border of the renal hilus in a caudal direction (Fig. 51-10) [9, 43]. This point is of importance in renal surgery because access to the renal pelvis is often from the posterior aspect of the kidney, and so the artery may be severed [3, 4, 41] (see Fig. 51-6). In hydronephrosis or in space-occupying lesions of the renal sinus, the displacement can rarely be appreciated in an anteroposterior view, whereas in a true lateral view of the kidney, vascular displacement is obvious (Fig. 51-11).

ARCUATE AND CORTICAL ARTERIES

In most angiograms, the arcuate arteries are the last branches of the renal artery that can be observed. In high-quality angiograms (particularly

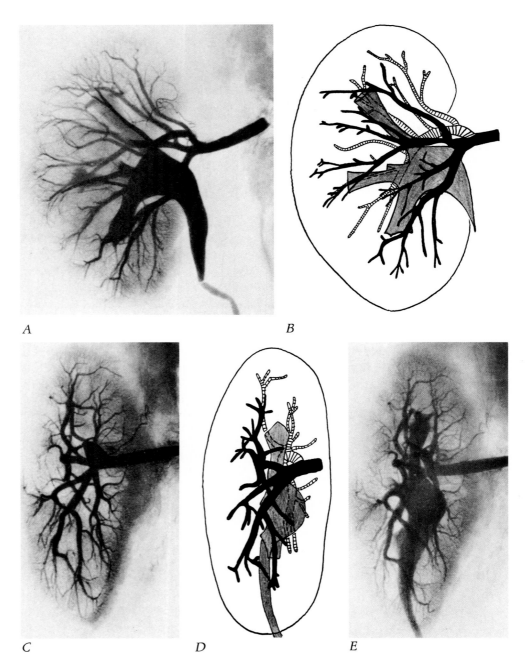

A

B

C

D

E

Figure 51-9. Autopsy specimen, right kidney. (A and B) True "frontal" projection. (C–E) True "lateral" projection of the kidney. Observe how close the ventral and dorsal arteries are to each other and to the renal pelvis in the renal sinus. The upper ramus is squeezed between the two vessels.

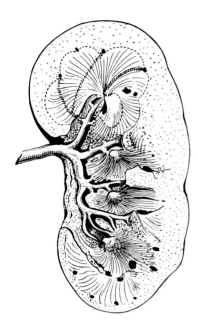

Figure 51-10. Course and ramification of the dorsal artery in the sinus according to Hou-Jensen [43]. (Reproduced by permission from *Z. Anat. Entwickl.*)

magnification angiograms), however, the summation effect of the interlobular arteries as well as the glomerular tufts is observed (Fig. 51-12; see also Fig. 51-1). The distance between the arcuate arteries running parallel to the renal surface and their closest distance to this surface give information about the amount of renal cortex present. (The interlobular arteries and the glomeruli are considered in the discussion of the nephrographic phase.)

CAPSULAR AND PELVIC ARTERIES

In the arterial phase, adrenal capsular and renal pelvic arteries are also observed (Fig. 51-13). The renal capsular artery system is composed of three basic pathways: superior, medial, and inferior capsular arteries. They very rarely all take their origin from the single renal artery. They are easy to define because the rate of flow through these arteries is slower than that through the renal

parenchymal arteries and because contrast material is more persistent in them during the nephrographic phase.

The superior capsular artery (see Fig. 51-3), which is observed in about one-third of all selective renal arteriograms, usually arises together with the inferior adrenal artery from the first part of the single renal artery and it follows a characteristic tortuous path over the superior pole of the kidney. It may arise together with all the adrenal arteries and the inferior phrenic artery as a common trunk from the first part of the renal artery, from the angle between the aorta and the renal artery, from a supplementary upper polar artery, or directly from the aorta.

The middle capsular arteries arise from the renal artery or its main branches, usually in the renal hilus. In order to reach the anterior and posterior aspects of the kidney, the middle capsular arteries pass medially before they spread in the perirenal fat (Fig. 51-14; see also Fig. 51-1).

The inferior capsular artery is rarely observed at selective renal angiography because it usually takes its origin from the gonadal artery or from an inferior polar artery arising from the aorta.

Perforating capsular arteries also exist. They arise from arcuate and interlobular arteries [9, 26] (Fig. 51-14). They may be important collateral pathways in occlusive disease. These arteries are most often observed in advanced nephropathy.

The pelvic arteries arise as tiny twigs from the branches of the renal artery in the renal sinus and form a network on the renal pelvis and calices [23]. They are too small to be seen at angiography, mainly because the accumulation of contrast medium in the nephrographic phase "hides" these very small vessels. In occlusive disease, they may enlarge markedly and then have a characteristic tortuous appearance (see Fig. 51-6). The ureteric or pelviureteric artery is usually observed as a very small artery running medially and caudally from one of the main branches of the renal artery (Fig. 51-14).

The importance of the perirenal and pelvic arterial supply of the kidney has been well demonstrated in anatomical dissection studies and in various disease entities [2, 10, 11, 26, 59, 60, 73].

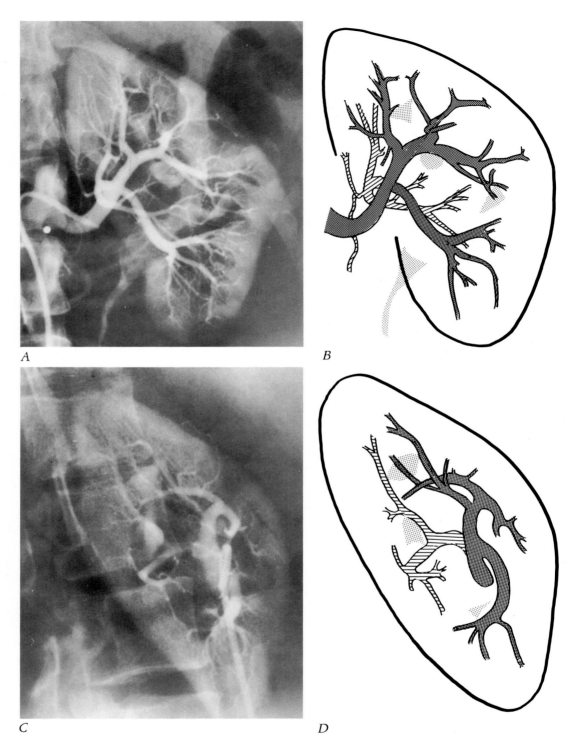

Figure 51-11. Abscess of the renal sinus that compresses the renal pelvis. (A and B) In the anteroposterior projection, displacement of the sinus branches can hardly be discerned. (C and D) In a true lateral view of the kidney, the segmental and interlobar branches are at a great distance from each other, and they are arch shaped owing to the expansive lesion in the sinus.

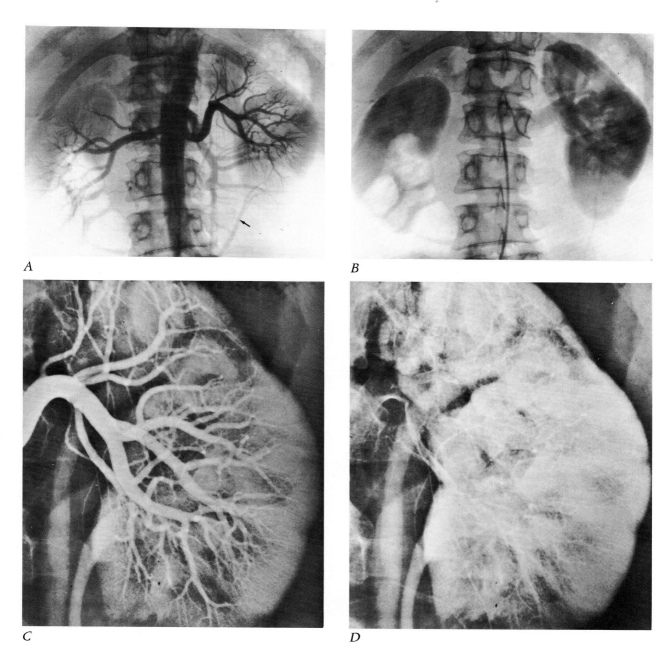

A

B

C

D

Figure 51-12. Double renal pelvis with hydrone-phrosis and parenchymal reduction of the left upper pole. (A and B) Semiselective renal angiography in the arterial and venous phases. Note the reduced width of the segmental branches to the upper pole, the lower polar artery from the common iliac artery on the left (*arrow*, A), and the early origin of a superior segmental polar artery on the right. (C and D) 3× magnification,

0.1-mm focal spot. Arterial and cortical glomerular nephrographic phases. The summation effect of the interlobular arteries and the glomerular tufts is well observed in the normal intermediate and lower parts. Slight cortical indentations are noted on the lateral surface, and there is marked reduction of the cortex in the upper pole. Pelvic and capsular arteries are seen.

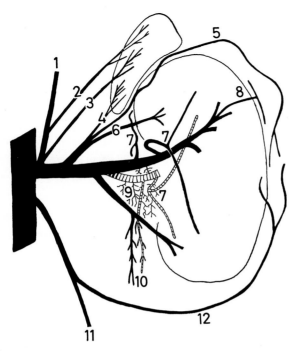

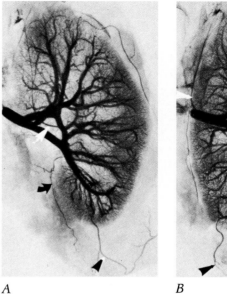

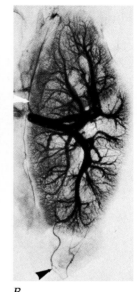

A   *B*

Figure 51-13. Diagram showing adrenal capsular and pelvic arteries that are frequently observed in the renal angiogram. Inferior phrenic artery (*1*); arteries to the adrenal gland (*2–4*); superior capsular artery (*5*); sublobular branch to the upper pole arising from the superior capsular–inferior adrenal artery (*6*); middle capsular arteries (*7*); perforating artery (*8*); pelvic and ureteric arteries (*9–10*); spermatic and inferior capsular arteries (*11–12*). (From Boijsen [9]. Reproduced by permission from *Acta Radiol.*)

Figure 51-14. Autopsy specimen. A view corresponding to in vivo (A) frontal and (B) true lateral views of the kidney. The middle capsular arteries (*white arrowheads*) arise from the dorsal artery and supply the fatty capsule posterior to the kidney. A wide perforating artery (*black arrowheads*) arises from an arcuate artery in the lower pole. The ureteric artery (*arrow*) branches from the lower polar artery. (From Boijsen [9]. Reproduced by permission from *Acta Radiol.*)

Nephrographic Phase

Four different stages of the nephrographic phase can be distinguished: the cortical arteriogram, the glomerulogram, the cortical nephrogram, and the general nephrogram.

The accumulation of contrast medium in the renal cortex appears simultaneously with the filling of the interlobular arteries. The *cortical arteriogram* (i.e., the point at which the contrast medium is observed in the interlobular arteries) lasts for less than 0.5 second because the vessels are quickly obscured by the increasing density of the cortex. The normal disappearance time of contrast medium from the renal arterial tree is approximately 1 second (0.5–2 seconds) after the end of the injection in selective renal angiography. Often the interlobular arteries cannot be seen in high-quality renal angiograms because the timing of the exposures is not correctly related to the short period they are visible. The interlobular

arteries arise at right angles from the arcuate arteries at approximately 3-mm intervals [17]. They run parallel and straight toward the renal surface. What is really seen in the cortical arteriogram is probably a composite of groups of interlobular arteries because of overlapping [1, 14].

With 3× magnification and with a fine focus of less than 0.2 mm the interlobular arteries and glomeruli more than 100 μm in diameter can be observed (see Figs. 51-1, 51-12). What is seen are not single glomeruli but a composite of glomerular tufts [14]. Thus with the magnification technique, in the early nephrographic phase a peppery appearance that depends on the filling of the glomeruli with contrast medium can be seen [70].

The *glomerulogram* lasts for about 1 to 2 seconds. The glomerulus acts as an aneurysm and stores the contrast medium temporarily because the diameters of the afferent and efferent arteriolae are one-third to one-fifth of the diameter of the glomerulus [17]. Because of overlapping, they seem to vary in size, being largest (2–3 mm) in the renal hilus and subcortically. By counting the glomeruli in certain areas, it seems possible to obtain highly accurate information about glomerular function. The glomerulogram represents only that part of the glomerular population that is most promptly perfused and that probably represents the fast component of the ^{133}Xe clearance curve [17].

After 1 to 2 seconds, the background density increases to such an extent that the glomeruli can no longer be seen. The *cortical nephrogram* becomes more homogeneous because the tubular filtrate, the cortical capillaries, and the peritubular spaces also become opacified. In normal kidneys, during the cortical nephrogram the cortex is well distinguished from the medulla and the renal surface is also well defined. The renal surface appears smooth, but shallow indentations between each lobe may be identified. Somewhat deeper fissures are often noted between the intermediate part and the superior and inferior poles. Fetal lobulation, represented by deep fissures between the lobes, is rarely observed [16, 68]. If marked lobulation is present, it is more often due to abnormal situations, such as central scarring or hyperplasia (see Fig. 51-6). This type of cortical fissure should be distinguished from the irregularities caused by cortical destruction.

The cortical width and the total cortical volume can be estimated and can be used to obtain accurate information about the amount of functioning parenchyma [39, 40]. The columns of Bertin are usually well outlined, giving good information about the position of the various lobes (see Fig. 51-3) [9]. The cortex is somewhat thicker in the poles (where it is about 10 mm) than in the intermediate parts (where it is 7–8 mm) [39].

The density of the cortical nephrogram depends on the amount and the rate of injection of contrast medium given and the functional capacity of the kidney. The high density of the cortical nephrogram lasts for about 4 seconds. It is followed by a *general nephrogram*, during which the density of the cortex steadily decreases over a period of 10 to 15 seconds. The border between the cortex and medulla then gradually disappears. During this period, the contrast medium is washed out of the cortical vessels and extracellular spaces, and it appears in the lumina of the pyramids and their vascular compartments. The slow disappearance rate has been said to be due partly to the relatively large amount of contrast medium in the tubular cells that is washed out to the peritubular capillaries and partly to the stagnation of the filtered contrast medium in the lumina of the nephrons [13]. It is more probable that the contrast medium is retrieved from the extracellular space. After about 20 seconds, a steady state of the nephrographic phase is observed for about 2 minutes, which is due to recirculation and to the slow transport through the lumina of the nephrons.

Venous Phase

Even if small intrarenal veins can sometimes be observed at magnification angiography [17], they usually cannot be distinguished in an angiogram performed with routine technique. The reason for this is that the high extraction of contrast medium from the blood results in a rather poor concentration of the medium in the veins. Furthermore, the dense cortical nephrogram prevents demonstration of the veins. Therefore the larger collecting veins in the renal sinus are also poorly demonstrated (see Figs. 51-3, 51-12).

The normal appearance time of the renal veins is approximately 3.5 seconds (1.75–5 seconds) after the onset of injection in the renal artery, with the peak density at 8 seconds (6–10 seconds). Contrast medium is retained in the veins for about 20 seconds [1]. The retardation of the contrast medium in the renal vein is in accordance with the slow disappearance of contrast medium from the cortex.

The normal anatomy of the intrarenal and extrarenal parts of the renal vein can usually not be defined with accuracy. With high doses of contrast medium, the extrarenal part may be reasonably well defined, but this technique can be accepted only in situations in which nephrectomy is planned. In selected cases, renal phlebography is a far better method for defining the anatomy.

Physiologic Considerations

Injection of contrast medium into the renal artery is an unphysiologic technique that is bound to cause changes in the renal blood flow [5, 15, 69]. The high viscosity and osmolality, the changes in the blood corpuscles, and the sudden increase in pressure at the injection are all factors of importance to remember when evaluating renal morphology and function by angiography. Nevertheless, an aortic or a selective injection of contrast medium gives information about renal function that cannot be obtained by other methods. Several of these parameters were mentioned before; they are briefly recapitulated:

1. The *size* of the renal artery and its branches is a crude but nevertheless good indication of renal function. It should be remembered, however, that in acute or subacute renal failure, the renal artery is of normal width. Also, in hypertension or atherosclerosis the renal artery may be of normal size despite the reduction in cortical flow.
2. The intrarenal arterial pattern shows so many variations that reliable information can be obtained only when local changes are present. General age-related changes are particularly difficult to evaluate.
3. A reflux of contrast medium to the aorta during selective injection at the rate of 8 to 10 cc per second usually indicates an increased resistance to flow. Use of a spillover flow meter combined with cinefluorography can give semiquantitative information [62].
4. The transit time of contrast medium through the renal arterial tree is another parameter that can be used to give certain information about the blood flow. In particular, local changes in blood flow may be appreciated, but these cannot be quantified.
5. The degree of accumulation of contrast medium in the cortical nephrogram and the cortical width is a crude but nevertheless practical and often-used method of quickly evaluating renal function. The cortical volume can be estimated [39, 40].
6. The number of glomeruli in a defined area can be counted to give quantitative information about renal functioning [17].
7. The appearance time of contrast in the renal vein and the width of the vein give less important information about renal function.

Counting the number of glomeruli, using the spillover technique and estimating the cortical volume can give some quantitative information about renal blood flow and functioning parenchyma, but on the whole, with this method, the renal arteriogram gives limited information. Since the arterial tree of the kidney responds in a rather limited manner to a variety of diseases, the renal arteriogram is not informative enough about early changes in the renal parenchyma. Age-related changes also have to be included in the evaluation, which makes a diagnosis of parenchymal disease even more difficult. One cannot predict, therefore, the state of the arteriolar bed based on angiographic data alone [19, 33]. During selective catheterization of the renal artery, quantitative information can be obtained by the dye dilution technique [35, 51] or with the radioactive gas washout technique [7]. Methods based on the linear velocity of the flow have been developed using either cinedensitometry or videodensitometry [21, 64, 67]. Another method is the videodensitometric measurement of iodine in the cortex [21, 28]. More recently, simpler techniques have been developed; one is the determination of the relative blood flow with a videodilution technique in which the renal blood flow is measured as a fraction of the cardiac output [50, 52]. The most recent method does not require renal catheterization [57]: An intravenous bolus injection gives enough opacification of the renal vasculature for computed videodensitometric measurement of blood flow to the organ, a method that holds great promise for the future.

References

1. Abrams, H. L. The kidney: Quantitative derivatives of renal radiologic studies: An overview. *Invest. Radiol.* 7:240, 1972.
2. Abrams, H. L., and Cornell, S. H. Patterns of collateral flow in renal ischemia. *Radiology* 84:1001, 1965.
3. Andersson, I. Renal artery lesions after pyelolithotomy. A potential cause of renovascular hypertension. *Acta Radiol.* [*Diagn.*] (Stockh.) 17:685, 1976.
4. Andersson, I., Boijsen, E., Hellsten, S., and Linell, F. Lesions of the dorsal renal artery in surgery for renal pelvic calculus. *Eur. Urol.* 5:343, 1979.
5. Aperia, A., Broberger, O., and Ekengren, K. Renal hemodynamics during selective renal angiography. *Invest. Radiol.* 3:389, 1968.
6. Aubertin, J., and Koumare, K. Variations of origin of the renal artery. *Eur. Urol.* 1:189, 1975.
7. Barger, A. C., and Herd, J. A. Physiology in medicine: The renal circulation. *N. Engl. J. Med.* 284:482, 1971.
8. Baum, S., and Gillenswater, J. Y. Renal artery impression on the renal pelvis. *J. Urol.* 95:139, 1966.
9. Boijsen, E. Angiographic studies of the anatomy of single and multiple renal arteries. *Acta Radiol.* [*Suppl.*] (Stockh.) 183:1959.

10. Boijsen, E., and Folin, J. Angiography in the diagnosis of renal carcinoma. *Radiologe* 1:173, 1961.
11. Boijsen, E., and Folin, J. Angiography in carcinoma of the renal pelvis. *Acta Radiol.* 56:81, 1961.
12. Boijsen, E., and Link, D. P. Arteriography before needle puncture of renal hilar lesions. *J. Urol.* 118:237, 1977.
13. Bolin, H. Contrast medium in kidney during angiography: A densitometric method for estimation of renal function. *Acta Radiol. [Suppl.]* (Stockh.) 257:1966.
14. Bookstein, J. J., Davidson, A. J., Hills, G. S., Hollenberg, N., and Sherwood, T. The Small Renal Vessels. In S. K. Hilal (ed.), *Small Vessel Angiography*. St. Louis: Mosby, 1973.
15. Caldicott, W. J. H., Hollenberg, N. K., and Abrams, H. L. Characteristics of response of renal vascular bed to contrast media. Criteria for vasoconstriction induced by renin-angiotensin system. *Invest. Radiol.* 5:539, 1970.
16. Cooperman, L. H., and Lowman, R. M. Fetal lobulation of the kidneys. *AJR* 92:273, 1964.
17. Cope, C., Raja, R. M., and Isard, H. J. Correlation of glomerulography and renal function in hypertension. *Radiology* 110:15, 1974.
18. Davidson, A. J. *Radiologic Diagnosis of Renal Parenchymal Disease*. Philadelphia: Saunders, 1977.
19. Davidson, A. J., and Talner, L. B. Lack of specificity of renal angiography in the diagnosis of renal parenchymal disease: A point of view. *Invest. Radiol.* 8:90, 1973.
20. Davidson, A. J., Talner, L. B., and Downs, W. M., III. A study of the angiographic appearance of the kidney in an aging normotensive population. *Radiology* 92:975, 1969.
21. Deininger, H. K., Heuck, F., and Vanselow, K. The determination of the circulation in normal human kidneys by means of angiocinedensitometry. *Ann. Radiol.* 21:365, 1978.
22. Doppman, J. An ectopic renal artery. *Br. J. Radiol.* 40:312, 1967.
23. Douville, E., and Hollinshead, W. H. The blood supply of the normal renal pelvis. *J. Urol.* 73:906, 1955.
24. Edsman, G. Angionephrography and suprarenal angiography. *Acta Radiol. [Suppl.]* (Stockh.) 155:1957.
25. Ekelund, L., Boijsen, E., and Lindstedt, E. Pseudotumor of the renal pelvis caused by renal artery aneurysm. *Acta Radiol. [Diagn.]* (Stockh.) 20:753, 1979.
26. Eliska, O. The perforating arteries and their role in the collateral circulation of the kidneys. *Acta Anat.* 70:184, 1968.
27. Engelbrecht, H. E., Keen, E. N., Fine, H., et al. The radiological anatomy of the parenchymal distribution of the renal artery. *S. Afr. Med. J.* 43:826, 1969.
28. Eriksson, U., Lörelius, L. E., and Ruhn, G. Determination of the renal blood flow by videodensitometry. *Ann. Radiol.* 21:363, 1978.
29. Fraley, E. E. Dismembered infundibulopyelostomy: Improved technique for correcting vascular obstruction of the superior infundibulum. *J. Urol.* 101:144, 1969.
30. Fraley, E. E. Vascular obstruction of superior infundibulum causing nephralgia. A new syndrome. *N. Engl. J. Med.* 275:1403, 1966.
31. Freed, T. A., Hager, H., and Vinik, M. Effects of intra-arterial acetylcholine on renal arteriography in normal humans. *AJR* 104:312, 1968.
32. Freed, T. A., and Vinik, M. Effects of acetylcholine on renal arteriography: Preliminary observations. *Invest. Radiol.* 3:81, 1968.
33. Gill, W. M., Jr., and Pudvan, W. R. Arteriographic diagnosis of renal parenchymal disease. *Radiology* 96:81, 1970.
34. Gold, J. M., and Bucy, J. G. Fraley's syndrome with bilateral infundibular obstruction. *J. Urol.* 112:299, 1974.
35. Göthlin, J., and Olin, T. Dye dilution technique with nephroangiography for the determination of renal blood flow and related parameters. *Acta Radiol. [Diagn.]* (Stockh.) 14:113, 1973.
36. Graves, F. T. The anatomy of the intrarenal arteries and its application to segmental resection of the kidney. *Br. J. Surg.* 42:132, 1954.
37. Graves, F. T. The anatomy of the intrarenal arteries in health and disease. *Br. J. Surg.* 43:605, 1956.
38. Hegedüs, V. Arterial anatomy of the kidney. A three-dimensional angiographic investigation. *Acta Radiol. [Diagn.]* (Stockh.) 12:604, 1972.
39. Hegedüs, V., and Faarup, P. Cortical volume of the normal human kidney. Correlated angiographic and morphologic investigations. *Acta Radiol. [Diagn.]* (Stockh.) 12:481, 1972.
40. Hegedüs, V., and Ravnskov, U. Cortical volume in apparently normal kidneys. *Scand. J. Urol. Nephrol.* 6:159, 1972.
41. Hellström, J. Über die Varianten der Nierengefässe. *Z. Urol. Chir.* 29:253, 1928.
42. Hodson, C. J. The Logic of the Blood Supply to the Kidney. In A. R. Margulis and C. A. Gooding (eds.), *Diagnostic Radiology*. San Francisco: University of California Press, 1978.
43. Hou-Jensen, H. Die Verästelung der Arteria renalis in der Niere des Menschen. *Z. Anat. Entwickl.* 91:1, 1930.
44. Idbohrn, H. Renal angiography in experimental hydronephrosis. *Acta Radiol. [Suppl.]* (Stockh.) 136:1956.
45. Kittredge, R. D., Hemley, S. D., Kanick, V., and Finby, N. The atrophic renal artery. *AJR* 92:309, 1964.

46. Köhler, R.   Incomplete angiogram in selective renal angiography. *Acta Radiol. [Diagn.]* (Stockh.) 1:1011, 1963.

47. Kreel, L., and Pyle, R.   Arterial impression on renal pelvis. *Br. J. Radiol.* 35:609, 1962.

48. Kupic, E. A., Gibbons, P. D., and Leavitt, T.   Angiographic studies of the canine kidney following intravenous injection of methedrine: A preliminary report. *Invest. Radiol.* 9:404, 1974.

49. Lantz, B.   Relative flow measured by roentgen videodensitometry in hydrodynamic model. *Acta Radiol. [Diagn.]* (Stockh.) 16:503, 1975.

50. Lantz, B. M. T., Foerster, J. M., Link, D. P., and Holcroft, J. W.   Determination of relative blood flow in single arteries: New video-dilution technique. *AJR* 134:1161, 1980.

51. Lingårdh, G., Muth, T., and Olin, T.   Renal blood flow in dogs studied by means of a dye-dilution technique. *Scand. J. Urol. Nephrol.* 3:281, 1969.

52. Link, D. P., Lantz, B. M. T., Foerster, J. M., Holcroft, J. W., and Reid, M. H.   New videodensitometric method for measuring renal artery blood flow at routine angiography: Validation in the canine model. *Invest. Radiol.* 14:465, 1979.

53. Ljungqvist, A.   The intrarenal arterial pattern in the normal and diseased human kidney. *Acta Med. Scand.* 174:1, 1963.

54. Löfgren, F.   Das topographische System der malpigischen Pyramiden der Menschenniere. University of Lund (Malmö) Thesis, 1949.

55. Ludin, H., Elde, M., Fehr, H., and Thoelen, H.   Correlation of renal size, renal artery calibre, and effective renal plasma flow in man. *Acta Radiol. [Diagn.]* (Stockh.) 6:296, 1967.

56. Lundius, B.   Intrathoracic kidney. *AJR* 125:678, 1975.

57. Meaney, T.   Digital angiography. Read at the Simposio Internazionale sulla Tomografia Computerizzata del Corpo. Rome, May 19–23, 1980.

58. Meiisel, P., and Apitzsch, D. E.   *Atlas der Nierenangiographie.* Berlin/Heidelberg/New York: Springer-Verlag, 1978.

59. Merklin, R. J., and Michels, N. A.   The variant renal and suprarenal blood supply with data on the inferior phrenic, ureteral, and gonadal arteries. *J. Int. Coll. Surg.* 29:41, 1958.

60. Meyers, M. A., Freidenberg, R. M., King, M. C., and Meng, C. H.   The significance of the renal capsular arteries. *Br. J. Radiol.* 40:949, 1967.

61. Newhouse, J. H., and Hollenberg, N. K.   Vascular characteristics of unilateral acute renal failure in the dog. Assessment with vasodilators and antagonists to angiotensin and norepinephrine. *Invest. Radiol.* 9:241, 1974.

62. Olin, T., and Redman, H. C.   Spillover flowmeter: A preliminary approach. *Acta Radiol. [Diagn.]* (Stockh.) 4:217, 1966.

63. Ozer, H., and Hollenberg, N. K.   Renal angiographic and hemodynamic responses to vasodilators. A comparison of five agents in the dog. *Invest. Radiol.* 9:473, 1974.

64. Pinet, A., Guey, A., and Lyonnet, D.   Mesure du débit de l'artère rénale par videodensitométrie. *Ann. Radiol.* 21:359, 1978.

65. Poisel, S., and Spängler, H.P.   Die Verästelungstypen der Arteria renalis in Hinblick auf die arterielle Blutversorgung des Parenchyms der Niere. Ein Beitrag zum Problem der sogennanten Nierensegmente. *Acta Anat.* 76:516, 1970.

66. Rusiewicz, E., and Reilly, B. J.   The significance of isolated upper pole calyceal dilatation. *J. Can. Assoc. Radiol.* 19:179, 1968.

67. Silverman, N. R.   Television fluorodensitometry: Technical consideration and some clinical application. *Invest. Radiol.* 5:35, 1970.

68. Sykes, D.   The correlation between renal vascularization and lobulation of the kidney. *Br. J. Urol.* 36:549, 1964.

69. Tadavarthy, S. M., Castaneda, W., and Amplatz, K.   Redistribution of renal blood flow caused by contrast media. *Radiology* 122:343, 1977.

70. Takaro, T.   Clinical renal glomerulography. *Radiology* 90:1203, 1968.

71. Widén, T.   Renal angiography during and after unilateral ureteric occlusion. *Acta Radiol. [Suppl.]* (Stockh.) 162:1958.

72. Wójtowicz, J.   Relationship of the surface parameters of the kidney to the size of the renal artery. *Invest. Radiol.* 2:231, 1967.

73. Yune, H. Y., and Klatte, E. C.   Collateral circulation to an ischemic kidney. *Radiology* 119:539, 1976.

Renal Tumor Versus Renal Cyst

HERBERT L. ABRAMS

The precise diagnosis of carcinoma of the kidney is of particular importance because renal mass lesions are frequently encountered that require nephrectomy if malignant and renal tissue conservation if benign. Although ultimate certainty is achievable only after a piece of tissue has been examined, imaging approaches to the kidney are so well developed that a high accuracy of diagnosis is now possible in most cases. Because multiple methods of radiologic investigation are available, it is essential that the contribution of each method be carefully defined. Intravenous urography, ultrasonography, computed tomography, radionuclide renography, angiography, renal venography, cyst puncture, and cyst biopsy are all relatively accurate methods of studying the kidney, and each makes its particular contribution. A carefully designed decision tree is required, one that takes into account the strengths and weaknesses of each method and the degree of certainty that is required before critical management decisions can be made.

This chapter, therefore, while emphasizing the application of angiography to the evaluation of the nature of renal mass lesions, also indicates the relative contributions of the other imaging methods.

Tumors

Tumors of the kidney account for about 1 percent of cancer deaths [47]. A number of intriguing features sometimes render diagnosis complex and therapy unexpectedly rewarding. Renal cell carcinoma may be characterized by such nonurologic symptoms and signs as polycythemia, fever, weight loss, hypertension, and hypercalcemia suggesting hyperparathyroidism. It is also one of the few tumors in which regression of the metastases has apparently been documented following removal of the primary carcinoma [35, 40].

Renal tumors are variously characterized as primary or secondary; benign or malignant; epithelial or nonepithelial; parenchymal, pelvic, or capsular; and mature or immature. While each of these classifications is useful, the relatively simple classification of Table 52-1 has the merit of placing the most important tumors in sharp focus. Wilms' tumor, renal cell carcinoma, and transitional cell carcinoma are the tumors of greatest clinical significance. Renal cell carcinoma

Table 52-1. Classification of Renal Tumors

Primary Tumors		Metastatic Tumors
Benign	Malignant	
Epithelial	Epithelial	Epithelial
Adenoma	Renal cell carcinoma (parenchymal)	Especially from lung and breast
Nonepithelial	Transitional or squamous cell carcinoma	carcinoma, but also from other primary
Fibroma	(pelvic)	carcinomas
Leiomyoma	Nonepithelial	Nonepithelial
Neurogenic tumor	Wilms' tumor	Lymphoma
Angioma	Sarcoma of different cell types	Melanoma
Hamartoma		Sarcoma

constitutes approximately 80 to 83 percent, transitional cell, 7 to 10 percent, Wilms' tumor, 5 to 6 percent, and miscellaneous tumors, 3 to 4 percent of clinically recognizable renal neoplasms [67, 83]. It is relatively uncommon that any other type of tumor is a clinically significant or life-threatening problem. On the other hand, in autopsy material, benign renal tumors of both epithelial and mesenchymal origin are found far more commonly than malignant tumors [28].

WILMS' TUMOR

Wilms' tumor (nephroblastoma, adenomyosarcoma) is derived from embryonal renal tissue and is a mixture of connective, epithelial, and muscular elements. It is by far the commonest renal tumor of infants and children; two-thirds of the cases of Wilms' tumor are observed before the age of 3, and three-fourths before the age of 5 (see also Chap. 75). This explains the unusual double-peak incidence of malignant renal tumors—in the first and the sixth decades of life. The tumor occurs twice as often in males as in females.

Pathology

These bulky tumors are the largest tumors of children, and they are characterized by rapid growth, early metastasis, and direct extension to neighboring organs. Metastases are found most commonly in the lung, but they also occur in the liver, bone, lymph nodes, and central nervous system (Table 52-2). Both kidneys are involved in 2 to 8 percent of cases, either with double primary tumors or by metastasis. By the time of clinical recognition, at least 20 percent of patients have metastases.

The tumors are usually solid in consistency, opaquely white on cut section, and lobular (Fig. 52-1). The larger tumors may have areas of necrosis, hemorrhage, and cyst formation. Histologically, the dominant cells are primitive spindle cells and round cells (resembling a sarcoma containing epithelial tubules), smooth and striated muscle cells, connective tissue, and sometimes cartilage and osseous tissue. Although the spindle-shaped cells resemble fibroblasts on light microscopy, their ultrastructure is such that some of them appear to be undifferentiated epithelial cells, such as those seen in the developing metanephros [95].

Symptoms and Signs

The commonest manifestation of Wilms' tumor that brings the patient to the physician's attention is *abdominal swelling or distention*, frequently observed by the mother or by the pediatrician on routine physical examination (Table 52-3). About one-half of cases are discovered in this way, but 90 percent of patients have a palpable mass on physical examination [93]. *Pain* is a less common presenting symptom in children; it probably depends on the mechanical effect of the tumor mass, stretching of the renal capsule, or bleeding into the tumor. *Fever and hematuria* may also sig-

Table 52-2. Extrarenal Metastases in 59 Patients with Wilms' Tumor

Site of Metastases	Number of Patients	Percentage of Patients
Lung	28	47
Liver	8	14
Bone	7	12
Spinal cord	1	2
Retroperitoneum	1	2

Adapted from Clark et al. [22] and Westra et al. [101].

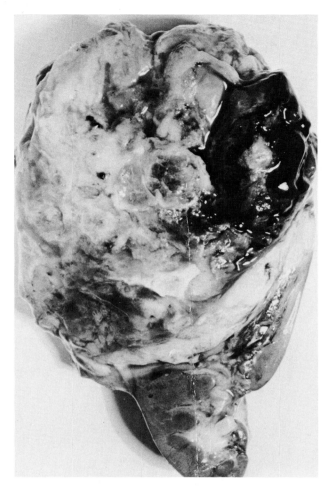

Figure 52-1. Gross pathologic appearance of Wilms' tumor. Most tumors are lobular and opaquely white on cut section. They may have areas of necrosis, hemorrhage, and cyst formation. Note that the tumor has virtually replaced the kidney in this case.

Table 52-3. Incidence of Symptoms and Signs in Wilms' Tumor

Symptom or Sign	Percentage of Patients Showing Symptom or Sign
Palpable mass	90
Hypertension	60
Abdominal pain	20
Anorexia, nausea, vomiting	16
Fever	10
Gross hematuria	6

Adapted from Snyder et al. [93].

nal the presence of the tumor. *Hypertension* has been noted rather commonly, perhaps on the basis of local ischemia caused by the renal mass.

On physical examination, the mass is commonly felt, enabling a presumptive diagnosis. Ascites and swelling of the limbs may be observed if the tumor is large enough to compress or invade the inferior vena cava. The child may seem somewhat ill and look emaciated by the time the tumor is suspected.

Diagnostic Evaluation

Intravenous Urography. Urography is the initial and most important confirmatory diagnostic procedure in suspected Wilms' tumor (Fig. 52-2; Table 52-4) [22, 61, 101]. The examination demonstrates in varying degrees in different patients: enlargement of the kidney by a mass; displacement, narrowing, flattening, elongation, bizarre distortion, or obliteration of the infundibula and calices; impingement on and compression of the renal pelvis; displacement and compression of the ureter, and at times a nonfunctioning kidney. Displacement of the adjacent viscera may be observed, depending on the size of the mass.

Ultrasound B Scanning. Ultrasound studies should be performed to determine whether the mass is solid or cystic. Infantile polycystic disease, multicystic kidney, and hydronephrosis of the kidney or of the upper pole of a double kidney may simulate Wilms' tumor, but all the masses are relatively anechoic or demonstrate complex patterns compared to solid tumors [44].

Computed Tomography. Recently body computed tomography (CT) has been increasingly used for numbers of children with abdominal mass lesions. CT delineates the size, location, texture, and extent of a mass and presents graphic information about its relationship with other viscera.

Renal Arteriography. Arteriography in Wilms' tumor may demonstrate a mass that is moderate sized (Fig. 52-2A–C) to huge (Fig. 52-2D–F) and that involves a variable volume of the kidney and sometimes displaces it strikingly. The tumor may appear to be well encapsulated (Fig. 52-2C, D) or diffusely infiltrating (Fig. 52-2E). Because Wilms' tumor may involve both kidneys, arteriography should always be done bilaterally. The important

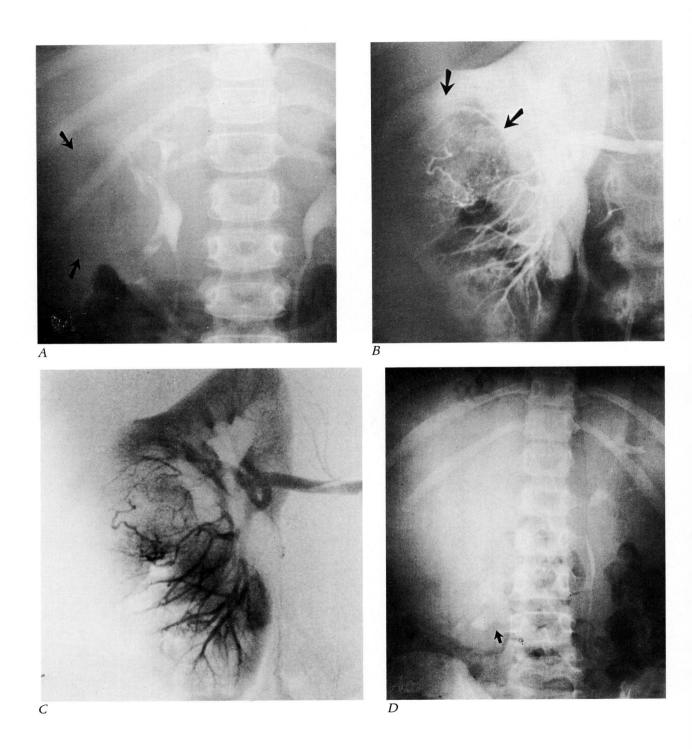

A

B

C

D

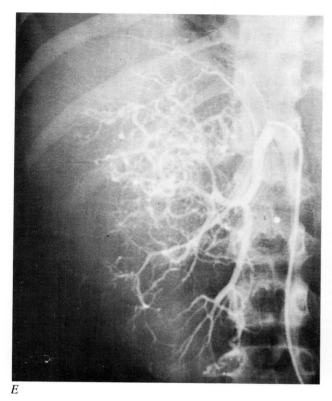

E

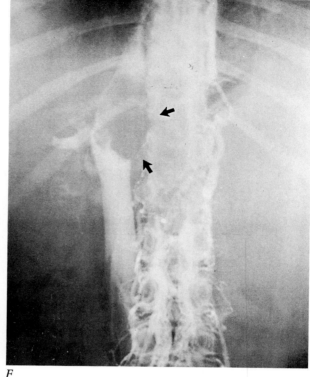

F

Figure 52-2. Wilms' tumor. (A, B, and C) Hypovascular localized mass. (A) Urogram. There are displacement and distortion of the middle and lower pole calices and clear evidence of a mass (*arrows*). (B and C) Angiogram. Although the tumor (*arrows*) is not highly vascular, irregular, coiled, randomly distributed tumor vessels are visible; they are particularly well shown on the subtraction film (C). (D, E, and F) Hypervascular Wilms' tumor invading the inferior vena cava. (D)

Urogram. The collecting system is displaced caudally (*arrow*), and a large mass fills the right upper quadrant. (E) Arteriography. A highly vascular renal tumor involves much of the total volume of the kidney. The renal artery is displaced to the left. (F) Inferior vena cavography. A large tumor embolus fills the suprarenal segment of the inferior vena cava (*arrows*). (Courtesy of Kenneth Fellows, M.D.).

Table 52-4. Urographic Signs in Wilms' Tumor

Sign	Number of Patients	Total Number of Patients	Percentage of Patients Showing Sign
Renal mass	48	50	96
Calcification	9	81	11
Nonfunctioning kidney	13	72	18
Distortion of calices or infundibula	4	12	33
Stretching of calices or infundibula	3	12	25
Compression of pelvis	2	12	—
Displacement and compression of pelvis and/or ureter	2	12	—
Hydronephrosis	2	12	—

Adapted from Clark et al. [22], Westra et al. [101], and Lalli et al. [61].

Table 52-5. Angiographic Signs in Wilms' Tumor

Sign	Number of Patients	Total Number of Patients
Tumor vessels	7	12
Avascular area	4	12
Stretching of intrarenal vessels	1	12
Hypovascular area	1	12

Adapted from Clark et al. [22].

arteriographic findings are as follows (Table 52-5; Fig. 52-2):

1. Stretching of vessels.
2. Narrowing of vessels.
3. Displacement of vessels.
4. Amputation of vessels.
5. Encasement of vessels.
6. Presence of tumor vessels. Wilms' tumor varies from a relatively avascular or hypovascular tumor (Fig. 52-2B, C) to a moderately hypervascular mass (Fig. 52-2E).
7. At times, metastases to the liver, retroperitoneal nodes, or other adjacent organs.

Arteriography is important not only in confirming the diagnosis but also in assessing the extent of tumor, liver metastases, bilaterality, response to therapy, and recurrence. Angiography usually distinguishes Wilms' tumor from hydronephrosis and multicystic kidneys (small, displaced, or widely spread vessels; no tumor vessels) [22, 70]. Although most cases of Wilms' tumor can readily be separated from neuroblastoma, in some instances it is difficult, if not impossible, to make the distinction, as noted below.

Chest films should always be obtained before angiography to determine the presence or absence of pulmonary metastases.

Inferior Vena Cavography and Renal Venography. Because these bulky tumors frequently invade the renal veins and the inferior vena cava when they are large (Fig. 52-2F), venography is useful in delineating the extent of involvement and the surgical requirements. Percutaneous transfemoral cavography should be done initially and then followed by selective renal venography if the cava is clear. The vein may be compressed, displaced, or invaded. With invasion, the wall is ragged and irregular.

Differential Diagnosis

Hydronephrosis produces renal enlargement, but a site of obstruction can usually be delineated on urography and the dilated collecting system of hydronephrosis is generally diagnostic. Arteriography may show the characteristic features: displaced, narrow vessels without encasement, amputation, or tumor vascularity.

Infantile polycystic disease may simulate Wilms' tumor. It is usually bilateral, and it involves most of both kidneys. Urography is helpful but not necessarily diagnostic. Ultrasonography may be useful.

While Wilms' tumor involves the intrarenal structures and alters the appearance of the renal pelvis and calices, *neuroblastoma* usually displaces the kidney because it is extrarenal in origin. Neuroblastoma may sometimes infiltrate the kidney, however, and Wilms' tumor may at times appear as a localized mass. The distinction, therefore, is not always clear-cut. Calcification is somewhat more common in neuroblastoma than in Wilms' tumor.

Other renal tumors, renal abscesses, and *intraabdominal masses* in infancy that arise from the liver, pancreas, retroperitoneum, and ovary must also be considered in the differential diagnosis.

Treatment

Surgical removal is the primary treatment of choice. Irradiation is useful in the postoperative period and is important in inoperable tumors, tumors that have metastasized, and bilateral tumors. Chemotherapy, particularly with actinomycin B, has demonstrated the importance of adjunctive therapy in these tumors and is now recognized as part of the management.

Prognosis

The overall survival for children with disease confined to the kidney, perinephric tissue, and abdominal lymph nodes is 78 percent at 2 to 4 years. Even with widespread metastatic disease, a 50 percent survival rate can be achieved [21].

RENAL CELL CARCINOMA

In 1883 Grawitz described renal cell carcinoma in the mistaken belief that it arose from the adrenal gland. The terms *hypernephroma* and *Grawitz' tumor* were applied to the tumor, and they have been difficult to dislodge. The concept that this tumor arises from renal tubular epithelial cells has received support from electron microscopic studies that demonstrate many striking similarities between the cells of renal cell carcinoma and normal epithelial cells of the proximal convoluted tubules [95]. This concept is now generally accepted, and the term *renal cell carcinoma* (or *renal adenocarcinoma*) seems most appropriate. This tumor constitutes 85 percent of renal malignancies [28, 31, 67], has a peak incidence in the sixth decade [31], and is more common in males. Its presence as a second primary carcinoma in elderly patients with carcinoma of other organs has been emphasized [47].

Pathology

Although the size varies greatly, often the tumor is bulky and larger than the remaining normal kidney (Fig. 52-3). The surface is usually white or yellow, knobby or irregular, and covered by dilated veins. The tumor usually appears to be well demarcated from adjacent renal tissue, even though it may have spread beyond its apparent capsule. On cut section, the highly vascular nature of the tumor is evident, and areas of necrosis

and hemorrhage are visible. Renal vein invasion, which is common, is a poor prognostic sign.

Microscopically, the tumor usually consists of clear cells or mixtures of clear and granular cells (Fig. 52-4) arranged variously, in sheets or tubules or in papillary fashion. Calcification is present in 5 to 10 percent of cases. In general, the more anaplastic and the larger the tumor is, the poorer the prognosis is.

Metastases are found in all sites, but they are commonest in the lung, bone, lymph nodes, liver, adrenal glands, and contralateral kidney, in descending order of frequency [5] (Table 52-6). At times, metastasis to the bone is the initial manifestation of the tumor [28].

Staging is important and is clearly related to the prognosis. A simple convenient approach to staging is that of Flocks and Kadesky [37]:

Stage I: Limited to renal capsule
Stage II: Invasion of the renal pedicle or perirenal fat
Stage III: Regional lymph node involvement
Stage IV: Distant metastases demonstrable

Figure 52-3. Gross pathologic appearance of renal cell carcinoma. The tumor is located in the midportion of the kidney. More medially, it has a somewhat meaty appearance, while laterally it is white and opaque (*arrows*), with an area of necrosis. Note the relatively well defined separation from the adjacent normal renal tissue despite the fact that the tumor has spread well beyond its apparent capsule. Multiple blood vessels are visible in the cut section.

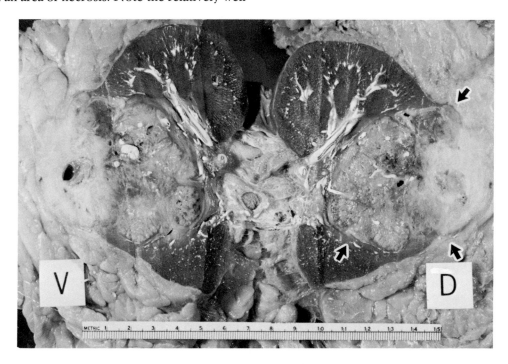

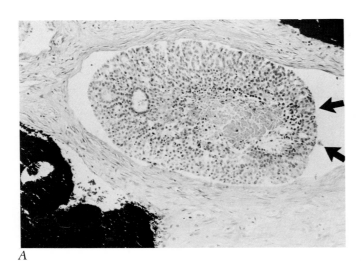

A   *B*

Figure 52-4. Renal cell carcinoma: microscopic pathology. (A) Low power. The large tumor embolus in the blood vessel (*arrows*) demonstrates the classic appearance of a renal cell carcinoma. The black mate-rial in the large vessels adjacent to the tumor embolus is postmortem injectate. (B) High power. Typical clear cells are visible throughout the section.

Table 52-6. Sites of Metastases of Renal Cell Carcinoma in 596 Proved Cases

Site of Metastases	Percentage of Patients
Lungs	44
Bone	26
Lymph nodes	23
Liver	18
Adrenal glands	12
Contralateral kidney	11

Adapted from Abrams et al. [5], Creevy [27], Crocker [28], Harvey et al. [50], Judd and Hand [54], Kozoll and Kirshbaum [58], and Wagle and Scal [99].

Symptoms and Signs

Hematuria, pain, and a mass (or "swelling") are the three common symptoms of renal cell carcinoma (Table 52-7). In the Peter Bent Brigham Hospital (PBBH) series, *hematuria*, the commonest symptom, was found in about one-half of the patients [28, 66]. It was usually gross, intermittent, and associated with blood vessel invasion or involvement of the renal pelvis or both.

Pain was noted slightly less often. It was commonly dull and continuous, but it was acute and severe when associated with hematuria. Pain was observed in over 40 percent of patients with renal capsular extension.

A *palpable mass* was detected in slightly less than 50 percent of patients. In this group, the patient noted the mass—which was the presenting symptom—25 percent of the time. No tumors

Table 52-7. Symptoms and Signs of Renal Cell Carcinoma in the Peter Bent Brigham Series

Symptom or Sign	Number of Patients	Total Number of Patients	Percentage of Patients Showing Symptom or Sign
Hematuria	36	80	45
Hematuria as first symptom	25	80	31
Painless hematuria	15	80	19
Pain	31	81	38
Pain as first symptom	11	81	14
Palpable mass	39	84	46
Palpable mass as first symptom	11	84	13
Polycythemia	3	84	4
Hypertension	19	57	33

Adapted from Crocker [28].

under 3 cm were felt; 35 percent of the tumors that were 3 to 10 cm and 70 percent of the tumors that were over 10 cm were palpable.

Nonspecific symptoms (e.g., weakness, fatigue, fever, weight loss, and anorexia) were common and frequently anteceded the development of hematuria, pain, or mass.

Polycythemia was found in 3.6 percent of PBBH patients, compared to 2 to 3 percent in the literature [91]. Since polycythemia may appear clinically as polycythemia vera, all such patients should probably have intravenous urography. The polycythemia is thought to be associated with the production of a factor stimulating erythropoiesis [96].

Hypertension was observed in one-third of the patients in the PBBH series, but its relationship to the tumor was uncertain.

Hypercalcemia is known to occur in patients with documented skeletal metastases but also (rarely) in the absence of bone involvement. In such patients, the tumor may secrete its own parathormone [28].

Besides polycythemia and hypercalcemia, other paraneoplastic syndromes include *pyrexia*, thought to be due to ectopic hormone secretion and observed in as many as 20 percent of patients [20, 66], and *hepatic dysfunction*, which occurs in as many as 15 percent of patients in whom liver metastases were not demonstrated [66, 97].

Left-sided varicocele, when present, is caused by left renal and testicular vein obstruction by the tumor.

Finally, *metastatic lesions* can give rise to manifestations (e.g., bone pain or central nervous system signs) that depend on the location of the secondary deposits. In 17 percent of the PBBH series, metastases were the source of the initial symptoms.

Renal cell carcinoma may also be asymptomatic. In the PBBH series, 19 patients (more than 20%) had no symptoms referable to their tumors. The tumors were found at autopsy in six, at surgery in three, on routine physical examination in six, at intravenous urography in three, and on laboratory analysis prompted by an elevated sedimentation rate in one [28]. In other series of patients examined during life, the rates of discovery in asymptomatic patients ranged from 5 to 31 percent, with most rates in the range of 8 to 15 percent [17, 18, 72, 88, 90, 94, 99, 100]. In autopsy series, asymptomatic renal cell carcinoma has been noted in as many as 66 percent of cases [19].

Diagnostic Evaluation

The sequence of the diagnostic procedures depends on the presenting symptoms. If significant hematuria is the first symptom, cystoscopy may be important in determining whether the source is above the bladder and, if so, from which ureter. In general, however, intravenous urography is the first and most useful special diagnostic procedure employed.

Intravenous Urography (Fig. 52-5). The preliminary film may show increased renal size, localized renal mass, an irregularly nodular surface, or calcification (Fig. 52-5A), which occurs in 5 to 10 percent of tumors examined pathologically [28] and radiologically (Table 52-8). Eccentric tumors may produce displacement and rotation of the kidney.

With opacification of the collecting system, the mass is better delineated by its effect on the calices. The following changes may be seen: displacement, narrowing, distortion, stretching, invasion, obliteration, and amputation of the calices and infundibula (Fig. 52-5B). Blunted calices may also be evident when the infundibulum is compressed or invaded by the renal mass (Table 52-9).

The renal pelvis may be displaced, flattened, distorted, elevated, depressed, or obliterated. It may contain filling defects that must be distinguished from renal pelvic neoplasms, clots, and stones. At times, the bizarre and distorted appearance of the collecting system simulates polycystic kidney, which is, however, invariably bilateral. If the tumor is localized and produces displacement and compression of the calices, it may be difficult to distinguish from a cyst on conventional urography. Nephrotomography may then be of value.

Isotope Imaging. While isotope imaging has its strong advocates [76, 78], we have found it of limited usefulness in the workup of patients with known renal masses because it is rarely accepted as the definitive diagnostic procedure. When the presence of a mass is uncertain and pseudotumor is suspected, isotope imaging may play an important role. Using chlormerodrin Hg 197, renal tumors or cysts larger than 2.5 cm in diameter can be identified (Fig. 52-6) [76]. Such pseudotumors as dromedary humps, fetal lobulation, lobular compensatory hypertrophy, and prominent columns of Bertin do not produce a defect (a cold spot) with this radionuclide. Thus, isotope imaging in this situation may confirm the innocuous nature of the urographic finding.

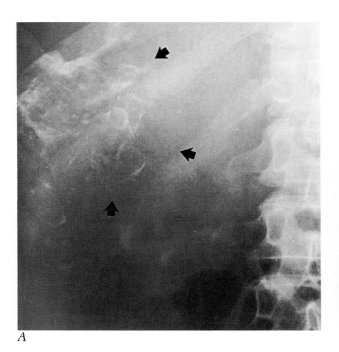

A

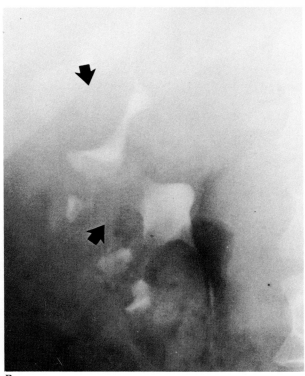

B

Figure 52-5. Renal cell carcinoma: plain films and urograms. (A) Calcification: plain film of the right kidney. There is an amorphous calcification that is more or less curvilinear but is irregularly placed in a large mass in the right kidney (*arrows*); it represents a renal cell carcinoma. (B) Infiltrating carcinoma, upper pole. This urogram demonstrates a mass in the right upper pole as well as compression and distortion of the calices and infundibula (*arrows*). (Compare with polycystic disease, Fig. 52-18A.)

Table 52-8. Plain Film in Renal Tumor

Sign	Number of Patients	Total Number of Patients	Percentage of Patients Showing Sign
Irregular renal outline	153	209	73
Obscuration of psoas shadow	14	35	40
Renal displacement	8	25	32
Renal enlargement or mass	35	176	20
Calcification	40	411	10

Adapted from Ettinger and Elkin [34], Kikkawa and Lasser [55], Graham [45], Folin [38], and Woodruff et al. [105].

Table 52-9. Urographic Signs in Renal Tumors

Sign	Number of Patients	Total Number of Patients	Percentage of Patients Showing Sign
Obliteration of pelvic or caliceal lumen	37	67	55
Extrinsic compression of calices or pelvis	93	209	44
Intraluminal filling defect	68	189	36
Diminished functioning	396	1,202	33
Caliectasis or pyelectasis	22	167	13
Hydronephrosis	28	251	11
Displacement of ureter	19	176	11
Nonvisualization of kidney	29	269	11
Elongation of pelvis and calices	17	167	10

Adapted from Ettinger and Elkin [34], Riches et al. [82], Kikkawa and Lasser [55], Köhler [57], Graham [45], Folin [38], and Woodruff et al. [105].

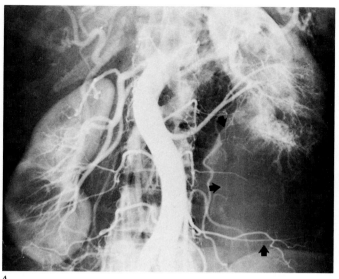

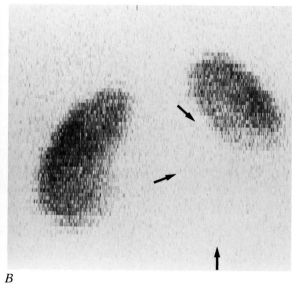

A

B

Figure 52-6. Renal carcinoma: renal isotope scan. (A) Renal arteriogram. A huge mass is present in the lower pole of the left kidney (*arrows*). Later films demonstrated multiple tumor vessels in the mass. (B) Isotope scan. The lower pole in the region of the tumor mass shows no perfusion and no function (*arrows*). This picture is consistent with that of a known renal mass replacing renal tissue, but it is by no means pathognomonic of carcinoma.

Figure 52-7. Renal carcinoma: ultrasound. (A) Ultrasonogram. (B) Diagram. Bilateral renal carcinoma. The normal kidney is better seen on the left side, with the collecting system centrally placed as a dark, mottled area. The tumors are medial and somewhat dorsal to the kidneys and show definite echoes, unlike the characteristic appearance of anechoic cysts. Ultrasonography has proved to be a useful adjunct in the diagnosis of carcinoma of the kidney and is a simple, noninvasive mode of delineating solid masses.

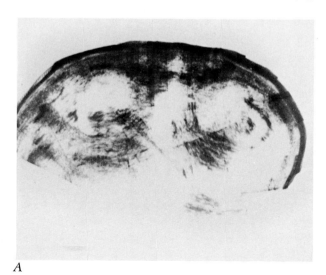

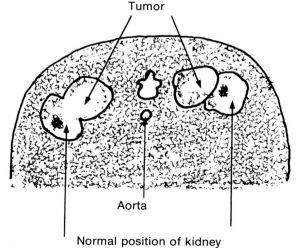

A

B

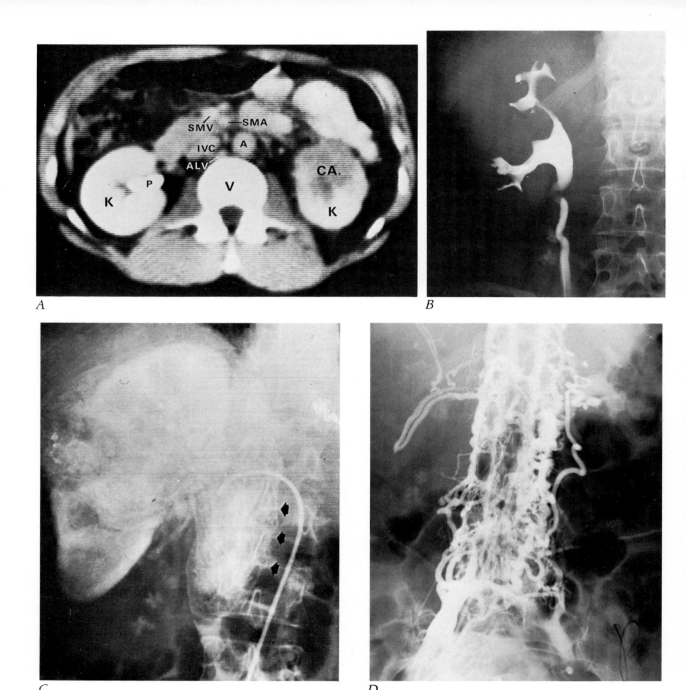

A

B

C

D

Figure 52-8. Renal carcinoma: computed tomogram. (A) A computed tomographic scan obtained in the supine position through the midportion of the kidneys. The right kidney is homogeneously opacified, and contrast material fills the renal pelvis. On the left side, however, only the lower pole shows normal opacification, while the upper pole and the midportions of the kidney demonstrate diminished concentration and an irregular mottled appearance (*CA*). This appearance is characteristic of renal neoplasm. *K* = kidney; *P* = pelvis of kidney; *A* = aorta; *ALV* = ascending lumbar vein; *IVC* = inferior vena cava; *SMV* = superior mesenteric vein; *SMA* = superior mesenteric artery; *V* = vertebral body. (B to I) Renal cell carcinoma with extension into the renal vein and the inferior vena cava. (B) Retrograde urogram. There is gross distortion of the infundibula, pelvis, and collecting system of the midportion and upper pole of the kidney. Complete amputation of the midpole infundibulum is visible. (C) Selective renal arteriogram, venous phase. The hypervascular renal cell carcinoma demonstrated in the earlier phase has invaded the renal vein and the inferior vena cava (*arrows*). Multiple striated contrast-filled tumor vessels are visible extending into a large tumor thrombus below the level of the renal hilus. (D) Femoral venogram. There is complete obstruction of the inferior vena cava, which is invaded by renal cell carcinoma. The vertebral venous plexuses and the ascending lumbar veins are opacified as the major avenues of blood return from the lower

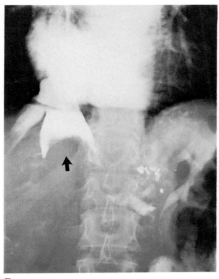

E

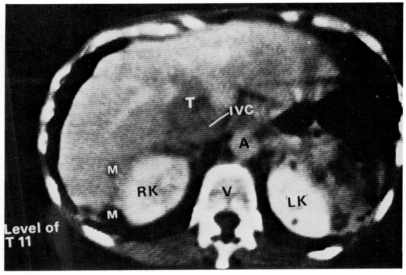

F

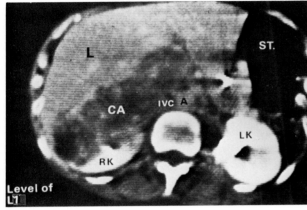

G

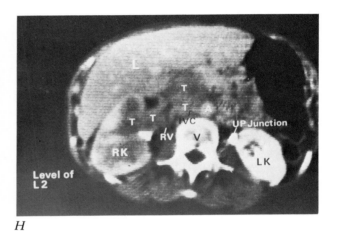

H

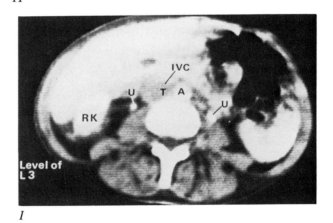

I

extremities. (E) Inferior vena cavogram. Opacification of the cephalic portion of the inferior vena cava has been accomplished through trans-right-atrial catheterization. In this way, the upward extent of the tumor is shown (*arrow*). This information may be of great importance to the surgeon because it tells precisely where resection of the cava is essential during nephrectomy and tumor removal. (F) Computed tomogram (CT) at the level of T11. The right kidney (*RK*) is opacified, but its ventral portion is invaded by a tumor (*T*) that extends into the inferior vena cava (*IVC*). Note the two metastases (*M*) in the adjacent liver. *A* = aorta; *LK* = left kidney; *V* = vertebral body. (G) CT at the level of L1. Extensive replacement of a large portion of the right kidney by the renal cell carcinoma (*CA*) is apparent. It extends into the retroperitoneum, with tumor thrombus in the inferior vena cava. *L* = liver; *ST* = stomach. (H) CT at the level of L2. Less involvement of the right kidney is visible, but the tumor mass extends well into the retroperitoneum (*T*) and involves the renal vein (*RV*). (I) CT at the level of L3. Although both ureters (*U*) are visible, the tumor thrombus (*T*) in the inferior vena cava is still clearly demarcated at the level of the lower pole of the right kidney.

1135

Table 52-10. Arteriographic Findings in Renal Cell Carcinoma

Finding	Number of Patients	Total Number of Patients	Percentage of Patients Showing Finding
Tumor vessels	278	312	92
Displacement of renal artery or its branches	96	105	91
Early venous filling	51	58	88
Enlarged renal artery	90	158	57
Enlarged capsular vessels	114	236	48
Nonvisualization of renal vein	158	347	46
Tumor stain	51	165	31
Venous collateral vessels	68	198	34
Distinct tumor edge	46	230	20

Adapted from Boijsen and Folin [15], Cornell and Dolan [26], Folin [39], and Watson et al. [100].

Ultrasonography. The main role of ultrasonography is to differentiate simple renal cysts from other renal masses and thus reduce the number of patients requiring arteriography. The solid ultrasonic pattern identifies a mass as a neoplasm with 90 percent accuracy because of the echoes generated by the solid tissue (Fig. 52-7) [36, 43, 44]. Complex patterns may be seen in a variety of lesions, including necrotic or hemorrhagic tumors, cysts, or hydronephrosis [76]. The classic anechoic pattern of simple cyst is quite reliable. Masses smaller than 2 to 3 cm cannot be reliably diagnosed by ultrasonography [14]. Ultrasonography may also be helpful in cyst puncture or renal biopsy and can readily define extension into the inferior vena cava.

Computed Tomography. CT is useful in distinguishing solid renal masses from cystic renal masses. The attenuation (or absorption) coefficient of tumor is significantly higher than that of fluid (cyst), so that the distinction can be made both on the basis of the image attained and on the quantitative assessment of x-ray absorption (Fig. 52-8). The method is clearly competitive with ultrasonography but has not yet been shown to be more accurate [6, 104]. On the other hand it may be of considerable value in demonstrating the precise extent and volume of the tumor, lymph node involvement, and involvement of

Table 52-11. Vascularity of Renal Cell Carcinoma As Judged by Angiography

Degree of Vascularity	Number of Cases
Avascular	6
Minimal vascularity	16
Moderate vascularity	16
Marked vascularity	62
Total	100

Adapted from Watson et al. [100].

adjacent tissues [65, 104]. Retroperitoneal and inferior vena caval involvement are delineated accurately, especially following contrast enhancement (Fig. 52-8B, C).

Angiography. The majority of renal cell carcinomas are hypervascular (Tables 52-10, 52-11), and they are readily diagnosed by angiography in 94 to 97 percent of cases (Fig. 52-9) [71, 100]. Characteristically, the angiogram will delineate the disordered tumor vascular bed and the limits of the renal mass lesion. The tumor size varies from a few centimeters to a huge mass, displacing the kidney and adjacent viscera. Bilateral arteriography should be performed because renal cell carcinoma may metastasize to the contralateral side or may occur as bilateral primary lesions.

The most characteristic finding on angiography is the presence of "tumor" vessels, which are irregular, tortuous, randomly distributed, variable in size, and unpredictable in branching. Although some tumors are hypovascular, the commonest findings are as follows:

1. Increased vascularity (Fig. 52-9A, B, E, G).
2. "Random" distribution of vessels, in contrast to the uniform distribution of normal renal vessels (Fig. 52-9E).
3. Tortuous vessels, with absence of normal tapering (Fig. 52-9B, C).
4. Dilated vessels, with pooling of contrast material in "lakes" (Fig. 52-9B, G).
5. Arteriovenous communications (Fig. 52-9B, C; see also Fig. 52-13A).
6. Encasement of arteries. The margins are irregular and appear fixed and unchanging during different phases of the heart cycle. This finding is more characteristic of transitional cell than of renal cell carcinoma.
7. Staining of the tumor mass during the capillary phase (Fig. 52-9D, F).
8. Pooling of contrast in venous lakes.
9. Neoplastic response to epinephrine (Figs. 52-10–52-12). If 6 to 10 μg of epinephrine is injected arterially prior to contrast injection, the normal renal vessels contract while the tumor vascular bed exhibits a lessened vasoconstrictor response. Thus, the tumor bed opacifies whereas normal kidney tissue does not. This selectivity provides better demarcation of the tumor mass, confirms the diagnosis when it is in doubt, and, at times, establishes a positive diagnosis when conventional arteriography is inconclusive (Figs. 52-10, 52-11) [16]. The relative lack of response by the tumor vascular bed is probably associated with the primitive muscular and elastic tissue in the walls of some tumor vessels [1, 3, 4].
10. Renal vein invasion and/or obstruction by tumor (Fig. 52-13; see also Fig. 52-9E, F).

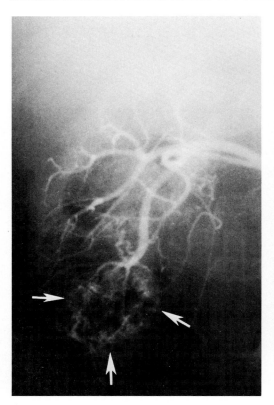

A

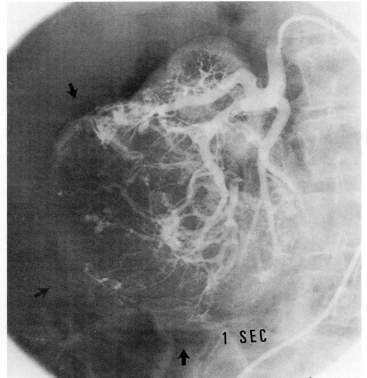

B

Figure 52-9

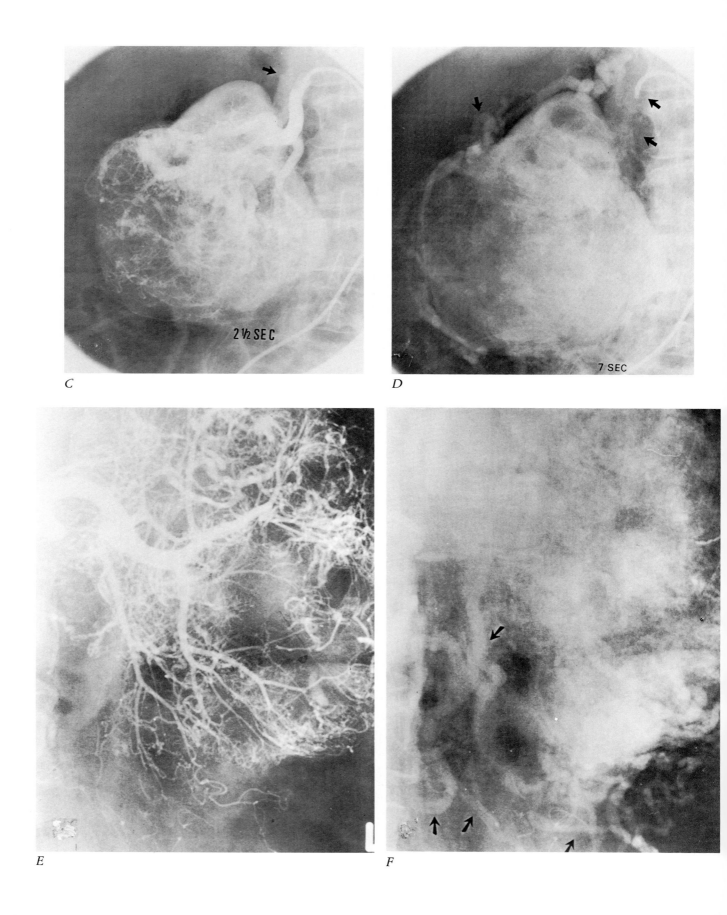

C

2½ SEC

D

7 SEC

E

F

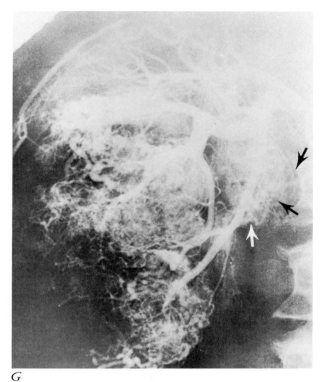

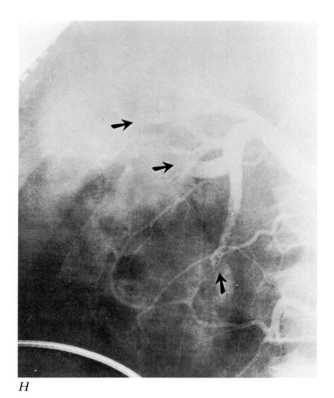

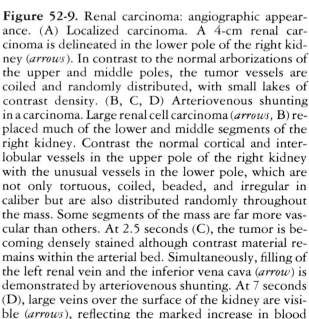

G

H

Figure 52-9. Renal carcinoma: angiographic appearance. (A) Localized carcinoma. A 4-cm renal carcinoma is delineated in the lower pole of the right kidney (*arrows*). In contrast to the normal arborizations of the upper and middle poles, the tumor vessels are coiled and randomly distributed, with small lakes of contrast density. (B, C, D) Arteriovenous shunting in a carcinoma. Large renal cell carcinoma (*arrows,* B) replaced much of the lower and middle segments of the right kidney. Contrast the normal cortical and interlobular vessels in the upper pole of the right kidney with the unusual vessels in the lower pole, which are not only tortuous, coiled, beaded, and irregular in caliber but are also distributed randomly throughout the mass. Some segments of the mass are far more vascular than others. At 2.5 seconds (C), the tumor is becoming densely stained although contrast material remains within the arterial bed. Simultaneously, filling of the left renal vein and the inferior vena cava (*arrow*) is demonstrated by arteriovenous shunting. At 7 seconds (D), large veins over the surface of the kidney are visible (*arrows*), reflecting the marked increase in blood

flow to the kidney rather than renal vein obstruction. Contrast this situation with that shown in (F). (E and F) Renal carcinoma with renal vein obstruction. The kidney's almost-complete replacement by a renal carcinoma diffusely spread throughout the parenchyma is reflected in the extensive network of tumor vessels and neovascularity in all segments of the kidney. The venous phase (F) shows no evidence of a discrete renal vein. Instead, there is a huge network of collateral channels (*arrows*), indicating renal vein obstruction by the tumor. This suspicion was confirmed at nephrectomy. (G and H) Large hypervascular carcinoma. The selective renal arteriogram (G) demonstrates remarkable hypervascularity in the renal cell carcinoma, with medial filling of a tumor mass adjacent to the pelvis of the kidney (*arrows*). Because this patient required nephrectomy and because it was desirable to diminish blood loss, Gelfoam was instilled through the selective catheter as multiple emboli (*arrows,* H). Thus the hypervascular mass was rendered ischemic, and the surgeon could work in a relatively bloodless field.

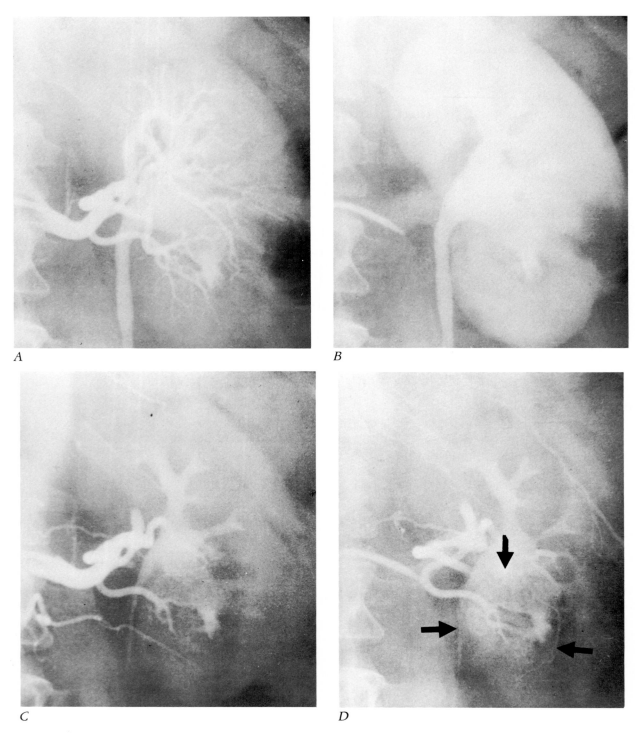

A

B

C

D

Figure 52-10. Renal cell carcinoma: epinephrine arteriography. (A) Selective renal arteriogram in a patient with hematuria. Arterial phase. No evidence of a neoplasm is visible. (B) Nephrogram. The nephrogram appears normal. (C) Epinephrine arteriogram, 2 seconds. Diminished flow is evident through all parts of the renal vascular bed, with only a few branches visible extending to the parenchyma, just caudal to the renal pelvis. (D) Epinephrine arteriogram, 4½ seconds. A discrete renal cell carcinoma impinging on the caudal margin of the pelvis is demonstrated (*arrows*). (Courtesy of Ronald Castellino, M.D.)

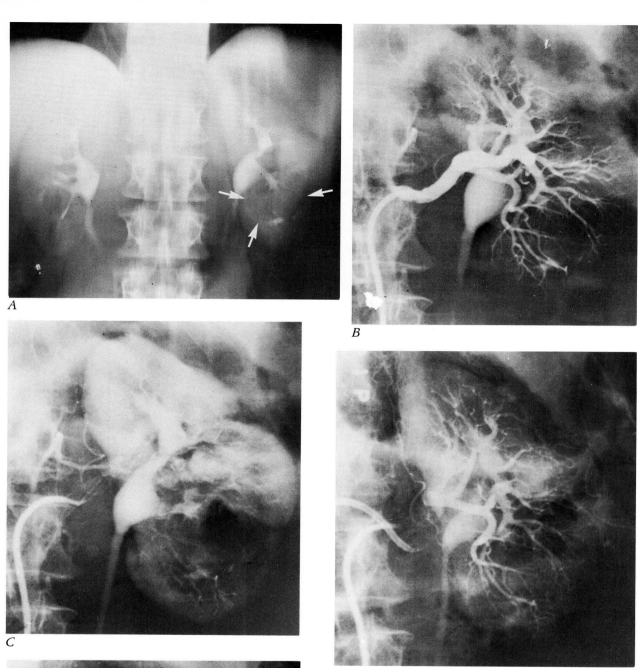

Figure 52-11. Renal carcinoma: epinephrine arteriogram. The patient entered the hospital for evaluation of hematuria. (A) Urogram. A mass is visible (*arrows*) in the lower pole of the kidney; its appearance is suggestive of a cyst. (B) Selective renal arteriogram. The vessels to the lower pole are displaced around a smooth, round mass. No tumor vessels or encasement is visible. (C) Nephrographic phase. A lucent area in the lower pole suggests a cyst. In addition, a localized invagination just above the midportion of the lateral border of the kidney resembles a prior infarct with scarring. (D) Epinephrine arteriogram, 1 second. There is no filling of the vessels to the cortex of the kidney. (E) Epinephrine arteriogram, 2.5 seconds. The interlobar renal arteries remain opacified, but now a small local area of increased density (*arrows*) extends beyond the margin of the kidney adjacent to the upper pole. Surgical exploration revealed that this lesion was a renal cell carcinoma. A benign simple cyst was present in the lower pole of the kidney. (Courtesy of Ernest Ferris, M.D.)

1141

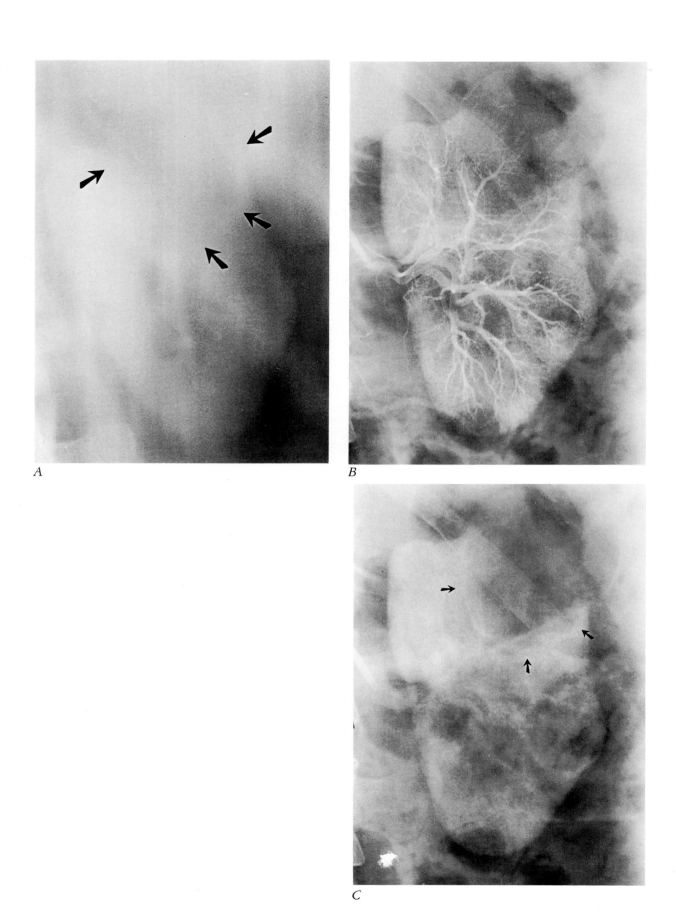

A

B

C

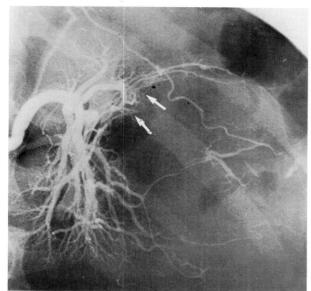

D

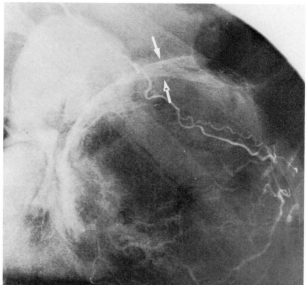

E

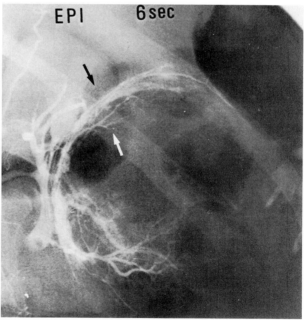

F

Figure 52-12. Renal carcinoma: cystic type. (A) Laminogram during intravenous urography. A bulge in the left upper contour of the left kidney (*arrows*) appears to be relatively lucent in character, similar to a cyst. (B) Selective renal arteriogram, arteriographic phase. The arteriogram reveals multiple fine vessels to the area of the mass in the left upper pole, some of them moderately tortuous and beaded in character. (C) Nephrographic phase. The mass (*arrows*) is certainly relatively lucent but has a somewhat thicker wall than the usual benign cyst. Exploratory surgery revealed a renal cell carcinoma. (D, E, and F) Large cystic carcinoma. (D) Arterial phase. There are obvious draping and stretching of vessels over a large mass in the lateral aspect of the left kidney (*arrows*). Multiple vessels are clumped together in the upper and lower margins of the mass, and a large capsular vessel runs over its surface and communicates with other capsular branches. (E) Nephrographic phase. At 7 seconds it is apparent (*arrows*) that the cyst wall is significantly thicker than that of a benign cyst and that there is contrast material in the vessels supplying tissue in the medial and caudal aspects of the cyst mass. (F) Post-epinephrine film. After administration of epinephrine, there is virtually no flow to the normal renal vessels. The vessels to the cystic mass (*arrows*) are relatively well filled with contrast agent, suggesting that they are neoplastic. Note staining of the medial caudal margin of the tumor. Surgery revealed an extensive cystic renal carcinoma.

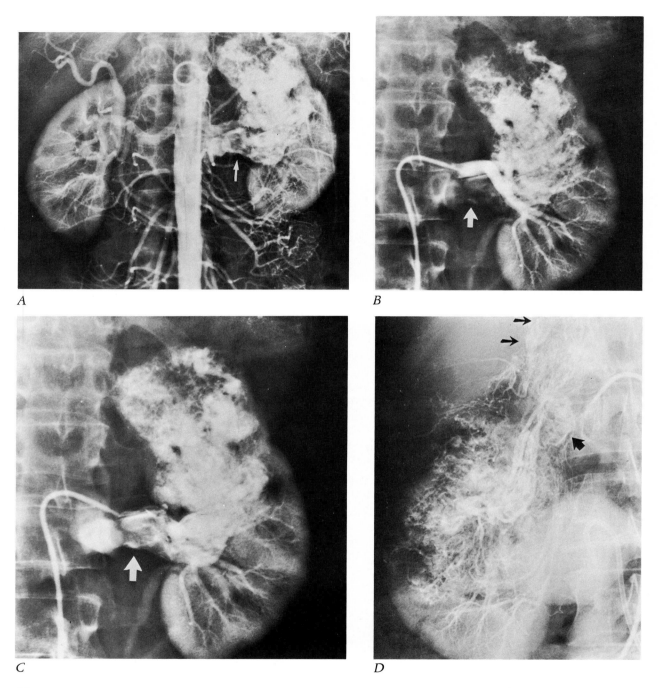

A

B

C

D

Figure 52-13. Renal cell carcinoma with renal vein invasion. (A) Aortogram. Dense staining of the neoplasm involving the upper two-thirds of the left kidney is apparent. In addition, the tumor has invaded the left renal vein (*arrow*). (B) Selective renal arteriogram, 1 second. While the artery is still opacified, arteriovenous shunting has occurred with renal vein opacification (*arrow*). (C) Selective renal arteriogram, 2 seconds. A large tumor thrombus is visible in the left renal vein (*arrow*). (D) Selective renal arteriogram in a patient with renal cell carcinoma, 2.5 seconds. Note the typical renal cell carcinoma extension into the vena cava as denoted by the malignant vessels extending far outside the kidney (*arrows*) and directly into the region of the inferior vena cava.

Once the diagnosis of carcinoma has been made, a large volume (25 cc) of contrast agent may be injected selectively to obtain better visualization of the veins since the kidney will be removed under any circumstances. Tumor vessels within the vein may be delineated and so establish the presence of invasion. Failure to opacify the renal vein is not conclusive evidence of tumor invasion; demonstration of a large venous collateral network is strongly suggestive [89]. It must be emphasized that large draining veins alone need not reflect renal vein invasion so much as the high vascularity of the tumor [62, 102].

Avascular renal cell tumors, although relatively few in number, may resemble benign cysts. Usually, tumor vessels will be apparent. Cyst puncture in these tumors demonstrates a thick, irregular wall if they are cystic neoplasms, and aspiration of cyst fluid may be positive for renal cell carcinoma on cytologic examination [106].

Renal tumors may invade renal arteries and produce massive hemorrhage, suggesting a huge renal tumor (Figs. 52-14, 52-15). At times, the tumor may be quite small (Fig. 52-15), and the mass effect may be predominantly that of the hematoma.

Aside from its diagnostic usefulness, renal arteriography furnishes the surgeon with important preoperative anatomic knowledge of the renal vascular bed. Its accuracy is high, approximately 95 percent [23, 62]. Its value in determining operability lies largely in its ability to detect metastases or widespread invasion. Even the demonstration of renal vein obstruction no longer precludes surgery although it is important to clarify its presence preoperatively.

Since angiography of the contralateral kidney is mandatory, the presence or absence of undetected abnormalities can also be determined. Once the diagnosis of renal carcinoma has been established, it is our custom to perform celiac arteriography to search for metastases. These are usually hypervascular, resembling the pattern of the primary tumor.

Inferior Vena Cavography and Renal Venography. Because of the common tendency of renal cell carcinoma to invade the renal vein and the inferior vena cava and because arteriography is not always conclusive with regard to renal vein involvement, cavography and renal venography may afford important information to the surgeon about the extent of the tumor [92] (see Chap. 59). The theoretical objection that renal venography may encourage the spread of tumor has not been borne out in our experience.

Other Radiologic Procedures. A chest examination for pulmonary metastases and a bone scan for osseous metastases are essential for the evaluation of patients with renal cell carcinoma. Bone scans are more accurate than radiographic skeletal surveys, and they improve the procedure of clinical staging [25].

Differential Diagnosis
The differential diagnosis of renal cell carcinoma includes all mass lesions of the kidney. In lymphomatous infiltration, a "palisadelike" appearance may be observed, with small abnormal arteries and a tumor blush [85]. In Hodgkin's disease, the appearance may resemble that of an infiltrative neoplasm, with abnormal vessels indistinguishable from those in hypovascular renal cell carcinoma [103]. The vascular tumors need to be differentiated from hamartomas (which is not always possible) and from other benign vascular tumors, such as those of neurogenic origin. The hypovascular and cystic tumors may resemble benign solitary cysts.

Inflammatory lesions, such as renal abscess (Fig. 52-16) and xanthogranulomatous pyelonephritis (Fig. 52-17), may mimic renal cell tumors. With abscesses or inflammatory masses, there are an increase in the size and number of capsular vessels, an abnormal intrarenal circulation manifested by slow and diminished blood flow, stretching of the interlobar branches, loss of the cortical-medullary border, and loss of the kidney outline (see Fig. 52-16). Typical tumor vessels of renal cell carcinoma are not observed, and no arteriovenous shunts are present. The distinction from cystic or hypovascular tumors may be difficult [56].

The urographic appearance of polycystic kidney may be similar to that of infiltrating carcinoma, but its angiographic appearance is quite different (Figs. 52-18, 52-19).

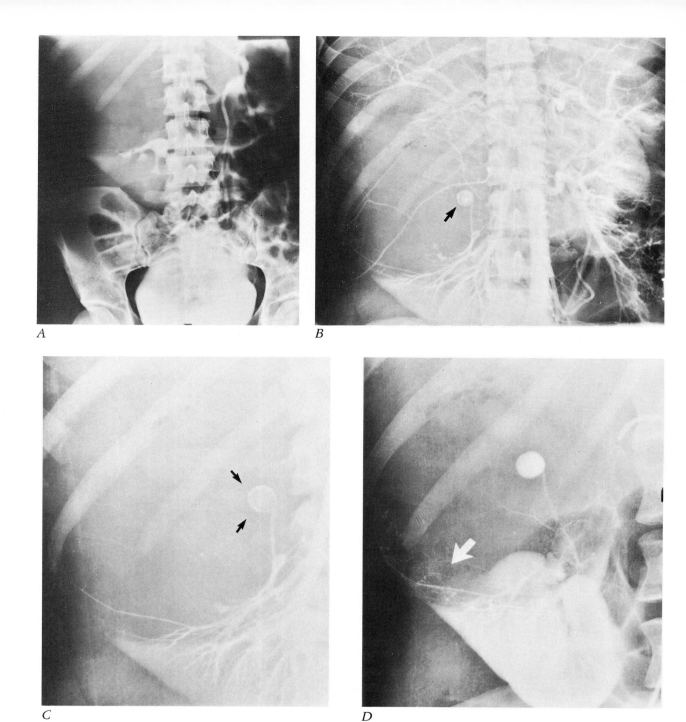

A

B

C

D

Figure 52-14. Renal cell carcinoma, with intrarenal hemorrhage. This patient entered the hospital with gross hematuria. (A) Urogram. The right kidney is markedly displaced and depressed by what appears to be a huge mass in its upper midportions. This area lacks the nephrographic effect. (B) Aortogram. The apparent mass lesion is generally avascular, except for a discrete collection of contrast material fed by a small branch vessel of the lower pole renal arteries (*arrow*). (C) Selective renal arteriogram. The collection of contrast represents a pseudoaneurysm (*arrows*), presumably in the middle of a large hemorrhagic mass. (D) Selective renal arteriogram, 3.5 seconds. The pseudoaneurysm is now densely opacified. In addition, abnormal vessels are seen (*arrow*) at the edge of the large mass, displacing and distorting the right kidney. A nephrectomy demonstrated a renal cell carcinoma with a massive intrarenal hematoma in the center of a necrotic area of tumor. (Courtesy of R. R. Freeman, M.D.)

Figure 52-15. Renal cell carcinoma with hemorrhage. This 35-year-old woman had a 24-hour history of severe left flank pain. An intravenous urogram revealed a nonfunctioning left kidney. (A) Retrograde left urogram. Extrinsic compression of the renal pelvis, with kinking of the ureteropelvic junction. No contrast ▶

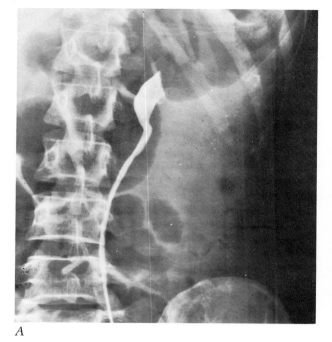

A

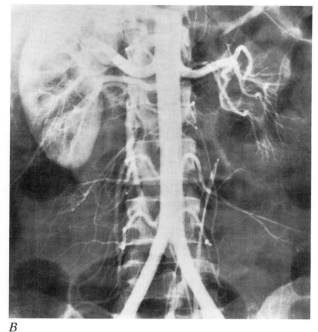

B

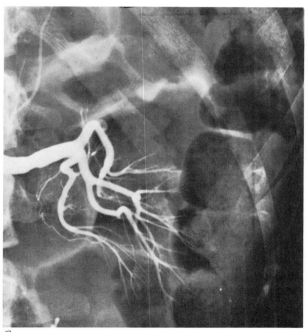

C

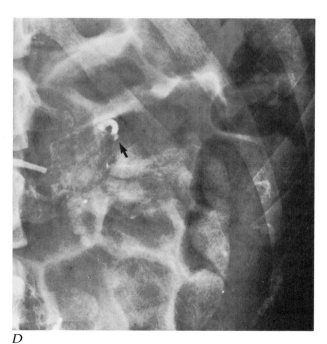

D

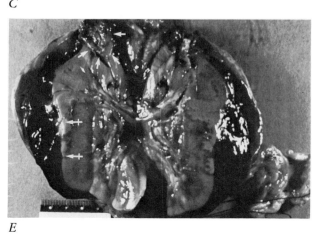

E

material fills the caliceal system. (B) Aortogram. There is profound slowing of the flow through the left kidney as compared to the right. (C) Selective renal arteriogram. The small vessels failed to fill, and the renal cortex is not opacified. No arterial filling to the upper pole of the kidney is apparent. (D) Nephrogram. At 8 seconds, the nephrogram is faint. Persistent contrast filling of a single arterial branch is visible (*arrow*). (E) Pathologic specimen. There was a 3-cm, highly vascular, infarcted upper pole renal cell carcinoma (*white arrows*) that had produced massive subcapsular hemorrhage. A large, tense, subcapsular hematoma (*barred arrows*) was present. Thus, although there was clearly a mass lesion, the findings were those of increased intrarenal resistance due to a large collection of blood within the renal capsule.

1147

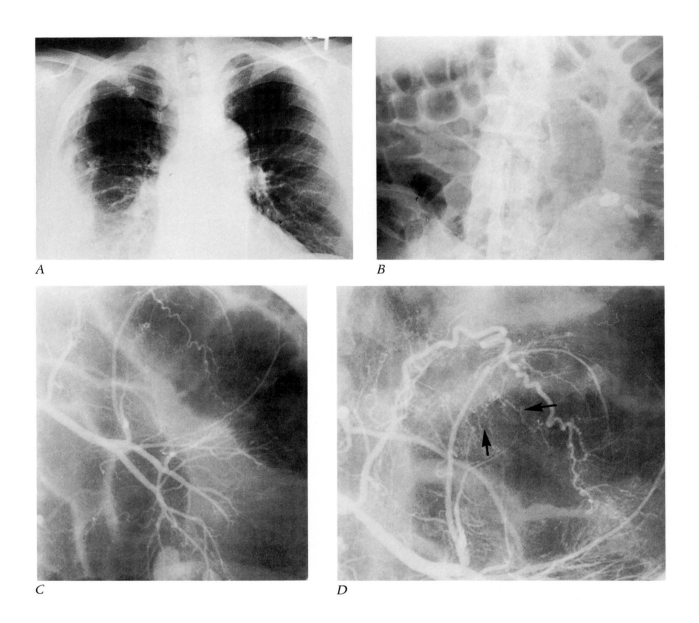

A

B

C

D

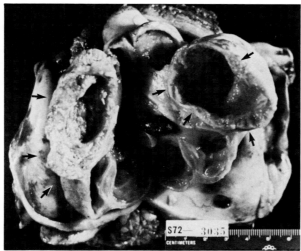

E

Figure 52-16. Infection versus neoplasm: chronic renal inflammation with abscess. This 60-year-old man entered the hospital because he had a low-grade fever, anorexia, and weight loss associated with left flank pain. (A) Chest film. There is marked pleural thickening on the right side associated with an episode of tuberculosis when the patient was 20 years old. A calcified tuberculous lesion is visible in the right upper lobe overlying the clavicle and the right posterior fourth rib. (B) Plain film of the abdomen. There are two large calcifications in the lower pole of the left kidney. Urography showed nonvisualization of the middle and upper pole calices. (C) Selective left renal arteriogram. There is marked displacement of upper pole vessels in a curvilinear fashion around a large mass in the upper portion and midportion of the kidneys. The vessels to the lower pole are somewhat narrowed and are slightly displaced in the region of the large calcific densities. (D) Magnified view of the left upper pole. In addition to the displacement of the vessels and the large feeder branches from the adrenal capsular artery, multiple thin, irregularly ramifying branches are visible within the mass lesion (*arrows*). A few irregularly coiled branches are also opacified. No lakes, no premature venous opacification, and no evidence of typical so-called malignant vessels can be seen. Nevertheless, an avascular renal cell carcinoma must be considered seriously, as must a large transitional cell carcinoma. Furthermore, in view of the known history of tuberculosis, the possibility of tuberculous pyonephrosis must be entertained (a diagnosis that is untenable without calcification in the involved area; in addition, the characteristic amputation of vessels associated with tuberculosis is not visible). Finally, the possibility that the picture is that of a chronic abscess in an individual with chronic pyelonephritis and calculus formation in the lower pole clearly requires serious consideration. Because of the continuing fever and the nonvisualization of the left kidney on urography, nephrectomy was performed. (E) Pathologic specimen. Pathologic examination revealed a large, thick-walled abscess in the left upper pole with inflammatory changes throughout much of the kidney (*arrows*).

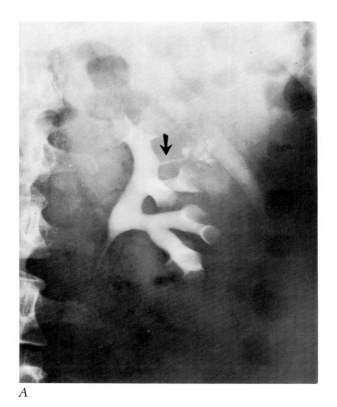

A

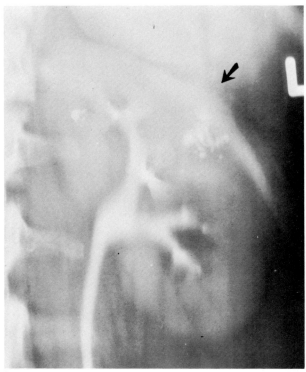

B

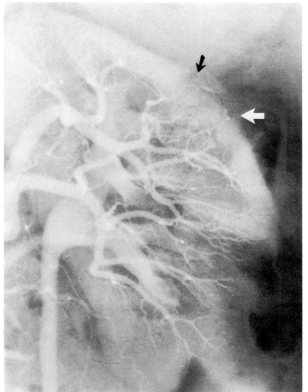

C

Figure 52-17. Localized xanthogranulomatous pyelonephritis. (A) Intravenous urogram. Calcification was present on the plain film, and the infundibulum extending to the area of amorphous calcification was stretched and narrowed (*arrow*). (B) Tomogram during urography. Extending from the region of the calcification, a small mass was apparent (*arrow*). (C) Selective renal arteriogram. Somewhat irregular vessels (*arrows*) are visible in the area of the mass, extending through the renal margin. Although these vessels are slightly irregular, they do not have the appearance of classic neoplastic vessels, but carcinoma could not be excluded. Pathologic examination of tissue obtained by a wedge resection of the area demonstrated a localized area of xanthogranulomatous pyelonephritis in association with calculi.

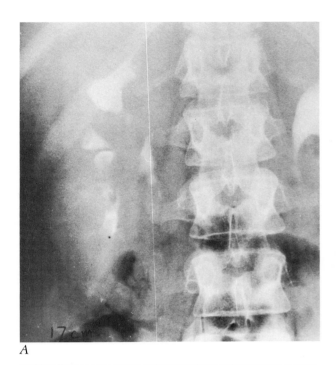

A

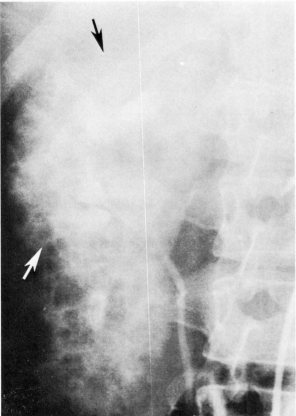

C

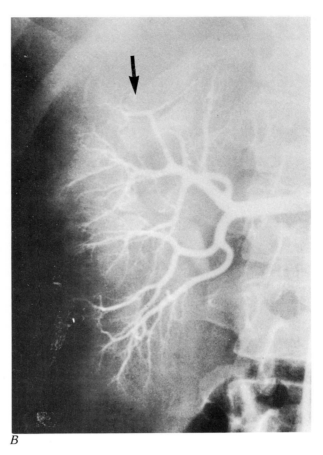

B

Figure 52-18. Polycystic kidney. (A) Urogram. There are dilatation and separation of the calices and rather marked deformity of the infundibula and the pelvis of the kidney. The appearance is not dissimilar to that in infiltrating carcinoma (compare with Fig. 52-8F, G). (B) Selective renal arteriogram. In multiple areas of the kidney, the renal arteries appear displaced and stretched around local small masses. In the upper pole, a larger mass (*arrow*) is apparent. (C) Nephrographic phase. The larger cyst in the upper pole (*black arrow*) is well defined. Multiple lucent areas visible throughout the kidney stretch from the upper pole to the lower pole and present a mottled appearance (*white arrow*). This is the classic appearance of polycystic kidney.

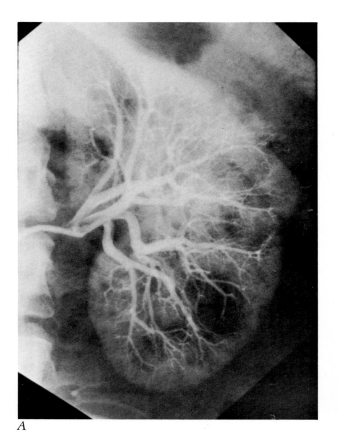

A

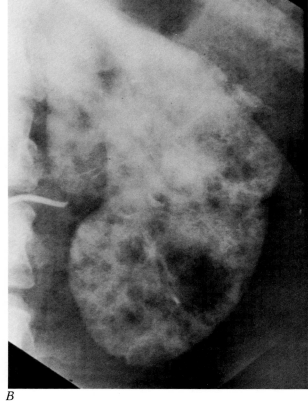

B

Figure 52-19. Polycystic kidney. The urogram was normal, except for the increased size of the kidney. (A) Selective renal arteriogram, 1.5 seconds. There is a slight displacement of multiple branches of the renal arteries throughout the kidneys. (B) At 3.5 seconds. Multiple lucent areas are visible, representing cysts of varying size and a polycystic kidney. Note that cysts may be so small that they do not necessarily cause major abnormalities of the collecting system in some patients.

Treatment

Radical nephrectomy is the treatment of choice. Irradiation plays a role in the management of the inoperable patient, the patient in whom surgery is known to have removed the tumors incompletely, and the patient who requires palliation of osseous or pulmonary metastases. Both nonhormonal and hormonal antitumor chemotherapies have been tried in carcinoma of the kidney with metastatic disease, but there is no evidence that objective tumor regression has occurred [66].

Prognosis

The overall survival rate is 30 to 50 percent at 5 years and 17 to 28 percent at 10 years [80]. If the tumor is localized to the kidney, a 5-year survival rate of 60 percent may be obtained, indicating the importance of the stage at the time of discov-ery. Renal vein invasion is a poor prognostic sign; with it, a 5-year survival rate of 29 percent may be anticipated, compared to 52 percent without it [12]. Anaplastic tumors have a poorer prognosis than have well-differentiated ones.

A fascinating aspect of renal cell carcinoma is the strong evidence of spontaneous regression both of the primary tumor and of metastases in the lung following nephrectomy [8, 9, 35, 40, 41, 68]. In a series of 82 patients at the Peter Bent Brigham Hospital, 45 underwent radical nephrectomy in the presence of metastatic disease in an effort to prevent anticipated intrarenal hemorrhage and to promote the possible regression of metastatic foci of tumor [66]. In no patient was objective regression of distant disease demonstrated. Nevertheless, a recent report documents regression of pulmonary metastases and analyzes 48 cases of such regression in the literature [40].

RENAL PELVIC TUMORS

Tumors of the renal pelvis, occurring mostly in the sixth and seventh decades of life, account for 7 to 8 percent of all malignant renal tumors. Although there are different histologic types, the transitional cell carcinoma predominates, accounting for over 80 percent of pelvic tumors.

Pathology

Transitional cell carcinoma is almost invariably papillary (Fig. 52-20). It is invasive and frequently reaches the lymphatics and invades the renal vein. It metastasizes to the retroperitoneum, lungs, liver, and bones. Squamous cell carcinoma (which comprises about 15% of renal pelvic tumors) is commonly papillary, but it may be solid and flat. It is frequently associated with calculus and infection. Mucin-producing adenocarcinoma is a much rarer tumor of the renal pelvis.

Symptoms and Signs

Hematuria, by far the commonest symptom [29], is found in more than 80 percent of patients with transitional cell carcinoma. It was the first symptom in 13 of 14 patients at the Peter Bent Brigham Hospital [28]. *Pain* was present in less than one-third of the patients, and none of the patients had a palpable mass. Squamous cell carcinoma and adenocarcinoma cause bleeding in the late stages and are sometimes discovered only because of the association with stone, infection, or hydronephrosis.

Diagnostic Evaluation

Intravenous Urography. The commonest urographic finding is a filling defect in the renal pelvis (Fig. 52-21) (Table 52-12). The defect varies in size and is associated with more or less deforming of the renal pelvis. Infundibular obstruction, mass, hydronephrosis, and nonvisualization of the collecting system are also observed (Fig. 52-22).

Ultrasonography and Computed Tomography. If the tumor has extended into the kidney, ultrasonography may be useful in demonstrating the presence of an echoic mass, leading to the presumptive diagnosis of carcinoma [36]. Computed tomography not only depicts the degree of involvement of the kidney but also may show the deformity of the renal pelvis of the mass lesion involving and surrounding the renal pelvis and, at times, the upper ureter.

Cystoscopy, Retrograde Pyelography, and Cytologic Examination of the Urine. If heavy bleeding is the initial symptom, cystoscopy may be helpful in determining whether the source is in the bladder or above it or, if no bladder source is defined, which ureter drains the blood. Because transitional cell carcinoma frequently seeds in the ureter, retrograde pyelography may be helpful if the ureter is not visualized. During cystoscopy and ureteral catheterization, urine samples should be collected for cytologic examination, which is helpful when positive.

Figure 52-20. Transitional cell carcinoma: gross appearance. Transitional cell carcinoma is almost invariably papillary. It is invasive and frequently reaches the lymphatics and invades the renal vein. It is visible in the bisected kidney as a verrucous mass in the renal pelvis (*arrows*). The patient's presenting symptom was hematuria.

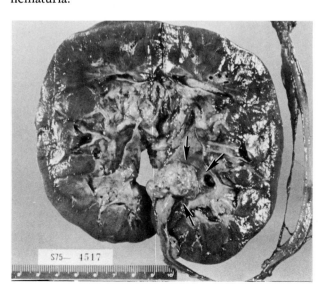

Table 52-12. Intravenous Urography in Renal Pelvic Carcinoma

Finding	Number of Patients
Filling defect	15
Infundibular obstruction	3
Mass	4
Hydronephrosis	5
Nonvisualization	8
Total	35

Adapted from Cummings et al. [29].

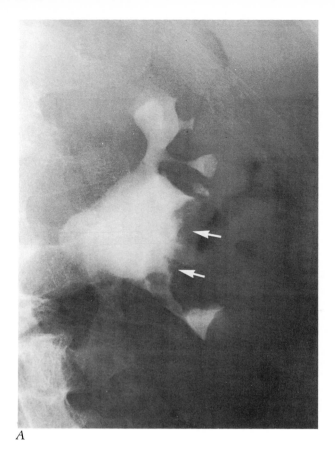

A

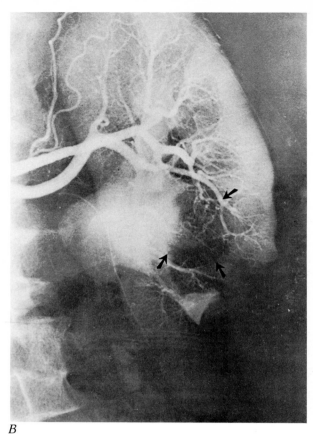

B

Figure 52-21. Renal pelvic carcinoma. (A) Urogram. An irregular mass apparently originates in the renal pelvis and presents an irregular margin laterally (*arrows*). It extends into the infundibulum to the lower pole with consequent slight dilatation of the calix to the lower pole. The appearance is strongly suggestive of a transitional cell carcinoma of the renal pelvis. (B) Selective renal arteriogram. This patient had two vessels to the kidney. Only the upper vessel is opacified; the supplementary artery supplying the lower pole is unfilled. Note that there are a number of small irregular vessels representing tumor vessels adjacent to the area of irregularity in the renal pelvis (*arrows*). The presence of these abnormal vessels demonstrates clearly that the tumor mass extends laterally into the parenchyma despite the fact that it has arisen in the renal pelvis.

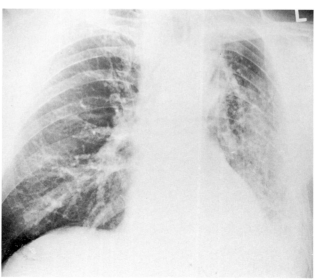

A

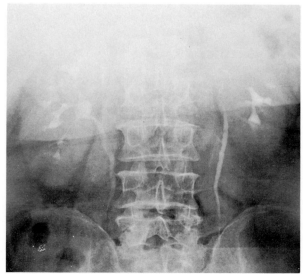

B

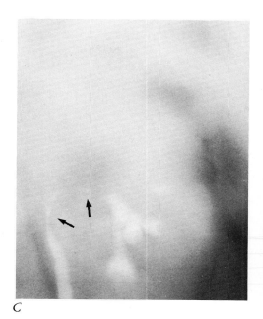

C

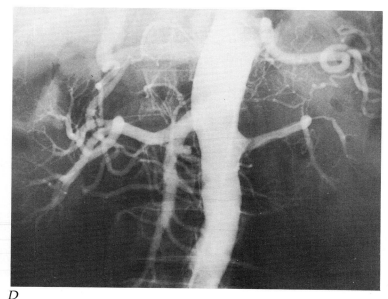

D

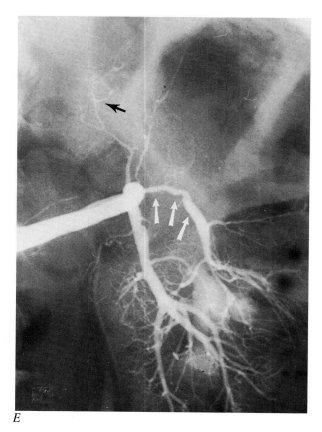

E

Figure 52-22. Transitional cell carcinoma of the kidney: differential diagnosis from tuberculosis. (A) Chest film. There is decreased volume of the left hemithorax associated with pulmonary fibrous lesions and pleural thickening as the residue of a tuberculous infection. (B) Urogram. The lower pole calices on the left are normal, but there is nonvisualization of the upper pole calices. The infundibulum to the middle calix is obliterated. (C) Laminogram. Marked narrowing of the pelvis of the kidney and of the upper ureter is seen (*arrows*). A single calix is seen in the midportion of the kidney, with no visualization of the infundibulum. (D) Abdominal aortogram. The right kidney appears normal. The left kidney demonstrates narrowed vessels, as to an atrophic kidney. (E) Selective renal arteriogram. Encasement of the central branches of the renal artery, particularly involving the branch to the midportion of the kidney (*white arrows*), is visible. Multiple small branches extend to the upper pole of the left kidney (*black arrow*). With the history of tuberculosis, the amputation of vessels, and the impingement on infundibula, the possibility of chronic tuberculous pyonephrosis in the upper portion of the kidney was considered. Epinephrine arteriography showed tumor vessels. Nephrectomy then was performed; the pathologic diagnosis was transitional cell carcinoma.

Angiography. Selective renal arteriography may be rewarding in establishing the diagnosis, clarifying the extent of the disease, and depicting the vascular anatomy preoperatively. Relatively few of these tumors are localized to the renal pelvis or collecting system. Frequently they infiltrate the kidney and, at times, produce the picture of an infiltrative disorder, without hypervascularity. Most of these tumors are hypovascular, but in many of them tumor vessels may be defined (see Fig. 52-21B), particularly if magnification and epinephrine arteriography are performed. Vascular encasement and a tumor blush are relatively common (Fig. 52-22) (Table 52-13), and arteriovenous shunting is never observed. The degree of main vascular involvement may be very extensive, and, at times, amputation of branch renal arteries is an important characteristic. In half of the cases, the pelviureteric artery is enlarged [79].

Renal Venography. Renal venography may be of great value in demonstrating venous encasement by renal pelvic carcinoma when the diagnosis is in doubt (Fig. 52-23). It also establishes the presence or absence of major renal vein invasion.

Differential Diagnosis

A filling defect in the renal pelvis may be a tumor, a blood clot, or a calculus. Although the distinction is usually readily made from the urogram, at times the diagnosis is unclear and arteriography may be required for a more definitive assessment. When the tumor extends into the parenchyma, it may resemble renal cell carcinoma, benign renal tumors, renal tuberculosis,

Table 52-13. Angiographic Findings in
22 Cases of Renal Pelvic Carcinoma

Finding	Number of Patients	Percentage of Patients with Finding
Prominent pelvico-ureteral artery	12	55
Neovascularity	18	82
Blush	18	82
Vessel encasement	16	73
Arteriovenous shunting	0	—

Adapted from Rabinowitz et al. [79].

and other chronic inflammatory processes. Infundibular narrowing may be produced by transitional cell carcinoma, by inflammation, or even by vascular imprints. Arteriography firmly establishes the relationship of the vascular bed to the involved infundibulum (Fig. 52-24).

TREATMENT

Nephrectomy and ureterectomy are the treatment of choice.

PROGNOSIS

The outlook is worse than with renal cell carcinoma: roughly 35 to 41 percent survive at 5 years and 10 to 18 percent survive at 10 years [81]. The prognosis depends on the stage at the time of discovery and the degree of tissue differentiation histologically.

OTHER TUMORS

Adenoma

The adenomas are the commonest benign renal tumors; many are found incidentally on examination of renal tissue at autopsy or in surgical specimens [107]. They are composed of small, uniform epithelial cells and have a papillary growth pattern. Preoperative distinction between large adenomas and renal cell carcinoma can be difficult because some adenomas have malignant features [21].

Adenomas rarely cause symptoms during life, but they may grow to considerable size and then be discovered as a mass on a urographic examination. A recent report of five cases indicated the presence of caliceal distortion in three, renal displacement in three, and calcification in one. Two of the tumors were lucent, and three were dense. Angiography in renal adenoma reveals increased vascularity in some cases, but with vessels less bizarre than in carcinoma; decreased vascularity may occur with a faint blush or the appearance of a cyst; and a third type of adenoma has a relatively normal appearance [52]. Since these tumors are benign, conservative therapy would be warranted if the diagnosis was established by percutaneous ultrasonically guided biopsy. In all five cases described by Holt et al., nephrectomy was performed [52].

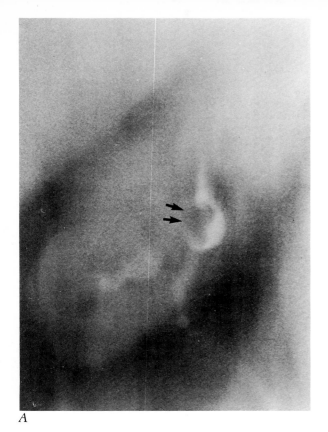

A

Figure 52-23. Renal venography in a renal pelvic carcinoma. The patient had entered the hospital because of hematuria. (A) Intravenous urogram: laminographic section. A lobulated filling defect is visible in the pelvis of the kidney (*arrows*). (B) Selective renal arteriogram. No definite abnormalities are visible, although there is a suggestion of a slight irregularity at the lateral edge of the dorsal renal arterial branch extending to the lower pole. (C) Selective renal venogram. Gross irregularity and encasement of the renal venous branch adjacent to the pelvis of the kidney is apparent (*arrows*). These findings confirm the malignant nature of the filling defect visible in the pelvis, which might otherwise have been a clot or stone on the basis of the radiographic appearance alone. (Courtesy of Stanley Baum, M.D.)

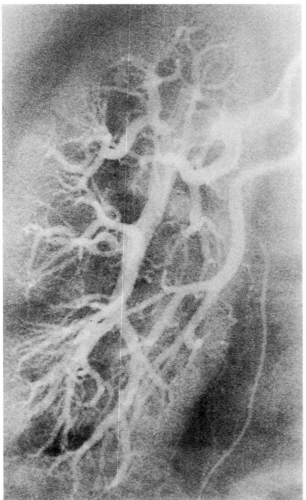

B

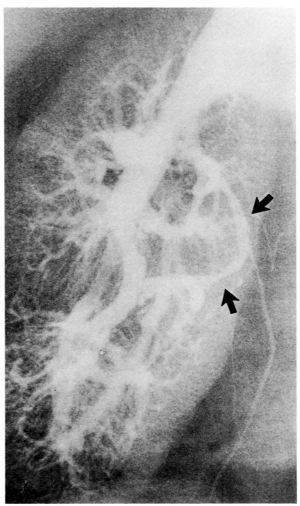

C

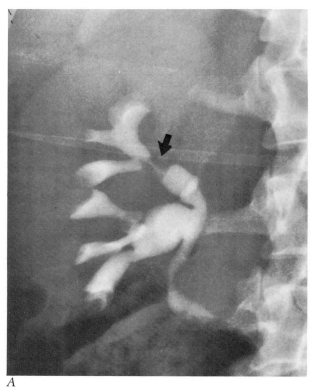

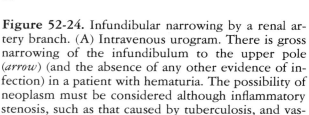

A

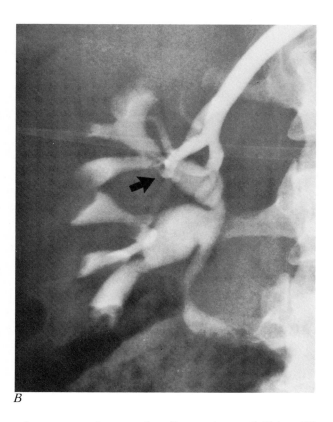

B

Figure 52-24. Infundibular narrowing by a renal artery branch. (A) Intravenous urogram. There is gross narrowing of the infundibulum to the upper pole (*arrow*) (and the absence of any other evidence of infection) in a patient with hematuria. The possibility of neoplasm must be considered although inflammatory stenosis, such as that caused by tuberculosis, and vascular compression are also diagnostic possibilities. (B) The narrowing of the infundibulum (*arrow*) represents a vascular impression, caused by the ventral branch of the renal artery. It could readily be eliminated with ureteral compression and altered positioning of the patient.

Hamartoma

Renal hamartoma (angiomyolipoma) is of greatest importance because it is difficult to differentiate from hypervascular clear cell carcinoma. The tumors associated with tuberous sclerosis present little diagnostic problem: 60 to 80 percent of patients with such tumors have multiple lesions in their kidneys in association with adenoma sebaceum and the classic features of the syndrome. Solitary tumors almost invariably come to surgery. Most occur in females. Pathologically, the tumor is composed of smooth muscle, fat, and angiomatous tissue.

The symptoms are usually vague, and the tumor is commonly found on a urogram as part of a general examination. Flank pain may be noted in some patients, and occasionally there may be hematuria. In a small percentage of cases, the presence of fat in a renal mass suggests the diagnosis on the plain film. Rarely, calcification may

be found. With filling of the collecting system during intravenous urography, a renal mass is defined, which displaces and distorts the calices but rarely amputates the calices and infundibula. When the hamartoma is associated with tuberous sclerosis or there are multiple hamartomas, the appearance is similar to that of adult polycystic disease. Conventional tomography may reveal low-density areas produced by fat (Fig. 52-25), and computed tomography of the tumor is also helpful in defining the invariable lipomatous component [48, 86].

The characteristic angiographic appearance is that of hypervascularity, a large feeder artery, tortuous vessels that may be circumferentially arranged in the arterial phase, and multiple aneurysms and a "sunburst" or "whorled" appearance in the nephrographic and venous phases (Fig. 52-25). Arteriovenous shunting is not observed, but filling of lakes is commonly in evidence. Although the findings have been said to be characteristic [69], hamartoma cannot be definitively distinguished from carcinoma on the basis of angiography.

Nephrectomy is usually performed for isolated hamartoma because of the difficulty of distinguishing it from renal cell carcinoma [10].

Other Tumors

Fibromas, leiomyomas, and neurogenic tumors, such as neurofibroma or schwannoma of the kidney (Fig. 52-26), sometimes reach considerable size and may be highly vascular, suggesting a malignant tumor.

Metastases

Ten percent of all patients who die of carcinoma have renal metastases [5]. The primary sites include the breast, lung, and other organs (Table 52-14). The metastases urographically appear as mass lesions and angiographically resemble the angioarchitecture of the primary tumor. Although metastatic renal tumors are at least twice as common as primary tumors at autopsy, they come to clinical attention far less often. The explanation is clear: Renal spread is part of a disseminated neoplastic process in which the involvement of other viscera frequently is the critical issue for the patient [13].

Renal Pseudotumors

A number of conditions mimic tumors of the kidney and require recognition if elaborate diagnostic procedures and surgery are to be avoided. Among these, prominent columns of Bertin, or focal cortical hyperplasia, represents a projection of normal renal cortical tissue into the renal sinus (Figs. 52-27, 52-28). The majority occur between the middle and upper pole calices and are marginated medially because of surrounding renal sinus fat. Caliceal stretching and deformity may be present, but arteriography demonstrates no tumor vessels, and there is a homogeneous, well-circumscribed nephrographic blush [77]. On [197]Hg chlormerodin renal scanning, pseudotumors do not show up as a cold spot or other defect [75].

Congenital lobulation is a common anatomic variant most often observed in the middle segment of the lateral margin of the kidney. It may mimic a renal mass and/or suggest cortical atrophy secondary to focal pyelonephritis or renal infarction.

Renal fibrolipomatosis is associated with excessive fat in the renal sinus producing pelvocaliceal deformities suggestive of tumor or cyst.

Focal or diffuse renal hypertrophy may follow infection, trauma, infarction, or obstruction and may suggest a mass on urography because of distortion of the calices or altered renal contour (Fig. 52-29). Such variants demonstrate no tumor vessels on angiography and frequently have associated signs of the predisposing conditions, such as chronic pyelonephritis, and a normal renal scan with [197]Hg chlormerodin.

The "dromedary hump" of the left kidney is now generally recognized as a normal variation, possibly caused by the adjacent spleen.

Other lesions that may simulate tumors, such as parapelvic cysts (Fig. 52-30), hydronephrosis of the upper pole of a duplicated collecting system [73], intrarenal abscess, intrarenal hematomas, and xanthogranulomatous pyelonephritis require careful and critical evaluation before a neoplasm can be excluded.

Table 52-14. Primary Site of Carcinomas Metastasizing to Kidney in 781 Consecutive Autopsied Cases

Primary Site	Number of Cases	Number of Cases with Renal Metastases	Percentage of Cases with Renal Metastases
Kidney	34	8	24
Lung	160	36	23
Breast	167	21	13
Stomach	119	12	11
Pancreas	32	3	9
Colon	118	9	8
Ovary	64	3	5
Rectum	87	3	3
Total	781	95	12

Adapted from Abrams et al. [5].

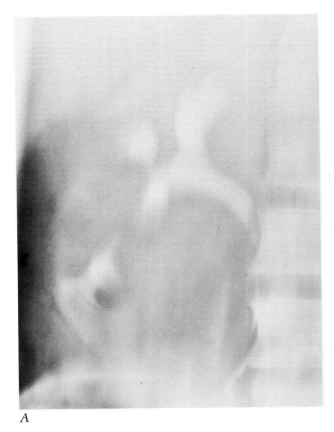

A

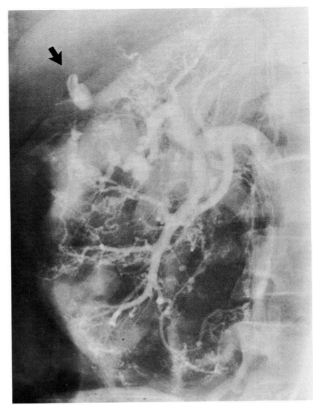

B

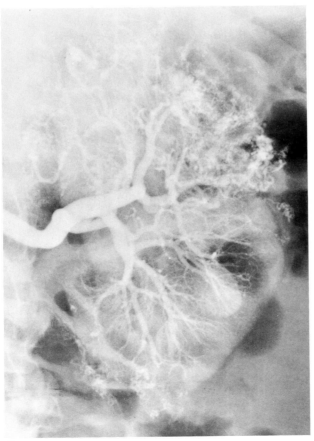

C

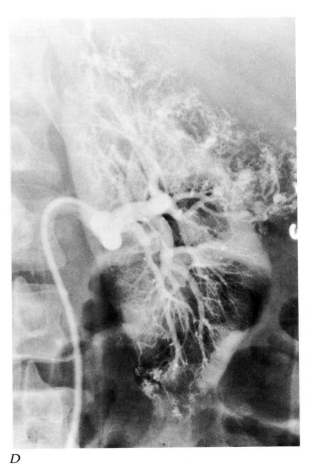

D

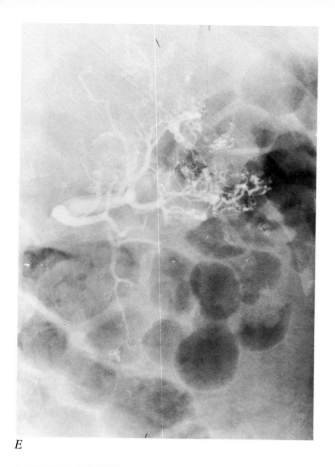

E

Figure 52-25. Renal hamartomas in a patient with tuberous sclerosis. (A) Tomogram of the right kidney during urography. The collecting system is grossly distorted, with the appearance of multiple masses. A number of lucent areas, in particular in the lateral aspect of the kidney, suggest the presence of fat. (B) Selective right renal arteriogram. A bizarre vascular pattern is apparent, characterized in particular by multiple sacular aneurysms (*arrow*) throughout the tumor masses. (C) Selective left renal arteriogram. Large vascular masses are present in both the upper and lower poles of the kidney, with the characteristically distorted vascular bed associated with hamartoma. Note that the multiple aneurysms demonstrated in particular in (C) are considered characteristic of the vascular pattern in hamartoma. (D) Selective left renal arteriogram, left posterior oblique position. The abnormal vessels are visible extending well outside the projected normal renal contour. (E) Selective epinephrine arteriogram. Only the abnormal vessels fill, while the normal renal arteries demonstrate failure of opacification in their midportion and distal portion. Because these vessels are relatively primitive and have relatively less muscle tissue than 20 normal vessels, they fail to respond the way normal vessels do to epinephrine. When multiple tumors of this type are seen in the presence of tuberous sclerosis, the diagnosis of hamartoma is readily made. An isolated hamartoma, on the other hand, may resemble renal cell carcinoma, and the high fat content shown on computed tomography in particular may be useful.

Figure 52-26. Neurogenic tumor of the kidney. The patient presented with increasing distention of his left lower abdomen and the sensation of a mass. Microscopic hematuria was present. The urogram demonstrated nonfunction of the left kidney, with a large mass apparently associated with the left kidney. (A) Aortogram, 1.5 seconds. There are gross displacement of the major renal arteries and the beginning filling of some abnormal vessels. (B) Aortogram, 3 seconds. A huge number of irregular, tortuous, randomly distributed vessels are opacified, a finding that is strongly suggestive of a malignant neoplasm. A nephrectomy was performed. The tumor demonstrated the classic histology of a schwannoma, a neurogenic tumor. Highly vascular neurogenic tumors are difficult to distinguish from classic renal cell carcinomas.

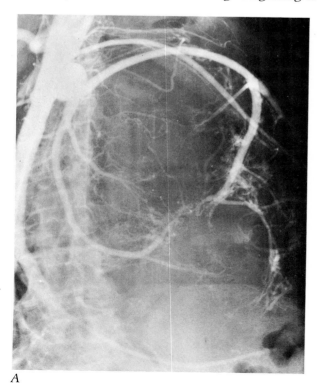

A

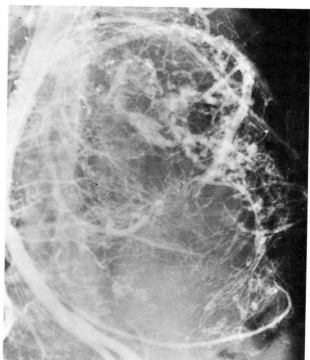

B

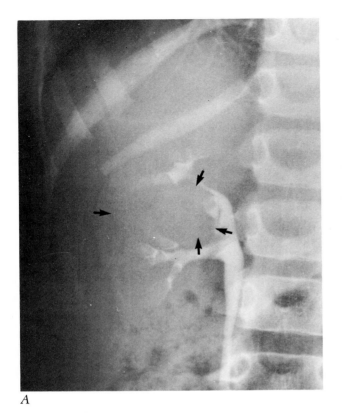

A

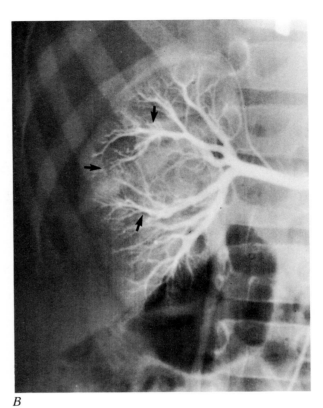

B

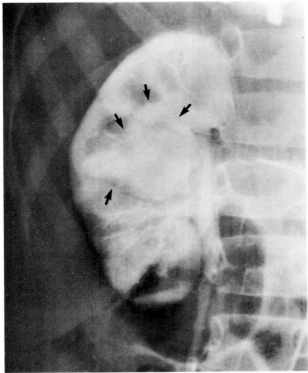

C

Figure 52-27. Renal pseudotumor. (A) Urogram. An apparent mass is visible on the right (*arrows*), separating the infundibulum to the midportion of the kidney from the infundibulum to the upper pole. (B) Selective renal arteriogram. There is separation of interlobar branches in the region of the "mass" shown on urography (*arrows*). No tumor vessels are visualized. (C) Nephrographic phase. A dense area in the midportion of the kidney (*arrows*) represents a large column of Bertin, an infolding of renal cortical tissue that has no pathologic significance. (Courtesy of H. Taybi, M.D.)

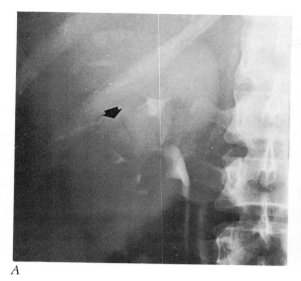
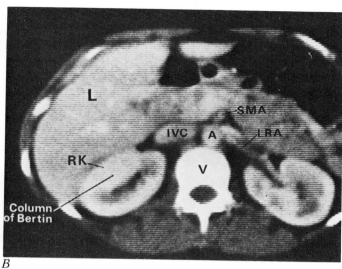

A   B

Figure 52-28. Renal pseudotumor. (A) Urogram demonstrates the separation of the upper pole and midpole calices by an apparent mass (*arrow*). (B) Computed tomogram. The "mass" lesion in the midportion of the right kidney is clearly defined as representing a column of Bertin, which is a normal variant.

Figure 52-29. Renal pseudotumor. (A) Selective arteriography. The ventral and dorsal vessels are widely separated by an apparent mass adjacent to the pelvis of the kidney. (B) Nephrographic phase. The mass is visible as an area of renal tissue (*arrows*), which represents compensatory hypertrophy in the presence of gross pyelonephritis involving the lower pole in particular but also the midportion of the kidney.

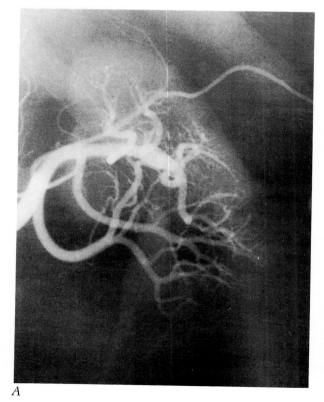
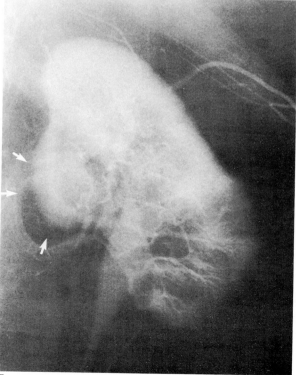

A   B

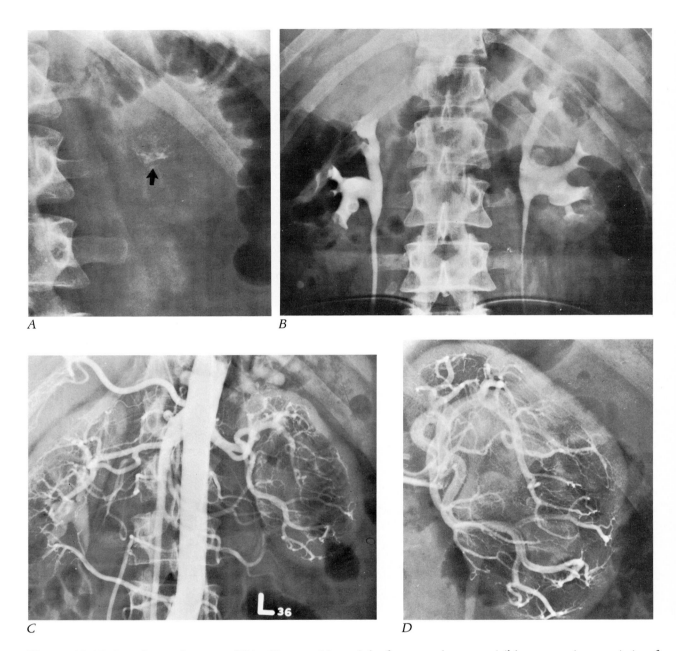

A

B

C

D

Figure 52-30. Renal pseudotumor. This 42-year-old man entered the hospital because of hematuria and hypertension. (A) Plain film. There is amorphous calcification in the left kidney (*arrow*). (B) Urogram. There was good concentration but evidence of a mass lesion on the left separating the upper and middle pole calices and compressing them. (C) Aortogram. The right kidney was normal, but the left kidney demonstrated splaying of vessels around a mass. (D and E) Selective renal arteriograms with magnification. Mul-tiple fine vessels were visible, none characteristic of renal cell carcinoma but presenting an unusual distribution for the renal circulation. (F) Specimen. On the assumption that the mass represented a renal tumor, a nephrectomy was performed. A 4-cm subcapsular posterolateral cyst showing fibrosis and focal calcification and ossification was found (*arrows*). It produced compression of the superior portion of the pelvis and calices.

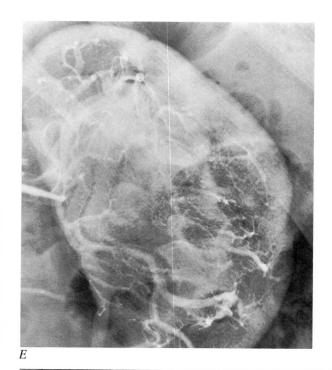

E

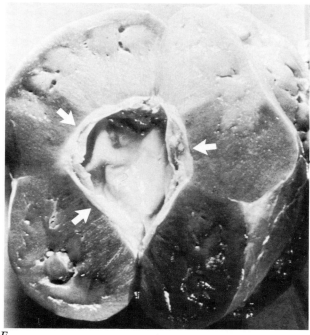

F

Renal Cysts

The subject of renal cystic disease is complex and beset with varying terms and classifications. Solitary renal cysts are of central importance in their resemblance, as renal masses, to renal neoplasms and therefore require detailed discussion. Congenital renal cystic disease presenting as renal mass lesions in infancy is covered in Chapter 75, while polycystic kidney is reviewed in the early pages of this chapter, in the discussion of the differential diagnosis of renal cell carcinoma.

INCIDENCE

Renal cysts are common in autopsies of adults over the age of 50 [51] but are observed in no more than 1 to 2 percent of patients at urography [11]. They are seen at all ages but most commonly in the sixth and seventh decades.

PATHOLOGY

The cysts are smooth, thin-walled masses that contain a clear serous fluid of low specific gravity (Fig. 52-31). More often located at the lower pole of the kidney, they vary markedly in size and volume and may contain up to a liter of fluid. Cysts are covered by the renal capsule, and they usually lie more or less laterally. As they enlarge, they

compress adjacent renal parenchyma. The cyst wall is no more than 1 to 2 mm in thickness and is lined with cuboidal epithelium. There has been much dispute as to the incidence of carcinoma arising from the cyst wall. Most observers consider the figure of 1 percent reliable [33], but estimates as high as 7 percent have been reported [42].

SYMPTOMS AND SIGNS

Small or modest-sized cysts rarely cause symptoms and are usually detected as incidental findings on the intravenous urogram. Large cysts may be associated with bulging of the flank and flank discomfort. Local pain may be produced by stretching of the renal capsule. Occasionally polycythemia [24] or hypertension [7] appear to be associated with simple renal cysts. One patient with a renal cyst had hypertension of six years' duration with a high ipsilateral renal vein renin value. Aspiration of the cyst was associated with a prompt remission in hypertension with a diastolic pressure of 80 mm throughout 9 months of follow-up [84].

DIAGNOSTIC EVALUATION

Intravenous Urography
The plain film demonstrates a smooth mass protruding from the renal border. So-called eggshell

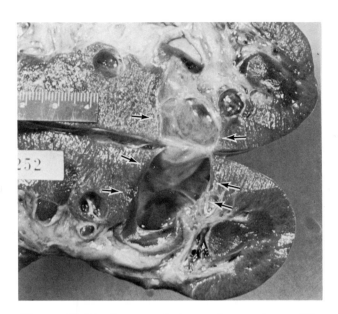

Figure 52-31. Gross pathology of a renal cyst. The kidney has been hemisected. The cyst (*arrows*) extends to the lateral edge of the kidney. It is smooth and thin walled and contained a clear, serous fluid of low specific gravity. In general, cysts vary markedly in size and volume and may contain up to a liter of fluid. Cysts are covered by the renal capsule and usually lie more or less laterally. As they enlarge, they compress adjacent renal parenchyma. The cyst wall is no more than 1 to 2 mm in thickness and is lined with cuboidal epithelium. There has been much dispute as to the incidence of carcinoma arising from the cyst wall. Most observers consider the figure of 1 percent reliable [31], but estimates as high as 7 percent have been reported [39].

calcification—a thin, smooth, curvilinear calcific density—is typical of simple renal cyst and is observed in 2 to 3 percent of cysts [30]. Unfortunately, it may also be observed (rarely) in carcinoma [60].

The early nephrographic film of 10 to 30 seconds is useful in depicting an avascular mass within the kidney. With contrast in the collecting system, varying degrees of deformity are demonstrated (Fig. 52-32). If the cyst is small, lateral, and partially extrarenal, the urographic appearance may be normal. More often, with moderate-sized-to-large cysts the calices are displaced, compressed, and "splayed," or spread. The infundibula may be narrowed or stretched. With large cysts, the caliceal system may be clumped or grouped in a relatively small portion of the kidney. The pelvis may be compressed,

flattened, or distorted. The axis of the kidney can be shifted in any direction, depending on the location and size of the cyst.

In general, no matter how great the impression on the collecting system, the calices remain delicate and sharp (unless infundibular obstruction occurs) and show no sign of irregularity or invasion. Similarly, the margins of the infundibula are smooth, even when narrowed, and are not irregular. Except for the nephrographic phase, which may strongly suggest the cystic character of the lesion, the urographic features cannot finally distinguish cyst from solid tumor.

Nephrotomography
Nephrotomography has been widely applied to evaluation of renal masses [11, 75, 76]. In approximately 85 percent of cases it establishes the diagnosis of renal cyst [46]. When the diagnosis of cyst is unequivocal, nephrotomography is highly accurate. Recent emphasis on the use of both the vascular and the nephrographic phases indicates the importance of the nephrographic phase for cyst evaluation and of the vascular phase for diagnosis of carcinoma [46].

Like ultrasonography, nephrotomography is a screening procedure, and to some extent it duplicates the diagnostic data derived from ultrasonography. Since our approach to renal masses ultimately involves cyst puncture or angiography or both as decisive procedures, we believe that nephrotomography provides useful supportive information but is rarely definitive, except in small, peripheral cysts, in which the appearance is unequivocal. In central cysts, it is useless, and it should not be performed.

Ultrasonography
B-mode ultrasound scanning is a major noninvasive advance in the evaluation of renal masses. It should follow the urogram as the next diagnostic step. The classic cyst is entirely lacking in internal echoes, at both high and low sensitivity levels (Fig. 52-33). The posterior cyst wall is smooth and well defined. Through transmission—the delineation of structures deep to the cyst—is characteristic. The accuracy of ultrasonography in simple cysts is approximately 90 to 95 percent [11, 32, 64, 78].

In some cystic lesions, such as abscesses, necrotic or hemorrhagic tumors, multiple cysts, and hydronephrosis, a complex sonographic pattern is observed with both cystic and solid (echoic) elements. Finally, the sonogram may indicate a solid mass, typical of tumor. If a solid or complex

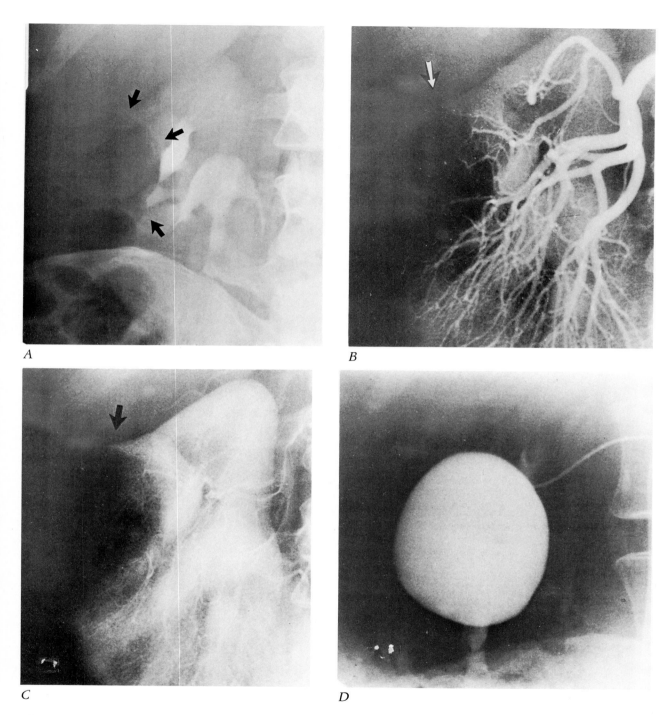

A

B

C

D

Figure 52-32. Renal cyst. (A) Urogram. A smooth, lucent mass at the lateral border of the right kidney (*arrows*) compresses and displaces the upper pole and midpole calices. (B) Selective renal arteriogram. The vessels to the lucent area are sharply displaced, and a so-called beak (*arrow*) characteristic of a renal cyst is seen. (C) Nephrographic phase. The beak (*arrow*) is well visualized, as are the striking lucency and absence of neoplastic vessels. Nevertheless, the entire wall of the cyst could not be visualized, and so a cyst puncture was undertaken. (D) Renal cyst puncture. The smoothly outlined ovoid collection of contrast agent represents a benign cyst. Fluid for cell and fat analyses was obtained, but no malignant cells were found. It is essential in cyst puncture that the area of the contrast-filled cyst fully account for any filling defect on the urogram.

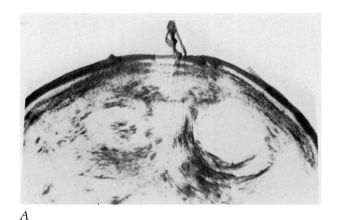

A

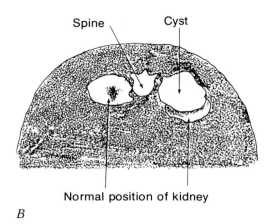

B

Figure 52-33. Renal cyst: ultrasonography. (A) Sonogram. (B) Diagram. A large mass is visible adjacent and dorsal to the left kidney, which is completely anechoic. Thus the diagnosis of cyst can be made confidently. The ultrasound study was followed by a cyst puncture, which revealed a smooth-walled collection of fluid. The cyst was collapsed, and a follow-up examination 6 months later failed to show any reaccumulation of fluid.

pattern is observed, selective renal arteriography should follow.

After the diagnosis of simple cyst is made, the next step is cyst puncture. Ultrasonography also is useful for cyst localization during cyst puncture and aspiration.

Computed Tomography

Because a cyst contains fluid, it attenuates the x-ray beam less than solid tissue does. This difference allows a reliable distinction of cyst from tumor to be made by computed tomographic scanning (Fig. 52-34).

Cyst Puncture

For many years we have used cyst puncture with injection of opaque contrast agent or, at times, injection of gas as a diagnostic method in cases of suspected renal cyst. The examination may be performed under fluoroscopic or ultrasound guidance. The initial step involves aspiration of fluid for cytologic examination and for analysis of the fat and enzyme content. The aspirate is replaced by the contrast agent, and films in multiple projections are obtained (Fig. 52-35; see also Fig. 52-32).

Demonstration of the typical smooth wall of the simple cyst in association with normal cytology and fat content is sufficient evidence of the benign character of the lesion to require conservative management [63]. It is essential that the entire volume of the mass visualized on the urogram be accounted for by the opacified cyst.

Figure 52-34. Renal cyst: computed tomography. A large mass is visible in the left kidney (*arrows*), displacing normal parenchyma medially. The right kidney, inferior vena cava, and aorta are clearly delineated. The mass in the left kidney has less density than does normal renal tissue and represents a renal cyst with a low mean value in Hounsfield units. In general, the density of a renal cyst is close to the density of water (i.e., 0), and the density of a renal tumor lies between that of a cyst and that of the normally opacified renal parenchyma after the intravenous injection of 50 to 100 cc of contrast agent. The normal parenchyma generally measures 80 to 100 Hounsfield units after opacification. (Courtesy of Stuart Segal, M.D.)

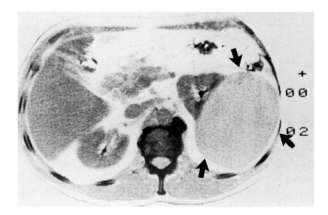

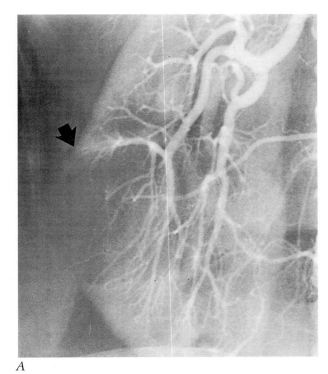

A

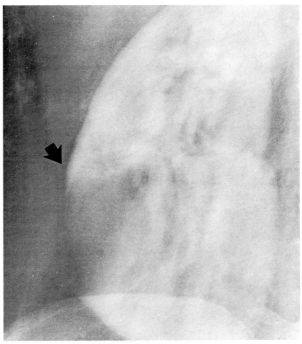

B

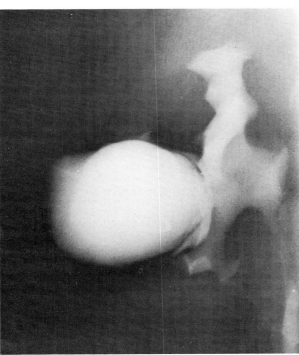

C

Figure 52-35. Renal cyst. (A) Arteriogram. Note the displacement of vessels and the avascular area (*arrow*). (B) Nephrogram. A "beak" (*arrow*) characteristic of a benign cyst is visible. (C) Cyst puncture. The cyst is opaque and accounts fully for the apparent mass seen on arteriography.

Although there is a possibility that a small carcinoma in the cyst may still be missed, the likelihood is very small [87] and must be balanced against the morbidity and mortality of surgery. Furthermore, the final step in cyst puncture, emptying the cyst as completely as possible, may be accompanied by permanent collapse and a lack of subsequent reaccumulation of cyst fluid.

The presence of old blood in the aspirate from a cyst poses a problem. Even if the cyst wall is smooth and the cytologic examination normal, such patients require arteriography. If there is no angiographic evidence of neoplasm and if all other criteria for benign cyst are present, conservative management is probably indicated [53, 87]. Harris et al. [49] have emphasized the need for surgical exploration in these cases, but in each of their three cases a significant element besides the bloody fluid was inconsistent with the diagnosis of simple renal cyst. In one case, there was an irregular cyst wall; in another case, there was a filling defect; and in another case, there were filling defects, irregular collection of contrast agent, and elevated lactic dehydrogenase levels. Many renal cysts are now discovered on CT sections of the abdomen for unrelated conditions. Although CT is clearly not infallible in the assessment of renal masses, cyst puncture is not always performed when the appearance on CT is classic.

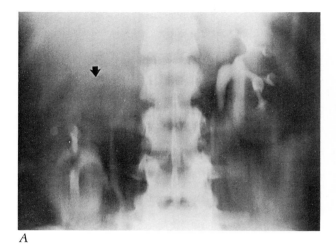

A

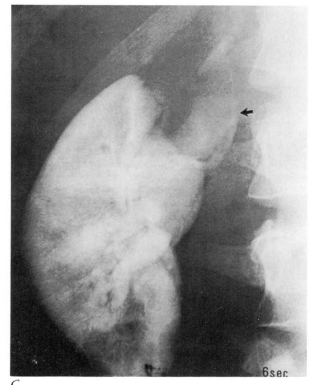

C

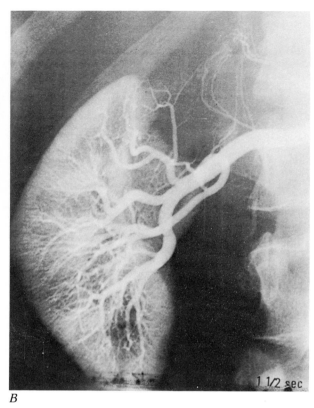

B

Figure 52-36. Hydronephrosis of the upper pole of a double collecting system. (A) Urogram. An apparent cyst (*arrow*) is visible in the upper pole in the kidney. Note that no calices extend above the midportion of the kidney and that there are fewer calices on the right side than on the left side. (B) Selective renal arteriogram, arterial phase. A few small vessels extend from the main renal artery and its branches to surround the apparent upper pole cyst. (C) Nephrographic phase. A thin but definite curvilinear density (*arrow*) surrounding the apparent cystic area medially represents compressed parenchyma. Surgical exploration revealed a hydronephrotic upper pole of a double collecting system on the right.

Angiography

The angiographic criteria of simple renal cyst are well established. A sharply defined radiolucent mass with a thin, smooth wall (1 mm in thickness) and an acute angle at the junction of cyst wall and renal cortex forming a "beak" is characteristic of a cyst (Fig. 52-35). Angiography has a high degree of accuracy, but it may be misleading (rarely) in the presence of avascular or cystic tumors. If any of the classic diagnostic criteria are lacking, epinephrine arteriography should be undertaken to enhance the demonstration of tumor vessels.

In addition, cyst puncture should be performed as the final diagnostic step if it has not been done.

DIFFERENTIAL DIAGNOSIS

Like renal cell carcinoma, renal cyst must be distinguished from all other renal masses. In particular, avascular or cystic renal cell carcinoma is the most important single diagnosis to establish because the treatment is radically different. Hydronephrosis of the upper pole of a kidney with a double collecting system is at times quite difficult to differentiate from a cyst (Fig. 52-36). Renal fibrolipomatosis may present a urographic image resembling that of either cyst or tumor.

TREATMENT

"Cysts should be explored surgically" [31]. There are still many urologists who feel uncomfortable even when the classic radiographic, sonographic, and computed tomographic criteria for simple cyst are definitely present. Our own concept is that when the diagnostic criteria for simple cyst are present, particularly following cyst puncture, conservative management is desirable. When the diagnosis is in doubt, exploration is mandatory.

Diagnostic Decision Tree in Renal Mass Lesions

All renal mass lesions must undergo special investigation. The stakes are reasonably high: the untreated tumor, mistakenly diagnosed as cyst, may spread locally, metastasize, and move the patient into the incurable group. The benign cyst, mistakenly taken to surgery, exposes the patient to significant morbidity and mortality. A mortality of 1.5 to 2.4 percent and a major morbidity of 30 percent have been reported [59, 74]. Pollack et al. [75] have compared the biologic and economic cost of the radiologic approach and the surgical approach to the diagnosis of renal cyst (Table 52-15). Not mentioned in Table 52-15 is the potential cost of leaving a renal carcinoma untreated, that is, failing to detect a carcinoma in the cyst. According to Sherwood and Trott, the likelihood is less than 1 in 1,000 [87]. Thus, the importance of a reasonable, systematic, and efficient approach to diagnosis must be emphasized.

Cyst puncture has been questioned on the grounds that tumor cells might be spread by the needle. This theoretical concern has not been substantiated in practice. No decrease in survival rate was observed in patients with renal cell carcinoma following needling as compared to those without needling [98].

Even the urologists are changing their approach to renal masses. "With modern radiologic techniques and analysis of cyst fluid, an asymptomatic renal mass can be diagnosed accurately. The non-operative approach is precise, has

Table 52-15. Comparison of Radiologic Diagnosis and Surgical Diagnosis of Renal Cyst

	Radiologic	Surgical
Diagnostic accuracy	100%*	100% (approx.)
Major morbidity	0%	30%
Mortality	0%	1.5%
Socioeconomic aspects		
Hospital days (av.)	0–1	7–10
Hospital costs (av.)	$130–180	$1,500–2,000
Lost wages (av.)	1 day	27 days

*8 percent of patients required an operation because of indeterminate results.
Adapted from Pollack et al. [75].

almost no morbidity and costs half as much as operative evaluation" [23].

The widening application of CT to the diagnosis of renal mass lesions is decreasing the need for arteriography in some cases. CT is also very useful in accurate staging of the tumor. Furthermore, for patients over the age of 60, CT depicts so many large cysts that fewer punctures are now being performed when the appearance is typical.

The problem of renal mass lesions is particularly acute in the aged. All too often the mass is discovered on the urogram performed for the patient with prostatic disease. In the older age group, the risk of renal exploration is higher. Scrupulous attention to the nonsurgical diagnostic management of such patients may forestall unnecessary surgery oriented not toward treatment so much as toward diagnostic confirmation.

ACKNOWLEDGMENT

Much of the material in this chapter appeared in *Cardiovascular Radiology* (1:59–75; 125–139, 1978). It is used here with the permission of the editor and the publisher.

References

1. Abrams, H. L. The response of neoplastic renal vessels to epinephrine in man. *Radiology* 82:217, 1964.
2. Abrams, H. L. Renal tumor vs. renal cyst. *Cardiovasc. Radiol.* 1:59, 125, 1979.
3. Abrams, H. L., and Obrez, I. Epinephrine in the Study of Renal Tumors. In H. L. Abrams (ed.), *Angiography* (2nd ed.). Boston: Little, Brown, 1971. P. 831.

4. Abrams, H. L., Obrez, I., Hollenberg, N. K., and Adams, D. F.   Pharmacoangiography of the renal vascular bed. *Curr. Probl. Radiol.* 1:1, 1971.

5. Abrams, H. L., Spiro, R., and Goldstein, N.   Metastases in carcinoma. Analysis of 1,000 autopsied cases. *Cancer* 3:74, 1950.

6. Alfidi, R. J., Haaga, J., Meaney, T. F., MacIntyre, W. J., Gonzalez, L., Tarar, R., Zelch, M. G., Boller, M., Cook, S. A., and Jelden, G.   Computed tomography of the thorax and abdomen; a preliminary report. *Radiology* 117:257, 1975.

7. Babka, J. C., Cohen, M. S., and Sode, J.   Solitary intrarenal cyst causing hypertension. *N. Engl. J. Med.* 291:343, 1974.

8. Bartley, O., and Helander, C. G.   Angiography in spontaneously healed hypernephromas. *Acta Radiol. [Diagn.]* (Stockh.) 57:417, 1962.

9. Bartley, O., and Hultquist, G. T.   Spontaneous regression of hypernephromas. *Acta Pathol. Microbiol. Scand.* 27:448, 1950.

10. Becker, J. A., Kinkhabwala, M., Pollack, J., and Bosniak, M.   Angiomyolipoma (hamartoma) of the kidney: An angiographic review. *Acta Radiol.* 14:561, 1973.

11. Becker, J. A., and Schneider, M.   Simple cyst of the kidney. *Semin. Roentgenol.* 10:103, 1975.

12. Beckmann, C. F., and Abrams, H. L.   Applications of renal venography. *Cardiovasc. Intervent. Radiol.* 3:45, 1981.

13. Ben-Menachem, Y., Marcos, J., Wallace, S., and Medelin, H.   Angiography of renal metastases. *Br. J. Radiol.* 47:869, 1974.

14. Bloom, H. N., Mattey, W. E., Arevalo, F. L., and Delguercio, L. R. M.   B-mode ultrasound scanning in the diagnosis of renal lesions. *Am. J. Surg.* 129:636, 1975.

15. Boijsen, E., and Folin, J.   Angiography in the diagnosis of renal carcinoma. *Radiologe* 1:173, 1961.

16. Bosniak, M. A., Ambos, M. A., Madayag, M. A., Lefleur, R. S., and Casarella, W. J.   Epinephrine-enhanced renal angiography in renal mass lesions: Is it worth performing? *AJR* 129:647, 1977.

17. Bosniak, M. A., Madayag, M. A., and Ambos, M. A.   Renal cell carcinoma determined by chance. Abstract presented at the 63rd Annual Meeting of the Radiological Society of North America, Chicago, Ill., Nov. 1977.

18. Böttiger, L. E., Blanck, C., and von Schreeb, T.   Renal carcinoma: An attempt to correlate symptoms and findings with the histopathologic picture. *Acta Med. Scand.* 180:329, 1966.

19. Böttiger, L. E., Hallberg, D., and von Schreeb, T.   Renal carcinoma as an accidental finding. *Acta Chir. Scand.* 127:158, 1964.

20. Chisholm, G. B., and Ray, R. R.   The systemic effects of malignant renal tumors. *Br. J. Urol.* 43:687, 1971.

21. Clark, P., and Anderson, K.   Tumors of the Kidney and Ureter. In J. Blandy (ed.), *Urology*. London: Blackwell, 1976. P. 391.

22. Clark, R. E., Moss, A. A., DeLorimer, A. A., and Palubinskas, A. J.   Arteriography of Wilms' tumor. *AJR* 113:476, 1971.

23. Clayman, R. V., Williams, R. D., and Fraley, E. E.   Current concepts in cancer: The pursuit of the renal mass. *N. Engl. J. Med.* 300:72, 1979.

24. Cohen, N. N.   Polycythemia associated with bilateral unilocular renal cysts. *Arch. Intern. Med.* 105:301, 1960.

25. Cole, A. T., Mandell, J., Fried, F. A., and Stabb, E. V.   The place of bone scan in the diagnosis of renal cell carcinoma. *J. Urol.* 114:364, 1975.

26. Cornell, S. H., and Dolan, K. D.   Angiographic findings in renal carcinoma: Analysis of 25 cases. *J. Urol.* 98:71, 1967.

27. Creevy, C. D.   Confusing clinical manifestations of malignant renal neoplasms. *Arch. Intern. Med.* 55:895, 1935.

28. Crocker, D. W.   Renal Tumors. In S. C. Sommers (ed.), *Kidney Pathology Decennial, 1966–1975*. New York: Appleton-Century-Crofts, 1975. P. 609.

29. Cummings, K. B., Correa, R. J., Jr., Gibbons, R. P., Stoll, H. M., Wheelis, R. F., and Mason, J. R.   Renal pelvic tumors. *J. Urol.* 113:158, 1975.

30. Daniel, W. W., Jr., Hartman, G. W., Witten, D. M., Farrow, G. M., and Kelalis, P. P.   Calcified renal masses: A review of ten years' experience at the Mayo Clinic. *Radiology* 103:503, 1972.

31. Demming, C. L., and Harvard, B. M.   Tumors of the Urogenital Tract. In M. F. Campbell and J. H. Harrison (eds.), *Urology*. Philadelphia: Saunders, 1970. P. 885.

32. Doust, V. L., Doust, B. D., and Redman, H. C.   Evaluation of ultrasonic B-mode scanning in the diagnosis of renal masses. *AJR* 117:112, 1973.

33. Emmett, J. L., Levine, S. R., and Woolner, L. B.   Co-existence of renal cyst and tumor. Incidence in 1007 cases. *Br. J. Radiol.* 35:403, 1963.

34. Ettinger, A., and Elkin, M.   Value of plain film in renal mass lesions (tumors and cysts). *Radiology* 62:372, 1954.

35. Everson, T. C.   Spontaneous regression of cancer. *Ann. N.Y. Acad. Sci.* 114:721, 1964.

36. Ferrucci, J. T., Jr.   Medical progress: Body ultrasonography. *N. Engl. J. Med.* 300:538, 590, 1979.

37. Flocks, R. H., and Kadesky, M. C.   Malignant neoplasms of the kidney: An analysis of 353 patients followed five years or more. *J. Urol.* 79:196, 1958.

38. Folin, J.   Conventional roentgenography and urography in the diagnosis of renal tumors. *Radiologe* 1:166, 1961.

39. Folin, J. Angiography in renal tumors. Its value in diagnosis and differential diagnosis as a complement to conventional methods. *Acta Radiol. [Suppl.]* (Stockh.) 267:1967.

40. Freed, S. L., Halperin, J. P., and Gordon, M. Idiopathic regression of metastases from renal cell carcinoma. *J. Urol.* 118:538, 1977.

41. Garfield, D. H., and Kennedy, B. J. Regression of metastatic renal cell carcinoma following nephrectomy. *Cancer* 30:190, 1972.

42. Gibson, T. E. Interrelationship of renal cysts and tumors: Report of three cases. *J. Urol.* 71:241, 1954.

43. Goldberg, B. B., Capitanio, M. A., and Kirkpatrick, J. A., Jr. Ultrasonic evaluation of masses in pediatric patients. *AJR* 116:677, 1972.

44. Goldberg, B. B., and Pollack, H. M. Differentiation of renal masses using A-mode ultrasound. *J. Urol.* 105:765, 1971.

45. Graham, A. P. Malignancy of the kidney. Survey of 195 cases. *J. Urol.* 58:10, 1947.

46. Greene, L. F., Fraser, R. A., and Hartman, G. W. Bolus nephrotomography in diagnosis of lesions of kidney. *Urology* 7:221, 1976.

47. Hadju, S. I., Berg, J. W., and Foote, F. W. Clinically unrecognized, silent renal-cell carcinoma in elderly cancer patients. *J. Am. Geriatr. Soc.* 18:443, 1970.

48. Hanse, G. C., Hoffman, R. B., Sample, W. F., and Becker, R. Computed tomography diagnosis of renal angiomyolipoma. *Radiology* 128:789, 1978.

49. Harris, R. D., Goergen, T. G., and Talner, L. B. The bloody renal cyst aspirate: A diagnostic dilemma. *J. Urol.* 114:832, 1975.

50. Harvey, N. A. Kidney tumors: A clinical and pathological study, with special reference to the 'hypernephroid' tumor. *J. Urol.* 57:669, 1947.

51. Heptinstall, R. H. *Pathology of the Kidney* (2nd ed.). Boston: Little, Brown, 1974.

52. Holt, R. G., Neiman, H. L., Korsower, J. M., and Newhouse, J. Angiographic features of benign renal adenoma. *Urology* 6:764, 1975.

53. Jackman, R. J., and Stevens, G. M. Benign hemorrhagic renal cyst: Nephrotomography, renal arteriography, and cyst puncture. *Radiology* 110:7, 1974.

54. Judd, E. S., and Hand, J. R. Hypernephroma. *J. Urol.* 22:10, 1929.

55. Kikkawa, K., and Lasser, E. C. 'Ring-like' or 'rim-like' calcification in renal cell carcinoma. *AJR* 107:737, 1969.

56. Koehler, P. R. The roentgen diagnosis of renal inflammatory masses—special emphasis on angiographic changes. *Radiology* 112:257, 1974.

57. Köhler, P. R. Correlation between vascular supply to the kidney and excretion as shown by urography in renal tumors. *Radiol. Clin.* 32:100, 1963.

58. Kozoll, D. D., and Kirshbaum, J. D. Relationship of benign and malignant hypernephroid tumors of kidney; clinical and pathological study of 77 cases in 12,885 necropsies. *J. Urol.* 44:435, 1940.

59. Kropp, K. A., Grayhack, J. T., Wendell, R. M., and Dahl, D. S. Morbidity and mortality of renal exploration for cyst. *Surg. Gynecol. Obstet.* 125:803, 1967.

60. Lalli, A. F. The roentgen diagnosis of renal cyst and tumor. *J. Can. Assoc. Radiol.* 17:41, 1966.

61. Lalli, A. F., Åhström, L., Ericsson, N. O., and Rudhe, U. Nephroblastoma (Wilms' tumor): Urographic diagnosis and prognosis. *Radiology* 87:495, 1966.

62. Lang, E. K. The accuracy of roentgenographic techniques in the diagnosis of renal mass lesions. *Radiology* 98:119, 1971.

63. Lang, E. K., Johnson, B., Chace, H. L., Enright, J. R., Fontenot, R., Trichel, B. E., Wood, M., Brown, R., and St. Martin, E. C. Assessment of avascular renal mass lesions: The use of nephrotomography, arteriography, cyst puncture, double contrast study and histochemical and histopathologic examination of the aspirate. *South. Med. J.* 65:1, 1972.

64. Leopold, G. R., Talner, L. B., Asher, W. M., Gosink, B., and Gittes, R. F. Renal ultrasonography: An updated approach to the diagnosis of renal cyst. *Radiology* 109:671, 1973.

65. Levine, E., Lee, K. R., Weigel, J. Preoperative determination of abdominal extent of renal cell carcinoma by computed tomography. *Radiology* 132:395, 1979.

66. Lokich, J. J., and Harrison, J. H. Renal cell carcinoma: Natural history and chemotherapeutic experience. *J. Urol.* 114:371, 1975.

67. Lucke, B., and Schlumberger, J. S. Tumors of the Kidney, Renal Pelvis, and Ureter. In *Atlas of Tumour Pathology*, Armed Forces Institute of Pathology, 1957. Sect. 8, Fasc. 33.

68. Markewitz, M., Taylor, D. A., and Veenema, R. J. Spontaneous regression of pulmonary metastases following palliative nephrectomy. *Cancer* 20:1147, 1967.

69. McCallum, R. W. The Pre-operative diagnosis of renal hamartoma. *Clin. Radiol.* 26:257, 1975.

70. McDonald, P. Retroperitoneal Tumors in Children. In H. L. Abrams (ed.), *Angiography* (2nd ed.). Boston: Little, Brown, 1971. P. 1201.

71. Meaney, T. F. Errors in angiographic diagnosis of renal masses. *Radiology* 93:361, 1969.

72. Newman, H. R., and Schulman, M. L. Renal cortical tumors: A 40-year statistical study. *Urol. Surv.* 19:2, 1969.

73. Olsson, O. Renal Malformation. In H. L. Abrams (ed.), *Angiography* (2nd ed.). Boston: Little, Brown, 1971. P. 823.

74. Plaine, L. I., and Hinman, F., Jr. Malignancy in asymptomatic renal masses. *J. Urol.* 94:342, 1965.

75. Pollack, H. M., Goldberg, B. B., and Bogash, M. Changing concepts in the diagnosis and management of renal cysts. *J. Urol.* 111:326, 1974.

76. Pollack, H. M., Goldberg, B. B., Morales, J. P., and Bogash, M. A systematized approach to the diagnosis of renal masses. *Radiology* 113:653, 1974.

77. Popky, G. L., Bogash, M., Pollack, H., and Longacre, A. M. Focal cortical hyperplasia. *J. Urol.* 102:657, 1969.

78. Pritchard, J. H., and Webber, M. Detection and diagnosis of renal masses with modern radioisotope and ultrasonic techniques. *CRC Crit. Rev. Diagn. Imaging* 5:423, 1974.

79. Rabinowitz, J., Kinkhabwala, M., Himmelfarb, E., Robinson, T., Becules, J. A., Bosniak, M., and Madayaz, M. M. Renal pelvic carcinoma: An angiographic re-evaluation. *Radiology* 102:551, 1972.

80. Riches, E. W. On carcinoma of the kidney. *Ann. R. Coll. Surg. Engl.* 32:201, 1963.

81. Riches, E. W. *Tumours of the Kidney and Ureter.* London: Livingstone, 1964.

82. Riches, E. W., Griffiths, I. H., and Thackray, A. C. New growths of the kidney and ureter. *Br. J. Urol.* 23:297, 1951.

83. Robbins, S. L. *Textbook of Pathology with Clinical Application* (2nd ed.). Philadelphia: Saunders, 1962.

84. Rockson, S. G., Stone, R. A., and Gunnells, J. C., Jr. Solitary renal cyst with segmental ischemia and hypertension. *J. Urol.* 112:550, 1974.

85. Seltzer, R. A., and Wenlund, D. E. Renal lymphoma: Arteriographic studies. *AJR* 101:692, 1967.

86. Shawker, T. H., Horváth, K. L., Dunnick, N. R., and Javadpour, N. Renal angiomyolipoma: Diagnosis by combined ultrasound and computerized tomography. *J. Urol.* 121:675, 1979.

87. Sherwood, T., and Trott, P. A. Needling renal cysts and tumors: Cytology and radiology. *Br. Med. J.* 3:755, 1975.

88. Siegleman, S. S., Sprayregen, S., and Bosniak, M. A. Serendipity in the diagnosis of renal carcinoma. *J. Can. Assoc. Radiol.* 23:251, 1972.

89. Simpson, A., Baron, M. G., and Mitty, H. A. Angiographic patterns of venous extension of hypernephroma. *J. Urol.* 111:441, 1974.

90. Skinner, D. G., Colvin, R. B., and Vermillion, C. D. Diagnosis and management of renal cell carcinoma: A clinical and pathologic study of 309 cases. *Cancer* 28:1165, 1971.

91. Smith, H., and Riches, E. Haemoglobin values in renal carcinoma. *Lancet* 1:1017, 1963.

92. Smith, J. C., Rösch, J., Athanasoulis, C. A., Baum, S., Waltman, A. C., and Goldman, M. Renal venography in the evaluation of poorly vascularized neoplasms of the kidney. *AJR* 123:552, 1975.

93. Snyder, W. H., Jr., Hastings, T. A., and Pollack, W. F. Retroperitoneal Tumors. In W. R. Mustard, M. M. Ravitch, W. H. Snyder, Jr., K. S. Welch, and C. D. Benson (eds.), *Pediatric Surgery* (2nd ed.). Chicago: Year Book, 1969. Vol. 2, p. 1020.

94. Steyn, J., and Morales, A. Clinical features of adenocarcinoma of the kidney. *S. Afr. Med. J.* 47:175, 1973.

95. Tannenbaum, M. Ultrastructural Pathology of Human Renal Cell Tumors. In S. C. Sommers (ed.), *Kidney Pathology Decennial, 1966–1975.* New York: Appleton-Century-Crofts, 1975. P. 647.

96. Thorling, E. B., and Ersbak, J. Erythrocytosis and hypernephroma. *Scand. J. Hematol.* 1:38, 1964.

97. Utz, D. C., Warren, M. M., Gregg, J. A., Ludwig, J., and Kelalis, P. P. Reversible hepatic dysfunction associated with hypernephroma. *Mayo Clin. Proc.* 45:161, 1970.

98. Von Schreeb, T., Arner, O., Skovsted, G., and Wikstad, N. Renal adenocarcinoma: Is there a risk of spreading cells in diagnostic puncture? *Scand. J. Urol. Nephrol.* 1:270, 1967.

99. Wagle, D. G., and Scal, D. R. Renal cell carcinoma—a review of 256 cases. *J. Surg. Oncol.* 2:23, 1970.

100. Watson, R. C., Fleming, R. J., and Evans, J. A. Arteriography in the diagnosis of renal carcinoma. *Radiology* 91:888, 1968.

101. Westra, P., Kieffer, S. A., and Mosser, D. G. Wilms' tumor. A summary of 25 years of experience before actinomycin-D. *AJR* 100:214, 1967.

102. Whitley, N. O., Kinkhabwala, M., and Whitley, J. E. The collateral vein sign: A fallible sign in the staging of renal cancer. *AJR* 120:660, 1974.

103. Williams, L. H., Anastopulos, H. P., and Present, C. A. Selective renal arteriography in Hodgkin's disease of the kidney. *Radiology* 93:1059, 1969.

104. Williamson, B., Jr., Hattery, R. R., Stephens, D. H., and Sheedy, P. F., II. Computed tomography of the kidneys. *Semin. Roentgenol.* 13:249, 1978.

105. Woodruff, J. H., Jr., Chalek, C. C., Ottoman, R. E., and Wilk, S. P. The roentgen diagnosis of renal neoplasms. *J. Urol.* 75:615, 1956.

106. Wright, F. W., and Walker, M. M. The radiological diagnosis of 'avascular' renal tumours. *Br. J. Urol.* 47:253, 1975.

107. Xipel, J. M. The incidence of benign renal nodules (in clinicopathologic study). *J. Urol.* 106:503, 1971.

Angiography of Renal Infection

MORTON A. BOSNIAK
MARJORIE A. AMBOS
RICHARD S. LEFLEUR

There is a wide spectrum of radiologic findings associated with renal inflammatory disease. The process may be acute, subacute, or chronic, and it may be either diffusely present throughout the kidney or localized. The disease may extend into the perirenal space or may be confined to the collecting system structures. The angiographic findings, which reflect this wide range of disease, depend on the stage of the inflammatory process, the etiologic agent, and the distribution of the disease in and around the kidney.

The following outline is used to organize the discussion of renal infection in this chapter:

1. Acute diffuse inflammation, including acute pyelonephritis, acute bacterial nephritis, and acute suppurative pyelonephritis (microabscesses)
2. Renal abscess, including acute localized abscess (carbuncle), subacute-to-chronic localized abscess, and perinephric abscess (either primary or due to extension from renal abscess)
3. Chronic inflammation, diffuse and localized
   a. Xanthogranulomatous pyelonephritis, tumefactive, and nontumefactive
   b. Tuberculosis
   c. Chronic atrophic pyelonephritis
4. Miscellaneous inflammatory conditions
   a. Infected cysts or caliceal diverticula
   b. Infected hydronephrosis, pyonephrosis (see Chap. 54)
   c. Fungous disease

Acute Pyelonephritis (Acute Bacterial Nephritis, Acute Suppurative Pyelonephritis)

Acute pyelonephritis is a renal parenchymal inflammation resulting from the spread of pathogenic organisms to the kidney, either by ascent up the ureter from the lower urinary tract or via the bloodstream. It has a wide range of radiologic and pathologic findings, depending on the severity of involvement [16, 54]. With acute infection, there is an inflammatory response in the renal parenchyma with secondary edema resulting in kidney enlargement [16, 50]. Gross examination of a kidney with acute pyelonephritis may reveal multiple microabscesses throughout the cortex. These range in size from approximately 1 to 5 mm and are most clearly seen on the subcapsular renal surface [16, 54]. Microscopically, there are interstitial edema, hyperemia, and infiltrates of neutrophilic leukocytes between the tubules [54]. In a more severe form of pyelonephritis, termed *bacterial nephritis* or *acute suppurative pyelonephritis*, the inflammatory process is more extensive, with increased leukocyte infiltration and focal areas of tissue necrosis. Pathologists refer to this latter condition as *phlegmon of the kidney* [54]. Another variant of acute renal infection has been termed *lobar nephronia* [45]. In this entity, one specific segment or lobe of the kidney is infected, generally by *Escherichia coli*. No true abscess exists since there is no liquefaction or necrosis. It is felt that lobar nephronia is probably secondary to reflux [45].

Histologic examination in cases of seemingly unilateral acute pyelonephritis has often revealed inflammatory changes in the contralateral kidney, suggesting that the infection is often bilateral but is subclinical on one side [50].

Acute pyelonephritis is most commonly seen in females between the ages of 15 and 40 [12]. Fever, chills, and flank pain are frequently present. Although the laboratory findings are variable, leukocytosis is often present, and analysis of the urine may show both white and red blood cells. The urine culture is frequently positive, and *E. coli* is often the offending organism, especially in patients with reflux [12, 45]. Bacterial nephritis, which represents a more severe infection than simple acute pyelonephritis, is frequently seen in diabetic females. In these patients, gram-negative organisms (most frequently *E. coli*) are cultured from both the urine and the blood [13, 14, 37, 54]. It has been postulated that bacterial nephritis rather than simple acute pyelonephritis develops in diabetics owing to an altered or diminished host response to infection.

In a patient with acute pyelonephritis, one of three courses occurs: (1) the inflammation may resolve completely, leaving a grossly normal kidney; (2) the inflammation may worsen into bacte-

Figure 53-1. Case 1. Acute diffuse inflammation with microabscesses in a 61-year-old man with fever and left flank pain. No visualization of the left kidney was noted on urography. (A) Selective left renal arteriogram, arterial phase. The vessels are stretched in the swollen kidney but no focal abnormalities are seen. (B) Selective left renal arteriogram, late arterial, early nephrographic phase. A diffusely mottled and decreased nephrogram is seen, with loss of the corticomedullary junction and the suggestion of slow flow through the arterial system. (C) Left renal venogram (epinephrine enhanced). Complete obstruction of the upper and middle pole veins can be seen, with attenuation and some stretching of the lower pole veins. It is evident that the findings on the venogram are more extensive than those on the arteriogram. Because of the left kidney's continued poor functioning, nephrectomy was performed. Pathologic examination of the removed kidney revealed a diffuse inflammatory process with several small focal abscesses, particularly in the upper portion of the kidney. (Reprinted with permission from Pingoud et al. [43].)

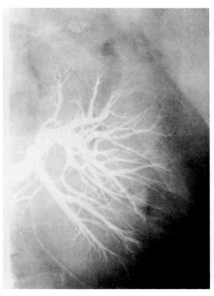

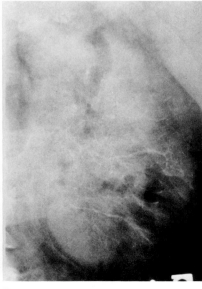

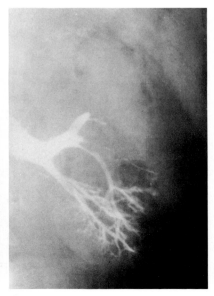

A   *B*   *C*

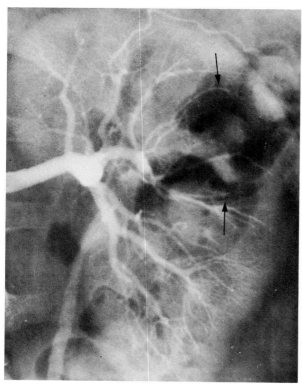

A

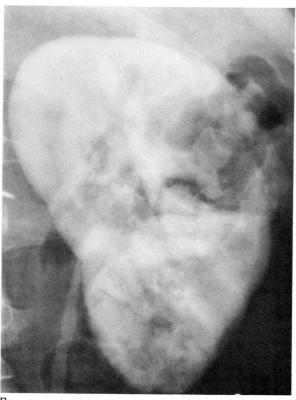

B

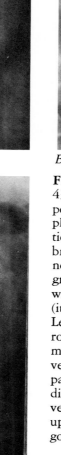

C

Figure 53-2. Case 2. Acute focal inflammation in a 43-year-old man with left renal colic and spiking temperatures. (A) Selective left renal arteriogram, arterial phase. A hypovascular mass is seen in the upper portion of the kidney with stretching of the interlobar branches around the mass (*arrows*), but there is no abnormal vascularity. (B) Selective left renal arteriogram, nephrographic phase. A diminished nephrogram with indistinct margins in the area of the mass is noted (it is somewhat obscured by overlying bowel gas). (C) Left renal venogram (epinephrine enhanced). Narrowed, irregular veins in area of the localized inflammatory mass are well seen (*arrows*). Note that the veins are much more affected than the arteries. The patient was treated with antibiotics, and his symptoms disappeared in about a week. Follow-up studies revealed no abnormality in the kidney, except for a small upper pole scar. (Reprinted with permission from Pingoud et al. [43].)

rial nephritis; or (3) the inflammation may go on to frank abscess formation [54]. The eventual outcome depends on a combination of therapy, host response, and organism involved.

Approximately 25 percent of patients having intravenous urography during an episode of acute pyelonephritis show one or more abnormal findings [12, 50, 54]. Urographic changes include focal or generalized renal enlargement, delayed filling of the collecting system, a decreased nephrogram, and a diminished density of contrast in the collecting system [16, 32, 54]. With appropriate antibiotic therapy, all these changes are reversible [45]. In the more severe cases of bacterial nephritis, there is often marked diminution in renal excretion of contrast material, with a faint nephrogram and a lack of caliceal visualization [13, 14, 37].

Arteriography may show a spectrum of changes in acute pyelonephritis, depending on the severity of the infection and whether it is generalized or segmental. There are often stretching and attenuation of the intrarenal arteries secondary to parenchymal edema, as well as loss of the corticomedullary junction [1] (Fig. 53-1). In the subgroup of acute lobar nephronia,

Figure 53-3. Case 3. Acute inflammation of the kidney in a 42-year-old woman with fever and flank pain. An intravenous urogram revealed swelling and fullness of the lower pole of the left kidney, as well as poor visualization of the lower pole calix. (A) Selective left renal arteriogram, arterial phase. Decreased vascularity in the lower pole of the kidney is noted, with areas of poor perfusion and slower flow of contrast medium. No distinct displacement of vessels is shown, however. (B) Selective left renal arteriogram, nephrographic phase. Multiple areas of decreased or absent nephrogram in the lower pole are seen, with loss of delineation of the corticomedullary junction and multiple defects in the contour of the kidney. At surgical exploration for possible drainage of abscess in the lower pole of the left kidney, a swollen, edematous kidney was noted. A left nephrectomy was performed because a neoplasm was suspected. Study of pathologic specimens revealed acute and chronic inflammation with edema and microabscesses but no gross collection of pus.

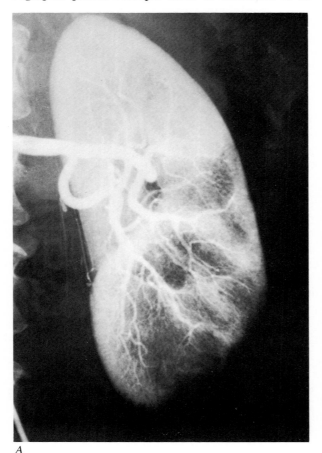

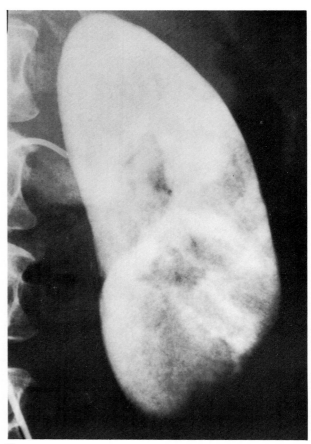

A

B

there is actual stretching of vessels around the infected lobe of tissue (Fig. 53-2) [45]. In the nephrogram phase of the angiogram in acute pyelonephritis, two patterns may be present. Multiple small lucencies, representing microabscesses, may be scattered throughout the parenchyma, giving the nephrogram a mottled appearance (Fig. 53-3). In other cases, there may be a series of alternately lucent and dense stripes in the cortex (striated nephrogram) [50, 54] (Fig. 53-4). In the milder forms of acute pyelonephritis, normal angiograms may be seen [50].

In the severe form of acute pyelonephritis (bacterial nephritis), arteriographic changes are consistently present and are more severe [12, 13]. The kidney is quite swollen, leading to marked stretching, splaying, and attenuation of the intrarenal arteries. The interlobar arteries and their branches are decreased in both number and caliber [13, 14, 54] (see Fig. 53-1), and slower flow is observed in the affected areas. In severe infection, the arteries are stretched around small inflammatory masses [12]. As in simple acute pyelonephritis, there is loss of the corticomedullary border, and the nephrogram may show mottled lucencies or cortical striations. In bacterial nephritis, the cortical striations are more consistently seen [13, 14]. It has been suggested that these striations are due to redistribution of blood flow away from the cortex as a result of obliteration of interlobular arteries by perivascular inflammatory cells [12, 13], whereas the loss of the corticomedullary border seen in acute pyelonephritis is due to cortical vasoconstriction [28, 50].

Follow-up urograms on patients with bacterial nephritis who were successfully treated with antibiotics reveal global wasting with caliceal clubbing but without focal scarring [13]. In another study, follow-up angiograms on patients with bacterial nephritis showed attenuation of the arterial tree [37].

Several groups have suggested that renal venography is more valuable than arteriography in

Figure 53-4. Case 4. Acute diffuse pyelonephritis in a 54-year-old man with right flank pain, fever, and leukocytosis. On urography a swollen right kidney was seen with faint visualization of the collecting system. (A) Selective right renal arteriogram, arterial phase. Stretching of the intrarenal branches and capsular artery is demonstrated. No focal abnormality is noted. (B) Selective right renal arteriogram, nephrographic phase. A diffusely swollen kidney is seen, with loss of delineation of the cortical-medullary junction. Note the striated nephrogram pattern throughout (best seen along outer margin of kidney).

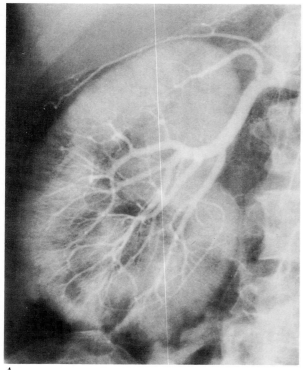

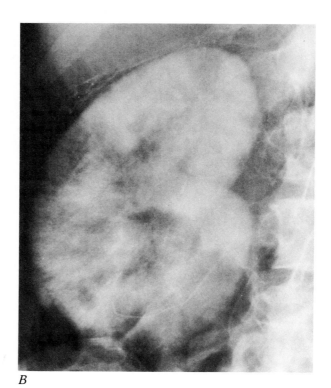

A

B

the diagnosis of acute pyelonephritis [1, 26, 43, 45]. Since the walls of veins are more sensitive to surrounding disease than are arterial walls, it is felt that they may reflect earlier changes in the kidney [45]. Epinephrine-enhanced venography in acute pyelonephritis may reveal smooth narrowing or total occlusion of intrarenal veins. As on the arterial side, the parenchymal edema leads to stretching and attenuation [43]. These venous changes are not diagnostic of infection but, with an appropriate history and laboratory findings, the changes are suggestive of infection [1]. Figures 53-1 and 53-2 demonstrate that the extent of the inflammatory disease is more clearly seen on venography than on arteriography.

Renal Abscess

Bacterial invasion of the renal parenchyma may, in certain cases, progress to abscess formation. When this occurs, the earliest stage of the infection is edema with multiple microabscesses. These abscesses may then coalesce into a suppurative mass that progresses to frank liquefaction or necrosis [12, 16]. At this point, a true abscess (renal carbuncle) is present, and it may follow one of three courses: (1) it may remain confined to the renal parenchyma; (2) it may break through into the perinephric space; or (3) it may extend into the renal collecting system [15, 16]. The radiologic findings will depend on the time at which the abscess is studied; that is, on whether the abscess is acute or chronic and whether it is confined to the parenchyma or has extended.

In the past, *Staphylococcus aureus* has been the commonest organism found in renal abscesses. It generally involves the kidney via the hematogenous route [7, 21, 27]. Ascending infections may also cause abscess formation, and in these cases gram-negative organisms are commonly found [33]. Ascending infections most commonly affect kidneys that were previously damaged by calculi or other causes of hydronephrosis [17]. The spectrum of organisms causing renal abscesses has changed in recent years because of the earlier treatment of infections with antibiotics and the increase in the abuse of intravenous drugs associated with drug addiction [27]. Today, gram-negative bacteria, especially *E. coli*, pseudomonas, and proteus, are increasingly found to be the cause of renal abscesses [34].

Whatever bacterium is involved, the most common pathway of infection is still the bloodstream. The bacteria lodge in the small intrarenal arteries and multiply there, forming microabscesses that may eventually coalesce to form a mass filled with pus [16, 29, 33, 34]. The abscess, when new, lacks a well-defined wall and is less a true mass than an area of inflamed parenchyma [29, 44]. At this early stage there may be an extension of the infection into the perirenal space or the renal collecting system [15, 34]. In cases in which the abscess remains confined to the renal parenchyma, a wall forms around it. This wall is the result of fibroblastic proliferation and vascularization around the periphery of the inflammatory mass. In time, the wall thickens into a pseudocapsule with quite vascular connective tissue [12]. The chronic renal abscess is actually a necrotic mass surrounded by a broad zone of granulation tissue [29].

CLINICAL FINDINGS

Two different clinical pictures may be seen in renal abscesses, depending on whether the process is acute or chronic. If it is acute, the patient complains of fever, chills, and flank pain. If the abscess is secondary to a staphylococcal skin or respiratory infection or to dental work, it usually becomes evident 1 to 8 weeks following the primary episode [17, 41, 44]. Laboratory findings may include leukocytosis and an elevated erythrocyte sedimentation rate. Unless the abscess breaks through into the collecting system, urine culture and urinalysis are often unremarkable [21, 54]. Chronic abscesses are more difficult diagnostic problems since they often develop insidiously, with minimal clinical and laboratory findings [36]. Localizing symptoms are rare, the history of a preceding infection is often overlooked, and the urine culture is usually negative [12, 14, 29]. Several reported series of chronic renal abscesses reveal that a correct preoperative diagnosis was made in only about 20 percent of cases [25, 49]. When the condition is correctly diagnosed, antibiotic therapy may be curative although larger abscesses often require drainage [17].

RADIOLOGIC FINDINGS

Radiologic findings in renal abscesses vary with the stage and extent of the process. The plain abdominal film often shows loss of the renal and psoas outlines on the affected side [10, 34, 35, 44]. If the renal outline is seen, it may reveal generalized or focal enlargement [10]. Intravenous urography often demonstrates a diminished excretion of contrast material with decreased opacification of all or parts of the collecting system [7, 29, 54]. In a series of 22 patients with renal abscess, the urogram showed enlargement of the kidney in 7 and a distinct mass effect in 12 [34, 36]. With chronicity, mass lesions are more commonly found [29]. Due to the necrosis within the abscess, an area of lucency may be seen on the urogram [54]. With extension into the perirenal space, the renal outline becomes hazy or blurred in the involved area [16]. Retrograde pyelography will show amputation or distortion of calices due to the abscess mass [35]. Ultrasonography of an acute abscess may show a sonolucent area, with few or no internal echoes; as time passes, the abscesses become more echogenic. Perinephric involvement may also be demonstrated by ultrasonography [33]. Computed tomography can also be helpful in the diagnosis of renal abscess. Perinephric extension may be more clearly seen (especially when the inflammatory exudate collects posterior to the kidney), and this finding may lead to a correct diagnosis. A chronic abscess in the parenchyma, however, cannot usually be distinguished from a necrotic neoplasm by computed tomography unless air can be seen within the lesion.

Angiographic findings in renal abscesses do, of

Figure 53-5. Case 5. Acute renal abscess in a 22-year-old heroin addict with fever, leukocytosis, and right flank pain. An intravenous pyelogram disclosed a mass in the lateral aspect of the midportion of the right kidney. (A) Selective right renal arteriogram, arterial phase. Poor visualization and flow in the vessels in the midportion of the right kidney in its lateral aspect is noted, with some elongation and straightening of the vessels on the outer margin of this hypovascular area. The capsular artery supplying the perinephric tissues adjacent to the hypovascular mass is hypertrophied. (B) Selective right renal arteriogram, nephrographic phase. There is loss of the nephrogram in the midportion of the kidney. Flattening of the lateral margin of the kidney in the involved area is noted, along with slight contrast staining in the perinephric space, which indicates subcapsular and perinephric extension of the abscess. At surgery, the abscess was drained.

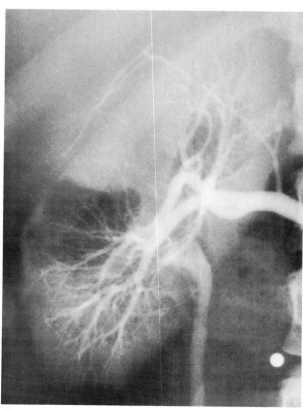

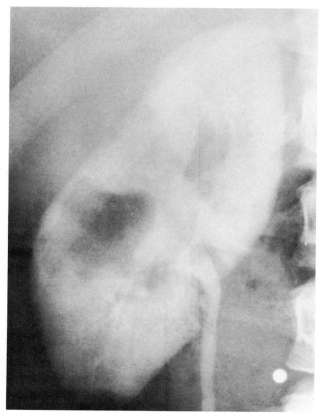

A   *B*

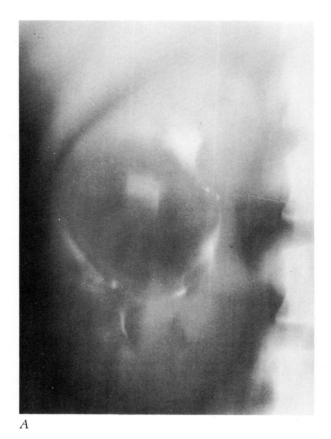

A

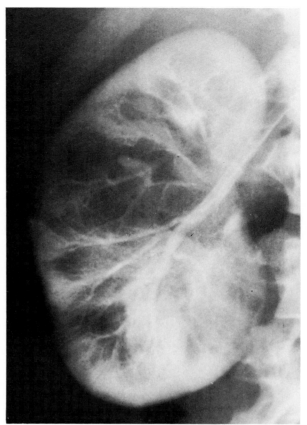

B

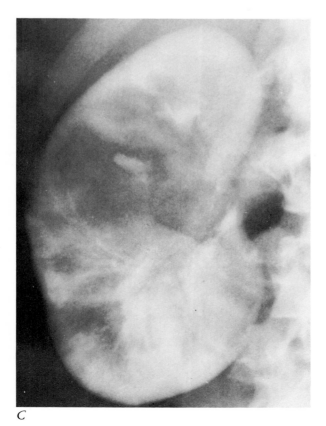

C

Figure 53-6. Case 6. Acute abscess of the kidney in a 24-year-old woman with juvenile diabetes who had acute right flank pain and a high fever. (A) Urogram with tomography of the right kidney. A large, fairly well-demonstrated lucent mass is seen in the midportion of the kidney. (B) Selective right renal arteriogram, arterial phase. The mass is shown to be hypovascular, and stretching of major vessels around the mass is seen. Two smaller avascular areas are demonstrated at the lower pole of the kidney laterally. (C) Selective right renal arteriogram, nephrographic phase. Loss of the nephrogram is evident in the large mass in the center of the kidney and in smaller areas in its lower portion. At surgery, a large abscess filled with purulent material was evacuated. A culture revealed *Escherichia coli*.

course, vary with the stage and extent of the process. Occasionally, a mass may not be appreciated angiographically, even when one is suggested on urography [29, 33]. An early, acute abscess suggests generalized edema rather than displaying a mass effect. Vessels are not displaced by the abscess but rather go through the involved area with some attenuation and stretching [11, 12, 29]. (The findings are similar to those described for acute, localized pyelonephritis.) There is slower flow through the vessels in the abscess and, as in other renal infections, loss of the corticomedullary junction [11, 44, 54].

If the therapy is inadequate, the inflammatory process will progress, localize, and liquefy, leading to an acute, localized abscess—a carbuncle. At this stage, the abscess appears radiographically as a renal mass (Fig. 53-5, 53-6). Angiographically, there are stretching of vessels about the mass and, often, a zone of increased density surrounds the abscess, representing compression of the surrounding renal parenchyma. There is often loss of the sharp renal margin adjacent to the area of the infection [33]. The nephrogram may show a hazy blush in the area of the abscess, depending on the duration of the inflammatory process. When the process is chronic, there is an increase in the neovascularity and hyperemia, both in and around the abscess. The degree of neovascularity is variable. Some abscesses remain quite hypovascular, while others show considerable hyperemia [29]. When neovascularity is present, it is of a fine or reticular type. While this pattern is not pathognomonic for infection, the vessels do tend to be more delicate and homogeneous than those seen in renal cell carcinoma [36, 47]. Reports of positive epinephrine studies and early venous filling in abscesses further emphasize the difficulty of ruling out tumor [8, 10, 31, 44]. Normal intrarenal arteries stretch around the abscess, as they do with any mass. Owing to central necrosis, the abscess is lucent during the nephrogram, but there is a blush around the border that becomes more prominent as the abscess becomes more chronic. This blush is due to hyperemia in the granulation tissue in the wall around the abscess [7, 12] (Figs. 53-7, 53-8).

EXTENSION INTO COLLECTING SYSTEM

If the acute abscess does not become walled off, it is free to break into either the collecting system or the perinephric space (Fig. 53-9). Extension into the collecting system usually occurs in chronic diseased kidneys with long-standing obstruction due to calculi. Angiography in these cases shows the changes of hydronephrosis; that is, stretching and attenuation of the arteries around the dilated calices. Because of the inflammatory process, however, neovascularity is often present around the dilated calices, which have hazy borders [35] (see Fig. 53-19).

PERINEPHRIC EXTENSION

More common than involvement of the collecting system is extension into the perinephric space with subsequent perinephritis. In fact, the perinephric process may often overshadow the parenchyma abscess (Figs. 53-10–53-12). With perirenal disease, the capsular vessels enlarge and are displaced away from the kidney. There is a distinct increase in both the size and number of capsular branches. A blush, often apparent in the perinephric space [12, 16, 34], is due to reactive hyperemia about the inflammatory process and possible leakage of small amounts of contrast medium into the inflamed tissues through diseased capillaries. While a perirenal abscess is generally secondary to a renal parenchymal abscess, it may arise either de novo or from other retroperitoneal infection. The perirenal process may be diffuse or localized. When localized, it generally occurs on the dorsolateral aspect of the kidney [16].

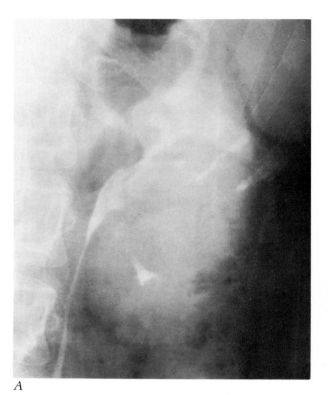

A

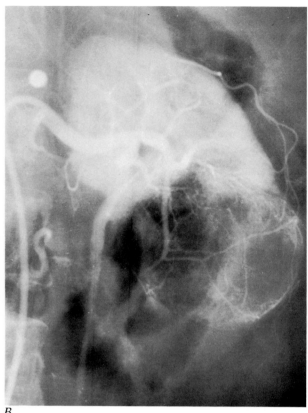

B

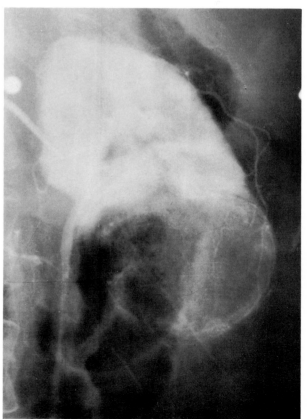

C

Figure 53-7. Case 7. Renal abscess in a 64-year-old woman with left flank pain and fever. (A) Urogram. A large mass is shown involving the middle and lower poles of the left kidney. (B) Selective left renal arteriogram, arterial phase. A hypovascular mass in the left kidney is well defined. Stretching of the vessels over and around the mass is evident, with hyperemia and neovascularity at the margin of the abscess. The lower margin of the kidney is not opacified because of the presence of an accessory renal artery. (C) Selective left renal arteriogram, nephrographic phase. A hypovascular mass in the lower pole of the left kidney is well defined. Some hyperemia along the margin of the abscess is seen, as well as slow flow and stasis of contrast material in the vessels along the abscess margin. A left nephrectomy was performed for acute and chronic abscess of the left kidney.

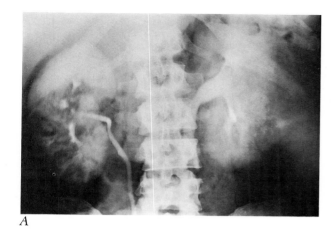

A

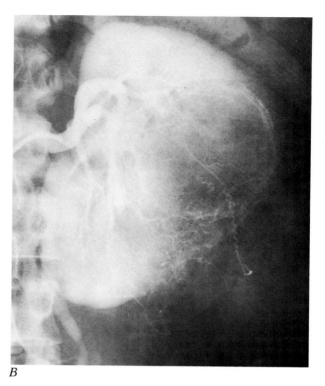

B

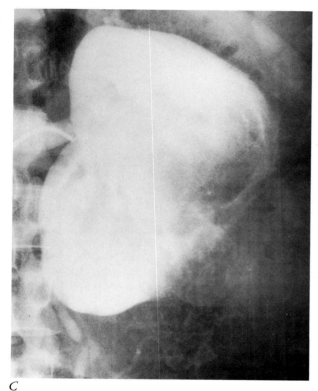

C

Figure 53-8. Case 8. Acute and chronic renal abscess angiographically indistinguishable from renal neoplasm. The patient, a 46-year-old man, had left flank pain but was without clear clinical symptoms or signs of infection. (A) Urogram. A large mass in the lateral aspect of the left kidney can be seen. (B) Selective left renal arteriogram, arterial phase. A large lucent mass occupies the lateral aspect of the left kidney. Vessels are stretched around the relatively hypovascular mass, with some hyperemia along the margins. Also seen are neovascularity with tortuous vessels inferior to the mass and some perforating capsular arteries extending into the perinephric space. (C) Selective left arteriogram, nephrographic phase. Extensive involvement of the kidney and extension into the perinephric space are seen. Some hyperemia and contrast blush are also seen. The mass has rotated the kidney and pushed the lower pole medially and anteriorly over the spine. The patient underwent a left radical nephrectomy after a preoperative diagnosis of renal cell carcinoma. The pathology examination revealed abscess of the left kidney with acute and chronic inflammatory changes.

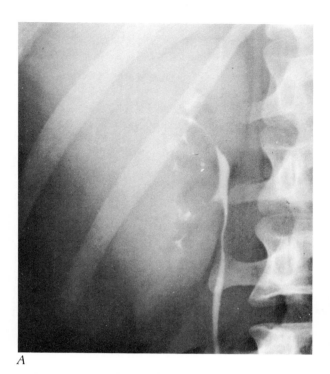

A

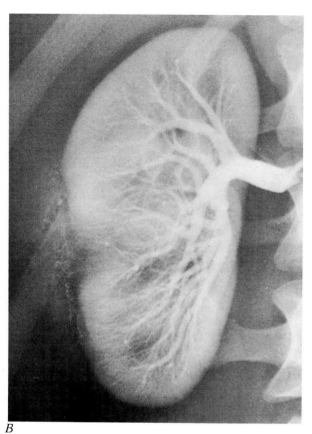

B

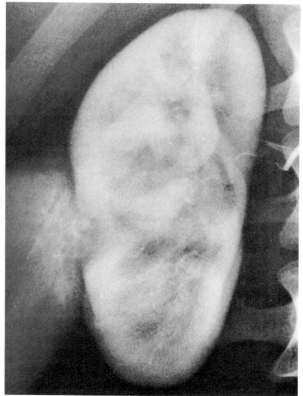

C

Figure 53-9. Case 9. Acute renal abscess with extension into the subcapsular and perirenal space. A 27-year-old man with flank pain and fever. (A) Urogram. A mass effect is noted along the lateral aspect of the right kidney. The lateral margin of kidney is poorly defined. (B) Selective right renal arteriogram, arterial phase. Flattening of the lateral aspect of the right kidney is seen. A defect in the cortex at this level is evident. Some delicate neovascularity is seen in the subcapsular and perirenal space in this area, with some tracking superiorly and inferiorly along the renal margin. (C) Selective right renal arteriogram, nephrographic phase. Flattening of the lateral aspect of the kidney is observed. A large blush of contrast medium is seen along the renal margin, indicating spread of the inflammation outside the cortex. Hyperemia and contrast blush are well demonstrated. An acute abscess was drained at surgery.

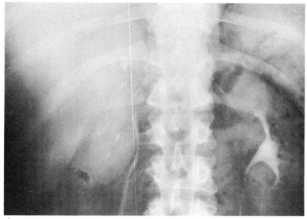

A

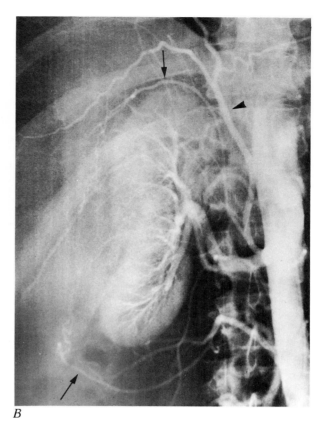

B

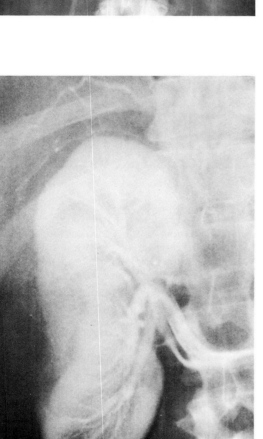

C

Figure 53-10. Case 10. Perinephric abscess. A 49-year-old man with flank pain and fever. (A) Urogram. A mass is seen flattening the lateral aspect of the right kidney and displacing the kidney medially. (B) Aortogram. Hypertrophy of a capsular artery (*upper arrow*), a branch of the inferior phrenic artery (*arrowhead*) (which in this case originates from the right renal artery), can be seen. The capsular artery inferior to the kidney is also visualized (*lower arrow*). Hyperemia and neovascularity lateral to the kidney are present. (C) Selective right renal arteriogram. Flattening of the lateral aspect of the kidney is apparent. No defect is present in the nephrogram, except for extrinsic pressure from the perinephric mass. Very little supply to the abscess from the renal vessels is visualized. (Some "flash filling" of the capsular vessels above the kidney can be seen since the catheter is deep within the renal artery, past the origin of the capsular vessels.) At surgery, a large perinephric abscess was drained.

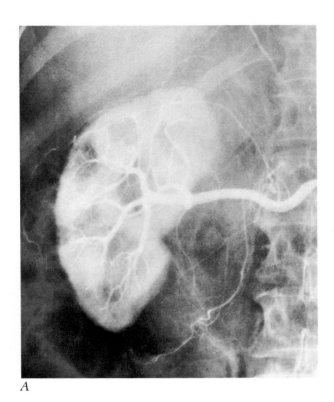

A

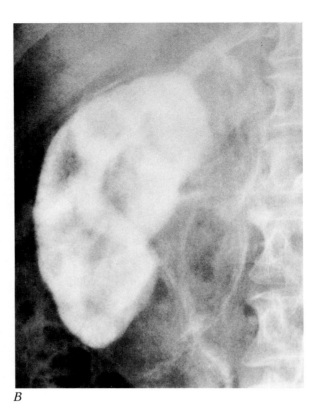

B

Figure 53-11. Case 11. Perinephric abscess. A 67-year-old diabetic with flank pain and fever. An intravenous urogram revealed nonvisualization of the right kidney. (A) Selective right renal arteriogram, arterial phase. The kidney is displaced laterally. The intrarenal vessels are intact, but there is increased filling of capsular vessels, which are stretched and separated from the kidney by the perirenal inflammatory mass. (B) Selective right renal arteriogram, nephrographic phase. The renal margin is hazy, particularly in the medial aspect of the kidney. Considerable blushing of the perirenal tissues is evident. At surgery, a large perinephric abscess was drained.

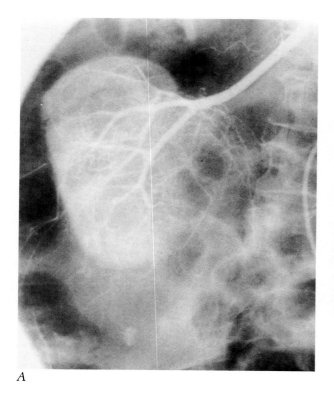

A

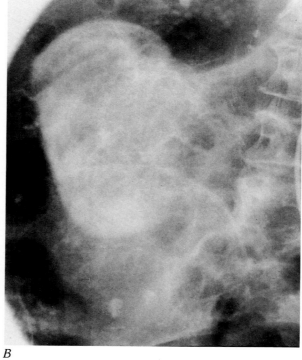

B

Figure 53-12. Case 12. Chronic abscess. A 56-year-old woman who had a fever and a palpable right-sided abdominal mass. Urography revealed nonvisualization of the right kidney. (A) Selective right renal arteriogram, arterial phase. Distortion and stretching of the intrarenal vessels are seen. Stretching, palisading, and hypertrophy of the medial capsular vessels over the area of the renal pelvis is evident, as is filling of the vessels in the perirenal space inferiorly. (B) Selective right renal arteriogram, nephrographic phase. An ir-regular spotty nephrogram is present. The renal margin is indistinct, particularly medially, and there is a contrast medium blush in the perirenal areas that indicates extension of the inflammatory process outside the kidney. A chronic abscess involving the right kidney and chronic inflammation in the perinephric space were found at surgery. Some foam cells were seen histologically, suggesting a diagnosis of xanthogranulomatous pyelonephritis. (Reprinted with permission from Caplan et al. [7].)

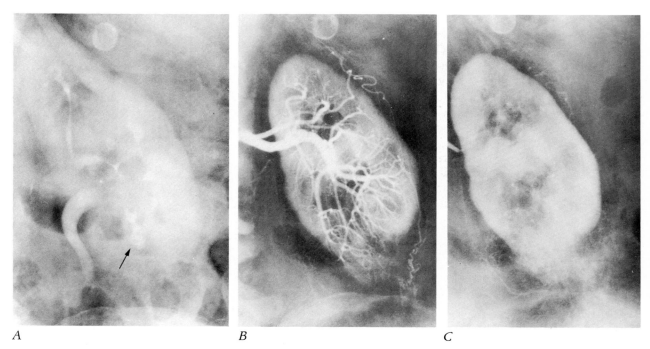

A   *B*   *C*

Figure 53-13. Case 13. Perirenal inflammation with abscess. A 61-year-old woman with left flank pain and fever. (A) Intravenous urogram. A calculus is present in the lower pole calix (*arrow*), and loss of the inferior renal margin is evident. A calcification in the splenic artery can be seen. (B) Selective left renal arteriogram, arterial phase. The intrarenal vessels are normal but slightly hypertrophied. A capsular artery feeding the perirenal tissues at the lower pole of the kidney is seen. Note the loss of margination of the kidney at the lower pole. (C) Selective left renal arteriogram, nephrographic phase. Hyperemia and blush at inferior margin of the kidney are present, indicating an inflammatory reaction. No mass is evident, however, indicating an inflammation without abscess. Because no distinct mass was demonstrated, the patient was treated with antibiotics; after one week, her symptoms resolved.

DIFFERENTIATION FROM RENAL CARCINOMA

Because chronic renal abscesses may have an insidious course, differential diagnosis may be a problem. The major entity to be ruled out is a cystic or necrotic renal cell carcinoma, which may so closely resemble an abscess angiographically that definite differentiation may not be possible. Chronic inflammatory vascularity and tumor vascularity, while quite different pathologically, can usually not be differentiated angiographically [36]. In both conditions, increased vascularity, hyperemia, and contrast staining can be seen (Fig. 53-13; see also Fig. 53-8). Since the "wild-looking" (aneurysmally dilated and corkscrew-shaped) vessels seen in neoplasms are not seen in inflammatory masses, inflammation can usually be excluded if these vessels are present. However, in necrotic neoplasms without such bizarre vessels, differentiation becomes difficult. The use of epinephrine angiography has not been helpful because inflammatory neovascularity, like neoplastic vessels, does not respond to epinephrine as normal vessels do. (There probably is a quantitative difference in the response of inflammatory and neoplastic vascularity to epinephrine, but the difference is not great enough to be used angiographically [31].)

It has been suggested that renal venography might be able to differentiate neoplastic from inflammatory disease by providing information about the venous involvement. Renal cell carcinoma tends to invade and extend into renal veins, while transitional cell carcinoma, squamous cell carcinoma, and other invasive neoplasms tend to constrict, encase, and amputate veins in the kidney [30, 51]. In inflammatory disease however, similar findings have been seen, including attenuation and occlusion of veins by extrinsic compression or by intraluminal thrombus formation [26, 43, 45]. Therefore, renal venography cannot be used to differentiate clearly severe inflammatory disease from neoplastic disease. On the other hand, if gross intraluminal occlusion of the main renal vein occurs, it is statistically likely that the disease is neoplastic.

Often a diagnosis of chronic abscess rather than carcinoma can be made only if there are clinical features that point to infection as the cause. *The possibility of abscess must be entertained if the diagnosis is to be made.* Often nephrectomy is the proper treatment for abscess as well as for carcinoma (if the abscess is large and has destroyed a large portion of the kidney); but simple nephrectomy is adequate for inflammatory disease whereas a radical approach must be taken for malignancy.

Xanthogranulomatous Pyelonephritis

Xanthogranulomatous pyelonephritis is a rare form of renal inflammation that is usually seen in patients with obstruction secondary to long-standing calculi [24, 52]. Why some patients with chronic obstruction develop not just simple hydronephrosis or even pyonephrosis but xanthogranulomatous pyelonephritis is not known. Clinically, these patients have flank pain and often a palpable mass. Because the process is generally severe and destroys the bulk of the kidney, nephrectomy is the usual therapy [2].

Xanthogranulomatous pyelonephritis may involve the kidney in two ways, either diffusely, replacing the entire kidney, or as a focal (tumefactive) disease. The diffuse form, which is by far the most common, develops behind an obstructing renal pelvic calculus [2, 12, 53]. In one study, more than 70 percent of those with diffuse disease had calculi [12]. With focal disease, a localized portion of the kidney is involved and a history of calculi is not as common [12]. Whether diffuse or focal, the pathologic process is the same. The renal parenchyma is replaced by xanthogranulomatous masses that have the gross appearance of yellow nodules scattered throughout the kidney. In addition to these masses, which are the hallmark of the process, small abscesses and areas of dense fibrous tissue may be seen. When diffuse involvement is present, all the calices are filled with purulent fluid and calculi [24, 52]. Microscopically, lipid-laden macrophages or foam cells are present. Occasionally, plasma cells, lymphocytes, and multinucleated giant cells are all seen [40, 52]. The glomeruli and tubules become atrophic [24]. *Bacillus proteus* is the most frequent pathogen found, but *E. coli* and *Staphylococcus aureus* have also been cultured in this disease [52].

The radiographic patterns of xanthogranu-lomatous pyelonephritis reflect the pathologic changes and are different in the diffuse and focal forms. In the diffuse disease, plain films of the abdomen often show enlargement of the renal outline and calculi [2, 24, 52]. The most common finding on intravenous urography is nonvisualization of the diseased kidney [2, 24]. Retrograde pyelography may demonstrate hydronephrosis or amputation of a portion of the collecting system [24], or it may show extravasation of contrast material into the parenchyma due to the friable urothelium (Fig. 53-14). In focal xanthogranulomatous pyelonephritis, the kidney is visualized on urography and a mass is seen. The mass may distort the collecting system or renal outline and may be indistinguishable radiologically from a renal neoplasm or a chronic renal abscess [2, 12, 52].

Angiography is performed to study further the nonvisualized kidney or to assess the solid renal mass [24]. With diffuse disease and hydronephrosis, the angiographic findings are similar in many ways to those of simple hydronephrosis (Fig. 53-15; see also Fig. 53-14), with stretching and attenuation of intrarenal vessels [2, 24, 46]. However, unlike simple hydronephrosis, neovascularity due to the inflammatory process is present [12]. During the later arterial phase, vessels are seen to be stretched around dilated calices and inflammatory masses [3]. The nephrogram may be either homogeneous or mottled. If it is mottled, the scattered lucencies again represent the calices and granulomas [2, 24, 52]. There may be areas of increased density in parts of the kidney representing residual normal parenchyma [22] or hyperemia due to the inflammatory reaction. The corticomedullary junction is not seen, and there may be prominent capsular and ureteric vessels [2, 3, 46]. These last changes are nonspecific and are seen with most chronic renal infections. Differential diagnosis of the angiogram in diffuse xanthogranulomatous pyelonephritis includes infected hydronephrosis or pyonephrosis [2]; however, the neovascularity is more prominent in xanthogranulomatous pyelonephritis. (Sonography is helpful in differentiating the fluid-filled hydronephrosis from the more solid xanthogranulomatous pyelonephritis.)

A more difficult diagnostic problem occurs in the focal or tumefactive form of xanthogranulomatous pyelonephritis. Here, even angiography is often unable definitely to rule out a hypovascular renal cell carcinoma [38]. The xanthogranulomatous mass, which closely resembles a chronic abscess, is generally avascular centrally

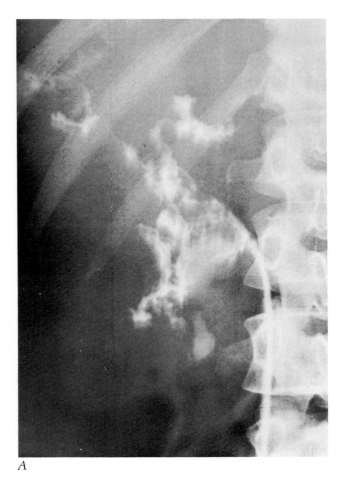

A

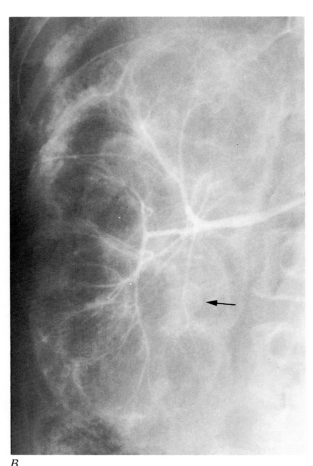

B

Figure 53-14. Case 14. Xanthogranulomatous py-elonephritis. A 44-year-old woman with right flank pain. An intravenous urogram revealed a nonfunctioning right kidney with staghorn calculi. (A) Right retrograde pyelogram. Extravasation of contrast material from the collecting system and into the kidney is noted. Large calculi in the right renal pelvis are some-what obscured by the contrast material. (B) Right renal arteriogram, arterial phase. Stretching of the intrarenal vessels over the hypovascular masses is seen. The pattern resembles hydronephrosis, except that more vascularity and hyperemia are present. The arrow points to calculi. A right nephrectomy revealed a xanthogranulomatous pyelonephritic kidney.

but often has neovascularity and blush on the periphery. Wild vascularity is not present [52, 53]. The problem is made more difficult because patients with the focal form of xanthogranulomatous pyelonephritis are often the ones without chronic calculus disease and infection. Nephrectomy is indicated in extensive xanthogranulomatous pyelonephritis as well as in renal cell carcinoma, so that differentiation may not be critical although a more radical approach should be taken with neoplasm. Localized disease can be treated by partial nephrectomy, but establishing this diagnosis preoperatively is difficult.

It should be noted that the diagnosis of xanthogranulomatous pyelonephritis is a pathologic diagnosis that often does not have relevance radiologically. Many cases of long-standing chronic inflammatory disease of the kidney show foam cells histologically and some yellow nodules of tissue on gross inspection, signs that permit a pathologic diagnosis of xanthogranulomatous pyelonephritis to be made. The lesions shown in Figures 53-7, 53-8, 53-12, and 53-19 contained foam cells as well as small areas of yellow xanthogranulomatous tissue, but they were considered chronic abscesses with some associated changes of xanthogranulomatous pyelonephritis. Varying gradations of disease exist, and a distinction should be made between (1) the more extensive tumefactive xanthogranulomatous pyelonephritis, in which the focal areas of interstitial inflammation become confluent, forming a parenchymal mass, and (2) the more common minimal changes of xanthogranulomatous pyelonephritis seen in many cases of chronic inflammatory disease of the kidney.

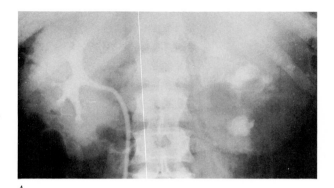

A

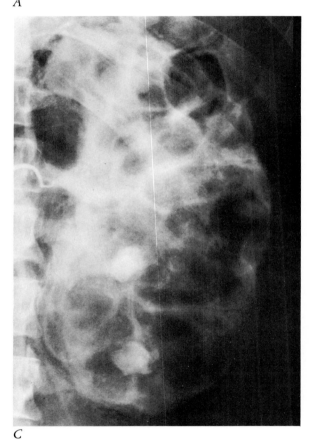

C

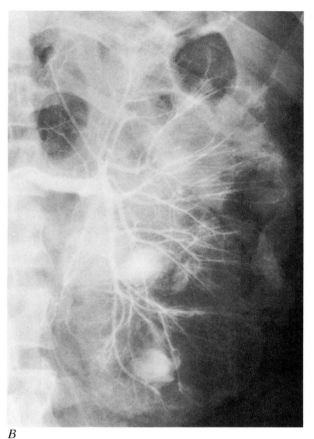

B

Figure 53-15. Case 15. Xanthogranulomatous pyelonephritis. A 48-year-old man with left flank pain and a palpable abdominal mass. (A) Intravenous urogram. Two large calculi are seen in a large, nonfunctioning left kidney. (B) Selective left renal arteriogram, arterial phase. Stretching of atrophic renal artery branches in an enlarged kidney is present. (C) Selective left renal arteriogram, nephrographic phase. Multiple hypovascular areas surrounded by hyperemic areas are seen. The pattern is similar to that in hydronephrosis, except for increased vascularity. A left nephrectomy revealed xanthogranulomatous pyelonephritis.

Tuberculosis

Tuberculosis usually involves the kidneys via the hematogenous route. The tuberculosis bacilli seed the kidneys, lodging in the glomerular and peritubular capillary beds. Often clinical symptoms do not occur, and healing takes place without residual effects. In some patients, however, there is erosion of the tuberculosis bacilli out of the vascular bed and into the tubules. From the tubules there may be extension into, and eventual erosion of, the renal papillae. Cavities of varying sizes occur with or without connection to the collecting system. Granulomas also may form and grow large enough that they appear as renal masses on urography—but this is an unusual finding. A definite diagnosis of renal tuberculosis requires microscopic demonstration of acid-fast bacilli or culture of bacilli on appropriate media [12].

The urographic findings in renal tuberculosis reflect the extent of the disease. In early renal involvement, the intravenous urogram is negative. The earliest urographic sign of renal tuber-

culosis is minimal irregularity of the minor calices due to papillary erosions. This irregularity may progress to extensive papillary necrosis with cavities of varying sizes filling on both intravenous urography and retrograde studies; however, not all cavities connect with the collecting system. Granulomatous masses or tuberculomas appear as solid masses distorting the collecting system or the renal outline. Calcification and fibrosis are the hallmarks of healing in tuberculosis and, as such, are often seen in the kidney. The fibrosis may lead to strictures of the infundibula or the renal pelvis and, if severe enough, will cause hydronephrosis as well as nonvisualization during urography [12].

Angiography in renal tuberculosis demonstrates a variety of findings, all of which are relatively nonspecific. The basic pathologic process that causes changes in the intrarenal arteries is a periarteritis and an endarteritis. This inflammation leads to irregularity and poor filling of the renal arteries on angiography. Changes are first seen in the smaller vessels (i.e., the arcuate and interlobular arteries), but, with progression, the

Figure 53-16. Case 16. Tuberculous right kidney. A 48-year-old man with hematuria. (A) Right retrograde pyelogram. Stricture of the lower pole infundibulum and nonfilling of the upper portion of the collecting system are demonstrated. (B) Selective right renal arteriogram, arterial phase. A decrease in the number of vessels in the upper pole of the kidney is seen. Am-

putation of some vessels (*arrows*) is evident, as is the loss of secondary branches. There is no evidence of a mass effect. (C) Selective right renal arteriogram, nephrographic phase. A greatly diminished nephrogram in the upper pole is noted. The tubercle bacillus was cultured from the urine.

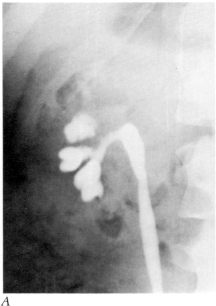
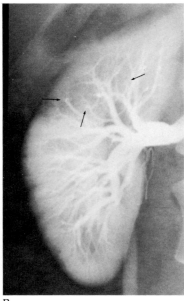
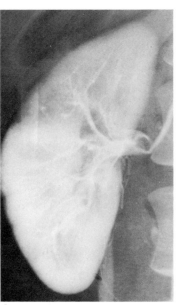

A   B   C

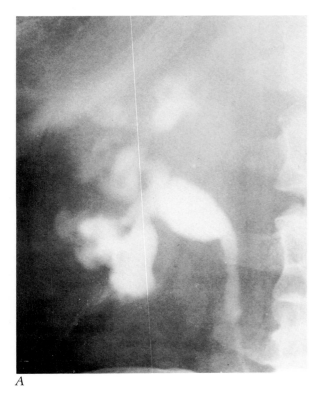

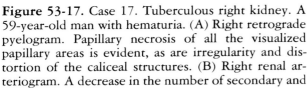

A

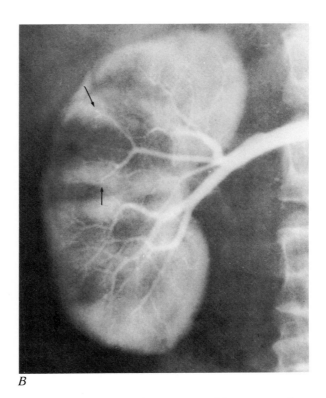

B

Figure 53-17. Case 17. Tuberculous right kidney. A 59-year-old man with hematuria. (A) Right retrograde pyelogram. Papillary necrosis of all the visualized papillary areas is evident, as are irregularity and distortion of the caliceal structures. (B) Right renal arteriogram. A decrease in the number of secondary and tertiary branches is evident, along with amputated vessels (*arrows*). Areas of diminished nephrogram are present. A right nephrectomy was performed. Extensive tuberculous destruction was noted in the excised specimen.

interlobar vessels are also affected [20, 25]. There may be a decrease in the number of vessels that fill during angiography and obliteration of portions of the arterial tree [5, 18] (Figs. 53-16, 53-17). If a tuberculoma is present, there is stretching of vessels around the mass, but no neovascularity within it. The nephrographic phase of the angiogram in renal tuberculosis is usually heterogeneous or patchy, with areas of diminished density due to obliteration of portions of the vascular tree. Tuberculous cavities may appear as discrete lucencies in the nephrogram [18]. While there is usually a general decrease in the renal vascularity, there may be hypertrophy of the peripelvic and capsular vessels secondary to the chronic inflammatory process [25]. When a part of the kidney or the entire kidney becomes hydronephrotic due to collecting system strictures, the arterial pattern is one of stretched and attenuated vessels. This is again nonspecific and can be seen in any hydronephrotic kidney, regardless of the cause [25].

The changes in renal tuberculosis that have been discussed are not consistently seen in all involved kidneys. In a series of 43 patients with renal tuberculosis, the most common angiographic findings were diminished vascularity in the involved portion of the kidney and pruning of the arterial tree. These findings were present in 74 percent; 65 percent showed parenchymal scarring, and 47 percent showed irregularity of the walls of the smaller arteries [6]. Again, it should be stressed that these angiographic findings are nonspecific and that the intravenous urogram is more diagnostic. Angiography is, therefore, generally not needed in the workup of a patient with renal tuberculosis, but it is useful in evaluating lesions that cannot be defined by other studies and in assessing more critically the extent of the disease process in the kidney.

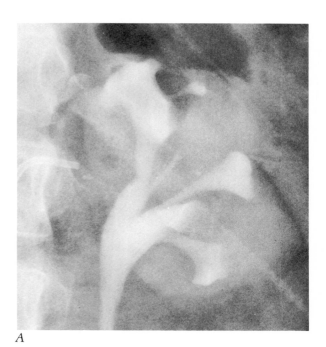

A

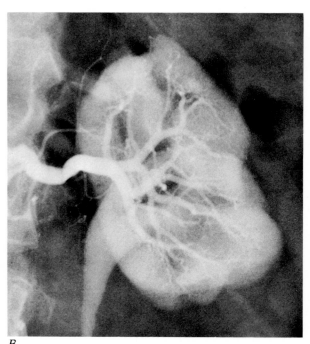

B

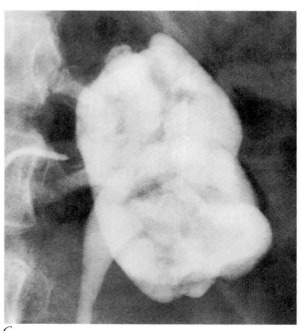

C

Figure 53-18. Case 18. Chronic pyelonephritis. A 42-year-old woman with a urinary tract infection. (A) Urogram. Scarring of the renal parenchyma can be seen associated with blunted calices. Some normal calices are seen and in these areas the parenchyma is normal. (B) Selective left renal arteriogram, arterial phase. Distortion of the renal vasculature in the scarred areas is evident, with abrupt tapering of the vessels and loss of peripheral branches. (C) Selective left renal arteriogram, nephrographic phase. Scarring of the parenchyma is well demonstrated. Areas of hypertrophied normal tissue give a lumpy contour to the renal margin.

Chronic Atrophic Pyelonephritis

While acute pyelonephritis generally affects the entire kidney, chronic atrophic pyelonephritis is a focal disease, involving a part or parts of one or both kidneys and sparing other portions. While the cause and pathogenesis of this disease have not been established, most studies suggest that a combination of infection and reflux in early infancy leads to focal areas of renal infection and subsequent atrophy. Although the infectious process is centered in the medullary portion of the kidney, the whole thickness of renal tissue is affected in scar formation [12]. Intravenous urography and angiography can demonstrate localized changes secondary to the scarring. Urography shows focal depressions in the renal outline, with distortion and clubbing of the underlying calices. These changes represent fibrosis and retraction of tissue [4, 19].

Angiography in chronic pyelonephritis shows arterial changes secondary to parenchymal loss and fibrosis (Fig. 53-18). There is a decrease in the size of the main renal artery commensurate with the decrease in functioning renal mass [18]. The intrarenal arteries, which are also diminished in caliber, are crowded together because of the loss of parenchyma, thus becoming tortuous or corkscrewed [18, 19, 28]. These changes are nonspecific and can be seen in any entity that leads to renal fibrosis and scarring, such as nephrosclerosis or radiation nephritis [28]. Some areas of the chronic pyelonephritic kidney may show diminished vascularity due to fibrotic occlusion of vessels. The nephrogram demonstrates cortical scarring and areas of increased density due to the crowding together of vessels [18]. Early venous filling, which was seen in 9 of 11 patients in one series, may be secondary to the shunting of blood through the larger medullary veins [4].

The renal scarring often leads to hypertrophy of uninvolved areas, which may then be confused with renal masses, so-called pseudotumors. Angiography can clearly show that the hypertrophied areas are normal renal parenchyma and not neoplastic. This conclusion can also be reached by nuclear medicine scanning in a less invasive fashion.

Miscellaneous Conditions

The remaining inflammatory conditions of the kidney include infected renal cyst, infected caliceal diverticulum, fungous disease, and infected hydronephrosis (pyonephrosis).

Infected renal cyst and *infected caliceal diverticulum* are comparatively rare phenomena. When a cyst becomes infected, the patient may have fever, chills, and flank pain. Sometimes leukocytosis or pyuria or both are present. The urographic appearance is usually identical to that of an uninfected cyst, but if higher doses of contrast material are used, the wall of the infected cyst may be seen to be hazier than expected. The ultrasound findings vary from an echo-free mass to a mass containing occasional low-level echoes [48].

Angiography demonstrates an avascular mass with a thin hypervascular rim. Inflammatory neovascularity is frequently seen around the rim, and the junction of cyst and normal parenchyma may be hazy. If the cyst is peripheral, there may be hypertrophy of a capsular artery [9]. If the lesion progresses and becomes extensive, however, the radiologic and pathologic findings are similar to those of an acute renal abscess.

Infected hydronephrosis, or *pyonephrosis*, which is depicted in Figure 53-19, has been covered in the section on hydronephrosis.

Fungous disease is a comparatively rare infection in the kidney. The offending organisms are most commonly candidia and aspergillus [23, 39, 42]. The patients affected are usually undergoing chemotherapy for malignancy, receiving steroid treatment while debilitated, or diabetic. The fungous disease usually involves the collecting system, with changes in the kidney usually secondary to obstruction. Occasionally, extensive involvement of the renal parenchyma occurs. Very little has been reported, however, about any angiographic findings, which would most closely resemble those existing in xanthogranulomatous pyelonephritis, infected hydronephrosis, or pyonephrosis.

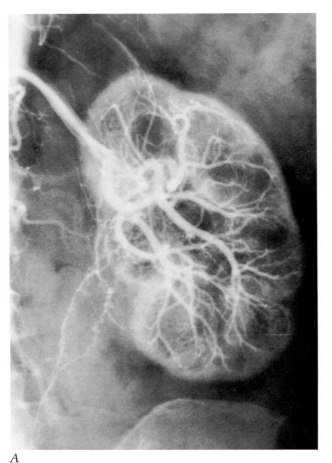

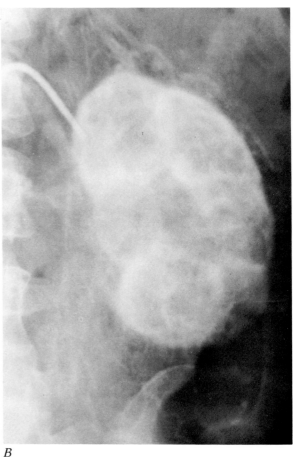

A

B

Figure 53-19. Case 19. Pyonephrosis (infected hydronephrosis). A 61-year-old woman with a high fever and left flank pain. No visualization of the right kidney was noted on intravenous pyelography. (A) Selective left renal arteriogram, arterial phase. Changes suggestive of mild hydronephrosis are seen, with some stretching of the interlobar branches over dilated caliceal structures. However, the usual atrophy of the peripheral vessels is not seen. In fact, there is a suggestion of increased vascularity. Prominent, enlarged, and tortuous pelvic arteries are seen supplying the pelvis and the upper ureter. (B) Selective left renal arteriogram, nephrographic phase. Hyperemia and staining in the perinephric spaces are present, along with filling of the capsular vessels. The changes of hydronephrosis, with irregular staining in the kidney, are seen. Contrast staining or blush in the wall of the pelvis is also seen. A left nephrectomy was performed for a diffusely infected and pyonephrotic kidney.

Role of Angiography in Renal Inflammatory Disease

The role of angiography in the workup of the patient with inflammatory disease has undergone considerable change as less invasive techniques, such as ultrasonography and computed tomography, have become available. The greater use of interventional techniques, such as percutaneous needle aspiration, has also had an effect on the need for angiography in some cases. However, angiography's role in helping establish the diagnosis and evaluating the extent of the inflammatory disease process when the other techniques are unable to do so is still valid. The use of angiography (both arteriography and venography) in conjunction with sonography or computed tomography is important in defining the correct treatment approach. For example, the radiologic findings can determine whether surgical or antibiotic therapy is indicated. Also, if intervention is contemplated, the type of interventional procedure to be used may be influenced by the radiologic findings. Whether needle aspiration with catheter drainage, surgical drainage, or nephrectomy is indicated can be determined by outlining the extent of the disease process. In summary, angiography along with other diagnostic techniques can help establish the diagnosis of inflammatory disease, determine the stage of disease and its extent, and thus greatly influence the treatment approach.

ACKNOWLEDGMENTS

We would like to thank Charles Smith, M.D., Babylon, New York, for Case 3; Marvin Hinke, M.D., Marshfield, Wisconsin, for Case 8; Richard Gordon, M.D., and Peter Sforza, M.D., New York, for Case 16; and Manuel Madayag, M.D., who performed many of the angiograms shown in this chapter.

References

1. Barth, K. H., Lightman, N. I., Ridolfi, R. L., and Catalona, W. J.   Acute pyelonephritis simulating poorly vascularized renal neoplasm. Non-specificity of angiographic criteria. *J. Urol.* 116:650, 1976.
2. Beachley, M. C., Ranniger, K., and Roth, F. J.   Xanthogranulomatous pyelonephritis. *AJR* 121:500, 1974.
3. Becker, J. A.   Xanthogranulomatous pyelonephritis: A case report with angiographic findings. *Acta Radiol. [Diagn.]* (Stockh.) 4:139, 1966.
4. Becker, J. A., Kanter, I. E., and Perl, S.   Rapid intrarenal circulation. *AJR* 109:167, 1970.
5. Becker, J. A., Weiss, R. M., and Lattimer, J. K.   Renal tuberculosis: The role of nephrotomography and angiography. *J. Urol.* 100:415, 1968.
6. Bjørn-Hansen, R., and Aakhus, T.   Angiography in renal tuberculosis. *Acta Radiol. [Diagn.]* (Stockh.) 11:167, 1971.
7. Caplan, L. H., Siegelman, S. S., and Bosniak, M. A.   Angiography in inflammatory space-occupying lesions of the kidney. *Radiology* 88:14, 1967.
8. Caro, G., Meisell, R., and Held, B.   Epinephrine-enhanced arteriography in renal and perirenal abscess. *Radiology* 92:1262, 1969.
9. Cho, K. J., Maklad, N., Curran, J., and Ting, Y. M.   Angiographic and ultrasonic findings in infected simple cysts of the kidney. *AJR* 127:1015, 1976.
10. Combs, J. A., Crummy, A. B., and Cossman, F. P.   Angiography in renal and pararenal inflammatory lesions: The significance of early venous filling. *Radiology* 98:401, 1971.
11. Craven, J. D., Hardy, B., Stanley, P., Orecklin, J. R., and Goodwin, W. E.   Acute renal carbun-

12. cle: The importance of preoperative angiography. *J. Urol.* 111:727, 1974.
12. Davidson, A. J.   *Radiologic Diagnosis of Renal Parenchymal Disease*. Philadelphia: Saunders, 1977. P. 237.
13. Davidson, A. J., and Talner, L. B.   Urographic and angiographic abnormalities in adult onset acute bacterial nephritis. *Radiology* 106:249, 1973.
14. Davidson, A. J., and Talner, L. B.   Late sequelae of adult onset acute bacterial nephritis. *Radiology* 127:367, 1978.
15. Doolittle, K. H., and Taylor, J. N.   Renal abscess in the differential diagnosis of mass in kidney. *J. Urol.* 89:649, 1963.
16. Evans, J. A., Meyers, M. A., and Bosniak, M. A.   Acute renal and perirenal infections. *Semin. Roentgenol.* 6:274, 1971.
17. Fair, W. R., and Higgins, M. H.   Renal abscess. *J. Urol.* 104:179, 1970.
18. Foster, R. S., Shuford, W. H., and Weens, H. S.   Selective renal arteriography in medical diseases of the kidney. *AJR* 95:291, 1965.
19. Friedenberg, M. J., Eisen, S., and Kissane, J.   Renal angiography in pyelonephritis, glomerulonephritis and arteriolar nephrosclerosis. *AJR* 95:349, 1965.
20. Frimann-Dahl, J.   Selective angiography in renal tuberculosis. *Acta Radiol.* (Stockh.) 49:31, 1958.
21. Gadrinab, N. M., Lome, L. G., and Presman, D.   Renal abscesses: Role of renal arteriography. *Urology* 2:39, 1973.
22. Gammill, S., Rabinowitz, J. G., Peace, R., Sorgen, S., Hurwitz, L., and Himmelfarb, E.   New thoughts concerning xanthogranulomatous pyelonephritis. *AJR* 125:154, 1975.
23. Gerle, R. D.   Roentgenographic features of primary renal candidiases. Fungus ball of the renal pelvis and ureter. *AJR* 119:731, 1973.
24. Gingell, J. C., Roylance, J., Davies, E. R., and Penry, J. B.   Xanthogranulomatous pyelonephritis. *Br. J. Radiol.* 46:99, 1973.
25. Giustra, P. E., Watson, R. C., and Shulman, H.   Arteriographic findings in various stages of renal tuberculosis. *Radiology* 100:597, 1971.
26. Goldman, M. L., Gorelkin, L., Rudé, J. C., Sybers, R. G., and O'Brien, D. P.   Epinephrine renal venography in severe inflammatory disease of the kidney. *Radiology* 127:93, 1978.
27. Goldman, S. M., Minkin, S. D., Naraval, D. C., Diamond, A. B., Pion, S. J., Meringoff, B. N., Sidh, S. M., Sanders, R. C., and Cohen, S. P.   Renal carbuncle: The use of ultrasound in its diagnosis and treatment. *J. Urol.* 118:525, 1977.
28. Hill, G. S., and Clark, R. L.   A comparative angiographic, microangiographic and histologic study of experimental pyelonephritis. *Invest. Radiol.* 7:33, 1972.
29. Himmelfarb, E. H., Rabinowitz, J. G., Kinkhab-

wala, M. N., and Becker, J. A. The roentgen features of renal carbuncle. *J. Urol.* 108:846, 1972.

30. Kahn, P. C. Selective venography in renal parenchymal disease. *Radiology* 92:345, 1969.

31. Kahn, P. C., and Wise, H. M., Jr. Simulation of renal tumor response to epinephrine by inflammatory disease. *Radiology* 89:1062, 1967.

32. Kass, E. J., Silver, T. M., Konnak, J. W., Thornbury, J. R., and Wolfman, M. G. The urographic findings in acute pyelonephritis: Non-obstructive hydronephrosis. *J. Urol.* 116:544, 1976.

33. Klein, D. L., and Filpi, R. G. Acute renal carbuncle. *J. Urol.* 118:912, 1977.

34. Koehler, P. R. The roentgen diagnosis of renal inflammatory masses—special emphasis on angiographic changes. *Radiology* 112:257, 1974.

35. Koehler, P. R., and Nelson, J. A. Arteriographic findings in inflammatory mass lesions of the kidney. *Radiol. Clin. North Am.* 14:281, 1976.

36. Levin, D. C., Gordon, D., Kinkhabwala, M., and Becker, J. A. Reticular neovascularity in malignant and inflammatory renal masses. *Radiology* 120:61, 1976.

37. Lilienfeld, R. M., and Lande, A. Acute adult onset bacterial nephritis: Long-term urographic and angiographic follow-up. *J. Urol.* 114:14, 1975.

38. Malek, R. S., and Elder, J. S. Xanthogranulomatous pyelonephritis: A critical analysis of twenty-six cases and of the literature. *J. Urol.* 119:589, 1978.

39. Michigan, S. Genitourinary fungal infections. *J. Urol.* 116:390, 1976.

40. Miller, H. L., Ney, C., and Puljic, S. Xanthogranulomatous pyelonephritis. *N.Y. State J. Med.* 76:919, 1976.

41. Moore, C. A., and Gangai, M. P. Renal cortical abscess. *J. Urol.* 98:303, 1967.

42. Myerson, D. A., and Rosenfield, A. T. Renal aspergillosis: A report of two cases. *J. Can. Assoc. Radiol.* 28:214, 1977.

43. Pingoud, E. G., Pais, S. O., and Glickman, M. Epinephrine renal venography in acute bacterial infection of the kidney. *AJR* 133:665, 1979.

44. Rabinowitz, J. G., Kinkhabwala, M. N., Robinson, T., Spyropoulos, E., and Becker, J. A. Acute renal carbuncle: The roentgenographic clarification of a medical enigma. *AJR* 116:740, 1972.

45. Rosenfield, A. T., Glickman, M. G., Taylor, K. J. W., Crade, M., and Hodson, J. Acute focal bacterial nephritis (acute lobar nephronia). *Radiology* 132:553, 1979.

46. Rossi, P., Myers, D. H., Furey, R., and Bonfils-Roberts, E. A. Angiography in bilateral xanthogranulomatous pyelonephritis. *Radiology* 90:320, 1968.

47. Salmon, R. B., and Koehler, P. R. Angiography in renal and perirenal inflammatory masses. *Radiology* 88:9, 1967.

48. Schneider, M., Becker, J. A., Staiano, S., and Campos, E. Sonographic-radiographic correlation of renal and perirenal infections. *AJR* 127:1007, 1976.

49. Shenoy, S. S., Culver, G. J., and Arani, D. T. Renal carbuncle: Stimulation of tumor response to epinephrine. *Urology* 10:601, 1977.

50. Silver, T. M., Kass, E. J., Thornbury, J. R., Konnak, J. W., and Wolfman, M. G. The radiological spectrum of acute pyelonephritis in adults and adolescents. *Radiology* 118:65, 1976.

51. Smith, J. C., Rösch, J., Athanasoulis, C. A., Baum, S., Waltman, A. C., and Goldman, M. Renal venography in the evaluation of poorly vascularized neoplasms of the kidney. *AJR* 123:552, 1975.

52. Strasberg, Z., Jacobson, S. A., Srolovitz, H., Sedlezky, I., and Schneiderman, C. Xanthogranulomatous pyelonephritis: Radiologic considerations. *J. Can. Assoc. Radiol.* 21:173, 1970.

53. Vinik, M., Freed, T. A., Smellie, W. A. B., and Weidner, W. Xanthogranulomatous pyelonephritis. Angiographic considerations. *Radiology* 92:537, 1969.

54. Wicks, J. D., and Thornbury, J. R. Acute renal infections in adults. *Radiol. Clin. North Am.* 17:245, 1979.

The Angiography of Hydronephrosis

MARJORIE A. AMBOS
RICHARD S. LEFLEUR
MORTON A. BOSNIAK

Although dilatation of the renal collecting system is usually the result of mechanical obstruction of the system somewhere along its course, nonobstructive causes, such as inflammation, atony, and neurogenic processes, may less frequently lead to the same changes [8]. With obstruction, the changes that are seen depend on the acuteness and duration of the pathologic process [9]. Animal experiments have shown that ligation of a ureter leads first to an increase in the pressure within the renal pelvis. Normal pelvic pressure is near zero; with total acute obstruction this pressure rises to 50 to 125 mm Hg. Glomerular filtration decreases but does not stop completely in the acute phase, so that if intravenous contrast material is administered it is still excreted, but its passage through the collecting tubules is slowed. Since water is resorbed and the contrast material becomes more concentrated, a dense nephrogram results [3, 7].

Patients with acute obstruction have radiographic changes that reflect this state. Urography classically demonstrates a swollen, enlarged kidney with delayed function, diminished excretion of contrast material, and a dense nephrogram [4]. Significant dilatation of the pelvis and calices and parenchymal atrophy only occur with time. The large kidney with saclike calices, a huge pelvis, and markedly diminished parenchyma is the result of long-term partial obstruction or multiple episodes of obstruction [9, 21]. The primary effect of the increased renal pelvic pressure of chronic obstruction is parenchymal atrophy. Two factors lead to this loss of tissue: (1) the relative ischemia of the kidney due to the increased pressure on the intrarenal arteries and (2) the direct effect of constant abnormal pressure on the renal parenchyma. Although this renal atrophy is global, it is first seen radiographically in the papilla. As the papilla atrophies, the corresponding calices enlarge, going from the classic Y configuration to a rounded shape and finally becoming clubbed. The end stage is a kidney with the merest shell of parenchyma, its major mass being saclike calices and a huge pelvis [8].

Most cases of chronic hydronephrosis are secondary to obstruction of the ureteropelvic junction due to a congenital abnormality. Pathologic studies of these kidneys have shown a deficient muscle layer or abnormal direction of muscle bundles at the ureteropelvic junction that, in

1201

turn, is felt to lead to submucosal fibrosis and secondary muscular hypertrophy. These changes may occasionally be associated with an aberrant vessel or accessory vessels in the area. Other common causes of chronic hydronephrosis are calculi, urothelial carcinoma, and retroperitoneal processes [5].

Findings on intravenous urography reflect the chronicity and severity of the obstructive process. In acute condition, function is compromised but no significant dilatation or atrophy occurs. With time there is progressively decreased excretion of contrast material and delay in filling of the collecting system so that films may have to be obtained up to 24 hours following administration of contrast material [3]. Eventually there is non-visualization of the kidney and collecting system [4, 8]. At that point, other techniques, such as retrograde pyelography, antegrade pyelography, ultrasonography, computed tomography, and angiography, may be necessary to evaluate the kidney further and to help decide on therapy.

In acute obstruction, leakage of urine from a renal calix into the renal sinus and into the retroperitoneum (or into the renal lymphatics) may occur, continuing until the obstruction is relieved. This phenomenon has been documented on urography in many cases, but how often this actually occurs is not known. In one series it was seen urographically in 22 to 33 percent of cases when higher doses of contrast material were used [2].

This extravasation may act as a protective mechanism to decrease intrapelvic pressure. The ability of the kidney to protect itself by leaking urine into its renal sinus or lymphatics might help explain the varied end results in cases of renal obstruction. In some patients with long-standing ureteral obstruction, large hydronephrotic sacs develop, while in others, small hydronephrotic sacs or atrophic small kidneys result. There are also various degrees of recovery of renal function when a long-standing ureteral obstruction is relieved.

Angiography

Angiographic findings in hydronephrosis are dependent on the severity and duration of the process. When selective renal angiography is performed on an acutely obstructed kidney, the findings are minimal, and often the angiogram is completely normal. However, the main renal artery branches can be stretched owing to renal swelling and enlargement [18]. There may also be delayed filling of the secondary and tertiary branches of the intrarenal arteries due to increased intrarenal pressure from the obstruction. These findings are best seen on a midstream aortic injection since it is by comparison to the normal arteries in the contralateral kidney that subtle differences in filling may be noted (Fig. 54-1).

The angiographic changes in chronic hydronephrosis are more constant and more severe than in the acute phase, reflecting the greater dilatation of the collecting system and the parenchymal atrophy (Figs. 54-2–54-6). The first vessels affected are the small distal arteries. These are tapered and show decreased branching. As the process worsens, changes proceed proximally [4, 24]. The intrarenal arteries are splayed, stretched, and narrowed as they pass around the dilated calices [4, 13, 27]. There is a decrease in the size and number of branches. Owing to increased intrarenal pressure, circulation time through the vessels is slowed [10]. If the renal pelvis becomes extremely dilated, as in a tight ureteropelvic junction obstruction, the dorsal and ventral branches of the main renal artery are spread over it, and the main renal artery itself is pushed upward over the large pelvis [22, 27] (Figs. 54-2–54-6).

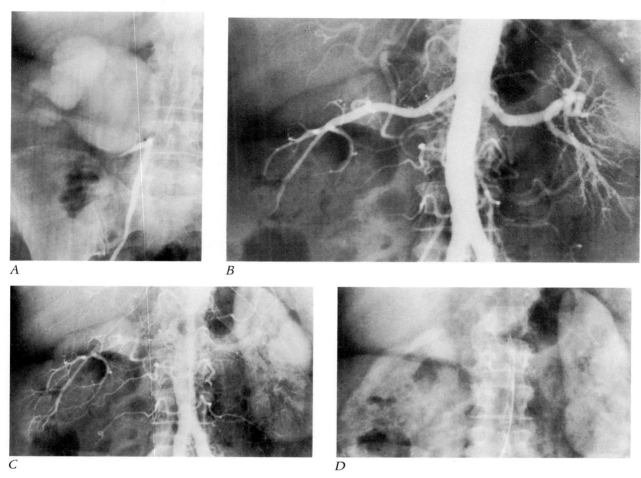

Figure 54-1. Case 1. Hydronephrosis with salvageable kidney in a 42-year-old woman with right-sided pain. (A) Retrograde pyelogram. A tight ureteropelvic junction obstruction with greatly dilated pelvis and calices is seen. (B) Aortogram, early arterial phase. The renal arteries are equal in size. The flow of contrast medium through the right kidney is slow as compared to its flow through the left. (C) Aortogram, later arterial phase. Delayed filling of the intrarenal vessels on the right can be seen. These vessels are stretched and somewhat attenuated. The nephrogram is already shown in the left kidney. (D) Aortogram, nephrogram phase. The nephrograms in both kidneys are similar. Surgical repair of the ureteropelvic junction obstruction on the right was performed, with return to normal function in the right kidney.

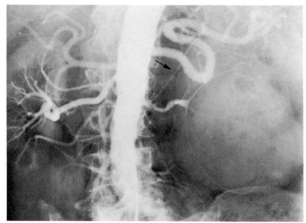

A

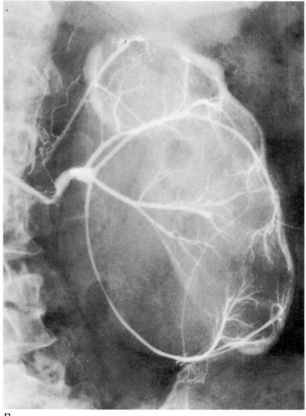

B

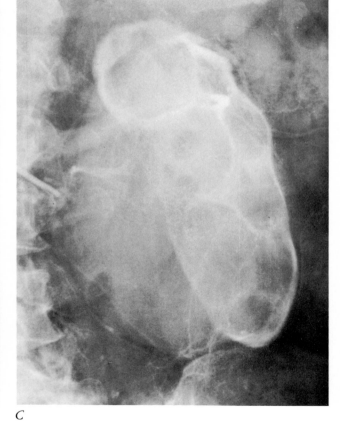

C

Figure 54-2. Case 2. Chronic hydronephrosis in a 59-year-old woman with a palpable left-flank mass. (A) Aortogram. An atrophic left renal artery is seen. Poor filling of vessels in the left kidney is noted, with sparse vascularity and stretching of filled vessels over a dilated pelvis. A superior polar artery is seen (*arrow*) supplying upper pole of left kidney. (B) Selective left renal arteriogram, arterial phase. Atrophic vascularity to the "shell" of the left kidney is well demonstrated. Diminished branches and stretching of vessels over a dilated collecting system are noted. Major branches of the renal artery are seen stretched over a dilated pelvis. (C) Selective left renal arteriogram, nephrogram phase. A minimal nephrogram in the remaining parenchyma is seen. Dilated calices are outlined by the opacified parenchyma. A left nephrectomy was performed.

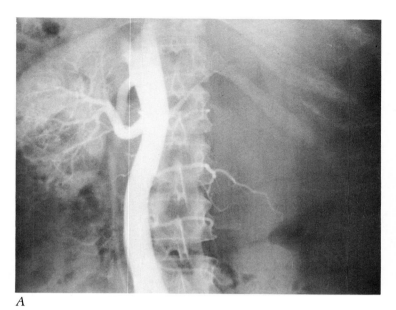

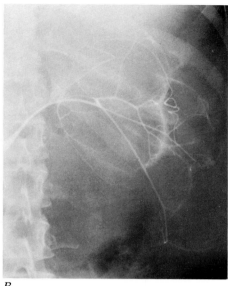

A

B

Figure 54-3. Case 3. Chronic hydronephrosis in a 45-year-old man with a palpable abdominal mass on the left. (A) Aortogram. Atrophy of the left renal artery is apparent, with minimal filling of the distal branches to the left kidney. A mass in the left flank is displacing the aorta to the right. (B) Selective left renal arteriogram. Marked stretching of an atrophic left renal artery and branches is apparent. This appearance is quite characteristic of chronic hydronephrosis. At surgery, a large hydronephrotic sac was removed.

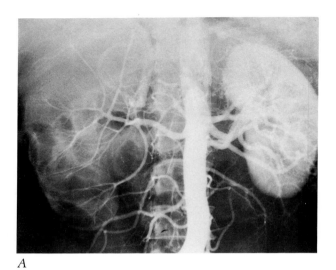

A

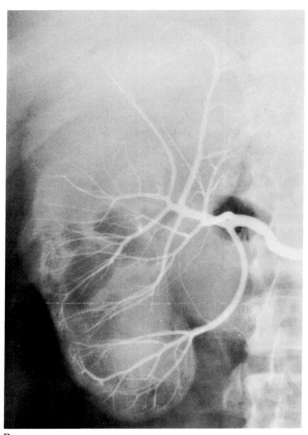

B

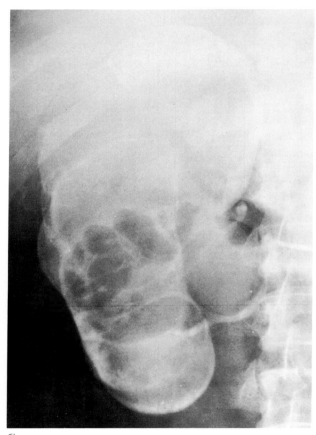

C

Figure 54-4. Case 4. Chronic hydronephrosis in a 31-year-old man with right flank pain. (A) Aortogram. An enlarged right renal contour and stretched atrophic vessels coursing over a hydronephrotic kidney are seen. (B) Selective right renal arteriogram, arterial phase. Characteristic stretching, splaying, and atrophy of branches of the right renal artery are noted coursing over dilated caliceal structures. (C) Selective right renal arteriogram, nephrogram phase. A thin rim of parenchyma is opacified. A right nephrectomy was performed. The parenchyma of the pathologic specimen was 1 to 2 mm thick.

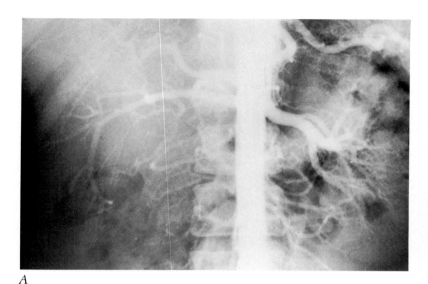

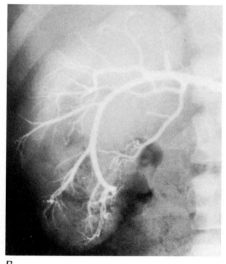

A   *B*

Figure 54-5. Case 5. Chronic hydronephrosis in a 22-year-old man with right flank pain. (A) Aortogram. Stretching of the right renal artery and its branches over a hydronephrotic right kidney is seen. (B) Selective right renal arteriogram. Stretching and atrophy of branches of the right renal artery can be seen, with some minimal parenchyma noted along the outer margin of the kidney. A right nephrectomy was performed. The parenchyma of the pathologic specimen was 0.1 to 1.0 cm thick.

The nephrogram reflects the amount of functioning renal tissue; its integrity is the key to determining whether a kidney is salvageable. In acute hydronephrosis, a good nephrogram is seen, but with time and atrophy it becomes progressively diminished, until eventually a nephrogram is no longer visualized. This decrease in functioning renal tissue is also reflected in the size of the main renal artery. As function diminishes, the renal artery and its branches atrophy [4, 12, 15]. In end-stage hydronephrosis, there is a small main renal artery, splayed and diminished intrarenal branches, and no functioning renal tissue.

The changes just mentioned are those of classic hydronephrosis; when they occur throughout the kidney, the angiographic diagnosis is obvious. However, hydronephrosis may be localized to one calix or segment of the kidney, appearing as a mass, and the condition may be more difficult to diagnose. In this localized form, the vessels are splayed and attenuated around the obstructed area. Although the appearance on urography is of a mass, the avascular nature, combined with contrast filling of the mass on delayed urogram films, will generally allow the correct diagnosis to be made [4] (Figs. 54-7–54-10).

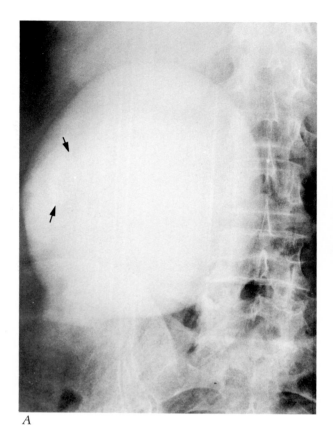

A

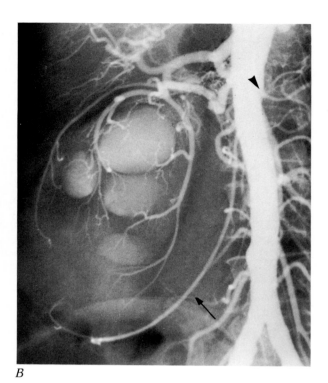

B

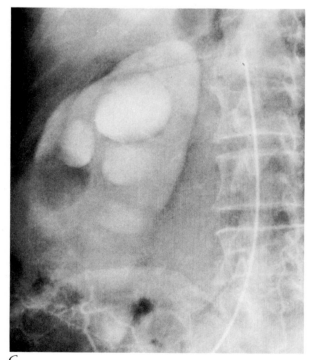

C

Figure 54-6. Case 6. Chronic hydronephrosis in a 66-year-old patient with right-sided pain and a palpable mass in the right side of the abdomen. (A) Delayed film (2 hours) of intravenous urogram. There is a greatly dilated right renal pelvis indicating a ureteropelvic junction obstruction. Some filling of the dilated calices (*arrows*) can be seen through the opacified pelvis. (B) Aortogram, arterial phase. A kinked right renal artery is shown supplying a hydronephrotic right kidney. Atrophy and stretching of the peripheral branches is seen. The accessory renal artery courses inferiorly (*arrow*) and stretches around the dilated pelvis. An accessory renal artery is not obstructing the pelvis but is being pushed by the pelvis. Also note an atrophic left renal artery (*arrowhead*). An atrophic kidney was present on the left. (C) Aortogram, nephrogram phase. A thinned parenchyma but some nephrogram is apparent, along with dilated calices. At surgery, a plastic repair of the renal pelvis was performed, with great improvement in the right renal function.

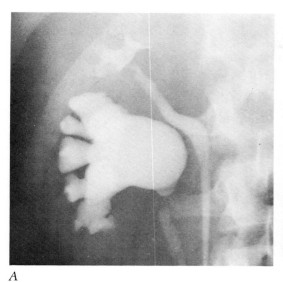

A

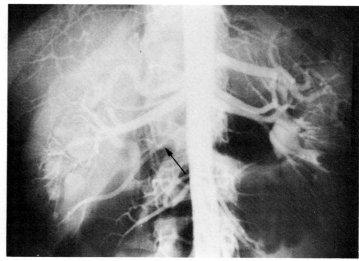

B

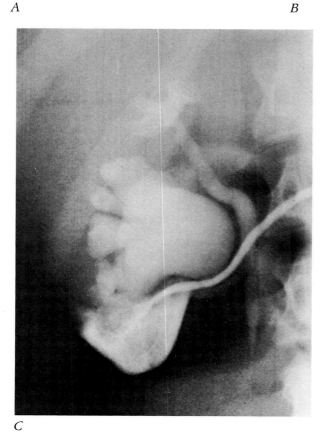

C

Figure 54-7. Case 7. Localized hydronephrosis caused by an accessory renal artery. A 19-year-old man with right flank pain. (A) Urogram, delayed film. A hydronephrotic lower collecting system is now opacified. A ureteropelvic junction obstruction is present. (B) Aortogram. Two renal arteries of about equal size to the left kidney are seen. A normal-sized right renal artery with a superior polar branch is filled. A smaller accessory renal artery is also seen (*arrow*) supplying the lower pole of the right kidney. (C) Selective study of the accessory right renal artery. The accessory artery to the lower pole crosses the pelvis of the lower pole collecting system, obstructing it. At surgery, a plastic repair of the obstruction was performed. The pelvis was placed anterior to the obstructing vessel.

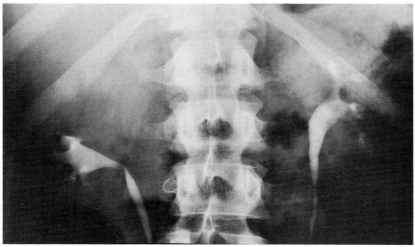

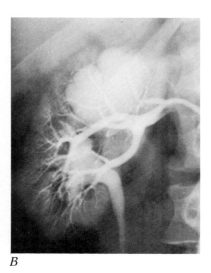

A

B

Figure 54-8. Case 8. Localized hydronephrosis in a duplicated collecting system. A 28-year-old woman with right-sided abdominal pain and infection. (A) Urogram. There is no visualization of the calices in the upper pole of the right kidney. (B) Selective right renal arteriogram. Localized hydronephrosis with dilated calices in the upper pole collecting system is seen. Atrophy of the branches to the upper pole is noted. Branches of the renal artery cross the upper pole collecting system and contribute to its obstruction. At surgery, a partial nephrectomy of the upper pole of the kidney was performed after it was determined that the plastic salvage would be technically difficult.

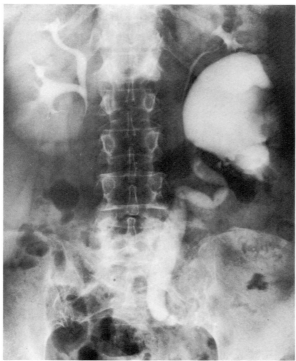

A

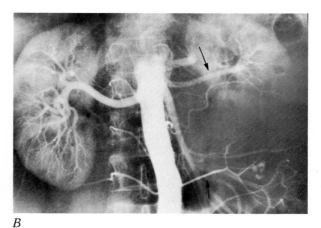

B

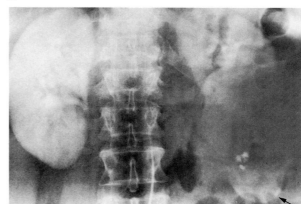

C

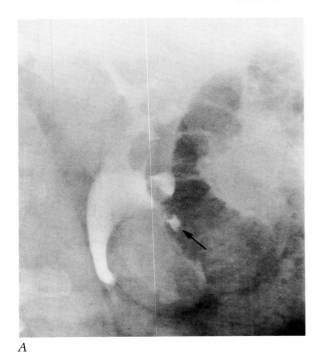

A

Figure 54-10. Case 10. Localized hydronephrosis due to a calculus. A 45-year-old man with left flank pain. (A) Urogram. A bulbous enlargement of the lower pole of the kidney is seen, with poor visualization of collecting system structures. The arrow points to a calculus seen on the preliminary film. (B) Selective left renal arteriogram, arterial phase. Atrophy and stretching of the branches to the lower pole of the kidney are seen. The upper pole vessels are normal. (C) Selective left renal arteriogram, nephrogram phase. A normal nephrogram is noted in the upper pole. Only the rim of the parenchyma is seen (*arrows*) surrounding the hydronephrotic lower lobe. A heminephrectomy of the lower pole of the left kidney was performed.

◄ **Figure 54-9.** Case 9. Localized hydronephrosis in a duplicated collecting system. A 50-year-old woman with left flank pain. The patient had had a hysterectomy 4 years previously. (A) Excretory urogram and antegrade pyelogram of a lower pole collecting system on the left. Hydronephrosis and hydroureter is seen in the lower pole collecting system of a duplicated system on the left. The right kidney and the upper pole left kidney are visualized secondary to the urogram. The hydronephrotic system on the left was not visualized on the urogram, and it was opacified by a percutaneous antegrade injection. The obstruction of the distal ureter on the left (by a surgical tie) is clearly seen. (B) Aortogram, arterial phase. The main renal artery to the left kidney is barely seen (*higher arrow*) on this film. A second atrophic renal artery (*lower arrow*) to the lower pole is noted. The atrophic branches are stretched. (C) Aortogram, nephrogram phase. The nephrogram of the normal upper pole is present intact. No nephrogram is seen in the lower portion of the kidney, except for a minimal rim at the lower pole (*arrow*) of the kidney. Note the overlying calcified mesenteric nodes. At surgery, the hydronephrotic lower pole was removed.

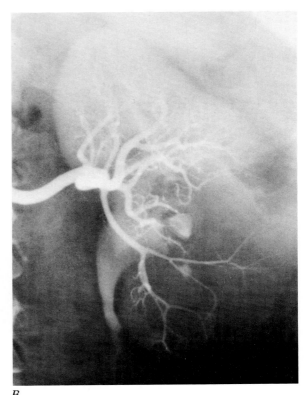

B

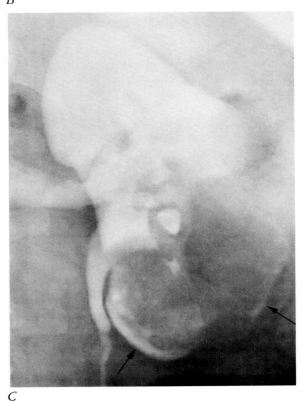

C

Angiography in Infected Hydronephrosis and Pyonephrosis

When the collecting system of a hydronephrotic kidney becomes infected, other radiographic findings are superimposed on those of dilatation and atrophy. Whatever the level of function of the kidney, infection generally worsens it. Visualization of an infected or a pyonephrotic kidney is poor or nonexistent on intravenous urography. With the use of high-dose infusion techniques, better visualization was reported and some nephrogram or rim of density around the dilated calices was seen in about half the patients in one study [28]. If a retrograde pyelogram is done in pyonephrosis, in which pus fills the collecting system, a shaggy, bizarre pattern is seen as the contrast material mixes with the exudate [8].

Angiography in pyonephrosis shows the previously described changes of hydronephrosis; i.e., atrophy of vessels, stretching and splaying of arteries around dilated calices, and a decrease in the number of terminal and parenchymal branches [17]. Added to this in many cases are inflammatory vascular changes. Small, fine tortuous neovascularity may be present around the infected collecting system structures. The borders of the calices are ill defined and hazy. Zones of abnormal vessels in the capillary phase lead to areas of abnormal "blush" on the nephrogram [1, 17, 29] (Fig. 54-11). As in other chronic renal infections, there may be hypertrophy and increased tortuosity of periureteric and capsular arteries as they give rise to some of these inflammatory vessels [17].

In summary, the angiographic picture reflects the pathologic picture and may range from a pattern like that of simple hydronephrosis to one of xanthogranulomatous pyelonephritis (see Chap. 53), with extensive inflammatory vascularity.

Figure 54-11. Case 11. Pyonephrosis. A 53-year-old woman with a high fever and right-sided discomfort. (A) Urogram. Calculi were seen on the preliminary film in the right kidney. No visualization of the contrast material is seen on the right. (B) Selective right renal arteriogram. The changes indicative of hydronephrosis are seen, with atrophy of the branches and stretching of the vessels over the hydronephrotic sacs. However, there is increased filling of the smaller branches, with hyperemia, and staining, which is indicative of an associated inflammation. A nephrectomy revealed a hydronephrotic sac filled with pus (pyonephrosis) and calculi.

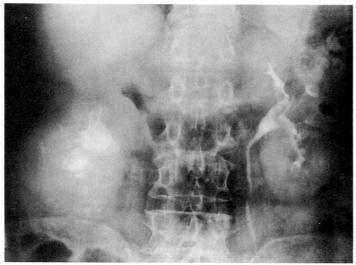

A

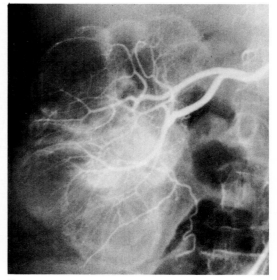

B

Use of Angiography to Determine the Cause of Hydronephrosis

A kidney that is not visualized on intravenous urography is generally assessed by the use of retrograde pyelography, ultrasonography, computed tomography, or, occasionally, antegrade pyelography. Ultrasonography has been found to be quite reliable in diagnosing chronic hydronephrosis, showing an echo-free mass with little surrounding parenchyma in the most severe cases or, in earlier stages, cystlike areas radiating out from the renal pelvis [19, 26].

Angiography on occasion may play a role in diagnosing the cause of hydronephrosis when other techniques are unable to do so. An example of this is depicted in Figure 54-12. In this case, a patient with hydronephrosis was unable to be studied with retrograde pyelography, and angiography demonstrated the hydronephrotic kidney and also tumor vascularity in the renal pelvis with extension into the ureter. In renal pelvic tumors, the artery to the renal pelvis and upper ureter may enlarge and give rise to this neovascularity. If the urothelial tumor invades the renal parenchyma, the previously normal intrarenal vessels in the involved area will be encased and often occluded [20, 25].

Another role of angiography in hydronephrosis is to determine whether an aberrant or accessory vessel, either artery or vein, is the cause of the obstruction [9, 22, 27]. Numerous angiographic studies of patients with hydronephrosis have shown that they have a higher-than-average incidence of accessory renal vessels (see Figs. 54-6, 54-7). The incidence of multiple renal arteries to a kidney is about 20 percent in the normal population. In patients with hydronephrosis due to structural congenital causes, the incidence is 40 percent [22]. Evidently, there is an embryologic association between the occurrence of ureteropelvic junction narrowing and the persistence of multiple renal vessels. While at first it was presumed that the accessory vessel was usually the cause of the obstruction, surgical correlation has now shown that it is uncommon for the accessory vessel to be responsible [5, 14, 23]. In one series of 39 patients with accessory renal arteries and hydronephrosis, an accessory vessel was found to be the cause of the obstruction in 14 patients. In another three patients in this series, the artery plus perivascular adhesions caused the narrowing, but in the other 22 patients the accessory vessel was in no way related to the hydronephrosis. In all cases in which the artery was a causal factor, it ran ventral to the renal pelvis and originated within 40 mm of the origin of the main renal artery. A polar branch with an early takeoff from the main renal artery may also cause obstruction, and aberrant veins are also capable of producing enough pressure on the collecting system to lead to obstruction [23].

Frequently, an accessory renal artery is present at an obstructed ureteropelvic junction but the vessel itself is not the cause of the obstruction (see Fig. 54-6). The vessel may merely contribute to the obstruction of an already enlarging renal pelvis or may merely limit its extent of dilatation. When it must be decided preoperatively whether an artery is associated with a point of obstruction, comparisons of the angiogram and the intravenous urogram should enable one to make the determination. This can be more clearly demonstrated by performing arteriography after initially filling the renal pelvis with contrast media. The point of obstruction and the crossing vessel can then be well correlated [27] (see Fig. 54-7).

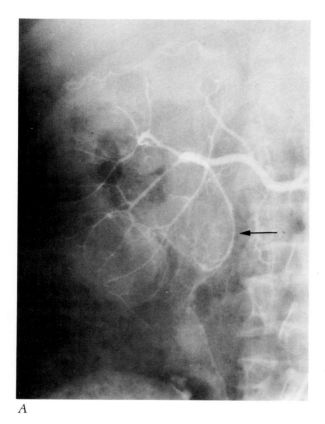

A

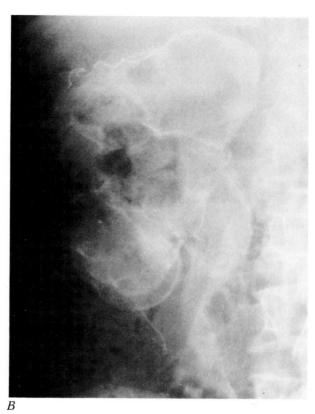

B

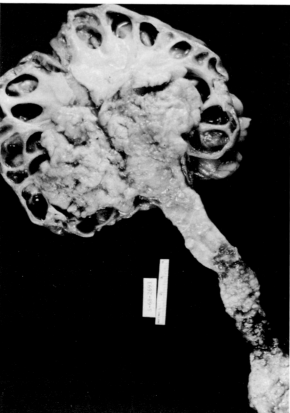

C

Figure 54-12. Case 12. Hydronephrosis secondary to renal pelvic carcinoma. A 65-year-old man with hematuria. A urogram revealed nonvisualization of the right kidney, and a right retrograde pyelogram could not be performed. (A) Selective right renal arteriogram, arterial phase. The typical changes of hydronephrosis, with atrophy and stretching of the intrarenal vessels over the dilated calices, is seen. A hypertrophied pelvic artery is seen (*arrow*); it gives off some tumor-like vessels in the renal pelvis and extends inferiorly to supply the ureter. (B) Selective right renal arteriogram, nephrogram phase. The hydronephrotic "shell" of the right kidney is seen. Also noted is a slight blush of tumor tissue in the renal pelvis and the upper ureter. (C) A pathologic specimen reveals hydronephrosis with extensive tumor in the renal pelvis and the ureter. (Reprinted with permission from J. A. Evans and M. A. Bosniak, *The Kidney* [*Atlas of Tumor Radiology* Series]. Chicago: Year Book Medical Publishers, 1971.)

Angiography in Treatment Planning

In situations of ureteropelvic junction obstruction, angiography has played a role in determining whether or not the chronically obstructed kidney is salvageable. If a plastic repair to relieve the obstruction will not result in a functioning kidney, a simple nephrectomy can be performed. Multiple animal experiments have shown that the size of the main renal artery is a guide to potential recovery of function [11, 13, 22, 24, 30]. When the ureter is totally occluded, there is a progressive decrease in both the size of the main renal artery and the intensity of the nephrogram. While these studies vary as to the exact length of time necessary for irreversible changes to occur, they generally agree that 30 to 40 days is the critical time. By this point, the artery has diminished in size to less than 50 percent of its original diameter. Once this critical value is reached, irreversible damage is done. No comparable data are available for humans; however, in cases of chronic hydronephrosis, diminution in the caliber of the renal artery has been a constant finding. When the main renal artery of the affected kidney has a caliber less than 50 percent of that of the contralateral vessel, there is little hope of restoring function to the hydronephrotic kidney [13, 22, 30]. However, if the decrease in the diameter of the main renal artery in the obstructed kidney has not reached 50 percent, release of the obstruction may result in a return of function of varying degrees (see Fig. 54-1). However, this is not necessarily true in every case. We have seen a number of examples of unsalvageable kidneys with main renal arteries greater than 50 percent of the original diameter in which at surgery no significant amount of renal tissue was present and in which nephrectomy was performed (see Figs. 54-4, 54-5).

The amount of functioning parenchyma left in the hydronephrotic kidney may also be well evaluated by selective renal angiography since the intensity of the nephrogram is in effect the amount of functioning renal tissue [6, 18, 27]. The same experiments that demonstrated increasing atrophy of the renal artery with increasing time of occlusion also showed decrease in the intensity of the nephrogram with time [13, 30]. The density of the nephrogram gives a better understanding of the amount of functioning parenchyma in the kidney than does the visualization of the collecting system structures by urography. However, nuclear medicine techniques, including the use of ^{99m}Tc–DMSA, are now being utilized increasingly to determine the amount of residual functional renal tissue in these cases [16].

Finally, the angiogram is an important roadmap for the surgeon, particularly if he contemplates plastic repair and salvage of the hydronephrotic kidney. Complete knowledge of the vascular anatomy is essential for the best surgical results.

References

1. Becker, J. A., Fleming, R., Kanter, I., and Melicow, M. Misleading appearances in renal angiography. *Radiology* 88:691, 1967.
2. Bernardino, M. E., and McClennan, B. High dose urography: Incidence and relationship to spontaneous peripelvic extravasation. *AJR* 127:373, 1976.
3. Bigongiari, L. R., Davis, R. M., Novak, W. G., Wick, J. D., Kass, E., and Thornbury, J. R. Visualization of the medullary rays on excretory urography in experimental ureteric obstruction. *AJR* 129:89, 1977.
4. Bosniak, M. A., Scheff, S., and Kaufman, S. Localized hydronephrosis masquerading as renal neoplasm. *J. Urol.* 99:241, 1968.
5. Chahlaoui, J., and Herba, M. J. Ureteropelvic junction obstruction in the adult. *J. Can. Assoc. Radiol.* 28:40, 1977.
6. Doss, A. K. Translumbar aortography: Its diagnostic value in urography. *J. Urol.* 55:594, 1946.
7. Elkin, M., Boyarsky, S., Martinez, J., and Kaplan, N. Physiology of ureteral obstruction as determined by roentgenologic studies. *AJR* 92:291, 1964.
8. Emmett, J. L., and Witten, D. M. *Clinical Urography* (3rd ed.). Philadelphia: Saunders, 1971. Vol. 1, p. 369; vol. 2, p. 800.
9. Frimann-Dahl, J. Angiography in Hydronephrosis. In O. W. Kincaid (ed.), *Renal Angiography*. Chicago: Year Book 1966. P. 209.
10. Herdman, J. P., and Jaco, N. T. The renal circulation in experimental hydronephrosis. *Br. J. Urol.* 22:52, 1950.
11. Hinman, F., and Morison, D. M. Experimental hydronephrosis: Arterial changes in the progressive hydronephrosis of rabbits with complete ureteral obstruction. *Surg. Gynecol. Obstet.* 42:209, 1926.
12. Idbohrn, H. Renal angiography in cases of delayed excretion in intravenous urography. *Acta Radiol.* 42:333, 1954.
13. Idbohrn, H. Renal angiography in experimental hydronephrosis. *Acta Radiol.* [*Suppl.*] (Stockh.) 136:1956.

14. Jewett, H. J. Accessory renal vessels. Their influence in certain cases of hydronephrosis. *Surg. Gynecol. Obstet.* 68:666, 1936.

15. Kauffmann, G., and Seib, U. C. Angiographische Differential diagnose der Hydronephrose. *Radiologe* 15:457, 1975.

16. Kawamura, J., Shinichi, H., Yosida, O., Fujita, T., Yashushi, I., and Torizuka, A. Validity of ^{99m}Tc dimercaptosuccinic acid renal uptake for an assessment of individual kidney function. *J. Urol.* 119:305,1978.

17. Koehler, P. R. The roentgen diagnosis of renal inflammatory masses—special emphasis on angiographic changes. *Radiology* 112:257, 1974.

18. Leary, D. J., Templeton, A. W., Thompson, I. M., and Sibala, J. L. Preoperative aortography in hydronephrosis. *J. Urol.* 107:542, 1972.

19. Marangola, J. P., Bryan, P. J., and Azimi, F. Ultrasonic evaluation of the unilateral nonvisualized kidney. *AJR* 126:853, 1976.

20. Mitty, H. A., Baron, M. G., and Feller, M. Infiltrating carcinoma of the renal pelvis. Angiographic features. *Radiology* 92:994, 1969.

21. Ney, C., Friedenberg, R. M. *Radiographic Atlas of the Genitourinary System.* Philadelphia: Lippincott, 1966. Pp. 114, 172.

22. Olsson, O. In H. L. Abrams (ed.), *Angiography* (2nd ed.) Boston: Little, Brown, 1971. Vol. 2, pp. 785, 815.

23. Olsson, O. Roentgen diagnosis of the urogenital system. Berlin: Springer-Verlag, 1973. Part 1, pp. 114, 319.

24. Petasnick, J. P., and Patel, S. K. Angiographic evaluation of the nonvisualizing kidney. *AJR* 119:757, 1973.

25. Rabinowitz, J. G., Kinkhabwala, M., Himmelfarb, F., Robinson, T., Becker, J. A., Bosniak, M., and Madayag, M. M. Renal pelvic carcinoma: An angiographic re-evaluation. *Radiology* 102:551, 1972.

26. Sanders, R. C., Bearman, S. B-scan ultrasound in the diagnosis of hydronephrosis. *Radiology* 108:375, 1973.

27. Siegelman, S. S., and Bosniak, M. A. Renal arteriography in hydronephrosis: Its value in diagnosis and management. *Radiology* 85:609, 1965.

28. Watt, I., and Roylance, J. Pyonephrosis. *Clin. Radiol.* 27:513, 1975.

29. Wicks, J. D., and Thornbury, J. R. Acute renal infections in adults. *Radiol. Clin. North Am.* 17:245, 1979.

30. Widen, T. Renal angiography during and after unilateral ureteric occlusion: A long-term experimental study in dogs. *Acta Radiol. [Suppl.]* (Stockh.) 162:1958.

Anomalies and Malformations

ERIK BOIJSEN

Multiple Renal Arteries

Multiple renal arteries are often present, particularly in malrotated and dystopic kidneys. In kidneys situated at a normal level, multiple arteries occur in anatomic dissection series in about 30 percent of cases [43]. In the angiographic literature, multiple renal arteries are reported to be observed in 20 to 27 percent of cases [6, 14, 22, 27], but lower figures (e.g., 12%) are on record [3]. The reason that the figures are lower at angiography than they are in dissection studies is mainly because very small sublobar branches that pass from the aorta directly to the upper pole [6] often arise together with the superior capsular artery and adrenal arteries; at aortography these branches are too small to be noted or are misinterpreted as capsular arteries. These branches pass directly to the parenchyma without passing the renal hilus (Fig. 55-1).

The branches that pass directly to the parenchyma are usually called *polar* or *aberrant arteries*, while those passing through the hilus are called *hilar arteries*. Polar arteries can arise directly from the aorta or from hilar branches (see Figs. 50-3, 51-12). The superior polar artery is most often encountered in dissection studies. In a thorough analysis, aortic superior polar arteries were found in 7 percent of cases and lower polar arteries were found in 5.5 percent. Polar branches from hilar arteries were found to the upper and lower pole in 12 percent and 1.4 percent, respectively [43]. In an angiographic series, extrahilar inferior polar arteries were found in 9 percent to arise from the aorta or the iliac arteries [6].

In kidneys with multiple arteries, usually one main stem arises from the aorta at a normal level. Usually the main stem supplies anterior parts of the kidney and, most often also, at least the dorsal intermediate part. The most common extra artery from the aorta, here called the *supplementary artery,* passes through the hilus to the lower pole. In a clinical angiographic series, 72.5 percent of all supplementary arteries pass to the lower renal pole [6]. In most cases, this artery behaves as a lower polar artery arising from the renal artery, and it originates usually close to the main stem (Fig. 55-2). This vessel is of particular clinical importance, because it usually passes on the anterior side of the ureteropelvic junction and may cause obstruction to the urinary flow. When it arises more distally from the aorta, the vessel has a horizontal course to the hilus and so does not cause mechanical obstruction. How-

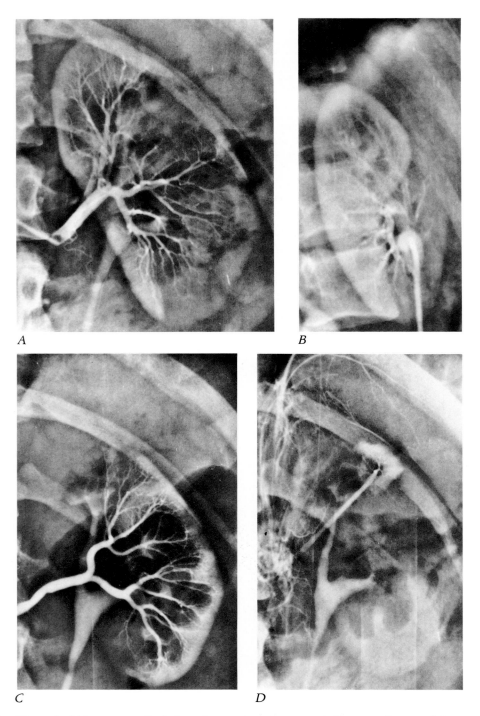

A

B

C

D

Figure 55-1. Normal kidney supplied by three branches arising from the aorta. (A and B) The arterial phase of a selective injection into the dorsal artery, which is the main renal artery; anteroposterior and lateral views. The entire posterior part and the anterior part of the superior lobe are supplied by the dorsal artery, except for a small area of the superior pole. (C and D) A selective injection (C) of the supplementary ventral artery and (D) of an artery with branches to the inferior phrenic artery, the adrenal gland, the renal capsule, and a small section of the upper pole.

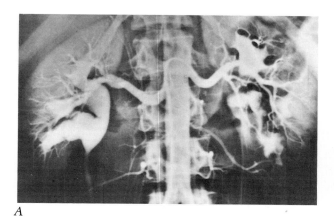

A

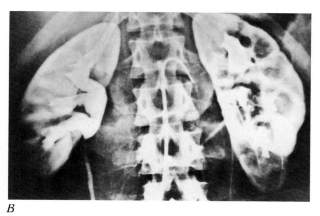

B

Figure 55-2. Hydronephrosis of the left kidney caused by a supplementary lower polar artery. (A and B) Semiselective left renal angiography, arterial and nephrographic phases. A lower polar artery arises from the aorta 3 cm below the main stem and is displaced in an arch, with convexity directed medially and distally.

Figure 55-3. Hydronephrosis of left kidney caused by a vein crossing the ureteropelvic junction. (A and B) Arterial and venous phases of semiselective renal angiography. The supplementary lower polar artery arises from the aorta 3.5 cm distal to the main stem. It passes almost horizontal to the lower part of the renal hilus. A concomitant lower polar vein (*arrow*) that is displaced in an arch, with convexity directed medially and distally, causes the obstruction.

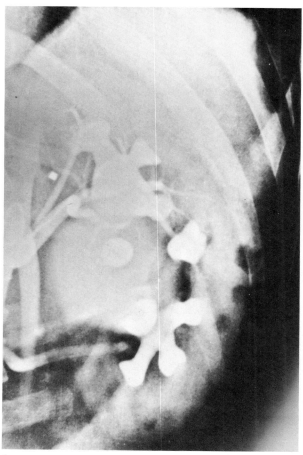

A

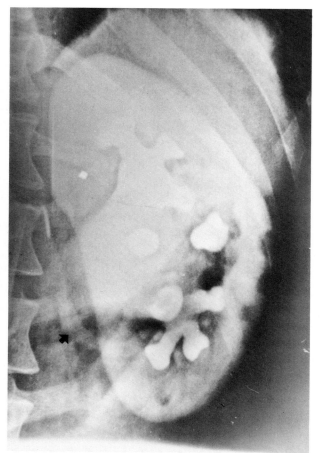

B

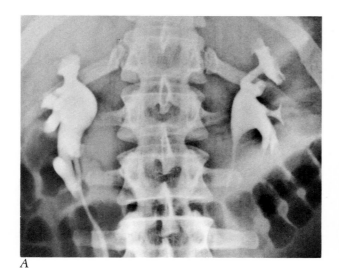

A

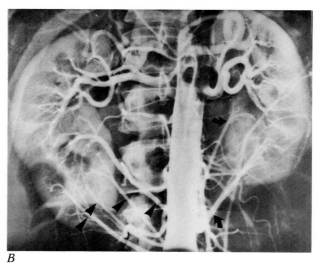

B

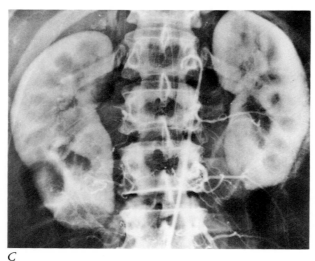

C

Figure 55-4. Incomplete rotation of the right kidney due to supplementary arteries. (A) Urogram. (B and C) Arterial and nephrographic phases. Both kidneys are at normal sites and are supplied by main stems that arise from the aorta at a normal level. The right kidney is long and is malrotated, with an atypical, broad lower pole that is supplied by four supplementary arteries (*arrowheads*) that arise from the lower aorta and the right iliac artery. The left lower pole is supplied by two supplementary arteries (*arrows*) that arise from the distal aorta, but the kidney is not malrotated.

ever, the concomitant vein may then cause the same type of obstruction (Fig. 55-3).

When the lower polar artery arises more distally from the aorta or the iliac arteries, it has a steep craniolateral course and may prevent the kidney from rotating to its final position (Fig. 55-4). The kidney is usually longer than normal but is situated at the normal place with the hilus directed anteriorly.

The supplementary arteries arising from the aorta are segmental or subsegmental arteries [6, 26]. The most important one is thus the lower polar artery. The next most common supplementary artery is the one to the upper pole, but that artery usually supplies only a minor part, and, as mentioned previously, it is not fully represented in clinical angiography. In a clinical series, the supplementary dorsal artery was present

as often as a superior polar artery (14%). A supplementary artery to the anterior intermediate segment was present in about 6 percent (see Fig. 55-1). The frequency of the supplementary arteries was above 100 percent in this series, because more than two arteries were present in 8 of the 152 kidneys with multiple arteries (Fig. 55-4; see also Fig. 55-1).

It is well known by anatomists that supplementary arteries may arise not only from the lumbar aorta and iliac arteries but also from a variety of abdominal vessels and supply kidneys at a normal level. Among others, the superior and inferior mesenteric, celiac, middle colic, lumbar, and middle sacral arteries are described [23, 43, 47]. In the angiographic literature, few observations of this kind have been reported. A supplementary artery arising from the contralateral renal artery has been observed [32, 38], as has a common trunk to the lower poles [37]. A lower polar artery from the inferior mesenteric is also reported [52].

The wide variations in the origin and course of multiple renal arteries can well be explained by the development of the mesonephric arteries

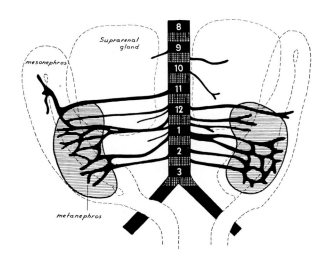

Figure 55-5. Diagram of the *rete arteriosum urogenitale*, formed by segmental arteries that supply the mesonephros and the later metanephros in early embryonal life. (After Felix [20].)

(Fig. 55-5) [20]. These arteries develop on each side of the aorta, and they are distributed from the sixth cervical to the third lumbar segments, where they form a network, the *rete arteriosum urogenitale*. In addition to the mesonephros, these arteries supply the adrenal, the metanephros (i.e., the final kidney), and the gonads. Eventually, some of the roots and part of the network degenerate, the area which they previously supplied being taken over by a neighboring root. Finally, only one mesonephric artery at the level of L1 takes over the entire supply of the kidney. The mesonephric arteries may reach down to the L3 segment and persist, which may explain the presence of supplementary arteries down to this level. Renal arteries distal to L3 represent vessels that arose during the ascent of the metanephros but for some reason were not obliterated. The appearance of vascular anomalies is thus the result of unusual paths in the primitive vascular plexuses and the persistence of vessels normally obliterated [1].

Renal Ectopy

The angiographic findings in malrotated and ectopic kidney have been presented in textbooks to a certain extent, but a comprehensive analysis is lacking. Besides the few case reports in which the cause of abdominal pain in ectopic kidney has been analyzed, only a few reports exist regarding the angiographic characteristics of these malformations [4, 6, 12, 45, 51]. The reason for this is, first, ectopic kidney is rare (fused kidney occurs in some 0.2% and ectopic kidney in 0.1% of all autopsies), and, second, angiography is performed only before a planned operation on such a kidney.

It is generally assumed that caudal ectopic kidneys have multiple arteries, but that is not necessarily the case. Thus, in *horseshoe kidney*, one single artery to each kidney, including the bridge, has been observed [5, 26]. Most often, however, multiple arteries are present in horseshoe kidney. The supplementary arteries arise below the main arteries from the lower aorta or iliac arteries, either as a single trunk to each side or as a main trunk to both sides of the bridge and the lower parts of the kidneys. Supplementary arteries arising above the main stem do also occur (Fig. 55-6). In horseshoe kidney, the distribution of the intrarenal arteries can still be traced [26]. The bridging part usually contains renal parenchyma, but an "avascular" connective tissue connection may be present. The bridge probably causes the anterior location of the renal hilus in the same manner that the supplementary lower polar artery does in malrotated kidneys at normal level [6].

The most common type of *fused kidney* is the horseshoe kidney, but a large variety exists, including crossed ectopia (Fig. 55-7), fused presacral kidney, and pelvic kidney (Figs. 55-8, 55-9). The vascular supply of these malformations is unpredictable. The main renal supply originates below L3, which means that the vessels do not belong to the segmental mesonephric system, and the intrarenal distribution can no longer be systematized. Multiple arteries originating from the lower aorta or pelvic arteries are usually present to supply each kidney, but this is not always so (Figs. 55-9, 55-10).

In *lumbar ectopia*, one artery may arise from the lower part of the aorta passing behind the kidney and one anterior to it, entering the laterally situated hilus, which may explain the renal colic present [33] (Fig. 55-10). In other situations, an artery passing from the iliac artery to the lower pole of the malrotated kidney may be stretched in a certain position and cause nephralgia [48].

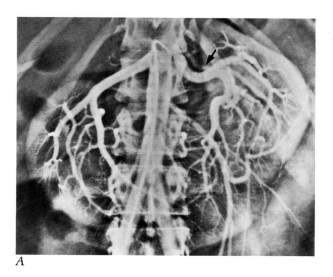

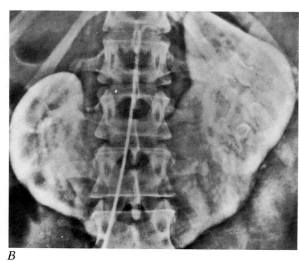

A

B

Figure 55-6. (A and B) Horseshoe kidney supplied by two main renal arteries that also supply the parenchymatous bridge. A small supplementary artery (*arrow*) arises from the aorta just above the main renal artery.

Figure 55-7. Lumbar ectopic, fused kidney on the right in a 38-year-old man with nephropathy and uremia. (A) At lumbar aortography, two arteries arising at the level of L4 supply the kidney, which measures 15 × 8 cm. No renal arteries are present on the left. (B) At selective angiography of the main artery, increased resistance of flow and poor cortical perfusion are observed.

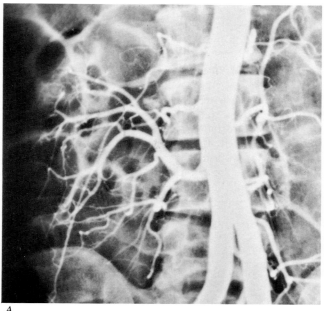

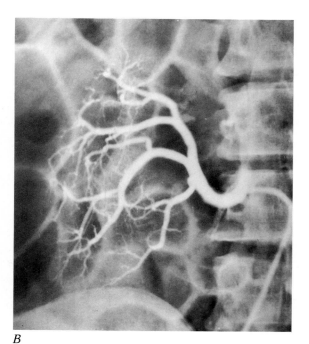

A

B

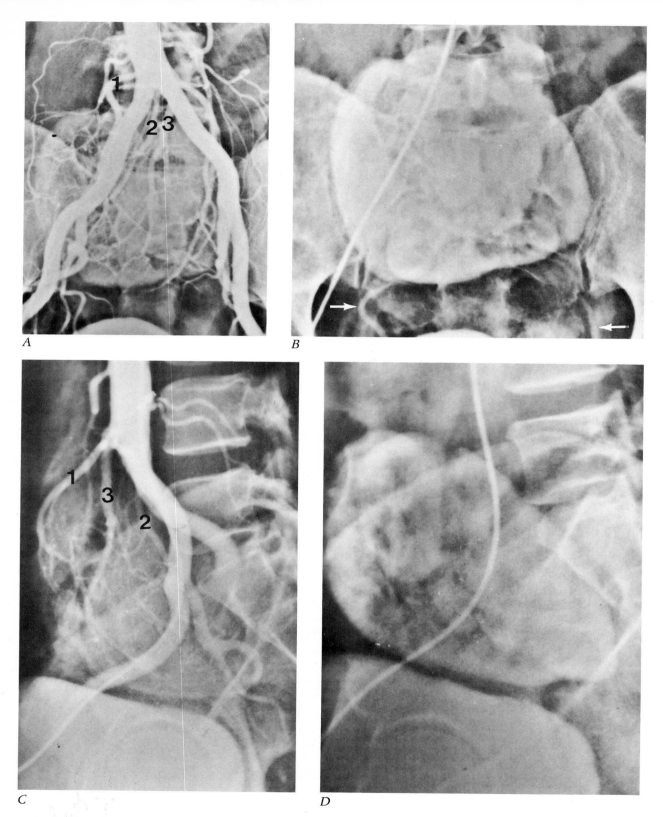

Figure 55-8. Sacral ectopic, fused kidney that measures 15 × 7 × 12 cm. (A and B) Lumbar aortography, anteroposterior view. Three arteries supply the conglomerated kidney, which does not seem to have a hilus. The arteries arise from the distal aorta at the level of the bifurcation (*1, 2, 3*). The normally coursing short ureters are observed in the nephrographic phase (*arrows*). (C and D) Lateral view. The kidney makes an impression on the fundus of the bladder.

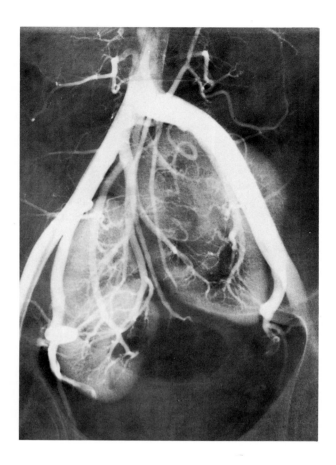

Figure 55-9. Partly fused pelvic kidney. Lower lumbar aortography, subtraction film. The right kidney is supplied by only one artery arising from the common iliac, and the left kidney is supplied by two arteries. The superior hemorrhoidal artery passes in a groove between the two kidneys.

Figure 55-10. Palpable tumor and pain on right side was the main indication for urography in this 51-year-old woman. At urography, a right lumbar ectopic kidney with the hilus directed laterally was observed. (A and B) Lumbar aortography, arterial and venous phases. The left kidney is supplied by one artery at a normal level. The right ectopic kidney is supplied by only one artery, which arises at the level of the disk between L3 and L4. Probably one branch passes anterior and one branch passes posterior to the kidney before entering the laterally oriented hilus. Probably also, the two draining veins follow the same course.

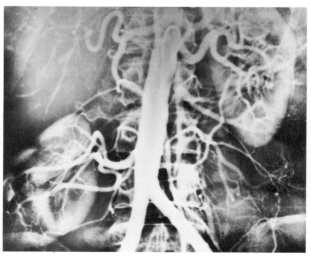

A

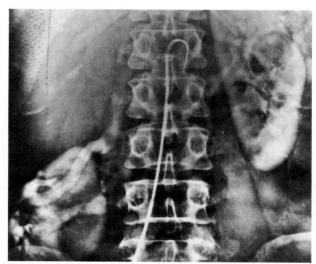

B

Malformation of the Renal Parenchyma

Absence of any fetal or metanephrogenic tissue (*agenesia*) or the presence of only fetal nephrogenic structures (*aplasia*) may be an indication for angiography when other methods fail to explain the absence observed at urography or scintigraphy [4, 30, 40, 45, 51]. If a small renal artery is observed at lumbar aortography, it usually represents an adrenal artery, but it may of course represent the very small blood supply of the *hypoplastic kidney* (Fig. 55-11). The acquired small kidney will also have a small renal artery. A distinction between this and the hypoplastic kidney could be that in acquired disease the origin of the renal artery retains its width [50]. The contralateral kidney is hyperplastic, and frequently multiple arteries are present [45] or abnormalities are present in the renal pelvis [Fig. 55-11]. Anuria in a newborn may be an indication for angiography to show the bilateral absence of renal arteries [45].

In *total renal dysplasia* of childhood, there is disturbed differentiation of nephrogenic tissue with persistence of structures inappropriate to the gestational age of the patient. It is the most common abdominal mass in the newborn infant and the most common cystic disorder of the kidney in children. At angiography, small renal vessels and poor perfusion have been observed [44].

Dysplasia may be localized to one small part or to several parts of the kidney. At angiography, no cortical vessels are observed and the renal pelvis reaches the renal capsule (Fig. 55-12).

Renal hypoplasia and *dysplasia* are controversial definitions from a pathoanatomic point of view [16, 17, 39]. The Ask-Upmark kidney is one such entity [2]. For the radiologist, there appears to be no definite way to decide whether the lesion is a congenital malformation or a lesion that occurred in early childhood or during intrauterine life. However, when the lesion is combined with other abnormalities regarded as malformations, it appears more justified to describe a localized absence of a lobe drained by a calix as a dysplasia (Fig. 55-12) and a very small kidney as a hypoplasia (see Fig. 55-11).

Many classifications of *cystic disease* of the kidneys exist, and the literature is controversial and confusing [8, 29, 31, 46]. It is not the purpose of this presentation to go into a deep analysis of

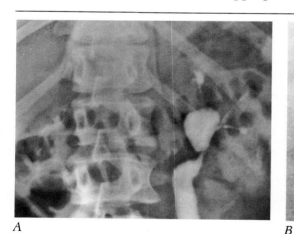

A

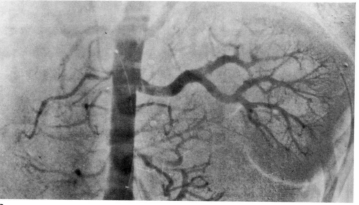

B

Figure 55-11. Hypoplastic right kidney and anomalous left renal collecting system in a hyperplastic kidney. (A) Urography. The 3-×-2-cm kidney on the right concentrates the contrast medium quite well. Three small infundibula with poorly developed calices drain into a wide confluent part of the renal pelvis on the left. (B and C) Lumbar aortography, subtraction film, arterial and capillary phases. One artery to each kidney arising at a normal level is demonstrated. The small right renal artery arises together with the inferior phrenic and adrenal arteries.

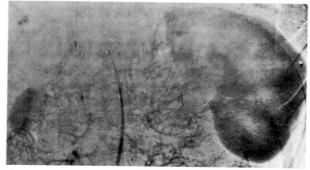

C

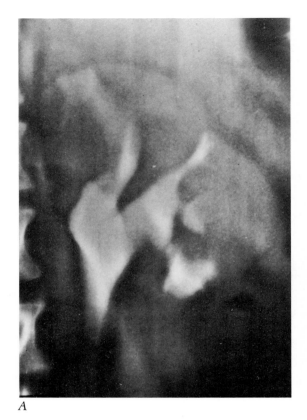

A

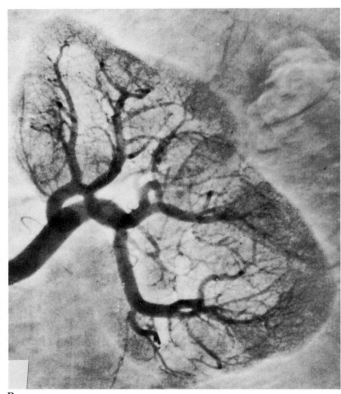

B

Figure 55-12. Congenital focal dysplasia with local absence of cortical structures and with the calices reaching the renal surface. (A) Urography, tomographic cut showing local absence of parenchyma in the superior pole and the intermediate part. (B) A selective renal angiogram, 2× magnification, subtraction film: localized absence of cortical vessels and glomeruli at the site of previously mentioned abnormalities but also in the lower pole. Marked localized hyperplasia between the absent cortical sections.

these entities. Suffice it here to say that with the combination of angiography and urography a distinction can be made among medullary cystic disease, the common type of adult hereditary polycystic disease, adult polycystic disease, type Potter 3, and the cystlike dilatation of the tubules in medullary sponge kidney.

In *medullary cystic disease,* or juvenile nephronophthisis, the kidneys are small. The renal arteries are thin, and in the nephrographic phase a marked cortical thinning is observed (Fig. 55-13). Filling defects of 1 to 2 mm in diameter are scattered through the kidney but spare the outermost cortical layer [42]. The lack of cortical interruption is thus the characteristic finding that is not observed in any other type of lesion.

The *common type of adult hereditary polycystic disease* differs completely from medullary cystic kidney disease (Fig. 55-14). The renal artery supplying a large kidney is reduced in caliber, and the cortical surface is interrupted by cysts of vari-

ous size, which gives the nephrographic phase an extremely irregular appearance, the extent of which varies with the stage of the disease [18, 31, 41].

In *adult polycystic disease, type Potter 3*, the cysts are not as numerous as in the common adult type, but the characteristic contrast-filled medullary cyst observed at urography is pathognomonic for this entity [13, 31]. Focal dysplasia often is present.

In *medullary sponge kidney*, or benign tubular ectasia, the renal angiogram is normal [15, 31]. Secondary pyelonephritis often occurs in this malformation of the papilla; when it does, angiography is, of course, abnormal.

Figure 55-14. Early stage of hereditary polycystic disease in a 31-year-old male. (A and B) Nephrographic phases of the right and left kidneys. There are a large number of cysts of varying size with typical cortical distribution in the moderately enlarged kidney.

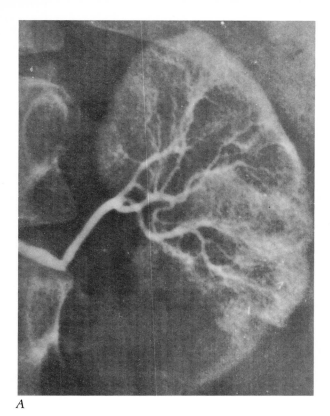

A

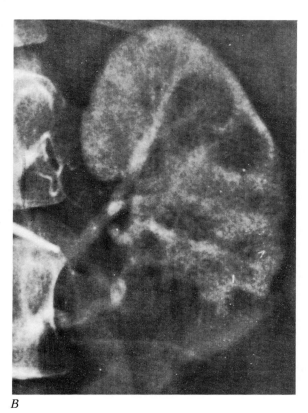

B

Figure 55-13. Medullary cystic disease, histologically verified in a 35-year-old uremic woman treated with hemodialysis for 4 years. (A and B) Selective left renal angiography of the main trunk, arterial and venous phases. The 7-×-3-cm kidney contains numerous small filling defects due to cystic dilatation of tubuli at the corticomedullary level, giving a honeycomb pattern. The cortical surface is not interrupted. Similar findings are observed on the right side.

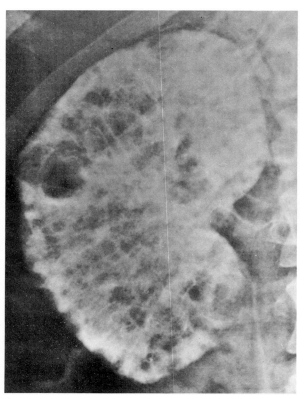

A

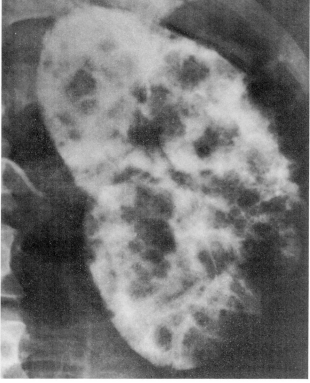

B

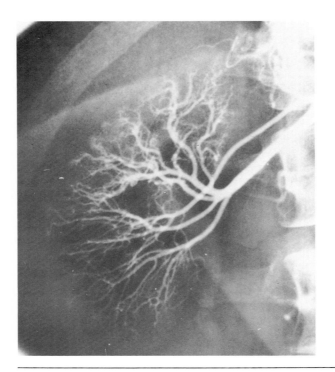

Figure 55-15. Hereditary nephritis (Alport's syndrome). Selective angiography of the right kidney, arterial phase. The intrarenal arteries are crowded and reduced in caliber. The cortex is reduced, and marked resistance to flow is present. Similar findings are observed in the opposite kidney.

In *hereditary nephritis* (Alport's syndrome), there are diffuse fibrosis and tubular atrophy, mainly in the corticomedullary junction. Angiographically, the lesion is not distinguishable from other types of nephropathy (Fig. 55-15) [11].

Pseudotumor is a blanket term for different types of normal variations of the renal pelvis or parenchyma, ranging from fetal lobulation to impressions made by adjacent organs, such as the spleen or the liver [9, 19, 21, 28, 34]. The cause may also be an unusually large column of Bertin, which causes splaying of the renal calices, the infundibula, and the associated interlobar arteries [7, 9, 10, 21, 25, 34]. At angiography, a well-circumscribed dense accumulation is observed

Figure 55-16. Arteritis in a 32-year-old woman with lupus. (A and B) At selective left renal angiography, arterial and nephrographic phases, the cortical surface is irregular because of small infarctions. In the inter- mediate part, the interlobar arteries (*arrows*, A) are slightly splayed by a pseudotumor, with central lucency. It is formed by a somewhat large column of Bertin.

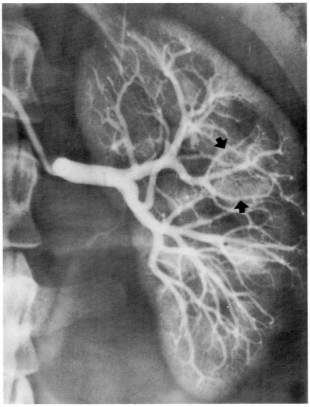

A

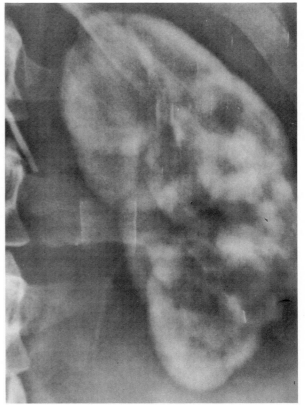

B

and, often, a central lucency (Fig. 55-16). Other causes of pseudotumor may be (1) traction applied to the lower pole by a supplementary lower polar artery in malrotated kidneys at the normal site [36] and (2) focal hyperplasia in a kidney with local destruction of parenchyma (see Fig. 55-12).

Malformation of the Renal Pelvis

Primary congenital anomalies of the renal pelvis, such as megacalices or renal pelvic duplication, do not influence the normal renal angiogram unless secondary disease affects the parenchyma [24, 35, 49] (see Fig. 51-12).

References

1. Arey, L. B. *Developmental Anatomy* (6th ed.). Philadelphia: Saunders, 1954.
2. Ask-Upmark, E. Über juvenile maligne Nephrosklerose und 1hr Verhältnis zu Störungen in der Nierenentwicklung. *Acta Pathol. Microbiol. Scand.* 6:383, 1929.
3. Aubert, J., and Koumare, K. Variations of origin of the renal artery. A review covering 403 aortographies. *Eur. Urol.* 1:182, 1975.
4. Bachmann, D., and Schäfer, P. Nierenmissbildungen: Angiographische Befunde. *ROEFO* 107:50, 1967.
5. Boatman, D. L., Cornell, S. H., and Kölln, C.-P. The arterial supply of horseshoe kidneys. *AJR* 113:447, 1971.
6. Boijsen, E. Angiographic studies of the anatomy of single and multiple renal arteries. *Acta Radiol.* [Suppl.] (Stockh.) 183:1959.
7. Chargi, H., Dessureault, P., Drouin, G., Gauthier, G. E., Perras, P., Roy, P., and Charbonneau, J. Malposition of a renal lobe (lobar dysmorphism): A condition simulating renal tumor. *J. Urol.* 105:326, 1971.
8. Cho, K. J., Thornbury, J. R., Bernstein, J., Heidelberger, K. P., and Walter, J. F. Localized cystic disease of the kidney. Angiographic-pathologic correlation. *AJR* 132:891, 1979.
9. Cooperman, L. R., and Lowman, R. M. Fetal lobulation of the kidney. *AJR* 92:273, 1964.
10. Dacie, J. E. The "central lucency" sign of lobar dysmorphism (pseudotumor of the kidney). *Br. J. Radiol.* 49:39, 1976.
11. Demetropoulos, K. C., Hoskins, P., and Rapp, R. Angiographic study of hereditary nephritis (Alport's syndrome). *Radiology* 108:539, 1973.
12. Dretler, S. P., Olsson, C., and Pfister, R. C. The anatomic, radiologic, and clinical characteristics of the pelvic kidney. *J. Urol.* 105:623, 1971.
13. Ebel, K.-D., and Olbring, H. Zur Röntgendiagnostik der polyzystischen Nierendegeneration im Kindesalter. *ROEFO* 110:28, 1969.
14. Edsman, G. Angionephrography and suprarenal angiography. *Acta Radiol.* [Suppl.] (Stockh.) 155:1957.
15. Ekström, T., Engfeldt, B., Lagergren, C., and Lindvall, N. *Medullary Sponge Kidney.* Stockholm: Almqvist & Wiksell, 1959.
16. Ericsson, N. O., and Ivemark, B. J. Renal dysplasia and pyelonephritis in infants and children: I. *Arch. Pathol.* 66:255, 1958.
17. Ericsson, N. O., and Ivemark, B. J. Renal dysplasia and pyelonephritis in infants and children: II. Primitive ductules and abnormal glomeruli. *Arch. Pathol.* 66:264, 1958.
18. Ettinger, A., Kahn, P. C., and Wise, H. M., Jr. The importance of selective renal angiography in the diagnosis of polycystic disease. *J. Urol.* 102:156, 1969.
19. Feldman, A. E., Pollack, H. M., Perri, A. J., Jr., Karafin, L., and Kendall, A. R. Renal pseudotumors: An anatomic-radiologic classification. *J. Urol.* 120:133, 1978.
20. Felix, W. Die Entwicklung der Harn- und Geschlechts-organe. In F. Keibel and F. P. Mall (eds.), *Handbuch der Entwicklungsgeschichte des Menschen.* Leipzig: Hirzel, 1911. Vol. 2, p. 732.
21. Felson, B., and Moskowitz, M. Renal pseudotumors: The regenerated nodule and other lumps, bumps and dromedary humps. *AJR* 107:320, 1969.
22. Fontaine, R., Kieny, R., Jurascheck, F., and Perez-Day, C. Étude angiographique des artères rénales accessoires (polaires supérieures et inférieures indépendantes des artères rénales normales) et leur signification pathologique. *Lyon Chir.* 61:685, 1965.
23. Gillaspie, C., Miller, L. J., and Baskin, M. Anomalous renal vessels and their surgical significance. *Anat. Rec.* 11:77, 1916.
24. Gittes, R. F., and Talner, L. B. Congenital megacalices versus obstructive hydronephrosis. *J. Urol.* 108:833, 1972.
25. Gooding, C. A. Childhood renal pseudotumor. A case report. *Radiology* 98:79, 1971.
26. Graves, F. T. Arterial anatomy of congenitally abnormal kidney. *Br. J. Surg.* 56:533, 1969.
27. Guntz, M. Radio-anatomie de l'artère rénale. Deductions chirurgicales. *C.R. Reun. Assoc. Anat.* 138:623, 1967.
28. Harrow, B. R., and Sloane, J. A. Dromedary or lumped left kidney: Lack of relationship to renal rotation. *AJR* 88:144, 1962.
29. Hatfield, P. M., and Pfister, R. C. Adult polycystic disease of the kidneys (Potter type 3). *J.A.M.A.* 222:1527, 1972.

30. Hynes, D. M., and Watkin, E. M. Renal agenesis—roentgenologic problem. *AJR* 110: 772, 1970.
31. Ivemark, B. J., Lagergren, C., and Lindvall, N. Roentgenologic diagnosis of polycystic kidney and medullary sponge kidney. *Acta Radiol. [Diagn.]* (Stockh.) 10:225, 1970.
32. Jeffery, R. F. Unusual origins of renal arteries. *Radiology* 102:309, 1972.
33. Jönsson, G., and Olsson, O. A case of renal ectopia with malrotation and vascular anomalies causing renal pain. *Acta Chir. Scand.* 123:447, 1962.
34. King, M. C., Friedenberg, R. M., and Tena, L. B. Normal renal parenchyma simulating tumor. *Radiology* 91:217, 1968.
35. Kittredge, R. D., and Levin, D. C. Unusual aspect of renal angiography in ureteric duplication. *AJR* 119:805, 1973.
36. Kyaw, M. M., and Newman, H. Renal pseudotumors due to ectopic accessory renal arteries: The angiographic diagnosis. *AJR* 113:443, 1971.
37. Levine, N. O. An unusual renal artery anomaly: Common origins of arteries to lower poles. *Br. J. Radiol.* 43:66, 1970.
38. Libschitz, H., Ben-Menachem, Y., and Kuroda, K. Unusual renal vascular supply. *Br. J. Radiol.* 45:536, 1972.
39. Ljungqvist, A., and Lagergren, C. The Ask-Upmark kidney. *Acta Pathol. Microbiol. Scand.* 56:277, 1962.
40. Love, L., and Des Rosier, R. J. Angiography of renal agenesis and dysgenesis. *AJR* 98:137, 1966.
41. Meaney, T. F., and Corvalan, J. G. Angiographic diagnosis of polycystic renal disease. *Cleve. Clin. Q.* 35:79, 1968.
42. Mena, E., Bookstein, J. J., McDonald, F. D., and Gikas, P. W. Angiographic findings in renal medullary cystic disease. *Radiology* 110:277, 1974.
43. Merklin, R. J., and Michels, N. A. The variant renal and suprarenal blood supply with data on the inferior phrenic, ureteral and gonadal arteries. *J. Int. Coll. Surg.* 29:41, 1958.
44. Newman, L., Simms, K., Kissane, J., and McAlister, W. H. Unilateral total renal dysplasia in children. *AJR* 116:778, 1972.
45. Olsson, O., and Wholey, M. Vascular abnormalities in gross anomalies of kidneys. *Acta Radiol. [Diagn.]* (Stockh.) 2:420, 1964.
46. Osathanondh, V., and Potter, E. L. Pathogenesis of polycystic kidneys. Historical survey. *Arch. Pathol.* 77:459, 1964.
47. Poisel, S., and Spängler, H. P. Über aberrante und accessorische Nierenarterien bei Nieren in typischer Lage. *Anat. Anz.* 124:244, 1969.
48. Schwartz, D. T., and Robbins, S. Nephralgia due to an aberrant renal capsular vessel: Case report. *J. Urol.* 109:761, 1973.
49. Talner, L. B., and Gittes, R. F. Megacalyces: Further observations and differentiation from obstructive renal disease. *AJR* 131:473, 1974.
50. Templeton, A. W., and Thompson, J. M. Aortographic differentiation of congenital and acquired small kidneys. *Arch. Surg.* 97:114, 1968.
51. Thiemann, K. J., and Wieners, H. Probleme der angiographischen Diagnostik von Agenesien, Aplasien, Fusionsanomalien und Ektopien der Niere. *Radiologe* 10:108, 1970.
52. Tisnado, J., Amendola, M. A., and Beachley, M. C. Renal artery originating from the inferior mesenteric artery. *Br. J. Radiol.* 52:752, 1979.

Renal Trauma

MARK H. WHOLEY
LAWRENCE A. COOPERSTEIN

Trauma is the fourth most common cause of death in the United States. More important, it is the single most common cause of death between the ages of 1 and 35 [1]. Trauma hospitalizes 11 million Americans annually and causes 110,000 to 150,000 deaths. It is apparent from the recent literature that a person who has been shot or stabbed in the abdomen—and who has not been killed outright—has a better chance of surviving than a person who has sustained a severe nonpenetrating blunt injury to the same area [2].

Because of the incidence and seriousness of trauma (often it involves multiple organ injury), the number of trauma units that have capabilities for not only routine radiography but also diagnostic and interventional angiography has been increasing. In these units, the patient is immobilized; the image intensifier and tube rotate in a "U-arm" concept.

Renal trauma is divided into blunt trauma and penetrating trauma. Blunt trauma is by far the more common type, and it is the causative factor in 60 to 70 percent of renal injury. The majority of blunt injuries result from automobile and motorcycle accidents and a variety of other kinds of crush injuries. The mechanism of injury has been related either to sudden deceleration or to direct compression with wedging of the kidney against the adjacent vertebrae or a lower rib fracture.

A penetrating injury to the kidney rarely presents diagnostic problems, because, with few exceptions, the wound is visible, and, when it is a significant wound, it is always explored [3–5]. Blunt renal trauma, however, can and often does present a much more subtle and difficult diagnostic problem [3, 4, 6–8], partly because of multiple organ involvement. In blunt injury to the abdomen, major disruption of every intraabdominal organ has been described. The viscera most frequently involved are the solid, high-tissue-density organs—the kidney, the spleen, and the liver.

Fifty percent of all intraabdominal injuries involve the kidneys as well as the liver and the spleen [9]. This incidence is understandable when the high tissue density of the kidneys, in addition to their relatively fixed position within the abdomen, is taken into account. The fixed position of the kidney is explained by its fascial and capsular ligamentous attachments and by the relatively fixed renal vascular pedicle. During deceleration injuries, herniation of the kidney occurs, with resultant avulsion injuries at the pedicle or

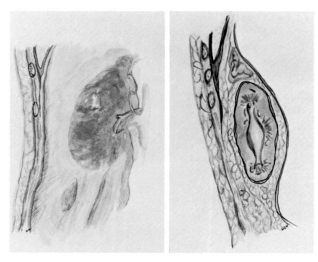

Figure 56-1. The renal capsule and the surrounding perinephric fat provide an effective tamponade against continuing blood loss. Note the fixed vascular pedicle.

Figure 56-2. Hydronephrotic, pathologically enlarged kidney with increased susceptibility to trauma.

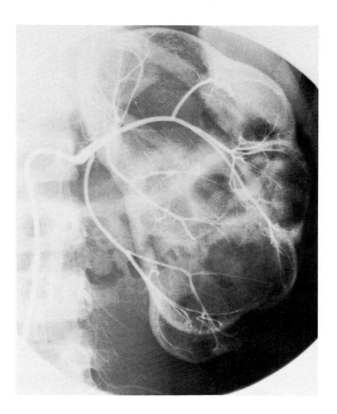

major capsular lacerations at the ligamentous attachment sites [3, 10–12].

On the other hand, the kidneys are relatively well protected against major injury since they are small, posteriorly placed, and relatively well protected by muscle and the adjacent rib cage. The true and false capsules and the surrounding perinephric fat add further physical protection, and, more important, they provide an effective tamponade against continuing blood loss (Fig. 56-1). Diseased kidneys are more easily injured, and considerably less violence is required for rupture of the diseased kidney. Sneezing, coughing, and muscular exertion have been responsible for significant hematuria in the hydronephrotic or neoplastic-involved kidney [9, 13–15] (Fig. 56-2).

Clinical Evaluation

Hematuria is present in 75 to 80 percent of all patients with renal trauma. Perirenal pain exists in 50 percent of the patients, and shock has been described in 10 percent of the patients. Leukocytosis, a palpable mass in the region of injury, albuminuria, and adynamic ileus are other findings [13]. Hematuria exists because of an interruption in the integrity of the renal parenchyma and the pelvocaliceal structures. Critical renal hilar injuries however, including traumatic occlusion or laceration of the renal artery, may appear without either macroscopic or microscopic hematuria [11, 12], especially if the renal parenchyma is intact. Diagnosis in such an instance is dependent on nonvisualization of the affected kidney during emergency intravenous urography. Occasionally, traumatic renal artery thrombosis is bilateral, and in those instances, anuria is present with nonvisualization of both kidneys during the survey radiographic studies [16–18].

Occasionally, traumatic renal vein thrombosis is associated with renal artery occlusion. The most frequent clinical features of traumatic renal vein thrombosis in adults is the nephrotic syndrome and associated thromboembolic phenomena. Proteinuria, hematuria, and local signs of kidney enlargement may exist. If the renal artery is also occluded, the nephrotic syndrome may not develop and the only clinical clue to the associated venous injury may be the signs of thromboembolism. Thromboembolism is likely to take the form of repeated pulmonary emboli. Since pulmonary embolism due to renal vein thrombosis may be fatal, renal vein thrombosis should be considered in all instances of major renal pedicle trauma. When the diagnosis is established, there should be no hesitation in removing the kidney that is a source of emboli. Although renal arteriography may show characteristic signs of renal vein thrombosis, the demonstration by means of renal venography is more definitive [10].

Classification

Over the last 20 to 30 years, a more conservative approach has developed toward the management of injuries involving the entire urinary tract [3, 14]. Controversy about the indication for operation on the injured kidney continues, but there is now uniform agreement that the very common renal contusion can be treated nonoperatively [5, 15]. There is also general agreement that hemorrhage from a renal injury alone rarely necessitates an immediate operation. Experiences include many instances of slight-to-moderate injury in which conservative therapy has resulted in a return to normal function. But "watchful waiting" in more extensive injuries has several major limitations. Irreversible shock may develop. Late complications secondary to extravasation of blood into the urine may occur, with associated abscess formation, hydronephrosis, pyonephrosis, pyelonephritis, hypertension, and, ultimately, complete loss of renal function. As early as 1950,

Table 56-1. Classification of Renal Trauma

Minor injury (75% incidence)
  Subsiding hematuria
Major injury
  Parenchymal damage
  Capsular rupture
  Progressive hematuria
Critical injury
  Shock
  Hemorrhage
  Rupture extension
  Pedicle avulsion
  Nonfunctioning kidney

classifications had been suggested [6, 19] to determine which renal injuries could be classified as surgical and which nonsurgical. In light of the advances that have occurred in diagnostic angiographic techniques and the development of sophisticated interventional methods for hemorrhage control, a proposed clinical-radiographic classification is suggested (Fig. 56-3) (Table 56-1).

The classification is based on the division of renal traumas into minor, major, and critical injuries. Our own survey using data from three major city referral hospitals and three community hospitals provided 54 cases for evaluation. Seventy-two percent of renal injuries could be categorized as minor, 20 percent as major, and 8 percent as critical. There was an 8 percent mortality in the critical category, a figure that was frequently related to the presence of associated injury of the central nervous system or a major visceral organ. There was a 10 percent incidence of nephrectomy overall. These figures are in keeping with those reported by others [3, 15, 20].

Minor Injuries

Fortunately, minor injuries are the most common ones; they constitute nearly 75 percent of renal trauma [9, 20]. Patients with minor injuries can be treated conservatively. Although some damage to the renal parenchyma has occurred, there has been no extension to the renal capsule and no involvement of the pelvocaliceal system. When present, shock is indicative that other organ damage exists. Although hematuria may be present in these patients and initially can be alarming, it subsides to microscopic level within a few days. Intravenous urography demonstrates either a

Figure 56-3. Diagrammatic illustration of angiographic classification of trauma into minor, major, and critical injuries. Note that critical injuries extend beyond the renal capsule and involve the renal pedicle.

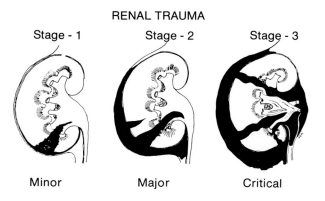

RENAL TRAUMA

Stage - 1   Stage - 2   Stage - 3

Minor   Major   Critical

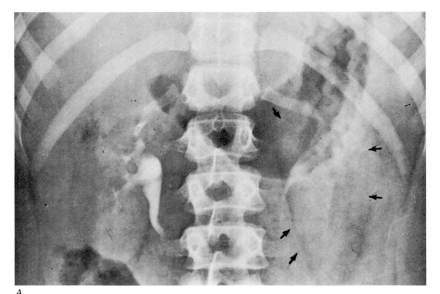

A

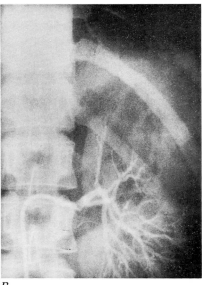

B

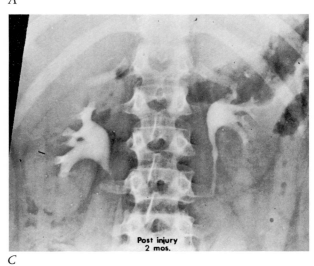

Post injury
2 mos.

C

Figure 56-4. (A) Minor renal trauma with an intact upper urinary tract demonstrating only minimal alteration in the function and in contour of the contused left kidney (*arrows*). (B) A renal arteriogram demonstrating intact arterial flow with only minor contusion and no visible extravasation in the upper pole. (C) An intravenous pyelogram done 2 months posttrauma demonstrates an essentially normal left kidney.

Major Injuries

In a major injury, there are parenchymal damage and capsular involvement that invariably result in a disruption of the gross renal collecting system [15, 20]. If present, a palpable mass usually indicates extravasated blood and urine in the perirenal tissues. Intravenous urography may demonstrate extravasation of contrast medium, a finding that places the injury in the major category. Hypovolemic shock may or may not be present, but generally the hematuria is progressive rather than subsiding (Fig. 56-5A–C).

These patients are best evaluated by arteriography to determine the exact extent of injury, the presence of multiple vessels, the status of the contralateral kidney, and the presence of additional organ involvement [13, 14, 21–23]. More recently, computed tomography (CT) has been used to evaluate certain of these patients with renal injuries, especially those with multiple organ damage [24]. The distinct advantage of CT is the ease with which multiple organs can be evaluated and retroperitoneal hemorrhage can be

completely intact upper urinary tract or a very minimal delay in function on the involved side. Demonstration of this integrity is the most important single criterion for considering these injuries minor. Satisfactory function is also an indicator that the renal artery is intact. These patients rarely need arteriography or interventional hemorrhage control, unless, as already indicated, the possibility of multiple organ injury is being considered. Minor defects in the caliceal system and minimal alteration in function will spontaneously resolve, and, in a matter of 1 to 2 months, the appearance of the kidney generally reverts to normal (Fig. 56-4A–C).

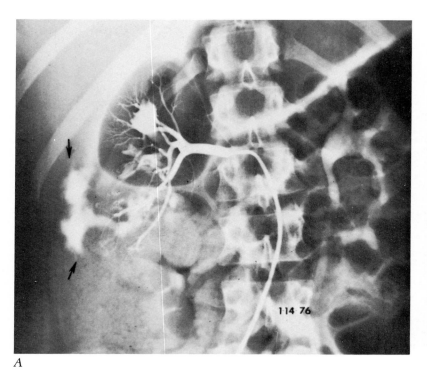

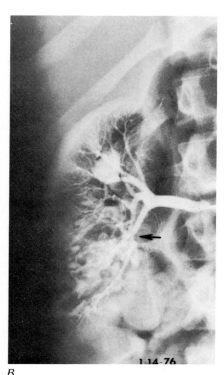

A   *B*

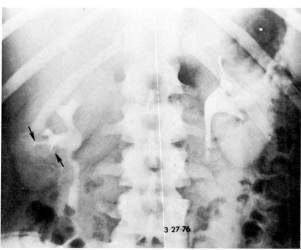

Figure 56-5. (A) A selective arteriogram in major injury with gross extravasation from the dorsal lower pole arterial branch (*arrows*). (B) Postembolization of the lower pole branch with control of the hemorrhage. Considerable intraparenchymal contusion remains (*arrow*). (C) An intravenous pyelogram 2 months after embolization and conservative management demonstrates a functioning intact right kidney with only minimal alteration in the lower pole caliceal structures (*arrows*).

C

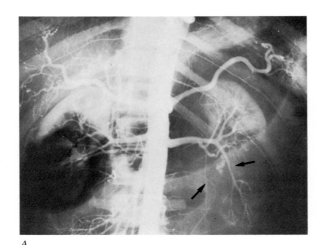

A

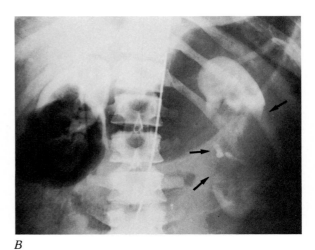

B

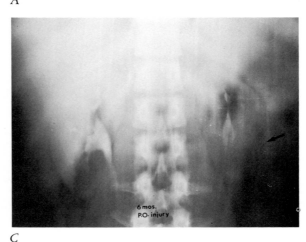

C

Figure 56-6. (A) Aortography that demonstrates a major laceration with wide separation of the renal parenchyma and free extravasation (*arrows*). (B) Nephrographic phase demonstrating the significant separation and fragmentation of the entire left kidney (*arrows*). (C) A patient managed conservatively for 6 months posttrauma demonstrates an intact and functioning left kidney with minimal residual alteration in the lower pole (*arrow*). (Courtesy of J. Copeland, M.D.)

arteriography, should classify these injuries more accurately and should eliminate unnecessary exploration [13, 21, 22, 26] (Fig. 56-6A–C).

Critical Injuries

Extension of the renal rupture into the pedicle is justification for placing the injury in the critical category. Major lacerations of the pedicle are not common; they occur in less than 10 percent of all renal injuries. When they do occur, however, the hemorrhage can be exsanguinating and frequently fatal in a very brief period of time [20]. An increase in the size of the palpable mass, hemorrhage, and shock signify that the lesion is severe. Sixty percent of the blood volume may have to be replaced in a 2-to-3-minute period.

Intravenous urography is obviously of value in determining the status of the contralateral kidney. The involved side rarely functions. If vital signs can be stabilized and if time permits, arteriography will demonstrate the laceration or the avulsed pedicle. Generally, when the patient survives, retraction and thrombosis of the mainstem renal artery have occurred [11, 12, 14, 20]

identified. In contrast, the use of ultrasonography in the evaluation of retroperitoneal structures may be technically limited [15, 24, 25]. Similarly, radionuclide scanning is limited because of its organ specificity [24]. During a period of watchful waiting, when there are no obvious signs of impending shock and when interventional hemorrhage control is not being considered, CT is a very useful noninvasive diagnostic method of detecting hemorrhage in the very early stages. When hemorrhage is apparent, early routine administration of antibiotics reduces the risk of infection in the surrounding hematoma and subsequent secondary bleeding.

In the past, as many as 25 percent of injured kidneys were removed, and in many of these cases the initial renal trauma may have been relatively minor. The routine use of intravenous urography, coupled with either CT or diagnostic

(Fig. 56-7). In the various stages before thrombosis has occurred, there may be actual extravasation of the contrast medium.

One should be continually aware of the existing adjacent organ involvement in severe pedicle injuries. The liver may be involved in 10 to 15 percent of these critical injuries to the right kidney and the spleen in 10 to 15 percent of left renal injuries. Injury to the contralateral kidney may also exist and may appear with confusing physical signs [3, 14, 15, 20]. Arteriography, when performed in these patients, should encompass an evaluation of all visceral organs, considering the incidence of involvement of multiple organs.

Complete thrombosis of the renal arterial system due to blunt trauma is surprisingly rare [11, 12, 17, 18]. Ordinarily, traumatic renal arterial thrombosis is unilateral and usually involves the left kidney. It has been postulated that this is because of the hypermobility of the left kidney as a result of its relatively long pedicle. Sudden deceleration might therefore cause acute angulation and traction on the artery at its point of fixation near the origin of the aorta, with consequent intimal fracture and subintimal dissection leading to arterial thrombosis with complete infarction of the kidney [11, 12]. It is obvious that renal angiography should follow immediately when the kidney is not visualized adequately on intravenous urography.

Surgical intervention in cases of renal artery thrombosis should take place within 12 hours of the time of injury (preferably earlier), with excision of the injured segment (Fig. 56-8A, B) and removal of the distal thrombus. An end-to-end anastomosis should be done in an effort to restore renal function. Although these repairs may restore renal blood flow, the ultimate success in restoration of normal renal function has not yet been achieved [11]. This failure is apparently related to delays in treatment, as evidenced by the fact that an 80 percent chance of restoring some

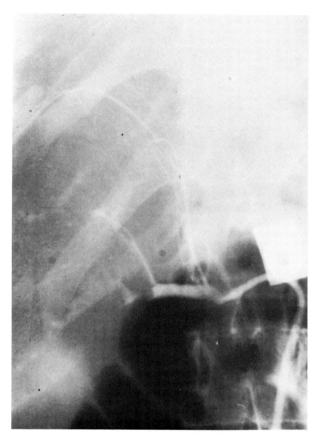

Figure 56-7. Major laceration of the renal pedicle with traumatic occlusion and thrombosis of the right renal artery. There is extensive perinephric hematoma, but thrombosis and retraction of the renal artery have prevented further hemorrhage.

function to the injured kidney is present at 12 hours, but only a 57 percent chance at 18 hours. The frequently associated splenic, hepatic, pancreatic, and duodenal injuries account for the overall mortality of 20 percent in renal artery injury. Although revascularization results are poor [11, 12, 17, 18], and the incidence of late hypertension is as high as 55 percent, an attempt at renal artery repair still seems indicated.

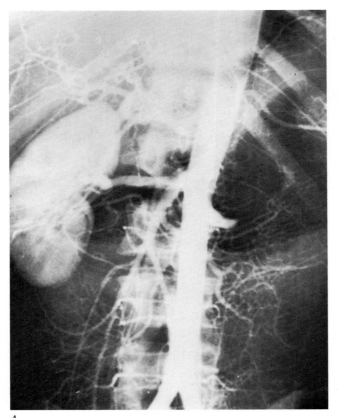
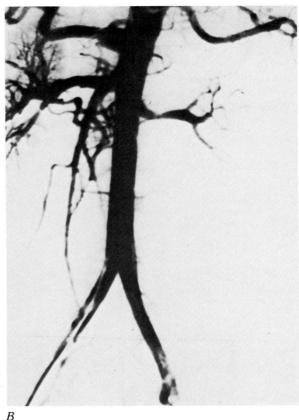

A

B

Figure 56-8. (A) Critical pedicle injury with complete thrombosis and associated laceration through the left renal artery. (B) Postsurgical reconstruction and end-to-end anastomosis of the lacerated renal artery with a functioning left kidney. (Courtesy of W. E. Goodwin, M.D.)

Interventional Hemorrhage Control

When massive hemorrhage exists at the time of diagnostic arteriography, the bleeding may be totally controlled by percutaneous balloon occlusion. During the occlusion, the patient's vital signs may be stabilized and the patient prepared for surgery. Similarly, with traumatic renal vein thrombosis and recurrent pulmonary emboli, balloon occlusion at the orifice of the renal vein may be established until more remedial surgical measures are available (Fig. 56-9A, B). In both these instances, for interval hemorrhage control, a 7 French double-lumen nondetachable latex polyethylene balloon catheter is appropriately positioned in the renal artery from either a femoral or transaxillary approach (Fig. 56-10A, B). Balloon expansion is monitored with dilute contrast medium under televised fluoroscopy.

While balloon occlusion prior to corrective surgery may be the applicable interventional technique in critical injuries, patients who have major injuries with angiographic evidence of continued bleeding or false aneurysm, for which exploration is not anticipated, may benefit from interventional embolization. If there is significant hematuria, balloon occlusion and then embolization can be done effectively before surgery [27–30] (Fig. 56-11A–D). When Gelfoam is used, 2-×-5-mm strips are injected through the double-lumen balloon catheter. A .035-inch guidewire is then passed through the catheter to displace any Gelfoam fragments at the catheter tip. This maneuver, with balloon expansion, eliminates the possible complication of Gelfoam reflux into the aorta. Other embolizing agents, including Avitene, Ivalon, isobutyl cyanoacrylate, autologous clot, and detachable balloons, may be used for hemostasis [31, 32]. The silicone detachable balloons are available with unexpanded diameters of approximately 1 mm and 2 mm and

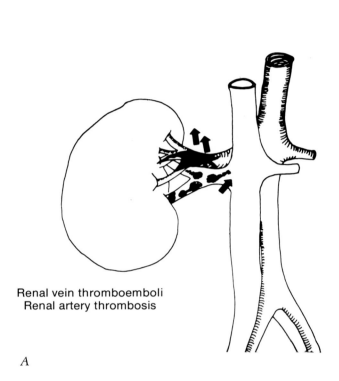

Renal vein thromboemboli
Renal artery thrombosis

A

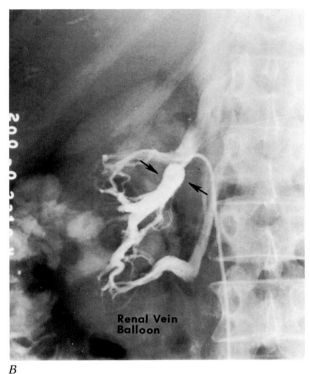

Renal Vein
Balloon

B

Figure 56-9. (A) Diagrammatic illustration of trau- matic renal vein thrombosis and the potential for a pulmonary thromboembolic source. (B) A balloon being used for occlusion of the renal vein (*arrows*).

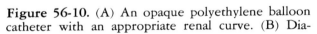

Figure 56-10. (A) An opaque polyethylene balloon catheter with an appropriate renal curve. (B) Dia- grammatic illustration of the correct positioning of the balloon prior to selective embolization.

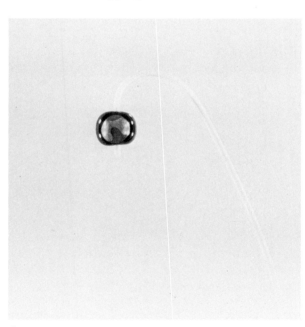

A

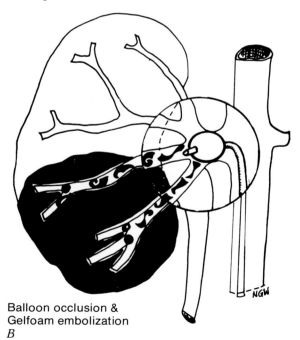

Balloon occlusion &
Gelfoam embolization

B

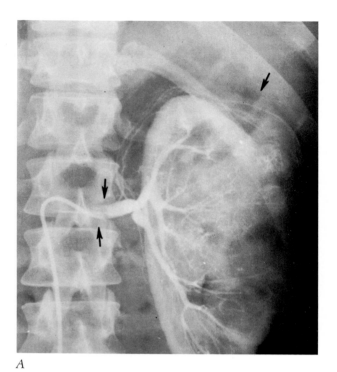

A

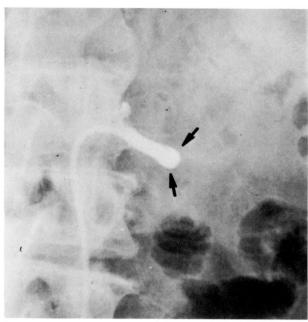

B

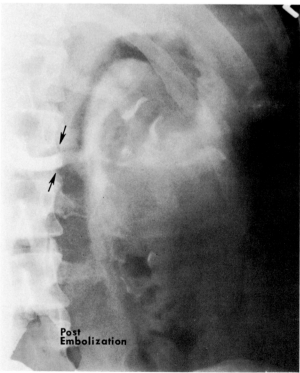

C

expansion capabilities approaching 4 mm and 8 mm, respectively. The balloons are introduced via a guiding catheter, which allows observation of the selective positioning of the balloon prior to detachment.

Absolute sterility in handling hemostatic agents is essential in view of the very high incidence of bacterial contamination during these interventional procedures, especially in patients who have already been compromised by hypovolemic shock. A variety of organisms have been cultured, the most prominent and persistent of which is the skin contaminant *Staphylococcus epidermidis* [32]. For that reason, the hemostatic agent is mixed with a systemic antibiotic and a radiopaque contrast medium. The patients are then routinely placed on systemic antibiotic therapy.

The delayed onset of hypertension in these patients with renal trauma and interventional hemorrhage control necessitates long-term observation [3, 33]. Posttraumatic renal hypertension has also occurred in other patients from parenchymal compression and perirenal hematoma [33]. Those patients also require long-term follow-up.

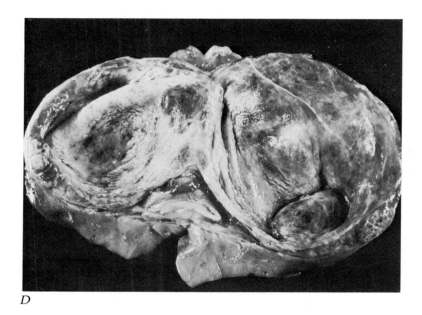

D

Figure 56-11. (A) A renal carcinoma showing massive hematuria following a minor trauma (*arrows*). (B) A balloon occlusion of the renal artery (*arrows*). (C) A postballoon occlusion and embolization with controlled hematuria (*arrows*). (D) A gross specimen with cystic renal cell carcinoma and a nodular hemorrhagic source.

Acquired Posttraumatic Arteriovenous Fistula

At present, three types of renal arteriovenous fistulas are recognized: (1) congenital, (2) idiopathic, and (3) acquired. The acquired fistulas can be subdivided into four etiologic groups: (1) traumatic, (2) surgical, (3) neoplastic, and (4) inflammatory [34, 35].

Penetrating wounds are the most common cause of traumatic fistulas. Blunt trauma rarely produces a fistula [22]. Occasionally, the diagnosis is not made until months or years after the initial injury, when the patient appears with symptoms of left-sided heart failure (Fig. 56-12). Fistulas develop in almost 15 percent of patients who have undergone percutaneous transluminal renal biopsy [36]; if a biopsy is considered as a penetrating wound, then postbiopsy fistulas would be the most common of traumatic fistulas. This incidence is related to the time between the biopsy and the angiographic procedure: The incidence may be higher when the arteriogram is performed within a month of the renal biopsy. Eighty percent of these fistulas close spontaneously within 18 months after the biopsy [36] (Fig. 56-13A, B). It is also apparent that the postpercutaneous-biopsy fistula is more likely to develop in a patient with existing hypertension [36, 37].

Figure 56-12. Significant arteriovenous fistula involving the entire dorsal division with a significant shunt and visualization of the vena cava during the earlier arterial phase.

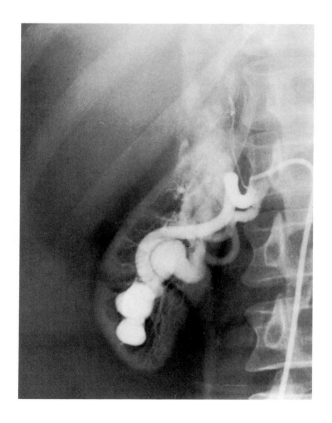

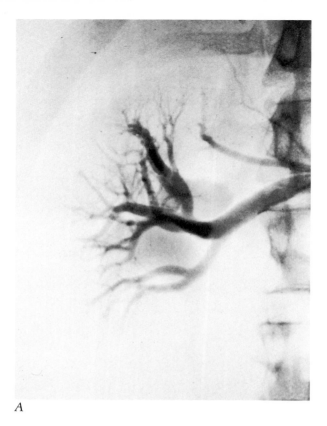

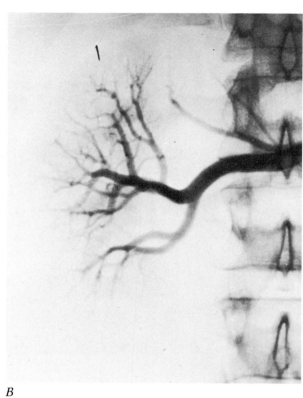

A

B

Figure 56-13. (A) A selective renal arteriogram demonstrating an arteriovenous shunt following a kidney biopsy. (B) A selective arteriogram 16 months later showing complete resolution of the previous fistula. (Courtesy of L. Ekelund, M.D.)

Figure 56-14. (A) An extensive arteriovenous fistula with associated hematuria (*arrow*). (B) A balloon occlusion of a fistula with total control of the renal flow during surgical excision (*arrows*).

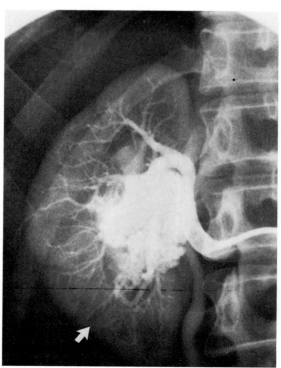

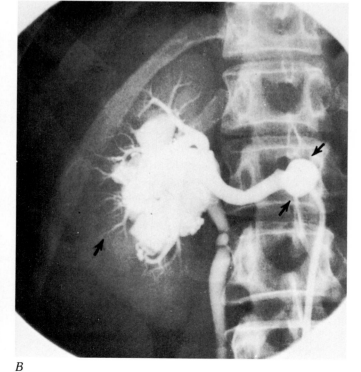

A

B

When the lesion persists and when an audible bruit exists with persistent hematuria, a diagnostic arteriogram should be performed [38]. If the lesion is enlarging and there are signs of cardiac decompensation, an interventional procedure with occlusion should be considered [39, 40]. Certain of these postbiopsy arteriovenous fistulas with functioning ipsilateral kidneys may be associated with diastolic hypertension. The hypertension may be related to localized ischemia causing activation of the renin-angiotensin system. However, accurate renal vein renin determinations are difficult to obtain; since the fistula allows such a large quantity of renal arterial blood to flow directly into the vein, a true increase in renin from an ischemic area can be significantly diluted. In the past, because of the intrarenal location of these fistulas, total or partial nephrectomy was necessary in symptomatic patients with renal vascular hypertension, high output failure, or bleeding. However, selective arterial occlusion can now be utilized as an alternative to surgery. Because of the very high incidence of spontaneous closure [37, 41], our approach has been periodic observation of the smaller postbiopsy fistulas. Persistent or expanding lesions in fistulas that are increasingly symptomatic require interventional embolization, with selective occlusion the procedure of choice (Fig. 56-14 A, B).

Other Complications

Unfortunately, the management of renal trauma is associated with a combination of both early and late complications. The early complications, including hemorrhage, sepsis, urinary extravasation, and perinephric abscess, as well as renal failure, invariably occur in the first 6 weeks after injury. The late complications, including hypertension, pyelonephritis, hydronephrosis, chronic renal insufficiency, arteriovenous fistulas, and a nonfunctioning kidney, are the late sequelae that tend to be chronically symptomatic and necessitate long-term observations (Fig. 56-15 A, B). With increasing sophistication in diagnostic modalities and continued improvement in surgical judgment and interventional methods of hemorrhage control, a decrease in both the immediate and the delayed complications of renal trauma can be anticipated.

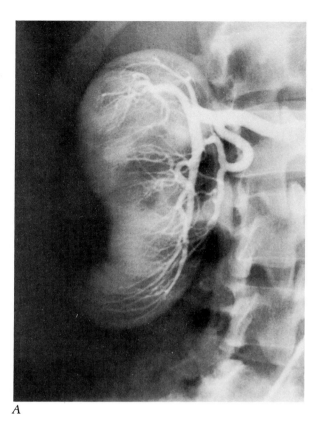

A

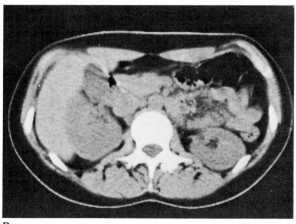

B

Figure 56-15. (A) A selective renal arteriogram of long-standing posttraumatic perinephric hematoma and associated hypertension (a "Page" kidney). (B) An unenhanced computed tomographic scan demonstrating alteration in the contour of the right kidney with associated perinephric hematoma.

ACKNOWLEDGMENTS

We would like to thank Norman D. Rabinovitz and Robert Lapiska, medical photographers, and Pamela Gaudio for their help in preparing this chapter.

References

1. Moylan, J. A. Office evaluation of blunt abdominal trauma. *Abdom. Trauma* 68:50, 1980.
2. Geelhoed, G. W. Blunt and penetrating abdominal trauma. *Am. Fam. Physician* 17:100, 1978.
3. Mendez, R. Renal trauma. *J. Urol.* 118:698, 1977.
4. Salvatierra, O., Rigdon, W. O., Norris, D. M., and Brady, T. W. Vietnam experience with 252 urological war injuries. *J. Urol.* 101:615, 1969.
5. Carlton, C. E., Jr., Scott, R., and Goldman, M. The management of penetrating injuries of the kidney. *J. Trauma* 8:1071, 1968.
6. Evins, S. C., Thomason, B. W., and Rosenblum, R. Nonoperative management of severe renal lacerations. *J. Urol.* 123:247, 1980.
7. Hodges, C. V., Gilbert, D. R., and Scott, W. W. Renal trauma—a study of 71 cases. *J. Urol.* 66:627, 1951.
8. Banowsky, L. H., Wolfel, D. A., and Lackner, L. H. Considerations in diagnosis and management of renal trauma. *J. Trauma* 10:587, 1970.
9. Hessel, S. J., and Smith, E. H. Renal trauma: A comprehensive review and radiologic assessment. *CRC Crit. Rev. Diagn. Imaging* 5:251, 1974.
10. Itzchak, Y., Adar, R., Mozes, M., and Deutsch, V. Occlusion of renal and visceral arteries following blunt abdominal trauma; angiographic observation. *J. Cardiovasc. Surg.* 15:383, 1974.
11. Maggio, A. H., and Brosman, S. Renal artery trauma. *J. Urol.* 11:125, 1978.
12. Clark, R. A. Traumatic renal artery occlusion. *J. Trauma* 19:270, 1979.
13. Taddei, L., Palma, F. D., and Selva, A. D. The role of urography in blunt trauma of the kidney. *Diagn. Imaging* 48:305, 1979.
14. Wein, A. J., Murphy, J. J., Mulholland, S. G., Chait, A. W., and Arger, P. H. A conservative approach to the management of blunt renal trauma. *J. Urol.* 117:425, 1979.
15. Ranking, G. N. Changing concepts in the diagnosis and treatment of closed renal injuries. *Can. Med. Assoc. J.* 116:617, 1977.
16. Griffen, W. O., Belin, R. P., Ernst, C. B., Sachatello, C. R., Daugherty, M. E., Mulcahy, J. J., Chuang, V. A., and Maull, K. I. Intravenous pyelography in abdominal trauma. *J. Trauma* 18:387, 1978.
17. Birkenstock, W. E., Rabkin, R., and Stables, D. P. Bilateral traumatic renal artery occlusion with survival after late reconstitution of arterial flow. *Br. J. Surg.* 59:915, 1972.
18. Steiness, I., and Thaysen, J. H. Bilateral traumatic renal artery thrombosis. *Lancet* 1:527, 1965.
19. Sargent, J. C., and Marquardt, C. R. Renal injuries. *J. Urol.* 63:1, 1950.
20. Mitchell, J. P. Trauma to the urinary tract. *Br. Med. J.* 2:567, 1971.
21. Elkin, M., Meng, C. H., and deParedes, R. G. Roentgenologic evaluation of renal trauma with emphasis on renal angiography. *AJR* 98:1, 1966.
22. Marks, L. S., Brosman, S. A., Lindstrom, R. R., and Fay, R. Arteriography in penetrating renal trauma. *Urology* 3:18, 1974.
23. Woodruff, J. H., Jr., Cockett, A. T. K., Cannon, R., and Swanson, L. E. Radiologic aspects of renal trauma with emphasis on arteriography and renal isotope scanning. *J. Urol.* 97:184, 1967.
24. Dury, E. M., and Rubin, E. B. Computed tomography in the evaluation of abdominal trauma. *J. Comp. Assist. Tomogr.* 3:40, 1979.
25. Stables, D. P. Unilateral absence of excretion at urography after abdominal trauma. *Radiology* 121:609, 1976.
26. Lang, E. K., Trichel, B. E., Turner, R. W., Fontenot, R. A., Johnson, B., and St. Martin, E. C. Renal arteriography in the assessment of renal trauma. *Radiology* 98:103, 1971.
27. Silber, S. J., and Clark, R. E. Treatment of massive hemorrhage after renal biopsy with angiographic injection of clot: *N. Engl. J. Med.* 292:1387, 1975.
28. Richman, S. A., Green, W. M., Kroll, R., and Casarella, W. J. Superselective transcatheter embolization of traumatic renal hemorrhage. *AJR* 128:843, 1977.
29. Chuang, V. P., Reuter, S. R., Walter, J., Foley, W. D., and Bookstein, J. J. Control of renal hemorrhage by selective arterial embolization. *AJR* 125:300, 1975.
30. Kalish, M., Greenbaum, L., Silber, S., and Goldstein, H. Traumatic renal hemorrhage treatment by arterial embolization. *J. Urol.* 112:138, 1974.
31. White, R. I., Strandberg, J. D., Gross, G. S., and Barth, K. H. Therapeutic embolization with long-term occluding agents and their effects on embolized tissues. *Radiology* 125:677, 1977.
32. Wholey, M. H., Chamorro, H. A., Rao, G., and Chapman, W. Splenic infarction and spontaneous rupture of the spleen after therapeutic embolization. *Cardiovasc. Intervent. Radiol.* 1:249, 1978.
33. Grant, R. P., Jr., Gifford, R. W., Jr., Pudvan, W. R., Meaney, T. F., Straffon, R. A., and

McCormack, L. J.   Renal trauma and hypertension. *Am. J. Cardiol.* 27:173, 1971.

34. Nelson, B. D., Brosman, S. A., and Goodwin, W. E.   Renal arteriovenous fistulas. *J. Urol.* 109:779, 1973.

35. Cosgrove, M. D., Mendez, R., and Morrow, J. W.   Traumatic renal arteriovenous fistula: Report of 12 cases. *J. Urol.* 110:627, 1973

36. Ekelund, L., and Lindholm, T.   Arteriovenous fistulae following percutaneous renal biopsy. *Acta Radiol. [Diagn.]* (Stockh.) 11:38, 1971.

37. Boijsen, E., and Kohler, R.   Renal arteriovenous fistulae. *Acta Radiol.* 57:433, 1962.

38. Clouse, M. E., and Adams, D. F.   Congenital renal arteriovenous malformation. Angiography in its diagnosis. *Urology* 2:282, 1975.

39. Bookstein, J. J., and Goldstein, H. M.   Successful management of postbiopsy arteriovenous fistula with selective arterial embolization. *Radiology* 109:535, 1973.

40. Goldman, M. L., Fellner, S. K., and Parrott, T. S.   Transcatheter embolization of renal arteriovenous fistula. *Urology* 3:386, 1975.

41. Halpern, M.   Spontaneous closure of traumatic renal arteriovenous fistulas. *AJR* 107:730, 1969.

Renal Arteriography in Hypertension

HERBERT L. ABRAMS

The widespread use of arteriography has clarified many of the underlying renal vascular changes in patients with hypertension. The primary focus of this chapter is on renovascular hypertension, but the chapter also reviews the alterations found in essential and malignant hypertension and in a number of other renal lesions associated with high blood pressure.

The relationship between hypertension and renal disease, suspected for many decades, was brought into focus by Goldblatt's report in 1933 that dogs subjected to nephrectomy and narrowing of the contralateral renal artery developed significant elevation of the blood pressure [47]. The renin-angiotensin system, studied by investigators for many years, has only slowly yielded to a systematic unraveling of its precise role in the hypertension associated with unilateral renal arterial disease in man. What is clearly known is that renin acts on renin substrate to produce angiotensin 1, which is metabolized by converting enzyme to angiotensin 2 in the lungs and other organs. Angiotensin 2 raises blood pressure both because of its direct vasoconstrictive effect and because it stimulates aldosterone production by the adrenal cortex. Aldosterone, in turn, raises blood pressure by increasing sodium reabsorption, with resultant elevation of blood volume.

It is now well established that unilateral elevation of renal venous renin activity is associated with a high likelihood of cure of hypertension when renal artery stenosis is present [7].

The enthusiasm for surgery for all patients with hypertension and demonstrated renal arterial disease has waxed and waned. The morbidity and mortality associated with such surgery is high, and investigators have provided unequivocal evidence that renal artery stenosis per se need not be causative of hypertension. In arteriographic studies of normotensive and hypertensive adults, Eyler found all types of major renal arterial stenosis in both the normotensive and the hypertensive groups [38]. Holley's series demonstrated that renal artery stenosis was present at autopsy in a significant percentage of patients who had been normotensive during life [59]. Except on rare occasions, therefore, the arteriogram should not be the sole determinant of whether surgery is undertaken: supporting physiologic data and renin assays are essential,

Supported by National Institutes of Health grants HL11668 and GM18674.

particularly in regard to patients whose hypertension can be controlled on drug therapy, without important side effects. Nevertheless, all patients under the age of 35 who have persistent hypertension probably deserve arteriography even if the hypertension is controlled by medication. Against the known failures and complications of surgery stand the marked variability of compliance with drug therapy, the possibility of progression of the renal vascular lesions, and the uncertainty about the long-term effects of sustained antihypertensive medication.

One other important factor that is decreasing the use of surgery is nonoperative renal artery dilatation, or angioplasty [92]. A large number of cases of renal artery stenosis have been successfully treated with catheter dilatation [64].

Estimates of the incidence of renovascular hypertension in the general population are without proper foundation. This inadequacy is due, at least partially, to the absence of a generally accepted definition of the disease. For some the definition is arteriographic; for others, functional. But the test of a purely renal etiology rests on one parameter: diastolic normotension 1 year after surgery in the patient with previously established diastolic hypertension. Such a definition is by no means all inclusive: it may eliminate individuals with operable lesions in whom reconstructive vascular surgery was technically inadequate, and it excludes patients with a significant lesion whose kidneys are the site of small-vessel disease so profound as to preclude any benefit from surgery. Nevertheless, if simple predictive indices are to be developed, the focus must be on cure. "Successful" surgery with persistent hypertension is a contradiction.

Angiography is the only method of demonstrating precisely the presence of stenosis of the renal artery or its branches prior to surgery. Although arteriography is sometimes less than 100 percent reliable in assessing the significance of such a lesion, it is a necessary preliminary to any more intensive search to define operable patients. It also discloses a significant group of other renal lesions in which ischemia may coexist with hypertension.

In 1967, we undertook the analysis of 340 arteriograms in hypertension [3] on which much of this chapter is based. Since that time, an additional 250 arteriograms of hypertensive patients have been reviewed. Xenon washout studies on many of these patients have permitted a comparison of flow studies with the appearance of the renal vascular bed.

Normal Renal Arteriogram

The position of the kidney is variable. In adults in the supine position, the upper pole is at T12, and the lower pole is at T3. The kidney drops about one vertebral body when the upright position is assumed [94]; it is not unusual to have considerably more mobility, especially in women. A useful centering point for the examination is a point halfway between the umbilicus and the xiphoid process. Usually the central ray will be just under the origin of the renal arteries.

The renal arteries, although described as dorsal branches, are usually lateral in origin and arise from the aorta at, slightly above, or slightly below the interspace between L1 and L2 (Figs. 57-1, 57-2) (see Chap. 50). Seventy-two percent of cadavers have single vessels bilaterally of approximately equal size [89]. The right renal artery may originate slightly anterior to the coronal plane. The inferior supplemental branches tend to originate somewhat anteriorly, especially on the right.

Occasionally the single main renal artery arises as high as the inferior aspect of T12 and as low as L2. The right renal artery may be either a little higher or a little lower than the left renal artery. This is in contrast to the usually lower position of the right kidney itself. The right renal artery generally follows a somewhat more caudal course than the left.

Supplemental renal vessels pose a problem for selective angiography because they are time consuming to find and to film, and, if they are small, they may easily be obstructed by the catheter tip. Their range of origin is wide, from T11 down to

Figure 57-2. Origin of the renal arteries. Normally, the right renal artery arises at a level somewhat lower than the left, and the right kidney is more caudal. The position is quite variable, however, and it is essential that these variations in anatomy be fully understood. (A and B) A higher origin of the left renal artery, the more common situation. (C) The origin of both right and left arteries at the same level. (D, E, and F) A more caudal origin of the left renal artery than of the right renal artery. In (E) and (F), the left kidney is lower than the right kidney, in contrast to the usual situation.

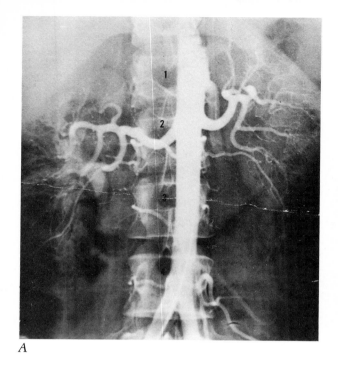

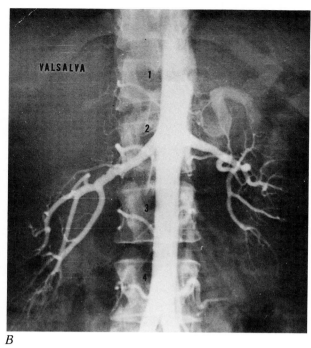

A

B

Figure 57-1. Normal renal arteriogram. (A) Expiration. The vessels arborize normally. There is minimal irregularity of the right renal artery. (B) Valsalva maneuver. The kidneys are now far more caudal than during the initial study. The renal arteries are stretched and uncoiled. The minimal fibromuscular hyperplasia of the right renal artery is of no dynamic significance. Split-function studies demonstrated equivalent renal plasma flows on both sides.

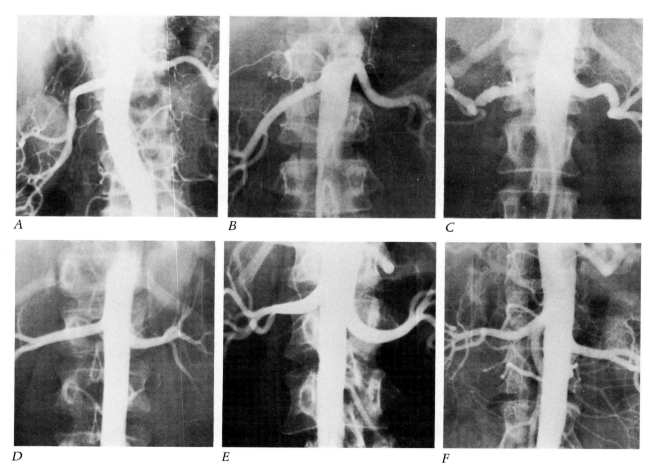

A

B

C

D

E

F

1249

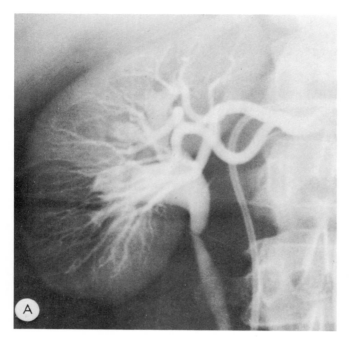

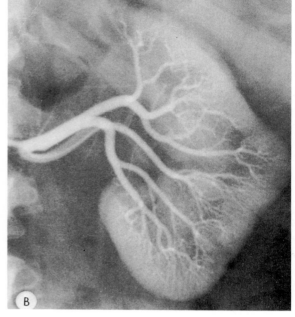

Figure 57-3. Normal selective renal arteriogram. (A) Right kidney. The cortex is well defined in the upper pole. There is an even, regular progression to smaller vessels, which have a straight or a mildly curved course. The tapering is uniform. (B) Left kidney. The catheter tip has been placed beyond the bifurcation of the main renal artery. As a consequence, there has been only flash filling of the dorsal renal arterial branch; the ventral renal artery is well filled. The artifactual lack of opacification of the central medial portion of the kidney and the upper pole might well have been interpreted as representing a large area of infarction.

the iliac vessels (Fig. 57-2; see also Figs. 57-21, 57-29). Rarely, supplemental branches arise from visceral aortic branches [49].

The kidney may be divided into dorsal and ventral segments and the arteries to these segments identified. Graves divides the kidney into five segments, recognizing two anterior and one posterior position in the middle of the kidney and a small apical segment and a larger caudal segment [48]. The orientation of the kidney is such that the dorsal arteries are medial and the dorsal segments and subsegments are not border forming at the lateral margin of the kidney in the true anteroposterior projection [13]. The ventral arteries are lateral, and the ventral subsegments are border forming along the lateral aspect of the kidney. The lower pole is usually supplied by the ventral vessel, and the dorsal vessel extends cephalad to supply a variable part of the superior pole.

A careful analysis of the normal arborization of the distal vessels demonstrates a reproducible, even, and regular progression to smaller and smaller vessels that have a straight or a mildly curved course. Normal vessels taper uniformly and evenly (Figs. 57-3, 57-4). The interlobar arteries branch repeatedly until they give rise to the arcuate arteries. The interlobular arteries of the cortex arise from the arcuate vessels, extend into the cortex in a more or less parallel fashion (Fig. 57-4), and may be defined with good-quality magnification [19]. As the cortex opacifies, it develops a granular pattern, thought to be produced by overlapping glomeruli [19].

In general, the nephrogram reflects the volume of flow to the kidney and is well appreciated within a few seconds after injection. With catheter injection into the abdominal aorta, however, the nephrogram frequently may reflect laminar flow rather than the total mixing of the contrast agent. Under the circumstances, a diminished nephrogram may be found in the absence of renal artery stenosis, and a relatively augmented nephrogram may be found in its presence. The 15-second film on the double-dose rapidly injected intravenous urogram is more reliable insofar as the nephrogram is concerned because total mixing is secured. During the nephrographic phase,

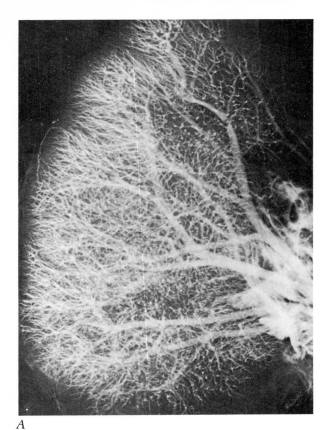

A

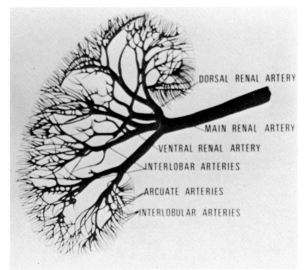

B

Figure 57-4. Normal renal vascular bed. (A) An injected specimen at autopsy. Note the progressive gradual tapering of the vessels and the multiple interlobular branches that arise from the arcuate arteries to enter the cortex of the kidney. (B) Diagrammatic representation of the renal arteries.

Figure 57-5. Standing waves in the renal arteries. (A) Main renal artery. Multiple serrated indentations are visible in the main renal artery (*arrow*), symmetrically distributed and at evenly spaced intervals. They have the characteristic appearance of "standing waves"; these have no pathologic significance and may represent a form of spasm. (B) Main and branch renal arteries. The standing waves in this patient extend from the main renal artery (*arrow, right*) to multiple interlobar branches (*arrows, left*) within the kidney itself. The appearance is characteristic of standing waves.

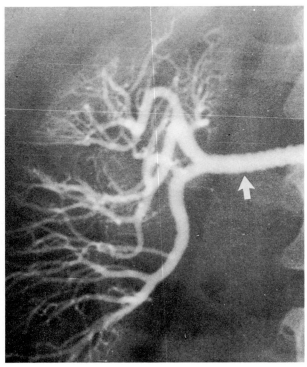

A

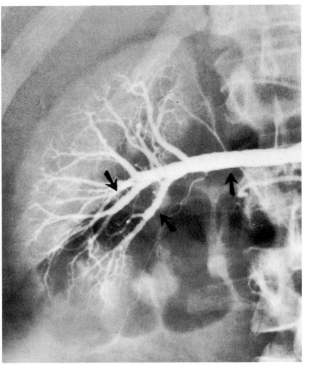

B

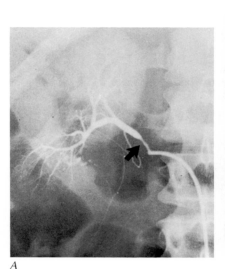
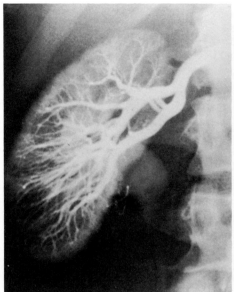
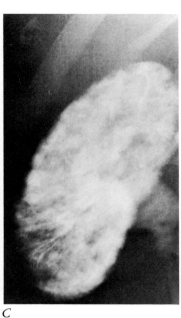

A   B   C

Figure 57-6. Renal artery spasm. (A) Localized. Precisely at the site of the catheter tip, the renal artery is profoundly narrowed (*arrow*). Removal of the catheter from the renal artery and an intraaortic injection demonstrate that the caliber of the renal artery is normal. (B and C) Spasm of the small renal arteries. Many distal vessels are narrowed in association with the selective injection. The nephrogram (C) demonstrates multiple lucent areas in the cortex, all of which disappeared following an intraaortic bolus injection. (Courtesy of David Levin, M.D.)

contrast material is present in the capillaries and in the renal excretory tissue. There is a general increase in density although the cortex is usually well defined—and its width measurable—as a dense homogeneous band around the kidney that is about 5 to 8 mm thick. The nephrogram is most useful when it demonstrates a local area of ischemia (see Figs. 57-21, 57-22, 57-30). Normally, the contrast-filled arteries have a smooth, even appearance throughout their course (see Fig. 57-2). Occasionally during aortography or selective arteriography, "standing waves" may be observed—regular, periodic, localized, symmetric indentations of the vessel wall thought to be caused by spasm (Fig. 57-5). Standing waves are important because they may be mistaken for dysplastic disease of the renal artery.

Another important finding to be recognized and understood is renal spasm during angiography (Fig. 57-6). Various types of spasm are visible: (1) concentric short-segment stenosis, which may resemble fixed stenosis; (2) long-segment fusiform narrowing; and (3) multiple small perfusion defects during the nephrographic phase of the angiogram, suggestive of renal parenchymal disease (Figs. 57-6B, C) [106]. Such confusing appearances may be better evaluated after the use of acetylcholine, which causes their elimination or sometimes simply by abdominal aortography without a selective study.

Renovascular Hypertension

The importance of renovascular hypertension in man lies precisely in the fact that, unlike the overwhelming number of cases of essential or malignant hypertension in the general population, it may be curable. Its incidence has not yet been finally established, but it is probably 3 to 10 percent of all cases of hypertension.

DIAGNOSIS

Perhaps the most important single clinical reference point is the patient's age: renovascular hypertension is frequently a disease of young adults.

On *physical examination*, aside from high blood pressure and, at times, cardiac enlargement and eye ground changes, the most conspicuous finding may be a bruit in the epigastrium. Although it has been claimed that bruits are heard in a high percentage of patients with renovascular hypertension, the figures are variable. In the presence of stenosis of above 50 percent, bruits are absent as often as they are present, and they do not reflect the degree of stenosis. In about 10 percent of patients, such bruits are heard in the absence of renal artery stenosis: this phenomenon may be related to aortic arteriosclerosis or to involvement of any of the other branch vessels of the aorta.

The most significant *urographic findings* that accompany a strongly positive arteriogram are disparities in size, appearance time, and concentration of the contrast agent in the collecting system [17]. In approximately 20 percent of patients with renovascular hypertension, these signs may be absent (and the study results false-negative), and, conversely, these signs may be present in 10 percent of patients with essential hypertension (and the study results false-positive).

Pathologically the kidney may demonstrate various degrees of nephrosclerosis as well as atrophic changes in the tubules. The juxtaglomerular apparatus is frequently increased in number, and the cellularity of the juxtaglomerular apparatus may be augmented. Although the ischemic kidney may have less arteriolar change than the nonischemic diseased kidney, the changes of arteriolar nephrosclerosis may be bilateral in a significant percentage of cases.

What is *significant arterial stenosis*? When the diameter of the vessel is reduced to 20 percent or less of its original size, the stenosis has a high chance of being causally related to hypertension known to be present. In practice, this implies a reduction in the diameter of the lumen to 1.0 to 1.5 mm [16]. The presence of stenosis, however, is not enough to guarantee the presence of hypertension [38], nor its causative role if hypertension is present. A developed collateral circulation is an important ancillary sign of the hemodynamic significance of arterial stenosis. Useful confirmatory evidence of significant stenosis lies in the renal vein renin assays. Lateralization of high levels of renin secretion to the underperfused kidney is associated with a 93 percent benefit rate following surgical correction [16, 65]. Even in the absence of lateralization, however, 50 percent of patients with renal artery stenosis and hypertension may respond to surgery [65], indicating that renin assays have a

high false-negative rate. Recent experience with Saralasin, a specific blocker of angiotensin 2, suggests that it has higher sensitivity and specificity in detecting renovascular hypertension than do assays of renal vein renins alone [65]. In the past, radioisotope renograms and split-function studies have provided useful information, but the renograms have many false-positive and false-negative results and split-function studies may be traumatic.

In patients cured of renovascular hypertension, the preoperative arteriogram almost invariably shows an apparently significant lesion. Nevertheless, a large group of patients with abnormal arteriograms are not cured because the lesion is not causative, contralateral disease is profound, surgery is inadequate, or operative death occurs [18]. Also, although split-function tests have been positive in most individuals cured of hypertension by nephrectomy or revascularization, many patients with positive split-function tests were not cured of hypertension by surgery. The prognosis for cure is worse when cardiac enlargement or advanced eye ground changes have developed.

ARTERIOSCLEROSIS

Arteriosclerosis is the most common cause of narrowing of the renal arterial lumen. It is usually observed in patients over 40 years of age and is more common in males. Because plaques develop most frequently at the origins or bifurcations of vessels, it is not surprising that renal artery stenosis due to arteriosclerosis usually is orificial or is located in the proximal one-third of the artery (Figs. 57-7–57-9). Furthermore, atherosclerotic involvement of the renal artery is frequently accompanied by aortic disease (Figs. 57-8, 57-9; see also Fig. 57-47) [53]. Aortic plaques may themselves cause stenosis or occlusion at the ostia of the renal artery.

Arteriosclerotic narrowing may be of any degree—from a small plaque to complete occlusion (Figs. 57-8, 57-9). It is usually more or less localized (see Fig. 57-7), and it may be eccentric (see Figs. 57-7A, 57-8) or circumferential (see Fig. 57-7A), but usually irregularly so [82]. The lesions may be single or multiple. In 30 to 50 percent of the cases, the lesions are bilateral (see Fig. 57-7A), with one side more severely affected [3, 53]. Immediately beyond the stenosis, marked poststenotic dilatation may be observed (see Fig.

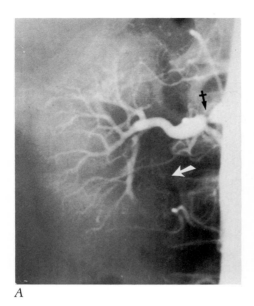

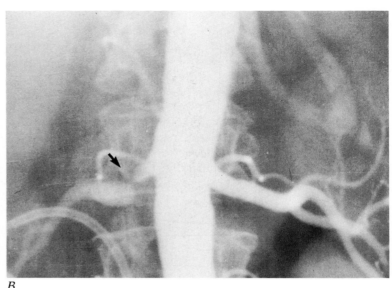

A   *B*

Figure 57-7. Arteriosclerotic stenosis of the renal artery. (A) Concentric stenosis. This 58-year-old man had a blood pressure of 180/110 mm Hg. Arteriography demonstrates a discrete zone of stenosis about 8 mm beyond the origin of the right renal artery, with circumferential narrowing and only minimal eccentricity (*barred arrow*). Poststenotic dilatation is visible. Both the radioactive renogram and the split-function studies were also abnormal. The appearance is typical of arteriosclerotic stenosis. Small collateral vessels are visible (*white arrow*). (B) Eccentric stenosis. Significant eccentric narrowing of the renal artery within the proximal third of the vessel strongly suggests the arteriosclerotic etiology. The lumen is no more than 1 mm in diameter (*arrow*). Note the dilatation beyond the stenosis.

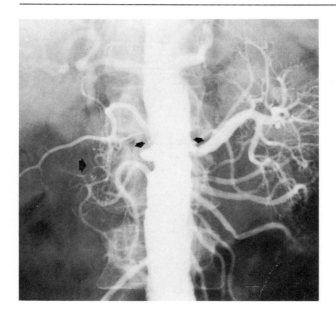

Figure 57-8. Arteriosclerotic stenosis and occlusion of the renal artery. This 56-year-old man had a 7-year history of hypertension (blood pressure of 228/100 mm Hg). A bruit was heard in the epigastrium, and there was hypertensive retinopathy. There is complete occlusion of the right renal artery approximately 8 mm beyond its origin (*right central arrow*). On the right, profuse collateral vessels fill from the lumbar arteries (*right lateral arrow*). Moderate renal artery stenosis is present in the left renal artery (*left central arrow*), and multiple irregularities indicate the presence of arteriosclerosis of the remainder of the main renal artery. Arteriosclerosis of the aorta is also visible, and there are large plaques immediately adjacent to the origin of the right renal artery.

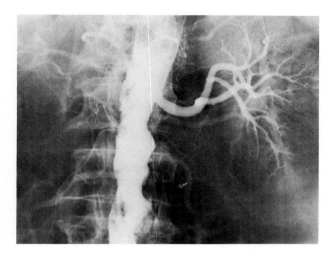

Figure 57-9. Arteriosclerotic occlusion of the renal artery. Bolus aortography demonstrates the left renal artery with normal bifurcations and multiple arteriosclerotic plaques in the aorta. The origin of the right renal artery is totally occluded by arteriosclerotic plaques.

57-7). This does not necessarily signify that the stenosis is dynamically important.

RENAL ARTERY DYSPLASIA

This intriguing lesion (also known as *fibroplasia* and *fibromuscular hyperplasia*) occurs predominantly in females [97], although we have seen many cases in young males as well. The female-to-male incidence is approximately 4 or 5:1 [35]. The youngest patient in our series was 6 months old. Most patients were in their 30s, 40s, and 50s. The disease is not localized to the renal arteries, and other visceral branches as well as the carotid arteries may be involved [12, 35, 98]. There is also an apparent association with cerebral aneurysms.

Histologically, there may be focal areas of intimal proliferation, possibly secondary to organized mural thrombi. The media is most often involved, usually by fibrous thickening, less commonly by muscular hyperplasia [77]. In some cases, there are two distinct medial layers: an inner muscular coat and an outer circular fibrous coat, distinct from the longitudinal adventitial investment of the vessel. A variable increase in the polysaccharide content of the media is present. The muscle cells are plump with decreased eosinophilia, and they may be difficult to differentiate from fibroblasts. Disruption and duplication of the elastic fibers are also apparent.

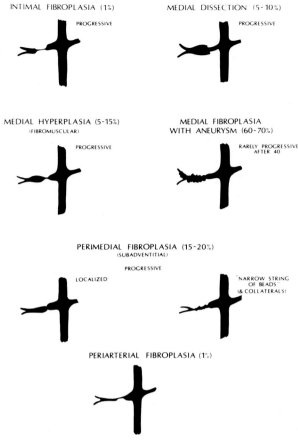

Figure 57-10. Dysplastic lesions of the renal artery. (Modified from McCormack et al. [76, 77] and from Kincaid [67].)

The classification of dysplastic lesions of the renal artery has been a focus of controversy for many years. On the basis of the studies of McCormack and his colleagues [76, 77], as well as those of Kincaid et al. [68], together with our own series of cases, we use the following classification, which combines the important pathologic and angiographic characteristics of these lesions. (Figure 57-10 delineates the angiographic findings of the different types of dysplastic disease.)

(1) Intimal fibroplasia. The intima is thickened by fibrous tissue. These lesions may be localized (Fig. 57-11), or they may involve a long segment of the renal artery. They account for a relatively small number of the total group of patients with fibroplastic disease.

(2) Medial dissection. This lesion also is characterized by the accumulation of collagen

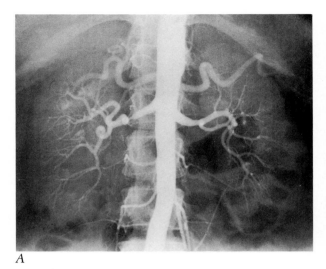

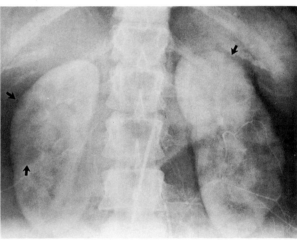

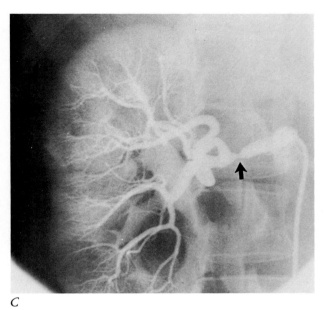

Figure 57-11. Renal artery dysplasia. Intimal fibroplasia. (A) Aortogram. A discrete area of narrowing in the midportion of the right renal artery is visible, about 1 cm in length with no other abnormalities of the main renal artery. Note that bilaterally the kidneys are large and the vessels appear somewhat spread. (B) Nephrographic phase. Multiple lucent areas are seen in both kidneys (*arrows*), representing small-to-moderate-sized cysts. The patient had polycystic disease coexisting with renal artery dysplasia. (C) Selective renal arteriogram, left posterior oblique projection. The single area of involvement (*arrow*) is symmetric and concentric in its appearance.

within the internal elastic lamina. It appears most frequently in the younger age group and is accompanied by fibroplasia of the intima and media, with degeneration of the media. As it progresses, a hematoma develops in the weakened media, and a communication between the lumen of the vessel and the media occurs because of the alterations in intima and media. The classic histologic and angiographic appearance of dissection may then be observed (Fig. 57-12) [91, 99]. This occurs in approximately 5 to 10 percent of all patients with fibroplastic disease.

3 Medial hyperplasia. Uncomplicated medial hyperplasia actually represents fibromuscular hyperplasia, with muscular as well as fibrous elements involved. The narrowing is frequently localized (Fig. 57-13) and sometimes tubular and involves the middle and distal thirds of the renal artery. It occurs in no more than 5 to 15 percent of patients with dysplastic disease.

4 Medial fibroplasia with aneurysm. Areas of thickened, fibrotic media alternate with thinned areas, the typical string-of-beads appearance that reflects the multiple concentric rings produced by the hyperplastic changes in the wall interspersed with local aneurysm formation at the site of elastic and muscle tissue degeneration in the media. The most common type of fibroplasia, it occurs in 60 to 70 percent of all patients with dysplastic disease. It is found in all age groups, and the angiographic appearance is quite characteristic (Fig. 57-14). It usually affects the renal artery in the middle and distal thirds to a variable degree, with localized constrictions alternating with aneurysmal dilatations. In contrast to perimedial fibroplasia, the aneurysms bulge beyond the expected diameter of the renal artery and appear to represent true aneurysms. This lesion is of particular importance, because, in contrast to the others, it is relatively stable and rarely

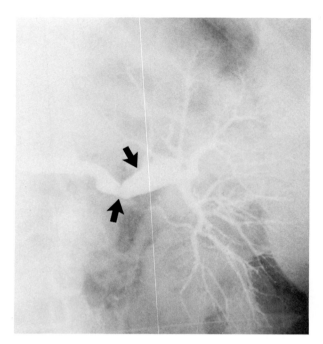

Figure 57-12. Renal artery dysplasia. Medial dissection. A selective left renal arteriogram demonstrates a normal proximal renal artery, a localized aneurysmal bulge just proximal to a stenotic area (*lower arrow*), and apparent dilatation of the vessel beyond (*upper arrow*). This dilatation extends into some of the branch arteries. Although the arteriographic change is not necessarily specific, it is suggestive. The false lumen represented by the dilated area is located in the media, which is markedly altered by the fibroplastic process. Disruption of the internal elastic lamina is also present, and intimal fibroplasia coexists. Compression of the normal lumen by the dissection produces renal ischemia, which may cause renin-dependent hypertension to develop.

progressive after the age of 40. Hence, the definition of the type of fibroplastic disease has important prognostic connotations. Conversely, medial hyperplasia with aneurysms has been shown to develop in individuals with angiographically normal renal arteries examined during adult life, strongly supporting the concept of renal artery dysplasia as an acquired disease [9].

(5) Perimedial fibroplasia, localized type. These lesions characteristically have a collagen collar of variable thickness between the media and the adventitia. When localized (Fig. 57-15), they are indistinguishable either from medial hyperplasia or from intimal fibroplasia.

(6) Perimedial fibroplasia, diffuse type (Figs. 57-16, 57-17). This type of lesion sometimes resembles medial fibroplasia with aneurysm, and has been called the *narrow-string-of-beads*. Char-

acteristically, the dilatations are smaller in caliber than the portions of the renal artery that are uninvolved, and therefore the appearance differs distinctively from that of medial fibroplasia with aneurysm.

(7) Periarterial fibroplasia. Fibrous thickening of the adventitia with cicatrix formation produces a relatively localized or (sometimes) diffuse area of narrowing in the main renal artery (Fig. 57-18), usually in the middle or distal thirds. This is a rare type of dysplastic disease but is equally capable of causing hypertension because of renal ischemia.

Thus the localized lesions of intimal fibroplasia, medial hyperplasia (or fibromuscular hyperplasia), and perimedial fibroplasia are difficult to distinguish from each other angiographically, and they have as an important aspect of their prognosis the capacity for being progressive in character. In contrast, the commonest single type of fibroplastic disease, medial fibroplasia with aneurysm, is rarely progressive after the age of 40. In 21 of 125 patients studied with fibroplastic disease, mixed lesions were noted that could not be categorized explicitly into a single pathologic type [68].

The proximal one-third of the main renal artery is usually spared in dysplastic disease, but the middle and distal thirds are typically involved (see Figs. 57-11–57-18). Much of the main renal artery and the interlobar branches may be the site of disease (see Figs. 57-15–57-17). When the process extends into the secondary branches, it may produce complete occlusion of vessels to the upper or lower pole, so that the total blood supply to the kidney segment may be derived from the collateral circulation. In about 40 to 70 percent of cases, the lesions are bilateral [35, 45, 68]. When unilateral, renal artery dysplasia is far more common on the right than on the left [18]. When the lesions are localized and nonrepetitive, and particularly if they are located in the proximal one-third, they may be difficult to distinguish from arteriosclerotic disease. The periarterial adventitial lesions may involve a long segment of the vessel, with a segment of smooth, tubular narrowing (Fig. 57-18).

Renal artery dysplasia has been demonstrated in the absence of hypertension and need not be causative of hypertension even when hypertension is present. Figure 57-13A illustrates the case of a young woman with hypertension and fibromuscular hyperplasia of the right renal artery. The Regitine test was positive and urinary

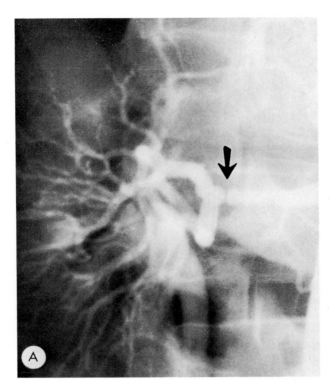

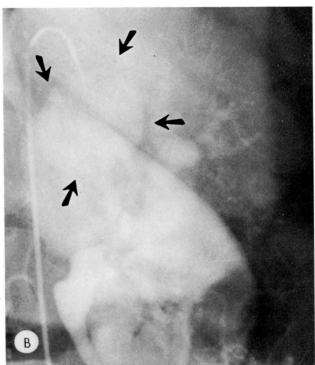

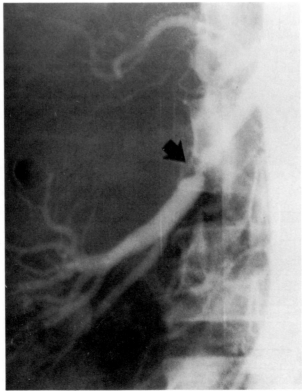

Figure 57-13. Renal artery dysplasia. Medial hyperplasia (fibromuscular). (A) Right side. The classic appearance of fibromuscular hyperplasia with an area of apparently significant stenosis (*arrow*) is visible. Despite this, there was no reduction of the blood flow to the right kidney. (B) Left side. A pheochromocytoma is well defined in the adrenal area (*arrows*), coexisting with the right renal artery stenosis. (C) Medial (fibromuscular) hyperplasia (*arrow*). The involvement is somewhat more tubular in character and is less localized.

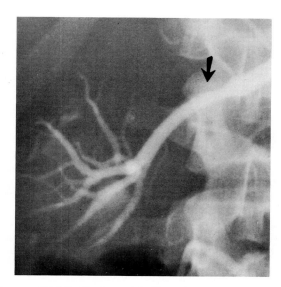

Figure 57-18. Periarterial fibroplasia. This 20-year-old woman had a 3-month history of hypertension (blood pressure of 220/140 mm Hg). The electrocardiogram showed left ventricular hypertrophy, and the hypertension ran a malignant course. The arteriogram demonstrates an area of smooth symmetric narrowing of the main renal artery beginning about 1.5 cm beyond its orifice (*arrow*). The funnellike constriction of the main renal artery is characteristic of one form of periarterial fibroplasia.

catecholamine levels were elevated. The split-function studies demonstrated equal blood flow to both kidneys. The patient's hypertension was cured when her pheochromocytoma was removed (see Fig. 57-13B). Aberrant pheochromocytoma may also involve the renal artery, and it may produce renal artery stenosis resembling dysplastic disease [6].

When renovascular hypertension is caused by renal artery dysplasia, a favorable response to surgery may be anticipated in over 70 percent of patients [18].

NEUROFIBROMATOSIS

A rare but important cause of renal artery stenosis is found in patients with neurofibromatosis [61, 87, 105, 112]. In most cases, the narrowing of the renal arteries is the direct effect of fibrous proliferation of the intima or the media. In other cases, neurofibromatous tissue has been demonstrated within the adventitia of the artery, producing periarterial fibrosis of a high degree, indistinguishable from that caused by the intimal lesions. In most patients, the site of stenosis is near the origin of the artery, and these lesions may be bilateral.

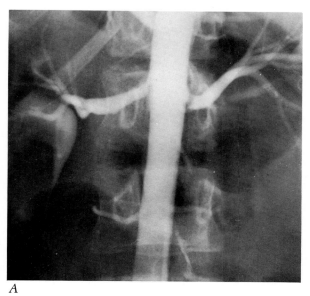

A

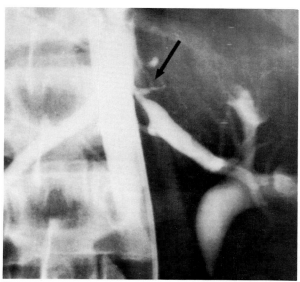

B

Figure 57-19. Renal artery stenosis. Neurofibromatosis. (A) Anteroposterior projection. (B) Left posterior oblique projection. Both renal arteries are involved, predominantly at the orifice, but also extending for about 1 to 2 cm beyond the orifice (*arrow*). The distal portion of the renal artery looks entirely smooth and normal. This appearance may be due either to a desmoplastic fibrotic involvement of the wall of the artery or to the actual presence of neurofibromatous tissue within the adventitia of the vessel, producing periarterial fibrosis. (Courtesy of Joseph Bookstein, M.D.)

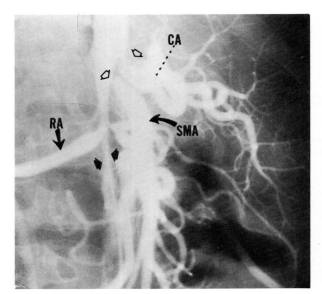

Figure 57-20. Congenital stenosis of the renal arteries. This 6-year-old girl had high blood pressure in the upper extremities (180/110 mm Hg) and lower blood pressure in the lower extremities (120/100 mm Hg). A thoracotomy had been done to look for coarctation, but none was found. A transfemoral abdominal aortogram demonstrates marked abdominal aortic narrowing beginning at the level of the celiac artery (*CA*). There is further reduction of the lumen (*black arrows*) at and below the origin of the superior mesenteric (*SMA*). The origins of these arteries (*open arrows*) are considerably narrowed. Both renal arteries (*RA*) are stenotic, with poststenotic dilatation.

Angiographically, there is a smooth stenotic segment usually at the orifice of the artery, with a tubular segment of dilatation beyond (Fig. 57-19). Thus, the appearance is different from that in dysplastic disease of the renal artery. The funnel-shaped appearance of poststenotic dilatation may be due to diffuse involvement of the arterial wall with thickening, disorganization and/or atrophy of the media and fibrosis of the adventitia [61]. The renal artery stenosis may be unilateral or bilateral, and it may be accompanied by renal artery aneurysm and, occasionally, by coarctation of the abdominal aorta as well. Rarely, iliac artery stenosis may be found. When aneurysms are present, it is because of localized fragmentation and atrophy of the media [61].

Hypertension in patients with neurofibromatosis may also be associated with the presence of pheochromocytoma. In patients below the age of 18, renal artery stenosis is a more common cause, while in patients over the age of 18, pheochromocytoma is the predominant factor [12].

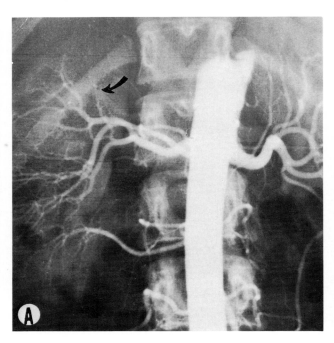

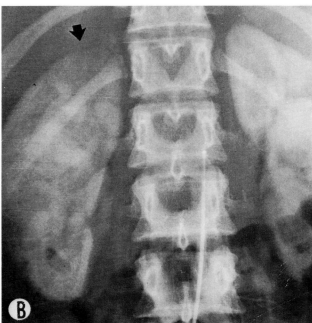

Figure 57-21. Renal artery branch stenosis. This 26-year-old woman had known hypertension of 4-years' duration. (A) Abdominal aortogram. Three renal arteries are visible on the right, and an occlusion of a small, somewhat tortuous, branch to the right upper pole is seen (*arrow*). The peripheral small branches to the upper pole are not adequately defined. (B) Nephrographic phase. The absence of contrast density in the upper pole of the right kidney reflects the segmental disease of the artery (*arrow*). The localized area of occlusion was caused by arteritis.

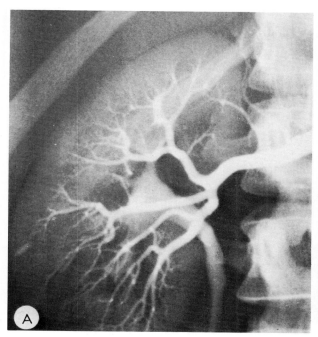

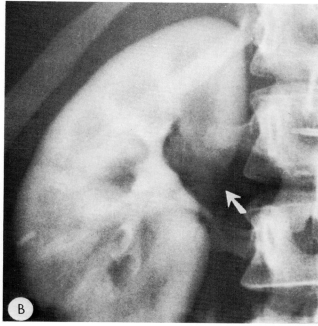

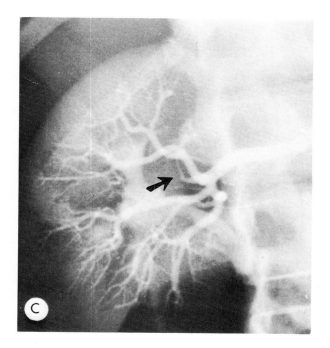

Figure 57-22. Renal artery branch stenosis. This 31-year-old woman had an episode of right flank pain about 3 months before her admission to the hospital. Increasing hypertension was then discovered; her blood pressure reached 220/140 mm Hg. Split-function data showed a 25 percent decrease in urine output on the right. A translumbar aortogram performed in another hospital was considered normal. (A) Selective renal arteriogram. The right kidney demonstrates a lack of the usual crossing vessels characteristically found in the normal arteriogram. A paucity of dorsal branches is apparent. This was also present, although not originally described, on the aortogram. (B) Nephrogram phase. There is decreased density in the medial, central aspect of the kidney (*arrow*). (C) Selective renal arteriogram, left posterior oblique view. A small, blind-end channel represents the proximal portion of the occluded dorsal arterial branch (*arrow*). At operation, a large area of infarction was found on the dorsal aspect of the kidney. Histologic examination demonstrated periarteritis nodosa.

CONGENITAL STENOSIS

Congenital stenosis, so-called coarctation of the renal artery, is a rare lesion that is assumed to be congenital because of its discovery in early life. The stenosis is relatively localized in the main renal artery [53]. It may coexist with coarctation of the abdominal aorta (Fig. 57-20) although some of these cases are probably the result of ar-

teritis of the aorta. Other cases may demonstrate the classic pathologic findings of renal artery dysplasia or neurofibromatosis [61, 105].

BRANCH STENOSIS

Branch stenosis may be due to arteriosclerosis, renal artery dysplasia, thrombus, embolus, or arteritis. In our experience, branch stenosis has been seen relatively commonly with fibroplastic disease although not necessarily as an isolated lesion. The importance of the isolated branch stenosis lies in the occasional difficulty of detecting it on the conventional arteriogram although aortography may at times be highly rewarding (Fig. 57-21A). It is essential to study both the arteriographic phase and the nephrographic phase because the latter may reveal ischemic areas with great clarity (Fig. 57-21B). If there is any question as to the presence of branch stenosis, the proper approach is a selective renal arteriogram. Multiple views may be required before the branch stenosis is detected (Fig. 57-22).

Essential Hypertension

In patients with essential hypertension of relatively short duration, there is no detectable alteration in the appearance of the major renal arteries or the intrarenal arterial branches. With the passage of time, minimal-to-moderate changes in

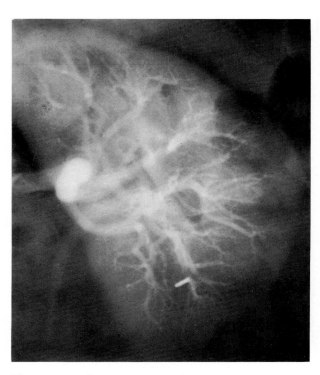

Figure 57-24. Slight-to-moderate arteriolar nephrosclerosis. There is more marked tortuosity of the arcuate vessels and, to a lesser extent, of the interlobar vessels. Diminished filling of the interlobular vessels is apparent. The metallic clip in the lower pole of the kidney represents the site of biopsy, which demonstrated arteriolar nephrosclerosis.

Figure 57-23. Mild arteriolar nephrosclerosis. Selective renal arteriography. Contrast material has been injected into one of the two vessels to the kidney. The interlobular and arcuate arteries are slightly tortuous, and there is present diminished filling of the interlobular vessels.

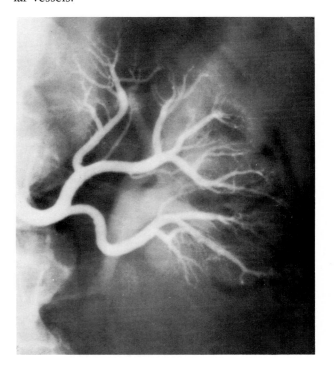

the appearance of the arterial bed appear, and these changes seem to be related to the mean renal blood flow [58]. In these selective arteriograms, the increasing tortuosity, irregularity, and narrowing of the arteries are related to the stage of the disease, the alterations in renal hemodynamics, and the mean renal blood flow (Figs. 57-23, 57-24). These findings may progress to those described in the following discussion.

Arteriolar Nephrosclerosis

Selective arteriography is usually necessary to obtain adequate detail of the small-vessel pattern of the kidney. In mild cases of nephrosclerosis, the arteriogram may be normal. As the disease progresses, histologically there is hyperplastic intimal proliferation in the small arteries and arterioles, with a reduction in luminal size. This is associated with a necrotizing arteriolitis and fibrinoid necrosis of the arteriolar wall [42]. An-

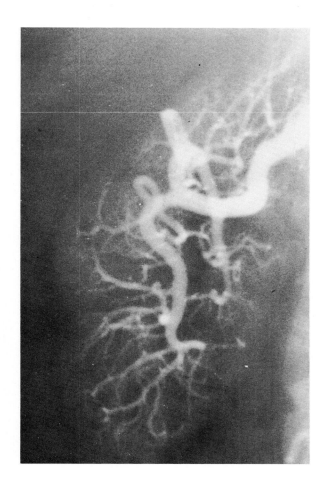

Figure 57-25. Severe arteriolar nephrosclerosis. This 47-year-old man entered the hospital because of right flank pain and hypertension. An intravenous urogram showed poor concentration and poor filling bilaterally. Selective renal arteriography demonstrates a slightly enlarged main renal artery. The interlobar and arcuate vessels are tortuous and irregular. They are somewhat diminished in caliber and have a curled or gnarled appearance. Sharp angulations of the small arteries are present. The peripheral vessels do not fill normally. The cortex is thin and irregular. The angiographic features are those of arteriolar nephrosclerosis. (Courtesy of Aaron J. Fink, M.D.)

giographically the main renal artery may be normal in size or even larger than usual, but the interlobar and arcuate vessels are reduced in caliber and have a curled or gnarled appearance, with irregularities and beading along their course (Fig. 57-25; see also Fig. 57-24). Normally these small vessels are smooth in outline and curve gently without tortuosity or narrowing; bifurcation in the periphery usually occurs with narrow angles. With disease, the gradual curvature is replaced by sharp angulations and tortuosity. Contrast flow into the periphery is delayed and results in an irregular pattern of small vessel filling. Because of a decrease in size and number of fine vessels opacified, the classic "pruned-tree" appearance is produced. Perhaps because the kidney size is reduced secondary to cortical atrophy, the subsegmental vessels bifurcate with broader angles, and the interlobar and arcuate arteries appear tortuous [20].

Hollenberg et al. [58] attempted to distinguish patients with essential hypertension from those with accelerated hypertension on the basis of the arteriographic findings. The arteriograms were graded 0 to 4. In the grade 4 arteriogram, there were few cortical vessels visible, marked tortuosity, abnormal vascular tapering, vessel irregularity with filling defects in the vascular lumen, and a prolonged vascular transit time of the contrast material (Fig. 57-26). These patients had a mean blood flow well below the lower limit of normal, and the cortical flow, as evaluated on the xenon washout, was significantly decreased. The transit time of the isotope, like that of the contrast material, was prolonged. Thus the arteriogram accurately reflected significant decreases in the renal blood flow and alterations in the distribution of the intrarenal blood flow. In uncomplicated essential hypertension, the renin secretion is low, whereas in the presence of accelerated hypertension and small-artery disease, the renin secretion is significantly increased [57].

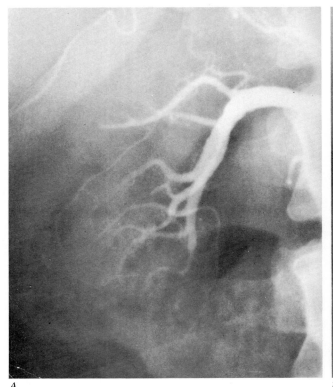
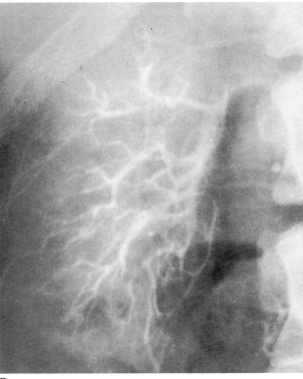

A   *B*

Figure 57-26. End-stage arteriolar nephrosclerosis. Selective renal arteriography. (A) Early phase. The main renal artery and the large branches are filled. The branches are strikingly thin. (B) Later phase. The intrarenal arteries are uniformly narrowed, and the distal terminations are tortuous. No filling of the interlobular vessels is apparent. A protracted transit time was observed. The nephrographic phase was very faint, and the cortex was markedly thin. The patient was uremic at the time of the study. Subsequently, bilateral nephrectomy and renal transplantation were done. An examination of the excised kidneys showed far-advanced nephrosclerosis.

Renal Hypertension Without Main Renal Arterial Stenosis

It has been apparent for some time that occasional cures of hypertension may be effected by nephrectomy when the kidney is small and contracted even though the main renal artery shows no evidence of stenosis [78]. McDonald, in a series of patients without renal artery stenosis, used only the split-function data of diminished urine volume associated with an elevated para-aminohippuric acid concentration as an indication for surgery in a group of patients. Of 18 patients with a small kidney and an ischemic functional pattern, 15 were cured of hypertension. Interestingly, among 10 patients who had a kidney that was 1 cm shorter than the other kidney and no ischemic functional pattern and who were subjected to nephrectomy, 3 became normotensive. It must be inferred that the group of patients with a small kidney and the ischemic functional pattern had small-vessel disease serious enough to cause local areas of ischemia.

Infarction of the Kidney

Infarction may result from embolism or thrombosis. Thrombosis, in turn, may be secondary to severe stenosis, arteritis, trauma, polycythemia, or aneurysm.

Initially the plain film shows a normal or a slightly enlarged kidney. The enlargement is due to severe edema. Nonspecific ileus, sometimes with localized small-bowel air adjacent to the affected kidney, may also be seen with various degrees of obliteration of the renal outline and psoas shadows. In chronic segmental renal infarc-

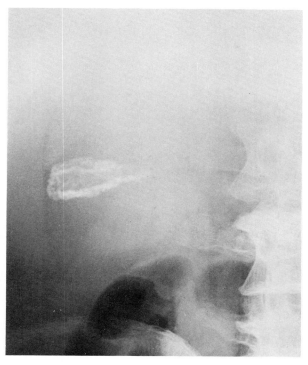

Figure 57-27. Renal infarction. A wedge-shaped area of calcification is visible on the plain film, with an indentation of the surface of the kidney precisely at the site of the calcification. The indentation represents a wedge-shaped infarction following arterial embolism in which the necrotic tissue has become heavily calcified.

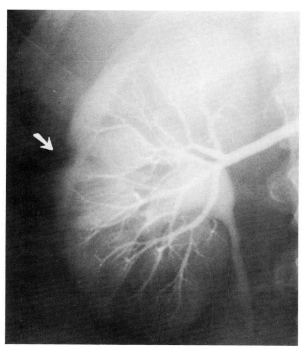

Figure 57-28. Renal infarction. Selective renal arteriogram. A localized area of underperfusion is visible adjacent to the surface of the kidney (arrow). The vessel to this area has been occluded, with consequent infarction, fibrosis, and retraction of renal tissue. This woman had hypertension, which was relieved by wedge resection of the area of infarction.

tion, a wedge-shaped area of calcification may sometimes be observed (Fig. 57-27).

The intravenous pyelogram may show normal or small calices, or lack of function. The local calix in segmental disease may be only faintly opacified. After infarction, the kidney becomes smaller, with local indentations reflecting areas with a loss of volume. The local calix may become distorted, and the appearance is similar to that in focal pyelonephritis, except that the loss of renal tissue appears excessive when compared to the degree of caliceal distortion. When the whole kidney is infarcted, there is a general decrease in size, and the kidney may resemble a congenitally hypoplastic kidney.

Angiography is helpful in elucidating the etiology. Cutoff or absence of normal vessels is visible and is associated with defects in the arteriogram and the nephrogram (Figs. 57-28–57-30). These defects may represent the infarcted tissue or the scar that has replaced it. Local increase in the circulation time is usually seen and may look like a

stain [63]. The disease is bilateral in half of the cases, and so both kidneys should be studied.

Embolism with consequent infarction may result in hypertension. Embolism of a single renal artery that leads to infarction of the entire kidney need not produce hypertension [113]. A supplementary renal artery or a collateral blood supply, however, commonly furnishes enough circulation to prevent the complete destruction of the kidney; the ischemic kidney may then cause hypertension. Similarly, if an embolus passes into a small secondary branch, only part of the kidney will be infarcted, and hypertension may well develop (Fig. 57-30). Pathologically, the source of the emboli is demonstrated at necropsy in 76 percent of the cases [60]. Clinically, the abrupt onset of constant flank pain with microscopic hematuria is typical of renal embolism although other causes of infarction cannot be excluded. When renal embolism causes incomplete infarction and hypertension or when segmental renal artery stenosis is associated with

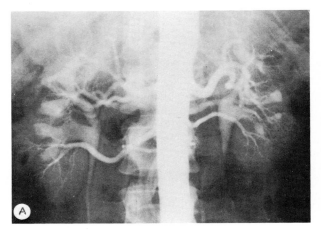 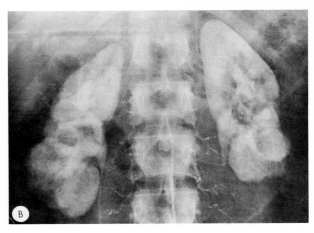

Figure 57-29. Renal infarction. This 39-year-old woman had mitral stenosis, a long history of atrial fibrillation, and multiple renal embolic episodes with recurrent bouts of flank pain and hematuria. (A) Aortogram. Double renal arteries are present bilaterally. The intrarenal branches demonstrate decreased arborization. The vessels to the midportion of the right kidney are truncated, as are those in the middle and lower portions of the left kidney. Incidentally noted is blunting of the calices bilaterally, resembling the appearance in pyelonephritis. (B) Nephrographic phase. On the left side, there are gross loss of cortex and marked irregularity in the lower part of the kidney. On the right side, similar findings are visible on the lateral aspect of the kidney and in the upper pole.

Figure 57-30. Renal embolism and infarction. Selective renal arteriography. (A) Arterial phase. Multiple emboli have occluded some of the small interlobar arteries (*arrows*). (B) Nephrographic phase. Localized areas of ischemia are visible (*arrows*) at the site of occlusion of the renal artery subserving these areas. These represent sites of infarction.

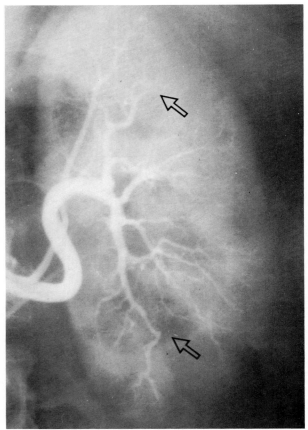 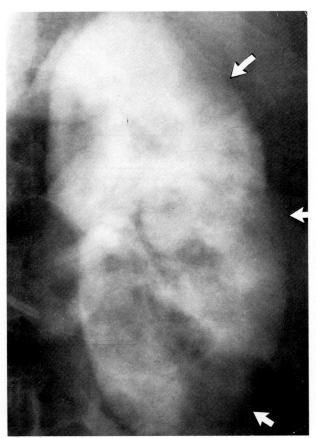

hypertension, deliberate therapeutic embolism may result in the infarction of the remaining viable tissue and so control hypertension [25, 101].

Renal Artery Aneurysm

Aneurysms of the renal artery are being diagnosed with increasing frequency as angiography becomes more widely used. The true aneurysm is defined as a localized dilatation of the renal artery retaining one or more of the original coats of the vessel wall (Figs. 57-31, 57-32). The primary pathologic process is weakening of the arterial wall due to degenerative changes particularly in the elastic tissue of the media. This weakening may be congenital, traumatic, inflammatory, or degenerative in origin; the process is accelerated by the persistence of the pulsatile arterial pressure. Aneurysms are usually unilateral but may also be found bilaterally. They can occur in chil-

dren but are most often found in patients between 50 and 70 years of age and are frequently associated with degenerative atherosclerotic disease of a generalized nature. The exception is renal artery dysplasia, in which aneurysms are frequently found in the fourth and fifth decades of life (Fig. 57-33).

Clinically, aneurysms are often asymptomatic but on occasion may cause pain and hematuria. Frequently, a wide variety of other renal pathologic changes may be present and actually may account for the pain and hematuria.

According to Boijsen and Köhler [15], hypertension was found to accompany renal aneurysms in about 15 percent of cases. Other authors have noted the presence of significant hypertension prior to death in 72 to 85 percent of patients with renal artery aneurysms [50, 67]. The hyperten-

Figure 57-32. Renal artery aneurysm. Selective right renal arteriogram. As in Figure 57-31, an aneurysm is present almost exactly at the bifurcation of the main renal artery into its dorsal and ventral branches. The patient was mildly hypertensive, and only the renal artery aneurysm was demonstrated as an abnormality in the renal vascular bed.

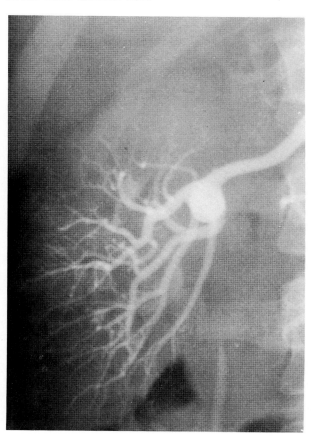

Figure 57-31. Renal artery aneurysm. Selective renal arteriography demonstrates a large localized sac filling with contrast agent just at the bifurcation of the main renal artery into dorsal and ventral renal branches (*arrow*). The patient had no evidence of a dysplastic disease of the renal arteries nor was there clinical evidence of a mycotic or a false aneurysm. It was assumed that the aneurysm was congenital.

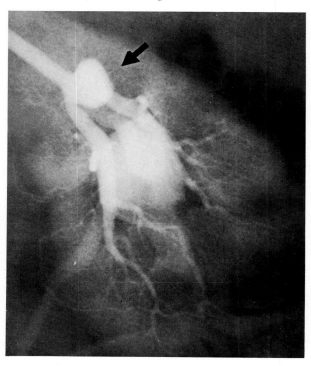

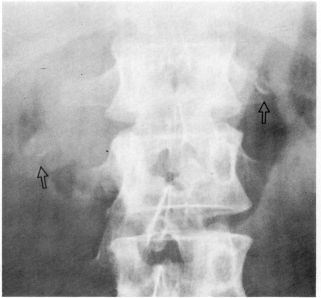

A

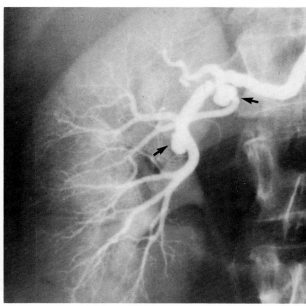

B

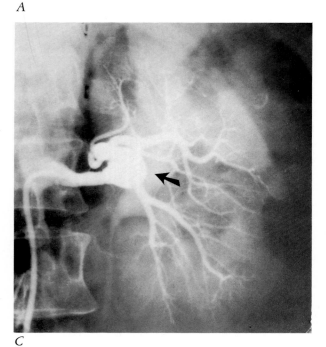

C

Figure 57-33. Renal artery aneurysm. This 47-year-old woman had hypertension of 15 years' duration. Her blood pressure was 190/130 mm Hg. An intravenous urogram was normal. (A) Plain film of the abdomen. Curvilinear calcific densities are visible in the region of the renal artery on the right and the left (*arrows*). (B) Selective renal arteriography. Renal artery dysplasia is present, with an aneurysm at the bifurcation of the main renal artery (*upper arrow*) and a second smaller aneurysm (*lower arrow*) at the division of the ventral renal arterial branch. It is this second aneurysm that is calcified. (C) Selective left renal arteriogram. A large aneurysm at the bifurcation of the left main renal artery is visible precisely at the site (*arrow*) where calcification was apparent on the plain films. On both sides there is early evidence of arteriolar nephrosclerosis, with cortical narrowing and tortuosity of the peripheral branches.

sion is presumably due to the decreased renal blood flow that may follow compression due to aneurysm. The reduction in blood flow may be segmental in location [32].

About 33 to 50 percent of renal artery aneurysms contain some calcium in their walls (Fig. 57-33), and recognition may be possible on plain radiographs of the abdomen. In general, calcified aneurysms do not tend to rupture, whereas those without calcium in their walls may

rupture spontaneously. The increased incidence of renal aneurysm rupture during pregnancy has been described by Burt et al. [23].

Angiographically, an aneurysm is either saccular (characterized by an outpouching from the artery, with an area of communication of variable width) (see Figs. 57-31–57-33) or fusiform (with circumferential and rather uniform dilatation of the arterial lumen over a variable distance). The fusiform type is more likely to be secondary to localized arteriosclerotic stenosis or renal artery dysplasia and occurs as a region of poststenotic dilatation also known as a *jet aneurysm*. The circulation time of contrast material within the aneurysm tends to be retarded, particularly in the saccular type, whereas the general circulation throughout the rest of the kidneys is normal. In some instances, however, the local circulation peripheral to an aneurysm may be markedly reduced and the peripheral vasculature rather sparse.

The association of hypertension and renal artery aneurysms has been well reviewed by Harrow and Sloane [54], Boijsen and Köhler [15], and Kincaid [67]. The best evidence suggests that cure of hypertension when aneurysms are present occurs only when renal artery stenosis and the physiologic stigmata of renovascular hypertension are present [28]. With hypertension and aneurysms but no evidence of renal ischemia, surgery is unlikely to be an effective treatment of hypertension [28].

Renal Arteriovenous Fistula

Renal arteriovenous fistulas were once believed to be rare but are now being identified with increasing frequency. They are thought to be a cause of renovascular hypertension because localized renal ischemia is produced by the "steal" of arterial blood shunted directly to the renal venous system. One of the characteristics of this lesion on physical examination is a continuous bruit over the upper abdomen. It should be noted, however, that there are numerous other causes of a continuous upper abdominal bruit.

Arteriovenous fistulas have been classified by Love [74] as:

1. Congenital fistula due to arteriovenous malformation
2. Acquired fistula
   a. Fistula following rupture of an arterial aneurysm
   b. Traumatic arteriovenous fistula resulting from penetrating trauma or trauma of the renal tissue in association with nephrolithotomy, partial nephrectomy, or percutaneous needle biopsy of the kidney
   c. Arteriovenous fistula in renal carcinoma, particularly where tumor has eroded the vein
   d. Stump fistula after nephrectomy

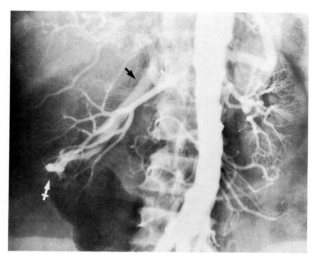

Figure 57-34. Renal arteriovenous fistula. Bolus aortogram. Simultaneous with opacification of the renal arteries is visualization of the renal vein (*black arrow*). An arteriovenous communication is readily defined in the lower pole (*white arrow*) as the source of immediate venous opacification.

Figure 57-35. Renal arteriovenous malformation. Selective right renal arteriogram. A cluster of small and large vessels in the lower pole of the right kidney is apparent (*white arrows*), with immediate venous opacification. Note that the inferior vena cava is opacified (*black arrow*).

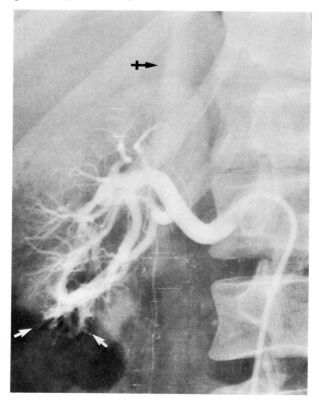

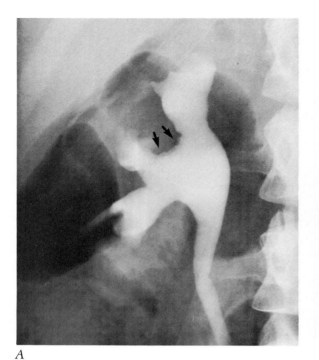

A

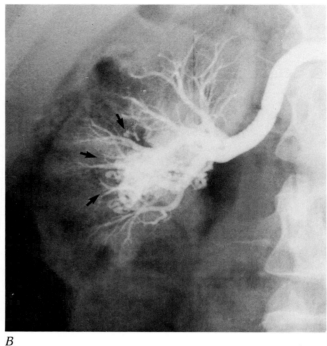

B

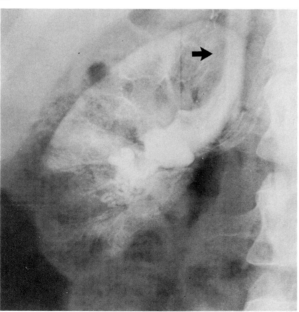

C

Figure 57-36. Renal arteriovenous fistula. The patient entered the hospital for evaluation of hematuria and hypertension. (A) Intravenous urogram. The collecting system appears normal, except for an irregular serration of the lateral aspect of the pelvis between the upper and middle pole calices (*arrows*). The appearance suggests a papillary tumor of the pelvis, extrinsic pressure on the pelvis from an intrarenal renal mass, or possibly, a vascular impression. (B) Selective renal arteriography. "Stationary waves" are visible in the distal one-third of the renal artery. A large cluster of vessels in and adjacent to the hilus of the kidney is opacified (*arrows*). (C) Nephrographic phase (4 seconds). There is early dense filling of the renal vein and the inferior vena cava (*arrow*) while some of the renal artery branches are still opacified. Note the absence of a nephrogram in the lower pole. Double renal arteries were present. The hypertension in this patient was thought to be associated with ischemia of the lower pole of the right kidney associated with the "steal" provoked by the direct arteriovenous communication.

Routine radiographic studies of the abdomen usually show no abnormalities although on occasion calcification may be visible.

The intravenous urogram may show some caliceal distortion, but differentiation from tumor or cyst is frequently impossible.

It is important to establish the diagnosis via angiography because there may eventually be cardiac complications due to hypertension or high-output cardiac failure. There is frequently physiologic evidence of increased cardiac output and blood volume and a decrease in the overall circulation time. The subject has been reviewed by Maldonado et al. [80], Boijsen and Köhler [14], and Love et al. [74].

Renal arteriovenous fistulas have been receiving increasing attention with the more widespread use of renal biopsy that has occurred in the last 15 years. Meng and Elkin demonstrated by arteriography immediately following percutaneous needle biopsy that the needle tract could be visualized, that perirenal extravasation occurred commonly, that arteriovenous communication was present in about 10 percent of patients, and that arterial occlusion, thrombus, or spasm was present in about 20 percent of patients [88]. In other series, the incidence of arteriovenous fistulas following renal biopsy has varied from 11 to 18 percent [10, 36, 71, 75]. Furthermore, in three recent papers [62, 95, 104], it has been emphasized that ablation or nephrectomy may produce cure of hypertension associated with arteriovenous fistula.

Angiographically, the renal artery and the renal vein may be normal in size or wider than normal. Rapid passage of contrast material directly from the artery to a vein can be visualized at the site of the arteriovenous communication (Figs. 57-34 to 57-36). Rapid passage of contrast material into the inferior vena cava may also be noted on serial angiographic studies (see Fig. 57-35). In cases in which the arteriovenous fistula is smaller and more localized, one may note enlargement and tortuosity or a "serpentine" appearance of the segmental arterial vessel and its branches. Vascularity of the renal parenchyma in the area adjacent to large fistulas is usually diminished. It may be difficult at times to differentiate numerous arteriovenous malformations from the arteriovenous shunts that occur in renal carcinoma, because wide, tortuous vessels and localized areas with rapid shunting to the venous system may be noted in both. In arteriovenous malformations,

there are, however, no pathologic vessels or displacement of vessels.

Angiography, therefore, is essential not only to establish the diagnosis but also to determine the location and extent of involvement. This assessment will aid in evaluating operability and planning the surgical approach.

Chronic Pyelonephritis

In mild cases of chronic pyelonephritis, no angiographic abnormality may be noted. With the destruction and subsequent fibrosis of renal tissue, the diameter of the main renal arteries tends to shrink, usually in proportion to the decrease in kidney size and function. Because the renal volume is diminished, the interlobar and arcuate vessels become crowded and tortuous (Fig. 57-37). There may be localized areas of reduced vascularity, and scar formation may so derange the vascular pattern that a mottled, irregular nephrogram is produced. The renal cortex is frequently irregular in outline, but the nephrogram may be disproportionately dense due to crowding of the vasculature secondary to a loss of interstitial renal tissue. The intrarenal vessels are small, and the cortex is thin (Fig. 57-38). Anastomoses between the parenchymal and capsular vessels may be demonstrated [20]. In addition, the renal veins may be visualized before the usual 6 to 12 seconds after contrast injection [42].

If renal size is reduced and there is atrophy of the renal artery, it may be very difficult to differentiate between chronic atrophic pyelonephritis and congenital hypoplasia of the kidney. Some authors feel that differentiation is impossible, but others conclude that in a majority of cases, small kidneys, particularly in young people, are the result of early infantile pyelonephritis and that congenital hypoplasia of the kidney is extremely rare. It is generally felt that pyelonephritis is often superimposed on congenital hypoplasia [69]. In the few cases of true congenital renal hypoplasia in which angiographic material is available, the arteries are smaller than normal, but the main vessels and branches retain the usual proportions and taper smoothly into the periphery. The flow of contrast material through the hypoplastic kidney is usually diminished, and opacification is less marked than in the normal kidney.

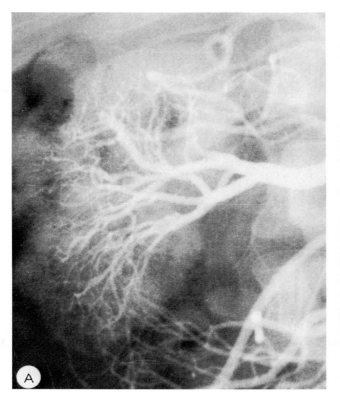

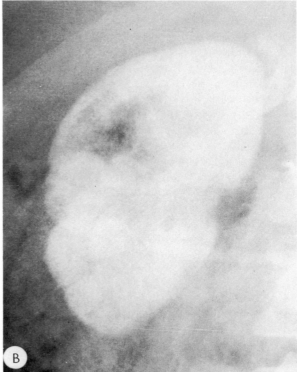

Figure 57-37. Pyelonephritis. This 31-year-old man had poor renal function and a history of pyelonephritis. (A) Renal arteriogram. The major renal artery is normal. The small branches are tortuous and irregular, and some are crowded together. Marked narrowing of the peripheral vessels is present. (B) Nephrographic phase. The kidney is small, and there is premature venous filling. The nephrogram is relatively dense but irregular. The cortex is grossly thin, particularly over the lower pole and the middle segment of the kidney laterally. The contour is deformed because of fibrosis secondary to chronic infection.

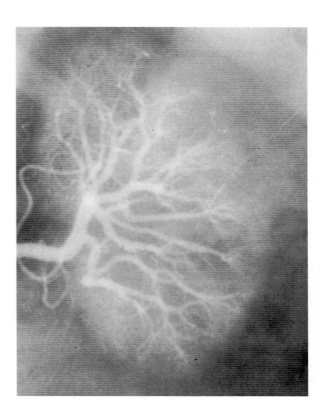

Figure 57-38. Chronic pyelonephritis. The kidney is small in association with a small main renal artery and small intrarenal branches. The arcuate vessels can be defined and reach virtually the edge of the kidney. They are moderately tortuous. There is a striking decrease in cortical tissue, which is somewhat more uniform than is usually seen in chronic pyelonephritis. The vessels are tortuous, and there are local areas of ischemia.

Chronic Glomerulonephritis

It may be difficult in the end stages to differentiate arteriolar nephrosclerosis from chronic glomerulonephritis or chronic pyelonephritis [43]. Examination of the nephrographic phase and the extent of overall involvement may be helpful. In glomerular nephritis, involvement is usually symmetrical bilaterally. There is prolonged opacification and abrupt attenuation of the larger vessels, whereas opacification of the smaller channels in the periphery may be markedly reduced. The nephrogram is usually homogeneous and relatively faint, but the cortical margin is smooth. The cortex is significantly thinned. Considerable tortuosity and irregularity of the vascular lumen are frequently important features (Fig. 57-39). In acute glomerular nephritis, the kidney, rather than being small, is frequently large, and the vessels are narrow but significantly separated from each other. At times,

Figure 57-39. Chronic glomerulonephritis. Selective renal arteriogram. The main renal artery is small. A local area of narrowing, caused by spasm, is visible near its origin. The intrarenal branches are attenuated, and there is marked tortuosity of the interlobular and arcuate vessels. The cortex is uniformly thin. The subsequent nephrographic phase was very faint, and the cortical edge appeared relatively smooth.

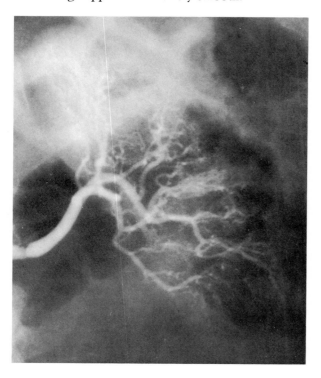

some of the vessels may appear to be crowded, depending on the degree of uniformity of disease throughout the kidney.

Extrinsic Compression of the Renal Artery

On rare occasions, the main renal artery may be compressed locally by a fibrous musculotendinous band, resulting in renal ischemia and hypertension that may be cured by appropriate surgery. This entity has been described in a small number of patients by D'Arbeau and Strickland [29], Kincaid [67], and Lampe [72]. Musculotendinous fibers of the psoas minor muscle or of the diaphragmatic crura are responsible for the renal artery compression. Compression by the crura of the diaphragm usually occurs when its insertion is abnormal and particularly when the renal artery takes off at a slightly higher position than normal. In all the cases reported to date, a normal blood pressure was restored after surgery. These lesions presumably are present from birth, with hypertension developing in adult life.

Angiographically, it may be difficult or impossible to differentiate this lesion from a localized stenosis due to an intrinsic abnormality of the renal artery. There is usually a very short segmental area of constriction near the renal artery origin, and the remaining renal vessels may be free of atheromatous disease. The bandlike area of stenosis may lie just lateral to the vertebral margin, an observation of potential diagnostic importance [109]. In some patients, the hypertension may be labile, and angiography may be required in varying positions and diaphragmatic contractions (supine and prone and with full inspiration and expiration). The effect of position and diaphragmatic contraction on the presence and degree of arterial narrowing and contrast filling of the renal vasculature can then be completely evaluated [29].

Extrinsic renal artery compression may also be produced by tumor. Lampe reported a case in which a hilar adenocarcinoma produced extrinsic pressure on the renal pedicle and impaired the renal blood flow [72]. The resulting hypertension was reversed by removal of the affected kidney. In another case, acceleration of preexisting hypertension occurred secondary to renal artery compression from a metastatic implant of a carcinoma of the colon. Other causes of pressure on the renal artery include lymphosarcoma, hydatid cysts, and abdominal aortic aneurysms.

Dissecting Aneurysm of the Renal Artery

In an analysis of the literature on primary renal artery dissecting aneurysm, Rao and Blavis found that hypertension was present in 89 percent of cases [99]. In those cases in which angiography was performed, the diagnosis was correctly made in most but not all cases. Following nephrectomy, most patients had a prompt remission of their hypertension. In one-fifth of cases, the dissection was bilateral, and as a consequence, nephrectomy was thought to be a hazardous procedure. Nevertheless, few of the lesions were suitable for revascularization. The typical appearance is demonstrated in Figure 57-40, in which the compression of the main renal artery, the intimal flap, and

the contrast material in the dissection itself are vividly demonstrated. This case also illustrates the impaired renal perfusion that may occur when dissection is present.

Probably the single most important cause of renal artery dissection is dysplastic disease of the renal artery (see Fig. 57-12) [91]. Dissection has also been reported in association with angiomatous malformation in the subadventitial layer of the renal artery [4].

Renal Trauma

Hypertension as a sequel of renal trauma, particularly of blunt trauma, has been reported [33], but the exact figures are unknown [56]. The mechanism by which hypertension results is probably varied: (1) there may be compression of the kidney by subcapsular and perirenal hematoma, with eventual fibrous thickening of the capsule; (2) thrombosis, spasm, or stenosis of

Figure 57-40. Renal artery dissection. Selective renal arteriography. (A) Early phase. There is compression of the proximal renal artery, with a curvilinear band extending across the vessel (*arrow*), representing the intima of the artery. Beyond the intimal flap, an irregular broad-based accumulation of contrast material is visible in the media, representing the dissection. Vessels to the midportion of the kidney are compressed. (B) Later phase. Contrast material persists in

the false lumen of the main renal artery for a protracted period of time. Portions of the upper pole of the kidney are well perfused, but there is virtually complete obstruction to branches to the midportion of the kidney. (Courtesy of Christos A. Athanosoulis, M.D.) In most patients, the dissection occurs in the media. The intramural hematoma collects between the media and the external elastic lamina. Renal infarction is a common accompaniment of dissection.

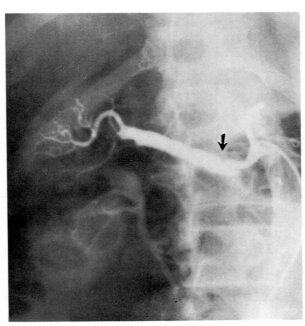

A

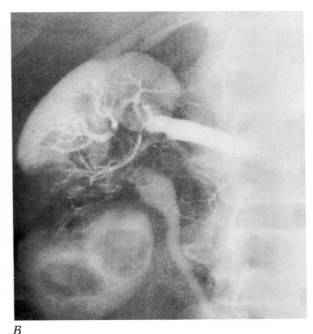

B

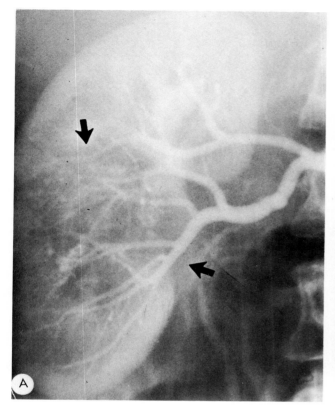

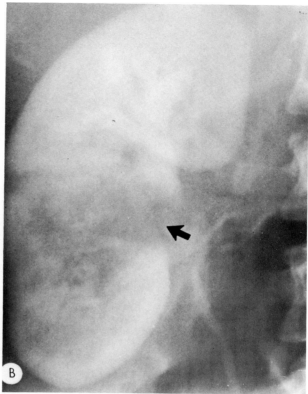

Figure 57-41. Renal trauma. This 51-year-old woman had fallen on her right flank, and pain and hematuria ensued. The plain film demonstrated a fracture of the right tenth rib and loss of the right psoas and kidney margin. The intravenous pyelogram showed poor opacification of the lower pole, with compression and distortion of the pelvis. (A) Selective renal arteriogram. The vessels are displaced around an area of intra-renal hemorrhage (*arrows*). The spotty areas of increased density may be caused by leakage of contrast material. (B) Nephrographic phase. An area of decreased opacification is visible (*arrow*). Its borders are irregular and extend to the lateral margin of the kidney. The appearance is that of a large intrarenal hemorrhage. (Courtesy of James McCort, M.D.)

the renal artery or the development of an arteriovenous aneurysm may be involved; (3) posttraumatic pyelonephritis, infection, nephrolithiasis, and stasis may occur [43]; or (4) large or small parts of the kidney parenchyma may be torn off without stopping the blood supply and thus remain vital but ischemic [96]. Retroperitoneal hematoma may produce rather localized constriction of the main renal artery with ensuing hypertension.

The history of a fall is usually elicited, and the physical examination shows flank tenderness and sometimes an obvious mass with tenderness. The kidney may suffer contusion, laceration, or rupture [41].

A plain film of the abdomen may demonstrate rib fractures, obscured renal and psoas outlines, evidence of a soft-tissue mass, and various degrees of localized and generalized ileus. The urogram generally shows a decrease in or a lack of contrast on the affected side and, possibly, extravasation. Crowding and displacement of the entire involved kidney and blood clots with filling defects in the kidney pelvis may be seen.

The renal arteriogram may disclose the following conditions [83]: (1) subcapsular hematoma (see Fig. 57-44); (2) intrarenal hematoma (Fig. 57-41); (3) rupture of the renal artery branches; (4) disrupted continuity of the renal outline, with abnormal straining of the traumatized tissue; and (5) so-called fractured kidney (Fig. 57-42). Displacement of the vessels is particularly common in the presence of intrarenal hematoma (see Fig. 57-41); the hematoma usually appears as an "avascular" site in the kidney in the absence of continued bleeding.

Posttraumatic renal vein thrombosis in association with pulmonary emboli in the nephrotic

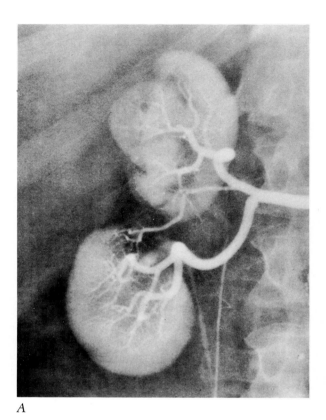

A

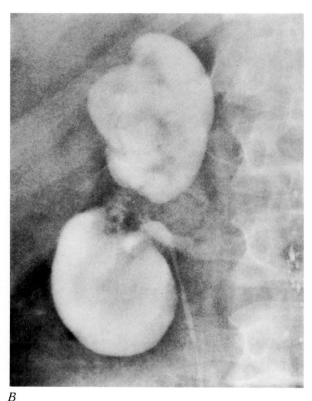

B

Figure 57-42. Renal trauma. This patient entered the hospital because of hypertension. Three years before, he had been in an automobile accident and thereafter had had a great deal of right flank pain. (A) Selective renal arteriogram. A fracture through the midportion of the right kidney is apparent. Although the visible portions of the kidney are subserved by branches of the renal arteries, there are gross distortion of the upper pole and a large area of dead tissue, which is not opacified. (B) Nephrogram. On the nephrogram, the distortion is apparent, and some areas in the midportion of the kidney, which seem lacking in vascular supply, appear to be faintly mottled, indicating that some contrast media and therefore blood are reaching this ischemic segment.

syndrome can be excluded if the renal vein is seen on the selective angiogram. Otherwise, renal venous opacification may be needed to establish this diagnosis [82].

Arteritis

Periarteritis nodosa is a relatively rare cause of renovascular hypertension, and only a few angiographic descriptions of this disease have been reported [22, 40, 51, 102]. The renal vessels are involved in about 80 percent of cases, and the pathologic lesion, a necrotizing inflammatory process, involves primarily the arterioles and the smaller intrarenal branches of the renal artery. The intravascular inflammatory process eventu-

ally results in the formation of granulation tissue and fibrosis intermingled with areas of vessel-wall destruction. Hemorrhage, thrombosis, and aneurysm formation, which is characteristic of the disease, result.

Angiographically the demonstration of multiple aneurysms in the small and medium-sized arteries is highly suggestive (Fig. 57-43), although we have seen the same appearance in lupus erythematosus. These aneurysms are most often of various sizes and shapes and are rather uniformly distributed throughout the renal parenchyma bilaterally. In addition, the medium and smaller sized intrarenal arteries may be stretched, attenuated, and diminished in number (probably as a result of thrombosis with secondary recanalization). This rather diffuse small-vessel throm-

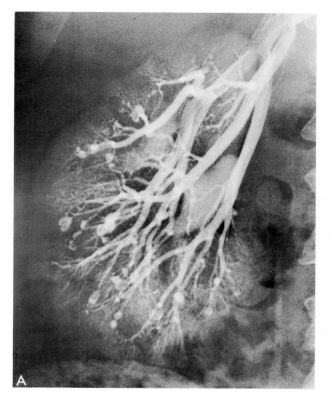

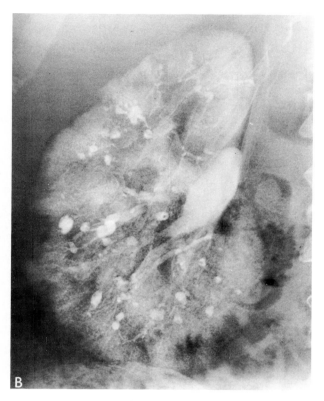

Figure 57-43. Periarteritis nodosa. The findings in the kidney are quite characteristic, with multiple renal artery aneurysms distributed throughout many segments of the kidney and affecting many branches of the renal artery. (A) Selective renal arteriogram. (B) Nephrographic phase. Note that in the nephrographic phase the aneurysms retain contrast agent and remain opacified long after the arteries have lost their contrast agent. Although this finding is characteristic of periarteritis nodosa, it has also been seen in Wegener's granulomatosis, drug-abuse patients, and disseminated lupus erythematosus. (Courtesy of Victor Millan, M.D.)

bosis results in variable degrees of cortical ischemia and in an irregular renal outline during the nephrographic phase due to scattered renal infarction (Fig. 57-43B). Abdominal aortography may also reveal numerous small aneurysms in the splenic, hepatic, and other visceral vessels.

There are numerous types of vasculitis in which the renal vascular bed may be involved [24, 51]. Drug abuse, ergot, and serum sickness may all produce similar blood vessel abnormalities in the kidney.

Wegener's granulomatosis is associated with a destructive arteritis of blood vessels and with granuloma formation. When it involves the kidney, it usually produces a focal necrotizing glomerulonephritis, with uncommon involvement of the large arteries [100]. At times, however, it may produce disruption of the arterial wall and pseudoaneurysms (Fig. 57-44). Intrarenal or subcapsular hematomas may then develop, and hypertension may be due to the presence of a "Page" kidney, with constriction and compression of the renal parenchyma [84].

Arteritis may also affect multiple vessels and produce an appearance in the renal arteries that is similar to that in renal artery dysplasia (Fig. 57-45). Together with aneurysm formation due to destruction of the media, fibrosis and cicatrix develop, and there may be profound narrowing or vascular occlusion as a result. The disease is similar to Takayasu's disease and to giant cell aortitis and arteritis of the Bantu type. Aside from the renal arteries, the aorta may be involved, as well as the celiac artery (Fig. 57-45B), the superior mesenteric artery, and many other aortic branches.

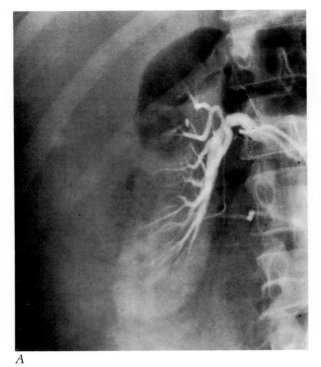

A

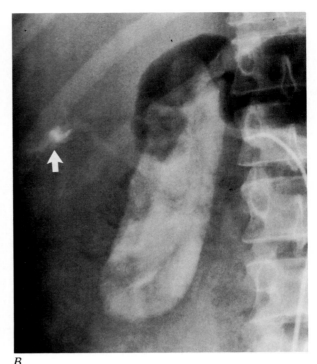

B

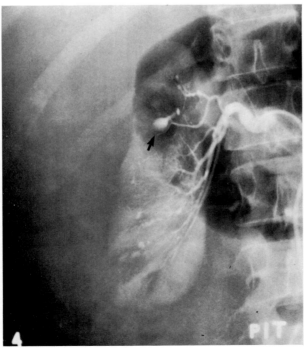

C

Figure 57-44. Wegener's granulomatosis. Involvement of the renal vessels. The patient entered with pain in the right flank and a falling hematocrit. Urography suggested the presence of a mass at the lateral aspect of the right kidney. (A) Selective renal arteriogram. There is obvious compression of the intrarenal vessels, which fill poorly. The kidney appears to be displaced medially by a large mass that extends to the lateral abdominal wall. (B) Nephrogram. The distorted appearance of the lateral aspect of the right kidney is clearly related to compression by a large collection of subcapsular fluid. Contrast agent has extravasated in a small tract into the center of the subcapsular hematoma (*arrow*). (C) Arteriogram following the administration of pitressin. The pitressin has produced narrowing of virtually all the intrarenal arterial branches. At the same time, local areas of extravasation are now delineated far better than on the conventional arteriogram, and there is a well-defined pseudoaneurysm in the upper portion of the kidney (*arrow*).

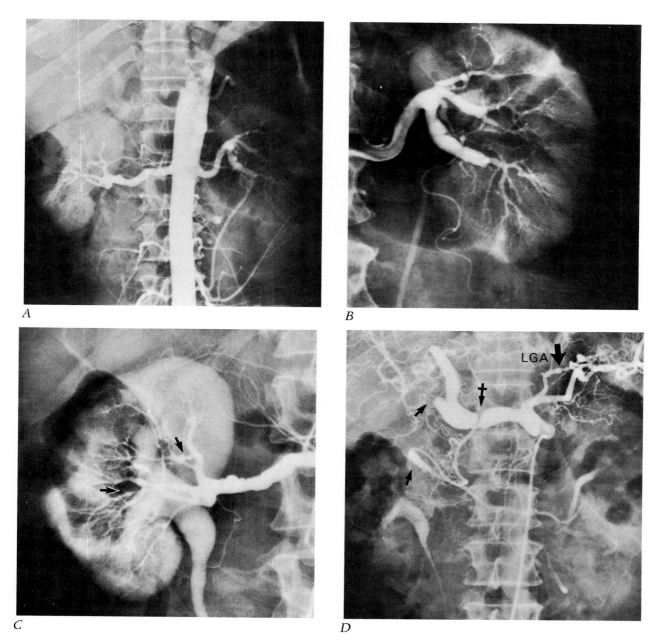

Figure 57-45. Arteritis involving the renal arteries and multiple other vessels. (A) Bolus arteriogram. Irregularity of the right main renal artery and its branches, together with localized areas of dilatation of the ventral branch of the left renal artery, is apparent. (B) Selective left renal arteriogram. Both main branches of the left renal artery at the hilus demonstrate localized areas of narrowing and dilatation and wall irregularity. (C) Selective right renal arteriogram. The appearance of the main renal artery resembles the appearance in renal artery dysplasia, with extension into multiple intrarenal arterial branches of localized areas of narrowing and dilatation (*arrows*). (D) Celiac arteriogram. There is a striking degree of stenosis in the common hepatic artery (*barred arrow*). In addition, areas of narrowing and dilatation (*arrow*) are visible in the left gastric artery (*LGA*) and the right gastroepiploic artery (*arrows*). Complete occlusion of a branch of the right hepatic artery is apparent. (Courtesy of R. Freeman, M.D.)

Unilateral Irradiation Damage

The deleterious effect of x-irradiation on the vascular system is well known and has been summarized by Asscher [8]. Crummy reported a case of unilateral irradiation damage that resulted in hypertension 24 years later and that was relieved by nephrectomy [27]. The average dose to the left kidney was 3,900 rems, and to the right kidney, 2,300 rems. The intravenous pyelogram failed to show any function on the left. Arteriography demonstrated a rapid tapering of arteries after a normal-sized origin on the left. Microscopically the left kidney showed postirradiation damage. After surgery, the patient's blood pressure fell gradually to normotensive levels.

The production of renal artery stenosis by irradiation has also been reported in man [44]. This phenomenon is understandable in view of the arterial damage previously reported, including thickening of the vascular wall, and damage with consequent fibrosis in the intima, media, and adventitia [107, 110].

A more recent report described a 12-year-old girl with renin-dependent hypertension and stenosis of the proximal right renal artery. After an end-to-side renal artery–aortic anastomosis, her blood pressure was normalized. The stenosis was thought to be caused by irradiation therapy administered at 7 months of age after left nephrectomy for Wilms' tumor. The right kidney was shielded when the radiation dose to the abdomen reached 2,200 rems. The authors note that while there have been numerous reports of large arteries injured after irradiation therapy, in only 2 of 24 cases were the renal arteries involved.

Other Renal Causes of Hypertension

The following factors have been discussed in association with renal hypertension:

(1) Oral contraceptives. A case report of hypertension thought to be caused by oral contraceptives described occlusion of two renal arteries on the right side as well as other arterial occlusions. No embolic source was discovered, and the hypertension was cured by nephrectomy [30].

(2) Umbilical artery catheterization. In six neonates with hypertension and elevated peripheral renin levels, renal artery stenosis or occlusion was shown in all. All these patients had had umbilical artery catheterization because of respiratory distress [90]. They became normotensive on conservative therapy.

(3) Dissecting aortic aneurysm repair. Although it is well known that acute hypertension may accompany dissection with compromise of the renal blood flow, a recent report describes surgical repair of a type 1 dissection in which hypertension developed with demonstrated stenosis of the left renal artery and a small left kidney. The surgical repair of the aneurysm had established a compromised flow through the left renal artery that had resulted in hypertension whereas a complete absence of blood flow before repair was consistent with normotension. Gelfoam embolization of both branches of the left renal artery was associated with the recovery of normal blood pressure [103].

(4) Solitary cyst. Most patients with solitary cysts are asymptomatic. Rarely, a large renal cyst may produce unilaterally increased plasma renin activity with elevation of the blood pressure. In one recent report, a patient was described in whom hypertension and a cyst coexisted, with left renal vein renin activity four times as high as that of the right. Aspiration of the cyst was accompanied by a return to normal blood pressure. Subsequently, a reaccumulation of fluid in the cyst was associated with hypertension. When the cyst was evacuated percutaneously a second time, the patient became normotensive [81].

(5) Polycystic disease. Hypertension is an important and known concomitant of adult polycystic disease. In relatively few patients has there been documentation of elevation of renin levels although the mechanism is thought to be ischemia due to compression by the multiple cysts [55].

(6) Renal cell carcinoma. Hypertension is found in a significant percentage of patients with renal tumors, including both renal cell carcinoma and Wilms' tumor. The mechanism in some patients is thought to be renal artery compression, in others arteriovenous shunting, and in rare cases actual release of renin from the tumor [26]. The hypertension may be the symptom that brings the patient to clinical attention [1].

(7) Page kidney. It has been shown that external renal compression may produce hypertension in the laboratory animal as well as in humans. Within recent years, a number of patients have been described in whom there was an apparent

causal relationship between hypertension and subcapsular hematomas with compression of renal parenchyma both by the hematoma and by the thickened capsule and subcapsular scar. Evacuation of the hematoma in one patient and nephrectomy in another patient were accompanied by cure of the hypertension [84].

(8) Other causes of renal hypertension that are relatively less common include hydronephrosis, renal tuberculosis, xanthogranulomatous polynephritis, and renal vein thrombosis.

Collateral Circulation in Renal Ischemia

Some years ago, we undertook a study of the collateral channels in 24 patients with renal artery stenosis [2] that is the basis for the discussion that follows.

The origin and termination of the collateral channels were found to be as indicated in Table 57-1. The first three lumbar arteries were the most common source of the collateral vessels to the ischemic kidney. Flow from the contralateral side was never demonstrated. The branches from the lumber arteries coiled in wormlike fashion and entered the peripelvic (Figs. 57-46A, 57-47A, 57-48C, 57-49B, 57-50B), periureteric (see Figs. 57-46B, 57-47A, 57-48D, 57-49C), or capsular branches of the kidney (see Figs. 57-46,

57-47). Most often, they communicated with the plexus of peripelvic vessels, but there were many capsular and periureteric anastomoses as well. Although the first, second, and third lumbar arteries communicated with both the superior and inferior capsular branches, the fourth lumbar artery branches were directed only to the inferior capsular collateral vessels. The course of these vessels was sometimes labyrinthine, but flow into the intrarenal branches could be demonstrated during the later phases of the examination in many cases.

Vessels arising directly from the aorta and communicating with the peripelvic or periureteric channels were often observed (see Fig. 57-47). Branches from the most proximal portion of the capsular artery, particularly the superior capsular vessel shortly after its origin from the renal artery, connected directly with peripelvic vessels and also bridged the gap to the main renal artery distal to the stenosis in five instances (Fig. 57-51). The inferior adrenal artery filled the capsular vessels and the peripelvic vessels in a significant number of cases (see Fig. 57-46). Collateral channels arising from the intercostal arteries, communicating with the capsular branches of the kidney (see Fig. 57-47), were also observed. The major flow to the periureteric circulation arose from the hypogastric artery in seven instances and ascended from the pelvis into the paraspinal area (see Fig. 57-48D). In some instances, the testicular or the ovarian artery was also a major source of collat-

Table 57-1. Origins and Communications of Collateral Vessels in 24 Cases with Renal Artery Stenosis or Occlusion

| Origin of Collaterals | Vessels Supplied | | | | | |
| | Capsular Arteries | | | | | |
	Superior	Inferior	Lateral	Peripelvic	Periureteric	Total
1st lumbar artery	2	2	2	6	—	12
2nd lumbar artery	4	1	—	5	4	14
3rd lumbar artery	4	3	—	6	6	19
4th lumbar artery	—	5	—	—	5	10
Aorta	—	—	—	7	3	10
Internal iliac artery	—	2	1	—	7	10
Testicular or ovarian artery	—	—	—	2	3	5
Intercostal artery	1	—	2	—	—	3
Inferior adrenal artery	3	—	3	4	—	10
Total	14	13	8	30	28	

From Abrams and Cornell [2]. Reproduced with permission from *Radiology*.

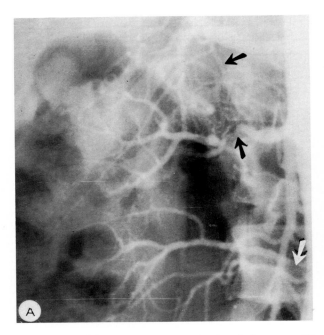

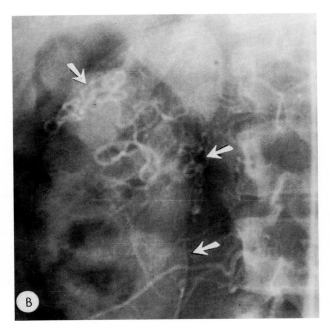

Figure 57-46. Renal collateral circulation. A 23-year-old woman with hypertension of 1 year's duration (blood pressure of 240/160 mm Hg). (A) Renal arteriogram at 1.5 seconds. There are profound narrowing of the main renal artery (*middle arrow*) and stenosis of the supplementary artery to the lower pole (*lower arrow*). The inferior adrenal branch, arising from the main renal artery, is opacified (*upper arrow*). (B) At 4 seconds, a periureteric collateral vessel fills from the internal iliac artery and anastomoses with peripelvic collateral vessels (*medial arrows*). The capsular collateral vessels that filled in part from the inferior adrenal artery (*lateral arrow*) empty into tortuous vessels that cross the midportion of the kidney.

eral flow to the periureteric channels and the capsular arteries (see Fig. 57-50).

The width and length of many of the collateral channels was striking. In a number of instances, segmental occlusion had occurred, and the intrarenal branches to a particular part of the kidney that had failed to fill initially were opacified late in the study from the collateral circulation (see Fig. 57-48).

Figure 57-52 is a diagrammatic sketch of the total collateral renal blood flow in man. Both Table 57-1 and Figure 57-52 fail to include the bridging collateral vessels direct from the proximal to the distal main renal artery. The proximal renal artery was also an occasional source of direct peripelvic collateral vessels. The stenosis was located in the middle third of the main renal artery in two-thirds of these patients.

The literature on the collateral circulation of the kidney is remarkably sparse, even though in 1906, ligation of the renal artery was found to be compatible with life in the dog if the renal capsule had previously been removed [85]. In 1940 Mason et al., in the course of experiments on hypertension in dogs, discovered a large

periureteric branch of the ovarian artery that supplied the kidney in one animal [86]. The renal artery had been completely occluded. Flasher et al., in a study of renal collateral blood flow in rabbits, emphasized that the collateral vessels represented dilatation of preexisting, nonfunctioning channels and that the initiation of collateral flow was related to the presence of renal ischemia [39]. Klapproth's morphologic study of the canine renal arterial circulation indicated that the ovarian and uterine arteries were the most frequent sources of collateral vessels and that the smaller branches came from the diaphragmatic, perirenal, and adrenal arteries [70]. More recently, attention has been focused on the periureteric collateral vessels because of the scalloped imprint that they produce on the ureter [9, 20, 52, 108, 111].

The vessels in man that supply the renal collateral vessels are largely the lumbar, internal iliac, testicular or ovarian, inferior adrenal, renal capsular, and intercostal arteries, as well as the aorta itself. Of all these vessels, the third lumbar artery is the commonest source of anastomotic flow to the kidney. Although it seems reasonable that the

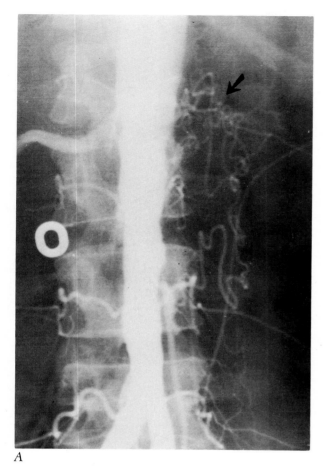

A

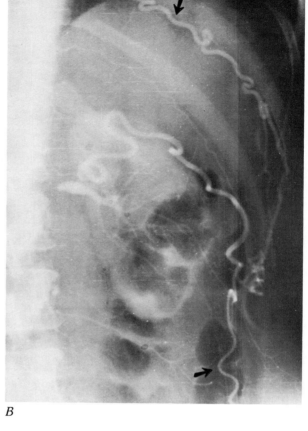

B

Figure 57-47. Renal collateral circulation. This 37-year-old woman had known hypertension for 3 years (blood pressure of 260/150 mm Hg). (A) Renal arteriogram 2 seconds after injection. There is complete occlusion of the left renal artery due to arteriosclerotic disease (*arrow*). Peripelvic and periureteric collateral vessels arise directly from the aorta, the adrenal artery, and the lumbar vessels. (B) At 18 seconds after injection. A tortuous collateral artery along the left flank (*lower arrow*) is visible anastomosing with a branch of the tenth intercostal artery (*upper arrow*). These two vessels join the dilated superior capsular artery and drain in a retrograde direction into the renal artery, which is reconstituted 1 cm to the left of the spine. A left nephrectomy was followed by profound lowering of the blood pressure but not to completely normal levels.

connections between the lumbar arteries and the renal circulation represent pathways already present but hitherto functionless, these anastomoses have not been demonstrated in postmortem injections in man in the absence of renal ischemia. Nevertheless, it is difficult to conceive of the development of such a multiplicity of vessels de novo.

The collateral channels are coiled, tortuous, and enormously lengthened in comparison with the normal. They are also conspicuously dilated. Although it is relatively easy to understand why thin-walled venous channels become grossly dis-

tended, as in the collateral system in portal hypertension or superficial leg varices, it is somewhat more difficult to explain why all collateral arterial beds have the serpiginous and characteristically elongated appearance so well demonstrated in coarctation of the aorta. The relatively thick-walled arteries should be able to distend without elongating but obviously do not. Instead, a striking increase in length is denoted by the multiple coils that are visible (see Fig. 57-51A). Because blood flow through an arterial collateral bed always requires, at some point in the delivery system, the reversal of the normal

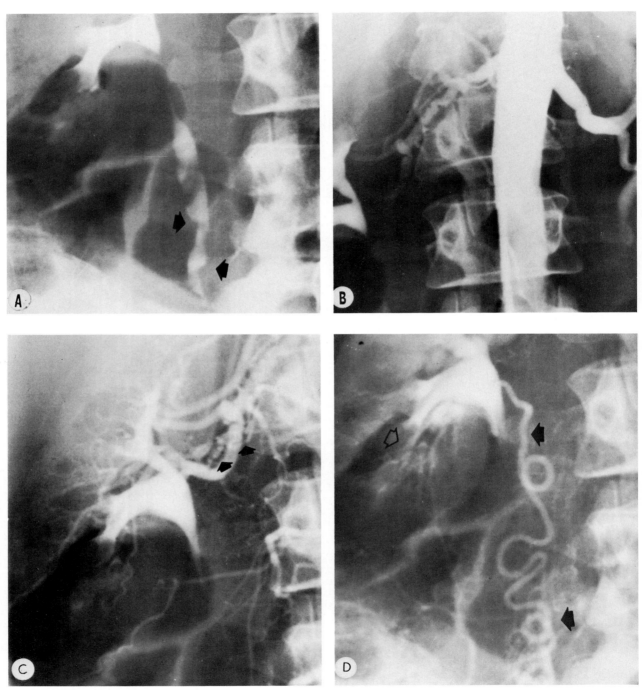

Figure 57-48. Renal artery dysplasia. Perimedial fibroplasia with florid renal collateral circulation. This 43-year-old woman had hypertension of 4 years' duration (blood pressure of 210/120 mm Hg). (A) Intravenous urogram. There are hyperconcentration and gross scalloping of the ureter (*arrows*). (B) Renal arteriogram, 0.5 second after injection. Both renal arteries show irregular narrowing, much more extensive on the right. (C) At 2 seconds, tortuous peripelvic collateral vessels are visible (*arrows*). No arterial branches are visible in the lower pole. (D) At 5 seconds, a dilated periureteric vessel (*black arrows*) is visible ascending in tortuous fashion and communicating with lower polar branches (*open arrow*). It impinges on the pelvis and the ureter, causing the shallow notching seen in (A). The pathologic lesion is perimedial fibroplasia.

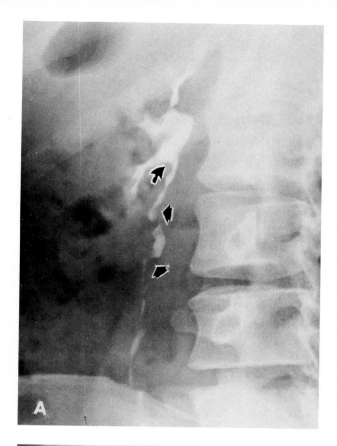

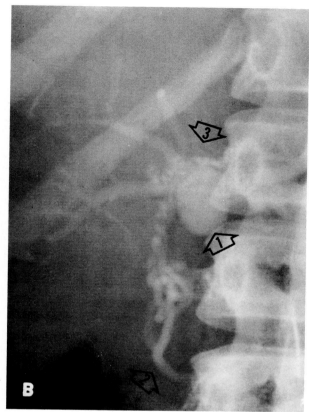

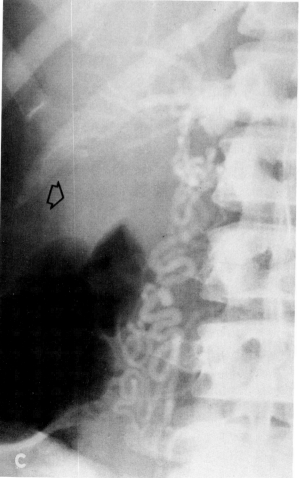

Figure 57-49. The collateral circulation in a renal artery aneurysm. A 24-year-old woman with known hypertension for 6 years (blood pressure of 160/110 mm Hg). (A) Intravenous urogram. An oblique 20-minute film shows extensive ureteral notching (*lower arrows*). A small notch in the caudal aspect of the renal pelvis is also seen (*upper arrow*). (B) Renal arteriogram, 1.5 seconds after injection. A large aneurysm of the right renal artery is opacified (*1*). A large collateral trunk arising from the aorta feeds the upper periureteric complex (*2*). A small branch of the proximal renal artery (*3*) gives rise to peripelvic collateral vessels. (C) Five-second film. Many tortuous, dilated periureteric collateral vessels arise from the lumbar and ovarian arteries. No lower pole intrarenal vessels are visible (*arrow*). These vessels filled later via a retrograde flow from the periureteric collateral chain. (From Abrams and Cornell [2]. Reproduced with permission from *Radiology.*)

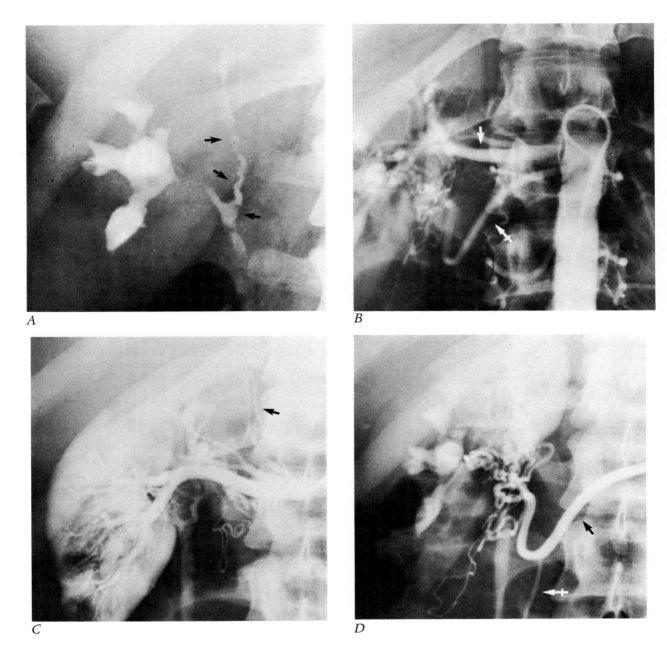

A   *B*   *C*   *D*

Figure 57-50. Renal collateral circulation. This young man entered the hospital becaue of hypertension. (A) Intravenous urogram. A bifid renal pelvis is present, with gross irregularity and notching of the pelvis to the upper pole of the kidney (*two upper arrows*) but notching as well of the renal pelvis (*lower arrow*). (B) Bolus aortogram. The main renal artery is visualized (*upper arrow*), and caudal to it a vessel of relatively large size is also opacified (*lower arrow*). Multiple peripelvic collateral vessels are visualized. (C) Selective right renal arteriogram. A normal distribution of vessels to the lower and midportions of the kidney is apparent, with a striking absence of branches to the upper pole. The adrenal-capsular branches are well visualized (*arrow*). Tortuous collateral vessels are seen adjacent to the spine. (D) Injection of the large caudally located arterial trunk to the kidney demonstrates that it is in fact the proximal portion of the gonadal artery (*black arrow*). This vessel supplies virtually all the blood to the upper pole of the kidney, produces a dense nephrogram, and is accompanied by multiple small collateral channels. Note that the normal gonadal artery (*white arrow*) extends caudally into the pelvis.

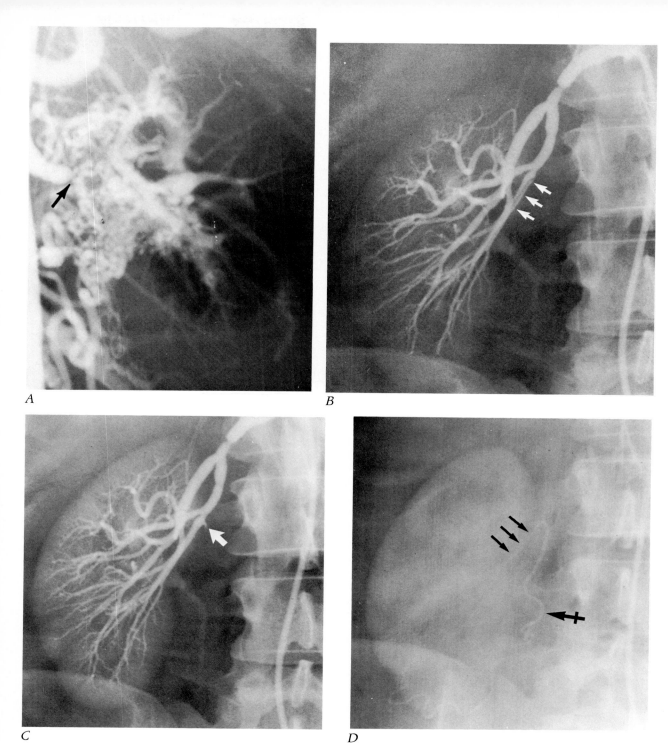

A

B

C

D

Figure 57-51. Renal collateral circulation. (A) This 20-year-old woman was studied because of hypertension. Arteriography demonstrates irregularity of the proximal renal artery, due to perimedial fibroplasia, with complete occlusion of the artery (*arrow*). An enormous cluster of peripelvic and periureteric collateral channels is opacified. The collateral pathways have carried the contrast agent into the renal artery beyond the area of occlusion so that the intrarenal branches are opacified. The appearance resembles that in an arteriogram. (B, C, and D) Reversal of the flow in a collateral channel. Medial hyperplasia. (B) A localized zone of narrowing produced by medial (fibromuscular) hyperplasia is visible in the right renal artery. In addition, a linear lucent band (*arrows*) is seen in a dorsal branch to the lower pole. This represents nonopaque blood entering the branch beyond the stenotic zone because of lower pressure. (C) With injection pressure at its height, the communication is revealed by contrast at its insertion (*arrow*), and a "dilution" defect is no longer apparent. (D) Late phase of an aortogram. A periureteric vessel (*lower arrow*), filling retrogradely, supplies the collateral branch visible in (B) and (C), after turning in a caudal direction (*three upper arrows*). **1289**

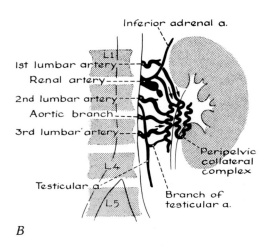

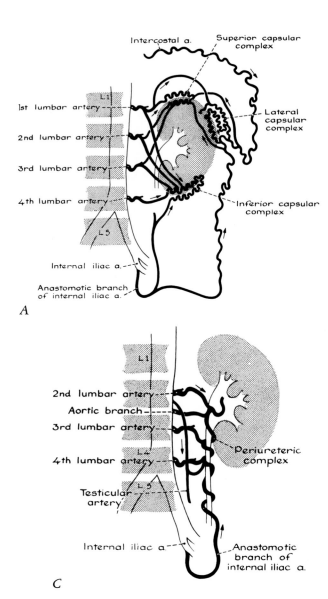

Figure 57-52. Diagrams of renal collateral circulation. (A) The capsular system. The first four lumbar arteries, branches of the internal iliac and the intercostal arteries, contribute significantly to the capsular complex. In addition (not pictured here), the inferior adrenal and capsular branches proximal to the stenosis also make major contributions. Note that a separate lateral capsular complex has been indicated; it represents a continuation of the superior capsular system but has been designated *lateral* because of its location and mode of filling. (B) The peripelvic system. The aorta, inferior adrenal, first three lumbar, and testicular (or ovarian) arteries each supplies branches to the peripelvic system. Other important pathways are the direct capsular branches from the renal artery proximal to the stenosis. (C) The periureteric system. The internal iliac artery is the single most common source of periureteric collateral vessels. The second, third, and fourth lumbar branches, the testicular branches, and the direct aortic branches are also large and important components of this collateral pathway.

direction, it is possible that retrograde flow itself may partially account for the elongation of the collateral vascular channels.

A developed collateral circulation on angiography implies a significant arterial lesion although significant stenosis need not be accompanied by visible collateral vessels [2]. Pharmacoangiographic methods have been employed and advocated for defining collateral vessels more frequently [21]. Epinephrine diminishes pressure gradients by producing distal vasoconstrictions; collateral flow is thus reduced, and the angio-

graphic injection may then opacify collateral vessels not previously visible by retrograde flow. Conversely, the vasodilatation produced by such drugs as acetylcholine augments the gradient, increases collateral flow, reduces retrograde collateral visualization during angiography, and may afford demonstration of nonopaque streams produced by collateral filling (see Fig. 57-51B–D) [21].

Sometimes a collateral circulation may develop that is sufficient to reduce renal ischemia, with a striking remission of hypertension in the presence of complete renal artery occlusion [31].

Angiography Following Surgery in Renovascular Hypertension

More often than not, angiography is performed in the postsurgical patient with renal artery stenosis because hypertension either has persisted, or, having responded to surgery, has recurred. It is not surprising, therefore, that in a large number of patients, changes are observed in the grafts. Ekelund et al. studied the postoperative appearance in 128 patients and found that with saphenous-vein bypass grafts there were 30 dilated grafts, 29 stenoses, 9 occlusions, 2 aneurysms, and 2 infarctions. When repeat angiograms were performed on patients with dilatation, progressive enlargement was usually found [10, 34].

In 19 patients with Dacron grafts, there were no abnormalities in 9, stenosis of the distal anastomosis in 6, and total occlusion in 4. In 13 patients with endarterectomies, 11 appeared normal, and there were stenosis in 1 and dilatation in another [34].

In one study, the postsurgical results in 35 pa-

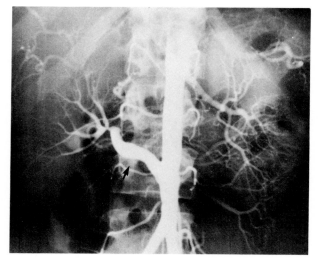

Figure 57-54. Renal artery bypass. Contrast material fills the intrarenal vessels, but there is stenosis at the site of anastomosis with the renal artery (*arrow*). Blood flow to the kidney is diminished, and the intrarenal branches are small.

Figure 57-53. Renal artery bypass in renal artery stenosis. The bypass (*arrow*) is functioning well, with a good-sized kidney, large intrarenal interlobar vessels, and excellent filling of the cortex. Note the widespread disease of the right main renal artery and some of the branches.

Figure 57-55. Bilateral renal artery bypass (*arrows*). Teflon prostheses are functioning very well to provide blood supply to the kidneys in the presence of bilateral renal artery stenosis.

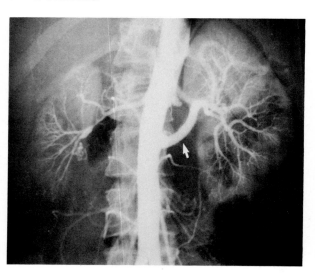

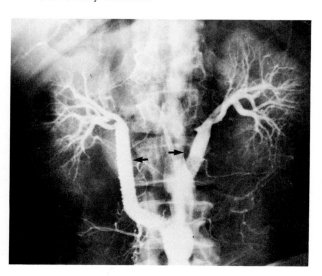

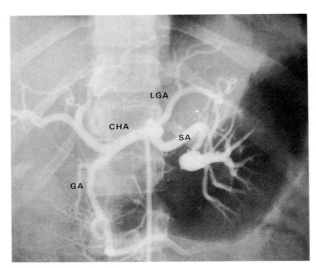

Figure 57-56. Renal artery stenosis after a splenic renal artery anastomosis. The catheter is in the celiac artery. The splenic artery (*SA*) has been anastomosed to the left renal artery beyond the area of renal artery occlusion. Although there is narrowing of the anastomotic site, good filling of the intrarenal arterial branches is demonstrated. Note the usual trifurcation of the celiac artery into the common hepatic artery (*CHA*) (with the gastroduodenal artery (*GA*) arising from it), the left gastric artery (*LGA*), and the splenic artery (*SA*).

tients with complete occlusion of the main renal artery were analyzed. Among these, nephrectomy was required in 14, and there were two deaths; in the remainder, the hypertension disappeared or improved. Follow-up studies in 20 patients showed continued patency of all revascularizations [73].

The ideal result is a widely patent graft or prosthesis that fully perfuses the kidney (Fig. 57-53). Unfortunately, even when the saphenous-vein graft is dilated, stenosis may be present at the anastomotic junction with the renal artery (Fig. 57-54). Occasionally bilateral renal artery stenosis requires bypass grafting with Teflon prostheses (Fig. 57-55). An alternative approach is to anastomose the splenic artery to the obstructed renal artery (Fig. 57-56). With vein grafts, stenosis need not occur at the anastomotic site itself, but may actually develop within the body of the vein (Fig. 57-57). Multiple projections and selective studies may be required before the anatomy can be unfolded completely, as is well illustrated in Figure 57-57, in which it is shown that 9 months after the initial study not only had the major visualized stenosis in the body of the vein graft become more profound but also there was a distal stenosing lesion at the site of

Figure 57-57. Arteriosclerotic occlusion of the renal artery. Vein bypass. (A) Aortogram, February, 1969. The renal artery on the right is occluded. The bypass extends from the level of the third lumbar vertebra to the dilated main renal artery. An area of narrowing is visible in the bypass (*arrow*). (B) Selective renal arteriogram, November, 1969. Stenosis of the bypass

adjacent to the aorta (*medial arrow*) and at the anastomosis with the renal artery (*lateral arrow*) is now visible. The distal stenosis was obscured in the aortographic study of February, 1969. The patient's hypertension responded well to surgery initially but then recurred later, probably in association with the narrowing of the saphenous-vein bypass.

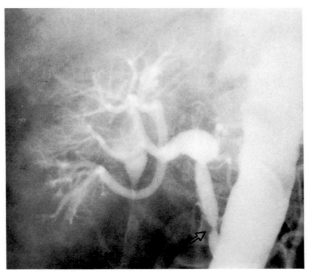

A

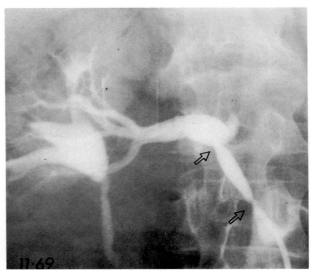

B

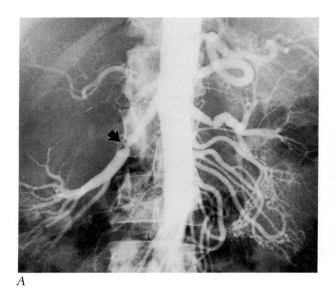

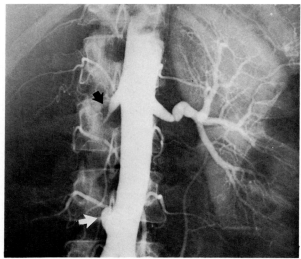

A

B

Figure 57-58. Renal artery vein bypass with subsequent occlusion of the renal artery and the bypass. (A) Aortogram. Bilateral renal artery dysplasia is visible, with involvement of both main renal arteries by perimedial fibroplasia. There is marked stenosis of the right renal artery (*arrow*). (B) Aortogram, 4 months after surgery. Venous bypass surgery was done in order to increase the renal blood flow. The bypass is occluded (*lower arrow*), and the main renal artery has now developed complete occlusion as well (*upper arrow*). Occlusion of the native circulation following bypass surgery may occur, with dominant flow moving through the bypass and with thrombosis of the aortic artery.

the saphenous-vein anastomosis to the renal artery. If thrombosis occurs after vein bypass, the native circulation may become occluded (Fig. 57-58), so that the patient may end up with a total absence of perfusion where it had been only diminished.

Finally, it should be emphasized that even in patients who have had renal artery reconstructive surgery with persistent improvement, restenosis or new lesions in the involved kidney may develop [37].

Interventional Radiology in Hypertension

Because the angiographic catheter has become so important a part of medical diagnosis, its application to medical therapy has been an expected advance, one that has developed over the past 15 to 20 years. Thus transcatheter thromboembolectomy with aspiration of emboli has been employed to treat acute renal artery obstruction, with successful application to uncontrollable hypertension [93].

Similarly, because surgical revascularization is a major operation with significant morbidity and mortality, it was natural that percutaneous transluminal angioplasty would be extended to the renal vascular bed [49, 64, 79, 92]. As described in Chapter 90, the results have been highly encouraging. Embolization of the kidneys in patients with uncontrollable hypertension has been used successfully although the experience is limited [5].

Because it is possible to occlude arteriovenous fistulas using such materials as cyanoacrylate [66], some patients with hypertension associated with renal arteriovenous fistulas may be treated by this nonsurgical method in the future.

ACKNOWLEDGMENTS

Some of the illustrations in this chapter are reproduced from H. L. Abrams, W. H. Marshall, and E. A. Kupric, The renal vascular bed in hypertension. *Semin. Roentgenol.* 2:157, 1967, by permission of the authors and publisher.

References

1. Abrams, H. L.   Renal tumor versus renal cyst. I and II. *Cardiovasc. Radiol.* 1:125, 1978.

2. Abrams, H. L., and Cornell, S. H.   Patterns of collateral flow in renal ischemia. *Radiology* 84:1001, 1965.

3. Abrams, H. L., Marshall, W. H., and Kupic, E. A.   The renal vascular bed in hypertension. *Semin. Roentgenol.* 2:157, 1967.

4. Acconcia, A., and Manganelli, A.   Dissecting aneurysm of renal artery owing to subadventitial angioma. *J. Urol.* 119:268, 1978.

5. Adler, J., Einhorn, R., McCarthy, J., Goodman, A., Solangi, K., Varanasi, U., and Thelmo, W.   Gelfoam embolization of the kidneys for treatment of malignant hypertension. *Radiology* 128:45, 1978.

6. Alvestrand, A., Bergstrom, J., and Wehle, B.   Pheochromocytoma and renovascular hypertension. A case report and review of the literature. *Acta Med. Scand.* 202:231, 1977.

7. Amsterdam, E. A., Couch, N. P., Christlieb, A. R., Harrison, J. H., Crane, C. H., Dobrzinsky, S. J., and Hickler, R. B.   Renal vein renin activity in the prognosis of surgery for renovascular hypertension. *Am. J. Med.* 47:860, 1969.

8. Asscher, A. W.   The delayed effects of renal irradiation. *Clin. Radiol.* 15:320, 1964.

9. Aurell, M.   Fibromuscular dysplasia of the renal arteries. *Br. Med. J.* 1:1180, 1979.

10. Bennett, A. R., and Wiener, S. N.   Intrarenal arteriovenous fistula and aneurysm. *AJR* 95:372, 1975.

11. Berlin, L., and Waldman, I.   "Scalloping" of the ureter: A urographic sign of renal artery disease. *J.A.M.A.* 187:680, 1964.

12. Black, H. R., Glickman, M. G., Schiff, M., Jr., and Pingoud, E. G.   Renovascular hypertension: Pathophysiology, diagnosis, and treatment. *Yale J. Bio. Med.* 51:635, 1978.

13. Boijsen, E.   Angiographic studies of the anatomy of single and multiple renal arteries. *Acta Radiol. [Suppl.]* (Stockh.) 183:1959.

14. Boijsen, E., and Köhler, R.   Renal arteriovenous fistulae. *Acta Radiol.* (Stockh.) 57:433, 1962.

15. Boijsen, E., and Köhler, R.   Renal artery aneurysms. *Acta Radiol. [Diagn.]* (Stockh.) 1:1077, 1963.

16. Bookstein, J. J.   Appraisal of arteriography in estimating the hemodynamic significance of renal artery stenoses. *Invest. Radiol.* 1:281, 1966.

17. Bookstein, J. J., Abrams, H. L., Buenger, R. E., Lecky, J., Franklin, S. S., Reiss, M. D., Bleifer, K. H., Klatte, E. C., Varady, P. D., and Maxwell, M. H.   Radiologic aspects of renovascular hypertension: II. The role of urography in unilateral renovascular disease. *J.A.M.A.* 220:1225, 1972.

18. Bookstein, J. J., Abrams, H. L., Buenger, R. E., Reiss, M. D., Lecky, J., Franklin, S. S., Bleifer, K. H., Varady, M. S., and Maxwell, M. H.   Radiologic aspects of renovascular hypertension: III. Appraisal of arteriography. *J.A.M.A.* 221:368, 1972.

19. Bookstein, J. J., and Clark, R.   *Renal Microvascular Disease.* Boston: Little, Brown, 1980.

20. Bookstein, J. J., and Stewart, B. H.   The current status of renal arteriography. *Radiol. Clin. North Am.* 2:461, 1964.

21. Bookstein, J. J., Walter, J. F., Stanley, J. C., and Fry, W. J.   Pharmacoangiographic manipulation of renal collateral blood flow. *Circulation* 54:328, 1976.

22. Bron, K. M., Strott, C. A., and Shapiro, A. P.   The diagnostic value of angiographic observations in polyarteritis nodosa. *Arch. Intern. Med.* (Chicago) 116:450, 1965.

23. Burt, R. L., Johnston, F. R., Silverthorne, R. G., Lock, F. R., and Dickerson, A. J.   Ruptured renal artery aneurysm in pregnancy: Report of a case with survival. *Obstet. Gynecol.* 7:229, 1956.

24. Christian, C. L., and Sergent, J. S.   Vasculitis syndromes: Clinical and experimental models. *Am. J. Med.* 3:385, 1976.

25. Chuang, V. P., Ernst, C. B., and Bhathena, D. B.   Evaluation of a new method for treating segmental renal disease. *Surg. Gynecol. Obstet.* 148:739, 1979.

26. Conn, J. W., Bookstein, J. J., and Cohen, E. L.   Renin-secreting juxtaglomerular cell adenoma. *Radiology* 106:543, 1973.

27. Crummy, A. B., Jr., Hellman, S., Stansel, H. C., Jr., and Hukill, P. B.   Renal hypertension secondary to unilateral radiation damage relieved by nephrectomy. *Radiology* 84:108, 1965.

28. Cummings, K. B., Lecky, J. W., and Kaufman, J. J.   Renal artery aneurysms and hypertension. *J. Urol.* 109:144, 1973.

29. D'Abreau, F., and Strickland, B.   Developmental renal artery stenosis. *Lancet* 2:517, 1962.

30. Delin, K., Aurell, M., Claes, G., Teger-Nilsson, A.-C., and Wallentin, I.   Multiple arterial occlusions and hypertension probably caused by an oral contraceptive: A patient in whom the development of renovascular hypertension has been followed. *Clin. Nephrol.* 6:453, 1976.

31. Dobrzinsky, S. J., Voegeli, E., Grant, H., Christlieb, A. R., Abrams, H. L., and Hickler, R. B.   Spontaneous re-establishment of renal function after complete occlusion of a renal artery. *Arch. Intern. Med.* 128:266, 1971.

32. Dodds, W. J., Noyes, W. E., Hinman, F., Jr., and Stoney, R. J.   Renal artery aneurysm: The cause of segmental alteration in renal blood flow and hypertension. *AJR* 104:302, 1968.

33. Downs, R. A., and Hewett, A. L.   Hyperten-

sion due to subcapsular renal hematoma. *J. Urol.* 88:22, 1962.

34. Ekelund, L., Gerlock, J., Jr., Goncharenko, V., and Foster, J. Angiographic findings following surgical treatment for renovascular hypertension. *Radiology* 126:345, 1978.

35. Ekelund, L., Gerlock, J., Molin, J., and Smith, C. Roentgenologic appearance of fibromuscular dysplasia. *Acta Radiol. [Diagn.]* (Stockh.) 19:433, 1977.

36. Ekelund, L., and Lindholm, T. Arteriovenous fistulae following percutaneous renal biopsy. *Acta Radiol. [Suppl.]* (Stockh.) 321:1972.

37. Ekeström, S., Liljeqvist, L., Nordhus, O., and Tidgren, B. Persisting hypertension after renal artery reconstruction. A follow-up study. *Scand. J. Urol. Nephrol.* 13:83, 1979.

38. Eyler, W. R., Clark, M. D., Garman, J. E., Rian, R. L., and Meininger, D. E. Angiography of the renal areas including a comparative study of renal arterial stenoses in patients with or without hypertension. *Radiology* 78:879, 1962.

39. Flasher, J., Drury, D. R., and Jacobson, G. Experimental arterial stenosis: Post stenotic dilatation and collateral blood flow. *Angiology* 2:60, 1951.

40. Fleming, R. J., and Stern, L. Z. Multiple intraparenchymal renal aneurysms in polyarteritis nodosa. *Radiology* 84:100, 1965.

41. Forsythe, W. E., and Persky, L. Comparison of ureteral and renal injuries. *Am. J. Surg.* 97:558, 1959.

42. Foster, R. S., Shuford, W. H., and Weens, H. S. Selective renal arteriography in medical diseases of the kidney. *AJR* 95:291, 1965.

43. Friedenberg, M. J., Eisen, S., and Kissane, J. Renal angiography in pyelonephritis, glomerulonephritis and arteriolar nephrosclerosis. *AJR* 95:349, 1965.

44. Gerlock, A. J., Jr., Goncharenko, V. A., and Ekelund, L. Radiation-induced stenosis of the renal artery causing hypertension: Case report. *J. Urol.* 118:1064, 1977.

45. Gill, W. M., Jr., and Meaney, T. F. Medial fibroplasia of the renal artery. *Radiology* 92:861, 1969.

46. Girl, J., and Tuhy, J. The development of hypertension after rupture of a kidney. *Circulation* 32:992, 1965.

47. Goldblatt, H., Lynch, J., Hanzal, R. F., and Summerville, W. W. The production of persistent hypertension in dogs. *Am. J. Pathol.* 9:942, 1933.

48. Graves, F. T. The anatomy of the intrarenal arteries and its application to segmental resection of the kidney. *Br. J. Surg.* 42:132, 1954.

49. Grüntzig, A. Treatment of renovascular hypertension with percutaneous dilatation of a renal artery stenosis. *Lancet* 1:801, 1978.

50. Hageman, J. H., Smith, R. F., Szilagyi, E., and Elliott, J. P. Aneurysms of the renal artery: Problems of prognosis and surgical management. *Surgery* 84:563, 1978.

51. Halpern, M., and Citron, B. P. Necrotizing angiitis associated with drug abuse. *AJR* 111:663, 1971.

52. Halpern, M., and Evans, J. A. Coarctation of the renal artery with "notching" of the ureter. A roentgenologic sign of unilateral renal disease as a cause of hypertension. *AJR* 88:159, 1962.

53. Halpern, M., Finby, N., and Evans, J. A. Percutaneous transfemoral renal arteriography in hypertension. *Radiology* 77:25, 1961.

54. Harrow, B. R., and Sloane, J. A. Aneurysm of renal artery: Report of five cases. *J. Urol.* 81:35, 1959.

55. Hatfield, P. M., and Pfester, R. C. Adult polycystic disease of the kidneys. *J.A.M.A.* 222:1527, 1972.

56. Hemley, S. D., and Finby, N. Renal trauma. A concept of injury to the renal artery. *Radiology* 79:816, 1962.

57. Hollenberg, N. K., Epstein, N., Basch, R. I., Couch, N. P., Hickler, R. B., and Merrill, J. P. Renin secretions in essential and accelerated hypertension. *Am. J. Med.* 47:855, 1969.

58. Hollenberg, N. K., Epstein, N., Basch, R. I., and Merrill, J. P. "No man's land" of the renal vasculature: An arteriographic and hemodynamic assessment of the interlobar and arcuate arteries in essential and accelerated hypertension. *Am. J. Med.* 47:845, 1969.

59. Holley, K. E., Hunt, J. C., Brown, A. L., Jr., Kincaid, O. W., and Sheps, S. G. Renal artery stenosis: A clinical-pathologic study in normotensive and hypertensive patients. *Am. J. Med.* 37:14, 1964.

60. Hoxie, H. J., and Coggin, C. B. Renal infarction: A statistical study of 205 cases and detailed report of an unusual case. *Arch. Intern. Med.* (Chicago) 65:587, 1940.

61. Itzchak, Y., Katznelson, D., Boichis, H., Jonas, A., and Deutsch, V. Angiographic features of arterial lesions in neurofibromatosis. *AJR* 122:643, 1974.

62. Jahnke, R. W., Messing, E. M., and Spellman, M. C. Hypertension and posttraumatic renal arteriovenous fistula: Demonstration of unilaterally elevated renin secretion. *J. Urol.* 116:646, 1976.

63. Janower, M. L., and Weber, A. L. Radiologic evaluation of acute renal infarction. *AJR* 95:309, 1965.

64. Katzen, B. T., Chang, J., Lukowsky, G. H., and Abramson, E. G. Percutaneous transluminal angioplasty for treatment of renovascular hypertension. *Radiology* 131:53, 1979.

65. Kaufman, J. J. Renovascular hypertension: The UCLA experience. *J. Urol.* 121:139, 1979.

66. Kerber, C. W., Freeny, P. C., Cromwell, L., Margolis, M. T., and Correa, R. J., Jr. Cyanoacrylate occlusion of a renal arteriovenous fistula. *AJR* 128:663, 1977.

67. Kincaid, O. W. *Renal Angiography.* Chicago: Year Book, 1966.

68. Kincaid, O. W., Davis, G. D., Hallerman, F. J., and Hunt, J. C. Fibromuscular dysplasia of the renal arteries: Arteriographic features, classification, and observations on natural history of the disease. *AJR* 104:271, 1968.

69. Kittredge, R. D., Hemley, S. D., Kanick, V., and Finby, N. The atrophic renal artery. *AJR* 92:309, 1964.

70. Klapproth, H. J. Distribution of renal arterial circulation in the dog. *J. Urol.* 82:417, 1959.

71. Köhler, R., and Edgren, J. Angiographic abnormalities following percutaneous needle biopsy of the kidney. *Acta Radiol.* [*Diagn.*] (Stockh.)15:514, 1974.

72. Lampe, W. T., II. Renovascular hypertension. A review of reversible causes due to extrinsic pressure on the renal artery and report of three unusual cases. *Angiology* 16:677, 1965.

73. Lawson, J. D., Hollifield, J. H., Foster, J. H., Rhamy, R. K., and Dean, R. H. Hypertension secondary to complete occlusion of the renal artery. *Am. Surg.* 136:648, 1978.

74. Love, L., Moncada, R., and Lescher, A. J. Renal arteriovenous fistulae. *AJR* 95:364, 1965.

75. Lundström, B. Angiographic abnormalities following percutaneous needle biopsy of the kidney. *Acta Radiol.* [*Suppl.*] (Stockh.) 321:1972.

76. McCormack, L. J., Dustan, H. P., and Meaney, T. F. Selected pathology of the renal artery. *Semin. Roentgenol.* 2:126, 1967.

77. McCormack, L. J., Poutasse, E. F., Meaney, T. F., Noto, T. J., Jr., and Dustan, H. P. A pathologic-arteriographic correlation of renal arterial disease. *Am. Heart J.* 72:188, 1966.

78. McDonald, D. F. Renal hypertension without main arterial stenosis. Function tests predict cure. *J.A.M.A.* 203:932, 1968.

79. Mahler, F., et al. Treatment of renovascular hypertension by transluminal renal artery dilation. *Ann. Intern. Med.* 90:56, 1979.

80. Maldonado, J. E., Sheps, S. G., Bernatz, P. E., DeWeerd, J. H., and Harrison, E. G., Jr. Renal arteriovenous fistula. A reversible cause of hypertension and heart failure. *Am. J. Med.* 37:499, 1964.

81. Mang, H. Y. L., Markovic, P. R., Chow, S., and Maruyama, A. Solitary intrarenal cyst causing hypertension: With plasma renin activity study before and after cyst aspiration. *N.Y. State J. Med.* 78:654, 1978.

82. March, T. L., and Halpern, M. Renal vein thrombosis demonstrated by selective renal phlebography. *Radiology* 81:958, 1963.

83. Marenta, V. E., and Schnauder, A. Angiographie und Nierentrauma. *Schweiz. Med. Wochenschr.* 94:1484, 1964.

84. Marshall, W. H., Jr., and Castellino, R. A. Hypertension produced by constricting capsular renal lesions ("Page" kidney). *Radiology* 101:561, 1971.

85. Martini, E. Ueber die Möglichkeit der Niere einen neuen collateralen Blutzufluss zu schaffen. *Arch. Klin. Chir.* 78:619, 1906.

86. Mason, M. F., Robinson, C. S., and Blalock, A. Studies on the renal arterial blood pressure and the metabolism of kidney tissue in experimental hypertension. *J. Exp. Med.* 72:289, 1940.

87. Mena, E., Bookstein, J. J., Holt, J. F., and Fry, W. J. Neurofibromatosis and renal vascular hypertension in children. *AJR* 118:39, 1973.

88. Meng, C.-H., and Elkin, M. Immediate angiographic manifestations of iatrogenic renal injury due to percutaneous needle biopsy. *Radiology* 100:335, 1971.

89. Merklin, R. J., and Michels, N. A. The variant renal and suprarenal blood supply with data on the inferior phrenic, ureteral and gonadal arteries. *J. Intern. Coll. Surg.* 29:41, 1958.

90. Merten, D. F., Vogel, J. M., Adelman, R. D., Goetzman, B. W., and Bogren, H. G. Renovascular hypertension as a complication of umbilical arterial catheterization. *Radiology* 126:751, 1978.

91. Meyers, D. S., Grim, C. E., and Keitzer, W. F. Fibromuscular dyplasia of the renal artery with medial dissection: A case simulating polyarteritis nodosa. *Am. J. Med.* 56:412, 1974.

92. Millan, V. G., Mast, W. E., and Madias, N. E. Nonsurgical treatment of severe hypertension due to renal-artery intimal fibroplasia by percutaneous transluminal angioplasty. *Med. Intelligence* 300:1371, 1979.

93. Millan, V. G., Sher, M. H., Deterling, R. A., Jr., Packard, A., Morton, J. R., and Harrington, J. T. Transcatheter thromboembolectomy of acute renal artery occlusion. *Arch. Surg.* 113:1086, 1978.

94. Moody, R. O., and Van Nyys, R. G. The position and mobility of the kidneys in healthy young men and women. *Anat. Rec.* 76:111, 1940.

95. Moore, M. A., and Phillippi, P. J. Reversible renal hypertension secondary to renal arteriovenous fistula and renal cell carcinoma. *J. Urol.* 117:246, 1977.

96. Olsson, O., and Lunderquist, A. Angiography in renal trauma. *Acta Radiol.* [*Diagn.*] (Stockh.) 1:1, 1963.

97. Palubinskas, A. J., and Wylie, E. J. Roentgen diagnosis of fibromuscular hyperplasia of the renal arteries. *Radiology* 76:634, 1961.
98. Perry, M. O. Fibromuscular disease of carotid artery. *Surg. Gynecol. Obstet.* 134:57, 1972.
99. Rao, C. N., and Blaivas, J. G. Primary renal artery dissecting aneurysm: A review. *J. Urol.* 118:716, 1977.
100. Reidbord, H. E., McCormack, L. J., and O'Duffy, J. D. Necrotizing angiitis: II. Findings at autopsy in twenty-seven cases. *Clev. Clin. Q.* 32:191, 1965.
101. Reuter, S. R., Pomeroy, P. R., Chuang, V. P., and Cho, K. J. Embolic control of hypertension caused by segmental renal artery stenosis. *AJR* 127:389, 1976.
102. Robins, J. M., and Bookstein, J. Percutaneous transcaval biopsy technique in the evaluation of inferior vena cava occlusion. *Radiology* 105:451, 1972.
103. Rose, E. A., McNicholas, K. W., Bethea, M. C., Casarella, W. J., and Bregman, D. Renovascular hypertension following surgical repair of dissecting aneurysm of the thoracic aorta. *Surgery* 83:235, 1978.
104. Sarramon, J. P., Cerene, A., Gorodetski, N., Bernadet, P., and Durand, D. Spontaneous renal arteriovenous fistula and arterial hypertension—conservative treatment and healing. *Eur. Urol.* 4:214, 1978.
105. Schurch, W., Messerli, F. H., Genest, J., et al. Arterial hypertension and neurofibromatosis: Renal artery stenosis and coarctation of abdominal aorta. *Can. Med. Assoc. J.* 113:879, 1975.
106. Spriggs, D. W., and Brantley, R. E. Recognition of renal artery spasm during renal angiography. *Radiology* 127:363, 1978.
107. Staab, G. E., Tegtmeyer, C. J., and Constable, W. C. Radiation-induced renovascular hypertension. *AJR* 126:634, 1976.
108. Stamey, T. A. *Renovascular Hypertension*. Baltimore: Williams & Wilkins, 1963.
109. Sutton, D., Brunton, F. J., Foot, E. C., and Gutherie, J. Fibromuscular, fibrous, and non-atheromatous renal artery stenosis and hypertension. *Clin. Radiol.* 14:381, 1963.
110. Thomas, E., and Forbus, W. D. Irradiation injury to aorta and lung. *Arch. Pathol.* 67:256, 1959.
111. Thomas, R. G., and Levin, N. W. Ureteric irregularity with renal artery obstruction. A new radiological sign. *Br. J. Radiol.* 34:438, 1961.
112. Tilford, D. L., and Kelch, R. C. Renal artery stenosis in childhood neurofibromatosis. *Am. J. Dis. Child.* 126:665, 1973.
113. Yuile, C. L. Obstructive lesions of the main renal artery in relation to hypertension. *Am. J. Med. Sci.* 207:394, 1944.

Renal Angiography in the Oliguric State

NORMAN K. HOLLENBERG
DONALD P. HARRINGTON
J. DANIEL GARNIC
DOUGLASS F. ADAMS
HERBERT L. ABRAMS

Renal angiography has been used primarily in the assessment of "surgical" diseases of the kidney, such as renal mass lesions, arterial stenosis, and trauma. The role of renal angiography in the evaluation of "medical" diseases of the kidney has received attention primarily in regard to hypertension [1, 27, 29, 43, 97]. Characteristic abnormalities in the renal angiograms also occur in patients with acute oliguric renal insufficiency in a number of clinical settings [2, 23, 38, 41]. The findings in the angiograms, interpreted in the light of simultaneous renal hemodynamic studies, suggest a pathogenic final common pathway of preferential renal cortical ischemia. There are, however, significant differences in the arteriograms of patients with different diseases. In this chapter, these changes are described and related to the pathophysiologic processes involved, and the clinical indications for renal angiography in the evaluation of selected patients with acute renal insufficiency are defined.

The Differential Diagnosis of the Acute Oliguric States

The sudden failure of the patient to elaborate urine is one of the most dramatic events in medicine. Because it is associated with a wide variety of causes, a specific diagnosis is required for appropriate therapy [28]. Aggressive volume therapy required to reverse prerenal azotemia can produce pulmonary edema in the patient with established acute renal failure. In other circumstances, emergency surgery is required, and a major delay in performing surgery may preclude recovery of renal function.

In most situations, the history, physical findings, characteristics of the urine, and other laboratory findings provide sufficiently strong evidence for a diagnosis, making more elaborate diagnostic procedures unnecessary. At times, however, further examinations must be carried out before a diagnosis or a prognosis can be made. Occasionally, the etiology of the renal failure remains obscure, even after such a specific study as renal biopsy or retrograde pyelography. Arteriography may play a vital role in clarifying the underlying problem and defining the proper management of the patient. In the following sections, the indications and potential usefulness of arteriography are considered in detail against the background of the differential diagnosis of the oliguric states and the role and limitations of other diagnostic methods.

PRERENAL AZOTEMIA

The commonest cause of the acute suppression of urine output is functional, secondary to depletion of extracellular and plasma volumes. Generally, prerenal azotemia develops in a patient whose history suggests volume depletion due to hemorrhage, diarrhea, burns, third-space factors in traumatized tissue or the gastrointestinal tract, overzealous diuretic therapy, prolonged vomiting, or gastrointestinal tract drainage. Frequently such patients show some physical signs of volume depletion and cardiovascular decompensation, but these signs may be absent. The diagnosis is frequently suggested by examination of the urine, which reveals an appropriate response to the physiologic stimulus of volume depletion. The urine shows a high specific gravity and osmolality and a very low concentration of sodium:

Figure 58-1. Effect of epinephrine on the renal arteriogram and xenon washout in the normal human kidney. (A) The control studies are shown. (B) After the injection of 6 μg of epinephrine into the renal artery, both the cortical vasculature visualized in the arteriogram and the rapid disappearance of xenon, which normally dominates the early portion of the tracing, are unrecognizable. Several lines of evidence suggest that the rapid flow component represents cortical perfusion. (From Hollenberg et al. [41]. Reproduced by permission from *Medicine*.)

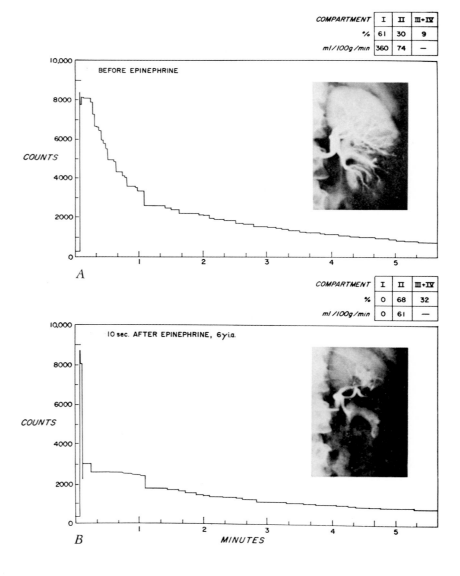

These characteristics all reflect the normal role of the kidney in repairing volume deficits. Patients with prerenal azotemia respond with a diuresis to prompt, vigorous replacement of the deficit, and they never require additional diagnostic studies.

ACUTE TUBULAR NECROSIS

Acute tubular necrosis (ATN) may develop in such patients if volume therapy is delayed. Nephrotoxins are also a common cause. The urine no longer shows the features of an appropriate response to a volume deficit. The specific gravity and the osmolality of the urine do not exceed the levels found in a plasma ultrafiltrate, the creatinine concentration in the urine does not exceed that in the plasma by a factor of more than three, and the urine sodium level is generally above 40 mEq per liter [28]. The patient no longer responds to intravenous therapy with a diuresis, and an attempt to induce a diuresis with intravenous fluids would result in fluid retention and pulmonary edema. Before this distinction was recognized, pulmonary edema was one of the common causes of death in ATN.

If the cause of acute renal failure was not obvious, retrograde catheterization of the ureter was once frequently performed to rule out obstruction as a factor. Renal biopsy is not routinely employed, generally being considered only if the onset or the course suggests the presence of irreversible cortical necrosis, an unusual and acute parenchymal disease, or previously undiagnosed chronic renal disease (Fig. 58-1).

VASCULAR ACCIDENTS

The presence of an acute arterial catastrophe, such as embolism, arterial dissection, or thrombosis of a renal artery, is the only absolute indication for renal arteriography suggested by the sudden onset of flank pain and hematuria [46]. These symptoms are much more likely to be followed by oliguria if a patient has only one functioning kidney. Frequently, the history suggests a source of the embolus, such as atrial fibrillation or a previous myocardial infarction. In some patients, the history may be vague, and the diagnosis of acute arterial catastrophe may be overlooked. Because emergency surgery is essential to reestablishing a renal blood supply and a delay may be dangerous, acute arterial catastrophe must be entertained as the diagnosis in any patient with acute renal failure of obscure etiology

once a functional cause of oliguria has been ruled out.

Other rare conditions in which arteriography may prove helpful include diseases in which the cortical vessels and the parenchyma may be spared (and so a relatively normal renal biopsy sample may be obtained) while the more proximal vessels show the predominant involvement. Thus polyarteritis or severe nephrosclerosis may at times involve primarily the arcuate and the more proximal arteries [2, 12, 18]. Bilateral renal artery stenosis is another condition to be considered in this category [62, 73, 90].

URETERAL OBSTRUCTION

Like acute arterial obstruction, ureteral obstruction does not cause oliguria unless the patient has only one kidney or unless the condition is bilateral. If the obstruction is complete, the urogram may fail to establish the diagnosis, although this failure has become much less common with high-dose urography and nephrotomography.

Moreover, ultrasonography and computed tomography (CT) have simplified the noninvasive diagnosis of ureteral obstruction [26, 85, 105]. Retrograde ureteral catheterization may be required under special circumstances, however. Patients with massive skeletal trauma involving the pelvis and the hips are poor candidates for retrograde catheterization, and diagnostic exploration and nephrostomy may be necessary. In patients with a kidney transplant in whom the ureteric anastomosis has been made at the level of the bladder rather than at the ureteropelvic junction, retrograde catheterization may be difficult or impossible. Arteriography may then be of value in defining the presence or absence of acute ureteric obstruction and in determining the need for exploration. In both of the above examples, ultrasonography or CT or both are the primary diagnostic choices.

Physiology and Pathophysiology of Renal Perfusion

The kidneys have one of the highest blood flow rates per gram of any organ in the body. Although they comprise less than 0.5 percent of the body mass, they receive about 20 percent of the cardiac output. This very high perfusion rate is not uniformly distributed throughout the kidney; the very high rates of blood flow are confined to the renal cortex [9, 11, 17, 64, 94, 97]. The very high cortical flow rate is ideally suited to delivering large volumes of plasma for glomerular filtration and to providing the hydrostatic pressure to promote filtration.

There is little controversy concerning the pathogenesis of functional renal failure in the patient with "prerenal azotemia" secondary to a volume deficit. In this setting, diminished plasma volume leads to a reduction in the cardiac output and thus to a decrease in renal perfusion.

The reduction in renal perfusion results in a plasma flow and a glomerular capillary pressure too low to sustain filtration. The outcome is a sharp reduction in urine output, generally to less than 15 cc per hour, and progressive azotemia. Restitution of the volume loss with saline, colloid, or blood results in reversal of the oliguria and a prompt and progressive improvement in renal function.

There is continued controversy about the pathogenesis of ATN. Although in acute renal failure induced with nephrotoxins in animals there is frequently evidence of severe tubular necrosis [70], in patients with acute renal failure such gross distortions of structure are much less common [24], and even electron microscopy may reveal only minimal damage [16, 24, 60, 71, 72]. These findings raise a nosologic problem. The failure of tubular lesions to account for the process suggests that the concept and term *acute tubular necrosis* should be abandoned [41]. A suit-

Figure 58-2. Acute tubular necrosis (ATN). (A) Selective renal arteriogram and xenon washout in a patient with ATN secondary to shock. (B) Studies repeated after recovery, when creatinine clearance had returned to normal. Note the striking similarity of the hemodynamic changes to those induced by epinephrine (see Fig. 58-1). The arteriographic features of acute renal failure are seen more clearly and are described in detail in Figure 58-7. (From Hollenberg et al. [41]. Reproduced by permission from *Medicine*.)

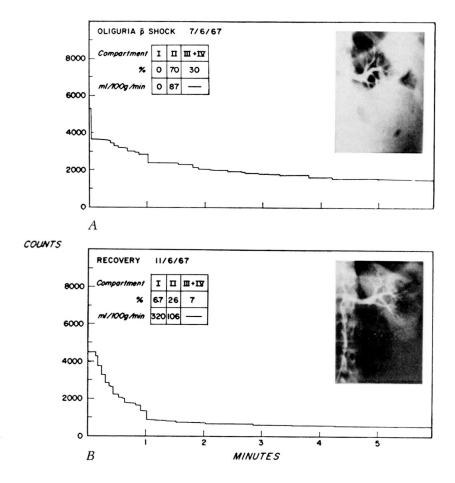

able alternative descriptive term, however, is not yet available. The generic term *acute renal failure* is potentially confusing because it may be used to denote all the clinical conditions covered in this chapter. We use the term *acute tubular necrosis (ATN)* in this chapter to avoid confusion, but we intend no pathophysiologic implications. Several hypotheses have been elaborated to account for the failure of function. One hypothesis is not based on the presence of tubular lesions but suggests rather that the loss of function is caused by a cessation of glomerular filtration, presumably resulting from some abnormality in renal hemodynamics [25, 84]. Renal perfusion is reduced to 30 to 50 percent of normal in most patients with ATN [59, 63, 75, 80, 100]. Many patients who have chronic renal failure have a similar reduction in total renal blood flow and yet have a normal urine output and a glomerular filtration rate adequate to maintain life. A simple reduction in the total renal blood flow could not account for the total disruption of renal function in ATN [63, 80].

According to a second hypothesis, the failure of filtration may reflect an abnormality of the filtering membrane in the glomerulus. A third hypothesis is that tubular obstruction is due to an accumulation of tubular debris within the lumen. The fourth hypothesis is that filtration continues but oliguria ensues because of the passive backleak to the circulation of the filtrate via the disrupted tubular walls [4, 25, 66, 74]. Although some experimental data support each of the hypotheses in animal models, it has been difficult to accept the last two hypotheses in patients with minimal morphologic renal damage [24, 60, 71, 72].

Observations in patients with minimal morphologic damage have suggested an alternative to account for the failure of glomerular filtration [41]. The application of renal arteriography and the xenon washout method to the determination of the intrarenal distribution of blood flow in man suggested the absence of the normally extremely high cortical blood flow in ATN [41, 43]. During recovery from ATN, cortical flow reappeared in approximate proportion to the recovery of glomerular filtration. The characteristics resemble those in the renal cortical ischemia induced by the injection of a large dose of epinephrine into the renal artery (Figs. 58-1, 58-2). In both situations, the decrease in cortical perfusion is out of proportion to the decrease in total renal blood flow (*preferential cortical ischemia*). A characteristic triad of changes in the selective renal arteriograms of patients with ATN, described in greater detail in following sections, supports the concept of a preferential and diffuse reduction in renal cortical perfusion. These changes are (1) the absence of a distinct cortical nephrogram, (2) the absence of identifiable arterial vessels beyond the arcuate arterial level (i.e., in the cortex), and (3) prolongation of the transit time of the contrast medium through the kidney.

In patients with chronic renal failure who had a similar reduction in total blood flow, there was a small but definite rapid flow component in the xenon washout curve, and patchy areas of cortical vascular filling were evident in the selective renal arteriogram, indicating that portions of the renal cortex are perfused at a rate that maintains glomerular filtration. Thus it appears that because of regional differences in perfusion in patients with ATN and chronic renal failure, the same overall blood flow rate results in differences in renal function.

There is strong supporting evidence that a selective but profound reduction in the renal cortical flow may occur on a functional basis due to active vasoconstriction [9, 11, 17, 39, 40, 42, 50, 54, 97]. Examples of the effects of hemorrhage on the renal arteriogram in man and the dog are shown in Figures 58-3 to 58-5. In these situations, perfusion in the medullary and juxtamedullary zones appears to be well maintained and therefore is probably under independent control [11, 17, 50, 54, 97].

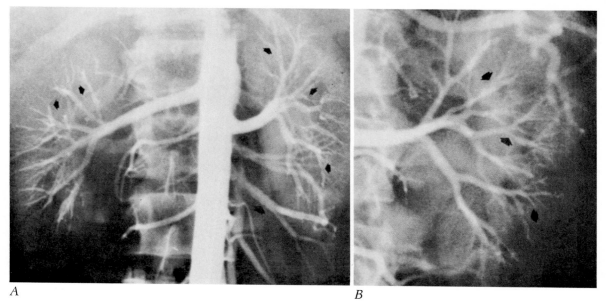

A   B

Figure 58-3. Renal arterial changes following acute hypotension in man. This arteriogram was performed 48 hours after an episode of shock following a gunshot wound of the head. (A) Abdominal aortogram. The main renal arteries are normal. There are numerous areas of narrowing and irregularity in the segmental arteries on both sides (*arrows*). The caliber of the ves- sels is quite variable, with alternating narrowing and dilatation. Note also the irregularity of an intestinal branch (*lower arrow, left*). (B) A detailed view of the left kidney. The arrows point to areas of marked nar- rowing, some of which are located at the bifurcations of the segmental branches.

Figure 58-4. Renal arteriography during hemorrhagic hypotension in the dog. (A) Control study. A selective left renal arteriogram has been performed. The mean aortic blood pressure was 150 mm Hg (film at 1 sec- ond after start of the injection). (B) Hypotension. The mean aortic blood pressure was maintained at 35 mm Hg for 15 minutes prior to the arteriogram. There is a decrease in the size of the segmental renal vessels as- sociated with localized areas of spasm (*small arrows*). Irregularities of the main renal artery (*large arrow*), presumably also due to spasm, were not visible on the control study (film at 1 second following start of the injection).

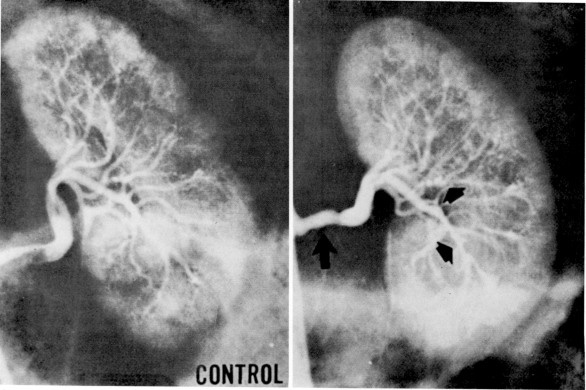

A   B

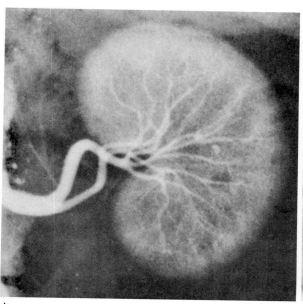

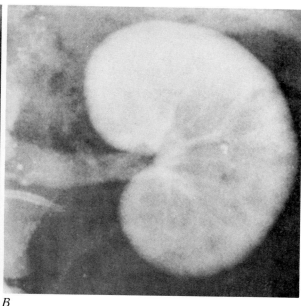

A

B

Figure 58-5. Renal arteriography after hemorrhagic hypotension in the dog. Control studies were performed at a mean blood pressure of 160 mm Hg. The mean blood pressure was then dropped to 50 mm Hg for 90 minutes and to 30 mm Hg for 30 minutes. (A) Control arteriogram, normal (film at 1 second after start of the injection). (B) Control nephrogram, normal (film at 3.5 seconds after start of the injection). (C) Arteriogram during hypotension. The major arteries have diminished strikingly in size, and cortical perfusion is profoundly diminished. The edge of the kidney is indicated (*arrows*) but the bulk of the contrast agent is in the inner cortical and medullary regions (film at 2 seconds after start of the injection).

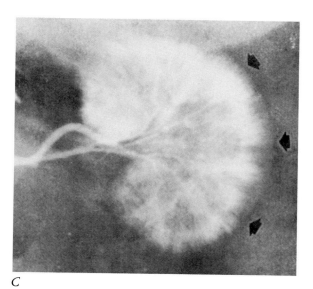

C

Trueta Phenomenon and Shunting

Trueta and his co-workers were the first to delineate clearly an independent control of the circulation through the renal cortex and medulla [96]. Certain terms these investigators used resulted in a continuing confusion about the nature of the hemodynamic changes associated with renal cortical ischemia. Their use of the terms *short circuit, bypass*, and *diversion* suggested that a shunt mechanism was operative, with an active diversion of an unchanged total renal blood flow from the cortex to the medullary circulation. (The term *shunt* appears only in Fulton's introduction to the monograph Trueta and his co-workers published.) These investigators offered two lines of evidence for such a bypass from their studies in the rabbit: the early appearance of

contrast material in the renal vein during angiographic studies and the "arterialization" of the renal venous blood [96].

No evidence of shunting was apparent with angiographic techniques in man [2, 23, 38, 41]. Studies with other indicators have also suggested that there is no quantitatively important short pathway for blood flow through the kidney in this setting [75, 80]. In addition, the normal renal venous effluent already has such a high oxygen saturation that an increase in the oxygen saturation would be extremely difficult to recognize by eye and, in fact, has not been demonstrated by measurement.

Preferential cortical ischemia associated with

the maintenance of juxtamedullary and medullary perfusion at normal levels occurs but is not what is now generally meant when the so-called Trueta phenomenon is cited [89]. In our experience, early renal venous opacification is evident in the selective renal arteriogram only when there is marked overall renal vasodilatation, especially in association with the infusion of a vasodilator drug, such as acetylcholine or dopamine, or with an arteriogram obtained during acute obturation of the renal artery.

Acute Organic Arterial Obstruction Leading to Renal Failure

The only absolute indication for renal arteriography in the patient with sudden oliguric renal failure is the possibility that an acute vascular catastrophe compromising the arterial blood supply has occurred. Because there is a clear relationship between the duration of ischemia and the extent of recovery of renal function, the arteriogram must be done as an emergency procedure [8, 15, 44, 46, 53, 64, 76, 90]. Reports of returned renal function after a renal artery embolectomy suggest that periods of ischemia of several days to several weeks may be tolerated by the kidney if a collateral blood supply for sufficient local nutrition is present [64, 76, 90]. An aortogram that reveals filling of intrarenal vessels despite arterial occlusion suggests that the collateral supply is sufficient for this purpose.

Illustrative Case
D. G., a 60-year-old woman, had the sudden onset of left flank pain and hematuria 24 hours prior to admis-

---

Figure 58-6. Renal embolism and oliguria (patient D. G.). This 60-year old woman had had her right kidney removed 20 years earlier. After a bout of atrial fibrillation, she developed anuria. Aortography was performed for evaluation of the circulation to the left kidney. (A) Anteroposterior study 1.5 seconds after the injection. The stump of the right renal artery, which had been ligated at the time of the nephrectomy, is clearly defined (*double arrow*). On the left, there is total occlusion of the left renal artery by embolus. A few small paraaortic collateral channels are visible. Single arrow points to occluded left renal artery at the interspace of L1 and L2. (B) Two seconds later. The intrarenal vessels are filled with contrast agent. They are attenuated, and the blood flow to the kidney is markedly reduced. Filling occurs via direct channels from the aorta as well as from the lumbar branches. The reconstituted renal artery (*single arrow*) indicates the length of the embolic obstruction, which was verified at surgery. The edge of the kidney (*double arrow*) is now defined by faint contrast staining, indicating the passage of contrast material (and therefore blood) into the peripheral circulation of the kidney.

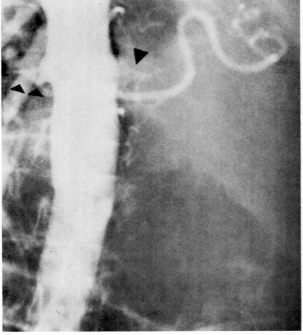

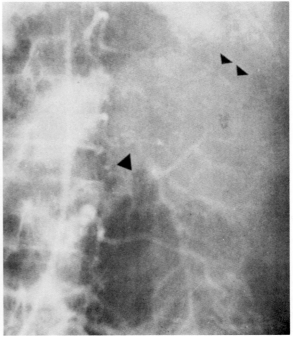

A   *B*

sion. A right nephrectomy had been carried out 20 years earlier, apparently for hydronephrosis, but the patient had had a normal blood urea nitrogen level of 20 mg per 100 cc 2 months before admission. In addition, she had a long history of rheumatic heart disease with mitral stenosis and atrial fibrillation and had suffered a mild cerebral vascular accident 1 year earlier. In the emergency room, she was found to have a ventricular tachycardia, which was reversed with lidocaine. She was not in gross congestive heart failure at the time. Although the patient had not voided in the preceding 24 hours, catheterization revealed no urine in the bladder. After 3 hours of absolute anuria and no response to 25 gm of mannitol given intravenously, the patient was taken to the angiography suite. Study revealed the absence of the right kidney and total occlusion of the left renal artery with evidence of more distal intrarenal arterial filling (Fig. 58-6).

An embolectomy of the left renal artery was performed approximately 30 hours after the onset of symptoms. After the Fogarty catheter was passed through the renal arteriotomy to clear the distal renal vessels of clot, a pulse reappeared in the distal renal artery, the needled renal cortex bled moderately well, and the kidney appeared to be viable. After surgery, the patient passed 200 cc of urine during the first day and 400 cc during the second day. Her blood urea nitrogen level continued to rise, however, and hyperkalemia resistant to conservative therapy developed. The patient developed ventricular fibrillation before dialysis could be carried out.

At postmortem examination, most of the kidney was clearly viable. The embolus had lodged in an area of moderate arterial narrowing adjacent to an atherosclerotic plaque.

Oliguria secondary to arterial occlusion is more likely to occur in the patient with only one kidney. Dissection of the aorta or extensive embolization, however, may involve both kidneys. Dissecting aneurysms usually begin in the ascending aorta and are suspected clinically from the characteristic history and from clinical evidence of obstruction of the blood supply to major vascular beds [20, 88].

Renal Causes of Acute Oliguric Renal Failure

The intrarenal causes of acute oliguric renal failure include the classic pathogenic factors in ATN (e.g., shock, sepsis, hemolysis, and nephrotoxins); the so-called hepatorenal syndrome; acute oliguric glomerulonephritis; vasculitis, including hypersensitivity angiitis and polyarteritis nodosa;

thrombotic thrombocytopenia purpura; scleroderma and accelerated nephrosclerosis; acute renal transplant rejection; and renal cortical necrosis. In the past, cortical necrosis most frequently followed an accident of pregnancy or sepsis, but now it is probably more common with hyperacute allograft rejection.

ACUTE TUBULAR NECROSIS

The renal angiographic features of ATN include an accentuated regular and smooth attenuation of the distal interlobar and arcuate arteries and failure of visualization of the more distal vessels; absence of the cortical nephrogram, indicating diminished delivery of contrast agent to this zone; and prolongation of the transit time of the contrast medium through the renal vasculature [38, 41, 70, 74, 87]. The last finding is best assessed on the basis of the rate of contrast agent washout from the arterial tree. No sign of early appearance in the renal vein has been recognized, and generally the renal vein is poorly visualized. Kidney size is variable, but only early in the course of the disease is there a suggestion of a reduction in size [38, 41, 70]. Edema, an inconstant feature, is apparently dependent primarily on the duration of the process. After several days, edema is generally present and results in an increase in renal size and in spreading and straightening of the intrarenal branches.

These observations and the findings in parallel renal hemodynamic studies reflect the absence of the normally preferentially high renal cortical perfusion. The failure of function on this basis is attributed to the absence of a head of pressure sufficient to promote glomular filtration. A tracing of a xenon washout study and an arteriogram from a patient in whom ATN followed a period of shock due to peritonitis is shown in Figure 58-2. Note the close similarity of the xenon washout tracing to that induced by epinephrine (see Fig. 58-1).

The course and the results of study in another patient with ATN were as follows:

Illustrative Case
A. H. was admitted to the hospital for mitral valve replacement because of recurrent mitral stenosis. He had moderate, progressive congestive heart failure despite aggressive medical therapy. Intermittent atrial fibrillation had been present for 15 years. Surgery was uneventful, but the patient's first postoperative week was complicated by disorientation, gross gastrointestinal bleeding without hypotension, and several epi-

sodes of acute pulmonary edema. During his second postoperative week, this man showed considerable clinical improvement. His renal function was well maintained. The blood urea nitrogen level ranged from 10 to 16 mg per 100 cc, and the daily urine output exceeded 2,000 cc.

In the third postoperative week, he developed a fever that rose to 39.4°C (103°F) and he had pyuria and difficulty in voiding. Because the infection did not respond to tetracycline, large doses of sodium colistimethate were added to the regimen. Two days later, the patient's urine output had dropped to 350 cc per 24 hours, the blood urea nitrogen level had risen to 66 mg per 100 cc, and the arterial pH had fallen to 7.28.

The patient developed a nodal rhythm apparently related to hyperkalemia, which was followed by cardiac arrest. Resuscitation was successful, and peritoneal dialysis was instituted. The patient received phenylephrine intermittently for blood pressure maintenance during the first 24 hours. The oliguria did not respond to the administration of mannitol or ethacrynic acid. The urine osmolality equalled the plasma osmolality, and the sodium concentration of the urine was 45 mEq per liter.

Because of the possible contribution of arterial embolization to the genesis of the acute renal failure and the very severe suppression of urine output, with 2 days of virtual anuria, arteriography was performed on

Figure 58-7. Acute tubular necrosis (patient A. H.). This 53-year-old man developed oliguria and azotemia 3 weeks after mitral valve replacement. Since a strong suspicion of renal embolism was entertained, arteriography was performed. (A) Arteriographic phase. The main renal artery and its large branches appear normal and show no evidence of embolus. The intrarenal branches are somewhat spread, and they fill poorly toward the periphery of the kidney, which is swollen and enlarged. (B) Nephrographic phase. The perfusion of the periphery of the kidney is grossly diminished, particularly in the middle and lower poles, and a clear corticomedullary demarcation is absent. The distribution of the contrast agent also appears to be nonuniform. There is no evidence of renal venous opacification. The patient's clinical course and the histologic features of the kidney suggested acute tubular necrosis, which was probably related to a nephrotoxin, colistimethate.

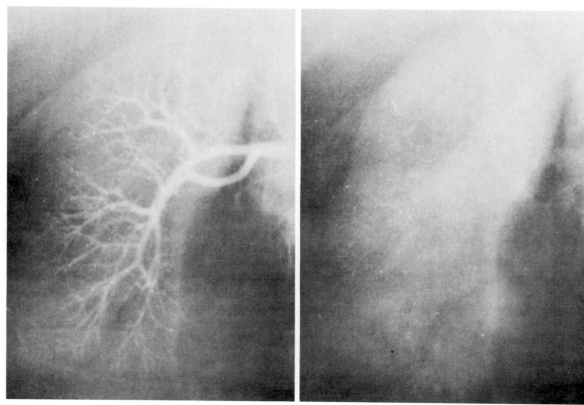

A   B

the third day. There was no evidence of intrarenal embolization. Instead, the arteriographic features of ATN were present (Fig. 58-7). Xenon washout revealed no rapid flow component, but the flow was sufficiently well maintained to suggest a reversible lesion. Two days after the study, the patient entered the diuretic phase of ATN, with urine outputs of 1,040 cc and 1,670 cc per day. At this time, he developed complete heart block with hypotension. Cardiac arrest occurred during an attempt to place a transvenous pacemaker, and efforts at resuscitation were unsuccessful.

Postmortem examination of the kidneys revealed healing ATN with minimal arteriolar nephrosclerosis. There was no evidence of embolization to the kidney. In retrospect, it seems likely that the ATN antedated the arrhythmias in the third week and was probably secondary to the administration of large doses of sodium colistimethate, a well-documented nephrotoxin [22].

THE HEPATORENAL SYNDROME

Patients with severe cirrhosis of the liver and hepatic failure develop a syndrome of acute oliguric renal failure that functionally differs from ATN in several respects. Despite progressive azotemia and oliguria, these patients frequently have a very low urinary sodium concentration and relatively good maintenance of the ability to concentrate the urine [23]. Although this combination of findings suggests a major prerenal component, responses to volume loading tend to be incomplete and evanescent.

The arteriographic abnormality in these patients is in many respects similar to that in ATN but is more severe. In addition to the loss of visualization of the peripheral arcuate and interlobular branches, there is severe attenuation of the interlobar arteries. With advanced renal failure, there is a further reduction in the size of the intrarenal branches, and an irregular, beaded appearance is frequently evident. The intensity of the nephrogram is considerably diminished, and the corticomedullary junction is no longer apparent. The transit time of the contrast medium is severely prolonged, and venous opacification is rarely demonstrable. The characteristic arteriographic abnormalities in these patients are well demonstrated in Figure 58-8, in which a postmortem injection study of the same kidney is also shown.

The reversibility of the angiographic abnormalities and the extremely labile blood flow found in the hemodynamic studies suggest strongly that the vascular abnormality is due to active vasoconstriction by a mediator that has yet to be defined. Sympathetic activity acting on the renal vasculature was at first an attractive hypothesis to account for the highly variable blood flow and severe abnormalities involving the proximal renal vasculature, particularly because catecholamines are well-documented vasoconstrictors of this order of kidney vessel (see Fig. 58-1). It was therefore disappointing that the intraarterial infusion of adequate doses of phentolamine, an alpha-adrenergic blocking agent, did not reverse either the blood flow reduction or the arteriographic changes [2, 25]. This approach is being pursued in the hope that suitable vasodilators will be found to make feasible treatment by the local infusion of the dilating agent at the time of selective arteriography.

ACUTE OLIGURIC GLOMERULONEPHRITIS

Glomerulonephritis usually involves the kidneys bilaterally and symmetrically. The arteriogram shows abrupt tapering of the larger intrarenal branches with so-called pruning of the more distal vessels. A characteristic feature is the considerable vessel tortuosity and irregularity of the vascular lumina of the more distal vessels. In patients with acute oliguric renal failure secondary to severe acute glomerulonephritis, the kidney is generally large and edematous. Many of the alterations associated with ATN, including failure of visualization of the peripheral vessels, the lack of a cortical nephrogram, and the prolongation of the transit time, are present [41]. The vascular changes are frequently sufficiently distinctive to suggest the diagnosis and to strengthen the indication for renal biopsy.

The following case example gives a history of such a patient; it is followed by a discussion of the angiographic features of acute oliguric glomerulonephritis.

Illustrative Case
G. E., a 45-year-old previously healthy man, was hospitalized because of fever, hematuria, and progressive azotemia. The initial evaluation revealed hypertension, anemia, and moderate azotemia. Protein and red cells were found in the urine, but no red cell casts were seen in the urine sediment.

In the subsequent 2 weeks, the patient became progressively more azotemic and oliguric. Renal angiography was undertaken because of the presence of severe hypertension and the possibility that a vascular

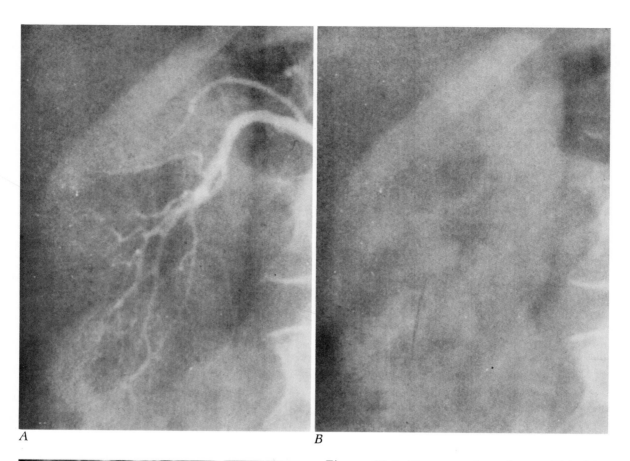

A

B

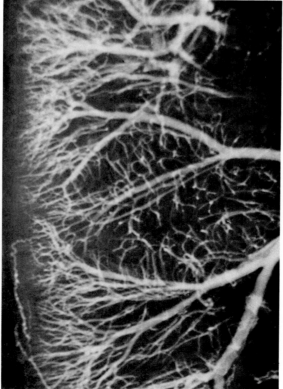

C

Figure 58-8. Hepatorenal syndrome. This 54-year-old woman had alcoholic cirrhosis and hepatorenal failure. Selective renal arteriography was performed in an effort to determine the status of the intrarenal vascular bed and to increase the renal blood flow pharmacologically if possible. (A) Arterial phase. The kidney is small, and the main renal artery and the intrarenal branches are diminished in caliber. The arcuate arteries are not visualized. The narrowing of the interlobar branches is profound, and there is mild tortuosity. (B) Nephrographic phase. The cortical flow is poor, spotty, and irregularly distributed, and corticomedullary differentiation is totally lacking. The renal vein is not opacified. (C) Injected specimen. The vessels are normal, as they were on histologic examination. The arcuate and the interlobular channels are sharply demarcated and show no evidence of organic obstruction.

lesion was contributing to his somewhat unusual down-hill course (Fig. 58-9A–C). The arteriogram showed swollen kidneys with spreading of the major branches and poor peripheral filling. Tortuosity, beading, and peripheral attenuation of the arteries were evident. The nephrogram was faint, and there was now poor cortical demarcation. The concurrent blood flow determination showed absence of the rapid flow component and a severe reduction in renal perfusion. Renal biopsy revealed acute necrotizing and proliferative glomerulonephritis.

The disease did not respond to immunosuppressive therapy, and the patient was placed on maintenance chronic hemodialysis. He received a kidney transplant from a well-matched cadaver donor 2 months later. Bilateral nephrectomy had not yet been carried out.

One month after transplantation, renal arteriography was repeated, primarily to study the transplanted kidney, which showed poor function associated with the recurrence of severe hypertension. A repeat study of the patient's intact diseased kidneys (Fig. 58-9D–F) showed a dramatic decrease in their size (see Fig. 58-9A–C). In addition, there was a striking increase in the vascular tortuosity and evidence of inceased renal ischemia. The glomerulonephritic kidneys were removed and studied; severe cortical atrophy was found. The patient is now 24 months posttransplant, and he is doing well clinically.

The characteristic irregularities apparent in the intrarenal vessels in the selective arteriogram suggested that vasculitis or glomerulonephritis was responsible for the renal failure. The follow-up angiographic studies showed the progression of the lesion to a chronic, irreversible stage. The final studies, especially, exemplified how angiography may be of value in identifying chronic renal disease in the patient who appears with an apparent acute illness of obscure origin. It is this possibility that leads to renal biopsy in some patients with the apparent acute onset of renal failure and an unusual clinical course when the plain film of the abdomen does not provide a clear indication of renal size. It is interesting in this regard that renal arteriography has been suggested by Junghagen et al. as a supplement to percutaneous renal biopsy to allow kidney localization in patients with renal failure [45]. Unfortunately, the arteriograms obtained in their extensive series were not described. It seems likely that the arteriographic findings in some of the cases would have made the subsequent biopsy unnecessary if they had suggested end-stage chronic renal disease. The angiographic findings in patients with acute renal failure due to accelerated nephrosclerosis and scleroderma are similar to those in acute oliguric glomerulonephritis.

Moreover advanced nephrosclerosis, when present, will interfere with recovery from acute renal failure (Fig. 58-10).

POLYARTERITIS NODOSA

A patient with vasculitis due to polyarteritis nodosa or hypersensitivity angiitis may appear with acute oliguric renal failure [12, 51]. The presence of hypertension, the protean clinical manifestations, and the characteristics of the urinalysis frequently suggest the diagnosis [18, 51]. In some patients, however, such clues may be absent [51]. The vasculitis generally involves the cortical vasculature and is diagnosed by renal biopsy, but in some patients the cortical vasculature is spared, and the involvement of more proximal vessels predominates [12, 18]. In such patients, the renal lesion can be demonstrated before death only by arteriography.

Polyarteritis nodosa produces in the renal arterial tree the same characteristic pattern of multiple small aneurysms seen elsewhere in the body [10, 57, 78]. Washout of contrast agent from the aneurysms may be delayed, and occluded vessels produce multiple scattered cortical infarcts of varying size, resulting in an irregular renal outline. The nonaneurysmal intrarenal arteries are attenuated and stretched. The multiple small aneurysms of polyarteritis nodosa must be differentiated from the severe but more uniformly distributed irregularities of the vessel wall seen in other diseases, such as malignant nephrosclerosis and glomerulonephritis. Reversal of aneurysmal changes with time has been documented by Robins and Bookstein [82]. These changes were unrelated to therapeutic maneuvers. Little has been documented on the angiographic appearance of hypersensitivity angiitis.

ACUTE RENAL TRANSPLANT REJECTION

Acute allograft rejection of sufficient severity to induce oliguric renal failure is characterized arteriographically by the slow transit of contrast medium throughout the kidney, loss of visualization of the more peripheral intrarenal arteries, and loss of the cortical nephrogram as seen in the syndromes described above [3, 41, 68, 92, 99]. The associated hemodynamic abnormalities are also similar [41, 83]. The difficulty in diagnosing acute allograft rejection in the early post-

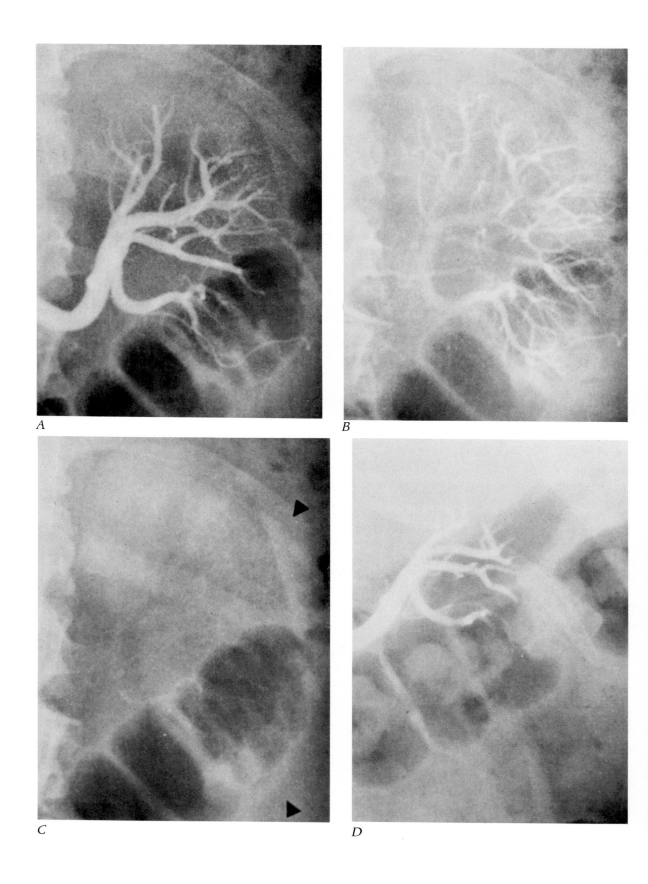

A

B

C

D

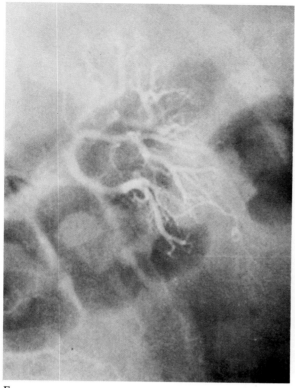

E

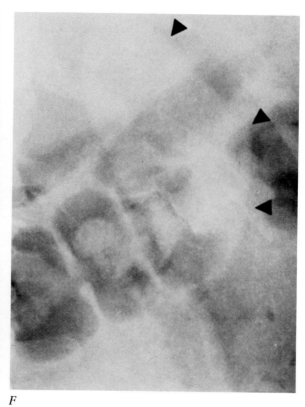

F

Figure 58-9. Acute oliguric renal failure in association with glomerulonephritis. This 45-year-old man was hospitalized because of fever, hematuria, and progressive azotemia. The renal failure became more profound in the following 2 weeks, and the patient became oliguric. Renal arteriography was undertaken because of associated severe hypertension. Subsequently, renal transplantation was undertaken, and the patient was restudied. (A, B, and C) Arteriography during the acute illness. (A and B) Arterial phase. The central vessels are large and spread out; there is an abrupt, striking tapering in the periphery. The kidney is grossly enlarged. The peripheral vessels, seen best in (B), show rather striking wall irregularity and moderate tortuosity. The arcuate vessels are poorly filled. Beading is also apparent in some of the intermediate vessels. (C) The nephrogram is relatively faint, and cortical perfusion is profoundly diminished although the edge of the kidney is defined (*arrows*). (D, E, and F) Selective renal arteriography of the same kidney, 2½

months later. At this time, no function had returned. (D and E) Arterial phase. The kidney has shrunk markedly in the interval, and the vessels have become significantly more tortuous. The interlobular vessels are not visible. Severe angulation and beading compare with (B). (F) Nephrogram. Faint, homogeneous opacification of kidney is apparent (*arrows*), with striking absence of corticomedullary differentiation. Compare with (C) and note the profound change in size in this end-stage kidney. The study during the acute phase, which was associated with marked swelling, a relatively large renovascular bed, and moderate irregularity and tortuosity of the vessels, suggests that a parenchymal lesion is responsible for the oliguria but that the renal failure need not be irreversible. By contrast, the later study (D, E, and F) clearly demonstrates a shrunken kidney with gross vessel abnormality, in which recovery of the renal function can no longer be expected.

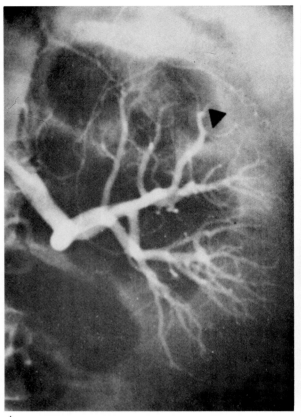

A

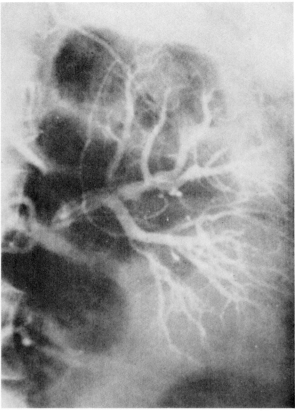

B

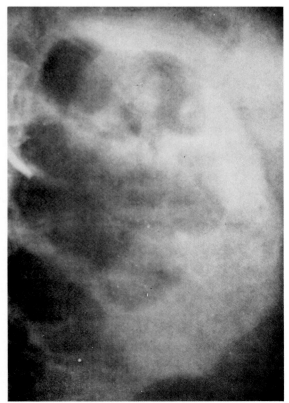

C

Figure 58-10. Nephrosclerosis complicating acute renal failure. This 53-year-old man developed postoperative acute oliguric renal failure, which failed to reverse. Biopsy suggested acute tubular necrosis (ATN) without healing and only slight arteriolar nephrosclerosis. (A) Arterial phase. The main renal artery and the major branches are normal. The interlobar arteries show some irregularity of the edge, but extreme narrowing is seen at the junction with the arcuate arteries (*arrow*) and in the arcuate vessels themselves. (B) Later arterial phase. The irregular narrowing and beading are better demonstrated with no filling of the interlobar vessels. (C) Nephrographic phase. The absence of a clearly defined cortical zone is the most striking finding. This patient's oliguria persisted for 3½ months, when transplantation was performed. The nephrectomy specimens revealed diffuse sclerotic lesions of the distal interlobar and arcuate arteries, with profound diminution in the lumen beyond, which explains the poor cortical perfusion and the failure to recover. Note that the changes in the arcuate and distal interlobar vessels are more striking than those seen in ATN. Because the biopsy yields tissue only from the cortex of the kidney, it fails to reveal nephrosclerotic change in the arcuate vessels.

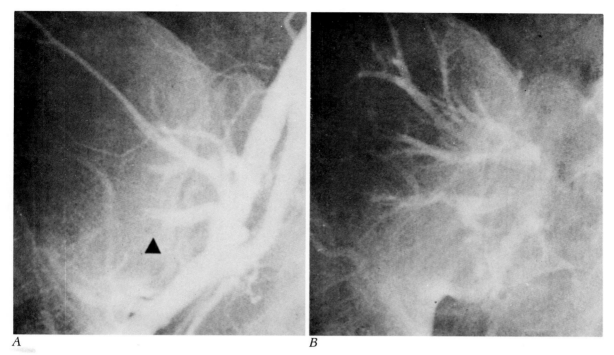

A   *B*

Figure 58-11. Hyperacute rejection with cortical necrosis in a transplanted kidney. This 43-year-old man had had a kidney transplantation 10 days prior to arteriographic study. After the transplantation, he was anuric. Arteriography was performed to define the status of the anastomosed main renal artery and the intrarenal arterial branches. (A) Early arterial phase. The internal iliac artery and the major renal artery are patent, excluding the possibility of thrombus at the site of the anastomosis. The large branches are truncated, and there is evidence of thrombus in a number of different branches (*arrow*). (B) Two and a half seconds later. Contrast material remains in the larger branches and in the interlobar branches of the kidney. No evidence of distribution of the contrast agent to the cortex can be seen. Later films demonstrated a total absence of the nephrographic phase, as a reflection of the failure to perfuse the small vessels of the kidney. Note that many of the branches are irregular, with small marginal defects. Pathologic examination of the kidney confirmed the presence of multiple clots in many small branches and total necrosis of the cortex of the kidney. In patients with acute oliguric nephropathy, total absence of the nephrographic phase has been found only in those who have acute cortical necrosis.

operative period has complicated the precise definition of the characteristic angiographic changes of rejection in man. Acute tubular necrosis is also a common complication of the ischemia associated with allograft placement and is associated with a similar reduction in flow.

Our clinical experience with studies in 25 kidneys oliguric from the time of transplantation suggests that a difference in the vascular pattern may be present. Patients with unequivocal rejection frequently show marginal irregularities in the vessel walls with irregular tapering apparently related in degree to the severity of the rejection phenomenon. The changes resemble those described above for glomerulonephritis and can be differentiated from the smooth and even tapering associated with ATN. The kidneys also generally show the manifestations of intrarenal edema. The

angiographic characteristics of the oliguric kidney, including the loss of the peripheral vasculature, the loss of the cortical nephrogram, and a delayed transit time, are present in all patients.

Studies of the renal angiographic changes associated with rejection unmodified by immunosuppressive therapy in the dog have not had consistent results [48, 98]. Further investigation is clearly required in this area, especially with immunosuppressive therapy in animal models, to slow the rate of rejection and to mimic the situation in man more closely.

RENAL CORTICAL NECROSIS

In patients with hyperacute rejection resulting in renal cortical necrosis, the renal angiographic and hemodynamic changes are extreme; and in most cases the diagnosis can be suspected strongly from the characteristics of the angiogram (Fig. 58-11). The interlobar arteries show marked filling defects that represent intravascular thrombus, and the arteries are strikingly diminished in size. The more distal vessels are unrecognizable. The nephrogram is much more abnormal than it is in the other states; it is essentially nonexistent. These angiographic features also characterize the cortical necrosis found in thrombotic thrombocytopenic purpura and other disease states.

Postrenal Cause of Acute Oliguric Renal Failure: Ureteral Obstruction

Ureteral obstruction as a cause of renal failure is most directly diagnosed by retrograde ureteral catheterization. Retrograde ureteral catheterization was once routinely carried out on one side in the patient with acute renal failure of obscure cause. In certain clinical settings, however, this approach was impossible: severe trauma with pelvic fractures made cystoscopy difficult. In kidney transplants, ureteral reimplantation often impeded retrograde catheter passage. Renal arteriography thus provided an approach to the assessment of obstruction. Recent refinements in nephrotomography with intravenous urography and advances in diagnostic ultrasonography and in CT have now provided first-line approaches to the diagnosis of ureteral obstruction once caliceal dilatation has ensued [26, 30, 85, 105]. We have studied two patients with oliguric renal failure after renal homotransplantation who had clinically unsuspected obstruction of the ureter that was identified by arteriography. Before the development of severe hydronephrosis, the vessels in the arteriogram appeared surprisingly normal for the degree of functional abnormality present. The kidney was large, the nephrographic phase was especially dense, and contrast medium appeared in the collecting system during the later phases of the arteriogram. In these patients, little or no opacification was evident in the intravenous pyelogram. The difference was presumably due to the higher concentration of contrast agent presented to the glomerulus for filtration during arteriography [36].

Illustrative Case

G. L., a 14-year-old girl with chronic glomerulonephritis, received a kidney transplant from her mother. The transplant procedure was apparently uncomplicated, with an ischemic interval of 43 minutes. The patient remained oliguric postoperatively. A transient diuresis occurred in response to increased immunosuppressive therapy with Imuran and prednisone in the second week. An intravenous pyelogram failed to visualize the kidney. Renal biopsy on the twenty-second day after the transplantation showed interstitial edema; a mild, patchy interstitial lymphocytic infiltrate; normal small arteries and arterioles; and viable parenchyma. There was no response to local irradiation of the kidney.

In the fifth postoperative week, after 10 days of absolute anuria and repeated unsuccessful attempts at retrograde ureteral catheterization, a renal angiogram was done (Fig. 58-12). The relatively normal intrarenal vasculature and the late appearance of contrast medium in the dilated renal calices suggested ureteral obstruction. Exploration 2 days later revealed ureteral obstruction secondary to a peritoneal fold. Correction of the obstruction was followed by a dramatic diuresis—daily urine outputs exceeding 2 liters—and a drop in the serum creatinine level to 0.8 mg per 100 cc without dialysis. Other than complications associated with a ureteral leak 2 weeks later, the patient's renal function has been well maintained.

In patients with chronic obstruction leading to severe hydronephrosis and parenchymal atrophy, the renal arterial system tends to be displaced around the dilated renal pelvis. There are considerable elongation and stretching of the intrarenal branches and a diminution in the size of the main renal artery in approximate proportion to the amount of parenchymal atrophy. The nephrogram is variable in quality and intensity, and in severe hydronephrosis it may be visible only as a thin, dense rim around the kidney.

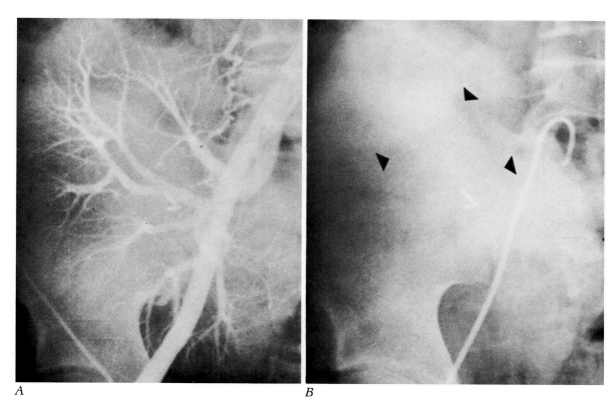

A   *B*

Figure 58-12. Acute anuria due to ureteral obstruction after transplantation. (A) Arteriographic phase. The large and small vessels are well defined and normal in appearance. Multiple interlobar, arcuate, and interlobular vessels are defined. The interlobular vessels are visualized well into the cortex of the kidney. (B) Nephrographic phase. The cortex is well perfused with the contrast agent. On the original films, the cortex of the kidney could be defined separately from the medulla. The nephrographic film was obtained after a second injection, so that contrast agent can now be seen in the collecting system of the kidney, which is grossly dilated (*arrows*). Both the calices and the pelvis are hydronephrotic and clearly indicated the presence of obstructive uropathy. Note the enlarged, swollen kidney. This patient appeared with the classic manifestations of acute rejection; if the underlying cause of her anuria had not been clarified, she might well have been subjected to aggressive immunosuppressive therapy. In such patients, it is critical to define the presence of obstructive uropathy as a remediable cause of anuria and so to obviate immunosuppressive therapy and its hazards.

Renal Vein Thrombosis

Patients with renal vein thrombosis generally appear with heavy proteinuria and the clinical features of the nephrotic syndrome. If the thrombosis is acute and bilateral, oliguric renal failure may develop. Renal failure generally ensues when there is inadequate collateral venous drainage because of propagation of the thrombus into the small renal veins or the collateral supply.

In the arteriogram, renal vein thrombosis characteristically results in deviation and stretching of the interlobar branches secondary to intrarenal edema. The density of the cortical nephrogram is reduced, and some swelling of the medullary pyramids may be evident [14, 37]. An important arteriographic manifestation of renal vein thrombosis is frequently evident during the venous phase, when multiple collateral veins draining the region of the kidney may be seen. This is not likely to be a useful sign in the patient with oliguric renal failure, however, because the renal failure occurs in this setting only when there is an inadequate collateral venous supply. It must be emphasized that the renal vein is so rarely demonstrated during arteriography in patients with acute renal failure that the absence of venous opacification is a poor indicator of renal vein thrombosis. Renal vein catheterization and venography make the diagnosis definitive.

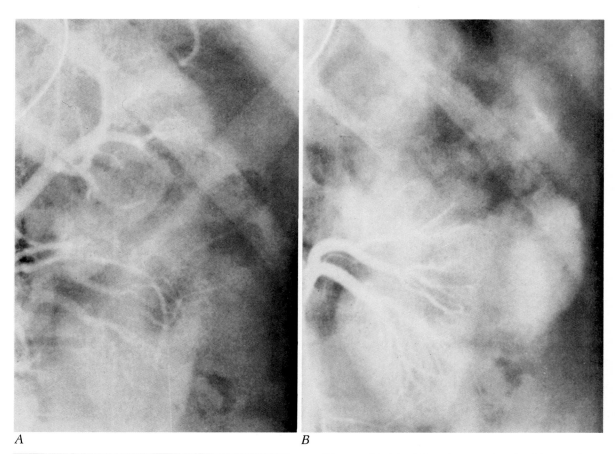

A   B

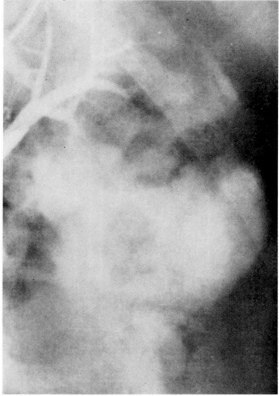

C

Figure 58-13. Oliguria associated with renal trauma (patient B. T.). This 20-year-old woman fell from a second-story balcony with resultant trauma to the kidney and spleen. She had significant blood loss. A preliminary intravenous urogram indicated the presence of blood in the left flank. There was no evidence of filling of the caliceal system on the left although faint ureteral opacification was observed. In addition, there was a suggestion of extravasated contrast agent. (A) Aortogram. Both renal arteries are opacified, the one to the upper pole far more densely. In addition, there is a central area with a conspicuous absence of renal arterial branches. No evidence of staining of the renal parenchyma in this midsegment of the kidney is noted. (B) Selective renal arteriogram, main left renal artery. This vessel supplies the lower segment and the midsegment of the kidney. The branches to the midsegment of the kidney are poorly filled, and no evidence of arcuate vessel opacification is present. By comparison, there is relatively good filling of the lower pole of the kidney, with good definition of the arcuate arteries and interlobular vessels. The collection of contrast agent that lies outside the kidney, adjacent to its midsegment, is particularly striking. Note that this was not present in (A) but has followed the bolus arteriogram, in which the kidney was presented with a relatively

Renal Nonfunction After Trauma

Oliguric renal failure is a common complication of massive trauma. Both prerenal azotemia due to volume depletion and established ATN frequently occur in this setting. Retroperitoneal hemorrhage or direct trauma to the lower urinary tract may result in ureteral obstruction. In the patient with only one kidney, direct trauma to the kidney may result in renal failure. Arteriography provides potentially important information, not only about the patient's renal status but also about the effects of the trauma on other intraabdominal structures. The patient described in the following case study did not present with oliguric renal failure, but her case is an excellent example of the clinically useful information that may be obtained by arteriography in this setting.

Illustrative Case

B. T., a 20-year-old woman, was admitted to the hospital with complaints of left flank pain and back pain after a fall from a second-story balcony. There were tenderness, rigidity, and guarding of the left side of the abdomen. Gross hematuria was present; four units of blood were required to produce a stable cardiovascular state and to raise the hematocrit from 28 to 40. An intravenous pyelogram failed to visualize the left kidney. In the ensuing 18 hours, sinus tachycardia developed and the hematocrit continued to fall, suggesting continued internal bleeding. Arteriography revealed a subcapsular splenic hematoma and a ruptured left kidney with spilling of filtered contrast medium into the retroperitoneal space from the torn renal pelvis (Fig. 58-13). The patient did well after a splenectomy and a left nephrectomy.

---

large volume of contrast agent. This collection is a reflection of the trauma to the kidney and represents extravasation into an opacified hematoma. (C) Selective arteriography, upper pole artery. The irregular linear density in the proximal portion of the artery represents subintimal injection. The branches to the upper pole are filled centrally, but there is relatively poor opacification in the periphery. Subsequent films showed irregularity of the cortical distribution of the contrast agent, and further arteriographic studies demonstrated that there was an associated rupture of the spleen. At surgery, nephrectomy and splenectomy were performed. The kidney was ruptured, with a large collection of blood communicating directly with the renal pelvis.

Relative Advantages and Disadvantages of Renal Arteriography

The decision to undertake renal arteriography in the evaluation of a patient with an acute failure of renal function can be based only on a weighing of the potential yield of clinically useful information against the potential morbidity of arteriography. If the probability of renal embolism or thrombosis is high, the importance of the information to be gained far outweighs any potential risk, and arteriography is the diagnostic procedure of choice, to be carried out without delay. In the patient with probable obstruction of the lower urinary tract, arteriography should be considered only when the cause of obstruction requires further definition or when retrograde ureteral catheterization is technically impossible and urography, ultrasonography, and CT do not establish the diagnosis.

When ATN runs an atypical course and when there is the possibility that acute renal parenchymal disease, vasculitis, cortical necrosis, or undiagnosed chronic renal failure contributes to the oliguria, the information yield and the morbidity of arteriography must be compared directly to the potential yield and risk of renal biopsy although the procedures are not mutually exclusive.

Renal biopsy is a well-established procedure for the evaluation of the kidney under these circumstances. In experienced hands, percutaneous renal biopsy is a procedure that has a measurable but low morbidity and an almost nonexistent mortality. In less experienced hands, however, as with other procedures, the morbidity and the other potential dangers of renal biopsy increase. In many centers, open renal biopsy rather than percutaneous renal biopsy is done. Although open renal biopsy may reduce the risk of severe hemorrhage, anesthesia is generally required. The major problem wih the diagnostic information available in a renal biopsy is that of patchy, nonuniformly distributed sampling. For example, it is not uncommon for a biopsy to miss areas of chronic pyelonephritis.

In the clinical problems discussed in this chapter, a major difficulty arises when an area of necrosis is sampled, suggesting that the kidney is not viable. In other patients, the biopsy may not be diagnostic. In the transplanted kidney, for example, the diagnosis of cortical necrosis may lead to nephrectomy. If the necrosis is local and the remainder of the kidney is viable, the biopsy may lead to an unwarranted therapeutic approach. Cortical necrosis in the nontransplanted kidney may also be local and compatible with the recovery of sufficient renal function to sustain life [32, 81, 101]. The following case study illustrates the sampling problem in renal biopsy.

Illustrative Case

E. C., a 29-year-old man with chronic glomerulonephritis, received a kidney from his brother. The period of ischemia was 2 hours. The kidney had an excellent appearance after the opening of the anastomosis, but it remained flaccid and initially no urine was passed. The urine output gradually increased to 100 cc per hour in the first several hours, but the patient had considerable bleeding both from the incision and in the urinary tract, requiring evacuation of clots. Twelve hours later the urine output decreased abruptly, and it was necessary to carry out a suprapubic cystostomy. A ureteral catheter did not reinitiate the brisk diuresis. During the next 3 days, the patient remained oliguric despite increased immunosuppressive therapy. On the fourth postoperative day, a renal arteriogram (Fig. 58-14) and an open renal biopsy were carried out. The kidney did not appear viable at surgery, and the histologic sections revealed cortical necrosis. Because of these findings and the patient's stormy clinical course, a nephrectomy was carried out. Study of the kidney revealed a central necrotic area fanning out from one column to the cortex. There was recent thrombus in the vessels supplying this region.

In retrospect, these findings were apparent in the arteriogram that was carried out primarily to assess the arterial anastomosis, which was intact. The implications of the arteriographic findings in the more distal renal vessels were not fully appreciated. The arterial supply to the central portion of the kidney was profoundly diminished, and a nephrogram was absent in this area. The vessels to the upper and lower poles were opacified, however, and were similar to those seen in ATN. Although it might ultimately have been necessary to carry out nephrectomy in this patient, it is also possible that the kidney would have survived and provided reasonable renal function.

Although it lacks the specificity of a positive renal biopsy, arteriography offers the distinct advantage of assessing the entire kidney, thus avoiding the sampling problem implicit in renal biopsy. It also appears that renal arteriography can provide information on many of the points for which a biopsy is carried out. The arteriographic findings may suggest the presence of an acute parenchymal disease, as opposed to un-

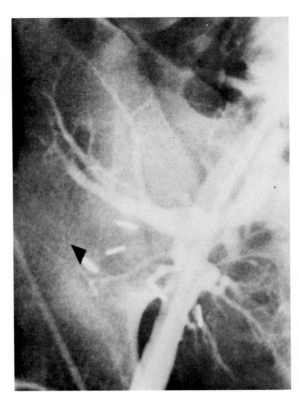

Figure 58-14. Localized cortical necrosis in a transplanted kidney (patient E. C.). This 29-year-old man with chronic renal failure had transplantation performed 5 days before the arteriogram. After surgery he developed oliguria and hematuria. Arteriography was performed to exclude the presence of renal artery obstruction and to determine the status of the intrarenal vascular bed. Arteriography showed no evidence of obstruction at the anastomotic site. The intrarenal vessels to the upper pole were well opacified, as were those to the lower pole. There was, however, poor flow to the midsegment of the kidney (*arrow*). In addition, films during the nephrographic phase demonstrated a nephrogram in the lower pole, and in the upper pole as well. Renal biopsy shortly after arteriography demonstrated acute cortical necrosis. The kidney was removed, and a localized area of cortical necrosis was found in the segment that appears ischemic on the arteriogram. The rest of the kidney, however, was pink and apparently viable. The sharp localization of this lesion had not been appreciated on the original arteriographic study. The presence of a cortical nephrogram in the upper and lower portions of the kidney should have indicated that the patient's oliguria was potentially reversible.

complicated ATN, and can rule out the presence of vascular or chronic parenchymal disease and, probably, cortical necrosis. In addition, previously unsuspected ureteral obstruction may be identified on the basis of a renal arteriogram. Another dividend of renal arteriography is the immediate availability of the diagnostic information it provides. Tissue processing after renal biopsy generally takes 1 to 2 days.

The renal arteriogram as a prelude to percutaneous transluminal angioplasty may also be useful in the treatment of patients with chronic renal failure when there is a strong clinical suspicion that renal artery occlusion contributes to the renal failure.

Percutaneous Transluminal Angioplasty

Dotter and Judkins in 1964 introduced the original approach to percutaneous transluminal angioplasty (PTA), which employed coaxial dilatation with progressively larger dilatation catheters [21]. Grüntzig in 1976 introduced a double-lumen catheter with an expansile balloon near its tip to dilate atherosclerotic and other obstructive lesions [34]. The first application of this technique to the renal arteries was reported by Grüntzig in 1978 [35]. In the past 2 years, numerous reports on the use of this technique for the treatment of atherosclerotic and fibromuscular diseases of the renal artery have appeared and have included detailed early results in approximately 150 patients [35, 47, 49, 55, 56, 61, 86, 91, 93].

The results suggest that PTA can (1) improve blood pressure control in patients with either atherosclerotic or fibromuscular disease, (2) improve renal excretory function, and (3) even restore renal function in patients with moderately advanced renal failure [103]. The advantages of PTA over surgery include reduced cost, reduced morbidity, immediate ambulation, and the possibility of easy repetition of the procedure. Percutaneous transluminal angioplasty does not preclude surgery. The complications reported to date include the anticipated embolization, femoral artery aneurysm, restenosis of a dilated artery, and contrast media–induced renal failure. The potential complications (anticipated but not yet reported) include rupture, thrombosis, and aneurysm of the renal artery.

With so few reported cases and the generally short follow-up (less than 2 years), it is far too early to predict precisely what role PTA will play in the attack on renovascular hypertension. But PTA, a moderately invasive approach whose early results have been extremely promising, will clearly have some impact. We can predict, by analogy with the surgical treatment of renovascular hypertension, that the initial reports on PTA will be positive, even enthusiastic, and that then a wave of negative papers will probably appear. The preliminary results suggest that PTA will be as effective as surgery in reversing hypertension and preserving renal function, will certainly be safer in high-risk patients, and perhaps will be the first approach in most patients in whom complete occlusion of the renal artery has not yet occurred.

Hazards of Arteriography

The hazards of arteriography are discussed in two sections in this text. The first (Chap. 2) gives a detailed analysis of the hazards of the contrast material. The second section (Chap. 23) deals with the hazards of the technique itself. Modern radiographic contrast material used for arteriography appears to be well tolerated in patients with normal renal function. The initial available reports on high-dose intravenous pyelography in patients with advanced renal insufficiency seemed to indicate that the procedure was relatively benign [5, 31, 33, 67]. Exceptions to the rule were noted in such specific instances as diabetes mellitus [17, 19, 104] and multiple myeloma [7, 61, 65]. More recent studies indicate that there is a higher incidence of increased renal failure in a broad spectrum of individuals with initial renal impairment after angiography or high-dose urography [58, 69, 79, 97]. The reason for the discrepancy between these various reports is not clear. Experimental work by Walsh et al., who used an animal model of renal failure that was supplemented by work using large doses of contrast agents, did not demonstrate a significant increase in the degree of renal failure induced by Renografin. When older types of contrast material (e.g., Urokon) were used, there was significant evidence of increased renal failure [102]. Renal impairment does not preclude angiography when it is indicated.

Summary

Useful information may be obtained from renal angiography in a number of conditions characterized by the acute onset of oliguric renal failure. In several circumstances, arteriography is the diagnostic method of choice in the evaluation of the patient. In other circumstances, the information available from renal arteriography can be useful in establishing a prognosis, deciding on the treatment, and assessing the sampling problem in a renal biopsy. Considerably more experience is required, however, before the use of angiography is advocated in any but special clinical situations in which its yield seems likely to be high.

Many features of the arteriogram are common to many of the conditions that result in oliguria. These features, such as a failure of visualization of cortical vessels, a decrease in the cortical nephrogram, and a decreased transit time, appear to reflect a preferential decrease in the cortical perfusion.

Other arteriographic features may provide clues to the specific etiology. Visible venous collateral vessels suggest renal vein thrombosis. Disruption of the renal contour suggests trauma. Normal cortical vessels and a dense cortical nephrogram, especially when coupled with visualization of dilated pelvic and caliceal structures, suggest ureteral obstruction. In the late phases of ureteral obstruction, hydronephrosis with stretching of the vessels and severe thinning of a dense cortex is diagnostic.

In the other diseases that cause oliguria, the differential features are in the interlobar and the arcuate vessels. If these vessels are smooth walled and taper rapidly, ATN is usually the cause. ATN in the renal transplant is also accompanied by smooth, rapidly tapered vessels. In the milder forms of hepatorenal syndrome, smooth tapering of the intermediate vessels may be present.

Multiple frank aneurysms are apparent in the intermediate vessels in polyarteritis nodosa. Severe attenuation and beading of the vessels with frank aneurysm formation are characteristic of the more severe forms of hepatorenal syndrome. Malignant nephrosclerosis, glomerulonephritis, and transplant rejection also show severe pruning of the peripheral vasculature, but marginal irregularity and tortuosity of the vessels may help to distinguish these conditions from ATN.

References

1. Abrams, H. L., Marshall, W. H., and Kupic, E. A. The renal vascular bed in hypertension. *Semin. Roentgenol.* 2:157, 1967.

2. Adams, D. F., Epstein, M., Berk, D. P., Hollenberg, N. K., Merrill, J. P., and Abrams, H. L. Renal circulatory alteration in the hepatorenal syndrome. *Radiol. Soc. North Am. Abstr.* 54:64, 1968.

3. Alfidi, R. H. L., Meaney, T. F., Buonocore, E., and Nakamoto, S. Evaluation of renal homotransplantation by selective angiography. *Radiology* 87:1099, 1966.

4. Bank, N., Mutz, B. F., and Aynedjian, H. S. The role of "leakage" of tubular fluid in anuria due to mercury poisoning. *J. Clin. Invest.* 46:695, 1967.

5. Bartley, O., Bengtsson, U., and Cederbom, G. Renal function before and after urography and angiography with large doses of contrast media. *Acta Radiol.* [*Diagn.*] (Stockh.) 8:9, 1969.

6. Bell, E. T. *Renal Diseases* (2nd ed.). Philadelphia: Lea & Febiger, 1950.

7. Berdon, W. E., Schwartz, R. H., Becker, J., and Baker, D. H. Tamm-Horsfall proteinuria: Its relationship to prolonged nephrogram in infants and children and to renal failure following intravenous urography in adults with multiple myeloma. *Radiology* 92:714, 1969.

8. Biachwal, K. S., and Waugh, D. Traumatic renal artery thrombosis. *J. Urol.* 99:14, 1968.

9. Block, M. A., Wakim, K. G., and Mann, F. C. Certain features of the vascular beds of the corticomedullary and medullary regions of the kidney. *Arch. Pathol.* 53:437, 1952.

10. Bron, K. M., Strott, C. A., and Shapiro, A. P. The diagnostic value of angiographic observations in polyarteritis nodosa. *Arch. Intern. Med.* 116:450, 1965.

11. Carriere, S., Thorburn, G. D., O'Morchoe, C. C. C., and Barger, A. C. Intrarenal distribution of blood flow in dogs during hemorrhagic hypotension. *Circ. Res.* 19:167, 1966.

12. Castleman, B., and McNeely, B. U. Case records of the Massachusetts General Hospital. Case 25-1968. *N. Engl. J. Med.* 278:1389, 1968.

13. Castleman, B., and McNeely, B. U. Case records of the Massachusetts General Hospital. Case 10-1969. *N. Engl. J. Med.* 280:550, 1969.

14. Chair, A., Stoane, L., Moskowitz, H., and Mellins, H. Z. Renal vein thrombosis. *Radiology* 90:886, 1968.

15. Cornell, S. H., and Culp, D. A. Acute occlusion of the renal artery demonstrated by angiography. *J. Urol.* 100:2, 1968.

16. Dalgaard, O. Z., and Pedersen, K. J. Ultrastructure of the kidney in shock. In Proceedings of the 1st International Congress of Nephrology, 1960. Amsterdam: Excerpta Medica, 1961. P. 36.

17. Daniel, P. M., Peabody, C. N., and Prichard, M. M. L. Cortical ischaemia of the kidney with maintained blood flow through the medulla. *Q. J. Exp. Physiol.* 37:11, 1952.

18. Davson, J., Ball, J. L., and Platt, R.   Kidney in periarteritis nodosa. *Q. J. Med.* 17:175, 1948.
19. Diaz-Buxo, J. A., Wagoner, R. D., Hattery, R. R., and Palumbo, P. J.   Acute renal failure after excretory urography in diabetic patients. *Ann. Intern. Med.* 83:155, 1975.
20. Dinsmore, R. E.   Angiography for dissecting aneurysm of the aorta. *N. Engl. J. Med.* 280:272, 1969.
21. Dotter, C. T., and Judkins, M. P.   Transluminal treatment of arterial sclerotic obstruction: Description of a new technique and a preliminary result of its application. *Circulation* 30:654, 1964.
22. Elwood, C. M., Lucas, G. D., and Muehrcke, R. C.   Acute renal failure associated with sodium colistimethate treatment. *Arch. Intern. Med.* 118:326, 1966.
23. Epstein, M., Berk, D. P., Hollenberg, N. K., Adams, D. F., Chalmers, T. C., Abrams, H. L., and Merrill, J. P.   Renal failure in the patient with cirrhosis: The role of active vasoconstriction. *Am. J. Med.* 49:175, 1970.
24. Finckh, E. S., Jeremy, D., and Whyte, H. M.   Structural renal damage and its relation to clinical features in acute oliguric renal failure. *Q. J. Exp. Physiol.* 37:11, 1952.
25. Flanigan, W. J., and Oken, D. E.   Renal micropuncture study of the development of anuria in the rat with mercury-induced acute renal failure. *J. Clin. Invest.* 44:449, 1965.
26. Forbes, W. St. C. Isherwood, I., and Fawcitt, R. A.   Computed tomography in the evaluation of the solitary or unilateral nonfunctioning kidney. *J. Comput. Assist. Tomogr.* 2:389, 1978.
27. Foster, R. S., Shuford, W. H., and Weens, H. S.   Selective renal arteriography in medical diseases of the kidney. *AJR* 95:291, 1965.
28. Franklin, S. S., and Merrill, J. P.   Acute renal failure. *N. Engl. J. Med.* 262:711, 1960.
29. Friedenberg, M. J., Eisen, S., and Kissane, J.   Renal angiography in pyelonephritis, glomerulonephritis and arteriolar nephrosclerosis. *AJR* 95:349, 1965.
30. Fry, K. I., and Cattell, W. R.   Radiology in the diagnosis of renal failure. *Br. Med. Bull.* 27:148, 1971.
31. Fulton, R. E., Witten, D. M., and Wagoner, R. D.   Intravenous urography in renal insufficiency. *AJR* 106:623, 1969.
32. Gormsen, H., Iversen, P, and Raaschou, F.   Kidney biopsy in acute anuria with case of acute bilateral cortical necrosis. *Am. J. Med.* 19:209, 155.
33. Grainger, R. G.   Renal toxicity of radiological contrast media. *Br. Med. Bull.* 28:191, 1972.
34. Grüntzig, A.   Die perkutane Rekanalisation chronischer arterieller Verschlüsse (Dotter-Prinzip) mit einem neuen doppellumigen Dilatationskatheter. *ROEFO* 124:80, 1976.
35. Grüntzig, A., Kuhlmann, U., Vetter, W., Lutolf, U., Meier, B., and Siegenthaler, W.   Treatment of renovascular hypertension with percutaneous transluminal dilatation of a renal-artery stenosis. *Lancet* 1:801, 1978.
36. Hare, W. S. C., and Rothfield, N. J. K.   Renal artery infusion urography. *Radiology* 90:565, 1969.
37. Hipona, F. A., and Crummy, A B.   Roentgen diagnosis of renal vein thrombosis: Clinical aspects. *AJR* 98:122,1966.
38. Hollenberg, N. K., Adams, D. F., Oken, D. E., Abrams, H. L., and Merrill, J. P.   Acute renal failure due to nephrotoxins: Renal hemodynamic and angiographic studies. *N. Engl. J. Med.* 282:1329, 1970.
39. Hollenberg, N. K., Epstein, M., Basch, R. I., and Merrill, J. P.   "No man's land" of the renal vasculature: An arteriographic and hemodynamic assessment of the interlobar and arcuate arteries in essential and accelerated hypertension. *Am. J. Med.* 47:845, 1969.
40. Hollenberg, N. K., Epstein, M., Basch, R. I., Merrill, J. P., and Hickler, R. B.   Renin secretion in the patient with hypertension: Relationship to intrarenal blood flow distribution. *Circ. Res.* 24 [Suppl. 1]:113, 1969.
41. Hollenberg, N. K., Epstein, M., Rosen, S. M., Basch, R. I., Oken, D. E., and Merrill, J. P.   Acute oliguric renal failure in man: Evidence for preferential renal cortical ischemia. *Medicine* 47:455, 1968.
42. Hollenberg, N. K., Epstein, M., Rosen, S. M., Dammin, G. J., and Merrill, J. P.   Vascular lesions of the transplanted human kidney—morphologic and hemodynamic studies in chronic rejection. *Trans. Assoc. Am. Physicians* 81:274, 1968.
43. Hollenberg, N. K., Rosen, S. M., O'Connor, J. F., Potchen, E. J., Basch, R. I., Dealy, J. B., Jr., and Merrill, J. P.   Effect of aortography on renal hemodynamics in normal man. *Invest. Radiol.* 3:92, 1968.
44. Janower, M. L., and Weber, A. L.   Radiologic evaluation of acute renal infarction. *AJR* 95:309, 1965.
45. Junghagen, P., Lindqvist, B., Michaelson, G., and Nyström, K.   Percutaneous renal biopsy on uraemic patients aided by selective arterial angiography and roentgen television. *Acta Med. Scand.* 184:141, 1968.
46. Kassirer, J. P.   Atheroembolic renal disease. *N. Engl. J. Med.* 280:812, 1969.
47. Katzen, B. T., Chang, J., Lukowsky, G. H., and Abramson, E. G.   Percutaneous transluminal angioplasty for treatment of renovascular hypertension. *Radiology* 131:53, 1979.
48. Knudsen, O. F., Davidson, A. J., Kountz, S. L., and Cohn, R.   Serial angiography in canine allografts. *Transplantation* 5:256, 1967.

49. Kuhlmann, U., Vetter, W., Furrer, J., Lotolf, U., Siegenthaler, W., and Grüntzig, A. Renovascular hypertension: Treatment by percutaneous transluminal dilatation. *Ann. Intern. Med.* 92:1, 1980.

50. Kupic, E. A., and Abrams, H. L. Renal vascular alterations induced by hemorrhagic hypotension: Preliminary observations. *Invest. Radiol.* 3:345, 1968.

51. Ladefoged, J. L., Nielsen, B., Raaschou, F., and Sorensen, A. W. S. Acute anuria due to polyarteritis nodosa. *Am. J. Med.* 46:827, 1969.

52. Ladefoged, J. L., and Pedersen, F. Renal blood flow, circulation times and vascular volume in normal man measured by intra-arterial injection: External counting technique. *Acta Physiol. Scand.* 69:220, 1967.

53. Lang, E. K. Arteriographic diagnosis of renal infarcts. *Radiology* 88:1110, 1967.

54. Lavender, J. P., Sherwood, T., and Russell, S. In vivo renal micro-angiography: An experimental technique to study renal cortical perfusion during hemorrhagic shock. *Br. J. Radiol.* 42:247, 1969.

55. Mahler, F., Krneta, A., and Haertel, M. Treatment of renovascular hypertension by transluminal renal artery dilatation. *Ann. Intern. Med.* 90:56, 1979.

56. Martin, E. C., Diamond, N. G., and Casarella, W. J. Percutaneous transluminal angioplasty in nonatherosclerotic disease. *Radiology* 135:27, 1980.

57. McClure, P. H., and Westcott, J. L. Periarteritis nodosa with perirenal hemorrhage: A case report with angiographic findings. *J. Urol.* 102:126, 1969.

58. McEvoy, J., McGeown, M. G., and Kumar, R. Renal failure after radiological contrast material. *Br. Med. J.* 4:717, 1970.

59. Meriel, P., Galinier, F., and Suc, J. M. Le débit sanguin rénal dans les états de choc. In Proceedings of the 1st International Congress of Nephrology, 1960. Amsterdam: Excerpta Medica, 1961.

60. Meriel, P., Moreau, G., Suc, J. M., and Putois, J. Lesions ultrastructurales de l'insuffisance rénale aigue. In Proceedings of the 1st International Congress of Nephrology, 1960. Amsterdam: Excerpta Medica, 1961.

61. Millan, V. G., Mast, W. E., and Madias, N. E. Nonsurgical treatment of severe hypertension due to renal-artery intimal fibroplasia by percutaneous transluminal angioplasty. *N. Engl. J. Med.* 300:1371, 1979.

62. Morris, G. C., Jr., DeBakey, M. E., Cooley, D. A., and Crawford, E. S. Experience with 200 renal artery reconstructive procedures for hypertension or renal failure. *Circulation* 27:346, 1963.

63. Munck, O. *Renal Circulation in Acute Renal Failure*. Oxford: Blackwell, 1958.

64. Mundth, E. D., Shine, K., and Austen, W. G. Correction of malignant hypertension and return of renal function following late renal artery embolectomy. *Am. J. Med.* 46:985, 1969.

65. Myers, G. H., and Witten, D. M. Acute renal failure after excretory urography in multiple myeloma. *AJR* 113:583, 1971.

66. Myers, J. K., Storrs, D., Miller, T. B., and Mueller, C. B. The role of renal tubular flow in the pathogenesis of traumatic renal failure. *Surg. Gynecol. Obstet.* 123:1243, 1966.

67. Neal, M. P., Jr., Howell, T. R., and Lester, R. G. Contrast infusion nephropyelography. *J.A.M.A.* 193:1017, 1965.

68. O'Connor, J. F., Dealy, J. B., Jr., Lindquist, R., and Couch, N. P. Arterial lesions due to rejection in human kidney allografts. *Radiology* 89:614, 1967.

69. Older, R. A., Miller, J. P., Jackson, D. C., Johnsrude, I. S., and Thompson, W. M. Angiographically induced renal failure and its radiographic detection. *AJR* 126:1039, 1976.

70. Oliver, J. Correlations of structure and function and mechanisms of recovery in acute tubular necrosis. *Am. J. Med.* 15:535, 1953.

71. Olsen, T. S. Ultrastructure of the renal tubules in acute renal insufficiency. *Acta Pathol. Microbiol. Scand.* 70:205, 1967.

72. Olsen, T. S., and Skoldborg, H. The fine structure of the renal glomerulus in acute anuria. *Acta Pathol. Microbiol. Scand.* 70:205, 1967.

73. Page, L. B., and Kimmelstiel, P. Long standing proteinuria, hypertension and gout in a young woman with progressive renal failure. *N. Engl. J. Med.* 274:1374, 1966.

74. Paster, S. B., Adams, D. F., and Hollenberg, N. K. Acute renal failure in McArdle's disease and myoglobinuric states. *Radiology* 114:567, 1975.

75. Pedersen, F., Baunoe, B. O., Berthelsen, H. C., Christiansen, P., Kemp, E. L., Ladefoged, J., and Winkler, K. Renal blood flow and mean circulation time for red cells and plasma in acute renal failure. *Proc. Eur. Dial. Transplant. Assoc.* 2:77, 1965.

76. Perkins, R. P., Jacobsen, D. S., Feder, F. P., Lipchik, E. O., and Fine, P. H. Return of renal function after late embolectomy. *N. Engl. J. Med.* 276:1194, 1967.

77. Pillay, V. K. G., Robbins, P. C., Schwartz, F. D., and Kark, R. M. Acute renal failure following intravenous urography in patients with longstanding diabetes mellitus and azotemia. *Radiology* 95:633, 1970.

78. Pollard, J. J., and Nebesar, R. A. Abdominal angiography. *N. Engl. J. Med.* 279:1035, 1968.

79. Port, F. K., Wagoner, R. O., and Fulton,

R. E.   Acute renal failure after angiography. *AJR* 121:544, 1974.

80. Reubi, F. C., Grossweiler, N., and Gurtler, R.   Renal circulation in man studied by means of a dye-dilution method. *Circulation* 33:426, 1966.

81. Riff, D. P., Wilson, D. M., Dunea, G., Schwartz, F. D., and Kark, R. M.   Renocortical necrosis. *Arch. Intern. Med.* 119:518, 1967.

82. Robins, J. M., and Bookstein, J. J.   Regressing aneurysms in periarteritis nodosa: A report of 3 cases. *Radiology* 104:39, 1972.

83. Rosen, S. M., Hollenberg, N. K., Dealy, J. B., Jr., and Merrill, J. P.   Measurement of the distribution of blood flow in the human kidney using the intraarterial injection of ^{133}Xe: Relationship to function in the normal and transplanted kidney. *Clin. Sci.* 34:287, 1968.

84. Ruiz-Guinazu, A., Coelho, J. B., and Paz, R. A.   Methemoglobin-induced acute renal failure in the rat. *Nephron* 4:257, 1967.

85. Sanders, R. C., and Jeck, D. L.   B-scan ultrasound in the evaluation of renal failure. *Radiology* 119:199, 1976.

86. Schwarten, D. E., Yune, H. Y., Klatte, E. C., Grim, C. E., and Weinberger, M. H.   Clinical experience with percutaneous transluminal angioplasty (PTA) of stenotic renal arteries. *Radiology* 135:601, 1980.

87. Shaldon, S., Sheville, E., and Rae, A. I.   Angiography in acute renal failure. *Clin. Radiol.* 15:123, 1964.

88. Shuford, W. H., Sybers, R. G., and Weens, H. S.   Problems in the aortographic diagnosis of dissecting aneurysm of the aorta. *N. Engl. J. Med.* 280:225, 1969.

89. Siegelman, S. S., and Goldman, A. G.   The Trueta phenomenon: Angiographic documentation in man. *Radiology* 90:1084, 1968.

90. Smith, H. T., Shapiro, F. L., and Messner, R. P.   Anuria secondary to renovascular disease. *J.A.M.A.* 204:176, 1968.

91. Sniderman, K. W., Sol, T. A., Sprayregen, S., Saddekni, S., Cheigh, J. S., Tapia, L., Tellis, V., and Veith, F. J.   Percutaneous transluminal angioplasty in renal transplant arterial stenosis for relief of hypertension. *Radiology* 135:23, 1980.

92. Staple, T. W., and Chiang, D. T. C.   Arteriography following renal transplantation. *AJR* 101:669, 1967.

93. Tegtmeyer, C. J., Dyer, R., Teates, C. D., Ayers, C. R., Carey, R. M., Wellons, H. A., Jr., and Stanton, L. W.   Percutaneous transluminal di-

latation of the renal arteries: Technique and results. *Radiology* 135:589, 1980.

94. Thorburn, G. D., Kapald, H. H., Herd, J. A., Hollenberg, M., O'Morchoe, C. C. C., and Barger, A. C.   Intrarenal distribution of nutrient blood flow determined with krypton^{85} in the unanesthetized dog. *Circ. Res.* 13:290, 1963.

95. Thurau, K.   Renal hemodynamics. *Am. J. Med.* 36:698, 1964.

96. Trueta, J., Barclay, A. E., Daniel, P. M., Franklin, K. J., and Prichard, M. M. L.   *Studies of the Renal Circulation.* Springfield, Ill.: Thomas, 1947.

97. Truniger, B., Rosen, S. M., and Oken, D. E.   Renale Haemodynamik and haemorrhagische hypotension. *Klin. Wochenschr.* 44:857, 1966.

98. Vinik, M., Smellie, W. A. B., Freed, T. A., Hume, D. M., and Weidner, W. A.   Angiographic evaluation of the human homotransplant kidney. *Radiology* 92:873, 1969.

99. Vinik, M., Smellie, W. A. B., Freed, T. A., Hume, D. M., and Weidner, W. A.   Renal ischemia and homograft rejection: Preliminary angiographic data in the dog. *Invest. Radiol.* 4:252, 1969.

100. Walker, J. G., Silva, H., Lawson, T. R., Ryder, J. A., and Shaldon, S.   Renal blood flow in acute renal failure measured by renal arterial infusion of indocyanine green. *Proc. Soc. Exp. Biol. Med.* 112:932, 1963.

101. Walls, J., Schorr, W. J., and Kerr, D. N. S.   Prolonged oliguria with survival in acute bilateral cortical necrosis. *Br. Med. J.* 4:220, 1968.

102. Walsh, P. C., Gittes, R. G., and Lecky, J. W.   Aortography in experimental renal failure: Evaluation of contrast media toxicity. *Radiology* 97:33, 1970.

103. Weinberger, M. H., Yune, H. Y., Grim, C. E., Luft, F. C., Klatte, E. C., and Donohue, J. P.   Percutaneous transluminal angioplasty for renal artery stenosis in a solitary functioning kidney. *Ann. Intern. Med.* 91:684, 1979.

104. Weinrauch, L. A., Healy, R. W., Leland, O. S., Goldstein, H. H., Kassissieh, S. D., Libertino, J. A., Takacs, F. J., and D'Elia, J. A.   Coronary angiography and acute renal failure in diabetic azotemic nephropathy. *Ann. Intern. Med.* 86:56, 1977.

105. Winston, M., Pritchard, M. D., and Paulin, P.   ARRT ultrasonography in the management of unexplained renal failure. *J. Clin. Ultrasound* 6:23, 1978.

Renal Venography

HERBERT L. ABRAMS

In the past, renal vein catheterization has been employed both in physiologic studies and in radiologic studies. Within recent years its usefulness has been emphasized particularly in the study of renal vein thrombosis in patients whose clinical and laboratory examinations are suggestive of that diagnosis. It has also been applied extensively to the investigation of patients with malignant disease of the kidney, and it has been helpful in confirming the presumptive diagnosis of renal agenesis, the presence of renal vein abnormalities in transplant patients, and the likelihood of closure of splenorenal shunts. It has been used in essential hematuria to search for renal vein varices and has played an important role in the determination of renin levels in the renal venous effluent. A relatively simple procedure technically, it may be highly rewarding when properly performed in selected cases.

Technique

A flexible, radiopaque catheter (Fig. 59-1A) large enough to permit a sufficiently rapid injection (e.g., a gray Kifa catheter) is passed percutaneously into the right femoral vein and advanced to the level of the renal vein. The catheter tip should be bent 130 degrees. The bent tip should be about 5 cm long on the right catheter and about 10 cm long on the left catheter; it is, however, possible to use the right catheter for both sides if a guidance system is used for placement into the distal left renal vein. Alternatively, a catheter with less curvature (e.g., an abdominal-visceral catheter) may be introduced into both renal veins with a controllable guidewire. The catheter should have two side holes within 1 cm of its tip. For selective catheterization of segmental veins, the tip may be deflected downward an additional 30 degrees. With different degrees of rotation, various portions of the intrarenal venous system may be catheterized. A coaxial catheter system or a controllable tip guidewire facilitates some examinations [89].

Total sustained opacification of the renal venous bed is best obtained with deliberate slowing of the renal blood flow by injecting 10 μg of epinephrine into the renal artery through a selectively placed arterial catheter [87]. Since tumor vessels are less responsive than normal vessels, epinephrine is often not useful in improving the visualization of the veins draining renal

1327

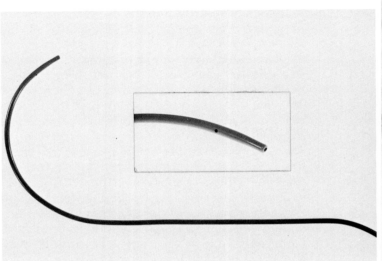

A

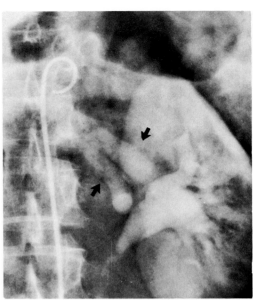

B

Figure 59-1. Technique of renal venography. (A) Renal vein catheter. The catheter has a curve of about 130 degrees, with two side holes 1 cm from the end. (B) Renal vein opacification during arteriography. Vi-sualization is adequate but not optimal. Two renal veins (*arrows*) unite medial to the kidney to form a single preaortic vein.

carcinomas [59]. Transient balloon occlusion of the corresponding renal artery achieves a similar result [40, 114] and may be an alternative if epinephrine is contraindicated, as it is in patients with arrhythmias. Excellent renal vein opacifica-tion is obtained by selective occlusive renal phlebography [85, 114]. In this method, a double-lumen catheter with distal side holes and a proximal balloon for occlusion of the renal vein are employed during selective venous injection, in addition to intraarterial epinephrine adminis-tration. If visualization of only the main renal vein is desired, epinephrine venography is not necessarily required; forceful countercurrent in-jection may be adequate.

The volume of contrast agent may be varied, depending on the reason for the examination. If good depiction of the intrarenal venous bed and the small veins is desired, 30 cc of Re-nografin-76 should be injected in 2 seconds, with the catheter tip placed in the renal hilus. If thrombus is suspected, 20 cc in 2 seconds may be injected. In renal carcinoma, the inferior vena cava (IVC) should be studied first, to rule out tumor thrombus extending into the IVC. The catheter tip is then positioned in the mouth of the renal vein, and a low pressure hand injection of 15 cc is made. With small peripheral lesions, the

catheter is placed more distally, and epi-nephrine-aided venography at 20 cc in 2 sec-onds is performed [60]. Generally the volume of contrast material used should be based on a pre-liminary test injection and the assessment of the renal venous flow.

Sometimes, the renal vein valves may interfere with venography and impede satisfactory vi-sualization. In such a case, venography should be repeated with adequate slowing of the renal blood flow; a normal renal venous bed may thus be displayed. The occasional failure to catheterize the renal vein and its branches selectively may well be explained by the presence of competent renal vein valves [13].

Many other methods of investigating the renal veins have been described. Inferior vena cavog-raphy, even when aided by the Valsalva maneu-ver, only rarely allows opacification of the renal veins [1, 14, 59]. More commonly, the dilution defects caused by the flow of nonopaque blood into the IVC are observed as signs of renal vein patency. Other methods described in the past in-clude transient balloon occlusion of the supra-renal IVC [31] and of the aorta during selec-tive renal vein injection [29]; parietal renal cavophlebography [16, 41, 42]; and spermatic vein injection [93]. These more complex approaches are neither necessary nor desirable in clinical practice. If the femoral vein cannot be used for catheter entry (because of IVC thrombosis), in an alternative method a catheter is passed from the antecubital vein, into the superior vena cava, through the right atrium, and into the IVC.

The renal veins may be visualized during arteriography, depending on the presence or absence of renal disease and on the amount of contrast material used (see Fig. 59-1B). Usually, opacification is not adequate for diagnostic purposes. Once a carcinoma has been demonstrated and a nephrectomy is anticipated, a larger than usual volume of Renografin-76 (25 cc or more) may be injected into the renal artery with a reasonable likelihood that the renal vein will be visualized if it is not occluded [18]. Nonvisualization of the renal veins and even demonstration of collateral vessels, however, do not necessarily mean tumor invasion; selective renal venography is usually required [68, 125] for optimal visualization of renal vein invasion.

Complications

In the last 11 years, only two complications have been reported in the literature in English. Takaro et al. [114] described a case of renal vein thrombosis that followed renal venography. A single case of intimal dissection without untoward sequelae to the patient has also been reported [6]. We encountered no complications in a series of 132 consecutive renal venograms.

Renal Vein Anatomy

Variations of the right and left renal veins can best be understood by reviewing their development (Fig. 59-2). In the embryo, three pairs of longitudinal veins provide drainage for the lower part of the body [24, 37, 47]. Posterior cardinal veins appear first, soon atrophy, and then are replaced by the anteromedially situated subcardinal veins. Subsequently, by 8 weeks, the supracardinal veins have appeared posterolateral to the aorta. The ringlike anastomoses at the renal level between the subcardinal and supracardinal veins form the circumaortic venous ring [37] (Fig. 59-2A). Two renal veins on each side connect the

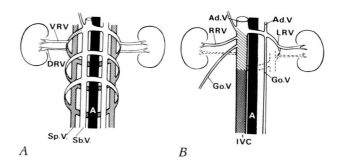

Figure 59-2. Development of the renal veins and the superior vena cava. Schematic drawing. (A) Patterns at the eighth week of fetal life. The posterior cardinal veins have already atrophied, and the venous drainage of the lower body is provided by the paired subcardinal and supracardinal veins, which are interconnected by venous rings. The venous ring at the renal level is called a renal collar. *VRV* = ventral renal vein; *DRV* = dorsal renal vein; *Sp.V.* = supracardinal vein; *Sb.V.* = subcardinal vein; *A* = aorta. (B) Adult pattern. The inferior vena cava develops out of the right supracardinal vein (*cross-hatching*), the right supracardinal anastomosis (*diagonal lines*), and portions of the intersubcardinal anastomosis and right subcardinal vein (*white areas*). Both the adrenal and the gonadal veins are derived from the subcardinal veins. *Go.V.* = gonadal vein; *Ad.V.* = adrenal vein; *A* = aorta; *IVC* = inferior vena cava; *RRV* = right renal vein; *LRV* = left renal vein.

kidneys with these anastomoses. The definitive right-sided IVC is then formed largely from portions of the right supracardinal vein, together with some elements of the right subcardinal veins (Fig. 59-2B). Normally, these veins atrophy on the left. On the right, one renal vein also atrophies, and the remaining vein connects directly with the future IVC. On the left, the retroaortic segment of the venous ring, together with the dorsal renal vein, which is closely connected to the left lumbar-hemiazygos system, normally atrophies. A single preaortic vein remains, formed from an anastomosis between the anterior subcardinal veins. This anastomosis receives the ventral embryonic renal vein and the adrenal and gonadal veins. Variations in the development of these venous channels are common and account for the different renal venous patterns encountered on renal venography [2, 37].

INTRARENAL VEINS

The intrarenal veins are larger than the arteries, but their distribution is similar (Fig. 59-3A, B).

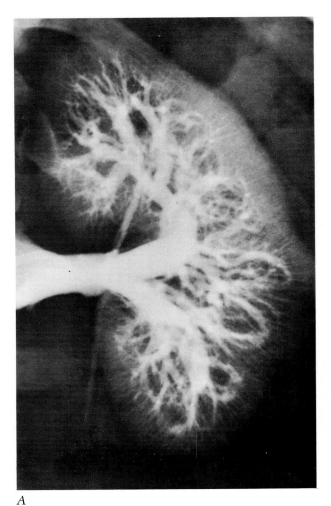

A

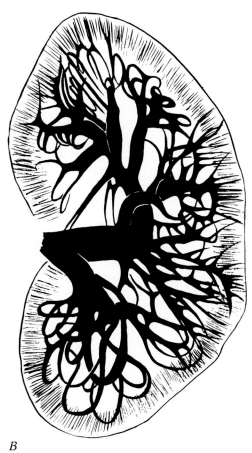

B

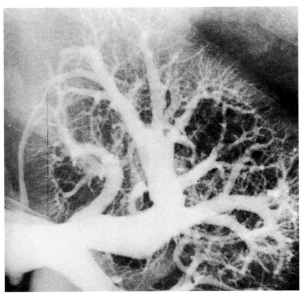

C

Figure 59-3. Intrarenal venous anatomy. (A) Normal left renal venogram. (B) Schematic drawing. The intrarenal veins, which are larger than the arteries, show multiple communications between segmental interlobar and, especially, arcuate veins. There is a single left renal vein in a typical location. (C) Normal magnification venogram. The fine detail of the interlobular venous anatomy may be appreciated.

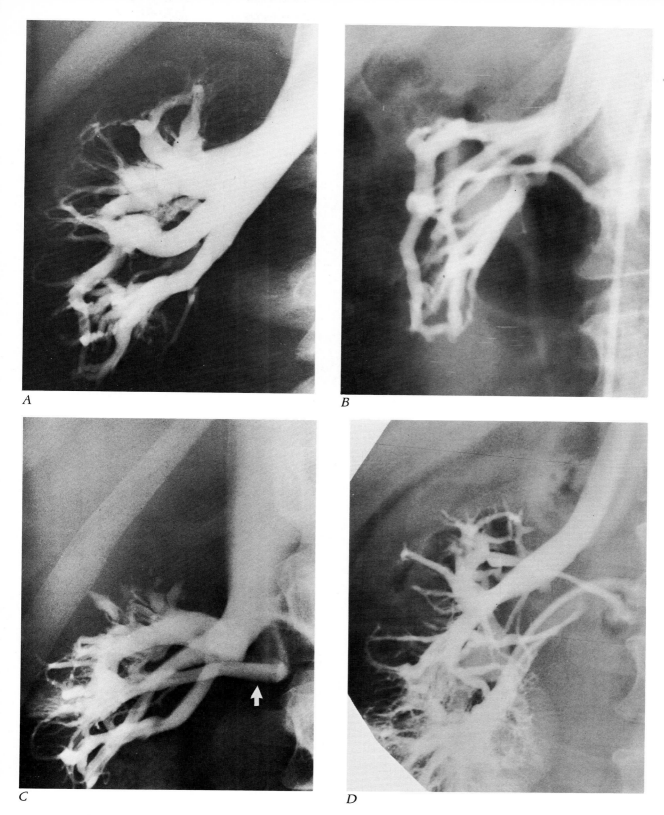

Figure 59-4. Variations of renal vein anatomy. (A) Single renal vein. Multiple branches communicate with larger interlobar veins. (B) Double renal veins. A small caudal vein enters the inferior vena cava (IVC) at the level of L2, well below the major vein entry. Note the plexoid configuration of the veins. (C) Double renal veins. A caudal vein (*arrow*) enters the IVC at virtually the same level as the major vein. (D) Triple renal veins. Three separate veins join the IVC.

1331

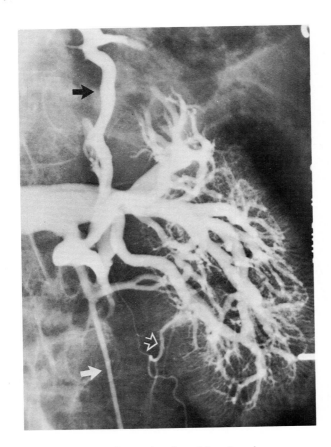

Figure 59-5. Left renal vein with a hemiazygos connection. There is confluence of the lobar veins outside the renal hilus. Both the gonadal vein (*solid white arrow*) and the hemiazygos vein (*black arrow*) communicate with the left main renal vein. In addition, a capsular vein (*open white arrow*) is seen extending from the intrarenal branches into the renal capsule.

Small interlobular vessels drain the renal cortex (Fig. 59-3C) and join medullary veins to form the arcuate veins, which run along the corticomedullary junction. The arcuate veins communicate with each other and drain into the interlobar vessels, which, in turn, form three or four lobar veins. These veins unite anterior to the renal pelvis to form the main renal vein. In contrast to the arteries, there are multiple communications between the segmental interlobar veins and the arcuate veins [31] (Figs. 59-3–59-5).

RIGHT RENAL VEIN (TABLE 59-1)

The right renal vein varies in length from 20 to 45 mm [7]; the average is 32 mm. The course of the vein is anterior and superior to the right renal artery [51]. It is single in 85 percent of people, while in 4 percent of people the single renal vein splits before joining the IVC. The spermatic artery may course through the hiatus formed by this split [92]. From two to four entirely separate renal veins are found in 15 percent of people. There is no correlation between the number of veins and the number of arteries [92]. In about 6 percent of people the renal vein is joined by the right gonadal vein; valves have been reported in the gonadal vein in 77 percent of men and 94 percent of women [3]. It may also be joined by an accessory branch of the adrenal vein (in 31% of people) [25]. Retroperitoneal veins join the renal vein in about 3 percent of people (Table 59-1). Ureteric and capsular veins join the renal vein in the hilar region.

Table 59-1. Variations of Right Renal Vein (Anatomic Literature)

Variation	Number of Positive Cases	Total Number of Patients Examined	Percent Positive	Percentage Range	References to Literature
Single RRV	762	897	85	73–89	92, 94, 124
Multiple RRV	135	897	15	11–28	92, 94, 124
Split of RRV at IVC entry	28	694	4	1.6–10	92, 94
Gonadal vein connected to RRV	49	764	6.4	3–15	4, 92, 94
Accessory adrenal vein connected to RRV	5	16	31	31	25
Retroperitoneal connections	7	258	2.7	2.7	35, 84

RRV = right renal vein; IVC = inferior vena cava.

Table 59-2. Radiographic Anatomy of the Right Renal Vein

Parameter	Present Series (56 patients)	Previous Series [1, 58] (72 patients)
Average length (range)	26 mm (4–51 mm)	22 mm (5–62 mm)
Number of renal veins		
1	72%	86%
2	23%	14%
3	5%	
Extrarenal confluence of lobar veins	27%	25%
Average diameter (range)	14 mm (7–23 mm)	15 mm (10–20 mm)
Angle to IVC (range)	59° (20–120°)	45° (15–85°)
Ureteric vein	4%	—
Demonstration of capsular and subcapsular veins	12%	—
Demonstration of gonadal vein connected to RRV	7%	9%
Demonstration of adrenal vein	4%	—
Usual site of entry into IVC	Lowest third of L1	Lowest third of L1
Variation in site of entry into IVC	Middle third of D12 to L2–L3 interspace	Upper third of L1 to mid-L2

IVC = inferior vena cava; RRV = right renal vein.

Radiographic Anatomy (Table 59-2)

Because of its anteriorly oriented course, the right renal vein appears foreshortened, and the angle of entry into the IVC varies with the degree of expiration.

In our series the average length of the right renal vein was 26 mm (the range was 4–51 mm), and the average diameter was 14 mm (the range was 17–23 mm) [15]. The right renal vein entered the IVC at the level of the lowest third of L1 (the range was the middle third of D12 to the interspace of L2 and L3) and formed an angle of 59 degrees with the infrarenal IVC (the range was 20–120 degrees). A single vein was found in 40 (72%) of 56 patients (see Fig. 59-4A), and in 15 patients it was formed by anastomoses of intrarenal venous branches outside the renal hilus. Two veins were found in 23 percent of patients and three veins were found in 5 percent of patients (see Fig. 59-4B–D), each with a separate caval entry. Usually one large vein predominates, with smaller accessory veins, but occasionally all are of equal size.

The gonadal vein joined the right renal vein in 7 percent of patients. Rarely, there was filling of the adrenal vein, which joined at the superior

Table 59-3. Variations of Left Renal Vein (Anatomic Literature)

Parameter	Number of Cases Positive	Total Number of Patients Examined	Percent Positive	Percentage Range	References to Literature
Single preaortic LRV	613	702	86	79–91	92, 94
Multiple LRV	6	694	1	0.8–1	92, 94
Circumaortic LRV	68	972	7	1.5–16.8	28, 92, 94
Retroaortic single LRV	24	972	2.4	1.8–3.4	28, 92, 94
Gonadal vein draining into IVC (all left-sided IVC)	5	765	0.7	0.4–1.2	4, 92, 94
Multiple gonadal veins	28	181	15.4	15.4	92
Adrenal vein draining into LRV	291	291	100	100	7, 8, 25
Persistent left-sided IVC	35	1,820	1.8	1–2.4	2, 4, 92, 94
Retroperitoneal venous connections	339	455	75	59–88	70, 84, 92

LRV = left renal vein; IVC = inferior vena cava.

point of the junction of the renal vein and the IVC. In 12 percent of patients, capsular and subcapsular veins were visualized that drained either through the renal cortex or to the renal hilus to join the main renal vein. This happens more frequently when the catheter is wedged in a small renal vein branch. In 4 percent of patients, the ureteric vein was opacified. The incidence of multiple renal veins was twice as high in our series as in other reported analyses [1, 58] (Table 59-2).

LEFT RENAL VEIN (TABLE 59-3)

The more complex embryology of the left renal vein compared to the right is associated with more anatomic variations. The left renal vein, which is longer than the right, varies from 60 to 110 mm in length; the average is 84 mm [7]. After crossing the aorta ventrally, it enters the IVC at about a 90-degree angle. Posteriorly it is near the third portion of the duodenum and the pancreas. A single preaortic left renal vein is seen in 86 percent of people [92, 94, 124], while a single retroaortic vein is described in 2.4 percent [28, 92, 94]. Multiple renal veins with separate renal origin and separate caval entry are rare (1% of people) on the left side [92, 94].

A circumaortic vein is found in 7 percent of people [28, 92, 94]. The renal vein splits in these people to form a preaortic component in the usual location and a retroaortic component that runs caudally to enter the IVC in the lower lumbar region. The preaortic and the postaortic components of the ring are frequently equal in size [28]. The retroaortic portion may receive lumbar veins [8] and may also split before entering the IVC. The hiatus formed by such a split may contain the left gonadal artery [92].

The adrenal vein, usually joined by the inferior phrenic and capsular veins, enters the left renal vein superiorly, just lateral to the lumbar spine. The gonadal vein joins inferiorly, lateral to the adrenal vein [8, 35, 92, 94]; if there is a periaortic venous ring, it joins either the preaortic portion or the unsplit renal vein trunk. Multiple gonadal veins occur in about 15 percent of people [92] but rarely number more than two. Gonadal vein valves have been described in 60 percent of men and 86 percent of women [3].

In addition, the left renal vein communicates with the retroperitoneal veins (e.g., the lumbar, ascending lumbar, and hemiazygos veins) in 75 percent of people [70, 84, 92] (Table 59-3). Communications occur directly through lumbar veins joining posteriorly or indirectly through the gonadal veins [8, 52]. The intrahilar portion of the left renal vein receives the ureteric vein [52]. The capsular veins drain into the adrenal and gonadal veins or directly into the renal vein [8,

Table 59-4. Radiographic Anatomy of the Left Renal Vein

Parameter	Present Series (76 patients)	Previous Series [1, 58, 71] (197 patients)
Average length (range)	68 mm (35–100 mm)	77 mm (55–120 mm)
Single preaortic vein	89%	91%
Extrarenal confluence of lobar veins	14%	2.5%
Periaortic venous ring	11%	9%
Single retroaortic vein	1%	1%
Average preaortic diameter		
Preaortic portion (range)	19 mm (11–25 mm)	—
Hilar portion (range)	13 mm (7–16)	—
Average angle to IVC (range)	74° (25–105°)	78° (50–90°)
Demonstration of adrenal veins	57%	49%
Demonstration of gonadal vein	83%	70%
Demonstration of retroperitoneal branches	55%	40%
Demonstration of capsular or subcapsular veins	34%	5%
Usual site of entry into IVC	L1–L2 interspace	L1–L2 interspace
Variation of site of entry into IVC (range)	Middle third of D12 to upper third of L3	Lowest third of D12 to lowest third of L2
Persistent left-sided IVC	None	2%

IVC = inferior vena cava.

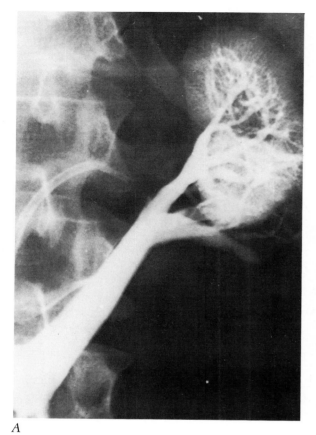

A

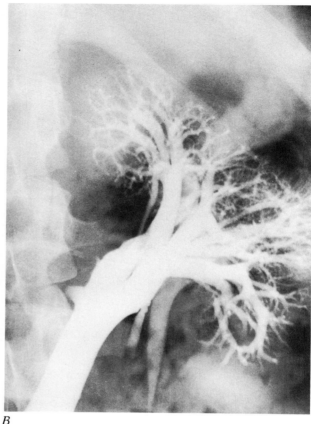

B

Figure 59-6. Solitary retroaortic renal vein. (A) The vein originates at the interspace between L1 and L2, and extends caudally from the kidney to enter the in-ferior vena cava in the region of L3. (B) In this case, the vein originates at the interspace between L2 and L3 and descends to the interspace of L3 and L4.

52]. A left-sided IVC occurs in less than 1 percent of the people [4, 92, 94]; the left gonadal vein then enters the left IVC directly.

Radiographic Anatomy (Table 59-4)

In a study of 76 consecutive left renal venograms performed at the Peter Bent Brigham Hospital, the average length of the left renal vein was found to be 68 mm (the range was 35–100 mm). In the preaortic portion, the average diameter was 19 mm (the range was 11–25 mm), and in the hilar portion, it was 13 mm (the range was 7–16 mm). Entrance into the IVC was typically at the interspace between L2 and L3 (the range was the middle third of D12 to the upper third of L3) with an angle of 74 degrees to the infrarenal IVC (the range was 25–105 degrees).

There was a single preaortic vein in 89 percent of patients (see Fig. 59-3); in 14 percent of patients it was formed by a confluence of renal veins outside the renal hilus (Fig. 59-5; see also Fig.

59-13A). Rarely, a single retroaortic vein was observed (Fig. 59-6). In 11 percent of the patients, there was a periaortic venous ring; that is, a preaortic vein in a typical location and a retroaortic limb that was always smaller and that entered the IVC in the low lumbar region (Figs. 59-7–59-9). In one instance, the retroaortic portion split before entering the IVC (Fig. 59-9). In six of eight patients, the retroaortic limb arose from an unsplit main renal vein trunk within 2 cm of the renal hilus (Fig. 59-9). In two patients, the bifurcation occurred within the renal hilus (see Figs. 59-7, 59-8) or at the confluence of the lobar veins, and the retroaortic vein seemed to drain parts of the lower pole preferentially. No patients had multiple renal veins. Computed tomography has been used to define circumaortic renal vein and other renal vein and caval anomalies [101, 115].

The adrenal vein was demonstrated in 57 percent of patients (see Fig. 59-8), and one or two

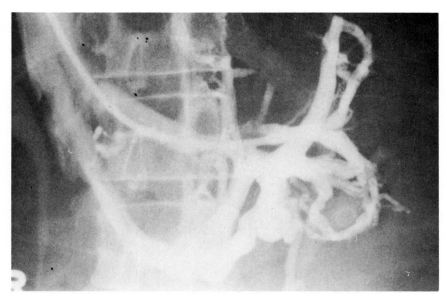

Figure 59-7. Circumaortic venous ring arising in the renal hilus. The veins of the lower pole drain preferentially into the retroaortic vein.

Figure 59-8. Circumaortic venous ring. Both the preaortic and the retroaortic renal veins (*open white arrow*) arise in the renal hilus. The latter vein seems to drain the lower pole preferentially. The adrenal vein (*solid white arrow*) joins the preaortic renal vein in the typical location. Note the valve of the preaortic vein (*black arrows*).

Figure 59-9. Circumaortic venous ring. The inferior vena cavogram demonstrates three communications of the ring with the vena cava. The retroaortic vein arises from an unsplit main renal trunk and splits before joining the inferior vena cava.

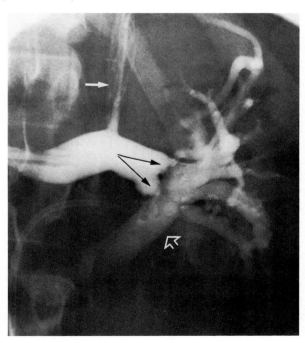

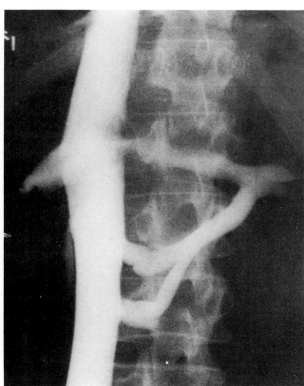

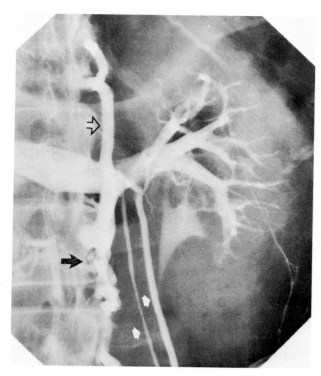

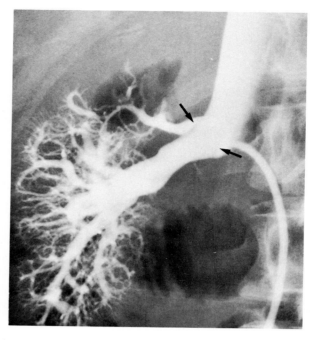

Figure 59-10. Azygos vein and gonadal vein opacification. Normal left renal venogram in a renal donor. Two left spermatic veins (*solid white arrows*) are opacified. Note the communications between the left main renal vein and the ascending lumbar vein (*black arrow*) and the hemiazygos vein (*open black arrow*).

Figure 59-11. Right renal vein valves. The valves are clearly defined (*arrows*) close to the entry of the renal vein into the inferior vena cava.

Figure 59-12. Right renal vein valves. These valves are located in the renal hilus. (A) The valve (*arrow*) has impaired the filling of the lower pole veins. (B) The valve (*arrow*) has impaired the filling of the upper pole veins.

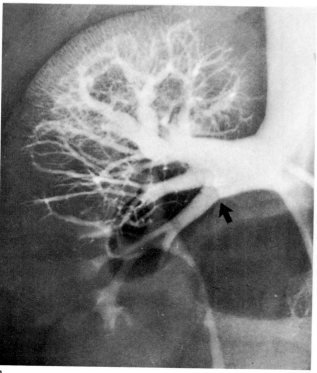

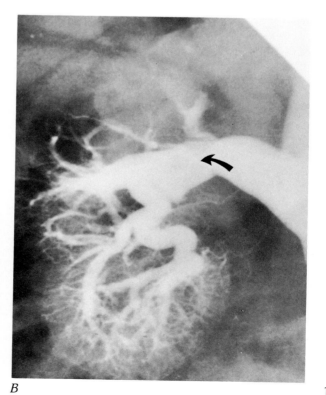

A

B

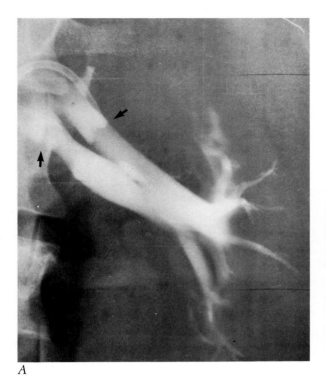

A

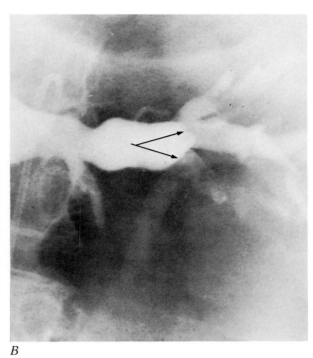

B

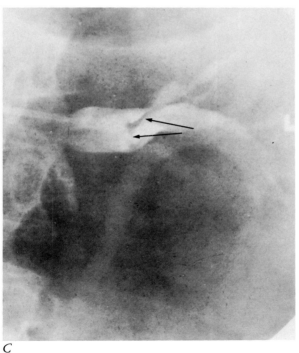

C

Figure 59-13. Left renal vein valves. (A) Two left renal veins, each with a valve (*arrows*), join ventral to the aorta. These valves may cause incomplete filling of the intrarenal branches. (B) The renal vein at the hilus (*arrows*) impedes renal venous filling. (C) Same as (B). With the termination of injection, the valve leaflets (*arrows*) are clearly delineated.

59-10; see also Fig. 59-5). In 34 percent of patients, capsular or subcapsular veins (see Fig. 59-5) joined intrarenal branches through the renal cortex or directly joined the adrenal vein, the gonadal vein, or the intrahilar portion of the renal vein.

Filling of side branches and demonstration of valves depends on the position of the catheter, the injection rate, and the blood flow. Our findings, with some exceptions, were similar to those of other authors (Table 59-4) [1, 58, 71].

RENAL VEIN VALVES

Autopsy studies have demonstrated renal vein valves in 28 to 70 percent of right renal veins and 4 to 36 percent of left renal veins [4, 114].

In our analysis of renal venograms, valves were visualized in 16 percent of dissections on the right; in only 4 percent of dissections they were almost equally distributed close to the entry into

gonadal veins were filled in 83 percent of patients (Fig. 59-10; see also Fig. 59-5). Filling varied, probably depending on the presence of competent venous valves. In 39 percent of patients, lumbar, hemiazygos, or ascending lumbar veins (retroperitoneal veins) were demonstrated (Fig.

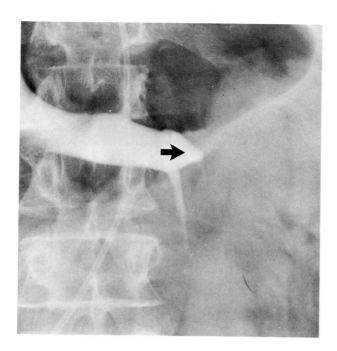

Figure 59-14. Competent left renal vein valve. A retrograde injection has closed the valve, which appears tent shaped and convex toward the renal hilus (*arrow*). This appearance must be differentiated from that in renal vein thrombosis (see Fig. 59-19) or renal vein invasion by carcinoma (see Figs. 59-15, 59-17).

the IVC (Fig. 59-11), or in the main renal vein, over 2 cm from the IVC, or in the renal hilus (Fig. 59-12).

On the left, valves were detected in 15 percent of dissections. Most valves were located in the main renal vein (Fig. 59-13A) or at the renal hilus (Fig. 59-13B, C).

Angiographically, renal vein valves appeared as thin, weblike structures that may block passage of the catheter or of contrast material and hence cause poor venographic filling (Figs. 59-11–59-13). There was a 12 to 31 percent higher incidence of inadequate venograms when valves were present. This inadequacy occurred more commonly when the renal blood flow was not slowed: the effect of the valve is then coupled with impedance of the contrast backflow by the normal antegrade flow of blood. Rarely, valves produced total obstruction to the retrograde flow of contrast material (Fig. 59-14), in which case they had to be distinguished from renal vein thrombus or neoplastic involvement.

Applications

CARCINOMA OF THE KIDNEY

Renal venography may be an invaluable method of assessing carcinoma of the kidney. The presence of renal vein invasion significantly affects the prognosis in patients with any renal malignancy [10, 27, 45, 48, 77, 82, 90, 96–98]. About 36 percent of patients undergoing nephrectomy for renal cell carcinoma exhibit invasion of the renal vein and, sometimes, the IVC; their 5-year survival is only 29 percent, compared to 52 percent for patients who do not have renal vein invasion (Table 59-5). Similarly, 36 percent of patients with carcinoma of the renal pelvis have renal vein invasion at surgery; their 5-year survival rate is even more markedly reduced (5%, as opposed to 43% in patients without renal vein invasion) (Table 59-6). Venous invasion is also found in Wilms' tumor in 22 percent (8–42%) of patients, with a worsened prognosis (Table 59-7).

Preoperatively it is important to know the extent of the tumor and whether it is operable. Instead of the traditional lateral incision, some authors [5, 30, 32] favor a transperitoneal approach in patients with renal vein invasion to enable early inspection of the renal vein and its medial clamping to prevent tumor embolization during surgical manipulation.

Renal venography may also be helpful in establishing the diagnosis in infiltrating avascular renal cell carcinoma [21, 99, 107] and transitional cell carcinoma [21, 40, 99, 107]. In these patients, the absence of typical arteriographic findings or the presence of only small abnormal arterial branches contrasts often with the striking abnormalities on the venogram (Fig. 59-15). At times, segmental renal vein involvement may be visualized (Fig. 59-16).

When the arteriogram does not allow differentiation between a renal tumor and an adrenal tumor, the renal venogram may show the drainage of the tumor veins either into the intrarenal veins (renal tumor) or into the adrenal veins (adrenal tumor), provided there is no proximal occlusion.

Because of the valuable information renal venography affords, most authors [21, 30, 40, 60, 68, 99, 106, 107] feel that the usefulness of the procedure outweighs the risk of tumor embolization during it. An inferior vena cavogram should be the first step, to rule out tumor thrombus extending into the IVC [68, 99], particularly with the advent of caval resection in such patients

Table 59-5. Renal Vein Invasion and Survival in Renal Cell Carcinoma

| Author | Year | Number of Patients with Renal Vein Invasion/Total Number | Percentage of Patients with Renal Vein Invasion | Number and Percentage with 5-Year Survival/Total Number | | | |
| | | | | With Invasion | | Without Invasion | |
				Number	%	Number	%
Hand and Broders [48]	1932	38/193	20	—	—	—	—
McDonald and Priestley [77]	1943	275/509	54	60/207	29	103/186	55
Griffiths and Thackray [45]	1949	23/80	29	2/10	20	13/26	50
Riches et al. [98]	1951	199/816	24	17/90	19	114/308	37
Riches [96]	1963	41/110	37	7/26	27	35/60	58
Riches [97]	1964	—	—	—	—	—	—
Arner et al. [10]	1965	51/172	30	15/51	29	62/121	51
Myers et al. [82]	1968	228/508	50	78/228	34	179/280	64
Crocker [27]	1975	31/84	37	—	—	—	—
Total		886/2,472	36	179/612	29	506/981	52

Table 59-6. Renal Vein Invasion and Survival in Carcinoma of the Renal Pelvis

| Author | Year | Number of Patients with Renal Vein Invasion/Total Number | Percentage of Patients with Renal Vein Invasion | Number and Percentage with 5-Year Survival/Total Number | | | |
| | | | | With Invasion | | Without Invasion | |
				Number	%	Number	%
McDonald and Priestley [77]	1943	31/76	40	1/21	5	15/35	43
Crocker [27]	1975	1/12	8	—	—	—	—
Total		32/88	36				

Table 59-7. Renal Vein Invasion and Survival in Wilms' Tumor and Sarcoma of the Kidney

| Author | Year | Number of Patients with Renal Vein Invasion/Total Number | Percentage of Patients with Renal Vein Involvement | Number and Percentage with 3-Year Survival/Total Number | | | |
| | | | | With Invasion | | Without Invasion | |
				Number	%	Number	%
Wilms' tumor							
McDonald and Priestley [77]	1943	13/31	42	—	—	—	—
Riches et al. [98]	1951	9/110	8	—	—	—	—
Perez et al. [90]	1973	17/40	42	4/17	24	16/23	70
Total		39/181	22				
Sarcoma							
McDonald and Priestley [77]	1943	2/20	10	—	—	—	—

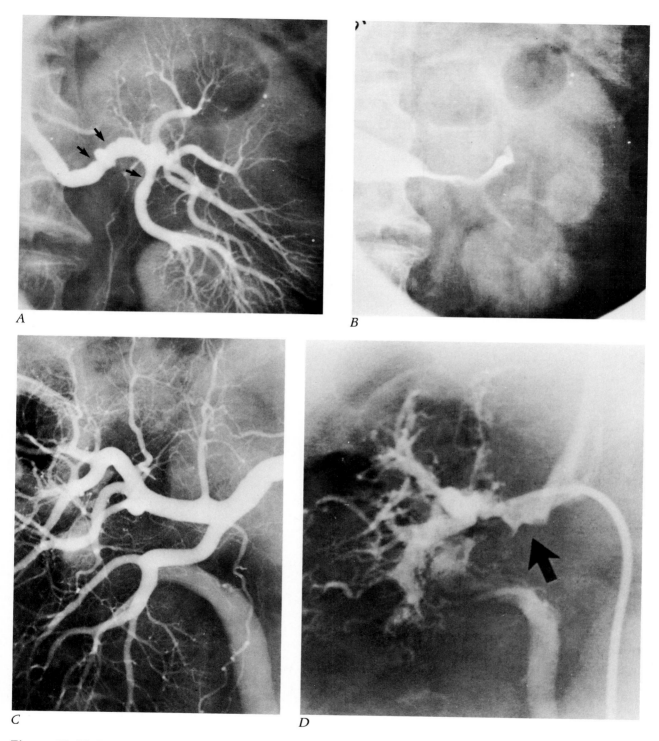

Figure 59-15. Renal vein invasion in carcinoma. (A) This patient had transitional cell carcinoma of the left kidney. Note the striking discrepancy between the arteriographic findings and the venographic findings. The arteriogram shows minimal encasement of the central renal arteries (*arrows*) but a striking absence of neovascularity. (B) Venogram. The left renal vein is occluded by a tumor. The irregularity of contour reflects a malignant invasion. (C) This patient, who had transitional cell carcinoma, has thin but definite tumor vessels close to the renal hilus but no major vessel involvement on the arteriogram. (D) Venogram, same patient as in (C). Gross tumor invasion (*arrow*).

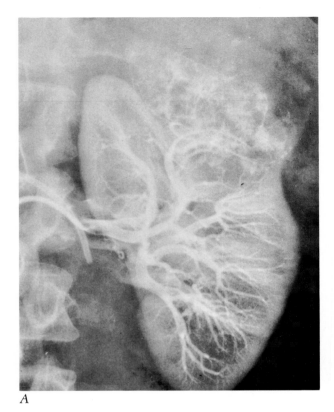

A

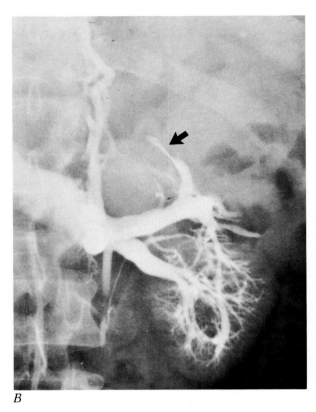

B

Figure 59-16. Renal cell carcinoma with segmental vein involvement. (A) Arteriogram. The area of neovascularity is confined to the upper pole. (B) Venogram. There is poor opacification of the upper pole branches. Note the narrowing, displacement, and occlusion of the upper pole branch (*arrow*) by the tumor.

[75]. Invasion of the IVC is usually accompanied by a persistent, sharply marginated and sometimes lobular filling defect originating from the renal vein [91, 121]. Tumor thrombus and bland thrombus are not always distinguishable [121], however, unless actual tumor vascularity is demonstrated in the thrombus on selective renal arteriography [36, 88] (Fig. 59-17). At times the IVC may be indented by metastatic nodes [88]. Both ultrasonography and computed tomography may demonstrate caval extension of renal carcinoma, but their reliability in defining the extent of renal vein invasion does not equal that of venography.

A normal inferior vena cavogram should be followed by a selective renal venogram (see p. 1327). Typical findings on renal venograms of invasion of the renal vein include irregular narrowing of renal vein (see Fig. 59-15B), vessel cutoffs (see Figs. 59-15B and D, 59-16B), indentations of the vessel wall, differences of contrast density, and filling defects within the renal veins (Fig. 59-17) [99]. In hypervascular tumors, however,

"functional" filling defects secondary to venous washout may be observed [99]. These can be indistinguishable from those secondary to tumorous extension into the venous system, and a positive diagnosis of renal vein invasion should be made only if the main renal vein or its major tributaries are involved [99].

RETROPERITONEAL TUMORS

In contrast to the right renal vein, the left renal vein may be an important vessel in the evaluation and staging of retroperitoneal disease. The left renal vein runs a course directly anterior to the pancreas and is located close to periaortic, mesenteric, and renal lymph nodes. Therefore, this vessel often shows early involvement in retroperitoneal tumors. The typical findings on venography include splaying and smooth narrowing of the vein when nodes or a mass is impinging on but not invading the renal vein and segmental irregular narrowing when there is

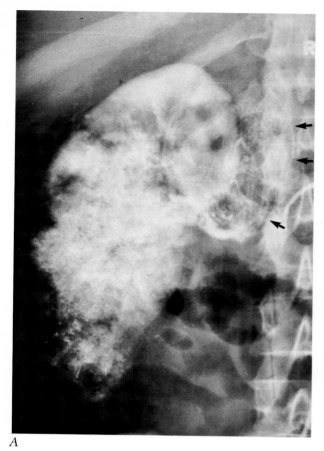

A

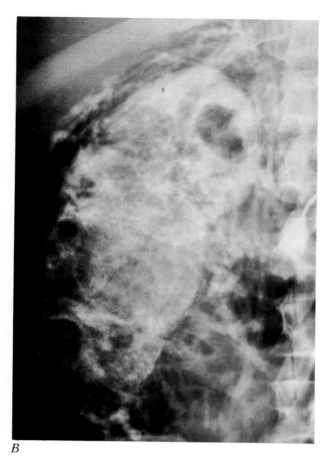

B

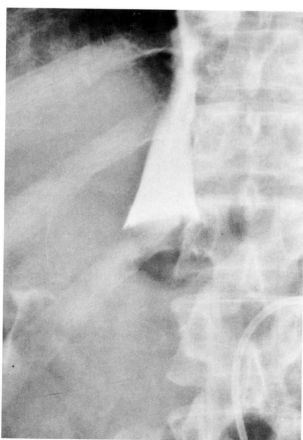

C

Figure 59-17. Renal vein and inferior vena cava invasion by renal cell carcinoma. (A) The late arterial phase film shows a large tumor of the lower half of the right kidney and an area of tumor vascularity in the region of the right renal vein and the inferior vena cava (*arrows*). (B) The venous phase film demonstrates multiple retroperitoneal collateral vessels. (C) An inferior vena cavogram demonstrates the upper extent of the caval occlusion, correlating with the tumor thrombus as seen on the arteriogram.

malignant invasion. Cope and Isard [26] found significant distortion of the left renal vein in 60 percent of patients in a series of 17 proved retroperitoneal tumors. In nine patients with cancer of the pancreas seven had invasion of the renal vein. Among these seven, three had little or no arteriographic evidence of malignancy.

RENOVASCULAR HYPERTENSION

Although arteriography can easily demonstrate a stenosis in the renal arteries, the functional significance of the stenosis may be uncertain unless collateral vessels are present [19, 34].

The renal venous washout time has been shown to reflect the rate of blood flow through the kidney and to be related to the renal plasma flow and to the presence of significant renal artery stenosis [1]. In the method used, contrast material was injected into the renal veins and the washout time was determined cineangiographically. With this method, both kidneys could be evaluated and compared. With significant renal artery stenosis and reduction in the renal blood flow, the washout time was usually prolonged.

RENAL VEIN RENIN DETERMINATION

The functional significance of arteriographically proved anatomic lesions and their potential surgical curability are commonly evaluated in the light of renal vein renin activity [20, 39, 53, 66, 102, 105, 117]. Renin, secreted in response to stimuli that compromise kidney perfusion, increases plasma angiotensin, which stimulates aldosterone secretion [69]. Vascular tone is regulated by an interaction between angiotensin levels and the available intravascular sodium ions. The two hormones, angiotensin and aldosterone, thus restore the sodium balance and the arterial pressure, thereby turning off renin release. Sealey et al. [104] showed that under steady-state circumstances, each kidney adds 24 percent more renin to the renal artery renin. They concluded that if the normal kidney is suppressed by high blood pressure, all the renin should be coming from the diseased kidney, which then will add at least 48 percent more renin to the renal artery level. The renal vein renin of the normal kidney should equal the renal artery renin. This line of reasoning supports the clinically established cri-

teria used in diagnosing renovascular hypertension and predicting surgical curability:

1. Increased renin production of the suspect kidney: $V - A/A > 0.48$ (V = venous renin activity; A = arterial renal activity) [116, 117]
2. Suppression of renin secretion on the contralateral, normal side: $V - A \sim 0$ [112, 117]
3. A renal vein renin ratio of 1.5:1 or more between the involved kidney and the uninvolved kidney [20, 102, 105, 112, 116]
4. Elevated plasma renin activity [112]

The renin-angiotensin-aldosterone system is easily influenced by many factors in both normal patients and hypertensive patients.

Upright posture leads to increased renin production [78]. In renovascular hypertension, Michelakis et al. [78, 79] found that the kidney with the stenotic artery produced excess renin, which led to a marked disparity in the renal vein renin concentrations between the involved side and the uninvolved side. If such a patient changes from an upright position to a recumbent one, exaggerated renin production is not stimulated for a time because of the high concentration of renin in the general circulation. As a result, the renal vein renin ratio between the involved kidney and the uninvolved kidney approaches unity and briefly loses its diagnostic usefulness [78, 79].

Salt depletion induced by diuretics or a low dietary intake of sodium increases the renin activity. The stimulus to increased renin production affects the involved kidney more than the contralateral kidney, leading to an exaggerated renin ratio [118].

Antihypertensive drugs [67, 69] influence renin release in both directions (Table 59-8). These drugs may increase renin release either by directly lowering the blood pressure or by their diuretic effect, with consequent decrease in the blood pressure [67]. The kidney with significant renal artery stenosis secretes disproportionately more renin than does the uninvolved kidney [61]. Other drugs suppress the plasma renin activity, probably by directly interfering with the physiologic pathways of renin release [67].

Technique of Venous Sampling for Renin Assay

The same catheter used for renal venography may be employed for renin sampling. For segmental vein sampling, an additional downward

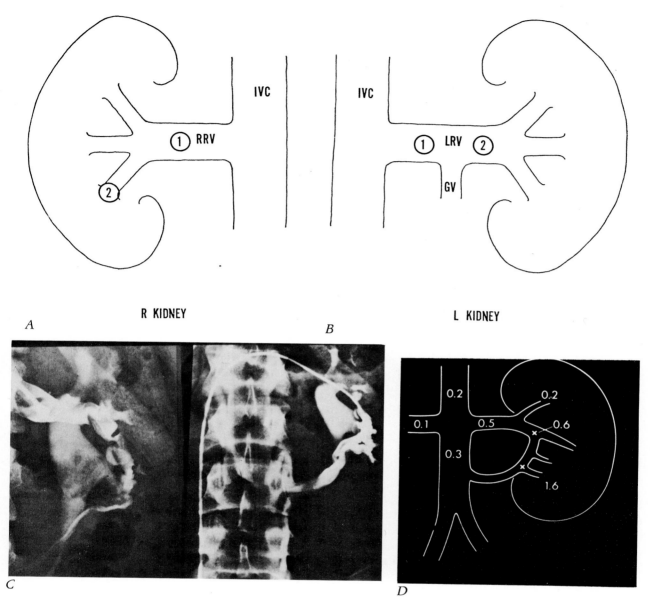

Figure 59-18. Renal vein renin determination. Importance of the catheter site. (A) A diagram of the right kidney in a 33-year-old woman with hypertension following surgical amputation of the right lower pole renal artery. Sampling showed lower renin values (3,636 ng/100 cc) at site 1 (the main renal vein) than at site 2 (the lower pole segmental vein) (4,916 ng/100 cc). This difference was due to dilution from the middle and upper pole veins at site 1. *IVC* = inferior vena cava; *RRV* = right renal vein. (B) A diagram of the left kidney in a 54-year-old man with hypertension following embolic occlusion of the left renal artery. Sampling showed lower renin values (2,381 ng/100 cc) at site 1 (the proximal renal vein) than at site 2 (the distal renal vein) (14,815 ng/100 cc). This difference was due to dilution from the gonadal vein at site 1. *IVC* = inferior vena cava; *LRV* = left renal vein; *GV* = gonadal vein. (C) Left renal venogram in a 16-year-old boy with posttraumatic hypertension and obstruction of a lower pole renal artery. A circumaortic venous ring is present. When the catheter was advanced through the preaortic vein, injection of contrast material into the lower pole vein showed preferential drainage into the retroaortic vein. (Courtesy of Christos A. Athanasoulis, M.D.) (D) Renin sampling. Samples from the retroaortic vein localize the ischemic focus to the lower pole.

Table 59-8. Antihypertensive
Drug Effect on Renin Release

Renin Inhibitors	Renin Stimulators
Propranolol	Aldosterone antagonists
Clonidine	Diuretics
Methyldopa	Vasodilators
Reserpine	Nitroprusside
Ganglionic blockers	Diazoxide
Guanethidine	Hydralazine

Adapted from Laragh [69].

deflection of 30 degrees should be incorporated in the catheter tip. At the Peter Bent Brigham Hospital, venous samples to be assayed for renin activity are taken from the main right renal vein, the main left renal vein peripheral to the entry of the gonadal vein, and the IVC above and below the renal veins. The lower caval sample value is interchangeable with the renal artery renin concentration, since there is no low inferior vena cava-abdominal aorta pressure gradient [117]. Correct localization of the catheter tip is essential for proper sampling (Fig. 59-18A, B) [89]. In the presence of a left circumaortic renal vein, the retroaortic vein can preferentially drain the lower poles (Fig. 59-18C, D); therefore samples should be taken from both veins. In branch stenosis or local infarction, the sample must be obtained from the draining renal vein branch, because venous blood from the nonischemic portions of the kidney may dilute the main renal vein renin and lead to false-normal values (Fig. 59-18A) [66, 89, 111]. The same holds true in those rare cases of locally circumscribed, renin-producing tumors of juxtaglomerular origin [103] or of a renal cyst compressing renal parenchyma and thereby creating focal ischemia. Samples should be drawn slowly to prevent aspiration from side branches [66, 89]. Simultaneous sampling of renal veins is unnecessary [49].

A rigid protocol should be followed for renin sampling. Samples should be obtained in hypertensive patients only after arteriographic demonstration of renal artery stenosis. This may follow abdominal aortography; Harrington et al. [49] found no significant change of renal vein renin activity 10 minutes after aortography in a series of 56 patients. Other authors, however, in a smaller series of animal experiments, found an increase of renin secretion after selective renal arteriography [62]. It is desirable, therefore, to obtain renin samples 15 to 20 minutes following selective renal arteriography. These patients should have no signs or symptoms of congestive heart failure and should preferably have received no diuretics or antihypertensive drugs [39]. Under standard conditions of recumbency and normal sodium intake, venous samples may then be drawn. If the results are normal or borderline, renin measurements should be repeated after stimulation by one of the following, alone or in combination:

1. Upright posture for 20 minutes [78] to 4 hours [39]
2. Sodium depletion by 3 days of severe sodium restriction at 10 mEq per day or administration of furosemide [39, 78]
3. Controlled hypotension [61]

Accuracy of Renin Assay

As a predictive index of the outcome of surgery in hypertensive patients with renal artery stenosis, the accuracy of renin activity varies between 70 and 95 percent [20, 39, 102, 105, 117]. The variability may be explained by the different criteria used and by the difference in how the patients are prepared. If the renal vein renin ratio between the involved kidney and the uninvolved kidney is used alone, the accuracy is approximately 85 percent (Table 59-9). The ratios between the two sides do not take into account the occult hypersecretion of renin (although to a lesser degree) on the presumably uninvolved side [116]. Such a finding suggests a nephrosclerotic kidney, and surgery might therefore be contraindicated. The additional demonstration of suppressed renin release or of an abnormally high peripheral plasma renin activity in relation to sodium excretion (indicating increased renin release) may increase the accuracy of predicting the surgical outcome to 95 percent [116, 117].

It is important to emphasize that absence of lateralization does not preclude a successful result from surgery; 21 percent of such patients with renovascular disease experience amelioration of hypertension [20].

RENAL VEIN THROMBOSIS

Renal vein thrombosis in adults differs from that in children [100]. In children, it is almost exclusively found in the presence of diarrhea and de-

Table 59-9. Accuracy of Lateralizing Renal Vein Renin Ratios (1.5:1 or Higher) in Predicting Cure of Hypertension in Unilateral Renal Artery Stenosis

Author	Year	Total Number of Patients	Number Cured	Percentage Cured
Bourgoignie et al. [20]	1970	124	107	85
Simmons et al. [105]	1970	21	19	90
Stockigt et al. [112]	1972	22	19	86
Schaeffer and Fair [102]	1974	17	12	71
Total		184	157	85

hydration, and the prognosis is grave. In adults, renal vein thrombosis is often associated with underlying renal disease, including both systemic diseases, such as lupus erythematosus and amyloidosis, and primary renal diseases, such as nephrosclerosis, chronic glomerulonephritis, pyelonephritis, and membranous glomerulonephritis [12, 46, 56]. Whether renal vein thrombosis is the cause or is an effect of membranous glomerulonephritis is not fully established; many authors consider it a consequence of the disease [9, 72, 113]. Patients with the nephrotic syndrome have a hypercoagulable state [63] that may account for a high incidence of peripheral thrombophlebitis, renal vein thrombosis, and pulmonary embolism (Table 59-10). Renal vein thrombosis may occur as an extension of thrombus within the IVC [74], or it may be associated with extrinsic pressure on the renal vein from an adjacent mass, such as a tumor or an aneurysm [95]. Trauma is a rare cause [23, 73, 110].

The response of the kidney to renal vein thrombosis depends on the rapidity and completeness of the occlusion and on the availability of collateral pathways [50, 65, 122]. If the occlusion is rapid and complete, hemorrhagic infarction may occur. If the occlusion is gradual, collateral vessels may develop. The balance between the speed with which this collateral system develops and the rapidity of the occlusion determines the outcome. If the collateral system cannot accommodate the renal blood flow, the kidneys become enlarged and congested; later they may atrophy. Ligation of the left renal vein may be accomplished with no long-term effects because of the collateral venous drainage although temporary renal dysfunction may be observed [76].

Renal vein thrombosis is twice as common in males as in females (Table 59-10). Clinically it is associated with the nephrotic syndrome and, frequently, with hematuria [110]. In addition, a third of these patients may develop pulmonary embolism (Table 59-10); at times, this may be the presenting symptom [110]. Patients with traumatic renal vein thrombosis and associated arterial occlusion do not exhibit the nephrotic syndrome but may present with recurrent pulmonary embolism [110]. Autopsy examination of patients with renal vein thrombosis has shown associated IVC thrombosis in 24 percent and iliofemoral vein thrombosis in 29 percent [74].

Among 39 patients with the nephrotic syndrome whom we have examined by renal venography, only seven had renal vein thrombosis.

Table 59-10. Incidence of Pulmonary Embolism and Sex Distribution in Patients with Renal Vein Thrombosis

Author	Number of Patients	Ratio of Female to Male	Number of Patients with Pulmonary Embolism
Llach et al. [72]	12	4:8	4
O'Dea et al. [86]	11	3:8	3
Chait [23]	6	2:4	2
McCarthy et al. [74]*	38	10:28	14
Rosenmann et al. [100]	15	8:7	7
Our series	7	1:6	1
Total	89	26:61 (31%:69%)	31 (35%)

*Autopsy series.

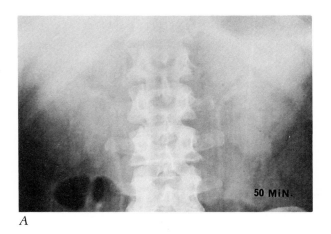

A

Figure 59-19. Renal vein thrombosis. (A) Intravenous urogram. At 50 minutes, the concentration of the contrast agent in the collecting system and ureters remains sharply decreased and the kidneys appear swollen. (B) Arteriogram at 3 seconds. The arterial branches are normal in caliber and appearance. (C) Arteriogram at 6 seconds. The transit time is markedly prolonged. (D) Arteriogram at 13 seconds. The main renal vein is not opacified. Capsular collateral veins are visualized (*arrows*). (E) Inferior vena cavogram. No thrombus is seen in the inferior vena cava. The usual dilution defects, visible at the points of union with the renal veins, are absent, suggesting renal vein thrombosis. (F) Right renal venogram. Chronic renal vein thrombosis with synechiae formation is apparent. A periureteric collateral vein fills. (G) Left renal venogram. Chronic left renal vein thrombosis is present.

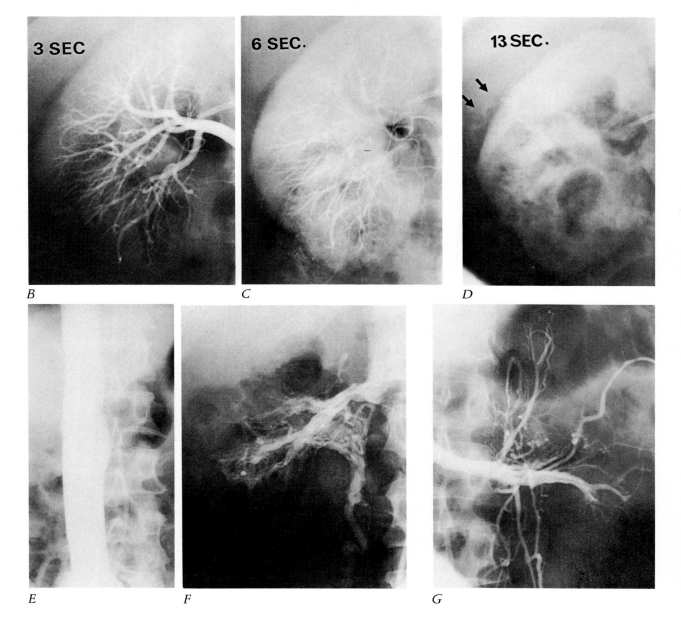

B   C   D

E   F   G

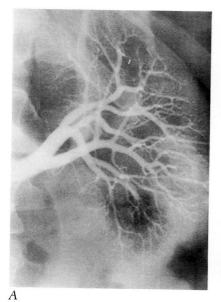 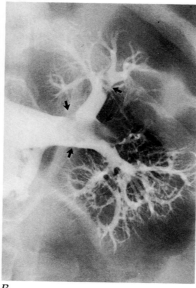 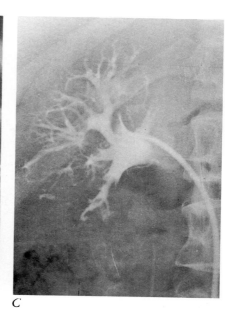

A   *B*   *C*

Figure 59-20. Bilateral renal vein thrombosis. (A) Left renal arteriogram. Stretching of branches is present in a moderately swollen kidney. (B) Left renal venogram demonstrating multiple thrombi (*arrows*).

(C) Right renal venogram. Multiple partially occluding intraluminal filling defects are visible both in the main renal vein and in the intrarenal branches.

Figure 59-21. Renal vein thrombosis. (A) Total occlusion. This patient had membranous glomerulonephritis. The thrombus within the main renal vein prevents opacification of the intrarenal branches. In contrast to competent renal vein valves (see Fig. 59-14), the thrombus is convex toward the inferior vena cava (*arrow*). (B) Segmental thrombus. This patient had biopsy-proved membranous glomerulonephritis. Bilateral renal venography revealed only one small

segmental thrombus (*arrow*) in the right kidney. (C) Organized thrombus. Twenty-nine-year-old woman with a 12-year history of systemic lupus erythematosus and a 4-year history of nephrotic syndrome. The left renal venogram shows peripheral occlusion. There are irregularly shaped filling defects in the central portion of the main renal vein, representing partially recanalized thrombus. This appearance is typical of chronic renal vein thrombosis.

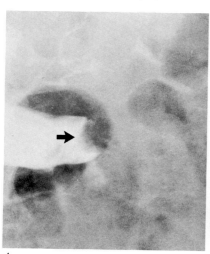 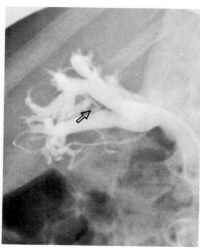 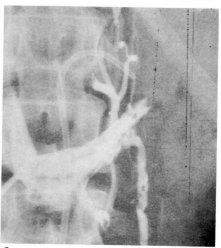

A   *B*   *C*

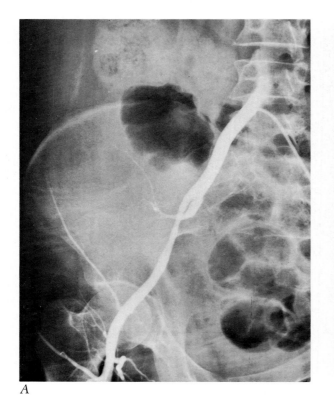
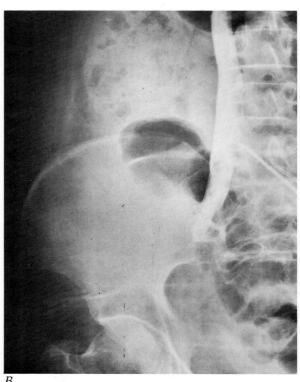

A   *B*

Figure 59-22. Renal transplant with renal vein thrombosis. This patient had marked oliguria in association with rejection. (A) Arteriogram. The intrarenal branches were profoundly narrowed, failed to fill adequately, and demonstrated a protracted transit time. (B) Common iliac venogram. Complete thrombosis of the common iliac vein adjacent to its anastomosis with the renal vein was present. A nephrectomy was performed; it demonstrated the pathologic changes of both rejection and renal vein thrombosis extending into the common iliac vein.

Table 59-11. Radiographic Findings in Patients with Renal Vein Thrombosis

| Author | Number of Patients with Thrombosis | Renal Vein Thrombus on Venography | | | Number of Patients Studied | Normal Urogram | Abnormal Urogram |
		Right	Left	Bilateral			
Llach et al. [72]	12	2	3	7	12	5	7
O'Dea et al. [86]	14	3	8	3	14	14	0
Rosenmann et al. [100]	10	0	2	8	14	9	5
Barclay et al. [12]	34	5	5	24	—	—	—
Our series	7	1	4	2	7	3	4
Total	77 (100%)	11 (14%)	22 (29%)	44 (57%)	47 (100%)	31 (66%)	16 (34%)

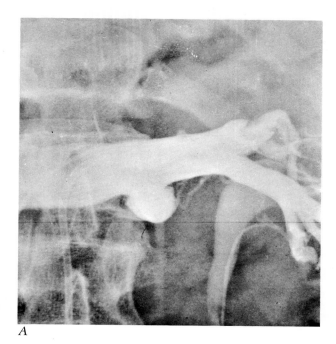

A

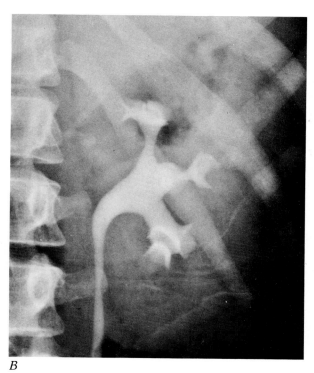

B

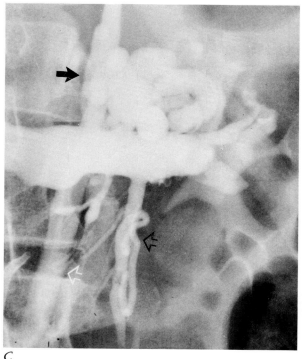

C

Figure 59-23. Renal vein varices. (A) Left renal venogram in an asymptomatic potential renal donor. There is a solitary varix at the entry of the spermatic vein. (B) Asymptomatic potential renal donor. An intravenous pyelogram shows a normal left collecting system. (C) Left renal venogram. A typical retroaortic vein (*open white arrow*) is seen arising from an unsplit main renal vein trunk. Note the network of varicose veins adjacent to the renal pelvis; there is opacification of the hemiazygos vein (*solid black arrow*) and of the ovarian vein (*open black arrow*). (D) A spontaneous portal vein–renal vein communication and varices in a patient with cirrhosis and portal hypertension, studied by transhepatic portography. An early-phase film of a selective coronary vein injection shows large gastric varices. (E) A late-phase film shows large varices in the region of the inferior phrenic and left adrenal veins that drain via the left renal vein (*open black arrows*) into the inferior vena cava (*arrowheads*). (Figure continued on p. 1352.)

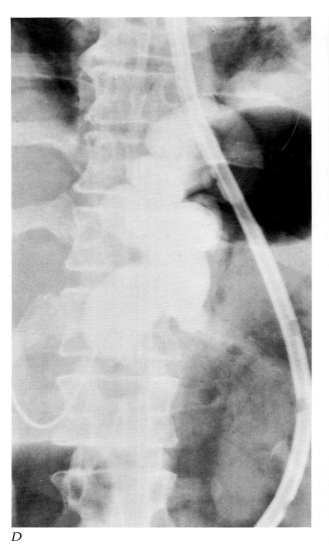

D

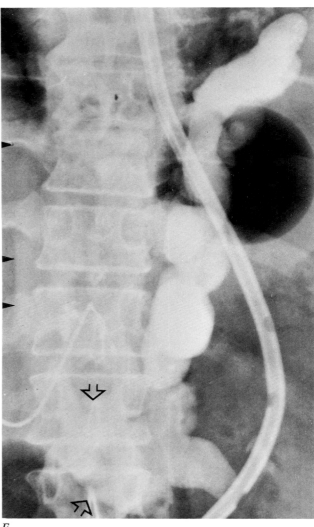

E

Urography may be negative; when it is positive, it is most often nonspecific. In the acute stage, the involved kidney is typically enlarged, with a moderate-to-marked reduction in function. Later, ureteral collateral vessels may produce notching of the renal pelvis and ureter. In the end stage, the kidney may be small and shrunken. These findings, either alone or together, are present in about one-third of patients; two-thirds have entirely normal urograms (Table 59-11).

Renal arteriography demonstrates stretching of the intrarenal arteries in the acute stage. During the venous phase, the main renal vein fails to opacify and retroperitoneal collateral vessels may be filled in total renal vein occlusion [55, 65]. These findings, although highly suggestive, are not diagnostic; they may be found in the absence of demonstrable renal vein thrombosis [38, 125].

An accurate diagnosis requires direct visualization of an intravascular thrombus by renal venography. One kidney is involved almost as often as both, the left kidney more commonly (Table 59-11). Both sides, therefore, should always be examined (Figs. 59-19, 59-20). The renal vein may be totally occluded near the entry to the IVC or adjacent to the kidney and thus prevent opacification of the intrarenal branches (Fig. 59-21A). In contrast to neoplastic invasion (see Fig. 59-15A, B), the thrombosed renal veins are distended and the central portion of the clot has a margin convex toward the IVC [13] (Fig. 59-21A). In some cases, the clot produces only partial obstruction and is seen as an intraluminal filling defect in the main renal vein (see Fig. 59-20B) or in intrarenal branches (Fig. 59-21B; see also Fig. 59-29A). Chronic or organized renal vein thrombus may be recognized by the demonstration of a

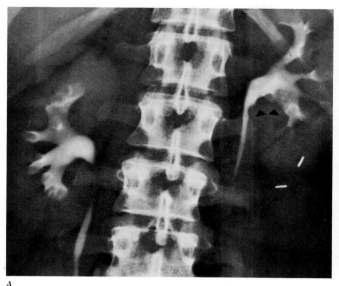

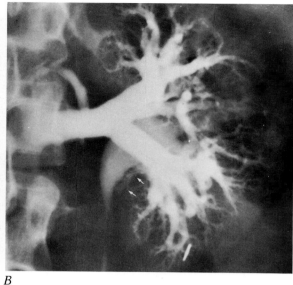

A   *B*

Figure 59-24. Renal vein varices. This 19-year-old woman had a history of recurrent hematuria. During prior surgery, varices had been ligated. (A) Intravenous pyelogram. There is notching of the renal pelvis and the proximal left ureter (*arrowheads*). (B) A left renal venogram shows a tortuous vein that notches the pelvis and the ureter (*arrows*).

narrow renal vein lumen with ill-defined outlines, linear bands representing synechiae, and peripheral occlusion (Fig. 59-21C; see also Fig. 59-19). In the transplanted kidney, oliguria, although most commonly caused by rejection, may also be associated with acute tubular necrosis, recurrence of glomerular nephritis, arterial stenosis or occlusion, renal vein thrombosis, and other causes. Venography is the only method of detecting renal vein thrombosis (Fig. 59-22). The early diagnosis of renal vein thrombosis is important; with appropriate anticoagulation therapy, pulmonary embolism may be prevented [9, 86].

In our experience, the risk of dislodging thrombus by the manipulation of a selective renal vein catheter is low. None of our patients developed pulmonary embolism after renal venography, an experience similar to that of other authors [86]. This low risk is amply justified if initial or repeated pulmonary embolism can be prevented.

RENAL VEIN VARICES

Pelviureteric varices are well documented as sequelae of renal vein thrombosis [33, 123]. Although there are few reports of idiopathic renal vein varices [17], they were found in eight (6%) of patients in the Peter Bent Brigham Hospital series. All were in the left renal venous system

and consisted of either a solitary varix of the left renal vein (Fig. 59-23A) or a network of veins (varicosities) adjacent to the renal pelvis (Fig. 59-23B, C). Renal vein varices are also formed in portal hypertension (Fig. 59-23D, E) [64]. Varices are probably more common than was previously reported, and the majority of the patients who have varices are free of symptoms. Rarely, varices may cause bleeding (Fig. 59-24). The urogram may be normal, even in cases in which varices are the source of bleeding [57, 81].

NONFUNCTIONING KIDNEY

In hypertensive patients, the differentiation of renal agenesis from a nonfunctioning hypoplastic kidney or a small, contracted kidney is clinically important. Diagnostic methods, such as abdominal aortography, cystoscopy, and retrograde pyelography, may be inconclusive and even misleading in these patients [11, 54]. Aortography may show the absence of a renal artery in both renal agenesis and small, shrunken kidneys [11]. In addition, the presence of a ureteral orifice on cystoscopy need not imply the presence of a kidney on that side [83].

On the other hand, the absence of a renal vein on venography is pathognomonic of agenesis of the kidney [11, 22, 54]. On the left side, the central portion of the renal vein (embryologi-

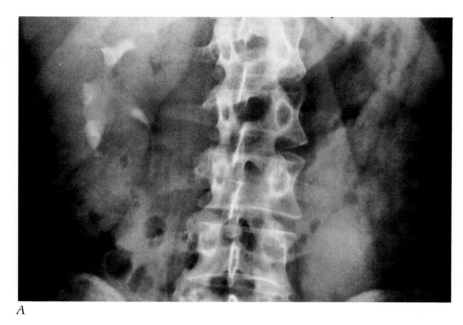

A

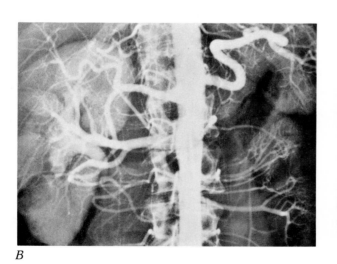

B

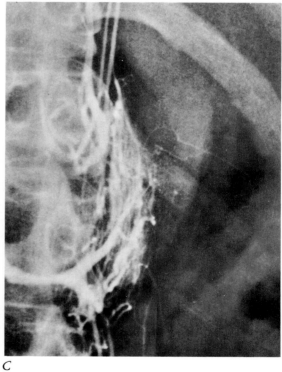

C

Figure 59-25. Agenesis of the left kidney. This patient had essential hypertension. (A) An intravenous pyelogram shows a large right kidney but no evidence of a left kidney. (B) On abdominal aortography, no left renal artery is seen. (C) Left renal venogram. In the expected location of the left renal vein, a small vein is seen draining both the left adrenal and the gonadal veins. The peripheral portion of the left renal vein, however, is absent. This appearance is pathognomonic for renal agenesis. (Courtesy of R. R. Freeman, M.D.)

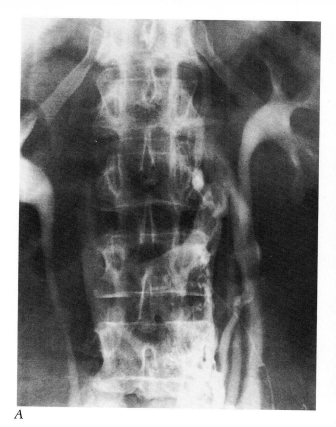

A

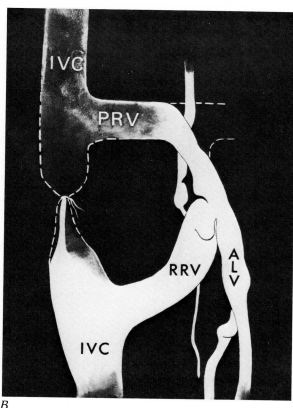

B

Figure 59-26. Caval ligation in a patient with a circumaortic venous ring. (A) Inferior vena cavogram (*IVC*) after the injection of contrast material into both iliac veins. (B) Explanatory drawing. The inferior vena cava is occluded in the region of L11. Opacified blood drains via the retroaortic renal vein (*RRV*) into the preaortic renal vein (*PRV*). *ALV* = ascending lumbar vein.

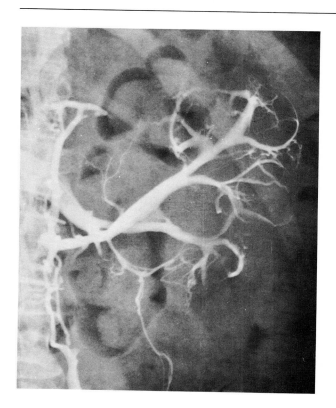

Figure 59-27. Venography in hydronephrosis. There are spreading and narrowing of the central veins, which are curved around the dilated renal calices. In contrast to intrarenal cysts (see Fig. 59-28), these veins are curved convex toward the periphery.

1355

cally, the preaortic portion of the renal collar) is still present, but it drains only the adrenal and the gonadal veins, thus creating a characteristic appearance on venography (Fig. 59-25). On the right side, if the kidney does not develop, there is no renal vein to catheterize.

The demonstration of a main renal vein with its lobar tributaries rules out renal agenesis. In contrast, in acquired diseases (i.e., shrunken kidneys), the main renal vein is of either normal size or only slightly diminished size, and the lobar veins are crowded and tortuous [22, 54]. In congenital hypoplasia, the main renal vein is small, and the intrarenal veins show an otherwise normal distribution [22]. In renal dysplasia [11, 22], venography shows the presence of a disordered venous architecture.

PREOPERATIVE AND POSTOPERATIVE EVALUATION OF THE RENAL VEINS

Prior knowledge of renal venous variations is important when retroperitoneal surgery is planned. A left circumaortic venous ring constitutes an instantaneous collateral pathway immediately after caval interruption [14] (Fig. 59-26); multiple right renal veins can serve as an alternative collateral route if the cava has been interrupted between these veins [44]. Therefore, a careful search for these frequent anatomic variations should be made by preoperative renal venography. If multiple right renal veins or a left circumaortic venous ring is found, the caval interruption must be below the orifice of these veins in the lower lumbar region.

During retroperitoneal surgery, the surgeon may visualize a preaortic vein but may be unaware of an additional retroaortic component and thus may involuntarily tear it while mobilizing the kidney or clamping the aorta [80]. Warren et al. [119, 120] have stressed the importance of preoperative angiographic evaluation of the left renal vein in preparation for splenorenal shunts for portal hypertension. Prior knowledge of the location, appearance, and possible variations of the left renal vein allows the procedure to be tailored to the needs of each patient and therefore results in less tissue manipulation at the operating table, to the advantage of the patients, who often are critically ill. Postoperatively, venography is important in evaluating the patency of these shunts. Even in the presence of occlusion of the left renal vein, however, these shunts might still be patent and drain into retroperitoneal collateral vessels [108].

BENIGN RENAL PARENCHYMAL DISEASE

Selective renal venography can be a useful but nonspecific method of evaluating diseases of the renal parenchyma.

In *acute glomerulonephritis*, the renal venogram is normal; however, in *chronic glomerulonephritis* there may be diffuse loss of cortex as documented by the distance between the arcuate veins and the renal surface. Similar diffuse findings may be seen in shrunken nephrosclerotic kidneys [59, 99].

Localized abnormalities are characteristic of *pyelonephritis*. Areas of closely approximated veins are found in pyelonephritic scars [59]. Pyelonephritic pseudotumors may produce displacement of both interlobar and arcuate veins [57, 109].

In *hydronephrosis* (Figs. 59-27, 59-28), there is spreading of the central veins, which appear narrowed, stretched, and curved [99], and the arcuate veins are irregularly filled and stretched. Rarely, anomalous renal veins may produce hydronephrosis [43]. In *polycystic disease* (Fig. 59-29), the interlobar veins primarily are stretched, narrowed, and curved around the centrally located cysts. Typically, however, the deformed veins have smooth outlines [99].

Renal fibrolipomatosis (Fig. 59-30) represents fatty replacement of destroyed or atrophic renal parenchyma. Although the urogram is suggestive and is frequently diagnostic when combined with tomography, the distinction from mass lesions is not always clear. The venogram may demonstrate a relatively normal distribution of venous tributaries when the urogram and the arteriogram are equivocal or suggestive of cysts or other mass lesions.

Renal venography is not required to establish the diagnosis of hydronephrosis, polycystic disease, or fibrolipomatosis. Nevertheless, when venography is indicated for other reasons (e.g., unexplained hematuria), familiarity with the venographic findings in these patients is important if the correct interpretation is to be made.

ACKNOWLEDGMENT

Some of the illustrations and text in this chapter are reproduced with permission from C. F. Beckmann and H. L. Abrams, Renal venography: Anatomy, technique, applications, analysis of 132 venograms, and a review of the literature. *Cardiovasc. Intervent. Radiol.* 3:45, 1980.

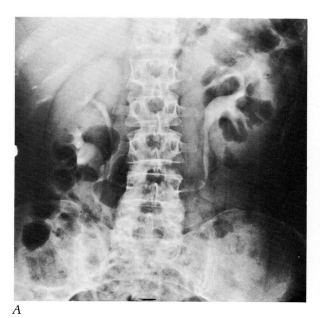

A

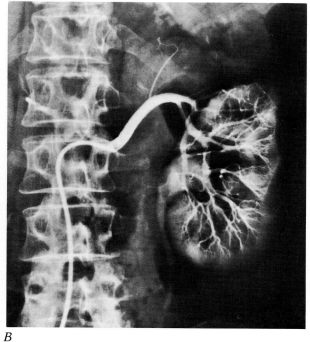

B

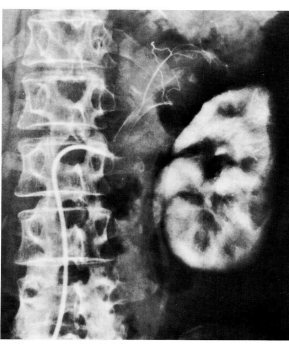

C

Figure 59-28. Venography in hydronephrosis of the upper pole of a double kidney. (A) Intravenous urogram. On the right, a bifid kidney is visible. On the left, the collecting system is normal insofar as it is visualized. No collecting system is visualized in the upper pole, which was thought to represent a mass. (B and C) Selective left renal arteriogram. Normal branches and nephrogram in the midsegment and the lower segment of the left kidney are apparent. An adrenal-capsular branch appears to supply the hypovascular upper pole. (D) Left renal venogram. The intrarenal veins in the midsegment and the lower pole appear normal. There is an unusual network of veins, including the adrenal vein, supplying the upper pole. The presence of an adrenal mass cannot be excluded on the basis of this study alone. (E) Selective upper pole renal venogram. Following injection, a network of veins is visible, arising from the renal vein and draped around the avascular "mass" in the pole of the kidney. It strongly suggests the renal origin of the apparent mass lesion. (F) Percutaneous puncture of the upper pole. A contrast injection demonstrates a hydronephrotic upper pole of a bifid collecting system, with gross hydroureter, which indicates obstruction in the distal ureter. (Courtesy of R. Hooshmand, M.D.)

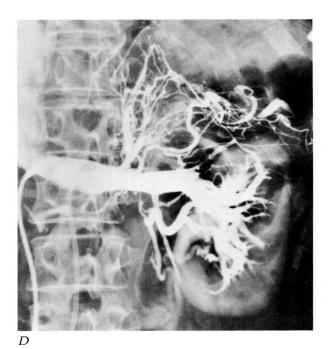

D

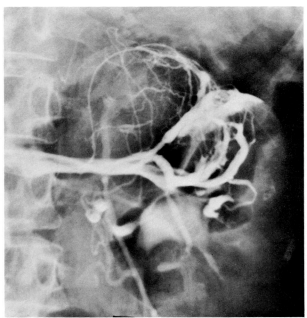

E

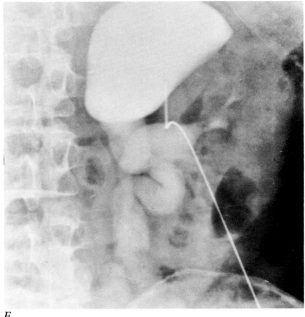

F

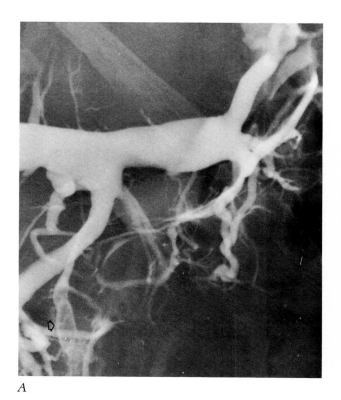

A

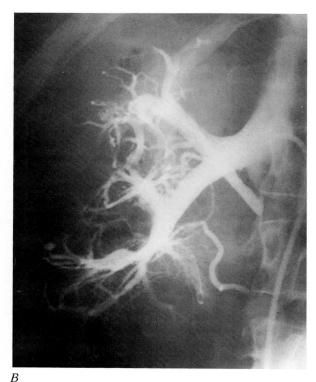

B

Figure 59-29. Polycystic disease. Bilateral renal venogram obtained because of suspected renal vein thrombosis in patients with known polycystic disease. (A) Left renal venogram. (B) Right renal venogram. The intrarenal veins are stretched and curved around the large intrarenal cysts in a fashion convex toward the renal hilus. Note the presence of two right renal veins and a capsular vein communicating with a lumbar branch. In (A), a small intravascular thrombus (*arrow*) is seen in a lower pole branch.

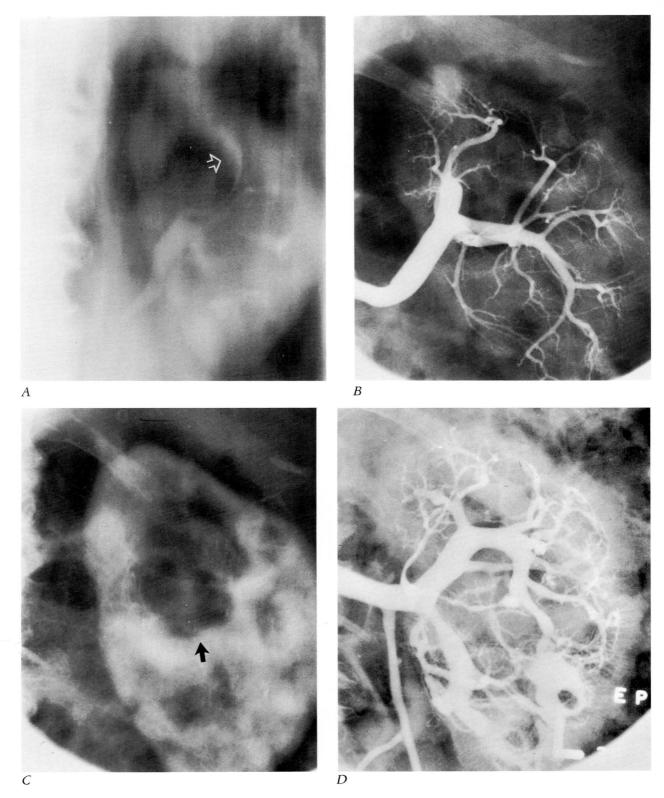

A

B

C

D

Figure 59-30. Renal fibrolipomatosis. (A) A tomographic section of the intravenous pyelogram suggests an upper pole mass indenting the upper pole infundibulum (*arrow*). The kidney of the periinfundibular areas suggests a lipomatous infiltration. (B) The early-phase film and (C) the late-phase film of a selective renal arteriogram again suggest the presence of a cystic avascular mass lesion of the upper pole (*arrow*). (D) The left renal venogram, however, shows a normal distribution of intrarenal venous branches, ruling out a mass lesion and supporting the diagnosis of renal fibrolipomatosis.

References

1. Abrams, H. L., Baum, S., and Stamey, T. Renal venous washout time in renovascular hypertension. *Radiology* 83:597, 1964.
2. Adachi, B. Cited by Reis and Esenther [94].
3. Ahlberg, N. E., Bartley, O., and Chidekel, N. Right and left gonadal veins, an anatomical and statistical study. *Acta Radiol. [Diagn.]* (Stockh.) 4:593, 1966.
4. Ahlberg, N. E., Bartley, O., and Chidekel, N. Occurrence of valves in the main trunk of the renal vein. *Acta Radiol [Diagn.]* (Stockh.) 7:431, 1968.
5. Ahlberg, N. E., Bartley, O., Chidekel, N., and Wahlquist, L. An anatomic and roentgenographic study of the communications of the renal vein in patients with and without renal carcinoma. *Scand. J. Urol. Nephrol.* 1:43, 1967.
6. Anatkow, J., and Kumanow, C. Selective Nephro-Phlebography. In L. Diethelm (ed.), *Symposium of the European Association of Radiology.* Mainz: Springer, 1972.
7. Anson, B. J., and Daseler, E. H. Common variations in renal anatomy, affecting blood supply, form, and topography. *Surg. Gynecol. Obstet.* 112:439, 1961.
8. Anson, B. J., Pick, J. W., Cauldwell, E. W., and Beaton, L. E. The anatomy of the pararenal system of veins, with comments on the renal arteries. *J. Urol.* 60:714, 1948.
9. Appel, G. B., Williams, G. S., Meltzer, J. J., and Pirani, C. L. Renal vein thrombosis, nephrotic syndrome and systemic lupus erythematosus. *Ann. Intern. Med.* 85:310, 1966.
10. Arner, O., Blank, C., and Schreeb, T. B. Analysis with references to malignancy grading and special morphological features. *Acta Chir. Scand. [Suppl.]* 346:1, 1965.
11. Athanasoulis, C. A., Brown, B., and Baum, S. Selective renal venography in differentiation between congenitally absent and small contracted kidney. *Radiology* 108:301, 1973.
12. Barclay, G. P., Cameron, H. M., and Loughridge, L. W. Amyloid disease of the kidney and renal vein thrombosis. *Q. J. Med.* 29:137, 1960.
13. Beckmann, C. F., and Abrams, H. L. Renal vein valves: Incidence and significance. *Radiology* 127:351, 1978.
14. Beckmann, C. F., and Abrams, H. L. Circumaortic venous ring: Incidence and significance. *AJR* 132:561, 1979.
15. Beckmann, C. F., and Abrams, H. L. Renal venography: Anatomy, technique, applications, analysis of 132 venograms, and a review of the literature. *Cardiovasc. Intervent. Radiol.* 3:45, 1980.
16. Beres, J. A., Zboralske, F. F., Wilson, S. D., and Amberg, J. R. Percutaneous transrenal venography in experimental renal vein obstruction and human renal vein thrombosis. *Radiology* 83:587, 1964.
17. Blaivas, J. G., Previte, S. R., and Pais, V. M. Idiopathic pelvic ureteric varices. *J. Urol.* 9:207, 1977.
18. Boijsen, E., and Folin, J. Angiography in the diagnosis of renal carcinoma. *Radiologe* 1:173, 1961.
19. Bookstein, J. J. Appraisal of arteriography in estimating the hemodynamic significance of renal artery stenosis. *Invest. Radiol.* 1:281, 1966.
20. Bourgoignie, J., Kurz, S., Catanzaro, F. J., Serirat, P., and Perry, H. M. Renal venous renin in hypertension. *Am. J. Med.* 48:332, 1970.
21. Braedel, H. U., Haage, H., Moeller, J. F., and Schindler, E. Differential diagnostic importance in cases of unusual ectasia and renal pelvic deformity. *Radiology* 119:65, 1976.
22. Braedel, H. U., Schindler, E., Moeller, J. F., and Polsky, M. S. Renal phlebography: An aid in the diagnosis of the absent or non-functioning kidney. *J. Urol.* 116:703, 1976.
23. Chait, A., Stoane, L., Moskowitz, H., and Mellins, H. Z. Renal vein thrombosis. *Radiology* 90:886, 1968.
24. Chuang, V. P., Mena, C. E., and Hoskins, P. A. Congenital anomalies of the inferior vena cava. Review of embryogenesis and presentation of a simplified classification. *Br. J. Radiol.* 47:214, 1974.
25. Clark, K. The blood vessels of the adrenal gland. *J. R. Coll. Surg.* 4:257, 1959.
26. Cope, C., and Isard, H. J. Left renal vein entrapment. *Radiology* 92:867, 1969.
27. Crocker, D. W. Renal Tumors. In S. C. Sommers (ed.), *Kidney Pathology Decennial 1966–1975.* New York: Appleton-Century-Crofts, 1975.
28. Davis, C. J., and Lundberg, G. D. Retroaortic left renal vein. *Am. J. Clin. Pathol.* 50:700, 1968.
29. Delin, N. A., and Haverling, M. Renal artery and vein flow during aortic and inferior vena caval occlusion and retrograde renal phlebography. *Invest. Radiol.* 1:148, 1966.
30. Dorr, R. P., Cerny, J. C., and Hoskins, P. A. Inferior venacavograms and renal venograms in the management of renal tumors. *J. Urol.* 110:280, 1973.
31. Dow, J. A., and Takaro, T. Anomalous tributary of the left renal vein diagnosed by selective renal phlebography: Case report. *J. Urol.* 98:150, 1967.
32. Duckett, J. W., Lifland, J. H., and Peters, P. C. Resection of the inferior vena cava for adja-

cent malignant disease. *Surg. Gynecol. Obstet.* 136:711, 1973.

33. Eisen, S., Friedenberg, M. J., and Klahr, S. Bilateral ureteral notching and selective renal phlebography in the nephrotic syndrome due to renal vein thrombosis. *J. Urol.* 93:343, 1965.

34. Ernst, C. B., Bookstein, J. J., and Moutie, J. Renal vein renin ratios and collateral vessels in renovascular hypertension. *Arch. Surg.* 104:496, 1972.

35. Fagarasanu, I. Recherches anatomiques sur la veine rénale gauche et ses collatérales; leurs rapports avec la pathogénie du variococèle essential et des varices du ligament large (Démonstrations expérimentales). *Ann. Anat. Pathol.* 15:9, 1938.

36. Ferris, E. J., Bosniak, M. A., and O'Connor, J. F. An angiographic sign demonstrating extension of renal carcinoma into the renal vein and vena cava. *AJR* 102:384, 1968.

37. Field, S., and Saxton, H. Venous anomalies complicating left adrenal catheterization. *Br. J. Radiol.* 47:219, 1974.

38. Folin, J. Angiography in renal tumors, its value in diagnosis and differential diagnosis as a complement to conventional methods. *Acta Radiol.* [*Suppl.*] (Stockh.) 267:30, 1967.

39. Genest, J., and Boucher, R. The Renin-Angiotensin System in Human Renal Hypertension. In G. Onesti (ed.), *Hypertension: Mechanism and Management*. New York: Grune & Stratton, 1971. Pp. 411–420.

40. Georgi, M., Marberger, M., Gunther, R., Orestano, F., and Halbsguth, A. Retrograde Nierenphlebographie bei Ballonverschluss der Nierenarterie. *ROEFO* 123:341, 1975.

41. Gilsanz, V., Anaya, A., Estrada, R., and Toni, P. Transparietal renal phlebography: A new method. *Lancet* 1:179, 1965.

42. Gilsanz, V., Estrada, R., and Malillos, E. Transparietal renal cavophlebography. *Angiology* 18:565, 1967.

43. Gilsanz, V., Rabadan, M., Leiva Galvis, O., and Estrada, V. A singular case of hydronephrosis produced by inferior left lobar renal vein demonstrated by transparietal renal phlebography. *Angiology* 23:311, 1972.

44. Greweldinger, J., Coomaraswamy, R., Luftschein, S., and Bosniak, M. A. Collateral circulation through the kidney after inferior vena cava ligation. *N. Engl. J. Med.* 281:541, 1969.

45. Griffiths, J. H., and Thackray, A. C. Parenchymal carcinoma of the kidney. *Br. J. Urol.* 21:128, 1949.

46. Hamilton, C. R., and Tumulty, P. A. Thrombosis of renal veins and inferior vena cava complicating lupus nephritis. *J.A.M.A.* 206:2315, 1968.

47. Hamilton, W. J., and Mossman, H. W. *Human Embryology* (4th ed.). Baltimore: Williams & Wilkins, 1972. Pp. 192–195.

48. Hand, J. P., and Broders, A. C. Carcinoma of kidney. *J. Urol.* 28:199, 1932.

49. Harrington, D. P., White, R. I., Kaufman, S. L., Whelton, P. K., Russell, R. P., and Walker, W. G. Determination of optimum methods of renal venous renin sampling in suspected renovascular hypertension. *Invest. Radiol.* 10:45, 1975.

50. Hipona, F. A., and Crummy, A. B. The roentgen diagnosis of renal vein thrombosis. Clinical aspects. *AJR* 98:122, 1966.

51. Hollinshead, W. H. Renovascular anatomy. *Postgrad. Med.* 40:241, 1966.

52. Hollinshead, W. H., and McFarland, J. A. The collateral venous drainage from the kidney following occlusion of the renal vein in the dog. *Surg. Gynecol. Obstet.* 97:213, 1953.

53. Hunt, J. C., and Strong, C. G. Renovascular hypertension. Mechanisms, natural history and treatment. *Am. J. Cardiol.* 32:562, 1973.

54. Itzchak, Y., Adar, R., Mozes, M., and Deutsch, V. Renal venography in the diagnosis of agenesis and small contracted kidney. *Clin. Radiol.* 25:379, 1974.

55. Itzchak, Y., Deutsch, V., Adar, R., and Mozes, M. Angiography of renal capsular complex in normal and pathological conditions and its diagnostic implications. *CRC Crit. Rev. Diagn. Imaging* 5:111, 1974.

56. Janower, M. L. Nephrotic syndrome secondary to renal vein thrombosis. *AJR* 79:911, 1962.

57. Jonsson, K. Renal angiography in patients with hematuria. *AJR* 116:758, 1972.

58. Kahn, P. C. Selective Venography of the Branches. In E. Ferris (ed.), *Venography of the Inferior Vena Cava and Its Branches*. Baltimore: Williams & Wilkins, 1969. Pp. 154–224.

59. Kahn, P. C. Selective venography in renal parenchymal disease. *Radiology* 92:345, 1969.

60. Kahn, P. C., Wise, H. M., and Robbins, A. H. Complete angiographic evaluation of renal cancer. *J.A.M.A.* 204:753, 1968.

61. Kaneko, Y., Ikeda, T., Takeda, T., and Ueda, H. Renin release during acute reduction of arterial pressure in normotensive subjects and patients with renovascular hypertension. *J. Clin. Invest.* 46:705, 1967.

62. Katzberg, R. W., Morris, T. W., Burgener, F. A., Kamm, D. E., and Fischer, H. W. Renal renin and hemodynamic responses to selective renal artery catheterization and angiography. *Invest. Radiol.* 12:381, 1977.

63. Kendall, A. G., Lohmann, R. C., and Dossetor, J. B. Nephrotic syndrome. *Arch. Intern. Med.* 127:1021, 1971.

64. Keshin, J. G., and Joffe, A. Varices of the upper urinary tract and their relationship to portal hypertension. *J. Urol.* 76:350, 1956.

65. Koehler, P. R., Bowles, W. T., and McAlister, W. H. Renal arteriography in experimental renal vein occlusion. *Radiology* 86:851, 1966.

66. Korobkin, M., Glickman, M. G., and Schambelan, M. Segmental renal vein sampling for renin. *Radiology* 118:307, 1976.

67. Kuchel, O., and Genest, J. Effect of Antihypertensive Drugs on Renin Release. In G. Onesti (ed.), *Hypertension: Mechanism and Management.* New York: Grune & Stratton, 1971. Pp. 411–420.

68. Lang, E. K. Arteriographic assessment and staging of renal-cell carcinoma. *Radiology* 101:17, 1971.

69. Laragh, J. H., Baer, L., Brunner, H. R., Buhler, F. R., Sealey, J. E., and Vaughn, E. D. Renin, angiotensin and aldosterone system in pathogenesis and management of hypertensive vascular disease. *Am. J. Med.* 52:633, 1972.

70. Lejar, R. C. Cited by Pick and Anson [92].

71. Lien, H. H., and Kolbenstvedt, A. Phlebographic appearances of the left renal and left testicular veins. *Acta Radiol. [Diagn.]* (Stockh.) 18:321, 1977.

72. Llach, F., Arieff, A. J., and Massey, S. G. Renal vein thrombosis and nephrotic syndrome. A prospective study of 36 adult patients. *Ann. Intern. Med.* 83:8, 1975.

73. March, T. L., and Halpern, M. Renal vein thrombosis demonstrated by selective renal phlebography. *Radiology* 81:958, 1963.

74. McCarthy, L. J., Titus, J. L., and Daugherty, G. W. Bilateral renal vein thrombosis and the nephrotic syndrome in adults. *Ann. Intern. Med.* 58:837, 1963.

75. McCullough, D. L., and Gittes, R. F. Vena cava resection for renal cell carcinoma. *J. Urol.* 112:162, 1974.

76. McCullough, D. L., and Gittes, R. F. Ligation of the renal vein in the solitary kidney: Effects on renal function. *J. Urol.* 113:295, 1975.

77. McDonald, J. R., and Priestley, J. T. Malignant tumors of the kidney. *Surg. Gynecol. Obstet.* 77:295, 1943.

78. Michelakis, A. M., and Simmons, J. Effect of posture on renal vein renin activity in hypertension. *J.A.M.A.* 208:659, 1969.

79. Michelakis, A. M., Woods, J. W., Liddle, G. W., and Klatte, E. C. A predictable error in use of renal vein renin in diagnosing hypertension. *Arch. Intern. Med.* 123:359, 1969.

80. Mitty, H. A. Circumaortic renal collar. A potentially hazardous anomaly of the left renal vein. *AJR* 125:307, 1975.

81. Mitty, H. A., and Goldman, H. Angiography in unilateral renal bleeding with a negative urogram. *AJR* 121:508, 1974.

82. Myers, G. H., Fehrenbaker, L. G., and Kelalis, P. P. Prognostic significance of renal vein invasion by hypernephroma. *J. Urol.* 100:420, 1968.

83. Ney, C., and Friedenberg, R. M. *Radiographic Atlas of the Genito-Urinary System.* Philadelphia: Lippincott, 1966.

84. Notkovich, H. Variations of the testicular and ovarian arteries in relation to the renal pedicle. *Surg. Gynecol. Obstet.* 103:487, 1956.

85. Novak, D. Selective renal occlusion phlebography with a balloon catheter. *Br. J. Radiol.* 49:589, 1976.

86. O'Dea, M. J., Malel, R. S., Tucker, R. M., and Fulton, R. E. Renal vein thrombosis. *J. Urol.* 116:410, 1976.

87. Olin, T. B., and Reuter, S. R. A pharmacoangiographic method for improving nephrophlebography. *Radiology* 85:1036, 1965.

88. Palmer, J., Barry, B., Williams, R., and Briscoe, P. Diagnosis of venous extension in renal cell carcinoma. The value of routine inferior venacavography. *Australas. Radiol.* 19:265, 1975.

89. Paster, S., Adams, D. F., and Abrams, H. L. Errors in renal vein renin collections. *AJR* 122:804, 1974.

90. Perez, C. A., Kaiman, H. A., Keith, J., Mill, W. B., Vietti, T. J., and Powers, W. E. Treatment of Wilms' tumor and factors affecting prognosis. *Cancer* 32:609, 1973.

91. Petasnick, J. P., and Patel, S. K. Angiographic evaluation of the nonvisualizing kidney. *AJR* 119:757, 1973.

92. Pick, J. W., and Anson, B. J. The renal vascular pedicle. *J. Urol.* 44:411, 1940.

93. Proca, E. Technique of renal phlebography through the left spermatic vein. An aid to the management of renal carcinoma. *Br. J. Urol.* 38:501, 1966.

94. Reis, R. H., and Esenther, G. Variations in the pattern of renal vessels and their relation to the type of posterior vena cava in man. *Am. J. Anat.* 104:295, 1959.

95. Renert, W. A., Rudin, L. J., and Casarella, W. J. Renal vein thrombosis in carcinoma of the renal pelvis. *AJR* 114:735, 1972.

96. Riches, E. On carcinoma of the kidney. *Ann. R. Coll. Surg.* 32:201, 1963.

97. Riches, E. W. Analysis of Patients with Adenocarcinoma in a Personal Series. In E. W. Riches (ed.), *Tumors of the Kidney and Ureter: Neoplastic Disease at Various Sites* (Vol. 5). Baltimore: Williams & Wilkins, 1964.

98. Riches, E. W., Griffiths, I. H., and Thackray, A. C. New growths of the kidney and ureter. *Br. J. Urol.* 23:297, 1951.

99. Rösch, J., Antonovic, R., Goldman, M. L., and

Dotter, C. T.   Epinephrine renal venography. *ROEFO* 126:501, 1975.

100. Rosenmann, E., Pollack, V. E., and Pirani, C. L.   Renal vein thrombosis in the adult: A clinical and pathologic study based on renal biopsies. *Medicine* 47:269, 1968.

101. Royal, S. A., and Callen, P. W.   CT evaluation of anomalies of the inferior vena cava and left renal vein. *AJR* 132:759, 1979.

102. Schaeffer, A. J., and Fair, W. R.   Comparison of split function ratios with renal vein renin ratios in patients with curable hypertension caused by unilateral renal artery stenosis. *J. Urol.* 112:697, 1974.

103. Schambelan, M., Howes, E. L., Stockigt, J. R., Noakes, C. A., and Biglieri, E. G.   Role of renin and aldosterone in hypertension due to a renin-secreting tumor. *Am. J. Med.* 55:86, 1973.

104. Sealey, J. E., Buhler, F. R., Laragh, J. H., and Vaughan, E. D.   The physiology of renin secretion in essential hypertension. Estimation of renin secretion rate and renal plasma flow from peripheral and renal vein renin levels. *Am. J. Med.* 55:391, 1973.

105. Simmons, J. L., and Michelakis, A. M.   Renovascular hypertension: The diagnostic value of renal vein renin ratios. *J. Urol.* 104:497, 1970.

106. Simpson, A., Baron, M. G., and Mitty, H. A.   Angiographic patterns of venous extension of hypernephroma. *J. Urol.* 111:441, 1974.

107. Smith, J. C., Rösch, J., Athanasoulis, C., Baum, S., Waltman, A. C., and Goldman, N.   Renal venography in the evaluation of poorly vascularized neoplasms of the kidney. *AJR* 123:552, 1975.

108. Sones, P. J., Rude, J. C., Berg, D. J., and Warren, W. D.   Evaluation of the left renal vein in candidates for splenorenal shunts. *Radiology* 127:357, 1978.

109. Sorby, W. A.   Renal phlebography. *Clin. Radiol.* 20:166, 1969.

110. Stables, D. P., and Thatcher, G. N.   Traumatic renal vein thrombosis associated with renal artery occlusion. *Br. J. Radiol.* 46:64, 1973.

111. Stockigt, J. R., Hertz, P., Schambelan, M., and Biglieri, E. G.   Segmental renal-vein renin sampling for segmental renal infarction. *Ann. Intern. Med.* 79:67, 1973.

112. Stockigt, J. R., Noakes, C. A., Collins, R. D., and Schambelan, M.   Renal-vein renin in various forms of renal hypertension. *Lancet* 1:1194, 1972.

113. Susin, M., Mailloux, L., and Becker, C.   Renal vein thrombosis in patients with membranous glomerulonephritis. *Kidney Int.* 6:103A, 1974.

114. Takaro, T., Dow, J. A., and Kishew, S.   Selective occlusive renal phlebography in man. *Radiology* 94:589, 1970.

115. Turner, R. J., Young, S. W., and Castellino, R. A.   Dynamic continuous computed tomography: Study of retroaortic left renal vein. *J. Comput. Assist. Tomogr.* 4:109, 1980.

116. Vaughan, E. D.   Renin sampling: Collection and interpretation. *N. Engl. J. Med.* 290:1195, 1974.

117. Vaughan, E. D., Buhler, F. R., Laragh, J. H., Sealey, J. E., Baer, L., and Bard, R. H.   Renovascular hypertension: Renin measurements to indicate hypersecretion and contralateral suppression, estimate renal plasma flow and score for surgical curability. *Am. J. Med.* 55:402, 1973.

118. Vermillion, S. E., Sheps, S. G., Strong, C. G., Harrison, E. G., and Hunt, J. C.   Effect of sodium depletion on renin activity of renal venous plasma in renovascular hypertension. *J.A.M.A.* 208:2303, 1969.

119. Warren, W. D., Salam, A. A., and Faislalo, A.   End renal vein-to-splenic vein shunts for total or selective portal decompression. *Surgery* 72:995, 1972.

120. Warren, W. D., Salam, A. A., and Hutson, D.   Selective distal splenorenal shunt. *Arch. Surg.* 108:306, 1974.

121. Watson, R. C., Fleming, R. J., and Evans, J. A.   Arteriography in the diagnosis of renal carcinoma. *Radiology* 91:888, 1968.

122. Wegner, G. P., Crummy, A. B., Flaherty, T. T., and Hipona, F. A.   Renal vein thrombosis, a roentgenographic diagnosis. *J.A.M.A.* 209:1661, 1969.

123. Weiner, P. L., Lim, M. S., Knudson, D. H., and Semekdjian, H. S.   Retrograde pyelography in renal vein thrombosis. *Radiology* 111:77, 1974.

124. Weinstein, B. B., Countiss, E. H., and Derber, V. S.   Renal vessels in 203 cadavers. *Urol. Cutan. Rev.* 44:137, 1940.

125. Whitley, N. O., Kinkhabwala, M., and Whitley, J. E.   The collateral vein sign, a fallible sign in the staging of renal cancer. *AJR* 120:660, 1974.

Renal Transplantation

JÜRI V. KAUDE
IRVIN F. HAWKINS, JR.

Renal transplantation is generally accepted as a definitive form of therapy for end-stage kidney disease. With better understanding of the immunologic problems of transplantation, the advances in immunosuppressive therapy, and the increasing use of kidneys from living related donors and because of the accumulated experience in transplant surgery, the success rate as well as the transplant survival time has increased steadily over the past 17 years [2, 3, 9, 144]. Nevertheless, both the transplanted kidney and its recipient may be endangered by a number of complications both surgical and medical, infectious and noninfectious [35, 69, 75, 85, 104, 112, 139]. These complications must be recognized early and treated properly to ensure the ultimate success of the transplant or at least to prolong its survival.

Indications for Angiography

Since the early days of transplantation surgery, angiography has been used extensively in the investigation of renal transplantation complications [4, 16, 17, 24, 28, 42, 43, 46, 67, 68, 84, 87, 94, 95, 97, 98, 100, 101, 106, 114, 118, 119, 125, 128, 134, 140, 142, 143]. In recent years, however, other imaging modalities (radionuclide studies, ultrasonography, and, to a lesser extent, computed tomography) have reduced the need to perform angiography [9, 28, 59, 71, 81, 133, 143, 151].

In our institution, Pfaff and his associates have transplanted more than 400 kidneys. We have conducted more than 230 angiographic examinations of these patients since 1966. We now perform angiography of a renal transplant on the following indications (and in most instances after radionuclide scans or ultrasonography has demonstrated the need for angiographic confirmation of a suspected pathologic condition):

1. Indications for arteriography
   a. Renal artery thrombosis
   b. Unrelenting rejection despite repeated boluses of intravenous methylprednisolone (20 mg per kilogram body weight)
   c. Progressive deterioration of renal function
   d. Uncontrollable hypertension (arteriography and venous sampling for the determination of plasma renin activity)

e. Hematuria
   (1) Unexplained
   (2) Persistent, following renal biopsy
2. Indications for venography
   a. Nephrotic syndrome (massive proteinuria), indicating renal vein thrombosis or chronic rejection
   b. Leg edema, indicating femoroiliac vein obstruction

Donor Angiography

Angiography is included in the preoperative workup of the kidney donor provided that the preceding urography did not reveal any abnormalities that would preclude renal transplantation. Preoperative donor angiography is performed to determine the vascular supply of the kidney (single or multiple arteries) and of the ureter; to make sure the renal veins are normal; to exclude vascular or renal pathology that may not be evident from the preceding urography (stenotic lesions or aneurysms of the renal arteries; small tumors or cysts; intrarenal vascular disease); and to determine whether atheromatosis of the aorta close to the renal arteries is present [26, 123, 132, 135].

Some authors believe that one or two aortic injections in different projections are sufficient for the preoperative evaluation of donor kidneys [123, 135]. The value of selective renal angiography in the detection of intrarenal vascular abnormalities and small or poorly vascularized renal lesions is, however, well documented and has been generally accepted. We believe that angiographic evaluation of donor kidneys should be performed as renal angiography in a patient thought to have renal disease. Therefore, we perform preoperative angiography with both aortic and selective renal artery injections using a single small catheter [50]. Alternatively, a semiselective technique for renal angiography can be used [13, 14, 66].

As many as 21 to 44 percent of the prospective donors have multiple renal arteries on at least one side, and abnormalities of the donor kidney or of vasculature that are of importance for transplant surgery or in the use of the kidney as a graft are detected in 9 to 17 percent of cases [26, 123, 132]. These findings include renal artery stenosis, aneurysms, nephrosclerosis, stone disease, py-

elonephritis, and tumors and cysts. Multiple renal arteries, although associated with a higher rate of transplantation complications [130], and ectopic kidneys [131] are not regarded as contraindications to transplantation [130, 132, 139]. Kidneys with simple cysts can also be used as grafts [132].

Technique of Transplant Angiography

The renal transplant recipients who are referred for angiography are often critically ill. Since they have been treated with steroids and other immunosuppressive agents, the risk for development of infections is generally higher for them than for other patients. In the early postoperative stage, they are heparinized, which increases the risk of bleeding during or after angiography. Finally, the possibility for the development of (additional) renal tubular damage from injected contrast medium must be considered. For all these reasons, scrupulous sterile technique must be observed, small catheters should be preferred to large ones, the examination must be performed quickly and with the least inconvenience to the patient but all diagnostic information needed for further treatment must be obtained, and the number of injections and the amount of contrast medium must be kept at a minimum.

ARTERIAL CATHETERIZATION

We prefer to puncture the contralateral femoral artery [67, 68] for the following three reasons:

1. We can stay away from the transplant, an incision from a recent operation, and drains, which may interfere both with the puncture and with compression of the artery following the withdrawal of the catheter.
2. Selective catheterization of the internal iliac artery or the renal artery is technically easier from the contralateral side, and a common iliac artery injection can be done in antegrade fashion with minimal or no reflux of contrast medium into the aorta.
3. The puncture site is farther away from the field of radiation and so the absorbed dose to the fingers of the angiographer during fluoroscopy is reduced.

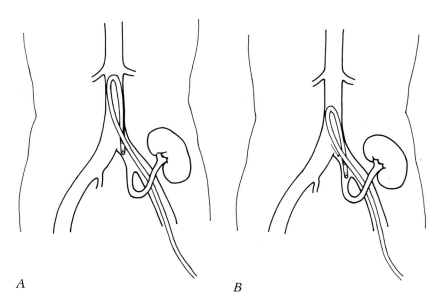

A   *B*

Figure 60-1. (A) After the direction of the catheter tip has been reversed in the lumbar or renal artery or with the aid of a deflector, the loop that is formed is retracted into the ipsilateral or the contralateral com-mon iliac artery. (B) After the initial common iliac artery injection, the catheter is retracted into the internal iliac artery for a selective injection.

Because in the great majority of cases, the kidney is transplanted into the right iliac fossa, the left femoral artery is punctured. The renal artery is usually anastomosed end to end with the internal iliac artery and can be catheterized with either a curved catheter or a straight catheter. The tip of the preformed catheter is reversed in one of the lumbar arteries or in the patient's own renal arteries. The formed loop is then retracted under continuous rotation, and the tip of the catheter is placed over the bifurcation into the common iliac artery on the side of the transplant. The catheter can be further advanced selectively into the internal iliac artery, occasionally with the help of a deflector (Fig. 60-1). Selective catheterization of the renal artery itself should not be performed in patients who have recently been operated on.

The straight catheter requires the use of a deflector (a pediatric deflector, with a curve radius of 0.5 cm) for selective catheterization (Figs. 60-2, 60-3). In recent years we have increasingly used a small (4.1 French) polyethylene catheter with three side holes [48, 50]. The vascular trauma from a puncture with a 19-gauge needle or a cannula with a Teflon sheath and from the small catheter is minimal. The catheter will deliver 12 cc per second of 60 percent contrast material or 10 cc per second of 76 percent contrast material without recoil.

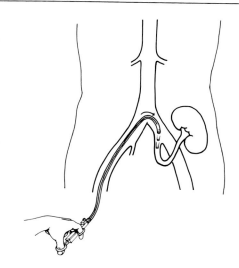

Figure 60-2. Minicurve (0.5-mm radius) deflector is advanced to the tip of the catheter, which is positioned at the aortic bifurcation. The deflector is anchored, and the catheter is advanced into the common iliac artery for the initial injection. After replacement of the deflector, the catheter is advanced into the internal iliac artery for a selective injection.

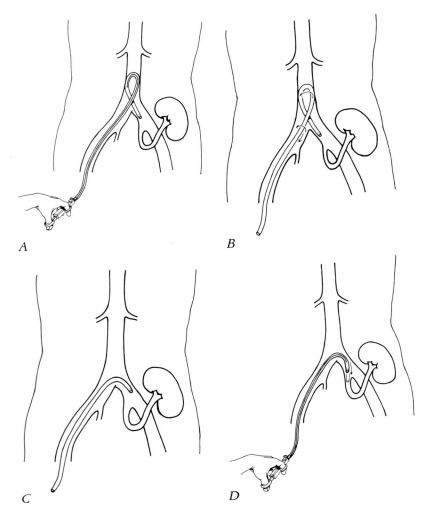

Figure 60-3. Frequently the deflector cannot be torqued into the common iliac artery. (A) The catheter is deflected several centimeters above the aortic bifurcation, and, with the deflector anchored, the catheter is advanced into the common iliac artery. (B) With counterclockwise rotation and retraction, the catheter is positioned for injection. (C) A common iliac artery injection. (D) The deflector is reinserted and anchored, and the catheter is advanced into the internal iliac artery.

If ipsilateral femoral artery catheterization is necessary (because contralateral artery pulsations are absent), the internal iliac artery catheterization is accomplished as shown in Figure 60-1 or with the sharply bent small-curve catheter that is used for selective bladder angiography [96].

In renal transplant angiography, an aortic injection is rarely necessary. For this purpose a "hook-tail" catheter [15, 62] that delivers 15 to 24 cc per second is suitable. If necessary, a longer hook-tail catheter (90–100 cm) is used for an axillary artery approach for an aortic injection (see Fig. 60-15B). In the presence of multiple stenotic lesions in the aorta and the iliac arteries, the area of bifurcation can be studied by retro-grade high-pressure injection into one of the iliac arteries (see Fig. 60-15A).

The catheters are heparinized [52], and intraluminal clotting is prevented by flushing the catheter with small amounts of contrast medium (about 2 cc per examination) [51].

For common iliac artery injection, we use Renografin-76 at a rate of 10 cc per second for a total of 20 cc. We inject into the internal iliac artery or the renal artery 8 cc per second for a total of 10 cc. A low aortic injection is made with 30 to 40 cc of contrast medium at 15 to 20 cc per second. At nonselective injection, a blood pressure cuff is applied on the thigh on the side of the transplant and inflated above the systolic pressure for better filling of the renal vessels [86] (see Fig. 60-10).

VENOUS CATHETERIZATION

The renal vein is usually anastomosed end to side with the common iliac vein. The renal vein is catheterized via an ipsilateral femoral vein puncture. Because thrombosis of the renal vein may extend into the common iliac vein, into the inferior vena cava (see Fig. 60-29), and, retrogradely, into the external iliac vein, a test injection with the tip of the catheter still in the femoral vein must be made. When thrombosis of the common iliac vein is suspected, the study is performed with an injection into the external iliac vein or the femoral vein (see Fig. 60-29A). When the flow is not obstructed, the catheter is advanced into the renal vein.

Although the size of the catheter is not as critical in the venous system, using smaller soft catheters should produce fewer complications (e.g., perforation or thrombosis). Usually an injection rate of 8 to 10 cc with a 4.1 French catheter is enough to opacify most of the venous system of the transplant, especially since the arterial perfusion of the rejecting kidney is decreased [4, 42].

If the distal veins are not opacified adequately with the above technique, the catheter may be advanced more distally into segmental veins and multiple injections performed at a rate of 5 to 10 cc per second, depending on the size of the vein and where the catheter is positioned. An alternative approach requires arterial blockage of the flow with 10 μg of epinephrine [99] (see Fig. 60-5). This technique involves injecting the main renal vein at a rate of 15 to 20 cc per second, which requires a 5 to 6 French catheter. Since contrast conservation is usually important, the injection time can be shortened to 0.5 to 1.0 second if rapid filming is employed (three films per second).

We have not found it necessary to perform intraosseous pertrochanteric venography [127] for renal transplant evaluation. In patients with uncontrollable hypertension, selective catheterization of the renal vein is frequently performed for determination of the plasma renin activity [11, 72, 88, 107].

Figure 60-4. Normal angiogram of a normally functioning transplant. (A) Arterial phase and (B) venous phase. There is slight narrowing at the arterial anastomosis (*arrow*).

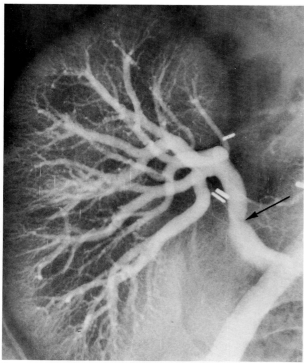

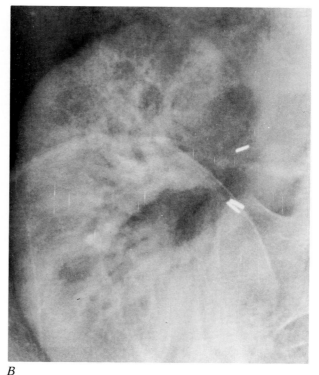

A

B

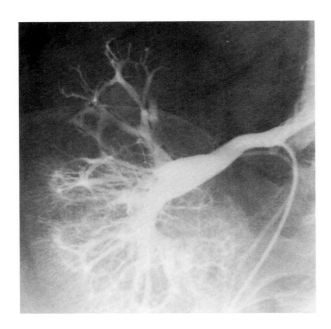

Figure 60-5. Venogram of a transplanted kidney after the intraarterial administration of 10 μg of epinephrine. Because of the catheter positioning, there is better venous filling (including the cortical veins) in the kidney's lower pole. (A cadaver transplant. Clinically there were massive proteinuria and a recent episode of rejection.)

POSITIONING OF THE PATIENT

The first film series is made in the anteroposterior projection for the best evaluation of the intrarenal vasculature (Figs. 60-4–60-6; see also Figs. 60-8, 60-12, 60-16 to 60-18, 60-20–60-23, 60-25, 60-28). Frequently, this position is sufficient also for the evaluation of the arterial anastomotic site for stenotic lesions (see Figs. 60-9–60-12). If the anastomosis cannot be demonstrated in the anteroposterior projection, a second injection is made in a steep posterior oblique position toward the side of the transplant (usually the right side). Biplane arteriography with alternate exposures [113] and the use of a lateral projection [78] have been recommended for the

Figure 60-6. Paradoxic vasospasm after the injection of 25 mg of Priscoline into the renal artery. (A) Arterial phase before Priscoline. The arteries are generally narrowed, and cortical perfusion is reduced in some areas. (B) Marked constriction of the intrarenal arteries after Priscoline; it is more severe in the lower pole, where some vessels are completely obliterated. (Moderate rejection. Clinically there was a bruit over the transplanted kidney.)

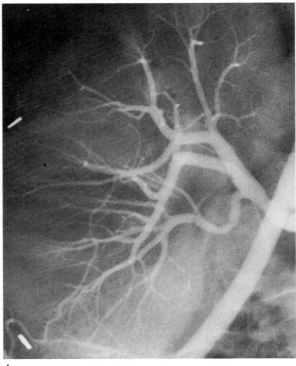

A

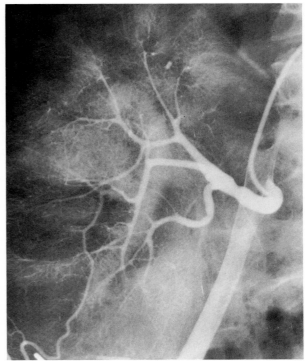

B

evaluation of the renal artery stenosis. These techniques have certain advantages in estimating the degree of the stenosis, and, with biplane radiography, the amount of contrast medium can be reduced because a second injection is not necessary. The clinical importance of an arterial stenotic lesion is, however, evaluated also by other parameters, and even with two injections, the total amount of injected contrast medium should not exceed 50 cc. Simultaneous biplane radiography makes the use of geometric magnification difficult.

SERIAL RADIOGRAPHY

The film sequence routinely used is the following one: two films per second for 3 seconds, one film per second for 3 seconds, and then three films in 6 or 9 seconds. The film rate is varied and the total time of serial radiography is prolonged when a test injection shows a delayed arterial washout time.

In renal transplant venography, the film rate is: three films per second for 1 second, one film per second for 3 seconds, and then finally two films in 6 seconds.

Xeroradiography has been recommended for renal transplant angiography for the better evaluation of the vascular detail [61], but it does not permit serial filming and it requires a much higher radiation dose. Instead, we use photographic subtraction, which is essential particularly where there is overlapping of the kidney by pelvic bone (see Fig. 60-19).

GEOMETRIC MAGNIFICATION

We use routinely an x-ray tube with a nominal focal spot of either 0.3-mm or 0.1-mm size for 1.8 or $\times 3$ geometric magnification, respectively [43, 67, 80, 122, 136, 149]. With this technique, small vascular detail is well demonstrated (see Figs. 60-22–60-24).

Pharmacoangiography

Except for the few occasions when epinephrine is administered for arterial constriction in venography, there is hardly any use for vasoactive agents in renal transplant angiography. Experimental studies suggest that in the early rejection period, increased vasomotor tone contributes to cortical ischemia [58, 117]. Therefore, we have tried to relieve the possibility of existing arterial

spasm in acute rejection with 12.5 to 25.0 mg of intraarterially administered tolazoline hydrochloride (Priscoline) [49]. In some patients, this drug has helped (1) to improve the angiographic appearance of acute rejection, as evidenced by better filling of the peripheral interlobar, arcuate, and cortical arteries; (2) to shorten the arterial emptying time; and (3) to reduce the reflux of contrast medium into the common iliac artery. In most patients, there has been no response to Priscoline, and in approximately 36 percent of cases we have encountered a spastic reaction of the renal arteries to Priscoline [67] (Fig. 60-6). This paradoxic vasospasm in response to a vasodilator has been observed also in the pulmonary arteries in the presence of pulmonary hypertension secondary to mitral valve disease [148]. In the transplanted kidney, it is possibly caused by inadequate postsynaptic blockage of the vascular alpha-receptors by Priscoline and by high circulating noradrenaline levels [18].

Complications of Renal Transplant Angiography

All patients undergoing angiography of a renal transplant must be hydrated; we limit the contrast medium to 50 cc per examination. In the 230 angiograms of renal transplants we have done (almost exclusively in patients with moderately or severely impaired renal function), we have encountered one complication—renal shutdown that developed after the injection of 10 cc of contrast medium selectively into the renal vein.

With the use of small catheters, we have not encountered any significant arterial bleeding or postangiography hematoma formation.

Normal Renal Transplant

A normally functioning transplanted kidney should not differ angiographically from a normally functioning nontransplanted kidney (see Fig. 60-4). Its size, however, may vary; on roentgenograms, a normal transplanted kidney may measure up to 16×9 cm [41]. Its size increases 10 percent in the month after transplantation and then 1 percent each month for the first year [19].

The arterial anastomosis (which is usually end to end between the renal and the internal iliac arteries) is smooth, the interlobar and arcuate arteries are regular, and the cortical vessels are well filled. The normal arterial washout time averages approximately 2 seconds (it should be less than 3 seconds after the onset of a 1-second injection at selective study) [1, 64, 67, 89]. The nephrogram is dense, with good demarcation of the corticomedullary junction. The renal vein is well filled 5 to 7 seconds after the onset of the injection, and the contrast medium is excreted by the kidney.

Pathologic Angiogram

RENAL ARTERY COMPLICATIONS

Arterial Thrombosis

Complete occlusion of the renal artery at the site of anastomosis occurs usually in the early postoperative period. The patient is anuric, and a radionuclide scan shows a total lack of perfusion of the kidney. Preoperative differentiation of arterial thrombosis from hyperacute rejection can be made by angiography (Fig. 60-7). Fortunately, occlusion of the renal artery is a rather rare postsurgical complicaton [35] (it occurs in less than 2% of cases), but it may also be related to acute rejection [16]. Its immediate recognition is important, because thrombosis of the renal artery requires an immediate operation and, frequently, graft nephrectomy. Occlusion of a smaller polar artery of the transplanted kidney (Fig. 60-8; see also Figs. 60-10, 60-22) results in partial renal infarction. Clinically it may simulate appendicitis [90]. Deterioration of renal function depends on the area of infarcted renal parenchyma.

Renal Artery Stenosis and Hypertension

An audible vascular murmur over the renal artery does not necessarily mean that the renal circulation is adequate, nor is it indicative of renal artery stenosis [108]. Angiographically, smaller irregularities at the arterial anastomosis are sometimes incidentally observed (see Fig. 60-4). They are not responsible for hypertension or renal graft dysfunction. Hypertension, a frequent and rather late complication of renal transplantation, is not always caused by renal artery stenosis but is often associated with intrarenal vascular or parenchymal disease with reduced cortical blood flow [11, 107, 128]. Hypertension that does not respond to medical treatment, in particular in a binephrectomized patient, is a definitive indication for angiography [12, 125].

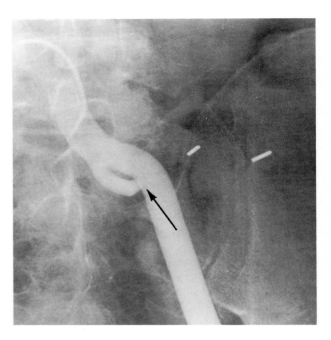

Figure 60-7. Arterial occlusion at the site of anastomosis (*arrow*) resulting in total kidney infarction. (From Kaude and Hawkins [67]. Reproduced by permission of *Radiol. Clin. North Am.*)

Figure 60-8. Occlusion of the upper pole renal artery (*arrow*) just distal to the anastomosis. Severe spasm in form of "standing waves" in the patent branch of the renal artery supplying the kidney's midportion and lower pole. There is occlusion of the distal branches of the interlobar arteries but no cortical perfusion. (Severe acute rejection.)

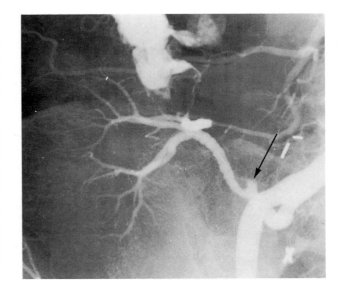

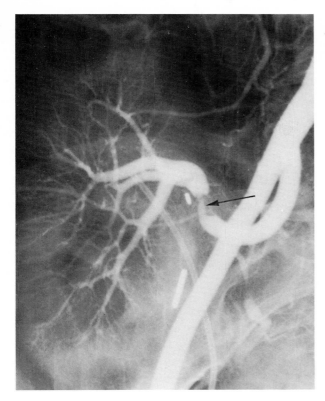

Figure 60-9. Stenosis at the anastomosis between the renal artery and the internal iliac artery in a patient with uncontrollable hypertension and increased plasma renin activity in the renal venous blood. The stenosis is eccentric and irregular (*arrow*). (From Kaude and Hawkins [67]. Reproduced by permission of *Radiol. Clin. North Am.*)

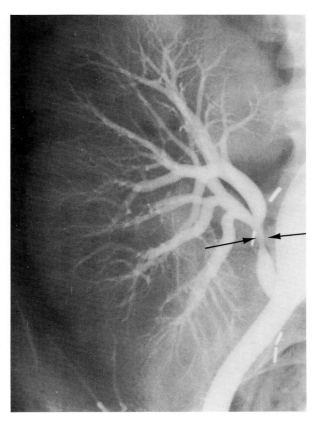

Figure 60-11. Smooth, approximately 60-percent stenosis of the renal artery at the site of anastomosis (*arrows*). The intrarenal vasculature is normal. (The patient was hypertensive.)

Figure 60-10. (A) The renal artery is anastomosed end to side with the external iliac artery. The first proximal centimeter of the renal artery is severely stenotic (*arrow*). All the interlobar arteries show severe irregular narrowing, several branches are occluded, and there is no filling of the arcuate or corti- cal vessels. (B) Late arterial phase. There is minimal retrograde filling of an occluded upper pole artery (*arrows*). (Severe acute rejection in a 2-month-old cadaver transplant. Angiography was performed with the blood pressure cuff on the upper thigh.)

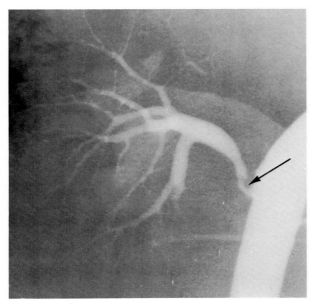

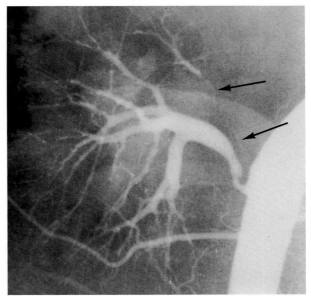

A

B

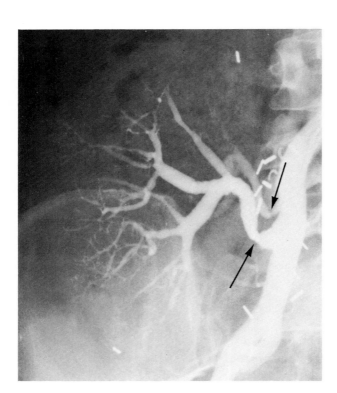

Figure 60-12. Both the main artery and an upper pole renal artery have been anastomosed end to side with the common iliac artery. Both renal arteries are stenotic (*arrows*). There is severe vasculitis, with irregular narrowing of the interlobar arteries and occlusion of multiple peripheral arterial branches. The lack of cortical perfusion is total. (Severe acute rejection.)

Renal artery stenosis with or without hypertension has been observed by almost all authors who have examined transplanted kidneys by angiography. Its incidence has been reported to be as high as 25 percent, and up to 95 percent of patients with renal artery stenosis are hypertensive [83, 91].

Significant renal artery stenosis occurs usually at the site of anastomosis, and it appears angiographically as rather short, circumferential, or eccentric [55] (Figs. 60-9–60-12).

There is some evidence that end-to-side anastomosis between the renal and common iliac arteries encourages the development of stenosis at the anastomotic site [91] (Figs. 60-10, 60-12). The stenosis may be caused also by surgical manipulations [120]; and the stenosis proximal [44] or distal to the anastomosis [91, 126, 146] is probably caused by clamping of arteries during the operation. Atheromatous plaques [83, 87] and rejection [120], periarterial fibrosis, and torsion or kinking of the renal artery [88, 143] are

other causes of renal artery stenosis. Sometimes the stenotic area has the appearance of fibromuscular dysplasia [91].

Renal artery stenosis may be responsible for the deterioration of renal function, and it may be associated with rejection or may simulate it clinically [111, 119, 120, 126] (Figs. 60-10, 60-12). Its significance for renovascular hypertension should be supported by renin assay, including selective sampling from the renal vein before surgical repair of the stenosis is attempted [11, 72, 88]. The determination of plasma renin activity may be particularly useful in the recognition of the role of the patient's own kidneys in sustained hypertension [107].

Surgical correction of renal artery stenosis is often successful [125, 139], but it may also be difficult or complicated [88, 120]. Therefore, percutaneous transluminal angioplasty could become an important modality for treatment of renovascular hypertension and/or reduced renal function secondary to arterial stenosis in renal transplant patients. Successful dilatation of a renal artery transplant has been reported [32, 129] (Fig. 60-13). It is noteworthy, however, that spontaneous regression of stenotic lesions in the artery of the transplanted kidney may also occur [138].

Occasionally, renal transplant dysfunction may be caused by compression of the iliac and renal arteries by a large hematoma [134, 143], or by atheromatous plaques in the common iliac artery (Fig. 60-14) or in the abdominal aorta above the bifurcation [67] (Fig. 60-15A). The last condition may require repair with an aortic graft (Fig. 60-15B).

Arteriovenous Fistula
Arteriovenous fistula between major renal vessels is apparently a surgical complication [108]. It may result in an ischemic kidney and cause systemic hypertension. Arteriovenous fistula secondary to rejection and as a complication of renal biopsy is discussed later in this chapter.

Renal Artery Aneurysms
Small arterial aneurysms may be found incidentally. Aneurysms in the interlobar branches of the renal artery may represent angiographic evidence of chronic rejection [22]. Pseudoaneurysms have been described at the site of arterial anastomosis, and ureteral compression by pseudoaneurysm causing hydronephrosis, reduced renal function, and hypertension has been also reported [133].

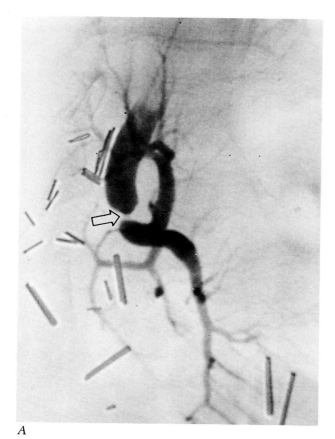

A

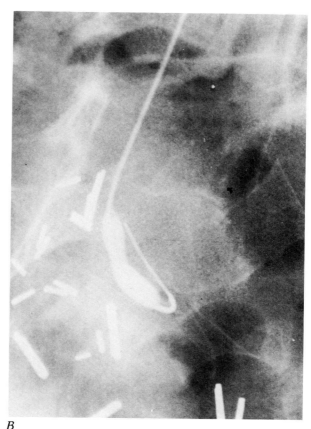

B

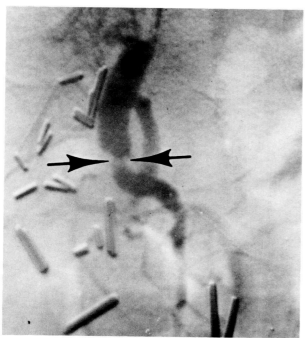

C

Figure 60-13. Angioplasty of a stenotic renal artery transplant in a patient with uncontrollable hypertension. The patient's blood pressure was 180/120 mm Hg although he was taking four drugs. (A) Stenosis of the renal artery before angioplasty (*arrow*). (Subtraction film.) (B) Catheter balloon in place. (C) Angiography after angioplasty. (Subtraction film.) There is marked improvement although moderate stenosis is still present (*arrows*). The patient was normotensive; he was taking two drugs. (Courtesy of Dan E. Wertman, M.D.)

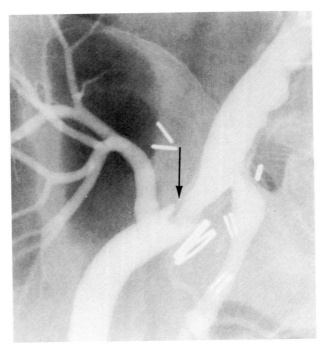

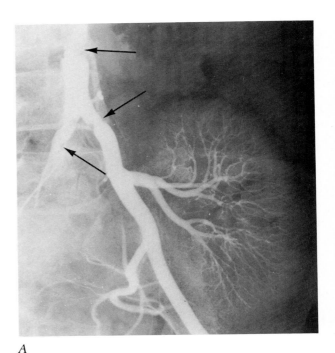

A

Figure 60-14. Membranelike atheromatous plaque causing severe stenosis in the common iliac artery (*arrow*), just proximal to the end-to-side anastomosis between the renal artery and the external iliac artery. (A 1-month-old cadaver transplant with clinically deteriorating renal function.)

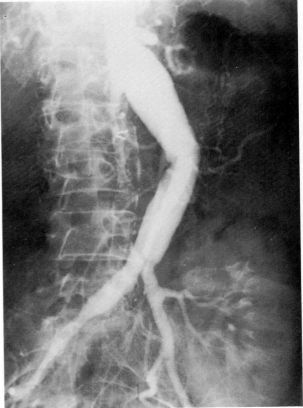

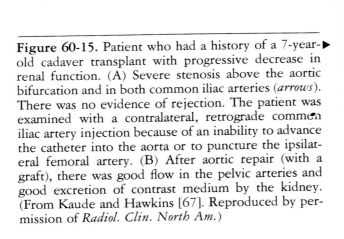

Figure 60-15. Patient who had a history of a 7-year-▶ old cadaver transplant with progressive decrease in renal function. (A) Severe stenosis above the aortic bifurcation and in both common iliac arteries (*arrows*). There was no evidence of rejection. The patient was examined with a contralateral, retrograde common iliac artery injection because of an inability to advance the catheter into the aorta or to puncture the ipsilateral femoral artery. (B) After aortic repair (with a graft), there was good flow in the pelvic arteries and good excretion of contrast medium by the kidney. (From Kaude and Hawkins [67]. Reproduced by permission of *Radiol. Clin. North Am.*)

B

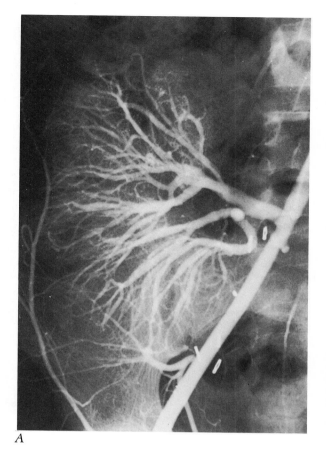
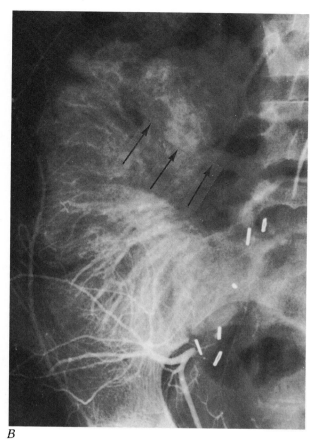

A *B*

Figure 60-16. Total cortical ischemia and infarction on the second day after transplantation. (A) Severe vasculitis. (B) Early venous filling in the upper pole of the kidney (*arrows*) is a sign of the redistribution of the intrarenal blood flow. In the lower pole, the arterial washout is retarded. (Cadaver kidney with hyperacute rejection resulting in renal death.) (From Kaude and Hawkins [67]. Reproduced by permission of *Radiol. Clin. North Am.*)

Large aneurysms may rupture, resulting in retroperitoneal hematoma [143].

PARENCHYMAL COMPLICATIONS

Rejection

Immunologic rejection is the most common complication of transplantation. Almost every kidney transplant undergoes a mild or a more severe rejection episode sometime during its lifetime.

Four types of rejection are distinguishable: hyperacute, accelerated, acute, and chronic. Hyperacute rejection is caused by preformed antibodies, and it develops almost immediately after the host-to-kidney circulation has been established. Hyperacute rejection is uncommon; it has a very poor prognosis since it destroys the kidney within 48 hours [7] (Fig. 60-16).

Accelerated rejection occurs within the first week after surgery; it is less severe than hyperacute rejection because of the lower antibody titer.

Acute rejection generally occurs between weeks 1 and 16 after transplantation, but it may develop at any time, even years later [7, 77]. Chronic rejection is a gradual process, with slow deterioration of renal function [77], often associated with hypertension and proteinuria. The primary site of immunologic rejection in renal transplants is the vascular endothelium [73, 76, 109–111], and rejection arteritis is a major cause of renal failure [21]. Depending on the severity and the stage of rejection, a whole spectrum of abnormal findings is present histologically: from interstitial and perivascular infiltrates of mononuclear cells to vascular thrombi and fibrinoid necrosis of small arteries, arterioles,

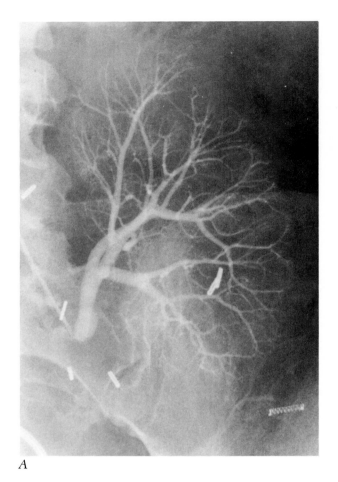

A

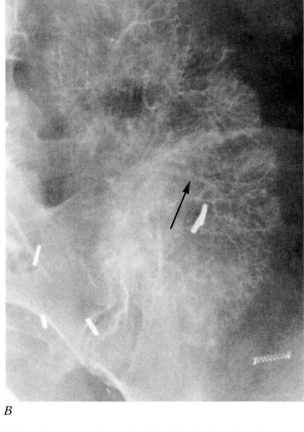

B

Figure 60-17. (A) Arterial phase. Severely stenotic constricted arteries throughout the kidney. Total ischemia of the cortex. (B) Delayed arterial washout (4 seconds after the injection). Simultaneous venous filling is present (*arrow*). Histologically, there is severe acute rejection, with cortical necrosis at nephrectomy. (From Kaude et al. [64]. Reproduced by permission of *ROEFO*.)

and glomerular capillaries [21, 31]. Vascular changes may lead to renal ischemia, resulting in cortical necrosis, tubular damage, hemorrhages, and infarcts [7]. Occasionally, severe acute rejection may lead to rupture of the kidney [35, 101].

Microangiographic studies in rejected human kidney transplants show poor or variable glomerular filling and tapering of cortical arteries [74]. In experimental studies with canine renal transplants it has been shown that the vascular obstruction in rejection develops from the outer cortex inward [25, 137, 140] and that the medullary vascular obliteration and hemorrhage necrosis develop subsequent to cortical changes [25]. Arteriovenous communications are observed in the late stage of rejection [25]. These communications are formed between the damaged arterioles and venules at the cortical, preglomerular, and postglomerular levels [5].

Acute Rejection. Angiographic findings in acute rejection reflect rather well the pathologic-histologic changes and the microangiographic findings of experimental studies (Figs. 60-17, 60-18; see also Figs. 60-8, 60-10, 60-12). The kidney is usually enlarged and edematous. The enlargement is more evident when the kidney is measured in three dimensions by ultrasonography [59]. There is no filling or only poor filling of the peripheral interlobar, arcuate, and cortical arteries. It has been our observation that for some unexplained reason the perfusion of the kidney in the presence of rejection may be poorer in the lower pole (in 31% of 131 patients with rejection). The arterial washout time is prolonged (>3 seconds) from the onset of a selective 1-second injection. The nephrogram is poor, and the impaired cortical perfusion is also evident from the ill-defined corticomedullary

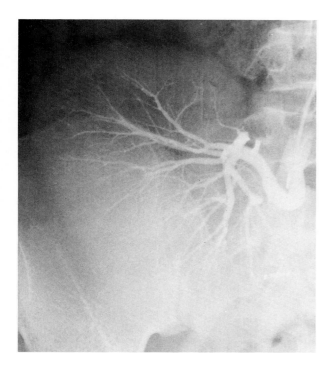

Figure 60-18. Acute renal transplant rejection, arterial phase. Edema of the kidney; irregular, stenotic or occluded arteries, no filling of cortical vessels. (From Kaude and Hawkins [67]. Reproduced by permission of *Radiol. Clin. North Am.*)

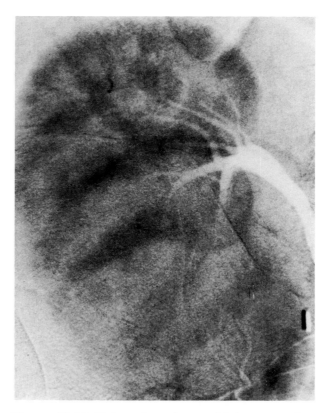

Figure 60-19. Enlarged renal pyramids in acute rejection. (Subtraction film.)

boundary. Medullary pyramids may be enlarged [119] (Fig. 60-19), or there may be hypovascularized areas in the kidneys, apparently representing areas of necrosis or hemorrhage (see Fig. 60-26). Concentration of contrast medium in the renal vein is low, or there is no appreciable venous filling at all. Arteriovenous shunting in rejection may occur [63, 64, 67, 82, 84, 92, 93, 147, 150] (see Figs. 60-16, 60-17). It is indicative of redistribution of the intrarenal blood flow and severe cortical ischemia [63, 64, 67, 93]. The total renal blood flow in patients with a decreased glomerular filtration rate, cortical ischemia, and arteriovenous shunting may, however, be normal, indicating that the shunting occurs at the juxtamedullary level [56, 64]. Renal infarcts secondary to vascular obliteration may occur [92, 93, 125] (see Figs. 60-8, 60-16, 60-21, 60-22). Finally, in severe acute rejection, no contrast medium is excreted by the kidney.

Acute rejection episodes are not always severe and do not always involve the whole kidney. In mild or focal rejection, only a few vessels may be obliterated or irregular, the arterial washout time is normal, the nephrogram and venous filling are

good, and some contrast medium is seen to be excreted by the kidney.

Chronic Rejection. The prominent histologic features of chronic rejection are fibrous endothelial thickening with vascular obliteration, glomerular deposits, basement membrane thickening, fibrosis of the interstitium, and tubular atrophy [77]. The kidney is of normal size or is smaller than a normally functioning renal transplant. Chronic rejection generally reflects the sequelae of earlier episodes of acute rejection, or the immunologic process may be slowly progressive [77]. Microangiography in chronic rejection reveals arterial narrowing and a lack of or the impaired perfusion of all segments of the kidney [74]. Angiographically, the number of filled vessels in the kidney is reduced, and both interlobar and smaller peripheral arteries in the whole kidney or in certain areas of the kidney are narrowed or irregular (Figs. 60-20–60-24). Smaller or larger infarcted areas may be present (see Figs. 60-21, 60-22). In less involved areas, cortical vascular filling may still be satisfactory. With ×3 magnification, the cortex frequently has a striate

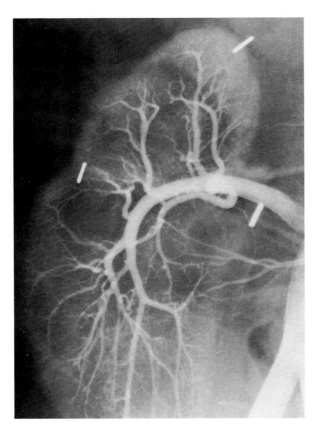

Figure 60-20. Chronic rejection. Reduced cortical thickness in the lateral upper pole of the kidney. Slightly narrowed peripheral interlobar arteries. Vessel displacement in the midportion of the kidney and in the kidney hilus by hydronephrosis. (Living related donor transplant; all the changes had developed after the pretransplantation donor angiography.)

appearance that is caused by the separation of the cortical vessels by ischemic areas (fibrosis, obliterated glomeruli and arterioles) [43, 140, 141] (see Figs. 60-22–60-24). In normally functioning kidneys, the linear cortical vascular structures that, we believe, represent rows of glomeruli rather than cortical arteries are also demonstrable, but they are not separated to the same extent as in a transplanted kidney that is undergoing rejection.

The arterial washout time in chronic rejection is usually normal or slightly prolonged, venous filling is appreciable, and (depending on the preserved functional parenchyma) the kidney excretes injected contrast medium. Arteriovenous shunts [20, 84] and intrarenal arterial aneurysms coexistent with stenotic segments caused by vascular fibrosis [22] occur in chronic rejection.

Chronic rejection is generally distinguishable from acute rejection by both microangiography [74] and clinical angiography. But both types of rejection may occur simultaneously, and when acute rejection is superimposed on a chronic state, the angiographic differential diagnosis between acute rejection and chronic rejection is difficult if not impossible.

Prognostic Value of Angiography in Rejection. Generally, the more severe the angiographic findings are, the more advanced the disease is [8, 43, 47] and the poorer the chances are that the transplant will recover from an acute rejection episode. Major-vessel obstruction [87], prolonged arterial washout time (> 4 seconds) [34, 79, 95], and cortical ischemia [43] have been found to be indicative of irreversible renal failure. It is, however, better to use all these parameters combined, in addition to poor demarcation of the corticomedullary junction, arteriovenous shunting, and a poor nephrogram, to predict the chances for survival of the transplant [63, 64]. Acute rejection episodes are usually treated with intravenously administered boluses of methylprednisolone (20 mg/kg body weight) [10]. From 1 to 6 boluses is given. High-dose immunosuppressive therapy is, however, associated with complications [6, 39, 40, 75]. To predict the reversibility of renal transplant rejection, sequential testing of the recipient's immune response has been suggested [45]; angiography is important in deciding whether therapy should be continued or discontinued in patients who have unrelenting acute rejection despite repeated boluses of methylprednisolone. It has been our experience that when four to six of the angiographic signs of acute rejection are present, more steroids will lead to more immunosuppressive complications and so an early graft nephrectomy must be considered [63, 64]. Cadaver transplants with unrelenting acute rejection have a significantly poorer prognosis than have transplants from a living related donor.

Acute Tubular Necrosis

Acute tubular necrosis is the most common cause of renal failure during the first days after transplantation. In studies in which only cadaver transplants were used, the incidence of postoperative acute tubular necrosis was reported to be 30 percent [71] and even as high as 48 percent [23]. With transplants from living related donors, acute tubular necrosis occurs less frequently (in

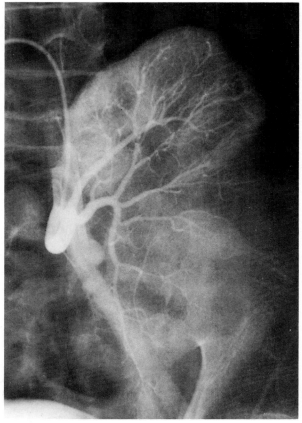

A

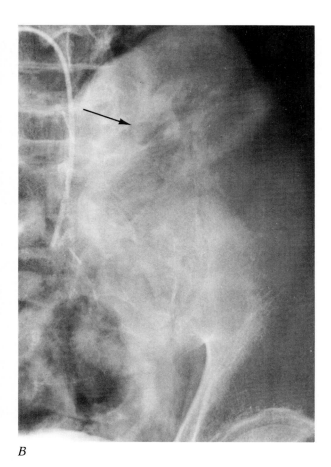

B

Figure 60-21. Chronic rejection. (A) Arterial phase and (B) venous phase. There is relatively well-preserved renal parenchyma in the upper pole of the kidney. Although the renal arteries are narrowed, there is perfusion of the cortex and filling of the veins (*arrow*). In the midportion and the lower pole of the kidney, only a few severely narrowed arteries are filled and there is marked loss of the renal parenchyma. (A 6-year-old cadaver transplant; proteinuria and reduced renal function.) (From Kaude and Hawkins [67]. Reproduced by permission of *Radiol. Clin. North Am.*)

11% of cases) [7]. In postoperative oliguria or anuria, radionuclide scans are preferred to angiography as the primary diagnostic procedure [9, 71, 133, 151]. For the past 8 years, we have no longer performed angiography in a patient with clinically suggested tubular necrosis.

In the past, there has been some disagreement about distinguishing acute tubular necrosis from acute rejection by angiography. In our opinion, and in the experience of several other authors, angiography in acute tubular necrosis is normal except for (1) the occasional presence of somewhat reduced cortical perfusion or mildly prolonged arterial washout time and (2) the absence of excretion of injected contrast medium [17, 28, 47, 67, 68, 92, 93, 98, 106, 141, 142] (Fig. 60-25).

Other authors [9, 20, 60, 80, 87, 101, 114]

have described in acute tubular necrosis at least one of the angiographic findings of acute rejection (arterial narrowing, cortical ischemia, a prolonged arterial emptying time, a poor nephrogram). Because vasoconstriction causing cortical ischemia plays some role in the development of both acute tubular necrosis and acute rejection [1, 43, 57, 58, 117], angiographic differential diagnosis between these two causes of renal transplant failure may be difficult in certain cases [9, 43]. It seems that at least some of the existing controversy about the angiographic diagnosis of acute tubular necrosis is related to the different stages of the disease at the time of examination [45, 67]. Most diagnostic difficulties arise when acute tubular necrosis must be differentiated from mild accelerated or acute rejection [9]. In more advanced or severely acute rejection, a

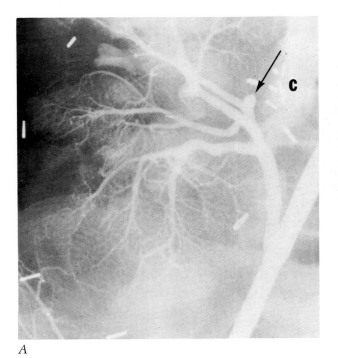

A

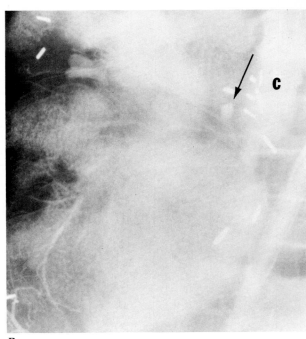

B

Figure 60-22. Chronic rejection with occlusion of the upper pole artery (*arrow*) and several peripheral interlobar branches. There are large areas of infarction and fibrosis but still partially preserved cortical perfusion in the lower pole of the kidney. (A) Arterial and (B) late arterial-capillary phase with ×3 geometric magnification. *C* = contrast medium in the ileal conduit. (A cadaver transplant; the renal scan had suggested infarction.)

Figure 60-23. Chronic rejection. All the arteries are markedly narrowed and irregular. Avascular spaces are seen throughout the kidney, apparently representing areas of fibrosis. Cortical perfusion is still preserved. (×2 geometric magnification.)

Figure 60-24. Angiogram obtained with 0.1-mm tube focus and ×3 geometric magnification. Chronic rejection. Irregularly stenotic arteries separated by avascular (fibrotic) spaces. In the cortex, the linear structures probably represent rows of glomeruli (*arrows*). (A 1-year-old living related donor transplant.)

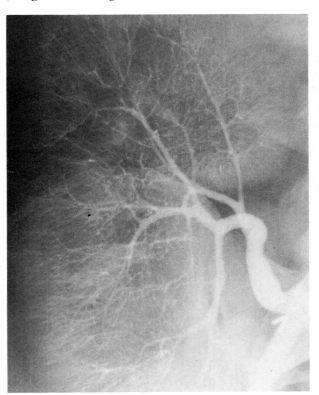

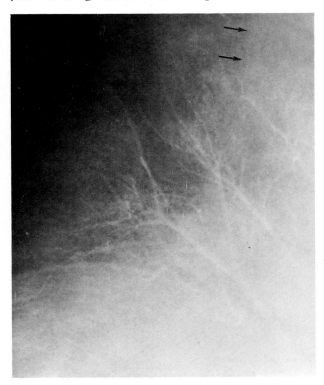

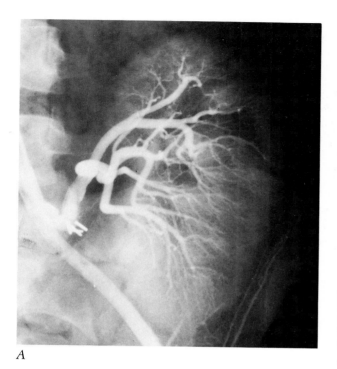

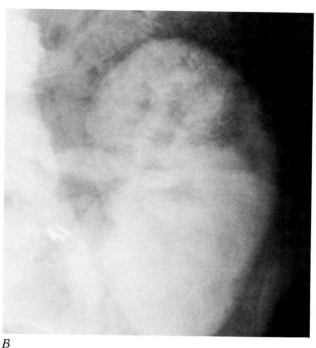

A   *B*

Figure 60-25. Patient with postoperative anuria after the transplantation of a cadaver kidney. Normal angiogram. (A) Arterial phase and (B) nephrographic-venous phase. The clinical course was consistent with acute tubular necrosis. (From Kaude and Hawkins [67]. Reproduced by permission of *Radiol. Clin. North Am.*)

markedly prolonged arterial washout time, pronounced cortical ischemia, arteriovenous shunting, and vasculitis make the angiographic differentiation from acute tubular necrosis easier. In cases in which acute rejection is superimposed on acute tubular necrosis, the latter diagnosis will probably be overlooked because the angiographic picture is dominated by diffuse or focal signs of rejection.

Graft Glomerulonephritis

Our experience with angiography in acute (recurrent) graft glomerulonephritis is limited. In one patient, we observed normal angiographic findings, except for minimal localized vasculitis (apparently a mild focal rejection) [67]. In another patient, there was enlargement of the kidney with cortical edema and reduced cortical perfusion, as described in acute glomerulonephritis in nontransplanted kidneys [37].

Graft glomerulonephritis may occur simultaneously with acute or chronic rejection, which, again, would confuse the angiographic picture.

In transplant glomerulopathy, normal angiographic findings have been reported [47].

Acute Pyelonephritis/Renal Abscess

The angiographic appearance of acute pyelonephritis with the formation of renal abscesses is that of an enlarged kidney with displacement of intrarenal vessels by edema [94]. Angiographically, it is difficult or impossible to differentiate an abscess from hemorrhagic or necrotic areas caused by rejection (Fig. 60-26).

Renal Papillary Necrosis

Renal papillary necrosis of the transplanted kidney is in some cases caused by ischemia secondary to earlier rejection episodes [69]. Occasionally a patient with renal papillary necrosis is referred for angiography because of transplant failure or persistent hematuria. Avascular areas adjacent to dilated and clubbed calices, apparently representing necrotic papillae in situ, may be seen angiographically (Fig. 60-27).

Graft Tumors and Cysts

Neoplasia occurs more often in transplant recipients than in the normal population [102, 103, 121]. Malignant tumors have been transmitted to the recipient with the kidney transplant [105] but

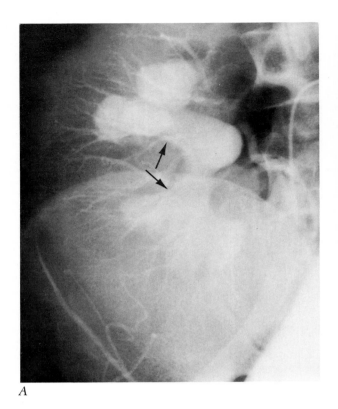

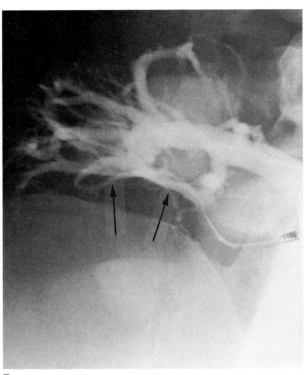

A   *B*

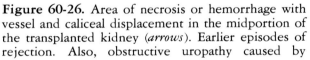

Figure 60-26. Area of necrosis or hemorrhage with vessel and caliceal displacement in the midportion of the transplanted kidney (*arrows*). Earlier episodes of rejection. Also, obstructive uropathy caused by stenosis at the ureteropelvic junction. (A) Late arterial phase and (B) a venogram with ×2 magnification. (The lower pole renal vein is not catheterized.)

we have not observed either such a tumor or a primary neoplasia.

Renal cyst is not considered a contraindication to transplantation [132]. A cyst may develop primarily also in a transplanted kidney [54], but ultrasonography should be preferred to angiography for cyst diagnosis.

Fibrolipomatosis of the transplanted kidney [65] causes vessel displacement in the renal sinus and must not be confused with an avascular tumor in the area.

Complications of Renal Biopsy

Percutaneous biopsy is an accepted procedure for histologic verification of parenchymal disease of the transplanted kidney [70]. In our institution, it is performed exclusively under ultrasonographic control. Because of the nature of the procedure, complications from renal biopsy cannot be totally avoided. Complications such as intrarenal or perirenal hematomas can be diagnosed by ultrasonography. Postbiopsy arteriovenous fistula [38] requires angiographic diagnosis. In renal transplant, arteriovenous communications have been demonstrated by angiography in several cases [8, 30, 33] (Fig. 60-28). Larger arteriovenous fistulas may cause ischemia of the kidney in involved areas, and clinical symptoms such as hypertension or reduced renal function, but smaller postbiopsy fistulas will often heal spontaneously [36].

VENOUS THROMBOSIS

Renal vein thrombosis is a relatively uncommon complication after kidney transplantation [4, 130, 139, 143]. Thrombi in the large veins (renal, femoral, and iliac) eventually extending into the inferior vena cava (Fig. 60-29) may occur, and venous obstruction may be secondary to vessel compression by hematoma [134, 139], lymphocele [67] (Fig. 60-30), or the graft itself [115]. Venous thrombosis has been observed also secondary to hypovolemia [143]. Femoroiliac venous thrombosis seems to occur more frequently on the left side with renal transplant in the left

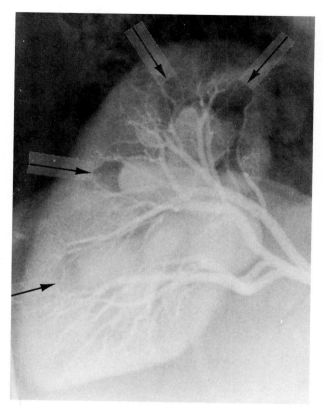

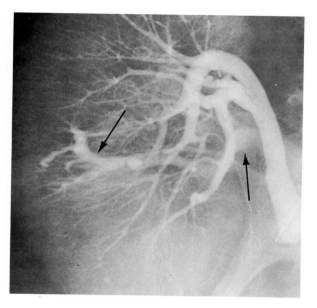

Figure 60-28. Postbiopsy arteriovenous fistula in a transplanted kidney. Simultaneous venous filling during the arterial phase (*arrows*). There is also evidence of acute rejection. (A 3-month-old transplant from a living related donor shows clinically decreased renal function.)

Figure 60-27. Papillary necrosis in a patient who had two previous rejection episodes. There are displacement of the arteries around dilated, grossly deformed minor calices, and adjacent avascular areas (*arrows*); they probably represent necrotic papillae in situ. (A 2-month-old living related donor transplant; hematuria, passing tissue.) (From Kaude and Hawkins [67]. Reproduced by permission of *Radiol. Clin. North Am.*)

fossa, probably because of the crossing of the iliac vein by the iliac artery [42] (see Fig. 60-29). Intrarenal venous thrombosis, eventually with extension into the main renal or iliac vein, can develop in association with rejection [4, 42, 68, 73, 101, 124, 143]. Nephrotic syndrome with massive proteinuria is also associated more frequently with chronic rejection [145] (see Fig. 60-21) than with recurrent membranous glomerulonephritis of the graft.

Early diagnosis of venous thrombosis is important so that anticoagulant therapy can be initiated or thrombectomy performed to relieve the clinical symptoms and to prevent further complications for the recipient and in the transplant.

Arterial injection in acute renal vein thrombosis in a nontransplanted kidney shows an enlarged edematous kidney, arterial spasm, poor cortical perfusion, prolonged arterial clearance time, and lack of venous filllng [27, 53]. Similar findings are seen in renal vein thrombosis in a transplanted kidney, but they are also part of the spectrum of angiographic findings in acute transplant rejection. A markedly prolonged arterial washout time suggests that renal vein thrombosis has developed secondary to rejection [68]. In any case, the diagnosis of venous thrombosis is verified by venography.

There has been one case report in which collateral veins from the transplant to the host had developed in the presence of obstructed flow through a stenotic renal vein [29] (Fig. 60-31).

URETERAL OBSTRUCTION

An occasional patient with the progressive or sudden onset of anuria or oliguria who has been referred for angiography may suffer from ureteral obstruction caused by stenosis at the site of ureterovesical anastomosis, calculus, sloughed necrotic papillary tissue, or blood clot in the ureter [24, 67, 68]. Angiography in these cases shows a prolonged nephrogram that may persist as long as 18 seconds after injection (Fig. 60-32).

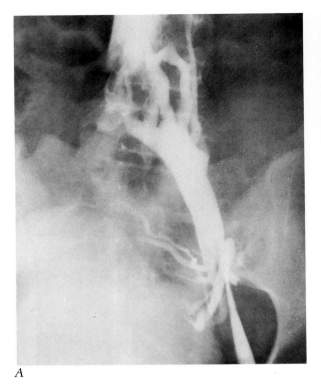

A

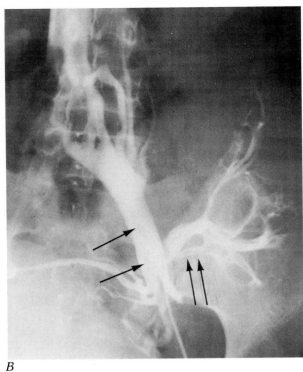

B

Figure 60-29. (A) External iliac vein injection. There is thrombosis of the left common iliac vein and the inferior vena cava just above the bifurcation. There are presacral collateral flow into the right common iliac vein and filling of the inferior vena cava via collat- eral vessels at the level of L4 to L5. (B) A renal vein injection shows multiple clots in renal veins and in the common iliac vein (*arrows*). (The patient had sig- nificant proteinuria and a creatinine clearance rate of 22 cc/min. A 3-year-old cadaver transplant.)

Figure 60-30. Lymphocele (*arrows*) compressing the common iliac vein and the bladder. Clinically progres- sive edema of the leg. Normally functioning graft. (From Kaude and Hawkins [67]. Reproduced by per- mission of *Radiol. Clin. North Am.*)

Figure 60-31. Stenosis of the renal vein with collat- eral vessels developed from the graft to the host. (Clinically proteinuria and decreased renal function.) (From Deal and Hawkins [29]. Reproduced by per- mission of *Radiology*.)

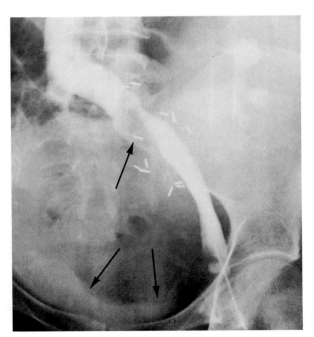

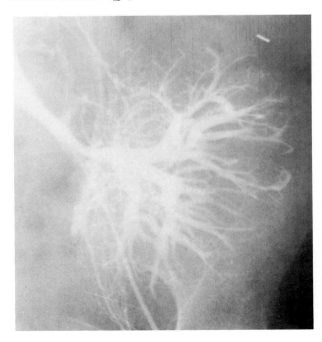

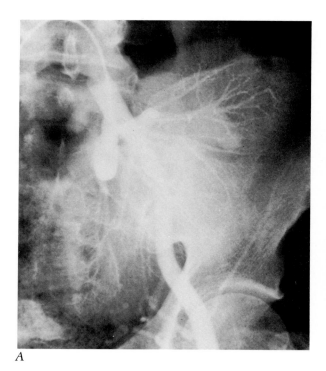

A

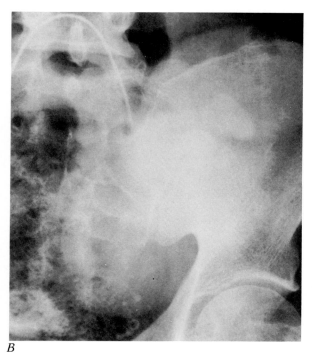

B

Figure 60-32. Acute ureteral obstruction. Renal papillary necrosis and a stone in the distal ureter (not seen on this film). (A) An essentially normal arterial phase and (B) a prolonged nephrogram. It persisted 15 seconds after the onset of the injection. (From Kaude and Hawkins [67]. Reproduced by permission of *Radiol. Clin. North Am.*)

Chronic ureteral obstruction resulting in hydronephrosis can be caused by a lymphocele, a hematoma, an aneurysm, or a urinoma that may also compress pelvic vessels [67, 133, 134, 139, 143] and the bladder (see Fig. 60-30).

Occasionally, an existent ureteral fistula can be demonstrated when contrast medium injected during angiography is seen to leak into the urinoma.

Summary

With the progressive use of ultrasound and radionuclide scanning, the role of angiography in the diagnosis of renal transplant complications has become somewhat less important. Angiography is currently performed mainly (1) in uncontrollable hypertension, (2) in rejection that does not respond to intravenous methylprednisolone treatment, (3) to verify arterial or venous stenosis or thrombosis, and (4) in the presence of persistent hematuria that cannot be explained by other diagnostic means. Small catheters should be used, and geometric magnification makes a better analysis of small vascular detail possible.

We expect that angioplasty will play a major role in the treatment of renovascular hypertension.

Addendum

Since the completion of this chapter, rapid development of radiologic technology has taken place in the field of digital subtraction angiography (see also Chapter 7). It is very likely that in many cases this procedure will be substituted for conventional angiographic techniques in both renal transplant donor and recipient angiography [56a]. A further advantage of digital subtraction angiography is that possible complications from injection of contrast medium in this high-risk group of patients can be prevented by the use of carbon dioxide arteriography [48a].

References

1. Abrams, H. L. Quantitative derivatives of renal radiologic studies. An overview. *Invest. Radiol.* 7:240, 1972.
2. Advisory Committee to the Renal Transplant

Registry.   The 12th report of the Human Renal Transplant Registry. *J.A.M.A.* 233:787, 1975.

3. Advisory Committee to the Renal Transplant Registry.   The 13th report of the Human Renal Transplant Registry. *Transplant. Proc.* 9:9, 1977.

4. Alfidi, R. J., Meaney, T. F., Buonocore, E., and Nakamoto, S.   Evaluation of renal homotransplants by selective angiography. *Radiology* 87:1099, 1966.

5. Almgård, L. E., Granberg, P. O., Lagergren, C., and Ljungqvist, A.   Arteriovenous anastomosis in the canine renal allograft. *Nephron* 3:295, 1966.

6. Bach, M. C., Adler, J. L., Breman, J., P'eng, F.-K., Sahyoun, A., Schlesinger, R. M., Madras, P., and Monaco, A. P.   Influence of rejection therapy on fungal and nocardial infections in renal-transplant recipients. *Lancet* 1:180, 1973.

7. Balch, C. M., and Diethelm, A. G.   The pathophysiology of renal allograft rejection: A collective review. *J. Surg. Res.* 12:350, 1972.

8. Beachley, M. C., Pierce, J. C., Boykin, J. V., and Lee, H. M.   The angiographic evaluation of human renal allotransplants. Functional graft deterioration and hypertension. *Arch. Surg.* 111:134, 1976.

9. Becker, J. A., and Kutcher, R.   The renal transplant: Rejection and acute tubular necrosis. *Semin. Roentgenol.* 13:352, 1978.

10. Bell, P. R. F., Briggs, J. D., Calman, K. C., Paton, A. M., Wood, R. F. M., MacPherson, S. G., and Kyle, K.   Reversal of acute clinical and experimental organ rejection using large doses of intravenous prednisolone. *Lancet* 1:876, 1971.

11. Bennett, W. M., McDonald, W. J., Lawson, R. K., and Porter, G. A.   Posttransplant hypertension: Studies of cortical blood flow and the renal pressor system. *Kidney Int.* 6:99, 1974.

12. Bodart, P., Dautrebande, J., Baert, A., Mathy, J., Pringot, J., Alexandre, G., and Van Ypersele, C.   Le radiodiagnostic dans les transplantations rénales. *J. Radiol. Electrol. Med. Nucl.* 56 [Suppl. 1]:352, 1975.

13. Boijsen, E.   Angiographische Diagnostik der nichttumorösen parenchymatösen Nierenerkrankungen. In O. Hug (ed.), *Deutscher Röntgenkongress 1970.* Stuttgart: Thieme, 1972. P. 93.

14. Boijsen, E.   Angiography in Renal Tumors: Indications and Technique. In E. Löhr (ed.), *Renal and Adrenal Tumors.* Heidelberg and New York: Springer, 1979. P. 78.

15. Boijsen, E., and Judkins, M. P.   A hook-tail "closed-end" catheter for percutaneous selective cardioangiography. *Radiology* 87:872, 1966.

16. Boltuch, R. L., and Alfidi, R. J.   Selective renal angiography: Its value in renal transplantation. *Urol. Clin. North Am.* 3:611, 1976.

17. Brücke, P., Pokieser, H., Piza, F., and Zaunbauer, W.   Angiographische Untersuchungen vor und nach Nierentransplantation. In K. E. Loose (ed.), *Angiographie und ihre Leistungen.* Stuttgart: Thieme, 1968. P. 162.

18. Brunner, H., and Gelzer, J.   Personal communication, 1980.

19. Burgener, F. A., and Schabel, S. I.   The radiographic size of renal transplants. *Radiology* 117:547, 1975.

20. Burgener, F. A., and Schabel, S. I.   Der Wert verschiedener radiologischer Untersuchungsmethoden für die Abklärung funktionsgestörter Nierentransplantate. *ROEFO* 129:679, 1978.

21. Busch, G. J., Garovoy, M. R., and Tilney, N. L.   Variant forms of arteritis in human renal allografts. *Transplant Proc.* 11:100, 1979.

22. Castaneda-Zuniga, W., Sibley, R., Zollikofer, C., Nath, P. H., Valdez-Davila, O., Coleman, C., and Amplatz, K.   Renal artery aneurysms: An angiographic sign of transplant rejection. *Radiology* 136:333, 1980.

23. Cho, S. I., Olsson, C. A., Bradley, J. W., and Nabseth, D. C.   Regional program for kidney preservation and transplantation in New England. *Am. J. Surg.* 131:428, 1976.

24. Choi, S., Gatzek, H., Kenny, G. M., and Murphy, G. P.   Techniques and results with arteriograms in human renal allotransplants. *AJR* 109:155, 1970.

25. Clark, R. L., Mandel, S. R., and Webster, W. P.   Microvascular changes in canine renal allograft rejection: A correlative microangiographic and histologic study. *Invest. Radiol.* 12:62, 1977.

26. Crummy, A. B., Jr., Atkinson, R. J., and Daves, M. L.   An analysis of the aortorenal angiograms of 66 prospective renal donors. *Radiology* 84:683, 1965.

27. Crummy, A. B., Jr., and Hipona, F. A.   The roentgen diagnosis of renal vein thrombosis. Experimental aspects. *AJR* 93:898, 1965.

28. Davidson, H. D., Loken, M. K., and Amplatz, K.   Isotope renography and renal arteriography in the evaluation of renal transplants. *AJR* 105:682, 1969.

29. Deal, P., and Hawkins, I. F., Jr.   Venous collaterals in a human renal allograft. *Radiology* 106:547, 1973.

30. Debruyne, F. M. J., Koene, R. A. P., Moonen, W. A., Renders, G. A. M., and Chatik, M. L.   Intrarenal arteriovenous fistula following renal allograft biopsy. *Eur. Urol.* 4:435, 1978.

31. Deodhar, S., and Benjamin, S. P.   Pathology of human renal allograft rejection. *Surg. Clin. North Am.* 51:1141, 1971.

32. Diamond, N. G., Casarella, W. J., Hardy, M. A., and Appel, G. B.   Dilatation of critical trans-

plant renal artery stenosis by percutaneous transluminal angioplasty. *AJR* 133:1167, 1979.

33. Diaz-Buxo, J. A., Kopen, D. F., and Donadio, J. V. Renal allograft arteriovenous fistula following percutaneous biopsy. *J. Urol.* 112:577, 1974.

34. Edgren, J., Laasonen, L., and Kuhlbäck, B. Diagnostic yield of angiography in renal transplants. *Ann. Radiol.* 21:384, 1978.

35. Ehrlich, R. M., and Smith, R. B. Surgical complications of renal transplantation. *Urology* 10 [Suppl. 3]:43, 1977.

36. Ekelund, L. Spontaneous closure of arteriovenous fistulae following percutaneous renal biopsy. *Acta Radiol* [*Diagn.*] (Stockh.) 11:289, 1971.

37. Ekelund, L., Kaude, J., and Lindholm, T. Angiography in glomerular disease of the kidney. *AJR* 119:739, 1973.

38. Ekelund, L., and Lindholm, T. Arteriovenous fistulae following percutaneous renal biopsy. *Acta Radiol.* [*Diagn.*] (Stockh.) 11:38, 1971.

39. Finkelstein, F. O., and Black, H. R. Risk factor analysis in renal transplantation: Guidelines for the management of the transplant recipient. *Am. J. Med. Sci.* 267:139, 1974.

40. Finkelstein, F. O., Lytton, B., Schiff, M., and Black, H. R. Rejection episodes and patient graft survival after renal transplantation. *Clin. Nephrol.* 3:217, 1975.

41. Fletcher, E. W. L., and Lecky, J. W. The radiological size of renal transplants—a retrospective study. *Br. J. Radiol.* 42:892, 1969.

42. Fletcher, E. W. L., Lecky, J. W., and Gonick, H. C. Selective phlebography of transplanted kidneys. *Clin. Radiol.* 21:144, 1970.

43. Foley, W. D., Bookstein, J. J., Tweist, M., Gikas, P. W., Mayor, G. H., and Turcotte, J. G. Arteriography of renal transplants. *Radiology* 116:271, 1975.

44. Frödin, L., Thorarinsson, H., and Willén, R. Preanastomotic arterial stenosis in renal transplant recipients. *Scand. J. Urol. Nephrol.* 9:66, 1975.

45. Gailiunas, P., Busch, G., Person, A., Carpenter, C. B., and Garovoy, M. R. Prediction of reversibility of renal allograft rejection. *Transplant. Proc.* 11:17, 1979.

46. Gedgaudas, T., White, R. I., and Loken, M. K. Radiology in renal transplantation. *Radiol. Clin. North Am.* 10:530, 1972.

47. Hamway, S., Novick, A., Braun, W. E., Levin, H., Banowsky, L., Alfidi, R., and Magnusson, M. Impaired renal allograft function: A comparative study with angiography and histopathology. *J. Urol.* 122:292, 1979.

48. Hawkins, I. F., Jr. "Mini-catheter" technique for femoral runoff and abdominal arteriography. *AJR* 116:199, 1972.

48a. Hawkins, I. F., Jr. Carbon dioxide digital subtraction arteriography. *AJR* 139:19, 1982.

49. Hawkins, I. F., Jr. Tolazoline for arterial enhancement in angiography. Excerpta Medica International Congress Series, No. 301. 13th International Congress of Radiology, Madrid, 1973. P. 244.

50. Hawkins, I. F., Jr. Haseman, M. K., and Gelfand, P. N. Single minicatheter technique for abdominal aortography for selective injection. *Radiology* 132:755, 1979.

51. Hawkins, I. F., Jr., and Herbert, L. Contrast material used as a catheter flushing agent—a method to reduce clot formation during angiography. *Radiology* 110:351, 1974.

52. Hawkins, I. F., Jr., and Kelley, M. J. Heparinized angiography catheters. *Radiology* 109:589, 1973.

53. Hellekant, C., and Kaude, J. Nierenvenenthrombose. *Radiologe* 12:349, 1979.

54. Henricks, D. G., Bluth, E. I., Figueroa, J. E., Schuler, S. E., and Brannan, W. Simple cyst arising in a transplanted kidney: A case report. *J. Urol.* 122:819, 1979.

55. Henriksson, C., Nilson, A. E., and Thorén, O. K. A. Artery stenosis in renal transplantation. *Scand. J. Urol. Nephrol.* [Suppl.] 29:89, 1975.

56. Herdman, R. C., Michael, A. F., Vernier, R. L., Kelly, W. D., and Good, R. A. Renal function and phosphorus excretion after human renal homotransplantation. *Lancet* 1:121, 1966.

56a. Hillman, B. J., Zukowski, C. F., Ovitt, T. W., Ogden, D. A., and Capp, M. P. Evaluation of potential renal donors and renal allograft recipients: Digital video subtraction angiography. *AJR* 138:921, 1982.

57. Hollenberg, N. K., Epstein, M., Rosen, S. M., Basch, R. I., Oken, D. E., and Merrill, J. P. Acute oliguric renal failure in man: Evidence for preferential renal cortical ischemia. *Medicine* 47:455, 1968.

58. Hollenberg, N. K., Retik, A. B., Rosen, S. M., Murray, J. E., and Merrill, J. P. The role of vasoconstriction of renal allograft rejection. *Transplantation* 6:59, 1968.

59. Jafri, S. Z. H., Kaude, J. V., and Wright, P. G. Ultrasound findings in renal transplant rejection. *Acta Radiol.* [*Diagn.*] (Stockh.) 22:245, 1981.

60. Jones, B. J., Palmer, F. J., Charlesworth, J. A., Shirley, D. V., MacDonald, G. J., Williams, R. M., and Robertson, M. R. Angiography in the diagnosis of renal allograft dysfunction. *J. Urol.* 119:461, 1978.

61. Kapdi, C. C., Silva, Y. J., and Wolfe, J. N. Xeroradiography in the angiographic evaluation of renal transplantation. *Radiology* 111:220, 1974.

62. Kaude, J. V. Advances in angiography. The catheter. *Int. Surg.* 59:563, 1974.

63. Kaude, J. V. Der Aussagewert der Angiographie bei akuter Abstossungsreaktion der transplantierten Niere. In K. E. Loose and D. A. Loose (eds.), *Aktuelle Ergebnisse der Angiographie und Angiologie.* Cologne: Deutscher Ärzteverlag, 1980. P. 402.

64. Kaude, J. V., Fuller, T. J., Hawkins, I. F., Jr., Juncos, L. I., and Pfaff, W. W. Prognostic value of angiography in management of severe acute renal transplant rejection. *ROEFO* 127:119, 1977.

65. Kaude, J. V., Fuller, T. J., and Soong, J. Fibrolipomatosis of the transplanted kidney. *ROEFO* 130:300, 1979.

66. Kaude, J. V., and Grotemeyer, P. Catheterization Technique. In K. E. Loose and R. J. A. M. van Dongen (eds.), *Atlas of Angiography.* Stuttgart: Thieme, 1976. P. 7.

67. Kaude, J. V., and Hawkins, I. F., Jr. Angiography of renal transplant. *Radiol. Clin. North Am.* 14:295, 1976.

68. Kaude, J. V., Slusher, D. H., Pfaff, W. W., and Hackett, R. L. Angiographic diagnosis of rejection and tubular necrosis in human kidney allografts. *Acta Radiol.* [*Diagn.*] (Stockh.) 10:476, 1970.

69. Kaude, J. V., Stone, M., Fuller, T. J., Cade, J. R., Tarrant, D. G., and Juncos, L. I. Papillary necrosis in kidney transplant patients. *Radiology* 120:69, 1976.

70. Kincaid-Smith, P. Histological diagnosis of rejection of renal homografts in man. *Lancet* 2:849, 1967.

71. Kjellstrand, C. M., Casali, R. E., Simmons, R. L., Shideman, J. R., Buselmeier, T. J., and Najarian, J. Etiology and prognosis in acute post-transplant renal failure. *Am. J. Med.* 61:190, 1976.

72. Klarskov, P., Brendstrup, L., Krarup, T., Jörgensen, H. E., Egeblad, M., and Palböl, J. Renovascular hypertension after kidney transplantation. *Scand. J. Urol. Nephrol.* 13:291, 1979.

73. Knudsen, D. F., Davidson, A. J., Kountz, S. L., and Cohn, R. Serial angiography in canine renal allographs. *Transplantation* 5:256, 1967.

74. Kormano, M., Kock, B., Brotherus, V., Lindfors, O., and Lindström, B. Microangiography of rejected human kidney transplants. *Invest. Radiol.* 12:74, 1977.

75. Kountz, S. L., Margules, R., and Belzer, F. O. Complications of renal transplantation. *Kidney* 5:5, 1972.

76. Kountz, S. L., Williams, M. A., Williams, P. L., Karpros, C., and Dempster, W. J. Mechanism of rejection of homotransplanted kidneys. *Nature* 199:257, 1963.

77. Kreis, H. Insuffisances rénales aiguës reject des reins transplantés. *Nouv. Presse Méd.* 8:2943, 1979.

78. Kyaw, M. M. Ideal radiographic projection for renal transplant angiograms. *Radiology* 107:275, 1973.

79. Laasonen, L. Prognostic value of angiography in early failure of renal transplants. *Acta Radiol.* [*Diagn.*] (Stockh.) 18:305, 1977.

80. Laasonen, L., Edgren, J., and Mattson, T. Magnification angiography in the evaluation of transplanted kidneys. *Acta Radiol.* [*Diagn.*] (Stockh.) 17:200, 1976.

81. Laasonen, L., and Kock, B. Angiography and isotope renography in acute rejection of renal transplant. *Scand. J. Urol. Nephrol.* 12:79, 1978.

82. Laasonen, L., Kock, B., and Nyberg, M. Early venous filling in transplanted kidneys. *Acta Radiol.* [*Diagn.*] (Stockh.) 18:593, 1977.

83. Lacombe, M. Arterial stenosis complicating renal allotransplantation in man: A study of 38 cases. *Ann. Surg.* 181:283, 1975.

84. Lecky, J. W., and Fletcher, E. W. L. Renal Homotransplant Angiography. In W. N. Hanafee (ed.), *Selective Angiography.* Section 18: L. I. Robbins (ed.), *Golden's Diagnostic Radiology.* Baltimore; Williams & Wilkins, 1972. P. 204.

85. Lee, D. B. N., Prompt, A. C., Upham, A. T., and Kleeman, C. R. Medical complications of renal transplantation: I. Graft and infectious complications in recipient. *Urology* [Suppl.] 9:7, 1977.

86. Lerona, P. T. Angiography of renal transplant using ipsilateral femoral artery compression. *Radiology* 114:737, 1975.

87. Levine, E., Meyers, A. M., Salant, D. J., Myburgh, J. A., Milne, F. J., Botha, J. R., and Goldberg, B. Angiography after renal transplantation. *S. Afr. Med. J.* 50:1295, 1976.

88. Lindsey, E. S., Garbus, S. B., Golladay, E. S., and McDonald, J. C. Hypertension due to renal artery stenosis in transplanted kidneys. *Ann. Surg.* 181:604, 1975.

89. Lingårdh, G., and Lundström, B. Renal blood flow determined by angiography. *Acta Radiol.* [*Diagn.*] (Stockh.) 15:529, 1974.

90. Matas, A. J., Mauer, S. M., Sutherland, D. E. R., Spanos, P. K., Simmons, R. L., and Najarian, J. S. Polar infarct of a kidney transplant simulating appendicitis. *Am. J. Surg.* 131:363, 1976.

91. Morris, P. J., Yadav, R. V., Kincaid-Smith, P., Anderton, J., Hare, W. S. C., Johnson, N., Johnson, W., and Marshall, V. C. Renal artery stenosis in renal transplantation. *Med. J. Aust.* 1:1255, 1971.

92. Müller, J. H., Schuldt, H. H., Hölzer, D. H., Kumm, K.-P., Waigand, J., and Althaus, P. Quantitative angiographische Unter-

suchungen zur Differentialdiagnose des frühen akuten Nierenversagens ischämieund rejektionsgeschädigter Transplantate. *Z. Urol. Nephrol.* 72:715, 1979.

93. Müller, J. H., Waigand, J., Schuldt, H. H., and Hölzer, D. H. Gefässveränderungen bei experimenteller Nierenischämie und nach Nierenhomotransplantation (Eine tierexperimentelle angiographische Studie). *Z. Urol. Nephrol.* 71:673, 1978.

94. Navani, S., Athanasoulis, C. A., Monoco, A. P., Cavallo, T., Lewis, E. J., and Hipona, F. A. Renal homotransplantation: Spectrum of angiographic findings of the kidney. *AJR* 113:433, 1971.

95. Nilson, A. E., Jacobson, B., Bergentz, S. E., and Westberg, G. Angiography of the transplanted kidney. *Scand. J. Urol. Nephrol.* 2:46, 1968.

96. Nilsson, J. Angiography in tumours of the urinary bladder. *Acta Radiol.* [*Suppl.*] (Stockh.) 263:58, 1967.

97. O'Connor, J. F., Couch, N. P., Lindquist, R., Dammin, G. J., and Murray, J. E. A correlation of arteriography, histology, and clinical course in kidney transplantation. *Ann. N.Y. Acad. Sci.* 129:637, 1966.

98. O'Connor, J. F., Dealey, J. B., Jr., Lindquist, R., and Couch, N. P. Arterial lesions due to rejection in human kidney allografts. *Radiology* 89:614, 1967.

99. Olin, T., and Reuter, S. R. A pharmacoangiographic method for improving nephrophlebography. *Radiology* 85:1036, 1965.

100. Otto, R., Pouliadis, G., and Uhlschmid, G. Angiographische Funktionsanlage bei der transplantierten Niere. In K. E. Loose and D. A. Loose (eds.), *Aktuelle Ergebnisse der Angiographie und Angiologie.* Cologne: Deutscher Ärzteverlag, 1980. P. 398.

101. Pastershank, S. P. Chow, K. C., Baltzan, M. A., Baltzan, R. B., Cunningham, T. A., and Cross, J. W. Renal homotransplantation: Angiographic features in first 180 days following surgery. *J. Can. Assoc. Radiol.* 24:104, 1973.

102. Penn, I. Cancer in immunosuppressed patients. *Transplant. Proc.* 7:553, 1975.

103. Penn, I. Tumors arising in organ transplant recipients. *Adv. Cancer Res.* 28:31, 1978.

104. Penn, I., Durst, A. L., Machado, M., Halgrimson, C. G., Booth, A. S., Jr., Putnam, C. W., Groth, C. G., and Starzl, T. E. Acute pancreatitis and hyperamylasemia in renal homograft recipients. *Arch. Surg.* 105:167, 1972.

105. Peters, M. S., and Stuard, I. D. Metastatic malignant melanoma transplanted via a renal homograft. A care report. *Cancer* 41:2426, 1978.

106. Pokieser, H. Röntgendiagnostische Aufgaben im Rahmen der Nierentransplantation (mit besonderer Berücksichtigung angiographischer Untersuchungen). *ROEFO* 114:1, 1971.

107. Pollini, J., Guttmann, R. D., Beaudoin, J. G., Morehouse, D. D., Klassen, J., and Knaack, J. Late hypertension following renal allotransplantation. *Clin. Nephrol.* 11:202, 1979.

108. Pool. R. Angiographic aspects in kidney transplantation. *Radiol. Clin.* (Basel) 47:22, 1978.

109. Porter, K. A., Dossetor, J. B., Marchioro, T. L., Peart, W. S., Randall, J. M., Starzl, T. E., and Terasaki, P. I. Human renal transplants: I. Glomerular changes. *Lab. Invest.* 16:153, 1967.

110. Porter, K. A., Marchioro, T. L., and Starzl, T. E. Pathological changes in 37 human renal homotransplants treated with immunosuppressive drugs. *Br. J. Urol.* 37:250, 1965.

111. Porter, K. A., Thomson, W. B., Owen, K., Kenyon, J. R., Mowbray, J. F., and Peart, W. S. Obliterative vascular changes in four human kidney homotransplants. *Br. Med. J.* 2:639, 1963.

112. Prompt, A. C., Lee, D. B. N., Upham, A. T., and Kleeman, C. R. Medical complications of renal transplantation. II. Noninfectious complications in recipient. *Urology* [Suppl.] 9:32, 1977.

113. Rankin, R. S., Crummy, A. B., and Belzer, P. O. Biplane arteriography for the evaluation of arterial stenosis in renal transplantation. *AJR* 128:330, 1977.

114. Raphael, M. J., Steiner, R. E., Shackman, R., and Ware, R. G. Post-operative angiography in renal homotransplantation. *Br. J. Radiol.* 42:873, 1969.

115. Reichert, J. R., and Tyson, I. B. Venophotoscintigraphy in renal transplant renograms: Demonstration of an unusual complication. *Radiology* 111:219, 1974.

116. Renigers, S. A., and Spigos, D. G. Pseudoaneurysm of the arterial anastomosis in a renal transplant. *AJR* 131:525, 1978.

117. Rosen, S. M., Retik, A. B., Hollenberg, N. K., Merrill, J. P., and Murray, J. E. Effect of immunosuppressive therapy on the intrarenal distribution of blood flow in dog renal allograft rejection. *Surg. Forum* 17:233, 1966.

118. Rosenberger, A., Munk, J., Better, O. S., Erlik, D., and Barzilai, A. The angiographic signs of rejection in cadaver kidney transplants. *Clin. Radiol.* 21:135, 1970.

119. Samuel, E. Radiology in the diagnosis of renal rejection. *Clin. Radiol.* 21:109, 1970.

120. Schact, R. A., Martin, D. G., Karalakulasingam, R., Wheeler, C. S., and Lansing, A. M. Renal artery stenosis after renal transplantation. *Am. J. Surg.* 131:653, 1976.

121. Shell, A. G. R., Mahoney, J. F., Horvath, J. S., Johnson, J. R., Tiller, D. J., May, J., and Stewart,

J. H. Cancer and survival after cadaveric donor renal transplantation. *Transplant. Proc.* 11:1052, 1979.

122. Sherwood, T., Lavender, J. P., and Greenspan, R. H. Renal magnification angiograms in the dog: Observations on response to vasodilators and surgical trauma. *Br. J. Radiol.* 42:241, 1969.

123. Sherwood, T., Ruuter, M., and Chisholm, G. D. Renal angiography problems in live kidney donors. *Br. J. Radiol.* 51:99, 1978.

124. Silverman, F. N. Radiologic contribution to organ transplantation. *J. Ky. Med. Assoc.* 65:1188, 1967.

125. Simma, W., Brücke, P., and Stadler, R. Zur Bedeutung der Nierenangiographie nach Transplantation. In K. E. Loose and D. A. Loose (eds.), *Aktuelle Ergebnisse der Angiographie und Angiologie.* Cologne: Deutscher Ärzteverlag, 1980. P. 394.

126. Simmons, R. L., Tallent, M. B., Kjellstrand, C. M., and Najarian, J. S. Renal allograft rejection simulated by arterial stenosis. *Surgery* 68:800, 1970.

127. Smellie, W. A. B., Vinik, M., Freed, T. A., and Hume, D. M. Pertrochanteric venography in the study of human renal transplant recipients. *Surg. Gynecol. Obstet.* 126:777, 1968.

128. Smellie, W. A. B., Vinik, M., and Hume, D. M. Angiographic investigation of hypertension complicating human renal transplantation. *Surg. Gynecol. Obstet.* 128:963, 1969.

129. Sniderman, K. W., Sos, T. A., Sprayregen, S., Saddekni, S., Cheigh, J. S., Tapia, L., Tellis, V., and Veith, F. J. Percutaneous transluminal angioplasty in renal transplant arterial stenosis for relief of hypertension. *Radiology* 135:23, 1980.

130. Spanos, P. K., Simmons, R. L., Kjellstrand, C. M., Buselmeier, T. J., and Najarian, J. S. Kidney transplantation from living related donors with multiple vessels. *Am. J. Surg.* 125:554, 1973.

131. Spanos, P. K., Weil, R., III, Simmons, R. L., and Najarian, J. S. Successful transplantation of ectopic kidneys from living related donors. *Am. J. Surg.* 131:360, 1976.

132. Spring, D. B., Salvatierra, O., Jr., Palubinskas, A. J., Amend, W. J. C., Jr., Vincenti, F. G., and Feduska, N. J. Results and significance of angiography in potential kidney donors. *Radiology* 133:45, 1979.

133. Stables, D. P., Klingensmit, W. C., III, and Johnson, M. L. Renal Transplantation. In A. T. Rosenfeld, M. G. Glickman, and J. Hodson (eds.), *Diagnostic Imaging in Renal Disease.* New York: Appleton-Century-Crofts, 1979. P. 167.

134. Staple, T. W., and Chiang, D. T. C. Arteriography following renal transplantation. *AJR* 101:669, 1967.

135. Strauser, G. D., Stables, D. P., and Weil, R., III. Optimal technique of renal arteriography in living renal transplant donors. *AJR* 131:813, 1978.

136. Takaro, T. Experimental renal glomerulography. *AJR* 101:681, 1967.

137. Truniger, B., Rosen, S. M., Kriek, H., and Oken, D. E. Die Rejektion der homotransplantierten Niere. *Urol. Int.* 21:163, 1966.

138. Van Cangh, P. J., Dautrebande, J., Pirson, Y., Van Ypersele de Strihou, C., and Alexandre, G. P. J. Reversible renal artery stenosis in renal transplantation. *Urology* 13:529, 1979.

139. Vidne, B. A., Leapman, S. B., Butt, K. M., and Kountz, S. L. Vascular complications in human renal transplantation. *Surgery* 77:81, 1976.

140. Vinik, M., Smellie, W. A. B., Freed, T. A., Hume, D. M., and Weidner, W. A. Angiographic evaluation of the human homotransplant kidney. *Radiology* 92:873, 1969.

141. Vinik, M., Smellie, W. A. B., Freed, T. A., Hume, D. M., and Weidner, W. A. Renal ischemia and homograft rejection. Preliminary angiographic data in dog. *Invest. Radiol.* 4:252, 1969.

142. Voegeli, V. E., Blaser, C., and Montandon, A. Die angiographische Abklärung funktionsgestörter Nierentransplantate. *ROEFO* 120:141, 1974.

143. White, R. I., Jr., Najarian, J., Loken, M., and Amplatz, K. Arteriovenous complications associated with renal transplantation. *Radiology* 102:29, 1972.

144. Williams, G. M. Progress in clinical renal transplantation. *Tranplant. Proc.* 11:4, 1979.

145. Williams, G. M., Lee, H. M., Weymouth, R. F., Harlan, W. R., Jr., Holden, K. R., Stanley, C. M., Millington, G. A., and Hume, D. M. Studies in hyperacute and chronic renal homograft rejection in man. *Surgery* 62:204, 1967.

146. Wilms, H., Halbfass, H.-J., Heinze, V., and Mittermayer, C. Die postanastomotische Nierenarteriestenose nach Nierentransplantation. *Dtsch. Med. Wochenschr.* 100:1376, 1975.

147. Wright, F. W., Fletcher, E. W. L., and Oliver, D. O. Arterio-venous shunting occurring with rejection in a renal transplant. *Br. J. Urol.* 44:395, 1972.

148. Yoran, C., and Glassman, E. The paradoxic effect of tolazoline hydrochloride on pulmonary hypertension of mitral stenosis. *Chest* 63:843, 1973.

149. Zeitler, E. Angiographische Probleme zur Diagnostik und Therapie der renovaskulären Hypertonie. *Radiologe* 11:43, 1971.

150. Zimmerman, R., and Sprayregen, S. Arteriovenous shunting in renal transplant rejection. *Angiology* 29:40, 1978.

151. Zum Winkel, K., Harlest, H., Das, K. B., and Newiger, T. Applications of radionuclides in renal transplantation. *Semin. Nucl. Med.* 4:169, 1974.

3. Adrenal Angiography

The Roles of Angiography in Adrenal Disease

JOSEPH J. BOOKSTEIN

Most diseases of the adrenal gland are associated with endocrine dysfunction and produce relatively characteristic clinical and biochemical abnormalities. Diagnosis of the basic disease process, therefore, is usually accomplished clinically, and angiography or other diagnostic imaging is generally reserved for localization of an adrenal or extraadrenal tumor, or for differentiating adrenal tumor from hyperplasia. A few adrenal diseases are not associated with endocrine dysfunction; in these circumstances, imaging methods are ordinarily intended to reveal the presence of an adrenal mass, such as a cyst or carcinoma.

Within the past several years, techniques for adrenal vascular catheterization have been considerably refined and now enable reliable evaluation by arteriographic, venographic, or sampling methods. More recently, alternative noninvasive diagnostic techniques, such as ultrasound, computed tomography, and isotope scintigraphy, have also undergone remarkable development. Thus, while diagnostic potential has advanced rapidly across a broad front, the relative roles of each diagnostic modality have fluctuated with time, and with the locally available expertise. The role of angiography vis-à-vis noninvasive methods requires individual assessment in each adrenal disease or condition. The conditions to be separately considered in this chapter include: (1) the normal adrenal gland, (2) aldosteronism, (3) Cushing's disease, (4) virilizing syndromes, (5) pheochromocytoma and Sipple's syndrome, (6) nonfunctioning adrenal tumors, (7) adrenal cysts, (8) hyperfunction after adrenalectomy due to remnants, (9) adrenal carcinoma, (10) Addison's disease, (11) miscellaneous diseases, (12) transcatheter adrenal ablation, and (13) instances in which angiography has advantages over computed tomography.

Vascular Anatomy

Each adrenal gland has three sources of arterial supply (Fig. 61-1): a superior adrenal artery that arises from the inferior phrenic artery, a middle adrenal artery that arises from the lateral aspect of the aorta at a level between the renal and celiac arteries, and an inferior adrenal artery that arises from the superior aspect of the ipsilateral renal artery. Each arterial trunk then breaks up into 10 to 20 smaller twigs that ramify and intercommunicate over the outer aspect of the gland. The

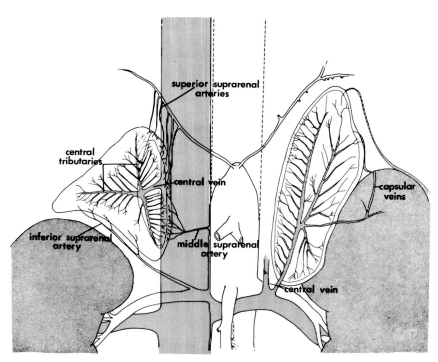

Figure 61-1. Artist's representation of arterial and venous anatomy of the adrenal gland. Note the three different sources of the arterial supply, representing inferior, middle, and superior adrenal arteries. There is but one central vein on each side; the right arises from the posterolateral aspect of the inferior vena cava, the left from the superior aspect of the left renal vein.

twigs terminate as perforating branches that pass perpendicularly through the cortex into the medulla. No direct arterial supply to the adrenal medulla seems to be present.

The perforating arteries gradually assume the histologic characteristics of veins as they pass centripetally into the medulla, and no other direct cortical venous supply is present. When these venules reach the central portion of the medulla, they join a central vein at right angles. The junction of perforating and central veins is deficient in medial musculature [16] and probably constitutes a site of predilection for rupture during adrenal venography [46].

On the left side the venous anatomy is quite constant. The central vein is valveless, usually solitary, and passes down the entire long axis of the gland. It generally joins an inferior phrenic vein just above the left renal vein, then joins the left renal vein as a phrenicoadrenal trunk. The junction of phrenicoadrenal trunk and renal vein usually occurs within 1 cm of a parasagittal plane passing through the left lateral aspect of the vertebral column. The phrenic vein is medial to the adrenal vein and generally contains a competent terminal valve. During left adrenal venography

and sampling, special manipulations or catheter shapes are sometimes necessary to direct the catheter from the inferior phrenic vein toward the central adrenal vein.

The central vein usually communicates, via large emissary veins, with an adrenal capsular vein, particularly via perforators at the apex of the gland. The adrenal capsular veins in turn communicate with renal capsular veins. Observation of these communications during adrenal venography is helpful in confirming proper catheter position.

On the right, three central tributaries are generally present, one from the superior aspect of the gland, another from the inferior aspect, and a third from the posterior aspect. These three tributaries join to form a short central trunk, which passes forward to join the right posterior aspect of the inferior vena cava. In about 10 percent of individuals, the right adrenal vein joins the posterior aspect of a hepatic vein near the inferior vena cava, rather than the inferior vena cava directly. Such an anatomic arrangement does not preclude successful right adrenal vein catheterization. Rarely, the right adrenal vein may drain into the right renal vein.

Angiographic Techniques

ARTERIOGRAPHY

Complete arteriographic depiction of both adrenal glands is likely to require selective injections of six arteries, three on each side. The minor communications that exist over the surface of the gland between the major arterial branches are not usually large enough to allow opacification of the entire gland from a single selective injection. To facilitate localization of the major adrenal arteries, an aortogram is obtained initially. For large or hypervascular tumors, aortography alone may provide sufficient information. If selective arteriography is necessary, the aortogram catheter is replaced with a "shepherd's crook" (see Fig. 61-2A), formed from a catheter with rather good torque characteristics. I use the pink Formocath material (U.S. Catheter and Instrument Co.) with OD 2.2 mm, ID 1.3 mm. The catheter tip is tightly tapered over a 0.028-inch guidewire to facilitate entry into the small adrenal arteries.

The catheter is initially passed above the celiac artery, and the correct reversed configuration within the aorta is obtained. The anterior aorta is then explored just above the origin of the celiac artery, and the inferior phrenic arteries are engaged from the aorta (see Fig. 61-20) or proximal celiac artery by exerting traction on the catheter. From 4 to 6 cc of 76 percent Renografin (E. R. Squibb & Sons) is injected at the rate of 3 cc per second for 2 seconds, during serial filming at the rate of 2 cc per second for 3 seconds, and then 1 cc per second for 3 seconds.

The catheter is then disengaged from the inferior phrenic artery while the downward angulation of the tip is maintained, and the lateral aspect of the aorta above the renal arteries is explored. When the middle adrenal artery is engaged, filming is performed as just discussed, except that the amount of contrast medium and rate of injection are reduced in proportion to the usual small size of this artery. Injection of contrast medium into the adrenal gland is associated with a fair amount of pain, which can be reduced by adding lidocaine to the contrast agent (final concentration, 0.2% lidocaine).

In order to catheterize the inferior adrenal artery, the catheter is disengaged from the middle adrenal artery, the downward angulation of the tip being maintained, and withdrawn until the tip enters the renal artery. Continued withdrawal will then direct the tip superiorly. As the tip is withdrawn medially toward the origin of the renal artery, small injections of contrast medium will indicate the point at which the inferior adrenal artery has been engaged. Filming and injection are the same as for the middle adrenal artery (see Fig. 61-11).

At times, selective adrenal arteriography may not be possible. Selective renal arteriography, after administration of 3 to 5 μg epinephrine, may provide an acceptable alternative. The epinephrine causes disproportionate constriction of renal microvasculature, diverting contrast medium into the inferior adrenal artery that usually arises from the renal artery (see Fig. 61-8C).

ADRENAL VENOGRAPHY

The catheter material is the same as that used for arteriography; the shapes are as indicated in Figure 61-2. Two tiny side holes are punched in the distal portion of the right adrenal vein catheter within 5 mm of the tip to facilitate aspiration of

Figure 61-2. Catheters for adrenal angiography. (A) Catheter shape for engaging superior, middle, or inferior adrenal arteries. (B) Right adrenal venous configuration. (C) Left adrenal venous configuration.

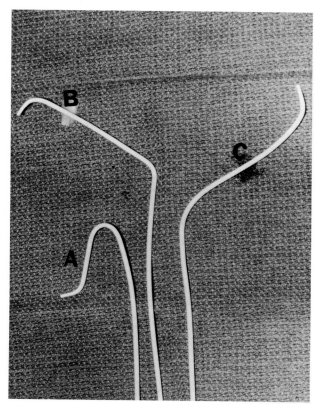

blood. I prefer to catheterize the right adrenal vein initially, using a catheter shaped as in Figure 61-2B. Search begins on the posterior aspect of the inferior vena cava, at the anticipated level of the center of the gland, i.e., just above the upper pole of the kidney. When minor advances and withdrawals at the shaft do not produce comparable motions at the tip, a test injection is performed to determine whether the adrenal vein has been entered. Considerable experience is required to recognize that the right adrenal veins have indeed been properly engaged. One looks for the typical stellate appearance, produced by two or three central tributaries opacifying from the short main trunk (see Fig. 61-4B). Small accessory hepatic veins are often encountered in the same region, but injection into a hepatic vein may be differentiated from adrenal injections by observing the following:

1. Injection into the adrenal gland is often somewhat painful, while injection into a hepatic vein is usually painless.
2. Injection into a hepatic vein often produces a homogeneous persistent blush, while a blush does not usually occur after adrenal venous injection.
3. Downward-coursing adrenal and renal capsular veins are often opacified after adrenal injections, while upward-curving hepatic veins may be well visualized after hepatic vein injections.

The catheter is not infrequently somewhat unstable in its position within the right adrenal vein. Minor adjustments in rotation, shallow respiration, slight adjustments in catheter shape, and conduct of the examination with alacrity are maneuvers that help maintain proper catheter position. Often during fluoroscopy it may be observed that the intraadrenal veins are much better opacified in one phase of respiration than another, and *that* respiratory phase should be selected for filming.

In experienced hands, the right adrenal vein can be successfully catheterized in about 90 to 95 percent [33] of cases. Difficulty is often due to entrance of the adrenal vein into the origin of a hepatic vein rather than directly into the inferior vena cava. This problem can be overcome by elongating the distal tip of the catheter so that it will reach through the hepatic vein to the adrenal vein. Alternatively, the shepherd's crook catheter can be utilized.

If adrenal venous sampling is to be performed,

it must be accomplished before definitive injections of contrast medium are made, inasmuch as the injections may affect the concentration of metabolites (personal unreported data).

In order to minimize the incidence of intraadrenal rupture and hemorrhage, gentle technique is required. The amount of contrast to be injected varies greatly and is best determined by noting the point at which the patient experiences the pain of glandular distention. I perform the injections by hand and generally have about 6 cc of contrast in the syringe. The patient is asked to hold his clenched fist in a visible position, usually near his ear, and to extend one finger when discomfort is noted. The injection is then begun slowly, during filming, and the injection rate gradually increased until the finger snaps open. At this point the injection is stopped. In most patients about 3 or 4 cc is injected, with the final injection rate often being about 2 cc per second. Sometimes, however, a much greater or lesser volume or rate is required. Filming is at the rate of 2 cc per second for 3 seconds and 1 cc per second for 3 seconds. Anteroposterior projections are used, usually with magnification technique; repeat injections or projections are performed infrequently, to minimize the incidence of extravasation.

Following completion of right adrenal catheterization, the right adrenal catheter is passed into the left renal vein. A guidewire is advanced far into the peripheral renal venous bed, and a catheter shaped as shown in Figure 61-2C is exchanged. The catheter is then slowly withdrawn while the tip is directed superiorly, until a sudden visible cephalic motion indicates entrance into the phrenicoadrenal trunk. Entrance into this trunk usually occurs within a centimeter of the left lateral vertebral margin. After engagement of the phrenicoadrenal trunk, test injection should show most of the contrast medium passing toward the central adrenal vein; if toward the phrenic vein, adjustment of the catheter shape or position may be necessary. Blood samples are then drawn, if indicated. Venography is performed in a manner similar to that described for the right adrenal vein. Often slightly larger amounts of contrast medium are required on the left before the discomfort of glandular distention is indicated by the patient.

VENOUS SAMPLING

Despite satisfactory catheterization of the adrenal veins, it may be difficult to aspirate the amounts of blood required for radioimmunoassay (about 5 cc at our institution). The problem is ordinarily due to obturation of the catheter end holes by venous walls and is much more frequent on the right side. Small side holes near the top of the right catheter are usually, but not always, helpful. Changes in respiration, or the Valsalva maneuver, are sometimes effective. Excessive force of aspiration on the syringe can be avoided by introducing 5 cc of air in the syringe, or by collecting the blood with gravity drainage. If all else fails, the adrenal vein wall can be displaced away from the catheter tip by passing a narrow guidewire (OD 0.020 inch) through and a little beyond the catheter tip, while a side-armed gasket-adapter around the externally protruding end of the guidewire prevents leakage and allows continued aspiration from the adrenal vein.

Complications

The major risk of adrenal vein catheterization is intraadrenal extravasation of contrast medium or blood. In experienced hands, this complication develops in about 4 percent of cases [7]. It is more prevalent in patients with aldosteronism or Cushing's disease, in whom the adrenal veins, as well as other systemic veins, are more fragile. Actual extravasation of contrast medium is evident in the minority of cases. More frequently the films are normal, but the patient will complain of persistent pain after the injection, which increases in intensity for a matter of 30 to 60 minutes. The pain may eventually become excruciating, requiring large doses of narcotic analgesics. Pain and fever usually persist for 24 to 36 hours and then subside. This sequence of events indicates intraadrenal hemorrhage and is almost invariably associated with complete and permanent destruction of glandular function. Hormonally active tumors within these injured glands may be temporarily or permanently ablated [18, 21, 36, 65, 66]. Radionuclide adrenal scans obtained days or months later will demonstrate total lack of uptake in the involved gland. If extravasation is bilateral, Addison's disease develops. Thus, extravasation occurring on one side is virtually an absolute contraindication to performance of the procedure on the other side, unless transcatheter adrenal ablation is the desired goal. Clinicians must be prepared to recognize and manage an acute addisonian crisis in any patient who has undergone adrenal vein catheterization.

Extravasation of contrast medium from *extraadrenal* venules is not infrequently observed during the course of the study. This complication is of little clinical significance and is accompanied by only minimal transient discomfort. Adrenal dysfunction does not occur. Differentiation from intraadrenal extravasation is easily accomplished by noting the extraadrenal location of contrast deposition.

Shortly after the introduction of adrenal venography, experienced surgeons began to note adhesions or edema around the glands, which they had not observed previously. These changes occurred despite lack of venographic or clinical evidence of extravasation at the time of the study [7]. Occult rupture of tiny paraadrenal veins during the venographic examination is presumed to be the responsible factor.

The Normal Angiogram

Normal adrenal arteriograms are demonstrated in Figure 61-3. Note that the gland is not usually entirely opacified after injection of any one artery. The parallel folds of the cortex produce a characteristic double density resembling railroad tracks. Each cortical track measures about 2 mm in thickness. The medulla is not distinctly opacified. Because only a portion of the gland is visualized after each injection, the overall appearance of the gland can be appreciated only by mental summation of separate injections, or sophisticated addition of photographic images.

Figure 61-4A illustrates the normal left adrenal venogram. Note the single central venule and the clear demonstration of the normal size, contour, and position of the left adrenal gland. The pinnate branching pattern of the central vein is particularly evident. The phrenic vein is seen medial to the adrenal vein. Because the venules lie within the medulla, the cortex is infrequently opacified. Communications with adrenal and renal capsular venules are noted.

A normal right adrenal venogram is illustrated in Figure 61-4B. Note two or three diverging branches from the short central vein. The pinnate branching pattern of the central venous tributaries is evident.

Planimetric determinations of projected areas of normal adrenal glands, as determined from venography, have demonstrated some direct correlation between patient weight and adrenal size. This correlation is indicated in Figure 61-8C.

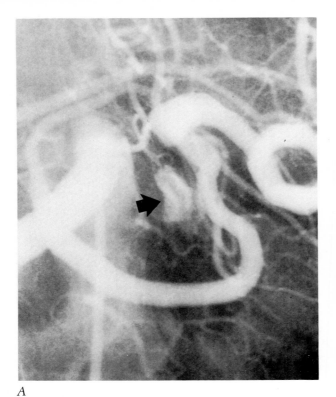

A

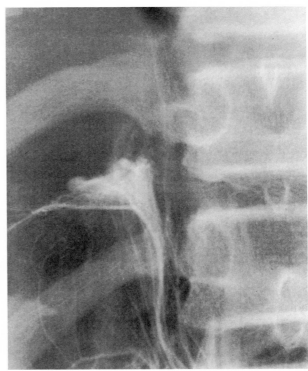

B

Figure 61-3. Arteriographic demonstration of normal adrenal glands. (A) Stain of superior pole of the left adrenal gland after celiac arteriography (*arrow*), with preferential injection into the left inferior phrenic artery. Note that only a portion of the gland is opacified, reaffirming the need to inject all adrenal arterial sources to opacify a normal gland completely. Also note the characteristic short parallel streaks, reflecting segments of cortical folds. (B) Selective inferior adrenal arteriogram of a normal right adrenal gland. Again, only the inferior portion of the gland is opacified.

Figure 61-4. Normal adrenal venograms. (A) Normal left adrenal venogram. Note the single central vein, a recurrent vein to the lower pole (*arrow*), and communications with adrenal and capsular veins. (B) Normal right adrenal venogram. Note the posterior origin of the central vein from the inferior vena cava, and its division into branches to the apex and the lower pole. The posterior branch is obscured in this case.

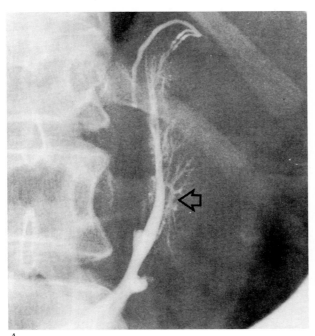

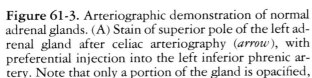

A

B

Other Methods of Adrenal Imaging

Detailed descriptions of techniques involved in adrenal scintigraphy, ultrasonography, and computed tomography are beyond the scope of the present chapter. Brief descriptions, however, are in order.

ADRENAL SCINTIGRAPHY

Development and evaluation of this method are primarily the work of William Beierwaltes, M.D., at the University of Michigan [3, 67]. The radionuclide used initially was ^{131}I-19-iodocholesterol. Intravenous injection of 2 mCi of this agent produced increasing activity over the adrenal cortex, which reached a maximum after 5 to 9 days. Serial computer-processed scans usually demonstrated the adrenal glands with fair resolution. The images predominantly reflect adrenocortical activity, rather than adrenal size. More recently, ^{131}I-6β-iodomethyl-19-norcholesterol [54, 57, 67] has produced images of even better quality.

ADRENAL ECHOGRAPHY

The staunchest proponent of adrenal echography was Frederick Sample, M.D., of the University of California, Los Angeles [55, 56]. By the exploitation of various projections to the fullest, satisfactory visualization of normal adrenal glands has been achieved in 90 percent of cases [55]. In my opinion, the technique requires unusual expertise and persistence, is not applicable in many patients, and will be largely supplanted by computed tomography. Adrenal echography certainly has a place in diagnosis of adrenal cysts (see Fig. 61-19C), and possibly in diagnosis of some other large masses of the adrenal gland (see Fig. 61-18B).

COMPUTED TOMOGRAPHY

The modern, fast computed tomographic abdominal scanner is capable of demonstrating the normal adrenal glands in almost all patients [75]. The normal size and configuration of the gland can generally be evaluated, and even small tumors or enlarged hyperplastic glands are usually depicted. Experience with the technique is still very limited, so that sensitivity, specificity, and overall accuracy in various lesions are not yet precisely known. Preliminary results, however, are highly encouraging [39, 56, 60], and it is likely that the technique will play a dominant role in radiographic evaluation of the adrenal gland.

Aldosteronism

Aldosteronism (hyperaldosteronism) may be secondary to renal disease or to primary adrenal disease. The major clinical manifestations are hypertension, hypokalemia, and increased serum and urinary aldosterone. Secondary aldosteronism is classically associated with elevated serum renin levels, while renin levels are depressed in the primary form. Thus, in evaluation of the cause of aldosteronism, serum renin determinations play a major role in directing investigation toward the kidney when the renin levels are high or toward the adrenal gland when they are low. Secondary aldosteronism is usually due to renal artery stenosis, or rarely to reninoma or other renal conditions, and will not be further considered here.

The primary form of aldosteronism is due to adrenal adenoma in about 75 percent of cases, bilateral multinodular adrenal hyperplasia in about 20 percent, and microscopic hyperplasia or carcinoma in the remainder [59, 73]. The adenomas are relatively small, usually only about 1.0 to 1.5 cm in diameter. There is a slight preponderance of left-sided involvement.

Treatment is usually required because of hypertension. Resection of solitary adrenal adenomas cures or significantly improves the hypertension in about 75 percent of cases [73]. Hypertension secondary to multinodular hyperplasia, however, responds poorly to adrenalectomy [73], and spironolactone is the therapeutic agent of choice. Differential diagnosis, therefore, is important and significantly influences therapy. Differentiation of adenoma and hyperplasia may sometimes be accomplished clinically, on the basis of the anomalous elevation of serum aldosterone that develops in patients with adenoma when they assume an upright position; this observation, however, is neither totally sensitive nor specific.

The angiographic method of choice is adrenal venography, with sampling of adrenal venous effluent for aldosterone concentration [33, 36, 47, 59]. Solitary adenomas are indicated venographically by arcuate displacement of one or more intraadrenal venules (Fig. 61-5A–D). Rarely, contrast medium refluxes into, and directly opacifies, the tumor itself (Fig. 61-6B).

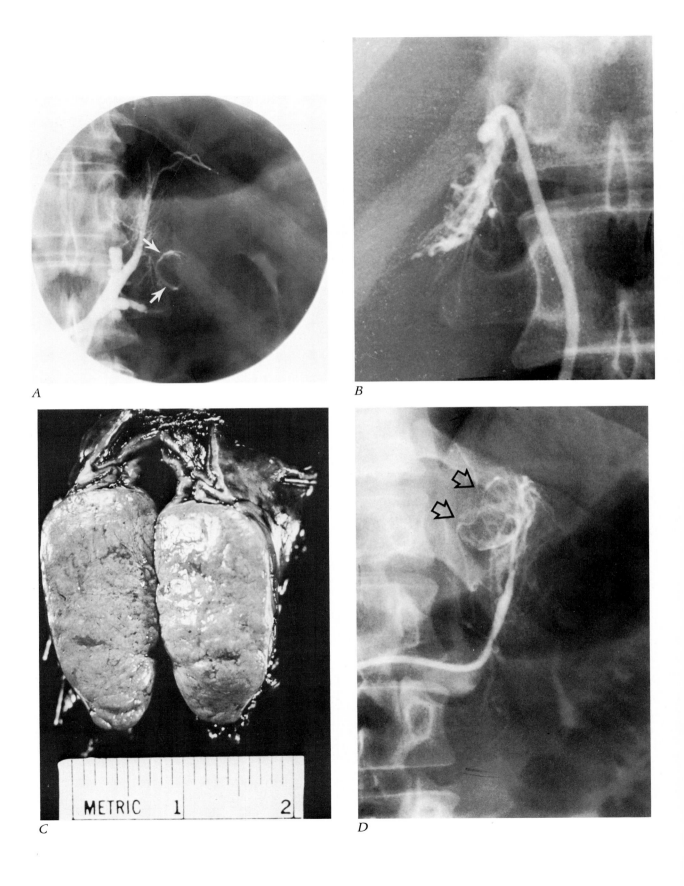

A

B

C

D

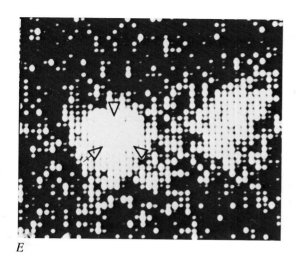

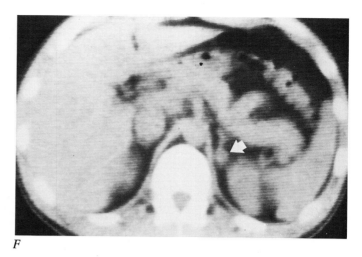

E   *F*

Figure 61-5. Aldosteronomas. (A) Typical 1-cm lesion in the lower lateral portion of the left gland (*arrows*). The adjacent adrenal veins are displaced in a parenthetic configuration and are slightly enlarged. (B) Right aldosteronoma, measuring about 1 × 2 cm on magnification venography. (C) Photograph of the gross specimen of (B). Note the excellent correlation between the tumor size on venography and gross ex- amination. (D) Aldosteronoma in upper portion of left adrenal gland (*arrows*). (E) Scintigraphy of same patient as in (D). Scan obtained several days after injection of [131]I-19-iodocholesterol. Area of increased activity, representing the aldosteronoma, is indicated by arrows. (F) Computed tomographic scan from another patient with a 1-cm left aldosteronoma (*arrow*). (Courtesy of Alvin Moss, M.D.)

Figure 61-6. Aldosteronoma, with some retrograde tumor stain. (Same patient as in Fig. 61-3A, showing normal left adrenal gland.) (A) Early film shows normal venographic anatomy of right gland, except for minimal opacification within the tumor. (B) On late films, stain of a bilobate tumor is clearly evident (*arrows*). Retrograde tumor stain is not infrequent.

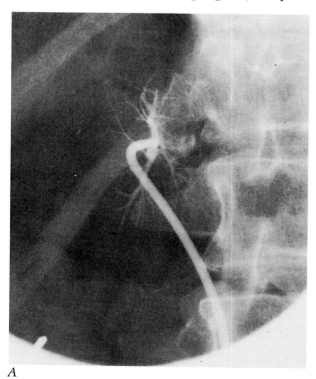

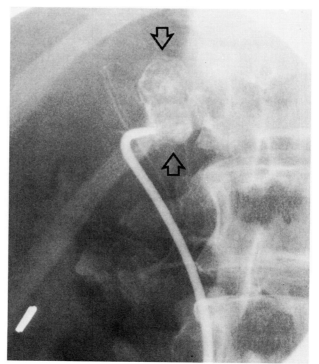

A   *B*

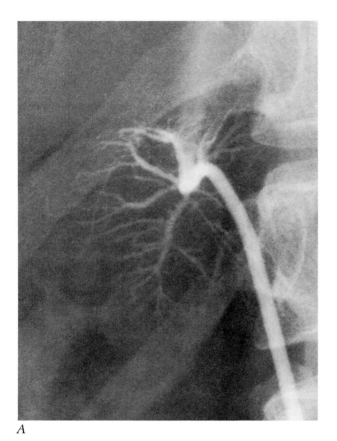

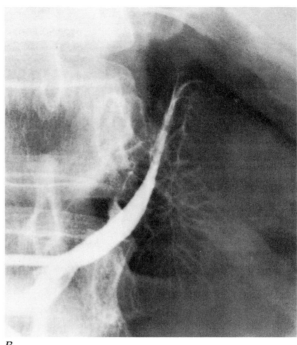

A   *B*

Figure 61-7. Aldosteronism due to adrenal hyperplasia in a 39-year-old woman with hypertension, hypokalemia, and elevated aldosterone excretion. Sampling from both adrenal veins indicated levels more than twice maximal upper normal levels. Sampling after venography demonstrated further doubling of aldosterone concentration on each side. (A) Right adrenal gland is enlarged, and intraadrenal venules are increased in caliber. The typical convergence of three veins to form the central vein is well shown. One vein leads inferiorly, another is arched posteriorly, and a small one supplies the upper portion of the gland. (B) The left gland is not so well opacified, but the rounded external contour can still be appreciated.

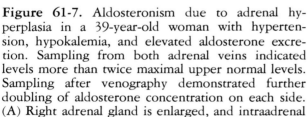

Tumors as small as 0.5 cm in diameter have been visualized [48], but most tumors detected venographically are 1.0 to 1.5 cm in diameter. Because the tumors are not hypervascular, the veins draining from, and displaced by, the tumors are usually of normal caliber or may be only slightly enlarged.

Venography will demonstrate the adenoma in 75 to 93 percent of cases [15, 47, 59]. In two studies that I have personally performed, good-quality venograms were negative in proved cases, even in retrospect. The normal venogram was explained by a central cylindrical adenoma in one case and by a very flattened one in a second case.

In multinodular hyperplasia, venography is usually near-normal. Occasionally there are multiple areas of mild curvilinear venous displacement, or the gland may be diffusely enlarged (Fig. 61-7).

Intraadrenal extravasation during venography has, in at least four cases, infarcted the gland harboring an aldosteronoma and cured the disease [21, 36, 65, 66].

Sampling of venous effluent is particularly rewarding in unilateral adenoma. Differences in concentration of aldosterone are usually great because of increased production on one side and depression on the other. Activity ratios of 20, 50, or even 100 to 1 are frequent [33, 47], so that positive results are obtained even when adrenal vein and caval blood are admixed. Accuracy of localization by biochemical assay in unilateral adenoma is approximately 90 to 95 percent [32, 33, 73], although Seabold et al. [59] found only

75 percent accuracy. In bilateral multinodular hyperplasia, evaluated concentrations are present in the effluent from both adrenal glands, and the ratios of concentrations may be as abnormal as in unilateral adenoma [73]. Thus, venous assay does not invariably distinguish unilateral adenoma from bilateral hyperplasia. The adrenal venous effluent should be assayed for cortisol, as well as aldosterone, in order to prove aspiration of adrenal, rather than hepatic or renal, venous blood.

Adrenal arteriography has occasionally demonstrated a stain of adenoma [2, 36], or the stain of multinodular hyperplasia [13]. Because venography is fairly accurate, and also allows biochemical assay, arteriography is performed infrequently in aldosteronism, and the incidence of positive arteriograms is not known.

Radionuclide adrenal scanning, with or without dexamethasone suppression, is an alternative method for localizing aldosteronoma. The method will detect a solitary adenoma in 47 to 67 percent of cases [59, 73]; false-positive results are not infrequent. Suppression scans, performed after adrenocortical function is suppressed with dexamethasone, accurately indicated the side of adenoma in 15 of 19 cases in the series by Seabold et al. [59]. A series by Hogan et al. [32] suggests somewhat greater accuracy of scintigraphy [32], but accuracy was not checked by venography or operation in patients with symmetric scans. Scintigraphy is probably somewhat less sensitive and less specific than venography but has the important advantage of being noninvasive. Relatively few institutions have the agents or equipment for performing adrenal scanning, and it is likely that the method will be largely supplanted by computed tomography.

Because most aldosterone-producing tumors are small, ultrasound examination of the adrenal glands has been relatively insensitive in diagnosis [15].

The value of computed tomography in aldosteronism is indicated in several series [39, 56, 60]. Since experience is still limited, the sensitivity and specificity of computed tomography are not yet precisely known. The wide applicability of computed tomography relative to adrenal scanning suggests that it will become the initial special imaging procedure in most suspected cases, with adrenal venography and sampling reserved for the equivocal or negative cases. For the time being, however, venography offers known accuracy, as well as the advantage of providing blood for biochemical assay, and continues to be performed for localization of adenoma and differentiation from multinodular hyperplasia.

Cushing's Disease

Cushing's disease is characterized clinically by truncal obesity, abdominal striae, hyperglycemia, hypertension, hirsutism, increased plasma corticosteroids, and increased urinary excretion of 17-hydroxycorticoids. In 75 percent of cases, bilateral cortical hyperplasia is responsible because of excessive ACTH production by pituitary basophilic cells or adenoma. The excessive ACTH production may rarely be secondary to extrapituitary tumor, particularly oat cell carcinoma of the lung, islet cell tumor of the pancreas [14], pheochromocytoma (Fig. 61-8) [58], or thymoma [62]. In 15 percent of cases, Cushing's disease is caused by adrenal adenoma, and in about 10 percent of cases, by adrenal carcinoma.

Biochemical features, particularly the presence of diurnal variations of cortisol excretion in hyperplasia, as well as the efficacy of dexamethasone suppression, generally enable differentiation of hyperplasia from tumor. Results, however, are sometimes equivocal. Thus, adrenal imaging may be indicated to differentiate hyperplasia from tumor, as well as to localize tumor.

Adrenal venography gained favor as the radiographic method of choice during the late 1960s. In 50 percent of cases of hyperplasia, both adrenal glands are enlarged, are excessively rounded, and demonstrate enlarged intraadrenal venules (Fig. 61-9A, B) [48, 50]. In the remaining cases of hypertrophy, the venograms are within normal limits. The hyperplasia not infrequently assumes a somewhat nodular character, but this is evident only occasionally by venography (Fig. 61-10). Adenomas, usually 3 to 5 cm in diameter, are indicated by the presence of displaced and enlarged adrenal veins (Fig. 61-11), and occasionally by stain of the tumor itself. The contralateral adrenal gland is almost invariably atrophic (Fig. 61-11C). Atrophy is reflected on the venogram by decreased size of the adrenal gland, as well as decreased caliber of adrenal venules. Because adenomas that produce Cushing's disease tend to be somewhat larger than those responsible for aldosteronism, venography has been invariably positive in my experience when the appropriate vein has been catheterized. In the presence of adrenal carcinoma, adrenal venog-

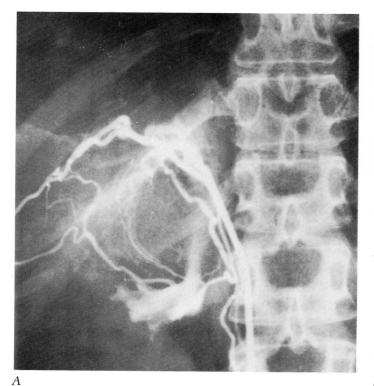

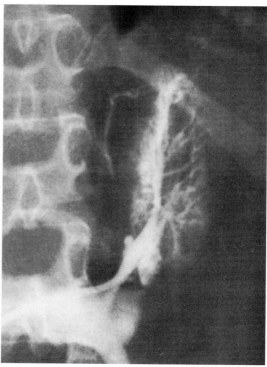

A

B

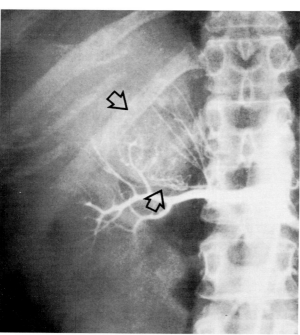

C

Figure 61-8. Cushing's disease and hyperpigmentation due to ectopic ACTH and beta-MSH production by an adrenal paraganglioma. (A) Right adrenal venogram demonstrates arcuate displacement of adrenal venules around a large mass. Sampling from this side indicated high concentration of ACTH and beta-MSH. (B) Left adrenal venogram demonstrates a slightly enlarged and rounded gland, with slight dilatation of intraadrenal venules. The absence of atrophy on this side was an important clue to the fact that the contralateral tumor was not cortisol-producing. Cortisol concentration was seven times as great on the left as on the right. (C) Selective right renal arteriography, after intrarenal administration of 7 μg of epinephrine, demonstrates a mildly hypervascular adrenal tumor (*arrows*). While awaiting operation, the patient developed an acute pneumonia and died. Autopsy revealed a right adrenal paraganglioma.

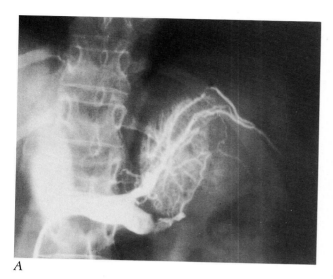

A

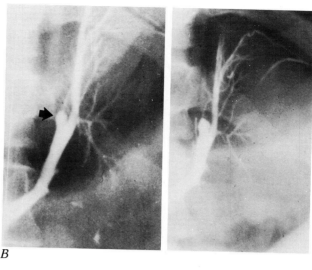

B

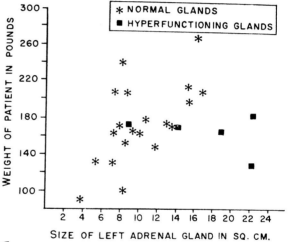

C

Figure 61-9. Cushing's disease due to adrenal hyperplasia. (A) Markedly hypertrophied, enlarged left adrenal gland. Note the abundant number and generous size of the intraadrenal veins. The gland has an excessively rounded contour. (B) Left adrenal hyperplasia in another patient with Cushing's disease (*left*), with regression after pituitary irradiation (*right*). Note valve of inferior phrenic vein (*arrow*). (C) Planimetered areas of 20 normal glands and 5 hypertrophied glands in 5 patients with Cushing's disease. Note that about one-half of the hypertrophied glands appeared enlarged venographically. (A, C from Reuter et al. [50]. Used by permission from *Radiology*.)

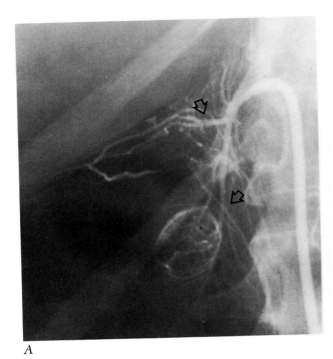

A

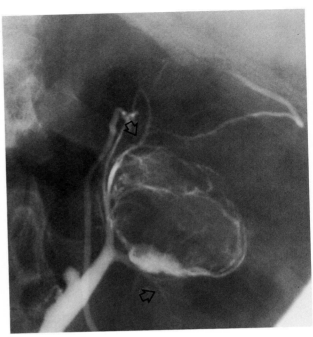

B

Figure 61-10. Cushing's disease due to rare bilateral nodular hyperplasia. Bilateral tumors were evident venographically. Adjacent portions of each gland, however, did not demonstrate the usual secondary atrophy. (A) Right gland demonstrating 1.5-cm nodule in lower portion and sizable venules elsewhere (*ar-* *rows*). (B) Left gland showing a 3-cm nodule and sizable venules elsewhere (*arrows*). At operation, the cortices contained the two large tumors shown, plus multiple 1- to 2-cm nodules elsewhere. The cortices were thickened throughout both glands.

raphy may partially demonstrate a large mass. More frequently, the adrenal veins are invaded and obstructed by tumor, so that the carcinoma is poorly demonstrated by venography. The contralateral gland is atrophic.

Adrenal arteriography is also usually diagnostic in Cushing's disease. Hyperplastic glands are often hypervascular, and their size and vascularity can be appreciated arteriographically in about 50 percent of cases [41]. Likewise, adenomas are sufficiently large and vascular to be visualized even if all appropriate adrenal arteries are not injected (Fig. 61-11A). Adrenal carcinomas are moderately hypervascular, as a rule, and tend to be much larger than adenomas (Fig. 61-12); consequently, arteriography almost always indicates a large mass in patients with adrenal carcinoma.

In Cushing's disease, angiography techniques are likely to be largely replaced by noninvasive methods, particularly computed tomography (CT). Since even normal glands are usually visible and measurable by CT, hyperplastic adrenal glands will almost always be demonstrable, when present. Further augmenting the reliability of CT is the large amount of retroperitoneal fat ordinarily present in patients with Cushing's disease. It must be emphasized, however, that in about 50 percent of cases of hyperfunction the glands are normal histologically and upon direct inspection [63]. Certainly the relatively sizable adenoma and the considerably larger carcinoma are within the size range that is easily depicted by CT. Biochemical assay of adrenal venous effluent, which would require adrenal venous catheterization, is seldom necessary.

Adrenal scintigraphy is also of high diagnostic accuracy in Cushing's disease and reflects both the size and the activity of the glands. Both adrenal glands show increased size and activity in virtually all cases with hyperplasia. In adenomas, there is marked unilateral uptake and contralateral suppression. Because of low specific activity, as well as contralateral suppression, carcinomas may show little uptake on either side.

In summary, then, despite the reliability of angiographic evaluation in Cushing's disease, noninvasive computed tomography or scintigraphy is usually sufficient for diagnosis.

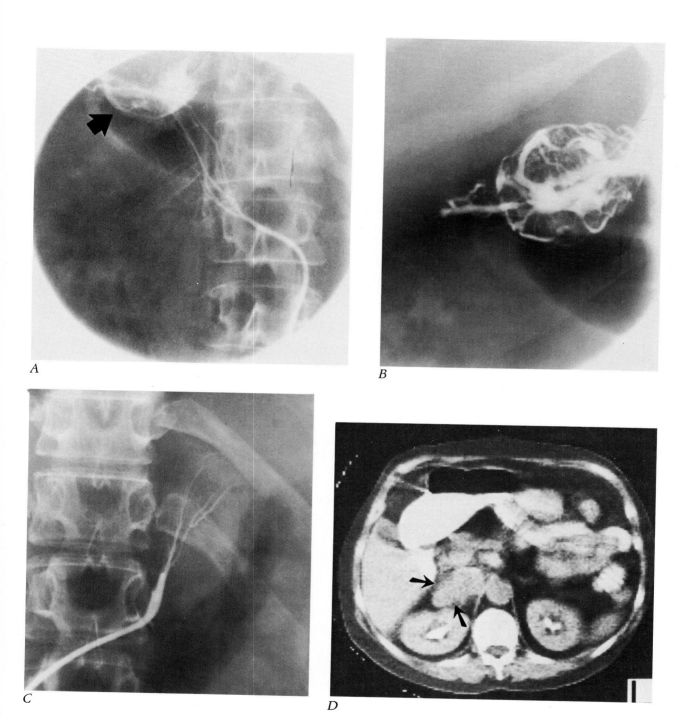

Figure 61-11. Cushing's disease secondary to right adrenal adenoma. (A) Inferior adrenal arteriogram shows portion of right adrenal adenoma (*arrow*). (B) Right adrenal venogram outlines a tumor 5 cm in diameter. This cortisol-producing tumor is larger than the tumors usually associated with aldosteronism. (C) The left adrenal venogram indicates glandular atrophy. Note the reduced size and number of intraadrenal venules and the reduced overall area occupied by the gland. Glandular atrophy contralateral to an adenoma indicates cortisol production and secondary depression of ACTH. In my experience, such atrophy occurs invariably in Cushing's disease and is not seen in aldosteronomas. (D) Computed tomography from another patient with Cushing's disease due to a large right adrenal adenoma (*arrows*).

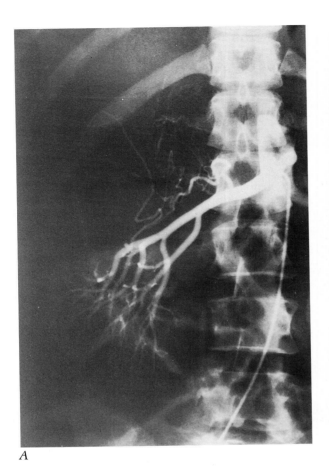

A

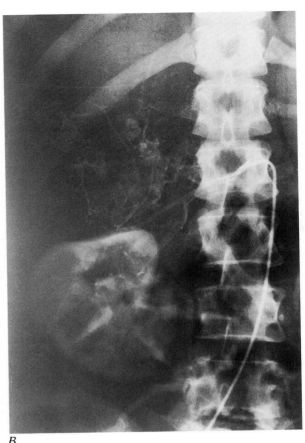

B

Figure 61-12. Cushing's disease due to carcinoma. (A) Selective right renal arteriography demonstrates enlargement of the right inferior adrenal artery, which supplies much of the moderately vascular carcinoma. (Courtesy of Lee Talner, M.D.) (B) Nephrogram phase nicely demonstrates the inferior and lateral displacement of the kidney, the impression upon the superior renal aspect, and the typical inhomogeneous whorled arterial pattern in carcinoma of the adrenal gland.

Adrenogenital Syndromes

Virilization in children is most commonly part of the adrenogenital syndrome, in which congenital deficiency of 21-hydroxylase [27], or other enzymes involved in steroid synthesis, leads to adrenal cortical hyperplasia. Although adrenal venography will often demonstrate enlarged glands, diagnosis is usually made clinically, and venography is infrequently indicated for childhood virilization. On the other hand, postpubertal virilization is often due to adrenal adenomas or carcinomas, or gonadal tumors, so that adrenal imaging is usually required. Adrenal venography is reliable in demonstrating the presence of adrenal tumor and may also demonstrate hyperplasia in many members of this older group (Fig. 61-13). Contralateral adrenal atrophy may be demonstrated in 30 percent of virilizing tumors [72]. Catheterization, sampling, and hormonal assay from the ovarian veins are often helpful in reaching a diagnosis of androgen-producing ovarian tumor [71].

Blair and Reuter performed routine adrenal venography and venous assay in 50 hirsute women [6]. In 20 percent, signs of adrenal hyperplasia were present.

Feminizing adrenal tumors may also occur. For obvious reasons, they are most readily recognized in males. The majority of the tumors are large and malignant.

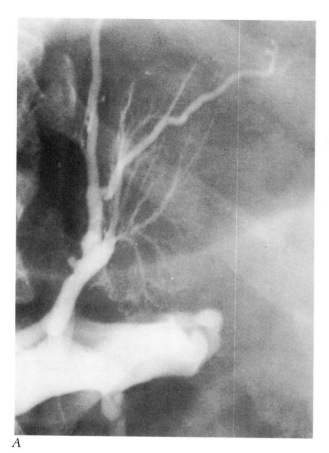

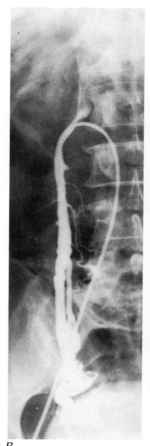

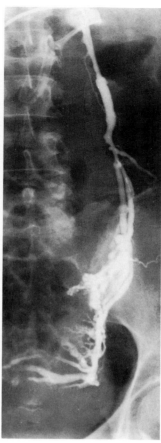

A

B

Figure 61-13. Virilization in a 25-year-old woman. Ovarian tumor was suspected, but adrenal venograms, as well as ovarian vein and adrenal vein assay, indicated adrenal hyperplasia. (A) Left adrenal venogram shows slightly enlarged adrenal gland, with intra-adrenal venules upper normal in caliber. (B) Both ovarian veins were catheterized for biochemical assay only. The venograms were obtained to document proper catheter position.

Pheochromocytoma

Pheochromocytoma is manifested clinically by hypertension, ordinarily paroxysmal but sometimes constant, tachycardia, flushing, and hyperglycemia. Elevated urinary vanillylmandelic acid (VMA) or methoxamine levels are prime diagnostic indices. Ninety percent of pheochromocytomas are situated within the adrenal gland, but about 10 percent are extraadrenal, in which case they are called paragangliomas. Paragangliomas may be located anywhere along the sympathetic chain of the abdomen or chest. Common sites outside the adrenal gland include the renal hilus, around the origin of the inferior mesenteric artery (organ of Zuckerkandl), or adjacent to the bladder (Fig. 61-14). In about 10 percent of cases of pheochromocytoma, multiple tumors are present, particularly in patients with neurofibromatosis or Sipple's syndrome [11, 12, 43, 61]. At least 10 percent of tumors are malignant [24]. The tumors are composed of chromaffin tissue. When located within the adrenal gland they ordinarily secrete epinephrine and norepinephrine; those located outside the gland generally secrete norepinephrine only.

Once diagnosis is made biochemically, preoperative localization is of great importance. Pheochromocytomas tend to be moderately large, usually more than 3 to 4 cm in diameter, and within the size range that can be demonstrated by computed tomography. In the future, it is likely that most lesions will be detected by this modality [19, 64].

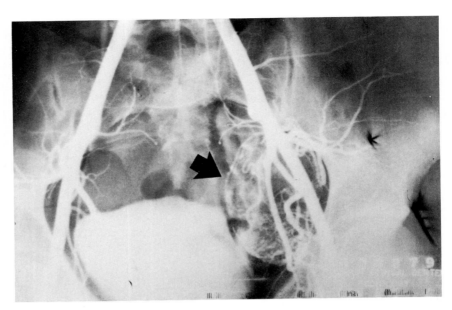

Figure 61-14. Pelvic paraganglioma (*arrow*). A lesion in this location cannot, of course, be shown by adrenal venography. Arteriography, CT, or ultrasound would be required for localization.

Angiography currently plays a major role in localization. Aortography is ordinarily obtained initially, as a survey procedure of the entire abdomen and pelvis. Subtraction techniques should be used because the tumor stain is often faint and easily overlooked (Fig. 61-15) [51]. Two series of exposures are usually required, one to include the upper abdominal and adrenal regions and the other to include the pelvis. Subsequently, selective studies are performed, depending on aortographic observations. Selective renal or adrenal arteriography will often demonstrate tumors missed by aortography. The tumors tend to be only moderately hypervascular. Typically, the adrenal arteries are somewhat enlarged and a fine network of arteries surrounds the tumor [52]. The tumor may stain homogeneously during the capillary phase. Central relative hypovascularity is common, however, and often reflects central necrosis [77]. In various series, 85 to 100 percent [2, 77] of pheochromocytomas have been detected by arteriography. Pheochromocytomas that occur adjacent to major renal arteries frequently produce focal functional arterial constrictions (Fig. 61-16) [70]. The combination of systemic hypertension and renal artery stenosis is then easily misinterpreted as renovascular hypertension.

In my experience, adrenal venography is more sensitive in detecting small intraadrenal pheochromocytomas than is arteriography. However, because venography is applicable to intraadrenal tumors only, it is used in complement to, rather than instead of, arteriography. Thus, adrenal venography is usually part of the angiographic workup in pheochromocytoma and is applied to those adrenal glands that do not demonstrate a tumor arteriographically. In the presence of pheochromocytoma, the adrenal veins are ordinarily somewhat enlarged, reflecting the usual moderate hypervascularity of the tumor (Fig. 61-17). Intraadrenal venules will be displaced around the tumor. I am unaware of any false-negative adrenal venograms in intraadrenal pheochromocytoma.

Because of the possibility of multiple pheochromocytomas in any given patient (sometimes more than a half dozen), both arteriography and venography are usually employed. Even so, there is no assurance that all tumors have been detected preoperatively, and the surgeon too must perform a search for additional lesions at the time of operation.

PREPARATION OF THE PATIENT

There is always some risk of precipitating a hypertensive crisis through diagnostic angiographic procedures. Indeed, in the absence of alpha-adrenergic premedication, mere aortography regularly causes significant rise in systemic

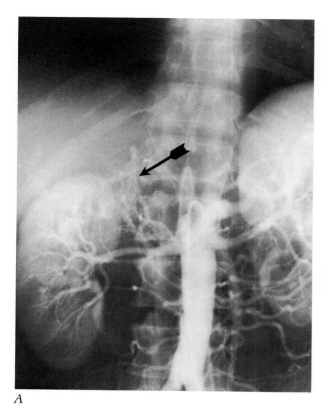

A

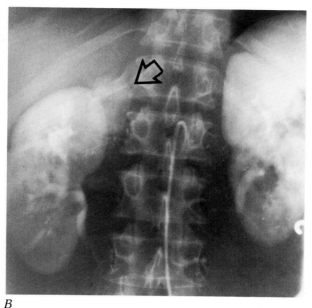

B

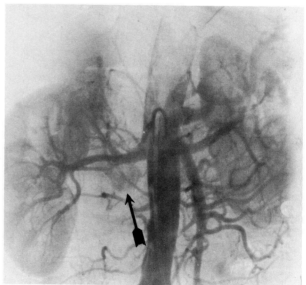

C

Figure 61-15. Pheochromocytoma, multiple tumors demonstrated by subtraction. (A) Aortogram showing some increased vascularity in the right adrenal region (*arrow*). (B) Capillary phase, with faint opacification of a right adrenal pheochromocytoma (*arrow*). (C) Subtraction film, now demonstrating an additional tumor adjacent to the right renal artery (*arrow*). (Courtesy of Stewart Reuter, M.D., and Lee Talner, M.D.)

pressure, apparently secondary to release of hormones from the tumor [44]. Hypertensive crises [25] and rarely death have occurred after arteriography; crisis but no death to my knowledge has occurred after venography [25]. Proper premedication of the patient is therefore mandatory. Furthermore, physicians capable of managing a hypertensive reaction should be in attendance during the procedure.

The patient is generally prepared with phenoxybenzamine, 1 to 2 mg per kilogram per day, divided into three or four doses, for several days before the procedure. Gittes and Mahoney [24] advise administration of the drug until the hematocrit decreases, reflecting the volume expansion secondary to vascular dilatation that occurs when the circulating vasoconstrictors are adequately blocked. During the procedure, phentolamine is kept readily available, in case of a reaction despite premedication. In the event of marked tachycardia reflecting excessive beta-adrenergic epinephrine effect, the patient is also premedicated with low doses (e.g., 15 mg qid) of the beta blocker propranolol.

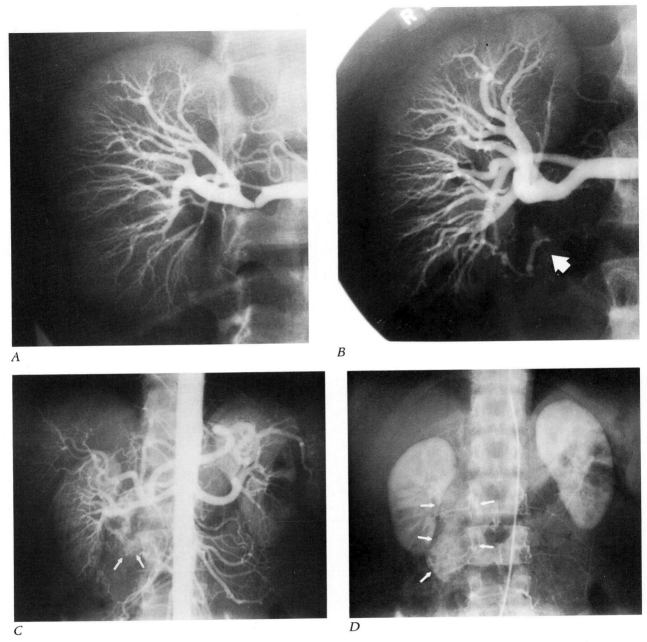

A

B

C

D

Figure 61-16. Pheochromocytoma demonstrating usual moderate hypervascularity and associated renal artery spasm that was relieved by Dibenzyline. (A) Selective renal arteriogram shows segmental renal arterial constrictions. (B) Subsequent arteriogram after administration of the alpha-blocking agent Dibenzyline shows that the stenoses have almost com-pletely disappeared, and a few tumor vessels are now evident (*arrow*). (C) Early phase of the aortogram shows a few fine tumor vessels in the region of the pheochromocytoma (*arrows*). (D) Late aortogram shows the typical stain of a large bilobulated pheochromocytoma (*arrows*). (From Velick et al. [70]. Used by permission from *Radiology.*)

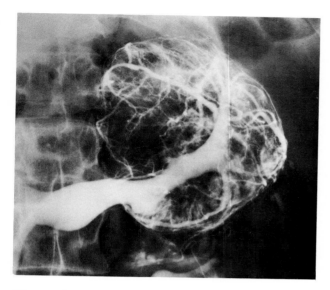

Figure 61-17. Large hypervascular left pheochromocytoma, shown by venography.

VENOUS SAMPLING FOR CATECHOLAMINE LEVELS

A few laboratories have the capacity to determine catecholamine levels in serum. Thus catecholamine assay of selective blood samples has been used to localize the side and level of chromaffin tumor [28, 29]. Arteriographic or venographic evidence of the presence or absence of intraadrenal tumors is usually reliable, and adrenal venous effluent is ordinarily not analyzed. In the absence of angiographic evidence of tumor, caval catheterization and sampling from multiple positions within the chest and abdomen have proved reliable in indicating the level of tumor but less reliable in indicating laterality.

It must be remembered that pheochromocytomas may be associated with tumors of brown fat, so-called hibernomas [20]. Hibernomas may occur in the retroperitoneum around the adrenal glands or kidneys and, because of their usual moderate hypervascularity, may simulate pheochromocytomas angiographically.

Pheochromocytoma is an integral part of a triad of multiple endocrine neoplasias known as Sipple's syndrome [11, 61]; the other two elements are parathyroid adenoma or hyperplasia and medullary carcinoma of the thyroid. A subtype includes alimentary tract ganglioneuromatosis as well [10, 12]; diarrhea, constipation, and megacolon may be dominant features. The pheochromocytomas are usually multiple and

often extraadrenal but almost always within the abdominal area [43]. Occasionally, the adrenal medullary overgrowth assumes the form of hyperplasia, rather than discrete pheochromocytoma [11]. Because of the risks of hypertension, the adrenal tumors should generally be localized and removed in Sipple's syndrome. The likelihood of multiple tumors requires application of multiple imaging techniques, including arteriography, venography, sampling, and computed tomography.

Nonfunctioning Tumors of the Adrenal Gland

Most adrenal tumors appear clinically with hormonal dysfunction. Some, such as neuroblastoma or ganglioneuroma, are not regularly associated with clinically apparent hormonal derangements, even though they may produce hormonal precursors. Some tumors, such as myelolipoma, almost never cause clinical manifestations. Others tend to appear relatively late, with symptoms due to effect of mass, tumor necrosis, or hemorrhage.

Venographic or arteriographic features are generally nonspecific. In hemangioma, arteriography may show characteristic punctate accumulations of contrast medium, often arranged in C- or O-shaped clusters, which retain contrast medium for prolonged periods [53]. The pattern is identical to that seen in liver hemangioma. Myelolipomas tend to be somewhat hypervascular and demonstrate peripheral vascularity with relatively little tumor stain [13]. They are often detected as incidental findings and probably would not require extirpation if somehow a correct preoperative diagnosis could be made. Neuroblastoma, carcinoma, and pheochromocytoma [5] are also generally hypervascular; their arteriographic patterns are described and illustrated in other sections of this chapter.

Metastases to the adrenal gland are frequent in patients who are dying of malignancy. In 1,000 consecutive autopsies of patients with carcinoma, Abrams et al. found adrenal metastases in 27 percent [1]; in patients with carcinoma of the breast or lung the incidence was 54 and 36 percent respectively. Renal carcinoma or melanoma [69] is also a frequent primary source (Fig. 61-18). The metastases are sometimes discovered during angiography of a retroperitoneal mass [31, 49] and

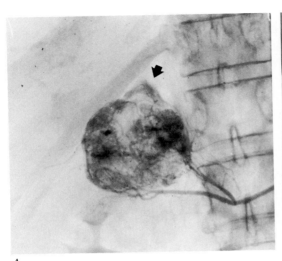
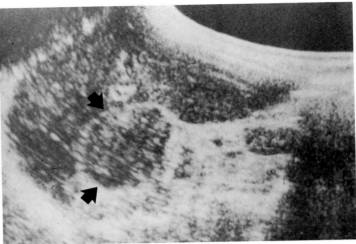

A   *B*

Figure 61-18. Adrenal metastases. (A) Arteriogram of a metastasis from a renal cell carcinoma. Overlying the metastasis is a normal adrenal remnant (*arrow*), exemplifying the usual persistence of functional adrenal tissue in metastatic disease and the infrequency of clinically evident Addison's disease. (Courtesy of L. Ekelund, M.D.) (B) Ultrasound demonstration of adrenal metastatic disease (*arrows*) in a patient with carcinoma of the lung.

are easily confused with a primary tumor. Knowledge of a primary tumor elsewhere should suggest the likelihood that the adrenal mass is metastatic.

Adrenal Cysts

Adrenal cysts are uncommon; approximately 250 had been reported by 1977 [37]. They are more frequent in women than men and are most often found between the third and fifth decades. In the series by Kearney and Mahoney [37], cysts were classified as follows:

Parasitic cysts (7%)
Epithelial cysts (9%)
   True glandular cysts
   Cystic adenomas
Endothelial cysts (45%)
   Lymphangiomatous
   Angiomatous
Hemorrhagic pseudocysts (39%)

Differentiation of simple adrenal cyst from solid, cystic, or necrotic adrenal tumor, or from pancreatic or renal cyst, is of obvious clinical importance. Ultrasound examination will ordinarily demonstrate a sonolucent mass, indicating the probable cystic nature and adrenal location of the lesion. Arteriography will demonstrate an avascular mass in the adrenal region, which displaces the adrenal arteries. Adrenal venography is usually very suggestive, demonstrating smooth arcuate displacement of normal-sized adrenal venules, without any veins within the mass (Fig. 61-19).

Percutaneous puncture is a valuable method for demonstrating the benign cystic nature, though not necessarily the intraadrenal location, of an adrenal cyst. Diagnostic cyst puncture of the adrenal gland may be used much the way renal cyst puncture is used. The cyst is punctured from a posterior approach, and fluid contents are analyzed for tumor cells, blood, and perhaps other elements. Injection of contrast medium can outline the usual smooth inner margin of the ordinary benign cyst. Cysts may disappear after puncture, and resection is usually unnecessary.

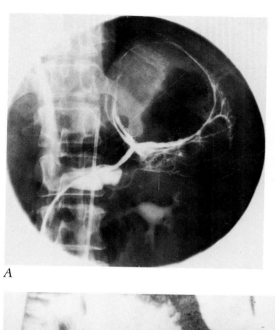

A

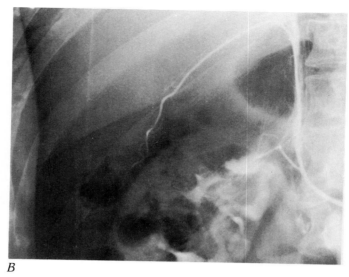

B

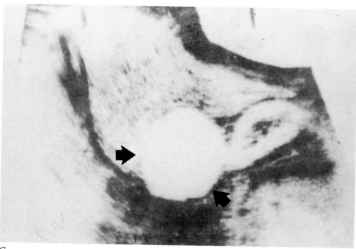

C

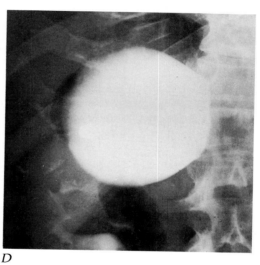

D

Figure 61-19. Adrenal cysts. (A) Multicystic adrenal gland. Mass was discovered above the left kidney during intravenous urography for hypertension. The patient had no evidence of hormonal dysfunction. Arteriography had shown an avascular mass in the adrenal region. The venogram demonstrates smooth arcuate displacement of adrenal venules above the central venule, suggesting a large adrenal cyst. Displacement of veins below the central venule reflects the association of several smaller cysts. (B) Selective arteriography from another patient with adrenal cyst. Note displacement of small adrenal arteries from the region of an avascular mass. (C) Ultrasound examination of the right adrenal cyst (*arrows*). (Courtesy of George Leopold, M.D.) (D) Cyst puncture and opacification of a right adrenal cyst. (Courtesy of Harvey Rosenkrantz, M.D.)

Neuroblastoma and Ganglioneuroma

Neuroblastomas are the second most common solid tumor of infancy and childhood, following behind cerebral tumors in this age group [17, 76]. They may arise anywhere along the sympathetic chain; 20 to 40 percent arise from the adrenal gland [17, 76]. Cure rate for abdominal neuroblastoma is 25 to 30 percent and seems to be favorably influenced by diagnosis at an early stage [9, 76].

Clinical presentation is prompted as a rule by abdominal mass. The tumors commonly secrete catecholamine precursors or metabolites [38], but hypertension develops only rarely [26]. Be-

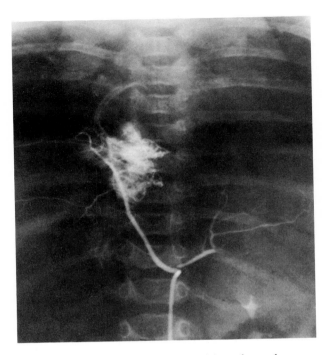

Figure 61-20. Neuroblastoma arising along the sympathetic chain above the right adrenal gland. Venous drainage was via a pulmonary vein. The tumor is markedly hypervascular and is supplied from the inferior phrenic artery.

cause of the usual large size of the tumor at the time of presentation, mass in the adrenal region is generally apparent on plain radiographs of the abdomen. Ultrasound or computed tomography may be required to further document the presence of tumor, or to further localize it to the adrenal glands. Angiography may also provide this information but is performed infrequently. The tumors are often somewhat hypervascular (Fig. 61-20), producing hypertrophy of the adrenal arteries and dense stain during the capillary phase [8]. Preoperative definition of the degree and source of vascularity would seem to facilitate surgery of large tumors, or to reveal signs of nonresectability, but this technique has not found wide favor.

Ganglioneuromas are benign tumors that may arise anywhere along the sympathetic chain; 60 percent of them appear in children or adolescents under the age of 20 [40]. Approximately 20 percent arise from the adrenal glands (medullary portion) [40]. Histologically they consist of mature nerve cells and fibers. A continuum exists between the immature cells of neuroblastoma, the intermediate maturity of ganglioneuroblastoma, and the mature cells of ganglioneuroma.

Ganglioneuromas are commonly small and are often discovered as incidental findings because of calcification apparent on plain abdominal films. Like neuroblastomas, ganglioneuromas usually produce catecholamine precursors [26], which may cause an intractable watery-diarrhea syndrome clinically indistinguishable from that due to islet cell tumor of the pancreas [14, 68]. Rarely, hypertension may also develop secondary to catecholamine excess [22]. Neuroblastomas may undergo maturation and convert to ganglioneuromas [22, 74]. Arteriographically, ganglioneuromas appear as hypovascular to moderately vascular masses [8].

Localization of Adrenal Remnants

Recurrent ACTH-responsive adrenal cortisol hyperproduction, usually reflecting persistent adrenocortical tissue, occurs occasionally after bilateral adrenalectomy for Cushing's disease. Localization of the adrenal residua can be a vexing problem. In the past, I have tried to localize such remnants by adrenal venography and venous sampling, with success in only one of three cases. A superior method is afforded by nuclear scanning. Beierwaltes and colleagues reported nuclear scans in 11 patients with residual hyperadrenalism after bilateral adrenalectomy [23]. Adrenal remnants could be localized in nine. Most commonly the remnant was thought to represent the upper tail of a gland, which is easily separated from the excised gland when surgical manipulation is vigorous or exposure is imperfect. On the right, this tail may retract into the liver; on the left, onto the diaphragm.

Adenocarcinoma

Adenocarcinoma of the adrenal gland comprises approximately 0.1 percent of human cancers [34]. The lesions are usually large (over 1,000 gm) when discovered [42, 62]. There are two peak periods of incidence, childhood and middle age [42], and two-thirds of the patients are female. The prognosis is relatively poor, the mean survival being 31 to 44 months [34, 42]. Histologic criteria of malignancy may be totally absent, and diagnosis of malignancy must sometimes be based solely on the size of the lesion or evidence of invasiveness at the margins.

The majority of patients with adenocarcinomas, in the range of 60 to 95 percent [34, 42], have clinical evidence of hormonal overproduction. Dysfunction may be manifested as virilization, feminization, Cushing's syndrome, or aldosteronism.

Because the mass is usually large, its presence may be demonstrated by multiple imaging modalities, including plain films of the abdomen, urography, computed tomography, and ultrasound. The intraadrenal origin of the tumor can be most reliably defined arteriographically. Neovascularity is ordinarily moderate (see Fig. 61-12), with tortuous arterial feeders often coursing over the surface of the tumor. Tumor stain is likely to be inhomogeneous, with some areas of hypovascularity probably reflecting necrosis. Extent of tumor can be evaluated, and invasion of the kidney, extension into renal veins or inferior vena cava [40], or hepatic metastases are frequently evident. Definition and preoperative embolization of the arterial supply may facilitate resection in selected cases but, to my knowledge, has not yet been described.

Because carcinomas are usually large, adrenal venography is not generally indicated. When occasionally performed, it tends to demonstrate only a portion of the large intraadrenal mass.

Addison's Disease

Addison's disease is commonly due to one of the following conditions [14]: (1) atrophy secondary to pituitary disease; (2) tuberculosis, histoplasmosis, or other infection; (3) Waterhouse-Friderichsen syndrome; (4) metastases; (5) iatrogenesis—adrenal venography or surgery; (6) anticoagulation; or (7) amyloidosis.

Although onset of Addison's disease is not generally an indication for adrenal angiography, we have in the past performed venography in a few cases. In a case of Sheehan's syndrome (postpartum pituitary necrosis), the glands were small and the intraadrenal venules narrow. Except for its bilaterality, the appearance was indistinguishable from the atrophy seen contralateral to a cortisol-producing adenoma. Adrenal glands devastated by tuberculosis would be expected to demonstrate total destruction of the gland

and marked distortion or virtual absence of the adrenal venous vasculature. Presumably this appearance would develop also in glands destroyed by other inflammatory disease, or by Waterhouse-Friderichsen syndrome. To my knowledge, angiography has not been reported in postinfectious or postinflammatory Addison's disease. In glands extensively infiltrated by metastatic disease, adrenal insufficiency develops only rarely. Angiographic appearances of adrenal metastases have already been described; presumably in Addison's disease the adrenal masses would be extensive and bilateral.

Miscellaneous Conditions

Infectious processes of the adrenal gland may be acute or chronic. Chronic tuberculous infection and histoplasmosis of the adrenal gland are relatively common causes of Addison's disease [62]. Acute infections are apparently very rare, and I have been unable to find any publications on this subject. I have, however, observed angiograms in two cases of acute suppurative adrenal infection secondary to *Escherichia coli*. In one case, marked enlargement of the gland and diffuse capillary blush were present. The other, a subacute abscess, resembled an adrenal neoplasm angiographically but was relatively lucent on computed tomography (Fig. 61-21).

Adrenal hemorrhage is not an uncommon condition [62]. Some degree of adrenal hemorrhage is frequently found at autopsy, and it is one of the commonest causes of abdominal mass in newborns. Adrenal hemorrhage may be due to a variety of causes, including birth trauma, hypoxia, sepsis (Waterhouse-Friderichsen syndrome), hemorrhage, transfusion reaction, and arterial or venous thrombosis [40], and may occur on one or both sides. The hemorrhage is usually asymptomatic, or dominated by symptomatology of the underlying cause, so that angiography is practically never indicated. Acute adrenal insufficiency is the exception, rather than the rule. Incompletely resorbed hemorrhage is thought to account for about 40 percent of adult adrenal cysts [37]. In infants, plain films of the abdomen may show unilateral or bilateral masses in the adrenal regions, and circumferential calcification may become apparent within a month. The appearance of chronic hematoma, namely, intraadrenal cyst, has been illustrated in Figure 61-19.

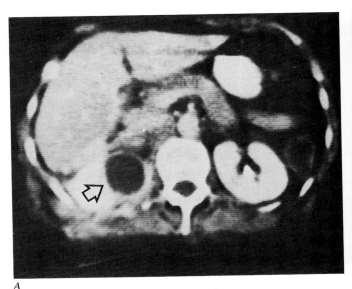
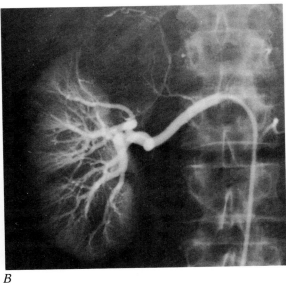

A   *B*

Figure 61-21. Adrenal abscess secondary to *Escherichia coli* in a 62-year-old woman with fever and back pain of 3 weeks' duration. (A) Computed tomography reveals a relatively lucent mass in the region of the right adrenal gland (*arrow*). (B) The arteriogram indicates a hypovascular mass supplied primarily from the inferior adrenal artery, and possibly also from small renal twigs. The mass was aspirated and grew a pure culture of *E. coli*. At operation, an adrenal abscess was found. (Courtesy of Stephan Dorros, M.D.)

Transcatheter Adrenal Ablation

So far, the value of adrenal angiography in depicting morphology of the normal or abnormal adrenal gland and the value of adrenal vein catheterization in assessing adrenal physiology have been discussed. Another potential of adrenal catheterization is transcatheter adrenal ablation.

Inadvertent destruction of normal adrenal glands after venography is the subject of numerous reports [7, 18, 45] and formerly occurred in 2 to 4 percent of cases [7]. Furthermore, venographic injury has produced permanent or temporary remission of hormonal overproduction in several patients with aldosterone- or cortisol-producing tumors [18, 21, 36, 65, 66].

Jablonski et al. [35] and Zimmerman et al. [78] have applied the ablative potential of venography therapeutically in patients with breast or prostatic cancer. The adrenal gland is injured by intentionally traumatic catheterization and forceful injection, producing intraadrenal extravasation of contrast medium and nitrogen mustard. Of six attempts by Zimmerman et al. [78], five were considered technically satisfactory, and in four of these adrenal function was markedly depressed after 6 weeks. The depression of adrenal function can last at least 6 months. The procedure produced only a very brief period of pain and was usually followed by 24 to 48 hours of nausea and sometimes vomiting. Three or four patients realized some regression of metastatic disease. Jablonski et al. [35] had similar results in eight patients with metastatic breast carcinoma.

Transcatheter embolization of adrenal neoplasms is another possible type of adrenal ablative procedure, but virtually nothing is to be found in the literature describing its use. The known occasional immunity to neuroblastoma, and the reported incidence of spontaneous remission (1–12%) [30] suggest that embolization of neuroblastoma may be worthy of trial when the entire tumor cannot be extirpated.

The technique of therapeutic transcatheter adrenal ablation has not been widely adopted, and its true efficacy and role are not yet defined. It must be regarded as an experimental procedure at the present time, available only at a few special centers.

Instances in Which Angiography Offers Advantage over Computed Tomography

With the emergence of computed tomography as a very safe and highly reliable diagnostic method, the question of the continued need for angiographic methods must be addressed. While experience is too limited to provide a definitive answer, it seems that angiography is still required in the following circumstances, or for the following reasons:

(1) It is likely that computed tomography will suffer from the limitations of all other imaging modalities and will provide equivocal or inadequate information in a significant number of patients. Presumably many of these patients will require further evaluation by angiographic methods.

(2) Aldosteronomas may be under 1 cm in diameter. The reliability of computed tomography in consistently demonstrating such small lesions has yet to be proved. The ability of venography and sampling to localize these lesions is well established.

(3) When small nonfunctional tumors, such as myelolipomas, are incidentally discovered by computed tomography, venographic sampling for hormonal production would be indicated. If no hormonal function is discovered, and the lesion is small, then an operation would probably be unnecessary.

(4) Angiography will be particularly indicated if bilateral tumors are suggested by computed tomography. Sampling and assay will be required to ascertain that both tumors are functional, and that one is not, for example, simply a myelolipoma (Fig. 61-22). Furthermore, venography will be very useful in differentiating bilateral hyperplasia from bilateral autonomous tumors. For instance, in Cushing's disease the presence of adrenal atrophy indicates contralateral tumor (see Fig. 61-11); in the presence of tumor nodules, the lack of atrophy of the nontumorous gland indicates nodular hyperplasia rather than benign or malignant tumor (see Fig. 61-10).

(5) In aldosteronism due to bilateral hyperplasia, ratios of aldosterone concentrations from adrenal effluent may be widely different, suggesting unilateral adenoma. Venography would be helpful in demonstrating bilateral

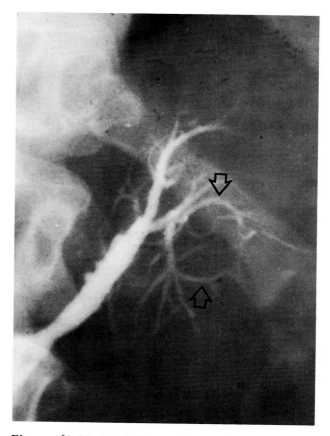

Figure 61-22. Myelolipoma in a patient with aldosteronism. Technically poor venogram, obtained in 1967. Venography showed a 1-cm mass in left adrenal gland (*arrows*). Right adrenal catheterization was unsuccessful, and at the time of this study aldosterone sampling was not performed. At operation, a 1-cm myelolipoma was found in the left gland, and an aldosteronoma was present in the right gland.

nodules or bilateral hyperplasia, or in confirming a unilateral tumor.

(6) Angiography will be incident to any transcatheter therapeutic procedures applied to the adrenal glands.

(7) Vascular mapping may be indicated to facilitate surgery, or to ascertain with confidence that a mass is supplied primarily by adrenal arteries and thus is intraadrenal in location.

(8) There are various other special situations. For example, I have had a patient with Cushing's disease due to hyperplasia on one side secondary to an ACTH-producing pheochromocytoma in the other adrenal gland. Correct diagnosis was made preoperatively by venography and sampling (see Fig. 61-8).

Summary

Arteriography and venography of the adrenal gland are reliable diagnostic methods for localizing functional or nonfunctional adrenal tumors, and for differentiating tumors from hyperplasia. The recent development of noninvasive methods for adrenal imaging, particularly computed tomography, will severely restrict the indications for angiography. Nevertheless, the potential for venous sampling and biochemical assay during venography offers a real advantage in selected instances. The therapeutic potential of the angiographic catheter has yet to be widely exploited.

References

1. Abrams, H. L., Spiro, R., and Goldstein, N. Metastases in carcinoma. Analysis of 1000 autopsied cases. *Cancer* 3:74, 1950.
2. Alfidi, R. J., Gill, W. M., and Klein, H. J. Arteriography of adrenal neoplasms. *AJR* 106:635, 1969.
3. Anderson, B. G., and Beierwaltes, W. H. Adrenal imaging with radioiodocholesterol in the diagnosis of adrenal disorders. *Adv. Intern. Med.* 19:327, 1974.
4. Anderson, E. E. Nonfunctioning tumors of the adrenal gland. *Urol. Clin. North Am.* 4:263, 1977.
5. Beckmann, C. F., Levin, D. C., and Phillips, D. A. Angiography of nonfunctioning pheochromocytomas of the adrenal gland. *Radiology* 124:53, 1977.
6. Blair, A. J., and Reuter, S. R. Adrenal venography in virilized women. *J.A.M.A.* 213:1623, 1970.
7. Bookstein, J. J., Conn, J., and Reuter, S. R. Intra-adrenal hemorrhage as a complication of adrenal venography in primary aldosteronism. *Radiology* 90:778, 1968.
8. Bosniak, M. A., Siegelman, S. S., and Evans, J. A. *The Adrenal, Retroperitoneum and Lower Urinary Tract.* Chicago: Year Book, 1976. P. 182.
9. Breslow, N., and McCann, B. Statistical estimation of prognosis for children with neuroblastoma. *Cancer Res.* 31:2098, 1970.
10. Carney, J. A., Go, V. L. W., Sizemore, G. W., and Hales, A. B. Alimentary-tract ganglioneuromatosis. *N. Engl. J. Med.* 295:1287, 1976.
11. Carney, J. A., Sizemore, G. W., and Tyce, G. M. Bilateral adrenal medullary hyperplasia in multiple endocrine neoplasia type 2. The precursor of bilateral pheochromocytoma. *Mayo Clin. Proc.* 50:3, 1975.
12. Cong, G. G., Beahrs, O. H., and Sizemore, G. W. Medullary carcinoma of the thyroid gland. *Cancer* 35:695, 1975.
13. Costello, P., Clouse, M. E., Kane, R. A., and Paris, A. Problems in the diagnosis of adrenal tumors. *Radiology* 125:335, 1977.
14. Cristy, N. P. *The Human Adrenal Cortex.* New York: Harper & Row, 1971. Pp. 329, 367.
15. Davidson, J. K., Morley, P., Hurley, G. D., and Holford, N. G. H. Adrenal venography and ultrasound in the investigation of the adrenal gland: An analysis of 58 cases. *Br. J. Radiol.* 48:435, 1975.
16. Dobbie, J. W., and Symington, T. The human adrenal gland with special reference to the vasculature. *J. Endocrinol.* 34:479, 1966.
17. Duckett, J. W., and Koop, C. E. Neuroblastoma. *Urol. Clin. North Am.* 4:285, 1977.
18. Eagan, R. T., and Page, M. I. Adrenal insufficiency following bilateral adrenal venography. *J.A.M.A.* 215:115, 1971.
19. Egdahl, R. W. Localization of pheochromocytoma by computed tomography. *N. Engl. J. Med.* 299:425, 1978.
20. English, J. T., Patel, S. K., and Flanagan, M. J. Association of pheochromocytomas with brown fat tumors. *Radiology* 107:279, 1973.
21. Fisher, C. E., Turner, F. A., and Horton, R. Remission of primary hyperaldosteronism after adrenal venography. *N. Engl. J. Med.* 285:334, 1971.
22. Fox, F., Davidson, J., and Thomas, L. B. Maturation of sympathicoblastoma into ganglioneuroma. *Cancer* 12:108, 1959.
23. Freitas, J. E., Herwig, K. R., Cerny, J. C., and Beierwaltes, W. H. Preoperative localization of adrenal remnants. *Surg. Gynecol. Obstet.* 145:705, 1977.
24. Gittes, R. F., and Mahoney, E. M. Pheochromocytoma. *Urol. Clin. North Am.* 4:239, 1977.
25. Gold, R. E., Wisinger, B. M., Geraci, A. R., and Heinz, L. M. Hypertensive crisis as a result of adrenal venography in a patient with pheochromocytoma. *Radiology* 102:579, 1972.
26. Greer, M., Anta, A. A., Williams, C. M., and Echevarria, R. A. Tumors of neural crest origin. *Arch. Neurol.* 13:139, 1965.
27. Handwerger, S., and Silverstein, J. H. Congenital adrenal hyperplasia. *Urol. Clin. North Am.* 4:193, 1977.
28. Harrison, T. S., and Frier, D. T. Pitfalls in the technique and interpretation of regional venous sampling for localizing pheochromocytoma. *Surg. Clin. North Am.* 54:339, 1974.
29. Harrison, T. S., Seaton, J. F., Cerny, J. C., Bookstein, J. J., and Bartlett, J. D. Localization of pheochromocytoma by caval catheterization. *Arch. Surg.* 95:339, 1967.

30. Hellström, K. E., and Hellström, I. Immunity to neuroblastoma and melanomas. *Annu. Rev. Med.* 23:19, 1972.

31. Hoevels, J., and Ekelund, L. Angiographic findings in adrenal masses. *Acta Radiol. [Diagn.]* (Stockh.) 20:337, 1979.

32. Hogan, M. J., McRae, J., Schambelan, M., and Biglieri, E. G. Location of aldosterone-producing adenomas with ^{131}I-19-iodocholesterol. *N. Engl. J. Med.* 294:410, 1976.

33. Horton, R., and Finck, E. Diagnosis and localization in primary aldosteronism. *Ann. Intern. Med.* 76:885, 1972.

34. Hutter, A. M., and Kayhoe, D. E. Adrenal cortical carcinoma. *Am. J. Med.* 41:572, 1966.

35. Jablonski, R. D., Meaney, T. F., and Schumacher, O. P. Transcatheter adrenal ablation for metastatic carcinoma of the breast. *Cleve. Clin. Q.* 44:57, 1977.

36. Kahn, P. C., Kelleher, M. D., Egdahl, R. H., and Melby, J. C. Adrenal arteriography and venography in primary aldosteronism. *Radiology* 101:71, 1971.

37. Kearney, G. P., and Mahoney, E. M. Adrenal cysts. *Urol. Clin. North Am.* 4:273, 1977.

38. Kogut, M. D., and Kaplan, S. A. Systemic manifestations of neurogenic tumors. *J. Pediatr.* 60:694, 1962.

39. Korobkin, M., White, E. A., Kressel, H. Y., Moss, A. A., and Montagne, J. P. Computed tomography in the diagnosis of adrenal disease. *AJR* 132:231, 1979.

40. Lecky, J. W., Wolfman, N. T., and Modic, C. W. Current concepts of adrenal angiography. *Radiol. Clin. North Am.* 14:309, 1976.

41. Lee, K. R., Lin, F., and Sibala, J. Adrenal adenoma and hyperplasia. Importance of arteriographic differential diagnosis. *AJR* 119:796, 1973.

42. Lewinsky, B. S., Grigor, K. M., Symington, T., and Neville, A. M. The clinical and pathologic features of "non-hormonal" adrenocortical tumors. *Cancer* 33:778, 1974.

43. Lips, E. J. M., Minder, W. H., Leo, J. R., Alleman, A., and Hackeng, W. H. L. Evidence of multicentric origin of the multiple endocrine neoplasia syndrome type 2A (Sipple's syndrome). *Am. J. Med.* 64:569, 1978.

44. Meaney, T. F., and Buonocore, E. Selective arteriography as a localizing and provocative test in the diagnosis of pheochromocytoma. *Radiology* 87:309, 1966.

45. Melby, J. C. Identifying the adrenal lesion in primary aldosteronism (editorial). *Ann. Intern. Med.* 76:1039, 1972.

46. Mikaelsson, C. G. The adrenal glands after epinephrophlebography. *Acta Radiol. [Diagn.]* (Stockh.) 10:1, 1970.

47. Mitty, H. A., Gabrilove, J. L., and Nicolis, G. L. Nontumorous adrenal hyperfunction: Problems in angiographic-clinical correlation. *Radiology* 122:89, 1977.

48. Mitty, H. A., Nicolis, G. L., and Gabrilove, J. L. Adrenal venography: Clinical-roentgenographic correlation in 80 patients. *AJR* 119:564, 1973.

49. Reuter, S. R. Demonstration of adrenal metastases by adrenal venography. *N. Engl. J. Med.* 278:1423, 1968.

50. Reuter, S. R., Blair, A. J., Schteingart, D. E., and Bookstein, J. J. Adrenal venography. *Radiology* 89:805, 1967.

51. Reuter, S. R., Talner, L. B., and Atkin, T. The importance of subtraction in the angiographic evaluation of extra-adrenal pheochromocytomas. *AJR* 117:128, 1973.

52. Rossi, P. Arteriography in adrenal tumors. *Br. J. Radiol.* 41:81, 1968.

53. Rothberg, M., Bastidas, J., Mattey, W. E., and Bernas, E. Adrenal hemangiomas: Angiographic appearance of a rare tumor. *Radiology* 126:341, 1978.

54. Ryo, U. Y., Johnston, A. S., Kim, I., and Pinsky, S. M. Adrenal scanning and uptake with ^{131}I-6β-iodomethyl-nor-cholesterol. *Radiology* 128:157, 1978.

55. Sample, W. F. A new technique for the evaluation of the adrenal gland with gray scale ultrasonography. *Radiology* 124:463, 1977.

56. Sample, W. F., and Sarti, D. A. Computed tomography and gray scale ultrasonography of the adrenal gland: A comparative study. *Radiology* 128:377, 1978.

57. Sarkar, D. S., Cohen, E. L., and Beierwaltes, W. H. A new and superior adrenal imaging agent, NP-59; evaluation in humans. *J. Clin. Endocrinol. Metab.* 45:353, 1977.

58. Schteingart, D. E., Conn, J. W., Otth, D. N., Harrison, T. S., Fox, J. E., and Bookstein, J. J. Secretion of ACTH and beta-MSH by an adrenal medullary paraganglioma. *J. Clin. Endocrinol. Metab.* 34:676, 1972.

59. Seabold, J. E., Cohen, E. L., Beierwaltes, W. H., Hinerman, D. L., Nishiyama, R. H., Bookstein, J. J., and Ice, R. D. Adrenal imaging with ^{131}I-19-iodocholesterol in the diagnostic evaluation of patients with aldosteronism. *J. Clin. Endocrinol. Metab.* 42:41, 1976.

60. Sheedy, P. F., Stephens, D. H., Hattery, R. R., Brown, L. R., and MacCarty, R. L. Computed tomography of abdominal organs. *Adv. Intern. Med.* 24:455, 1979.

61. Sipple, J. H. The association of pheochromocytoma with carcinoma of the thyroid gland. *Am. J. Med.* 31:163, 1961.

62. Sloper, J. C. The Adrenal Glands. In W. St. C. Simmers (ed.), *Systemic Pathology*. Edinburgh: Churchill Livingstone, 1976.

63. Soffer, L. J., Innaccone, A., and Gabrilove, J. L. Cushing's syndrome. Study of fifty patients. *Am. J. Med.* 30:129, 1961.

64. Stewart, B. H. Localization of pheochromocytoma by computed tomography. *N. Engl. J. Med.* 299:460, 1978.

65. Taylor, H. C., Sachs, C. R., and Bravo, E. L. Primary aldosteronism: Remission and development of adrenal insufficiency after adrenal venography. *Ann. Intern. Med.* 85:207, 1976.

66. Teixeira, P. E., Dwyer, D. E., and Voil, G. W. Remission of primary hyperaldosteronism consequent on adrenal venography. *Can. Med. Assoc. J.* 117:789, 1977.

67. Thrall, J. H., Freitas, J. E., and Beierwaltes, W. H. Adrenal scintigraphy. *Semin. Nucl. Med.* 8:23, 1978.

68. Trump, D. C., Livingston, J. W., and Baylis, S. B. Watery diarrhea syndrome in an adult with ganglioneuroma-pheochromocytoma. *Cancer* 40:1526, 1977.

69. Twersky, J., and Levin, D. C. Metastatic melanoma of the adrenal. *Radiology* 116:627, 1975.

70. Velick, W. T., Bookstein, J. J., and Talner, L. B. Pheochromocytoma with reversible renal artery stenosis. *AJR* 131:1069, 1978.

71. Weiland, A. J., Bookstein, J. J., Cleary, R. E., and Judd, H. L. Preoperative localization of virilizing tumors by selective venous sampling. *Am. J. Obstet. Gynecol.* 131:797, 1978.

72. Weinberg, T. Contralateral adrenal atrophy associated with cortical adrenal neoplasms. *N.Y. State J. Med.* 41:884, 1941.

73. Weinberger, M. H., Grim, C. E., Hollifield, J. W., Kem, D. C., Arunabha, G., Kramer, N. J., Yne, H. Y., Wellman, H., and Donahue, J. P. Primary aldosteronism. *Ann. Intern. Med.* 90:386, 1979.

74. Willis, R. A. *The Pathology of the Tumours of Children.* Springfield, Ill.: Thomas, 1962. Pp. 9–17.

75. Wilms, G., Baert, A., Marchal, G., and Goddeeris, P. Computed tomography of the normal adrenal glands: Correlative study with autopsy specimens. *J. Comput. Assist. Tomogr.* 3:467, 1979.

76. Wilson, L. M. K., and Draper, G. J. Neuroblastoma, its natural history and prognosis. A study of 487 cases. *Br. Med. J.* 3:301, 1974.

77. Zelch, J. V., Meaney, T. F., and Belhobek, G. H. Radiologic approach to the patient with suspected pheochromocytoma. *Radiology* 111:279, 1974.

78. Zimmerman, C. E., Eisenberg, H., and Rosoff, C. B. Transvenous adrenal destruction: Clinical trials in patients with metastatic malignancy. *Surgery* 75:550, 1974.

4. Pancreatic, Hepatic, and Splenic Arteriography

Pancreatic Angiography

ERIK BOIJSEN

A quarter of a century has passed since Ödman published his first experience with selective angiography of the main branches of the aorta [185]. This work was soon followed by more detailed reports by him on celiac angiography and pancreatic angiography, the latter as a chapter in the first edition of *Angiography* [186–188]. During the following 10 years angiography of the pancreas became a well-established, safe, and reliable method for diagnosing pancreatic disease, as documented in the second edition [33]. In the most recent decade further development in angiographic technique, especially improvements in superselective catheterization of pancreatic arteries and pharmacoangiography, has made pancreatic angiography the most reliable way to detect pancreatic disease. During the last few years, however, a remarkable change has occurred as newer, less invasive diagnostic methods replace angiography as the primary technique for diagnosis of pancreatic disease. Today ultrasonography, computed tomography (CT), and endoscopic retrograde cholangiopancreatography (ERCP) have largely, but not completely, replaced angiography as a diagnostic method. Angiography is not outdated, but the indications for its use have changed. It is as important as ever to know what type of vascular changes can be observed in a patient with pancreatic disease and what significance these abnormalities have for the patient's future.

Vascular Anatomy

ARTERIES

Dissection studies of the pancreatic vasculature by Pierson [200], Woodburne and Olsen [275], Michels [169], and others form the basis of roentgenologic angiographic anatomy (Fig. 62-1). The following description of the pancreatic arterial pattern is based on reports on angiographic studies in vivo and on specimens [65, 119–121, 138, 153, 167, 173, 186, 188]. Unlike other organs, the pancreas has no hilus and no main artery supplying it. It is encircled by arteries originating from the celiac axis and superior mesenteric arteries. The splenic and common hepatic arteries are in close contact with the upper border of the organ; the gastroduodenal artery and the pancreaticoduodenal arcades form an incomplete lateral and inferior border of the head of the pancreas; and the transverse pancreatic artery follows

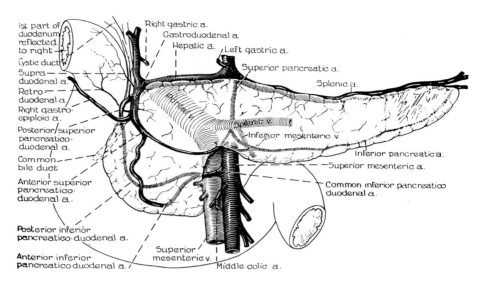

Figure 62-1. The arterial supply of the pancreas, anterior view. (From Pierson [200]. By permission of *Surgery, Gynecology and Obstetrics*.)

the inferior margin of the body and tail of the pancreas. Large anatomic variations exist, but these arteries can usually be defined if contrast medium is injected into both the celiac axis and the superior mesenteric artery (Fig. 62-2).

From cadaver specimens it is obvious that the pancreas has a rich vascular network with large interarterial anastomoses. In the pancreatic tail, however, the anastomoses may be absent—an important consideration when ligation of the splenic artery is performed for splenectomy [119, 120]. The small ramifications of the intrapancreatic arteries preclude the use of lumbar aortography for demonstration of this vasculature [138, 153, 173]. Only high-quality celiac and superior mesenteric angiography gives acceptable information about the pancreatic arteries, and sometimes even superselective injection of contrast medium into hepatic, splenic, or pancreatic arteries is the only method by which to obtain the necessary information (Figs. 62-2, 62-3).

In order to demonstrate the complete pancreatic arterial supply by angiography, the arteries described here should be well defined because they are usually involved in pancreatic disease.

Celiac Axis

Best observed in the lateral view, the celiac axis has a varying course in the anterior direction [34, 153, 186] (Fig. 62-4).

Splenic Artery

The splenic artery usually arises from the celiac axis, but occasionally it stems from the aorta or superior mesenteric artery. Great variations occur in the course of this vessel because of its inconstant degree of tortuosity. According to Kupic et al. [138], it can be divided into four main segments: the suprapancreatic, which is the first 1 to 3 cm of the vessel; the pancreatic, which is usually the most tortuous and lies on the dorsal surface of the pancreas; the prepancreatic, which runs on the anterior surface of the tail of the pancreas; and the prehilar, which courses between the pancreas and the spleen.

Common Hepatic Artery

The common hepatic artery has a variable course along the cranial border of the body and head of the pancreas, and tortuosity is usually not observed. Anatomic variation is common. Most often this occurs as an aberrant right hepatic artery, which can traverse the pancreatic head during its passage from the superior mesenteric artery to the liver and give off branches to the pancreas. Also the common hepatic artery may arise from the superior mesenteric artery and traverse the pancreas [55]. These anatomic variations are particularly important to define prior to pancreaticoduodenectomy or pancreatic resection [157, 172].

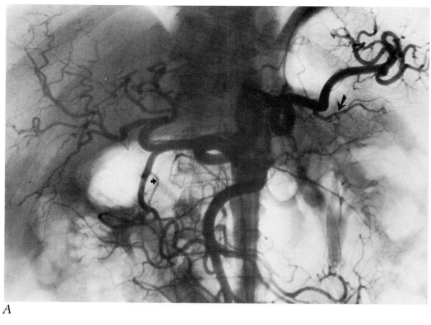

A

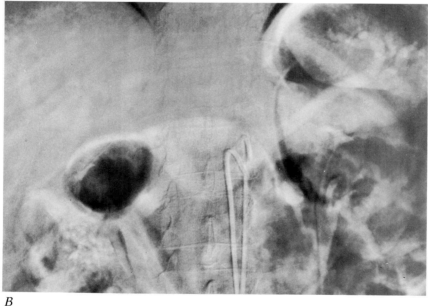

B

Figure 62-2. Normal pancreas. Simultaneous injection of contrast medium into celiac and superior mesenteric arteries. Arterial (A) and venous (B, subtraction) phase in frontal projection without drugs; in right posterior oblique projection (C and D) after injection of 25 mg tolazoline into the superior mesenteric artery. The superior mesenteric vein is best observed in the latter series. All pancreatic arteries are demonstrated by these two series but are far better outlined after injection of contrast medium into the gastroduodenal artery (E, subtraction). The catheter deforms the gastroduodenal artery. Observe the increased width of the pancratic arteries with the exception of the superior posterior pancreaticoduodenal artery (*short arrow*). This artery is not distended because the tip of the catheter is positioned distal to the origin. The transverse pancreatic artery (*long arrowhead*) arises from the gastroduodenal artery and communicates with the dorsal pancreatic artery (*short arrowhead*) and the artery of the pancreatic tail. The pancreatic magna artery (*long arrow*) is observed only at celiac injection (A–C).

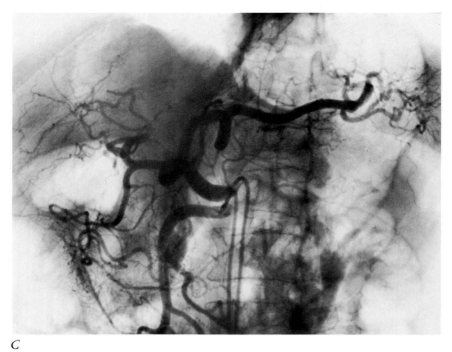

C

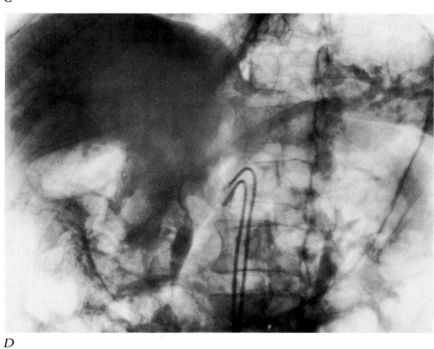

D

Figure 6-2 (Continued)

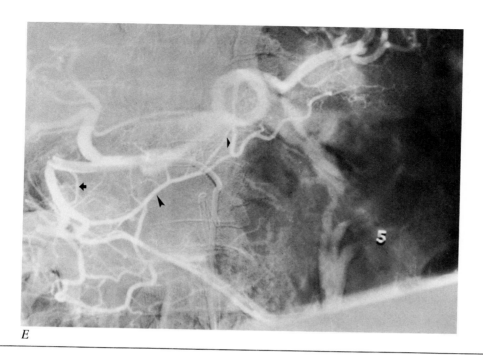

E

Gastroduodenal Artery

The gastroduodenal artery arises from the common hepatic artery in most cases but may take its origin from an aberrant right or left hepatic artery. It has a variable course in a caudal direction that depends largely on the degree of filling of the stomach and on the size and position of the liver and gallbladder.

Pancreaticoduodenal Arcades

The pancreaticoduodenal arcades are represented by the superior and inferior pancreaticoduodenal arteries with wide interconnections via posterior and anterior branches forming single or double arcades on the posterior and anterior aspects of the pancreas. The superior arteries arise separately from the gastroduodenal artery; the posterior artery is consistently the first branch, and the anterior artery arises a few centimeters further distally. The inferior arteries arise as a common branch directly from the posterior aspect of the superior mesenteric artery or, more often, from the first branch of the jejunal artery passing behind the superior mesenteric artery (Fig. 62-4).

Arterial anastomoses between the pancreaticoduodenal arteries and the dorsal pancreatic artery are regularly observed. Often, direct anastomoses with the transverse pancreatic artery are also noted (Fig. 62-5; see also Fig. 62-2).

Dorsal Pancreatic Artery

The dorsal pancreatic artery usually arises from the hepatic or splenic artery, but an origin from the superior mesenteric artery is not uncommon. Branches to the uncinate process and the superior pancreaticoduodenal arteries are frequently observed. The transverse pancreatic artery usually takes its origin from this vessel (see Figs. 62-3–62-5). Wide communication with the superior mesenteric artery is sometimes shown. The middle colic or left colic arteries may originate from the dorsal pancreatic artery.

Transverse Pancreatic Artery

Although not regularly observed, probably because it is too small [153], the transverse pancreatic artery usually originates from the dorsal pancreatic artery. Other common origins are from the superior mesenteric or the gastroduodenal artery. When arising from the latter, the vessel may be wide and may not anastomose with arteries in the tail of the pancreas coming from the splenic artery. This feature is important to note when a right-sided pancreatic resection is contemplated [121].

Splenic Branches to the Body and Tail of the Pancreas

These branches vary in appearance and are often the most difficult to define on the angiogram.

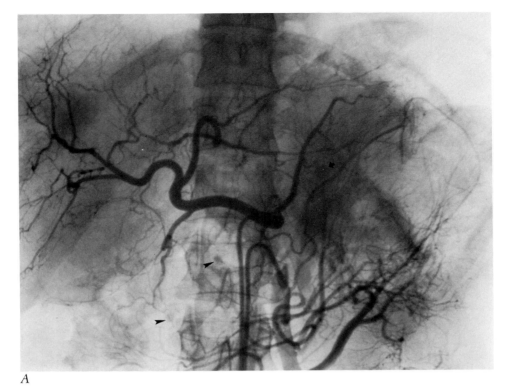

A

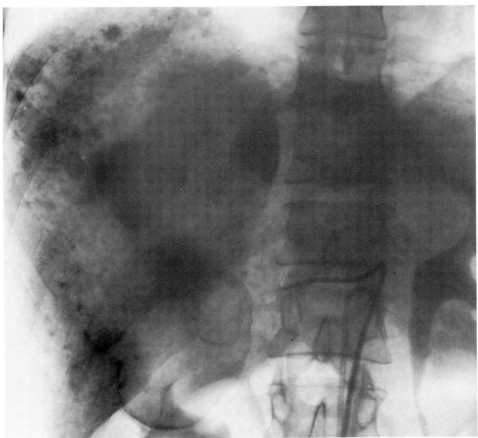

B

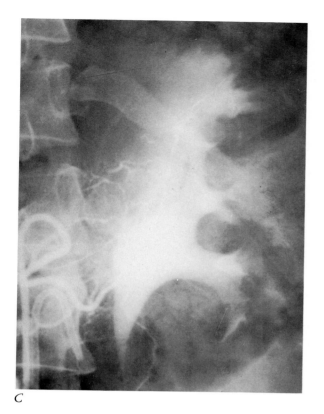

C

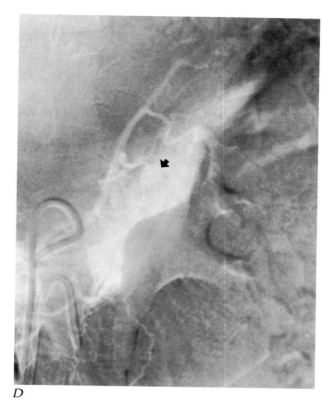

D

Figure 62-3. Multiple malignant gastrinomas in the pancreas and hepatic metastases in a patient with previous operation for hyperparathyroidism and the Zollinger-Ellison syndrome. Gastrectomy, splenectomy, and enucleation of a gastrinoma in the head of the pancreas had been performed previously. At celiac and superior mesenteric angiography (A) two 4-mm tumors (*arrowheads*) are observed in the head of the pancreas and one 6-mm tumor was suspected in the tail of the pancreas (*arrow*). The richly vascularized small hepatic metastases were not observed until hepatic artery injection of contrast medium was performed (B). Selective injection of contrast medium into the dorsal pancreatic artery (C and D) shows that the transverse pancreatic and small pancreatic tail arteries communicate with the small splenic artery, and in late arterial phase a small tumor in the tail of the pancreas is verified (*arrow*).

Usually the largest one is called the pancreatic magna artery (see Fig. 62-2). In addition, numerous small branches originate from the splenic artery. They run in a more or less vertical direction and can be the only vessels demonstrated to the left part of the body and the tail of the pancreas. One more constant branch is the caudal pancreatic artery, which arises from the splenic artery in the hilus of the spleen or from the left gastroepiploic artery.

Superior Mesenteric Artery

The superior mesenteric artery arises from the aorta posterior to the body of the pancreas. Its first part is usually not shown with the commonly employed angiographic procedures because of its course, which is almost perpendicular to the central ray. For complete information a lateral view is necessary (see Fig. 62-4).

VEINS

The pancreatic veins are normally not observed at celiac and superior mesenteric angiography. Because veins adjacent to the pancreas are liable to change in pancreatic disease, the angiographic study should demonstrate and outline the splenic, portal, and superior mesenteric veins clearly (see Fig. 62-2). Pharmacoangiography is therefore recommended as an additional procedure to the more conventional celiac and superior mesenteric arteriogram [45].

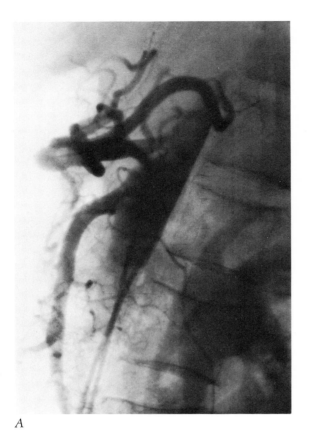

A

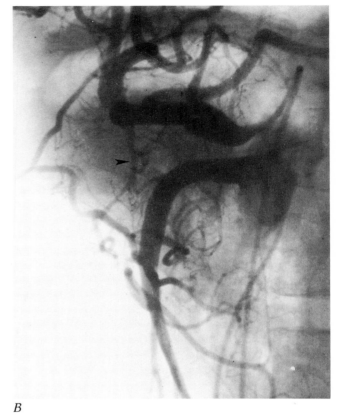

B

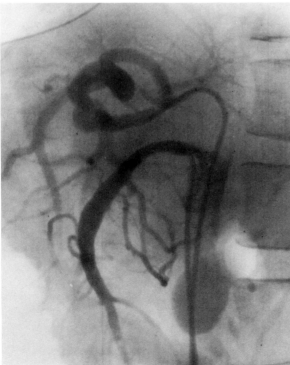

C

Figure 62-4. Lateral view of combined celiac and superior mesenteric arteries after 0.5 IU vasopressin (Pitressin) and then 20 cc of contrast medium were selectively injected into each artery. (A) Normal course of vessels in a thin patient. (B) Stenosis of celiac axis at origin by atherosclerosis. Infiltration of gastroduodenal artery (*arrowhead*) by carcinoma of the head of the pancreas. (C) Infiltration of the celiac and superior mesenteric arteries by carcinoma of the body of the pancreas. Observe that the inferior pancreaticoduodenal arcade arises from the posterior aspect of the superior mesenteric artery.

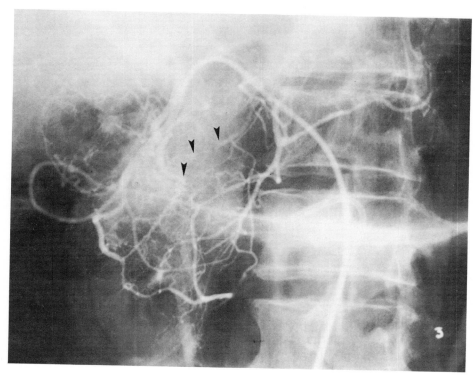

Figure 62-5. Gastroduodenal angiography in a patient with carcinoma of the head of the pancreas causing jaundice and intra- and extrahepatic bile duct dilatation. At operation the tumor was believed to have a diameter of about 5 cm, but pathologic examination of specimen proved the tumor to have a diameter of less than 1 cm. Angiography reveals several abrupt arterial occlusions within a small area (*arrowheads*), i.e., the site of the tumor. Marked hypervascularization around the tumor is a secondary reaction due to ductal obstruction. Dorsal and transverse pancreatic arteries communicate with anterior superior arcades.

Technique

Various methods are recommended for pancreatic angiography. The original cutdown technique of the brachial artery, including antegrade catheterization of the splanchnic arteries [26, 175–177], has been replaced by the percutaneous femoral retrograde [185, 186] or the axillary antegrade approach [32, 226].

The radiopaque polyethylene catheters introduced by Ödman for percutaneous use facilitated the procedure and reduced the complications [187]. The retrograde technique became the routine procedure and is still regarded as the method of choice. The technique of retrograde catheterization has not changed since the report in the first edition of this book, except for minor modifications (see Chaps. 64 and 68 for a discussion of the technique of celiac arteriography). Boijsen and Olin [44] recommended using one of the renal arteries to reverse the tip of the catheter to enter the splanchnic arteries when direct catheterization proved difficult. It has been

shown on dogs that the reversal of the catheter in the renal arteries involves an increased risk of aortic or renal intimal lesions and subintimal bleeding with possible consequent renal infarctions [272]. The original technique recommended by Ödman caused the same complications to a lesser degree except that no renal complications were observed [186]. The aortic intima of the dog as well as that of young patients is more vulnerable than the aortic wall in patients with atherosclerosis. Because the problems of splanchnic artery catheterization occur in the older age group, the risks with the reversal technique using the renal arteries seem small. Even though no complications of this kind have been observed in vivo, the increased risk should be recognized during angiography.

To reduce the complication rate, a smaller catheter than that originally recommended by Ödman should be used. With the development of image amplification, thin-walled catheters are now recommended. In comparison to the standard-wall catheters, the outer diameter has been reduced to 2.2 mm but the inner diameter remains the same (1.5 mm). Thus contrast medium may be injected at the same high rate [37].

SIMULTANEOUS AND SEQUENTIAL APPROACHES

Because the pancreas is supplied from both celiac and superior mesenteric arteries, most authors agree that angiography of both arteries should be performed. The use of two catheters, previously introduced through bilateral femoral artery punctures with injection of contrast medium simultaneously into the celiac and superior mesenteric arteries through a Y connection, has been recommended [44, 152, 153, 191, 195, 207, 211]. Nevertheless, most authors prefer sequential catheterization of the arteries with one catheter [125, 180, 222, 227, 268]. Proponents of the sequential technique suggest that there is less trauma to the femoral arteries because only one vessel is punctured and that the delineation is better because there are fewer superimposed contrast-filled arteries in the pancreatic area. Gastric insufflation [153, 186], stereoscopic filming, and vasoconstrictive drugs, however, reduce these problems when the simultaneous technique is employed [46]. Both methods are acceptable and should be regarded as screening procedures.

ROUTINE TECHNIQUE

As mentioned previously, there are many variations in the routine technique, depending upon the policy of the institution and the experience of the angiographer. But the routine technique also varies with indications, which have changed over the years. Angiography is today seldom used as a diagnostic method because ultrasonography, CT, percutaneous transhepatic cholangiography (PTC), and ERCP have high diagnostic accuracy in pancreatic disease. One or several of these methods should be used before angiography is contemplated. Thus, angiography is mainly used for preoperative mapping of the pancreatic vasculature, for predicting resectability and prognosis in patients with carcinoma, for defining vascular abnormalities in a patient with severe pancreatitis, and after severe trauma to the pancreas. It is therefore only in exceptional cases that the superselective technique is required, as in pa-

tients suspected of having islet cell tumors of the pancreas. This does not mean that the quality of the angiographic examination should be inferior; it means that the procedure can be carried out faster and with fewer complications.

Anteroposterior Projection

In University Hospital, Lund, Sweden, the simultaneous technique is used. A total of 60 cc of 76 percent contrast medium is injected at a rate of 20 cc per second simultaneously into the celiac and superior mesenteric arteries (30 cc at a rate of 10 cc/second into each artery). Exposures are made at a rate of two per second for 5 seconds, one per second for 5 seconds, and then one every other second for 10 seconds (10/5, 5/5, 5/10) (see Fig. 62-2A, B).

Right Posterior Oblique Projection

A second series always follows in the RPO projection after injection of a vasodilating substance into the superior mesenteric artery (bradykinin 5–10 μg [24]; tolazoline 25–50 mg [144]); 80 to 100 cc of the contrast medium is injected simultaneously at a rate of 25 cc per second (10/5, 10/20). The patient is turned only slightly to the right in order to have maximum information on the venous system (see Fig. 62-2C, D).

If the expected information is obtained with the AP and RPO views, no further injections are made and the examination is concluded. On the other hand, if the information is not in agreement with other diagnostic data or if there is clinical reason to suspect an islet cell tumor, or if the two series mentioned give incomplete or inadequate information, pharmacoangiographic methods and/or superselective angiography should be employed at the same time.

PHARMACOANGIOGRAPHY

Vasoconstricting Drugs

Injection of small doses of vasoconstrictors into the celiac and superior mesenteric arteries before the injection of contrast medium will usually improve the visualization of the pancreatic arteries. Epinephrine (5–10 μg), norepinephrine (5–10 μg), and vasopressin (0.5–1.0 IU) are those most extensively used [13, 39, 46, 64, 132, 183]. These drugs, when injected intraarterially in small doses, cause a marked constriction of all splanchnic arteries, but the effect is different on different vascular beds, and the main stems of the celiac and superior mesenteric arteries are not

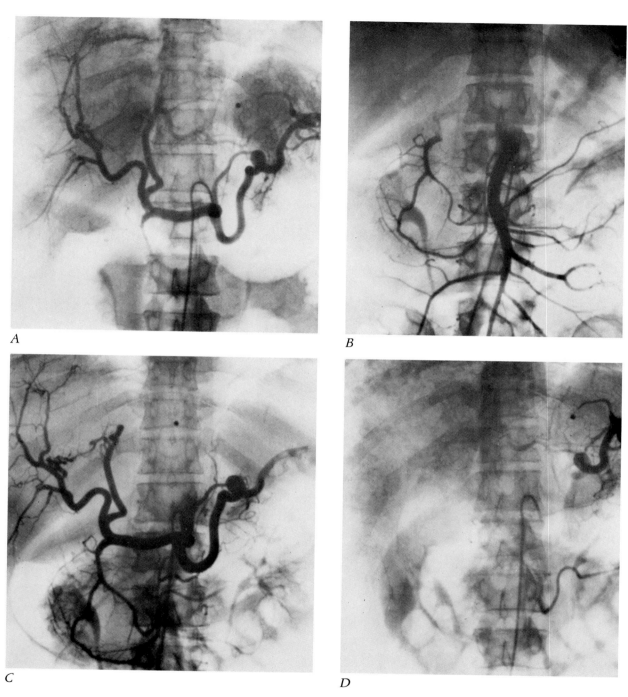

A

B

C

D

Figure 62-6. Cystic carcinoma of the head of the pancreas with nodular lesions within the liver proved to be abscesses. (A and B) Sequential celiac and superior mesenteric angiography performed without any previous drug. (C and D) Celiac angiography after 1 IU of vasopressin was injected. Increased vascular supply of the liver secondary to bile stasis and abscesses caused a reversal of flow in the gastroduodenal artery; tumor of the head of the pancreas is therefore not demonstrated in the control study. Decreased flow in the hepatic artery after injection of vasopressin permitted complete filling of gastroduodenal and pancreatic arteries, and the tumor is well demonstrated. Displacement of pancreatic arteries and tumor vessels is observed, but there is no infiltration of the arteries. In the capillary phase abscess formation was demonstrated after vasopressin injection (D) but not in the control study. At superior mesenteric angiography, tumor is demonstrated by reverse flow through the pancreaticoduodenal arteries (B).

influenced. Thus, the pancreatic vasculature reacts less than the gastric and splenic vasculatures. The density of the contrast medium therefore increases in the pancreatic arteries, and previously superimposed gastric arteries are eliminated. Because of the higher density of the contrast medium in the arteries and probably also because neoplastic and collateral vessels do not constrict, the scanty tumor vessels of pancreatic carcinoma or the collateral arteries around infiltrated or occluded arteries are better observed (Fig. 62-6). In patients with obstructive jaundice a reverse flow is often observed in the gastroduodenal artery because of an increased arterial supply to the liver. Regular celiac angiography will then not fill the pancreaticoduodenal arteries (Fig. 62-6). Arterial collaterals are not affected by the vasoconstrictive drug; therefore, far better demonstration of the pancreatic arteries is obtained in those cases after injection of vasoconstrictors.

Because of the improvement in angiographic technique (superselectivity, magnification), pharmacoangiography is now rarely performed to obtain diagnostic information about the pancreas. However, vasoconstrictors are often of great support in the evaluation of the first parts of the celiac and superior mesenteric arteries in a lateral view (see Fig. 62-4). This method is used in patients with an angiographically normal pancreas who have upper abdominal pain but otherwise normal pancreatic tests. Stenosis or infiltration of the arteries is best observed in this view, which therefore may show that the cause of the upper abdominal pain is abdominal angina.

Vasodilating Drugs

Experimental and in vivo angiographic studies have been performed after intraarterial injection of vasodilating substances employed to increase pancreatic blood flow and enhance the accumulation of contrast medium in the pancreas. Priscoline, bradykinin, papaverine, trypsin, histamine, acetylcholine, secretin, and cholecystokinin have given somewhat varying results in terms of their usefulness for demonstrating the pancreas and pancreatic lesions [24, 45, 131, 146, 148, 188, 224, 230, 234, 253, 264, 265]. So far the most promising results have been obtained with secretin injected in high doses intraarterially or intravenously, but the results are not consistent. Injection of these substances in the superior mesenteric artery increases the circulation through the bowel and results in better filling of the superior mesenteric vein (see Fig. 62-2; Fig. 62-7). In this respect bradykinin, tolazoline, secretin, prostaglandin E_1 and F_2-alpha have been found useful without causing any complications [45, 78, 79, 208, 264]. For angiographic demon-

Figure 62-7. (A) Carcinoma of the head of the pancreas. At celiac angiography the gastroduodenal, superior anterior, and posterior pancreaticoduodenal arteries and the first part of the gastroepiploic artery are seen to be infiltrated by tumor. Abnormal tumor vessels. (B) Venous phase of superior mesenteric angiography. Compression of the vein at the level of the tumor is demonstrated. The high density of the contrast medium in the vein was obtained by injecting 10 μg of bradykinin immediately before the contrast-medium injection.

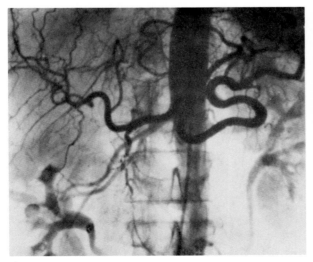

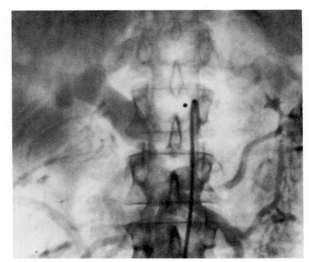

A

B

stration of the splenic vein an increased dose of contrast medium in the celiac artery is usually sufficient [179, 180], but it has been shown that a combination of alpha-blocking and beta-stimulating drugs improves opacification of the portal venous system [267]. From a diagnostic point of view, superselective injection of tolazoline has been found to give the best information about the pancreas and its arteries [118, 154].

Combined Vasodilating and Vasoconstricting Drugs

A combination of vasodilating and vasoconstricting drugs has also been tested with good results, from a diagnostic point of view, in celiac angiography. Thus, Udén [266] combined secretin and epinephrine and improved the technical quality.

SUPERSELECTIVE ANGIOGRAPHY

Superselective pancreatic angiography is a selective catheterization of splenic, common hepatic, gastroduodenal, or separate pancreatic arteries. In 1958 Morino et al. [174], using the cutdown brachial antegrade technique, demonstrated its great potential. Later investigations [6, 9, 10, 31, 32, 61, 88, 98, 118, 154, 155, 179, 180, 199, 211, 223, 250–252] have proved that better information is obtained about the pancreatic vasculature with this technique. Reuter [211] showed in a large series that this technique can be performed consistently with relative ease, is safe, and adds minimally to the time required for conventional pancreatic angiography. The method should first of all not be utilized if the conventional technique has shown a pancreatic abnormality, unless there is an islet cell tumor. In the latter case, more than one endocrine tumor may be present, and therefore superselective angiography should be performed (see Fig. 62-3). Superselectivity does indeed increase accuracy in diagnosis of pancreatic carcinoma to more than 94 percent [9, 88, 118]. Pharmacoangiography increases information about pancreatic vasculature, and so does magnification technique [88, 98, 118, 154, 155]. Because of its high resolution, the magnification technique can in fact replace the superselective one in most instances [43] (Fig. 62-8). No doubt, in experienced hands the superselective technique is a quite satisfactory method, but often the examination time and consequently the complications are unduly high

with this technique. It is therefore recommended only on very specific indications, as in patients with endocrine tumors. It should also be stated that a normal pancreatic angiogram of the highest quality does not rule out a pancreatic lesion.

In order to have complete filling of all pancreatic arteries, injection into gastroduodenal, dorsal pancreatic, and splenic arteries is required, but this is only occasionally feasible [211]. Where it is impossible to reach the pancreatic arteries by superselective technique, modification of the pancreatic blood flow may be obtained by balloon catheters with consequent improvement in the density of the pancreatic arteries [212].

CONTRAST MATERIAL AND FILMING

The amount and type of contrast medium used for pancreatic angiography vary. The most commonly used medium is a sodium methylglucamine salt of diatrizoate, metrizoate, or iothalamate acid, administered in a 76 percent solution when given into main stems. Medium amount and injection rates used in conventional technique have already been presented. The amount and rate of contrast medium injection in specific pharmacoangiographic studies, superselective studies, or combinations thereof, vary. There is a tendency to use larger amounts and higher rates since no complications caused by the contrast medium per se have been observed. The total amount of about 300 cc of contrast medium is well tolerated by an adult patient who is well hydrated and has normal renal function [84]. The procedure usually takes about 1 hour. If the procedure is prolonged, up to 500 cc can be utilized [118].

The film series should cover the various phases of the angiogram. The transit of the contrast medium through the arteries to the capillary bed should be followed at a rate of two frames per second unless the circulation is slowed down by a vasoconstrictor or balloon. The appearance of contrast in the portal system varies, and therefore the whole series must cover about 20 seconds; during the capillary phase one frame per second is adequate, followed later by one frame every other second. The pancreatic veins are sometimes observed after administration of secretin or a combination of secretin and epinephrine in celiac angiography [253, 266] but are even better observed after administration of secretin in superselective angiography [118]. In most cases the main interest is to image the maximum den-

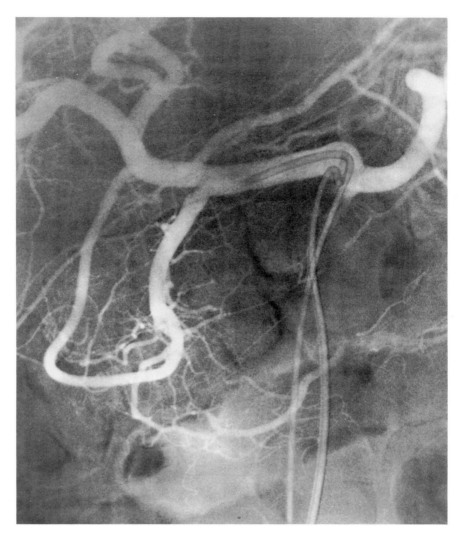

Figure 62-8. Carcinoma of the head of the pancreas. Magnification angiography shows infiltration and abrupt occlusion of branches of the posterosuperior pancreaticoduodenal artery.

sity of the portal venous system, which will be obtained after vasodilating drugs have been given according to the regimen previously mentioned.

Complications

Acute pancreatitis has been observed after injection of contrast medium at translumbar aortography [160, 219]. The contrast media used were more toxic than those now employed and were the probable cause of this complication. Dogs with normal pancreases and with experimentally induced pancreatitis were found not to have any histopathologic changes after contrast-medium injection into the celiac axis and superior mesenteric artery [272]. Amounts and concentration of medium were comparable to those used in vivo. Extensive experience with pancreatic angiography gives the same impression that the method does not cause any complications as far as the pancreas is concerned. At first there was some hesitance at the superselective injection of pancreatic arteries, but later experience showed that even 20 to 50 cc of contrast medium may be injected at a high rate (up to 10 cc/second), especially after vasodilation with tolazoline (12.5 mg).

Intimal and subintimal lesions in the aorta and the visceral arteries can be kept at a minimum with adequate technique [211]. However, in a prospective study of a consecutive series such le-

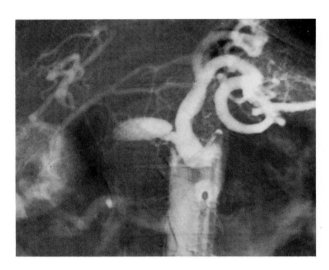

Figure 62-9. Subintimal dissection of the common hepatic artery after attempts to catheterize the vessel. Collateral circulation to the liver is observed via the left gastric artery.

sions were found to occur more often than expected [129, 239]. Nevertheless they are rarely of any significance within the branches of the celiac artery because of the collateral circulation (Fig. 62-9).

Complications at the puncture site are unusual with good technique and with the small catheters recommended.

Angiography in Pancreatic Disease

PANCREATIC CARCINOMA

Selective angiography in carcinoma of the pancreas (Fig. 62-10; see also Figs. 62-4–62-8) became a frequently used method soon after the new technique with radiopaque catheters became established [186]. In the following years a few case reports appeared on the angiographic findings [44, 75, 103, 166, 181, 201], but it was not until 1965 that the real breakthrough occurred. Lunderquist [153] presented a series of 26 patients with pancreatic carcinoma who had had angiography with the simultaneous technique. Abnormal angiograms were observed in retrospect in 92 percent of the cases. Numerous reports during the next decade dealt with various aspects of diagnostic importance in angiography of pancreatic carcinoma [7, 14, 18, 19, 22, 32, 52,

59, 63, 90, 96, 138, 140, 141, 143, 151, 161, 165, 180, 191, 193, 194, 196, 201, 204, 207, 216, 221, 222, 226, 227, 247, 258, 259, 268, 270].

During this period the superselective technique for diagnosis of pancreatic carcinoma was developed and proved to be a remarkable improvement in the diagnosis of this lesion [31, 88, 118, 154, 199], as was pharmacoangiography, with special emphasis on arterial and venous contrast medium enhancement [46, 47, 125, 132, 146, 208]. At the same time the value of angiography as a method for predicting resectability and prognosis increased [109, 229, 244–246, 248, 261]. Even though some negative reports on the accuracy of pancreatic angiography as a method for diagnosis of pancreatic carcinoma were published in the first years of this period, it became apparent that experience and high quality gave a sensitivity better than what Lunderquist reported in his retrospective analysis [9, 88, 109, 118]. It is not to be inferred that routine preoperative angiography in pancreatic disease will reach these very high levels of accuracy in all institutions. In a review of preoperative reports in 116 patients with pancreatic carcinoma Tylén [258] found a correct diagnosis noted in 68 percent. In a recent report Mackie et al. [157] found a sensitivity of 72 percent and a specificity of 71 percent in a series of 103 patients including 40 with carcinoma. The high rate of false-positive findings in their material was due partly to the fact that periampullary and other tumors were included as false-positive results, a procedure that is not usually followed. Nevertheless, false-positive diagnoses of pancreatic carcinoma are not rare and result mainly from misinterpretation of vascular changes caused by pancreatitis or pseudocysts [91, 240].

Since 1975 new diagnostic methods have reduced the importance of angiography as a diagnostic tool. It is true that the combination of angiography and other diagnostic methods (PTC, cytology, pancreatic function tests, pancreatic scintigraphy) were used before this time [42, 47, 87, 110]. ERCP became the first serious alternative to angiography, but in most reports, where both methods were used it became obvious that ERCP and angiography were complementary [11, 36, 70, 73, 243, 257]. To rely entirely on ERCP as a way to diagnose pancreatic carcinoma seems impossible after a study of observer variation and error in interpretation of the pancreatogram [210]. During the last few years, gray-scale ul-

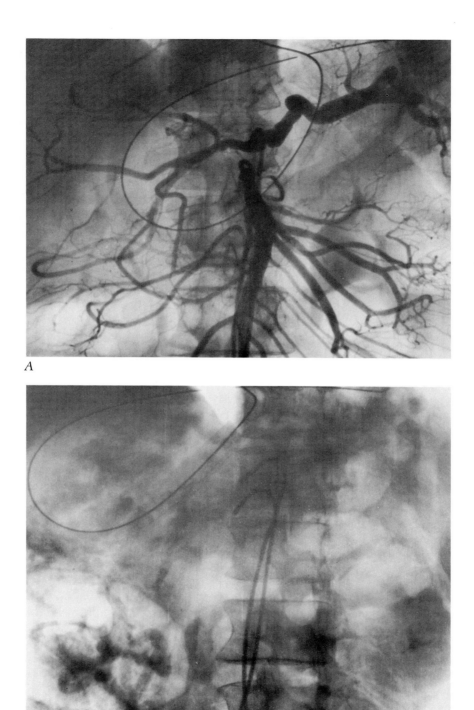

A

B

Figure 62-10. (A) Inoperable carcinoma of the body of the pancreas with typical infiltration of the common hepatic, splenic, and superior mesenteric arteries observed in simultaneous celiac and superior mesenteric angiography. Infiltration of celiac and superior mesenteric arteries is best observed in lateral projection (see Fig. 62-4C). (B) In the venous phase, after administration of tolazoline, occlusion of superior mesenteric, splenic, and portal veins is observed with collateral circulation to intrahepatic portal system via the veins of the gallbladder and stomach.

trasonography, CT, and pancreatic scintigraphy have been evaluated and compared with angiography [82, 91, 98, 133, 155, 156, 235]. Since a pancreatic scan is regarded as nonspecific, most investigators agree that with the present technique it is unnecessary in pancreatic disease. Both ultrasonography and CT have high sensitivity in pancreatic cancer, and clearly they should be used as primary methods in patients suspected of having this disease [144]. In a well-controlled series of 73 patients with pancreatic carcinoma Mackie et al. [155] found a higher sensitivity of ultrasonography and ERCP (96 and 87 percent, respectively, in resectable cancers and 83 and 89 percent in nonresectable cancers), as compared with angiography, which had a sensitivity of 75 and 78 percent, respectively, in the two groups. On the other hand, in other prospective series, ultrasonography was found to have a relatively low sensitivity (68%) compared with CT (87%) in patients evaluated for pancreatic disease [126]. It is well known that neither CT nor ultrasonography will show tumors less than 2 cm. Therefore, it can be debated whether ultrasonography and/or CT is indicated in patients with obstructive jaundice where PTC has to be performed anyhow [107], especially since PTC combined with percutaneous biopsy is the simplest way to arrive at a diagnosis [41].

The main indication for angiography today is therefore not primarily diagnostic, but it still has an important place in pancreatic disease. In carcinoma of the pancreas angiography is used chiefly in patients who are regarded as being operable—i.e., those in whom no metastases have been observed at CT or ultrasonography and the size of the tumor does not preclude its removal (see Fig. 62-5). Thus, while angiography is still of assistance for diagnosis, it is particularly useful for management [82, 98, 157, 172].

There are three principal indications for preoperative angiography in a patient with pancreatic carcinoma. The first is to provide a vascular map for the surgeon. It is most important for the surgeon to know whether there is a vascular anomaly. This can of course be searched for during operation, but sometimes the pulsations in an accessory right hepatic artery passing over or through the head of the pancreas are impossible to palpate [55, 172]. Some 25 percent of the patients have an anomaly of the celiac and superior mesenteric vessels, and in about 90 percent of these the arteries supplying the liver are involved. This is of importance since, as has been

noted by Mackie et al. [157]: "In our experience ligation of a major hepatic artery, in the presence of jaundice, uniformly leads to fatal hepatic necrosis." Also, in patients with complete celiac stenosis, ligation of collateral arteries of the superior mesenteric artery is hazardous [33].

The second indication for preoperative angiography is to define the site and extent of the tumor, thereby predicting resectability [9, 33, 157, 229, 245, 246, 248, 261]. With few exceptions [157], it is agreed that if no vascular abnormalities are observed in a patient with pancreatic carcinoma there are good prognostic signs of resectability. As has been pointed out by Suzuki et al. [243], lesions that cause ductal abnormalities but have small or no vascular changes have a better prognosis for resectability because the lesions are in the center of the gland. Most of the pancreatic arteries we observe at routine angiography are located on the surface of the gland; thus if any of them are infiltrated, the carcinoma has probably passed through the capsule. Consequently, even though only one of the pancreaticoduodenal arcades is infiltrated, the tumor may have passed the resectable stage, particularly if the tumor is positioned on the posterior aspect of the head of the pancreas [246, 248]. With increasing numbers of vessels infiltrated, the chance of resectability is decreased and, if the tumor is nevertheless resectable, the possibility of recurrence rises. Veins should always be well demonstrated. Even if the tumor can be resected when the mesenteric or portal veins are deformed by the tumor, the risk of recurrence is very high. The possibility of predicting survival time from the angiographic findings is another reason for showing the local extent of tumor by angiography [244, 261].

The third indication for angiography is to verify or exclude a strongly suspected carcinoma of the pancreas. With superselective technique combined with magnification, angiography has a very high sensitivity, better than that of any other method available. ERCP may show short strictures of the pancreatic duct that are benign but that may look like pancreatic carcinoma [11]. In those cases angiography is of particular importance to avoid unnecessary operation. Neither ultrasonography nor CT will be of any assistance in this situation.

The typical angiographic findings in a patient with pancreatic carcinoma are irregular stenosis or occlusions of arteries within or adjacent to the pancreas (see Figs. 62-5, 62-7, 62-10). Stenoses of arteries adjacent to the pancreas may also be

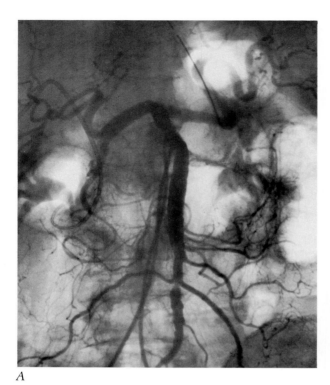

A

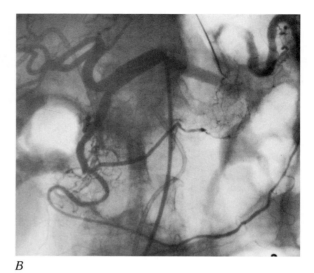

B

C

observed in atherosclerosis, chronic pancreatitis, arteritis, and fibromuscular dysplasia [21, 121, 136, 198, 221, 227] (Fig. 62-11). These changes may simulate tumor encasement, but in atherosclerosis and chronic pancreatitis the arterial wall usually has a different appearance, with single-plaque formation in the former and a smooth outline in the latter. Nevertheless, these changes may at times be impossible to differentiate from carcinoma (Figs. 62-12, 62-13).

Displacement of vessels in and around the pancreas may occur in carcinoma but usually cannot be appreciated because of the frequent congenital variations. When it is present, there will often be an abrupt change of direction different from the arc-shaped displacement observed in pancreatitis and other tumors. There are, however, exceptions to this rule (see Fig. 62-6).

Accumulation of contrast medium within the carcinoma may occur but is not a reliable finding with current methods. On the contrary, in superselective pharmacoangiography, tumors of about

Figure 62-11. Arteritis or severe arteriosclerosis in splanchnic arteries in a 76-year-old patient with silent jaundice and known temporal arteritis. At PTC, stones were seen to be present in the common bile duct. Pancreatic angiography (A) reveals marked irregularities in the arteries surrounding the pancreas. The superior mesenteric artery is severely stenosed at its origin and in its distal part. (Drainage catheter in common bile duct after PTC.) Gastroduodenal angiography (B and C) also shows marked narrowing in small pancreatic arteries, and the pancreas is hypervascularized. The splenic and portal veins are intact.

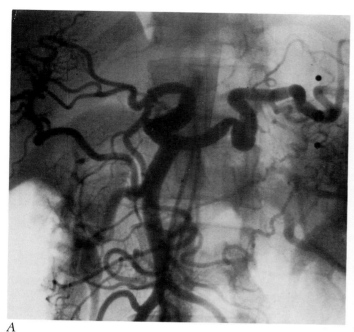

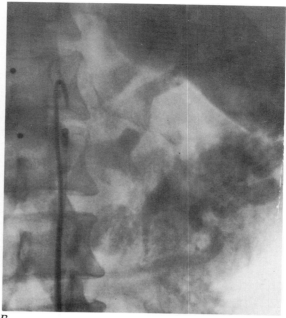

A   *B*

Figure 62-12. (A) Chronic pancreatitis with marked irregular changes in splenic, transverse pancreatic, and middle colic arteries observed in arterial phase. (B) Venous phase showing splenic vein compressed by the tortuous splenic artery; collaterals noted over the gastroepiploic veins.

Figure 62-13. Chronic pancreatitis with pseudocyst in the tail of the pancreas with irregular stenoses and tortuosity of pancreatic and peripancreatic arteries noted at celiac (A) and superior mesenteric (B) angiography. The cyst extends lateral to the spleen, displacing the latter medially. Beading of distal part of splenic artery is observed.

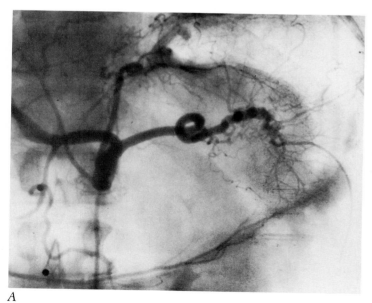

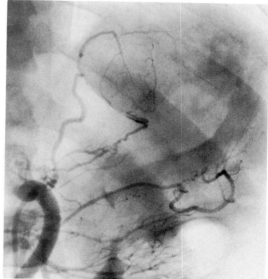

A   *B*

1 cm in diameter are observed as filling defects in the parenchyma, and often there are no vascular abnormalities at all. Tumor vessels have been observed in as many as 60 percent of the cases of pancreatic carcinoma [153]. These abnormal vessels are probably not of the same type as observed in richly vascularized malignancies like renal carcinoma. The scirrhous carcinoma is almost avascular and infiltrates or occludes vessels. The abnormal vessels observed are therefore probably infiltrated arteries or collateral arteries caused by occlusion. This situation may also explain the improved filling of these vessels after administration of vasoconstrictive drugs because collateral arteries are not influenced by vasoconstrictors.

Compression or occlusion of veins is commonly seen [63, 236] and should, if present, be demonstrated by angiography (see Figs. 62-7, 62-10).

While the prognosis of carcinoma of the pancreas is poor, with greater clinical awareness and with trained radiologic-surgical teams to attack this disease the prognosis should improve [172].

ISLET CELL TUMORS

The islet cells of the pancreas are said to be part of a neuroendocrine system [232]. The cells of this system all have the ability to concentrate and decarboxylate precursors of biogenic amines and are called APUD cells (*a*mino *p*recursor *u*ptake and *d*ecarboxylation). They include endocrine cells in the pituitary, pancreatic islets, gastrointestinal tract, adrenal medulla, lungs, urogenital tract, and carotid body.

Tumors originating from the islet cells of the pancreas (Fig. 62-14; see also Figs. 62-17, 62-18) may produce symptoms caused by an overproduction of insulin, gastrin, glucagon, or a vasoactive peptide [29, 56, 111, 163, 277, 278]. The tumors may be benign or malignant. There are also islet cell tumors that do not give evidence of endocrine activity. Tumors with endocrine activity are most often benign adenomas, while nonactive tumors are usually malignant.

Insulin-producing tumors originate from the beta cells and are somewhat more common in the body and tail of the pancreas [56]. Multiple tumors are present in 10 percent of cases. Most tumors reported as being diagnosed by angiography were located in the head of the pancreas, and of those reported in the body and tail, angiographic diagnosis more often failed [22, 48,

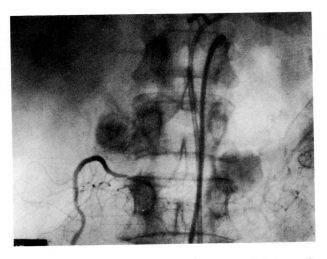

Figure 62-14. Two insulinomas, 1.5 and 2.0 cm in diameter, in the head and uncinate process of the pancreas, respectively. The latter was not seen or palpated during operation until incision of the parenchyma was made.

51, 62, 146, 158, 163, 165, 180, 189, 190, 192, 218, 222, 233, 268, 271]. The opposite has, however, also been observed [100, 241].

Bookstein and Oberman [51] were originally of the opinion that only 20 percent of insulin-producing tumors could be found by selective angiography. Their figures were based on the histologic findings and their own angiographic experience. Later they found, however, a higher detection rate, since 15 of 40 insulinomas (38%) were discovered preoperatively [218]. This is still not in agreement with most other reports. Thus, we found in our series of nine tumors only one that was not detected preoperatively [48]. In another consecutive series of 14 patients no false-negatives were obtained [242]. In the largest series presented [122], a correct diagnosis was obtained in 63 out of 82 patients (77%), a frequency that is in good agreement with other recent reports of smaller series [5, 72, 80, 81, 89, 100, 101, 112, 162, 202, 241]. The relatively low detection rate in the new series of Robins, Bookstein, et al. [218] can be explained by the high rate of multiple tumors (40 tumors in 26 patients), a high rate of benign lesions, and the fact that 16 of the tumors were less than 1 cm in diameter and 9 of these were below 0.3 cm. In three patients there was general adenomatosis of the gland, and in general hyperplasia, angiography has so far been negative [122, 128]. The malignant insulinomas are found more often by angiography than the benign tumors [122]. It may be assumed that the second or third smallest tumors of the islet cells were detected by detailed dissection of the operation specimen not performed in other series. It is also probable that the tumors must reach a certain size before any endocrine symptoms appear, as is true of the small carcinoids of the bowel.

The symptoms of hyperinsulinism, though often dramatic, are nevertheless frequently misinterpreted and the diagnosis delayed. In a recent review of 31 patients with insulinoma, 25 patients had to wait more than a year before the correct diagnosis was made, and four patients had to wait more than 10 years [12]. When, however, hypoglycemia has been detected, the diagnosis of hyperinsulinism is not difficult. If the clinical diagnosis of hyperinsulinism is firm, angiography is at present the most reliable and rewarding method. If possible, every patient should have not only celiac and superior mesenteric angiography but also selective study of separate pancreatic arteries for maximum information [5, 48, 72, 112, 213, 218, 238, 242]. Pharmacoangiography (angiotensin) [218] and magnification, if available, should be used. As mentioned, the tumors may be multiple and very small, but with high-

quality studies, lesions with a diameter of 5 mm or more should in most cases be found and localized for surgery. Tumor vessels are often observed in tumors of only 1 cm. Dense, long-lasting accumulation and early-draining veins are frequent findings (Fig. 62-14).

Differential diagnostic problems may occur. Thus, an accessory spleen [48, 124, 134, 137, 215], metastatic nodes close to the pancreas [80, 137], bleeding into intrapancreatic pseudocysts [137], or angioma of the pancreas [80, 124, 184, 215] (Figs. 62-15, 62-16) may simulate an insulinoma. Superselective injection into the splenic artery or pancreatic branches [48, 213] may simulate an insulinoma of the tail of the pancreas.

If the angiographic results are negative, the surgeon will rarely find the tumor [53]. In this event, venous sampling from the pancreatic veins has proved quite rewarding [128].

Gastrin-producing lesions may occur not only in the pancreas but also in the duodenum and antrum of the stomach. Reports of single or few cases have given the impression that these lesions could be demonstrated by angiography with the same characteristics and with the same frequency as the insulin-producing tumors [30, 48, 71, 83,

Figure 62-15. Splenic angiography in a patient with Rendu-Osler-Weber disease. Multiple angiomatous lesions are present in the tail of the pancreas. Shunting to the splenic vein is noted (subtraction).

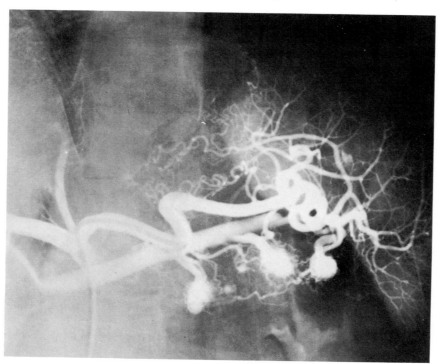

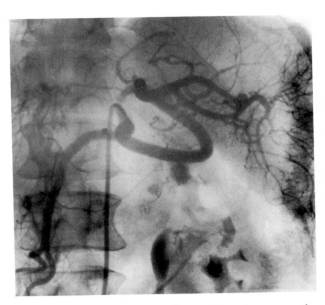

Figure 62-16. Metastases of a renal carcinoma to the tail of the pancreas.

93, 112, 117, 124, 137, 197, 202, 238, 255, 274, 276] (see Fig. 62-4). Early [151] as well as recent reports [171, 225, 238], however, also indicate that even with the best available technique angiography very often fails. In series with unequivocal clinical and laboratory signs of gastrin-producing lesions, tumors within the pancreas were observed in only 1 out of 6 [225] and 3 out of 20 patients [171], respectively. Richly vascularized metastases were observed somewhat more often than pancreatic gastrinomas. The inferior results are ascribed to the fact that diffuse hyperplasia and microadenomatosis are more often present in the Zollinger-Ellison syndrome than in hyperinsulinism. Furthermore, an intense "blush" of the hypervascular bowel mucosa may obscure details [171, 238]. It is of interest to note that the primary tumors may degenerate and even calcify [54, 225].

The metastases may be partly calcified and partly active and hence demonstrated at angiography [54]. This condition may explain why some of the patients with a Zollinger-Ellison syndrome had richly vascularized hepatic metastases observed at angiography while the primary tumor was not found. Despite the fact that small gastrinomas may pass unnoticed at angiography, the method is still worthwhile. If the tumor is observed and localized by angiography, the surgeon is in a better position to find the lesion. Furthermore, angiography may demonstrate that the tumor is outside the pancreas—in the duodenal wall, for example [164].

Tumors producing a vasoactive intestinal polypeptide (VIPoma) cause severe watery diarrhea, hypokalemia, and anacidity (the WDHA syndrome) [29]. The angiographic characteristics are the same as for the other endocrine tumors of the pancreas [8, 15, 106, 111, 254].

Glucagon-producing tumors cause the glucagonoma syndrome. A pancreatic islet cell tumor results in elevated glucagon in the serum, intolerance for glucose, and migrating necrolytic erythema of the skin [159]. The first case diagnosed by angiography was reported in 1966 [163]. The tumor had the same profuse vascular supply as other islet cell tumors, a finding that was later verified in a few reports [15, 209]. In our own series of three patients, positive angiographic studies and positive venous sampling results were most rewarding for tumor diagnosis and localization of the lesions (Fig. 62-17).

Inactive islet cell tumors are said to represent approximately one-quarter of the published cases of endocrine tumors. Only a few authors have commented on their angiographic characteristics [3, 15, 16, 35, 48, 80, 81, 94, 112, 165, 180, 222], most in reports of single cases. The lesions may have a characteristic appearance: large pancreatic tumors, richly vascularized, often causing vascular incasement or venous occlusion, and small, richly vascularized metastases of the liver (Fig. 62-18). Many other varieties occur. Thus, an avascular, calcified tumor has been observed [35]. With the richly vascularized tumors, differentiation between cystadenoma and rare retroperitoneal tumors such as leiomyosarcoma is not always possible.

CYSTIC NEOPLASMS

Cystadenoma and cystadenocarcinoma are rare pancreatic tumors (Figs. 62-19, 62-20). Of the 26 cases reported in the literature in which angiography was performed, 19 were benign and 7 malignant [99]. From an angiographic point of view the cystadenoma cannot be distinguished from the malignant tumor unless metastasis or arterial infiltration is present. The tumors tend to be large when detected, and arterial displacement is therefore almost always observed. Most cases recorded in the literature have been highly or moderately vascular with neovascularity and tumor staining [2, 17, 21, 25, 99, 103, 117, 146, 206, 207, 249] (Fig. 62-19). Irregular uptake of

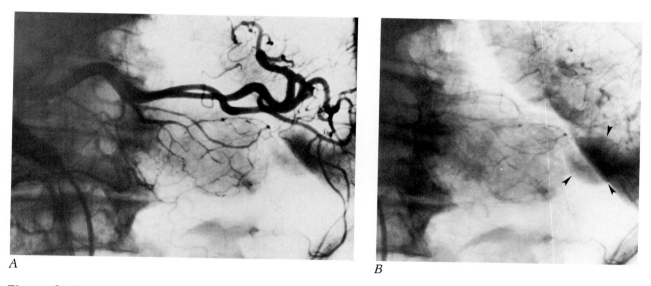

A   B

Figure 62-17. Arterial (A) and late arterial (B) angiography of a moderately vascularized glucagonoma with a diameter of 3 cm in the tail of the pancreas. Adjacent to the tumor is an accessory spleen (*arrowheads*).

Figure 62-18. Nonactive malignant insulinoma of the head of the pancreas. The highly vascularized, well-circumscribed, large tumor is a characteristic finding.

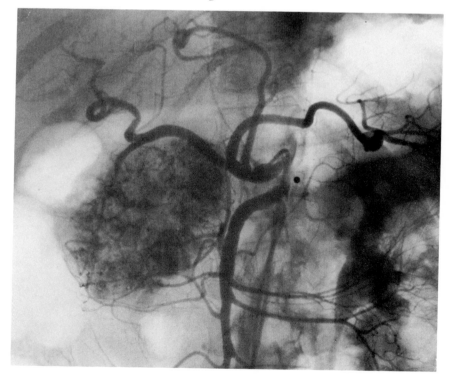

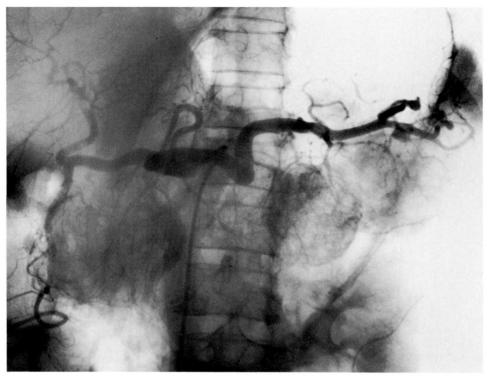

A

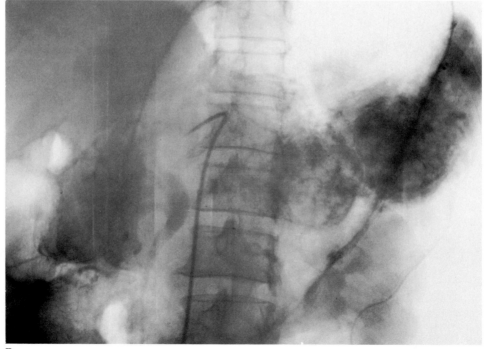

B

Figure 62-19. (A and B) Multiple benign cyst-adenomas of the pancreas. At celiac angiography multiple richly vascularized tumors with cystic components are found in the body and tail of the pancreas. Additional tumors were present in the head and body of the pancreas, supplied from the common hepatic and superior mesenteric arteries.

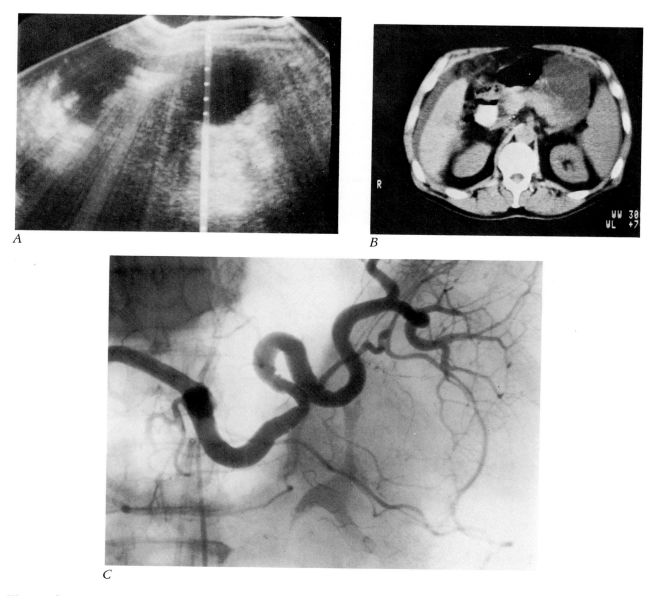

Figure 62-20. A palpable mass was thought to represent a pancreatic pseudocyst at ultrasonography (A). CT proved the lesion to have an irregular attachment to the tail of the pancreas (B). At celiac angiography (C) a poorly vascularized lesion was observed. The splenic artery has a local constriction. Percutaneous biopsy verified a malignant lesion, which proved to be a cystadenocarcinoma.

the contrast medium, which is often observed, causes a heterogeneous appearance of the tumor corresponding to the cystic and solid tissue components in the tumor. Compression or occlusion of the portal venous system is often noticed. This type of lesion may be difficult or impossible to distinguish from nonactive endocrine tumors of the pancreas or leiomyosarcoma originating in or infiltrating the gland.

A low grade of vascularization has been observed in benign tumors [2, 249] as well as in cystadenocarcinomas [99, 117]. In this situation the tumors will be difficult to distinguish from pancreatic pseudocysts or even cystic adenocarcinoma (Fig. 62-20; see also Fig. 62-6). Ultrasonography or CT including biopsy will, however, give the necessary information about the lesion.

UNCOMMON TUMORS

Angiomatous lesions of different types occur in the pancreas: telangiectasia of the hereditary type as a manifestation of Rendu-Osler-Weber disease, true hemangiomas, or an unspecific type of angiodysplasia [11, 67, 76, 115, 121, 123, 139, 184, 215, 222]. From a differential point of view these lesions, when small and well circumscribed, may have an appearance similar to that of an insuloma, but the draining veins are observed earlier and better in the angiomatous lesions (see Fig. 62-15). In their more diffuse form the lesions may resemble the hypervascular types of pancreatitis [23, 27, 145, 220].

Leiomyosarcoma [44, 99], reticulum cell sarcoma [4, 182, 260], and other retroperitoneal tumors [121, 180] may invade the pancreas and cause angiographic abnormalities. Sometimes, when richly vascularized, they simulate a cystadenocarcinoma; at other times they infiltrate arteries as in adenocarcinoma. Usually, however, they cause more prominent changes than the scirrhous ductal carcinoma. Also, invasion from gastric cancer [50, 222] or metastatic nodes [58, 216] may produce abnormalities, as in ductal cancer. Lymphomatous abnormalities usually cause only displacement of vessels [182, 260].

PANCREATITIS

Until a few years ago angiography, in experienced hands, was regarded as a valuable method in the diagnosis of pancreatitis (Figs. 62-21–62-25; see also Figs. 62-12, 62-13) when characteristic, although not pathognomonic, abnormalities could be observed in the pancreatic vasculature. These vascular abnormalities occurred often in both acute and chronic pancreatitis but were most prominent in patients who had had the disease for more than 2 years [217, 262]. Particularly ERCP, but also ultrasonography and CT have drastically reduced the indications for angiography in pancreatitis and its sequelae. Nevertheless, there is still reason to be aware of the vascular changes that can be observed because the newer methods can fail. Another important indication for angiography in pancreatitis is gastrointestinal hemorrhage as a dominant symptom.

Acute Pancreatitis

In the uncomplicated form of acute pancreatitis the angiogram usually appears normal, but a widening and stretching of the pancreatic arteries

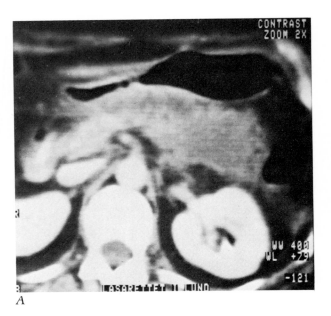

A

Figure 62-21. Abscess of the tail of the pancreas following blunt trauma in a patient with chronic alcoholism. (A) CT showing tail of pancreas expanded by a poorly outlined lesion. (B) Angiography showing vascular changes typical of pancreatitis with smooth narrowing of the distal part of the splenic artery. (C) Venous phase showing splenic vein compressed by pancreatic abscess and venous collaterals.

due to edema may be observed [1, 217, 262]. If angiography is performed after the acute attack has subsided, tortuosity and arterial irregularities may be seen as well as venous compression or occlusion [262]. Also, aneurysms of the splenic or gastroduodenal arteries have been observed after an acute attack of pancreatitis.

Recurrent Acute or Chronic Pancreatitis

Recurrent acute or chronic pancreatitis (relapsing pancreatitis) almost always shows vascular abnormalities of the same kind as previously described. There is a continuous progression of the vascular changes depending on how long the disease has been present and on the severity of the attacks. Sequelae, such as pseudocysts and abscesses, can cause marked vascular displacement and venous compression or occlusion (see Figs. 62-12, 62-13, 62-21). Hypervascularization of the pancreas may be present but is not regularly observed (Fig. 62-22).

Chronic Pancreatitis

The characteristic finding first described by Reuter et al. [217] is the beaded appearance of smaller pancreatic arteries, with short dilated

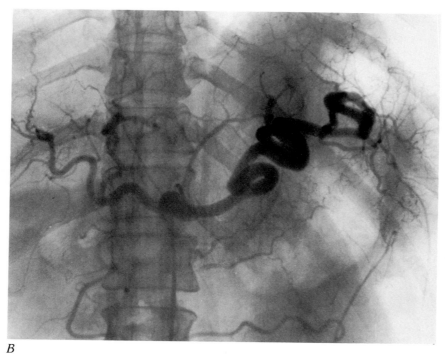

B

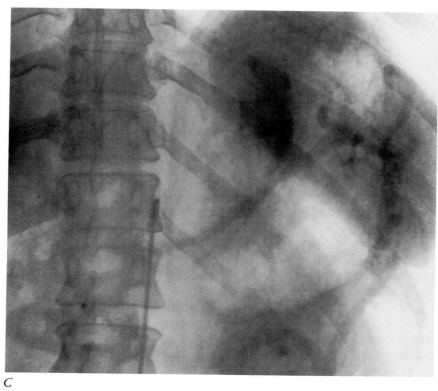

C

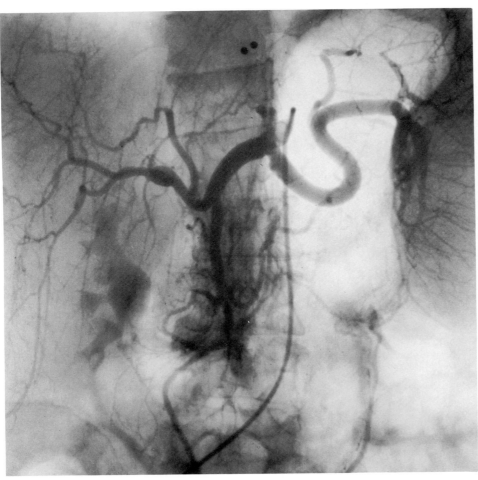

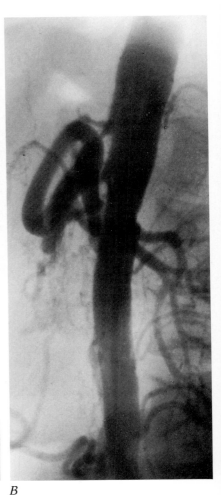

A   *B*

Figure 62-22. Chronic recurrent calcifying pancreatitis. At celiac angiography (A) and lumbar aortography (lateral view) (B) marked stenosis of the celiac axis and occlusion of the superior mesenteric artery are observed. Local short constriction typical of pancreatitis is seen in the splenic artery. Marked hypervascularization and irregular, tortuous pancreatic arteries are other typical findings.

segments alternating with stenosed parts. Short diaphragmlike stenoses are frequently observed in the larger arteries [121, 123]. Smooth regular stenoses of arteries surrounding the pancreas are typical in a high percentage of cases. Changes resembling fibromuscular dysplasia may also be noted (see Fig. 62-13). Stenoses of the celiac and/or superior mesenteric arteries are often encountered [142, 262]. Arterial aneurysms may be observed in the spleen and in the hepatic, gastroduodenal, and jejunal arteries. Displacement of arteries sometimes occurs with pseudocysts or abscesses but is also due to retraction secondary to peripancreatic fibrosis [49, 262]. The vascularization of the pancreas varies from markedly increased [23, 27, 220] to markedly decreased [121, 123]. Occlusion or compression of the splenic, superior mesenteric, or portal veins is a common finding.

It appears obvious that the vascular changes observed in the various forms of pancreatitis depend largely on when the angiographic procedure is performed and also on the intensity of the disease and whether pseudocysts or abscesses have occurred. It is likewise clear that in chronic pancreatitis the duration of the disease is of importance [217, 220, 262]. This may explain the somewhat contradictory reports of findings in chronic pancreatitis, ranging from an increased vascular supply to hypovascularization, from normal arteries to various forms of arterial stenoses, tortuosity, beading, displacement, etc. [21, 44, 59, 142, 146, 161, 178, 180, 207, 220, 222, 227].

Celiac and/or superior mesenteric arterial stenosis is found more often in patients with pancreatitis [59, 142, 262] than in unselected series of patients examined with angiography [57]. Arteriosclerosis or compression from the crura may cause the constriction [85, 86, 214]. It is, however, conceivable that the close relationship of these vessels to the pancreas is of importance and could explain the increased frequency of abnormalities (Fig. 62-22).

The most important angiographic observation in patients with pancreatitis is aneurysms, which in collected series are found in approximately 10 percent of patients [49, 262, 273]. Numerous reports of single or a few cases of aneurysms that have ruptured and caused gastrointestinal hemorrhage, ordinarily in combination with cysts or abscesses, have appeared [20, 38, 40, 74, 95, 108, 113, 127, 147, 149, 150, 237, 269, 273]. Most aneurysms occur in the splenic or gastroduodenal arteries, but aneurysms have been observed in other arteries as well, such as the jejunal and left gastric arteries (Fig. 62-23). One can expect that in a patient with severe pancreatitis, the enzymes will first attack the arteries within or close to the pancreas.

The so-called blood cysts of the pancreas are probably the result of destroyed small intrapancreatic arteries (Fig. 62-24). Later on, when the pancreatic enzymes pass out into the "mesenteric planes" [168] destruction of more peripherally situated arteries can be expected (Fig. 62-25). Aneurysms in these areas can of course have other etiologies than pancreatitis [40, 116]. Tylén did not find any aneurysms in patients with calcifying chronic pancreatitis [262], and he thought the explanation lay in the fact that peripancreatitis is not so prominent in this type of disease. A bleeding arterial aneurysm has, however, been found even in calcifying pancreatitis [66, 113, 231]. Angiography is rewarding in such a case because today it is possible not only to find the aneurysm but to treat it with electrocoagulation or embolization [105]. In severe attacks of pancreatitis, both arterial wall destruction and thrombosis, with consequent bowel infarction, may occur [263].

Another important and frequent sequela of pancreatitis is venous compression or occlusion by thrombosis. Like other vascular structures in or around the pancreas, the veins showed progression of the disease when they were later followed up by repeat angiography [49].

Vascular abnormalities may thus occur both in carcinoma of the pancreas and in pancreatitis. In most cases high-quality angiography can distinguish between these two entities [52, 216, 259], but there are clearly cases in which it is not possible to make a distinction between them. Most often the angiographic changes caused by chronic pancreatitis are said to be the result of a carcinoma, but the opposite error also occurs. With the modern angiographic methods previously mentioned, such errors are infrequent today [156].

Pseudocysts and Abscesses

Ultrasonography and CT are more reliable methods than angiography for disclosing pseudocysts and abscesses (see Figs. 62-13, 62-21, 62-24, 62-25), but it is in patients with this condition that angiography is particularly important, mainly because of the severe vascular complications that often occur [263]. Levin et al. [147] noted four reasons for performing angiography when pseudocysts have been diagnosed. The primary indication should be because of the particularly high frequency of aneurysms in patients with pancreatitis and pseudocysts. Operation on a pseudocyst without knowledge of the vasculature adjacent to it may cause a massive hemorrhage [231]. The aneurysms may be clinically silent and they may even close [69]. Thus there is every reason to follow the patients closely if operation or intraarterial therapy is not contemplated (see Fig. 62-24).

A second reason for angiography is the fact that the pseudocysts may be secondary to pancreatic carcinoma obstructing the duct. Neither CT nor ultrasonography may show the true cause for the cyst formation, and therefore ERCP and/or angiography should give complementary information.

Third, in cases of cystadenoma ultrasonography and CT may not reveal the true lesion but only suggest the presence of a cystic tumor. Abundant tumor vessels may disclose the true nature, but it should be emphasized that the hypovascular cystadenoma might very well simulate a pseudocyst or an abscess. In one case recently observed, CT and percutaneous biopsy gave reliable information while ultrasonography and angiography gave the impression of a pseudocyst (see Fig. 62-20).

The fourth reason for angiography in pseudocysts or abscesses is the extrahepatic portal hypertension that is frequently observed and always possible to show with angiography.

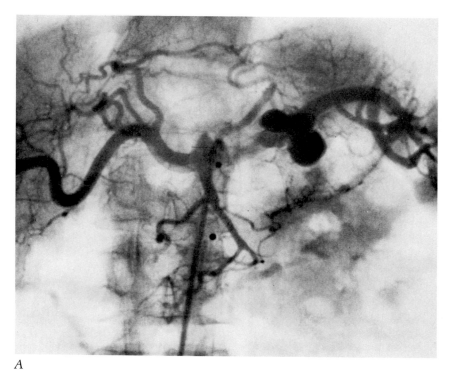

A

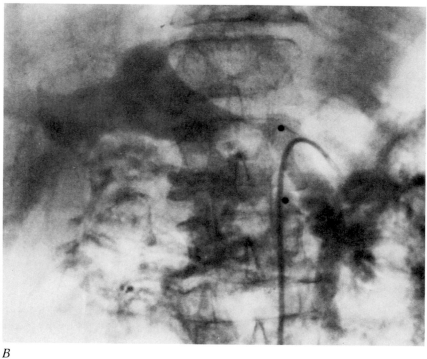

B

Figure 62-23. (A) Chronic pancreatitis with aneurysm of the splenic artery rupturing into the pancreatic duct with gastrointestinal bleeding. (B) Celiac angiography showing a 16-mm aneurysm of the splenic artery penetrating the pancreas with hypervascularization of the tail of the pancreas. Marked constriction of the portal vein due to peripancreatic fibrosis is observed in the venous phase of superior mesenteric angiography. Bradykinin was used to increase the flow rate.

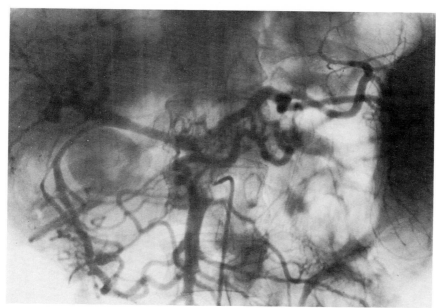

Figure 62-24. Recurrent chronic pancreatitis with complete occlusion of celiac axis and a blood cyst in the head of the pancreas. Since there was no severe bleeding in the gastrointestinal tract, no operation was performed. At control angiography 6 months later the aneurysm had disappeared.

Figure 62-25. Pseudocyst in the lesser sac and in the small bowel mesentery secondary to chronic pancreatitis. Aneurysms are present in splenic and jejunal arteries (*arrowheads*).

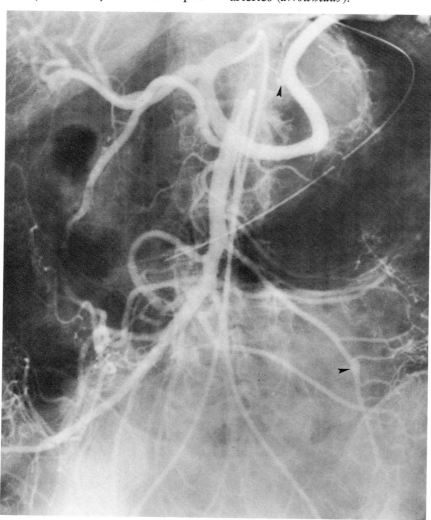

TRAUMA

Direct contusion of the pancreas by a steering wheel or in bicycle accidents is not rare. The close relationship of the pancreas and the spine forms the anatomic basis for blunt traumatic lesions of the gland (see Fig. 62-21). Occlusion of pancreatic arteries and impaired circulation of the organ are common angiographic findings in the acute phase. Displacement of arteries adjacent to the pancreas and spleen occurs when hematoma is present [28, 114]. Rupture of the splenic artery with extravasation has also been observed [102]. Compression or occlusion of the portal venous system as well as displacement secondary to hematoma formation may be observed. Portal venous thrombosis is a known complication of pancreatic trauma [68].

The most frequent complication of pancreatic trauma is pseudocyst or abscess formation, which may appear within a few weeks [60]. The lesions of posttraumatic pancreatitis and pseudocysts are the same as in other types of pancreatitis.

References

1. Aakhus, T., Hofsli, M., and Vestad, E. Angiography in acute pancreatitis. *Acta Radiol. [Diagn.]* (Stockh.) 8:119, 1969.
2. Abrams, R. M., Berenbaum, E. R., Berenbaum, S. L., and Ngo, N. L. Angiographic studies of benign and malignant cystadenoma of the pancreas. *Radiology* 89:1028, 1967.
3. Adler, O., Kaftori, J. K., Rosenberger, A., and Ben Arieh, J. Non-functioning islet cell tumors of the pancreas: A review of radiological literature and a report of two cases. *ROEFO* 127:559, 1977.
4. Albrechtsson, U., and Tylén, U. Angiography in reticulum cell sarcoma. *Acta Radiol. [Diagn.]* (Stockh.) 18:210, 1977.
5. Alfidi, R. J., Bhyun, D. S., Crile, G., Jr., and Hawk, W. Arteriography and hypoglycemia. *Surg. Gynecol. Obstet.* 133:447, 1971.
6. Almén, T. A steering device for selective angiography and some vascular and enzymatic reactions observed in its clinical application. *Acta Radiol. [Suppl.]* (Stockh.) 260:1966.
7. Anacker, H. Pankreas-Karzinom—Angiographische Diagnostik. *Langenbecks Arch. Chir.* 339:239, 1975.
8. Andersson, H., Dotevall, G., Fagerberg, G., et al. Pancreatic tumor with diarrhea, hypokalemia and hypochlorhydria. *Acta Chir. Scand.* 138:102, 1972.
9. Ariyama, J., Shirakabe, H., Ikenobe, H., Kurosawa, A., and Owman, T. The diagnosis of the small resectable pancreatic carcinoma. *Clin. Radiol.* 28:437, 1977.
10. Ariyama, J., Shirakabe, H., Ikenobe, H., Kurosawa, A., and Sumida, M. Angiographic diagnosis of pancreatic carcinoma. *Stomach and Intestine* 11:1605, 1976.
11. Ariyama, J., Shirakabe, H., Sumida, M., and Bartram, C. I. Angiographic evaluation of the abnormal endoscopic pancreatogram. *Gastrointest. Radiol.* 4:231, 1979.
12. Arnesjö, B., Ihse, I., Lilja, P., Ljungberg, O., and Petersson, B.-G. Insuloma—a neglected diagnosis? *Lakartidningen* 73:51, 1976. (In Swedish.)
13. Aronsen, K.-F., and Nylander, G. Angiographic studies of the action of vasopressin in the dog. *Vasc. Dis.* 1:127, 1964.
14. Artigas, V., and Sala, E. La arteriografia selectiva en el diagnostico de las afecciones hepaticas y pancreaticas. *Rev. Int. Hepat.* 15:359, 1965.
15. Auerbach, R. C., and Koehler, P. R. The many faces of islet cell tumors. *AJR* 119:133, 1973.
16. Baghery, S., Alfidi, R. J., and Zelch, M. G. Angiography of non-functioning islet cell tumors of the pancreas. *Radiology* 120:57, 1976.
17. Bång, I. Ein angiographisch diagnostizierter Fall von Cystadenoma Pancreatis. *Radiologe* 5:287, 1965.
18. Baron, M. G. Carcinoma of the pancreas demonstrated by selective celiac angiography. *Mount Sinai J. Med. (N.Y.)* 33:97, 1966.
19. Baron, M. G., Mitty, H. A., and Wolf, B. S. The arteriographic appearance of carcinoma of the uncinate process of the pancreas. *AJR* 101:649, 1967.
20. Baum, S., Greenstein, R. H., Nusbaum, M., and Blakemore, W. Diagnosis of ruptured non-calcified splenic artery aneurysm by selective celiac arteriography. *Arch. Surg.* 91:1026, 1965.
21. Baum, S., Kuroda, K., and Roy, R. H. The value of special angiographic techniques in the management of patients with abdominal neoplasms. *Radiol. Clin. North Am.* 3:583, 1965.
22. Baum, S., Roy, R., Finkelstein, A. K., and Blakemore, W. S. Clinical application of selective celiac and superior mesenteric arteriography. *Radiology* 84:279, 1965.
23. Bennet, J., Bigot, R., Monnier, J. P., Goldlust, M., and Doyon, D. Les hypervascularisations pancréatiques. *J. Radiol. Electrol. Med. Nucl.* 52:485, 1971.
24. Bennet, J., Chérigié, E., Caroli, J., Doyon, D., Economopoulos, P., Plessier, J., and Stoopen, M. La pancréatographie après stimulation par la sécrétin intra-artériell (à propos de 33 cas). *Ann. Radiol.* (Paris) 10:617, 1967.
25. Bieber, W. P., and Albo, R. J. Cystadenoma of

the pancreas: Its arteriographic diagnosis. *Radiology* 80:776, 1963.

26. Bierman, H. R., Miller, E. R., Byron, R. L., Jr., Dod, K. S., Kelly, K. H., and Black, D. H. Intra-arterial catheterization of viscera in man. *AJR* 66:555, 1951.

27. Bigot, R., Lagadec, B., Monnier, J.-P., and Doyon, D. Artériographie d'une pancréatite subaiguë. *Ann. Radiol.* (Paris) 14:801, 1971.

28. Bléry, M., Etienne, J., Farah, A., and Bismuth, V. Le traumatisme du pancréas. Intérêt de l'artériographie sélective. *Sem. Hop. Paris* 48:473, 1972.

29. Bloom, S. R., Polak, J. M., and Pearse, A. G. E. Vasoactive intestinal peptide and watery-diarrhoea syndrome. *Lancet* 2:14, 1973.

30. Boijsen, E. Selective hepatic angiography in primary and secondary tumors of the liver. *Rev. Int. Hepat.* 15:383, 1965.

31. Boijsen, E. Selective pancreatic angiography. *Br. J. Radiol.* 39:481, 1966.

32. Boijsen, E. Selective visceral angiography using a percutaneous axillary technique. *Br. J. Radiol.* 39:414, 1966.

33. Boijsen, E. Pancreatic Angiography. In H. L. Abrams (ed.), *Angiography* (2nd ed.). Boston: Little, Brown, 1971.

34. Boijsen, E. Angiography in Pancreatic Disease. In M. M. Forell (ed.), *Handbuch der inneren Medizin,* III/6, Berlin, Heidelberg, New York: Springer-Verlag, 1976.

35. Boijsen, E. Inactive malignant endocrine tumors of the pancreas. *Radiologe* 15:177, 1975.

36. Boijsen, E. Pancreatic Angiography and ERCP in Patients with Pancreatic Carcinoma. In A. R. Margulis and C. A. Gooding (eds.), *Diagnostic Radiology.* New York: Masson, 1979. P. 319.

37. Boijsen, E., and Bron, K. M. Visceral arteriography. *Ann. Rev. Med.* 15:273, 1964.

38. Boijsen, E., and Efsing, H.-O. Aneurysm of the splenic artery. *Acta Radiol.* [*Diagn.*] (Stockh.) 8:29, 1969.

39. Boijsen, E., and Göthlin, J. Abdominal angiography after intraarterial injection of vasopressin. *Acta Radiol.* [*Diagn.*] (Stockh.) 21:523, 1980.

40. Boijsen, E., Göthlin, J., Hallböök, T., and Sandblom, P. Preoperative angiographic diagnosis of bleeding aneurysms of abdominal visceral arteries. *Radiology* 93:781, 1969.

41. Boijsen, E., Lunderquist, A., and Isper, J. The relative value of radiologic imaging methods in patients with obstructive jaundice. In press.

42. Boijsen, E., Lundh, G., and Stormby, N. Roentgenologic, secretoric and cytologic diagnosis of cancer of the pancreas. *Acta Chir. Scand.* [Suppl.] 332:104, 1965.

43. Boijsen, E., and Maly, P. Vergrösserungstechnik in der abdominellen Angiographie. *Radiologe* 18:167, 1978.

44. Boijsen, E., and Olin, T. Zöliakographie und Angiographie der Arteria mesenterica superior. In H. R. Schinz, G. Glauner, and A. Rüttiman (eds.), *Ergebnisse der medizinische Strahlenforschung Neue Folge.* Stuttgart: Thieme, 1964.

45. Boijsen, E., and Redman, H. C. Effects of bradykinin on celiac and superior mesenteric angiography. *Invest. Radiol.* 1:422, 1966.

46. Boijsen, E., and Redman, H. C. Effect of epinephrine on celiac and superior mesenteric angiography. *Invest. Radiol.* 2:184, 1967.

47. Boijsen, E., and Reuter, S. R. Combined percutaneous transhepatic cholangiography and angiography in the evaluation of obstructive jaundice. *AJR* 99:153, 1967.

48. Boijsen, E., and Samuelsson, L. Angiographic diagnosis of tumors arising from the pancreatic islets. *Acta Radiol.* [*Diagn.*] (Stockh.) 10:161, 1970.

49. Boijsen, E., and Tylén, U. Vascular changes in chronic pancreatitis. *Acta Radiol.* [*Diagn.*] (Stockh.) 12:34, 1972.

50. Boijsen, E., Wallace, S., and Kanter, I. E. Angiography in tumors of the stomach. *Acta Radiol.* [*Diagn.*] (Stockh.) 4:306, 1966.

51. Bookstein, J., and Oberman, H. A. Appraisal of selective angiography in localizing islet-cell tumors of the pancreas. *Radiology* 86:682, 1966.

52. Bookstein, J. J., Reuter, S. R., and Martel, W. Angiographic evaluation of pancreatic carcinoma. *Radiology* 93:757, 1969.

53. Bourgeon, R., Ghnassia, J.-P., Audoly, P., Navarro, B., and Kermarec, J. Adénome langerhansien et artériographie. *J. Chir.* (Paris) 103:509, 1972.

54. Bozymski, E. M., Woodruff, K., and Sessions, J. T., Jr. Zollinger-Ellison syndrome with hypoglycemia associated with calcification of the tumor and its metastases. *Gastroenterology* 65:658, 1973.

55. Braasch, J. W., and Gray, B. N. Technique of radical pancreatoduodenectomy with consideration of hepatic arterial relationships. *Surg. Clin. North Am.* 56:631, 1976.

56. Breidahl, H. D., Priestly, J. T., and Rynearson, E. H. Hyperinsulinism: Surgical aspects and results. *Ann. Surg.* 142:698, 1955.

57. Bron, K. M., and Redman, H. C. Splanchnic artery stenosis and occlusion: Incidence; arteriographic and clinical manifestations. *Radiology* 92:323, 1969.

58. Bron, K. M., and Sherman, L. Arteriography in evaluating retroperitoneal mass lesions. *N.Y. State J. Med.* 67:1875, 1967.

59. Bücheler, E., Boldt, I., Frommhold, H., and Käufer, C. Die angiographische Diagnostik der Pankreastumoren und der Pankreatitis. *ROEFO* 115:726, 1971.

60. Bücheler, E., Raschke, E., and Felix, R. Abs-

zess in der Bursa omentalis nach traumatischer Pankreasruptur. *ROEFO* 107:293, 1967.

61. Bücheler, E., and Thelen, M. Angiographie der Äste des Truncus coeliacus. *Roentgenblaetter* 24:11, 1971.

62. Buonocore, E., Meaney, T. F., Skillern, P. G., and Crile, G., Jr. Functioning pancreatic islet-cell adenoma diagnosed preoperatively by means of splanchnic arteriography. *Arch. Intern. Med.* 116:824, 1965.

63. Buranasiri, S., and Baum, S. The significance of the venous phase of celiac and superior mesenteric arteriography in evaluating pancreatic carcinoma. *Radiology* 102:11, 1972.

64. Cen, M., and Rosenbusch, G. Zöliakographie mit Adrenalin. Möglichkeiten der Pharmakoangiographie in der Pankreasdiagnostik. *ROEFO* 111:82, 1970.

65. Chérigié, E., Mellière, D., Bennet, J., Doyon, D., and Chenard, J. C. Anatomie radiologique de la vascularisation du pancréas. *J. Radiol. Electrol. Med. Nucl.* 48:346, 1967.

66. Chermet, J., Bigot, J.-M., and Monnier, J.-P. Les hémorrhagies digestives par érosions artérielles au cours des pancréatites. Diagnostic pré-opératoire par l'artériographie en urgence. *J. Radiol. Electrol. Med. Nucl.* 55:117, 1974.

67. Chuang, V. P., Pulmano, C. M., Walter, J. F., and Cho, K. J. Angiography of pancreatic arteriovenous malformation. *AJR* 129:1015, 1977.

68. Chvojka, J. Ein Beitrag der gezielten Angiographie zur Diagnostik der Pankreasverletzungen. *ROEFO* 113:336, 1970.

69. Chvojka, J. Ungewöhnliche Komplikation akuter Pankreatitis im angiographischen Bild. *ROEFO* 124:131, 1976.

70. Classen, M., Koch, H., and Rösch, W. Duodenoskopische Diagnose des Pankreaskarzinoms. *Leber Magen Darm* 4:222, 1974.

71. Clemett, A. R., and Park, W. M. Arteriographic demonstration of pancreatic tumor in the Zollinger-Ellison syndrome. *Radiology* 88:32, 1967.

72. Clouse, M. E., Costello, P., Legg, M. A., Soeldner, S. J., and Cady, B. Subselective angiography in localizing insulomas of the pancreas. *AJR* 128:741, 1977.

73. Clouse, M. E., Gregg, J. A., and Sedgwick, C. E. Angiography vs pancreatography in diagnosis of carcinoma of the pancreas. *Radiology* 114:605, 1975.

74. Corbeau, A., Sahel, J., Fraissinet, R., et al. Wirsungorragie, diagnostic artériographique en urgence. A propos d'un cas. *J. Radiol. Electrol. Med. Nucl.* 59:275, 1978.

75. Cortesini, R. L'arteriografia selettiva del tripode celiaco e delle arterie renali. *Policlinico* [*Prat.*] 70:817, 1963.

76. Couinaud, Jouan, Prot, Chalut, and Schneider.

Hémo-lymphangiome de la tête du pancréas. *Mem. Acad. Chir.* (Paris) 92:152, 1966.

77. Creutzfeldt, W. Klinik der chronischen Pancreatitis. In K. Heinkel and H. Schön (eds.), *Pathogenese, Diagnostik, Klinik und Therapie der Erkrankungen des exokrinen Pankreas.* Stuttgart: Schattauer, 1964.

78. Davis, L. J., Anderson, J. H., Wallace, S., Gianturco, C., and Jacobson, E. D. The use of prostaglandin E_1 to enhance the angiographic visualization of the splanchnic circulation. *Radiology* 114:281, 1975.

79. Dencker, H., Göthlin, J., Hedner, P., Lunderquist, A., Norryd, C., and Tylén, U. Superior mesenteric angiography and blood flow following intra-arterial injection of prostaglandin $F_{2\alpha}$. *AJR* 125:111, 1975.

80. Deutsch, V., Adar, R., Jacob, E. T., Bank, H., and Mozes, M. Angiographic diagnosis and differential diagnosis of islet-cell tumors. *AJR* 119:121, 1973.

81. Diard, F., Tavernier, J., Delorme, G., and Rabin, A. Diagnostic angiographique des nésidioblastomes. *Ann. Radiol.* (Paris) 17:101, 1974.

82. Di Magno, E. P., Malagelada, J.-R., Taylor, W. F., and Go, V. L. W. A prospective comparison of current diagnostic tests for pancreatic cancer. *N. Engl. J. Med.* 297:737, 1977.

83. Dodds, J., Maddison, F. E., Hogan, W. J., and Schulte, W. J. Arteriographic demonstration of two islet cell tumors in a patient with Zollinger-Ellison syndrome. *Radiol. Clin.* (Basel) 42:110, 1973.

84. Doust, B. D., and Redman, H. C. The myth of 1 ml/kg in angiography. *Radiology* 104:551, 1972.

85. Drapanas, T., and Bron, K. M. Stenosis of the celiac artery. *Ann. Surg.* 164:1085, 1966.

86. Dunbar, J. D., Molnar, W., Beman, F. F., and Marable, S. A. Compression of the celiac trunk and abdominal angina: Preliminary report of 15 cases. *AJR* 95:731, 1965.

87. Eaton, S. B., Fleischli, D. J., Pollard, J. J., Nebesar, R. A., and Potsaid, M. S. Comparison of current radiologic approaches to the diagnosis of pancreatic disease. *N. Engl. J. Med.* 279:389, 1968.

88. Eisenberg, H. Angiography of the Pancreas. In S. K. Hilal (ed.), *Small Vessel Angiography. Imaging, Morphology, Physiology, and Clinical Applications.* St. Louis: Mosby, 1973.

89. Epstein, H. Y., Abrams, R. M., Berenbaum, E. R., and Localio, S. A. Angiographic localization of insulinomas. High reported success rate and two additional cases. *Ann. Surg.* 169:349, 1969.

90. Evans, J. Techniques in the detection and diagnosis of malignant lesions of the liver, spleen and pancreas. *Radiol. Clin. North Am.* 3:567, 1965.

91. Fitzgerald, P. J., Fartner, J. G., Watson, R. C., et al. The value of diagnostic aids in detecting pancreas cancer. *Cancer* 41:868, 1978.
92. Fontaine, J.-L., Piétri, J., and Babin, S. De l'utilité de l'angiographie sélective d'urgence pour le diagnostic des hémopéritoines. *Presse Med.* 75:655, 1967.
93. Fontaine, R., Kieny, R., and Lang, G. Découverte par l'angiographie sélective d'une tumeur ulcérogène du pancréas à symptomatologie atypique. *Mem. Acad. Chir.* (Paris) 91:896, 1965.
94. Fontaine, R., Lampert, M., Babin, S., and Philippe, E. Quelques refléxions sur les tumeurs du pancréas endocrine, à propos d'une observation nouvelle de nésidioblastome malin, nonfonctionelle, de la tête du pancréas, traité par duodenopancréatectomie avec une survie prolongée. *Ann. Chir.* 22:1285, 1968.
95. Francillon, J., Grandjean, J. P., Vignal, J., Tissot, E., and Moulay, A. Hemorrhagie artérielle dans l'évolution des pseudokystes pancréatiques. *Lyon Chir.* 70/3:192, 1974.
96. Fredens, M., Egeblad, M., and Holst-Nielsen, F. The value of selective angiography in the diagnosis of tumors in pancreas and liver. *Radiology* 93:765, 1969.
97. Freeny, P. C., and Ball, T. J. Evaluation of endoscopic retrograde cholangiopancreatography and angiography in the diagnosis of pancreatic carcinoma. *AJR* 130:683, 1978.
98. Freeny, P. C., Ball, T. J., and Ryan, J. Impact of new diagnostic imaging methods on pancreatic angiography. *AJR* 133:619, 1979.
99. Freeny, P. C., Weinstein, C. J., Taft, D. A., and Allen, F. H. Cystic neoplasms of the pancreas: New angiographic and ultrasonographic findings. *AJR* 131:795, 1978.
100. Fujii, K., Yamagata, S., Sasaki, R., Ohneda, A., Shoji, T., and Suzuki, J. Arteriography in insuloma. *AJR* 120:634, 1974.
101. Fulton, R. E., Sheedy, P. F., II, McIlrath, D. C., and Ferris, D. O. Preoperative angiographic localization of insulin-producing tumors of the pancreas. *AJR* 123:367, 1975.
102. Geindre, M., Marty, F., Fournet, J., Baudain, Ph., and Champetier, M. Aspects angiographiques des contusions du pancréas. *Ann. Radiol.* 16:341, 1973.
103. Glenn, F., Evans, J. A., Halpern, M., and Thorbjarnarson, B. Selective celiac and superior mesenteric arteriography. *Surg. Gynecol. Obstet.* 118:93, 1964.
104. Glenn, F., and Halpern, M. Celiac and superior mesenteric angiography. *Rev. Int. Hepat.* 15:337, 1965.
105. Gold, R. E., Blair, D. C., Finlay, J. B., and Johnston, D. W. B. Transarterial electrocoagulation therapy of a pseudoaneurysm in the head of the pancreas. *AJR* 125:422, 1975.
106. Gold, R. P., Black, T. J., Rotterdam, H., and Casarella, W. J. Radiologic and pathologic characteristics of the WDHA syndrome. *AJR* 127:397, 1976.
107. Gold, R. P., Casarella, W. J., Stern, G., and Seaman, W. B. Transhepatic cholangiography: The radiological method of choice in suspected obstructive jaundice. *Radiology* 133:39, 1979.
108. Goldlust, D., Chalut, J., and Rault, J. J. Un cas d'anéurysme de l'artère pancréatique dorsale. *J. Radiol. Electrol. Med. Nucl.* 51:519, 1970.
109. Goldstein, H. M., Neiman, H. L., and Bookstein, J. J. Angiographic evaluation of pancreatic disease. A further appraisal. *Radiology* 112:275, 1974.
110. Göthlin, J., Mansoor, M., and Tranberg, K.-G. Combined percutaneous transhepatic cholangiography (PTC) and selective visceral angiography (SVA) in obstructive jaundice. *AJR* 117:419, 1973.
111. Goulon, M., Rapin, M., Charleux, H., Baguet, J.-C., Kuntziger, H., Nouailhat, F., Barois, A., and Breteau, M. Diarrhée aqueuse et hypokaliémie associées à une tumeur langerhansienne non insulino-sécrétante: Discussion nosologique de ce syndrome avec celui de Zollinger et Ellison. *Presse Med.* 74:2345, 1966.
112. Gray, R. K., Rösch, J., and Grollman, J. H., Jr. Arteriography in the diagnosis of islet cell tumors. *Radiology* 97:39, 1970.
113. Greenstein, A., deMaio, E. F., and Nabseth, D. C. Acute hemorrhage associated with pancreatic pseudocysts. *Surgery* 69:56, 1971.
114. Haertel, M., and Fuchs, W. A. Angiography in pancreatic trauma. *Br. J. Radiol.* 47:641, 1974.
115. Halpern, M., Turner, A. F., and Citron, B. P. Hereditary hemorrhagic telangiectasia: An angiographic study of abdominal visceral angiodysplasia associated with gastrointestinal hemorrhage. *Radiology* 90:1143, 1968.
116. Harris, R. D., Anderson, J. E., and Coel, M. N. Aneurysms of the small pancreatic arteries: A cause of upper abdominal pain and intestinal bleeding. *Radiology* 115:17, 1975.
117. Hawkins, I. F., Jr., and Kaude, J. V. Angiographic findings in some rare pancreatic tumors. *ROEFO* 125:521, 1976.
118. Hawkins, I. F., Kaude, J. V., and MacGregor, A. Priscoline and epinephrine in selective pancreatic angiography. A comparison study using high-pressure injection, Valsalva maneuver and geometric magnification. *Radiology* 116:311, 1975.
119. Hentschel, M. Pankreas-Anatomie. *Langenbecks Arch. Chir.* 313:233, 1965.
120. Hentschel, M. Die Oberbauch-Chirurgie im lichte neurer anatomischer Untersuchungen. *Fortsch. Prax. Fortbild.* 18:647, 1967.
121. Hepp, J., Hernandez, C., Moreaux, J., and Bismuth, H. *L'artériographie dans les affections*

chirurgicales du foie, du pancréas et de la rate. Paris: Masson, 1968.

122. Hernandez, C.   Angiographie des hypoglycémies organique. *Ann. Gastroenterol. Hepatol.* 13:145, 1977.

123. Hernandez, C., Ecarlat, B., and Bismuth, V. L'artérioportographie des affections pancréatiques. *J. Radiol. Electrol. Med. Nucl.* 48:327, 1967.

124. Hernandez, C., and Hélénon, C.   Les tumeurs pancréatiques langerhansiennes (exploration vasculaire). *J. Radiol. Electrol. Med. Nucl.* 48:339, 1967.

125. Hernandez, C., Morin, G., and Ecarlat, B. L'embole pulsé en artériographie sélective digestive. *Presse Med.* 73:2889, 1965.

126. Hessel, S., Siegelman, S. S., Adams, D. F., et al. Prospective Analysis of Computed Tomography and Ultrasound in Evaluating the Pancreas. Presented at the Radiological Society of North America meeting in Atlanta, November, 1979.

127. Hughes, E. S. R., and Joske, R. A.   Aneurysm of the splenic artery and chronic pancreatitis, with a report of successful surgical resection. *Med. J. Aust.* 2:188, 1955.

128. Ingemansson, S., Kühl, C., Larsson, L.-I., Lunderquist, A., and Lundquist, I.   Localization of insulomas and islet cell hyperplasias by pancreatic vein catheterization and insulin assay. *Surg. Gynecol. Obstet.* 146:725, 1978.

129. Jonsson, K., Lunderquist, A., Pettersson, H., and Sigstedt, B.   Subintimal injection of contrast medium as a complication of selective abdominal angiography. *Acta. Radiol.* [*Diagn.*] (Stockh.) 18:55, 1977.

130. Kadell, B. M., and Riley, J. M.   Major arterial involvement by pancreatic pseudocysts. *AJR* 99:632, 1967.

131. Kahn, P. C., and Callow, A. D.   Selective vasodilatation as an aid to angiography. *AJR* 94:213, 1965.

132. Kahn, P. C., Frates, W. J., and Paul, R. E.   The epinephrine effect in angiography of gastrointestinal tract tumors. *Radiology* 88:686, 1967.

133. Karp, W., Lunderquist, A., Tylén, U., and Ihse, I.   Angiography and ultrasonography in the evaluation of pancreatic lesion. *Acta Radiol.* [*Diagn.*] (Stockh.) 21:169, 1980.

134. Kaude, J.   Angiographischer Nachweis eines Insuloms und einer akzessorischen Milz. *ROEFO* 111:130, 1969.

135. Khademi, M., Lazaro, E. J., and Rickert, R. R. Selective arteriography in the diagnosis of chronic inflammatory pancreatic disease. *AJR* 119:141, 1973.

136. Kincaid, O. W., Davis, G. D., Hallermann, F. J., and Hunt, J. C.   Fibromuscular dysplasia of the renal arteries: Arteriographic features, classification and observations on natural history of the disease. *AJR* 104:271, 1968.

137. Korobkin, M. T., Palubinskas, A. J., and Glickman, M. G.   Pitfalls in arteriography of islet cell tumors of the pancreas. *Radiology* 100:319, 1971.

138. Kupic, E. A., Marshall, W. H., and Abrams, H. L.   Splenic arterial patterns: Angiographic analysis and review. *Invest. Radiol.* 2:70, 1967.

139. Lande, A., Bedford, A., and Schechter, L. S. The spectrum of angiographic findings in Osler-Weber-Rendu disease. *Angiology* 27:223, 1976.

140. Lang, E. K.   Angiographic demonstration of carcinoma of the tail of the pancreas. *J. Indiana State Med. Assoc.* 59:252, 1966.

141. Laurijssens, M. J., and Galambos, J. T.   Selective abdominal angiography. *Gut* 6:477, 1965.

142. Lechner, G., and Pokieser, H.   Ergebnisse angiographischer Untersuchungen bei Pankreatitis. *ROEFO* 114:49, 1971.

143. Lechner, G., Pokieser, H., Zaunbauer, W., and Brücke, P.   Zur angiographischen Diagnose des Pankreaskarzinoms. *ROEFO* 113:340, 1970.

144. Lee, J. K. T., Stanley, R. J., Nelson, G. L., and Sagel, S. S.   Pancreatic imaging by ultrasound and computed tomography. A general review. *Radiol. Clin. North Am.* 17:105, 1979.

145. Legre, J., Guien, C., Clément, J. P., and Piétri, H.   Tumeurs pancréatiques a caractère angiomateux revelées par angiographie sélective. *J. Radiol. Electrol. Med. Nucl.* 50:229, 1969.

146. Lenarduzzi, G., Romani, S., and Zacchi, C.   La stimulazione farmacologica della funzione esocrina nella contrastografia opaca del pancreas. *Radiol. Med.* (Torino) 54:97, 1968.

147. Levin, D. C., Eisenberg, H., and Wilson, R. The role of arteriography in the evaluation of pancreatic pseudocysts. *AJR* 129:243, 1977.

148. Lewicki, A. M., Kupic, E. A., and Kohatsu, S. Selective visceral canine angiography for pancreatic visualization. Use of pharmacodynamic agents. *Invest. Radiol.* 2:119, 1967.

149. L'Herminé, C., Gautier-Benoit, C., Vankemmel, M., and Lemaitre, G.   Les érosions artérielles des pseudokystes pancréatiques. Etude angiographique de six observations. *Ann. Radiol.* (Paris) 14:55, 1971.

150. Lower, W. E., and Farrel, J. I.   Aneurysm of the splenic artery: Report of a case and review of the literature. *Arch. Surg.* 23:182, 1931.

151. Ludin, H., Enderlin, F., Fahrländer, H. J., and Scheidegger, S.   Failure to diagnose Zollinger-Ellison syndrome by pancreatic arteriography. *Br. J. Radiol.* 39:494, 1966.

152. Ludin, H., Fahrländer, H. J., and Maurer, W. Arteriographische Diagnostik von Karzinomen des Pancreaskörpers und schwanzes. *Schweiz. Med. Wochenschr.* 96:871, 1966.

153. Lunderquist, A.   Angiography in carcinoma of the pancreas. *Acta Radiol.* [*Suppl.*] (Stockh.) 235:1, 1965.

154. MacGregor, A. M. C., and Hawkins, I. F., Jr. Selective pharmacodynamic angiography in the diagnosis of carcinoma of the pancreas. *Surg. Gynecol. Obstet.* 137:917, 1973.

155. Mackie, C. R., Blackstone, M. O., Dhorajiwala, J., Bowie, J., and Moossa, A. R. Value of new diagnostic aids in relation to the disease process in pancreatic cancer. *Lancet* 2:385, 1979.

156. Mackie, C. R., Cooper, M. J., Lewis, M. H., and Moossa, A. R. Non-operative differentiation between pancreatic cancer and chronic pancreatitis. *Ann. Surg.* 189:480, 1979.

157. Mackie, C. R., Lu, C. T., Noble, H. G., Cooper, M. B., Collins, P., Block, G. E., and Moossa, A. R. Prospective evaluation of angiography in the diagnosis and management of patients suspected of having pancreatic cancer. *Ann. Surg.* 189:11, 1979.

158. Madsen, B. Demonstration of pancreatic insulomas by angiography. *Br. J. Radiol.* 39:488, 1966.

159. Mallinson, C. N., Bloom, S. R., Warin, A. P., Salmon, P. R., and Cox, B. A glucagonoma syndrome. *Lancet* 2:1, 1974.

160. McAfee, J. G. A survey of complications of abdominal aortography. *Radiology* 68:825, 1957.

161. McConnell, F., Thompson, A. G., and Kiss, J. Selective celiac and superior mesenteric arteriography. *Can. J. Surg.* 9:15, 1966.

162. McGarity, W. C., Miles, A. E., and Hoffman, J. C. Angiographic diagnosis and localization of endocrine tumors. *Ann. Surg.* 173:583, 1971.

163. McGavran, N. H., Unger, R. H., Recant, L., Polk, H. C., Kilo, C., and Levin, M. E. A glucagon-secreting alpha-cell carcinoma of the pancreas. *N. Engl. J. Med.* 274:1408, 1966.

164. McKinnon, C. M., Brant, B., and Rösch, J. Angiography in the diagnosis and management of extrapancreatic islet-cell tumors. *Ann. Surg.* 177:381, 1973.

165. Meaney, T. F., and Buonocore, E. Arteriographic manifestations of pancreatic neoplasm. *AJR* 95:720, 1965.

166. Meaney, T. F., Winkelman, E. I., Sullivan, B. H., and Brown, C. H. Selective splanchnic arteriography in the diagnosis of pancreatic tumors. *Cleve. Clin. Q.* 30:193, 1963.

167. Mellière, D. Cited in Hepp et al. [121].

168. Meyers, M. A., and Evans, J. A. Effect of pancreatitis on the small bowel and colon: Spread along mesenteric planes. *AJR* 119:151, 1973.

169. Michels, N. A. *Blood Supply and Anatomy of the Upper Abdominal Organs, with a Descriptive Atlas.* Philadelphia: Lippincott, 1955.

170. Mikal, S. Operative criteria for diagnosis of cancer in a mass of the head of the pancreas. *Ann. Surg.* 161:395, 1965.

171. Mills, S. R., Doppman, J. L., Dunnick, N. R., and McCarthy, D. M. Evaluation of angiography in Zollinger-Ellison syndrome. *Radiology* 131:317, 1979.

172. Moossa, A. R., Lewis, M. H., and Mackie, C. R. Surgical treatment of pancreatic cancer. *Mayo Clin. Proc.* 54:468, 1979.

173. Moretti, S. Studio-anatomo-radiografico del circolo arterioso pancreatico. *Radiol. Med.* (Torino) 51:16, 1965.

174. Morino, F., Olivero, S., and Tarquini, A. Arteriografia selettiva del tronco celiaco e delle sue branche. (Studio-anatomo-morfolgico). *Minerva Chir.* [Suppl.] 13:279, 1958.

175. Morino, F., and Tarquini, A. Cateterismo attraverso l'arteria omerale per l'arteriografia dei rami collaterali dell'aorta addominale. *Minerva Med.* 47:935, 1956.

176. Morino, F., Tarquini, A., and Olivero, S. Artériographie abdominale sélective par le cathétérisme de l'artère humérale. *Presse Med.* 64:1944, 1956.

177. Morino, F., Tarquini, A., and Quaglia, C. Unsere Erfahrungen mit einer neuen Methode der selektiven abdominellen Arteriographie. *Chirurg* 28:152, 1957.

178. Moskowitz, H., Chait, A., and Mellins, H. Z. "Tumor encasement" of the celiac axis due to chronic pancreatitis. *AJR* 104:641, 1968.

179. Nebesar, R. A., and Pollard, J. J. Advances in abdominal angiography. *Postgrad. Med.* 37:504, 1965.

180. Nebesar, R. A., and Pollard, J. J. A critical evaluation of selective celiac and superior mesenteric angiography in the diagnosis of pancreatic diseases, particularly malignant tumor: Facts and "artefacts." *Radiology* 89:1017, 1967.

181. Nebesar, R. A., Pollard, J. J., Edmunds, L. H., Jr., and McKahn, C. F. Indications for selective celiac and superior mesenteric angiography: Experience with 128 cases. *AJR* 92:1100, 1964.

182. Neiman, H. L., Goldstein, H. M., Silverman, P. J., and Bookstein, J. J. Angiographic features of peripancreatic malignant lymphoma. *Radiology* 115:389, 1975.

183. Nylander, G. Vascular response to vasopressin as reflected in angiography: An experimental study in the dog. *Acta Radiol.* [Suppl.] (Stockh.) 266:1, 1967.

184. Nyman, U. Angiography in hereditary hemorrhagic telangiectasia. *Acta Radiol.* [Diagn.] (Stockh.) 18:581, 1977.

185. Ödman, P. Percutaneous selective angiography of the main branches of the aorta. *Acta Radiol.* (Stockh.) 45:1, 1956.

186. Ödman, P. Percutaneous selective angiography of coeliac artery. *Acta Radiol.* [Suppl.] (Stockh.) 159:1, 1958.

187. Ödman, P. The radiopaque polythene catheter. *Acta Radiol.* (Stockh.) 52:52, 1959.

188. Ödman, P. Pancreatic Angiography. In H. L. Abrams (ed.), *Angiography* (1st ed.). Boston: Little, Brown, 1961.

189. Olivier, C., Hélénon, Epfelbaum, Toumieux,

Favre, Rettori, and Baur, O. Adénome langerhansien hypoglycémiant, l'image artériographique. *Presse Med.* 74:2313, 1966.

190. Olsson, O. Angiographic diagnosis of an islet cell tumor of the pancreas. *Acta Chir. Scand.* 126:346, 1963.

191. Olsson, O. Angiographie bei Pankreastumoren. *Radiologe* 5:281, 1965.

192. Olsson, O. Angiographie in drei Fällen von Insuloma Pancreatis. *Radiologe* 5:286, 1965.

193. Olsson, O. Le diagnostic radiologique du pancréas. *J. Radiol. Electrol. Med. Nucl.* 46:860, 1965.

194. Olsson, O. Die radiologische Pankreasuntersuchung. *Radiol. Clin.* (Basel) 35:14, 1966.

195. Olsson, O., Boijsen, E., and Olin, T. Portography by Simultaneous Catheterization of the Celiac and Superior Mesenteric Arteries. In X. *International Congress Book of Abstracts,* Montreal, 1962.

196. Olsson, O., and Tylén, U. Angiography in carcinoma at the papilla of Vater. *Acta Radiol.* [*Diagn.*] (Stockh.) 12:375, 1972.

197. Otto, H., Reschke, H., and Ewe, K. Arteriographischer Nachweis und operative Behandlung einer ulzerogenen Pankreastumors (Zollinger-Ellison-Syndrom). *Dtsch. Med. Wochenschr.* 94:486, 1969.

198. Palubinskas, A. J., and Ripley, H. R. Fibromuscular hyperplasia in external arteries. *Radiology* 82:451, 1964.

199. Paul, R. E., Jr., Miller, H. H., Kahn, P. C., Callow, A. D., Edwards, T. L., Jr., and Patterson, J. F. Pancreatic angiography, with application of subselective angiography of the celiac and superior mesenteric artery to the diagnosis of carcinoma of the pancreas. *N. Engl. J. Med.* 272:283, 1965.

200. Pierson, J. M. The arterial blood supply of the pancreas. *Surg. Gynecol. Obstet.* 77:426, 1943.

201. Pirker, E. Angiographische Röntgendiagnostik der Oberbauchorgane. *Radiol. Austria.* 12:79, 1961.

202. Pistolesi, G. F., Frasson, F., Fugazzola, C., Taddei, G., and Caresano, A. Angiographic diagnosis of endocrine tumors of the pancreas. *Radiol. Clin.* (Basel) 46:401, 1977.

203. Plessier, J., Doyon, D., Bennet, J., Stoopen, M., Economopoulos, P., Chérigié, E., and Caroli, J. Effets de la sécrétine intra-artérielle en angiographie coeliaque (artériographie couplée avec le tubage duodénal). *Arch. Fr. Mal. App. Dig.* 56:852, 1967.

204. Pokieser, H. Angiographie bei Pankreaserkrankungen. *Roentgenblaetter* 24:281, 1971.

205. Pressman, B. D., Asch, T., and Casarella, W. J. Cystadenoma of the pancreas. A reappraisal of angiographic findings. *AJR* 119:115, 1973.

206. Pyrah, L. N., and Cowie, J. W. Two unusual aortograms. *J. Fac. Radiol.* 8:416, 1957.

207. Ranniger, K., and Saldino, R. M. Arteriographic diagnosis of pancreatic lesions. *Radiology* 86:470, 1966.

208. Redman, H. C., Reuter, S. R., and Miller, W. J. Improvement of superior mesenteric and portal vein visualization with tolazoline. *Invest. Radiol.* 4:24, 1969.

209. Reichardt, W., Ericsson, M., Holst, J., Ingemansson, S., and Lunderquist, A. Glucagonomproduzierende endokrine Pankreastumoren. *Chirurg* 50:754, 1979.

210. Reuben, A., Johnson, A. L., and Cotton, P. B. Is pancreatogram interpretation reliable? A study of observer variation and error. *Br. J. Radiol.* 51:956, 1978.

211. Reuter, S. R. Superselective pancreatic angiography. *Radiology* 92:74, 1969.

212. Reuter, S. R. Modification of pancreatic blood flow with balloon catheters: A new approach to pancreatic angiography. *Radiology* 95:57, 1970.

213. Reuter, S. R. Potential overdiagnosis of pancreatic islet cell adenomas. *J. Can. Assoc. Radiol.* 22:184, 1971.

214. Reuter, S. R., and Olin, T. Stenosis of the celiac artery. *Radiology* 85:617, 1965.

215. Reuter, S. R., and Redman, H. C. *Gastrointestinal Angiography* (2nd ed.). Philadelphia: Saunders, 1977.

216. Reuter, S. R., Redman, H. C., and Bookstein, J. J. Differential problems in the angiographic diagnosis of carcinoma of the pancreas. *Radiology* 96:93, 1970.

217. Reuter, S. R., Redman, H. C., and Joseph, R. R. Angiographic findings in pancreatitis. *AJR* 107:56, 1969.

218. Robins, J. M., Bookstein, J. J., Oberman, H. A., and Fajans, S. S. Selective angiography in localizing islet-cell tumors of the pancreas. *Radiology* 106:525, 1973.

219. Robinson, A. S. Acute pancreatitis following translumbar aortography: Case report with autopsy findings seven weeks following aortogram. *Arch. Surg.* 72:290, 1956.

220. Roe, M., and Greenough, W. G. Marked hypervascularity and arteriovenous shunting in acute pancreatitis. *Radiology* 113:47, 1974.

221. Rösch, J. *Roentgenology of the Spleen and the Pancreas.* Springfield, Ill.: Thomas, 1967.

222. Rösch, J., and Bret, J. Arteriography of the pancreas. *AJR* 94:182, 1965.

223. Rösch, J., and Grollman, J. H., Jr. Superselective arteriography in the diagnosis of abdominal pathology: Technical considerations. *Radiology* 92:1008, 1969.

224. Rosenbusch, G., and Cen, M. Zöliakographie mit Sekretin. Möglichkeiten der Pharmakoangiographie in der Pankreasdiagnostik. *ROEFO* 110:639, 1969.

225. Rosenbusch, G., Lamers, C. B. H., van Tongeren, J. H. M., Boetes, C., Snel, P., and Lubbers,

E. J. C. Röntgendiagnostik beim Zollinger-Ellison-Syndrom. *ROEFO* 129:168, 1978.

226. Roy, P. Percutaneous catheterization via the axillary artery: A new approach to some technical roadblocks in selective arteriography. *AJR* 94:1, 1965.

227. Sammons, B. P., Neal, M. P., Jr., Armstrong, R. H., Jr., and Hager, H. G. Ten years experience with celiac and upper abdominal superior mesenteric arteriography. *AJR* 101:345, 1967.

228. Sarles, H., Muratore, R., Sarles, J.-C., Guien, C., and Camatte, R. Die chronischen Pankreatiden. *Dtsch. Med. Wochenschr.* 87:125, 1962.

229. Sato, T., Saito, Y., Koyama, K., and Watanabe, K. Preoperative determination of operability in carcinomas of the pancreas and the periampullary region. *Ann. Surg.* 168:876, 1968.

230. Scatliff, J. H., Simarak, S., Cutler, L., and Larsen, P. B. Angiography of the celiac axis: Experimental evaluation of methods. *Radiology* 78:215, 1962.

231. Schechter, L. M., Gordon, H. E., and Passaro, E., Jr. Massive hemorrhage from the celiac axis in pancreatitis. *Am. J. Surg.* 128:301, 1974.

232. Schein, R., DeLellis, R. A., Kahn, C. R., Gorden, P., and Kraft, A. R. Islet cell tumors: Current concepts and management. *Ann. Intern. Med.* 79:239, 1973.

233. Scheinin, T. M., and Tala, E. Diagnosis and treatment of pancreatic islet cell adenomas. *Acta Chir. Scand.* 132:590, 1966.

234. Schmarsow, R. Angiography of the pancreas following the administration of secretin, trypsin and histamine. *Acta Radiol. [Diagn.] (Stockh.)* 12:175, 1972.

235. Schmarsow, R., Kiefer, H., Linhart, P., Gruner, H. J., and Hammes, P. H. Sonographie und Pharmakoangiographie des Pankreas. *ROEFO* 131:392, 1979.

236. Serebro, H. A diagnostic sign of carcinoma of the body of the pancreas. *Lancet* 1:85, 1965.

237. Sheps, S. G., Spittel, J. A., Jr., Fairbairn, J. F., II, and Edwards, J. E. Aneurysms of the splenic artery with special reference to blind aneurysms. *Mayo Clin. Proc.* 33:381, 1958.

238. Siegelman, S. S. Current Perspectives on Zollinger-Ellison Syndrome. In A. R. Margulis and C. A. Gooding (eds.), *Diagnostic Radiology 1977.* San Francisco: University of California Printing Department, 1977. Pp. 27–40.

239. Sigstedt, B., and Lunderquist, A. Complications of angiographic examinations. *AJR* 130:455, 1978.

240. Sigstedt, B., Lunderquist, A., Tylén, U., and Boijsen, E. Angiography in pancreatic disease revisited: A prospective and blind evaluation. *Acta Radiol. [Diagn.] (Stockh.)* 22:235, 1981.

241. Skjoldborg, H., and Madsen, B. Selective angiography in surgical management of pancreatic insulomas. *Acta Chir. Scand.* 137:169, 1971.

242. Skjoldborg, H., Steen Olson, T., Lundbaek, K., and Madsen, B. Diagnosis and Treatment of Pancreatic Beta-Cell Tumor. In L. M. Nyhus (ed.), *Surgery Annual.* New York: Appleton-Century-Crofts, 1975.

243. Suzuki, T., Imamura, M., Tamura, K., Sumiyoshi, A., Sakanashi, S., Nishimura, Y., and Tobe, T. Correlative evaluation of angiography and pancreatoductography in relation to surgery for cancer of the pancreas. *Surgery* 85:644, 1979.

244. Suzuki, T., Kawabe, K., Imamura, M., and Honjo, I. Survival of patients with cancer of the pancreas in relation to findings on arteriography. *Ann. Surg.* 176:37, 1972.

245. Suzuki, T., Kawabe, K., Nakayasu, A., Takeda, H., Kobayashi, K., Kubota, N., and Honjo, I. Selective arteriography in cancer of the pancreas at a resectable stage. *Am. J. Surg.* 122:402, 1971.

246. Suzuki, T., Kuratsuka, H., Uchida, K., et al. Correlation between clinical aspects and location of lesions in carcinoma of the head of the pancreas. *Am. J. Surg.* 125:546, 1973.

247. Suzuki, T., Kuratsuka, H., Uchida, K., Matsumoto, Y., and Honjo, I. Carcinoma of the pancreas arising in the region of the uncinate process. *Cancer* 30:796, 1972.

248. Suzuki, T., Tani, T., and Honjo, I. Appraisal of arteriography for assessment of operability in periampullary cancer. *Ann. Surg.* 182:66, 1975.

249. Swanson, G. E. A case of cystadenoma of the pancreas studied by selective angiography. *Radiology* 81:592, 1963.

250. Takashima, T., and Shin, M. Transfemoral superselective celiac catheterization. Technical considerations. *AJR* 113:280, 1971.

251. Takashima, T., Yamamoto, I., Mitani, I., and Shin, M. Transfemoral superselective celiac angiography. *AJR* 110:813, 1970.

252. Tavernier, J., Delorme, G., and Fagola, M. L'artériographie "super-sélective" du pancréas. *Ann. Radiol. (Paris)* 14:555, 1971.

253. Taylor, D. A., Macken, K. L., and Fiore, A. S. Angiographic visualization of the secretin-stimulated pancreas. *Radiology* 87:525, 1966.

254. Thomas, M. L., Lamb, G. H. R., and Barraclough, M. A. Angiographic demonstration of a pancreatic "Vipoma" in the WDHA syndrome. *AJR* 127:1037, 1976.

255. Thomas, R. L., Robinson, A. E., Johnsrude, I. S., Goodrich, J. K., and Lester, R. G. The demonstration of an insulin and gastrin producing pancreatic tumor by angiography and pancreatic scanning. *AJR* 104:646, 1968.

256. Tillander, H. Selective angiography of the abdominal aorta with a guided catheter. *Acta Radiol. (Stockh.)* 45:21, 1956.

257. Triller, J., Voegeli, E., Halter, F., Witzel, L., and Wanger, F. Die selektive Pankreas-Angiographie und retrograde Pankreas-Cholangiogra-

phie als Kombinationsuntersuchung. *ROEFO* 122:138, 1975.

258. Tylén, U. Accuracy of angiography in the diagnosis of carcinoma of the pancreas. *Acta Radiol. [Diagn.]* (Stockh.) 14:449, 1973.

259. Tylén, U. Angiographic differentiation between inflammatory disease and carcinoma of the pancreas. *Acta Radiol. [Diagn.]* (Stockh.) 14:257, 1973.

260. Tylén, U. Angiography in disease of the peripancreatic lymph nodes. *Acta Radiol. [Diagn.]* (Stockh.) 16:625, 1975.

261. Tylén, U., and Arnesjö, B. Resectability and prognosis of carcinoma of the pancreas evaluated by angiography. *Scand. J. Gastroenterol.* 8:691, 1973.

262. Tylén, U., and Arnesjö, B. Angiographic diagnosis of inflammatory disease of the pancreas. *Acta Radiol. [Diagn.]* (Stockh.) 14:215, 1973.

263. Tylén, U., and Dencker, H. Roentgenologic diagnosis of pancreatic abscess. *Acta Radiol. [Diagn.]* (Stockh.) 14:9, 1973.

264. Udén, R. Effect of secretin in celiac and superior mesenteric angiography. *Acta Radiol. [Diagn.]* (Stockh.) 8:497, 1969.

265. Udén, R. Cholecystokinin-pancreozymin in celiac and superior mesenteric angiography. *Acta Radiol. [Diagn.]* (Stockh.) 12:363, 1972.

266. Udén, R. Secretin and epinephrine combined in celiac angiography. *Acta Radiol. [Diagn.]* (Stockh.) 17:17, 1976.

267. Van Heertum, R. L., Cioffi, C. M., and Ruzicka, F. F. The use of alpha blocking and beta stimulating drugs in combination to improve opacification of the portal venous system. *Radiology* 100:679, 1971.

268. van Voorthuisen, A. E. *Ervaringen met Selectieve Arteriografie van de Arteria Coeliaca en de Arteria Mesenterica Superior.* Leiden: Stafleu's Wetenschappelijke Uitgeversmaatschappij N.V., 1967.

269. Warter, J., Kempf, F., Sibilly, A., and Brechenmacher, J. C. Dissection pseudo-anéurysmale de la paroi duodénale au cours d'une poussée de pancréatite. *J. Radiol. Electrol. Med. Nucl.* 51:639, 1970.

270. Weissleder, H., Baumeister, L., Fischer, P., and Renemann, H. Die selektive Darstellung der Arteria coeliaca und mesenterica superior in der abdominalen Diagnostik. *ROEFO* 104:137, 1966.

271. Wenz, W. Selektive Arteriographie der Oberbauchorgane. *Dtsch. Med. Wochenschr.* 90:643, 1965.

272. Weyer, K. H., van de, Kössling, F. K., Habighorst, L. V., and Albers, P. Experimentelle Untersuchungen zu Technik und Risiko der Pankreasangiographie. *ROEFO* 108:733, 1968.

273. White, A. F., Baum, S., and Buranasiri, S. Aneurysms secondary to pancreatitis. *AJR* 127:393, 1976.

274. White, T. T., and Kavlie, H. Hormone-producing pancreatic islet-cell tumor and hyperplasia. *Acta Chir. Scand.* 138:809, 1972.

275. Woodburne, R. T., and Olsen, L. L. The arteries of the pancreas. *Anat. Rec.* 111:255, 1951.

276. Zboralske, F. F., and Amberg, J. R. Detection of the Zollinger-Ellison syndrome: The radiologist's responsibility. *AJR* 104:529, 1968.

277. Zollinger, R. M. Islet cell tumors and the alimentary tract. *AJR* 126:933, 1976.

278. Zollinger, R. M., and Moore, F. T. Zollinger-Ellison syndrome comes of age. *J.A.M.A.* 204:361, 1968.

Pancreatic Venography

ANDERS LUNDERQUIST
TORBEN OWMAN
WOLFGANG REICHARDT

Previously, the pancreatic veins have received little attention. However, the availability of the portal vein and its tributaries for selective catheterization has opened up a new way to localize pancreatic tumors. It has also given hope for earlier detection of pancreatic carcinoma as veins are invaded earlier by the tumor than are arteries. Selective catheterization of pancreatic veins and sampling of pancreatic venous blood is possible only if the pancreatic venous anatomy is well known. Lack of knowledge of the mode of drainage and intervenous communications may cause erroneous interpretations.

Anatomy

The distribution of the pancreatic veins corresponds roughly to that of the arteries (Fig. 63-1). The pancreatic head is drained to the main stem of the portal vein and to the superior mesenteric vein [3, 9, 11].

The posterior aspect of the pancreatic head is drained by one or several posterior superior pancreaticoduodenal veins (Fig. 63-2). These veins empty into the dorsal circumference of the portal vein 1.5 to 3.0 cm from the confluence of the splenic, the superior mesenteric, and the portal veins.

A dorsal pancreatic vein is often present draining the mediodorsal part of the pancreatic head, and ending in the dorsal aspect of the confluence of the splenic, superior mesenteric, and portal veins. It is interesting that both the posterior superior pancreaticoduodenal vein and the dorsal pancreatic vein do not empty into the most adjacent part of the portal vein but turn around to empty into its dorsal aspect [3, 11].

The posterior superior pancreaticoduodenal vein or the dorsal pancreatic vein may form an arcade with the posterior inferior pancreaticoduodenal vein. This venous arcade runs in the pancreaticoduodenal sulcus, receiving tributaries from the pancreas as well as from the duodenum, and empties into the first jejunal vein, second jejunal vein, or directly into the superior mesenteric vein, thus corresponding to the dorsal pancreatic arterial arcade.

The anterior aspect of the pancreatic head is drained mainly by the anterior superior pancreaticoduodenal vein (Fig. 63-3) as one stem or as multiple branches that empty into the gastrocolic trunk. The gastrocolic trunk itself, 1467

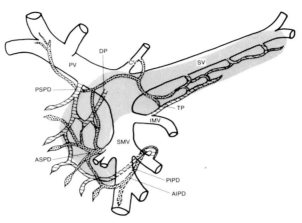

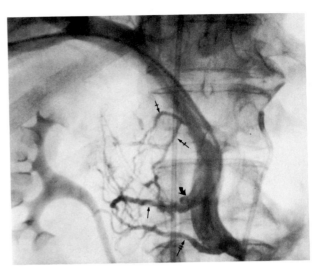

Figure 63-1. Venous anatomy of the pancreas, schematic. *PV* = portal vein; *SV* = splenic vein; *SMV* = superior mesenteric vein; *IMV* = inferior mesenteric vein; *PSPD* = posterior superior pancreaticoduodenal vein; *ASPD* = anterior superior pancreaticoduodenal vein; *PIPD* = posterior inferior pancreaticoduodenal vein; *AIPD* = anterior inferior pancreaticoduodenal vein; *TP* = transverse pancreatic vein; *DP* = dorsal pancreatic vein; *CV* = coronary vein. The dotted veins are anterior, the striped veins posterior to the pancreas. (From Reichardt and Ingemansson [13].)

Figure 63-3. Injection of contrast into anterior superior pancreaticoduodenal vein (*straight arrow*). Over collaterals the anterior inferior pancreaticoduodenal vein (*double-barred arrow*), gastrocolic trunk (*curved arrow*), and two branches of the posterior superior pancreaticoduodenal vein (*barred arrows*) are demonstrated.

Figure 63-2. Selective injection of contrast into the posterior superior pancreaticoduodenal vein (PSPD). (A) Anteroposterior view. (B) Lateral view. Two PSPDS are demonstrated (*arrows*). Over collaterals the anterior superior (*barred arrows*) and posterior inferior pancreaticoduodenal veins (*double-barred arrows*) are filled.

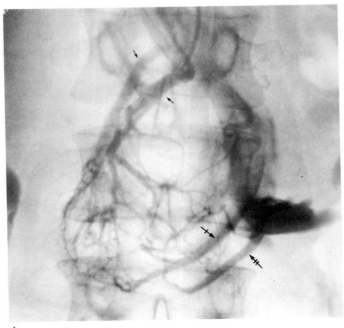

A

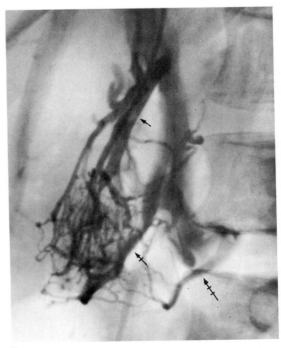

B

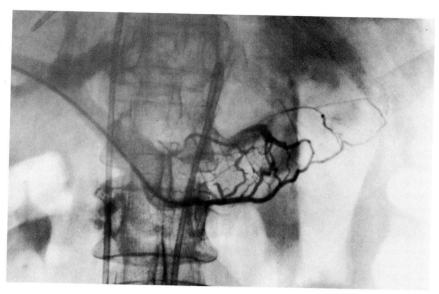

Figure 63-4. Injection of contrast into transverse pancreatic vein. Over collaterals a faint filling of splenic vein is received. (From Reichardt and Cameron [11].)

moreover, receives the right gastroepiploic vein and a middle colic vein and empties into the right side of the superior mesenteric vein 1 to 3 cm from its junction with the splenic vein. Sometimes the cranioventral aspect of the pancreatic head is drained by a vein ending in the ventral circumference of the portal vein 3 to 4 cm from the confluence of the superior mesenteric, splenic, and portal veins [2].

An anterior inferior pancreaticoduodenal vein

Figure 63-5. Selective injection of contrast into pancreatic vein draining to the splenic vein. Transverse pancreatic vein is filled over collaterals.

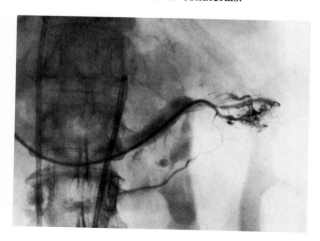

(AIPD) drains the lower ventral aspect of the pancreatic head and empties into the first jejunal vein or directly into the superior mesenteric vein. A posterior inferior pancreaticoduodenal vein drains the lower dorsal aspect of the pancreatic head (see Fig. 63-2) and usually joins the AIPD in its last course.

Most of the larger pancreatic vein branches draining the pancreatic head run on the surface of the gland and not into the parenchyma. This is an important feature to be aware of when lesions of this part of the pancreas are studied.

The body of the pancreas is drained by several rather small branches, the largest being the transverse pancreatic vein (Fig. 63-4). This vein runs along the inferior border of the pancreatic body and empties into the inferior mesenteric vein, the upper part of the superior mesenteric vein, the medial part of the splenic vein, or the confluence of the splenic, superior mesenteric, and portal veins. Other veins draining the body empty into the posterior superior pancreaticoduodenal vein, the left gastric vein, or directly into the confluence of the large venous trunks [11].

The tail of the pancreas is drained by a large number of small short veins emptying into the caudal aspect of the splenic vein (Fig. 63-5). Anastomoses are seen between several of these veins and the transverse pancreatic vein. The most distal part of the pancreatic tail is often drained into the lower polar vein of the spleen.

Catheterization and Sampling Technique

The catheterization technique of the portal vein is described in Chapter 65. Here we will be concerned only with the technique of catheterization of the pancreatic veins and problems related to the blood sampling for hormone assay [13].

The key to a successful catheterization of the pancreatic veins is the choice of guidewire. We have found essential a 0.9-mm guidewire in which not too soft a tip is used and a curve can be formed by hand. (This guidewire is now available from Cook Co., Copenhagen; Surgimed Co., Copenhagen; and Biotrol Pharma, Paris.) The catheter (inner diameter, 1.0 mm; outer diameter, 1.6 mm) is radiopaque and is the same as that on the needle for transhepatic puncture of the portal vein. The length of the catheter is enough for catheterization of the veins draining the pancreatic head.

If we start with catheterization of the posterior superior pancreaticoduodenal vein, we use the straight catheter without side holes but with a curved guidewire (Fig. 63-6A). The tip of the catheter is left in the main stem of the portal vein close to its bifurcation into right and left branches. The guidewire is introduced beyond the catheter with the curved tip caudally and dorsally. The guidewire is moved along the wall of the portal vein until its tip enters the posterior superior pancreaticoduodenal vein and is slowly advanced about 1 cm. The catheter is pushed over the guidewire until it is end to end; then the guidewire is removed. Slow injection of 6 to 8 cc of contrast medium is performed, and eight films are exposed, two per second. It has to be remarked that if the catheter is advanced beyond the tip of the guidewire the wall of the vein can easily be penetrated.

When the anterior superior pancreaticoduodenal vein is to be catheterized, another curve of guidewire is necessary (Fig. 63-6B). This shape of the guidewire suggests a complicated catheterization, but in fact the anterior superior pancreaticoduodenal vein is one of the easiest of the pancreatic veins to catheterize. With the tip of the catheter in the portal vein at the entrance of the superior mesenteric vein, the guidewire is advanced. Because of its shape it follows the right wall of the superior mesenteric vein, enters the gastrocolic trunk, and turns up into the anterior superior

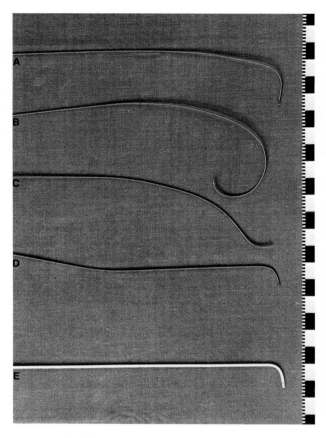

Figure 63-6. Different shapes of guidewire and catheter for pancreatic vein catheterization. (From Reichardt and Ingemansson [13].)

pancreaticoduodenal vein. The catheter is then advanced until it is end to end with the guidewire, and the guidewire is removed. If the posterior superior pancreaticoduodenal vein cannot be found during the first trials, it will ordinarily be demonstrated when contrast medium is injected into the anterior superior pancreaticoduodenal vein (see Fig. 63-3). With the knowledge of its opening into the portal vein, the posterior superior pancreaticoduodenal vein can then in most cases be catheterized.

In order to catheterize veins draining the pancreatic tail into the splenic vein, a longer catheter with the same diameter has to be used. This catheter has a short bend at its tip (Fig. 63-6E) and a side hole very close to the tip. A similar curve is used on the guidewire (Fig. 63-6D). With the catheter and the guidewire end to end in the splenic vein at the hilus of the spleen, the curved tip is directed caudally and slowly moved medially. The guidewire is intermittently advanced a few millimeters beyond the tip of the catheter, and the point at which it enters a pancreatic vein as it passes beyond the margin of the splenic vein is easily recognized. The catheter is then slowly pushed over the guidewire into the vein and the guidewire removed. A slow injection by hand of contrast medium (2–8 cc) will show the distribution of this vein and usually adjacent veins because of collateral filling. When the adjacent veins are demonstrated, they are later easily catheterized. Injection of contrast medium into veins draining the lateral part of the pancreatic body into the splenic vein often also demonstrates the transverse pancreatic vein (see Fig. 63-5).

If the transverse pancreatic vein drains into the proximal part of the inferior mesenteric vein, another shape guidewire is used (Fig. 63-6C). This shape fits the anatomy in such a way that the guidewire easily enters the inferior mesenteric vein and its tip turns toward the lateral wall of the inferior mesenteric vein where the transverse pancreatic vein often enters (see Fig. 63-4).

When blood is to be sampled for hormone assay, one catheter is introduced into the celiac artery and one into the hepatic vein in addition to the pancreatic vein catheter. Blood samples are taken from all three catheters at the beginning of the examination, once or several times during the procedure, and at the end of the examination. In between, blood is withdrawn only from the pancreatic veins. Because of the size of the pancreatic veins, the aspiration of blood has to be performed very slowly. This is the most time-consuming part of the whole procedure, usually taking 2½ to 3 hours. From each vessel 10 cc of blood is taken and collected in ice-chilled tubes. Blood samples for radioimmunoassay of gastrin, vasoactive intestinal polypeptide, and insulin are then centrifuged and sera stored at −20° C until assayed. Blood samples for radioimmunoassay of glucagon and somatostatin are collected in tubes containing trasylol and heparin until centrifuged and stored at −20° C [13].

Pancreatic and Common Bile Duct Carcinoma

Pancreatic carcinoma is known to invade the veins early. When Göthlin, Lunderquist, and Tylén reported the first clinical phlebographies of the pancreas in 1974 [4], they expressed the hope that this method could be useful in the diagnosis of carcinoma of the pancreas. The dominant diagnostic phlebographic findings are occluded veins in the region occupied by the tumor [10]. Irregularity of the pancreatic veins is often observed but is not a diagnostic indication of carcinoma and can be found in association with chronic pancreatitis. The most obvious finding of intrapancreatic venous occlusion in patients with carcinoma of the head of the pancreas is the absence of collateral flow from the posterior superior to the anterior superior pancreaticoduodenal vein and vice versa when a selective injection of contrast medium into one of these veins is performed (Fig. 63-7).

The majority of pancreatic veins run on the surface of the organ [11], and the phlebographic appearance is dominated by these superficial veins. This is the reason the reported minimum size of demonstrable tumors is as large as 3 cm. However, 5-cm tumors can present relatively discrete phlebographic findings. When main branches of

Figure 63-7. Nonresectable carcinoma. Injection into the anterior superior pancreaticoduodenal vein. No collateral flow to the posterior superior pancreaticoduodenal vein. The lines represent the shape of the obstructed common bile duct at percutaneous transhepatic cholangiography. (From Reichardt [10].)

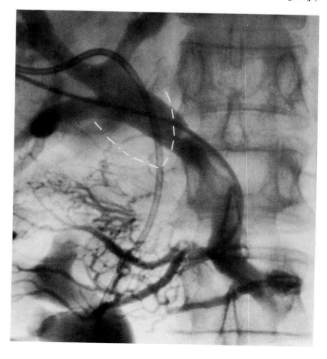

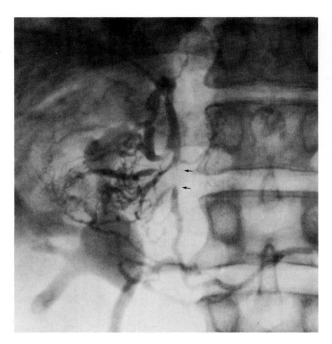

Figure 63-8. Nonresectable carcinoma. Injection into the posterior superior pancreaticoduodenal vein. Main branches are obstructed (*arrows*).

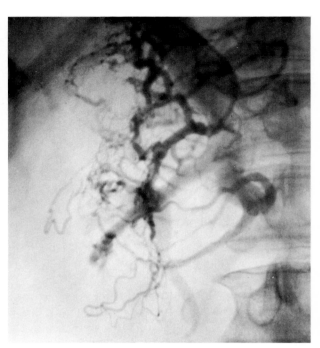

Figure 63-10. Bile duct carcinoma in the hilus of the liver. Common bile duct veins are widened and tortuous. Pancreatic veins are patent. (From Reichardt [10].)

Figure 63-9. Nonresectable carcinoma. Injection into the superior mesenteric vein. Severe stenosis with a pressure gradient of 13 cm H_2O. Widened pancreaticoduodenal veins serve as collaterals. (From Reichardt and Ihse [12].)

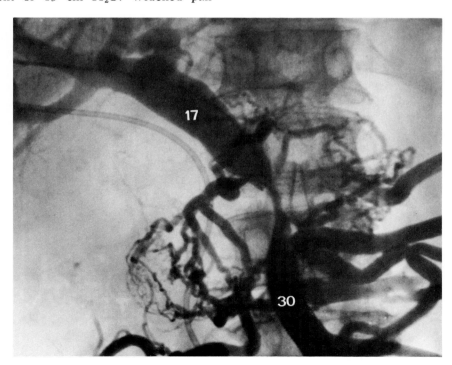

the superficial veins are involved, the changes cannot be overlooked (Fig. 63-8).

In most patients with pancreatic carcinoma the tumors are nonresectable at the time of diagnosis. In such a case the superior mesenteric vein, the splenic vein, or the portal vein is often partially obstructed. The superficial pancreaticoduodenal veins can serve as collateral pathways and become considerably dilated (Fig. 63-9). Demonstration of encasement of the superior mesenteric or the portal vein can be a valuable—and in some cases the only—angiographic sign of nonresectability of the tumors [12].

The veins of the common bile duct are often visualized by selective phlebography of the head of the pancreas. In patients with carcinoma of the common bile duct proximal to the pancreas, the veins of the head of the pancreas are patent and appear normal. If the common bile duct veins can be demonstrated, they show dilatation, tortuosity, and even obstruction (Fig. 63-10).

Endocrine Tumors

The insulin-producing adenoma is the commonest endocrine tumor of the pancreas. As it is usually less than 3 cm in size, it cannot be demonstrated by morphologic changes at pancreatic phlebography [10].

In patients with rare endocrine tumors such as glucagonomas, vipomas, and somatostatinomas, the diagnosis is often established late and the detected tumors are larger. If the tumor exceeds 4 cm in diameter, an expanding lesion with displacement of the veins can be found at phlebography (Fig. 63-11). In smaller tumors no venous changes are seen [10]. Selective pancreatic phlebography is therefore not a useful way to localize endocrine pancreatic tumors.

On the other hand, catheterization of pancreatic veins is essential if blood sampling and hormone assay for localization of endocrine pancreatic tumors are performed [5–8] (Table 63-1). Blood sampling in the main portal vein tributaries only does not allow a correct localization of all endocrine tumors [13] (Table 63-2). Selective phlebography has to be performed because the venous anatomy varies considerably and must be investigated individually. The sites

for blood sampling have to be documented to obtain a proper interpretation of hormone analyses regarding tumor localization (Fig. 63-12). For this purpose, too, selective phlebography is necessary. As the main pancreatic veins are to be found on the surface of the organ, the veins can be dissected and located during operation, and the phlebographic anatomy can be identified. According to the results from the hormone assay, the surgeon thus can find even nonpalpable adenomas or islet cell hyperplasia by following the tumor-draining vein [13].

Gastrinomas are often multiple. In these cases a generally elevated gastrin concentration in all the veins may indicate multiplicity of gastrin-releasing tumors but does not allow a distinct localization of the tumors [7]. If the gastrin-producing tissue is limited to one part of the pancreas, a curative resection may be possible [1].

Figure 63-11. Islet cell tumor in the head of the pancreas, 5 cm in diameter. Only displacement of the posterior superior pancreaticoduodenal vein (*arrow*) is found at phlebography. (From Reichardt [10].)

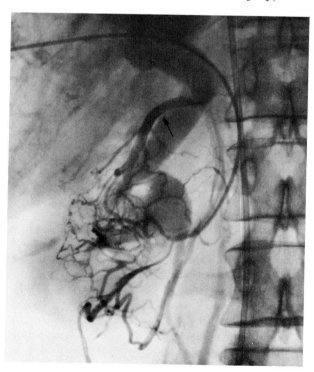

Table 63-1. Patients with Islet Cell Tumors or Islet Cell Hyperplasia Examined with Angiography and Selective Pancreatic Catheterization for Hormone Assay—University Hospital, Lund, Sweden, Series

Patient Number	Angiography	Hormone Assay	Final Diagnosis
1	+	+	Insulinoma
2	—	+	B-cell hyperplasia
3	—	+	B-cell hyperplasia
4	+	+	Insulinoma
5	—	+	Insulinoma
6	—	+	Insulinoma
7	—	—[a]	Insulinoma
8	+	+	Glucagonoma
9	(+)[b]	+	Glucagonoma
10	+	+	Tumor producing glucagon, insulin, and serotonin
11	+	(+)[b]	Somatostatinoma
12	+	—	D-cell tumor
13	(+)[c]	(+)[d]	Multiple gastrinomas
14	(+)[c]	(+)[d]	Multiple gastrinomas
15		(+)[d]	Multiple gastrinomas
16	+	+	Gastrinoma, not verified

+ = correct localization.
[a]Venous abnormality.
[b]Found retrospectively.
[c]One of multiple tumors demonstrated.
[d]Generally elevated gastrin concentration. No distinct localization of tumors possible.

Table 63-2. Hormone Concentrations in Tumor-Draining Veins Compared with Main Portal Vein Tributary Outside the Tumor-Draining Veins

Tumors	Hormone Concentration		Range of Concentrations in Main Portal Vein Tributaries
	In Tumor-Draining Vein	In Main Portal Vein Tributary at Tumor Level	
	(μU/cc)		
Insulinomas			
1	—	865	93–260
2	600	300	13–58
3*	1,130	45	11–165
4*	245	14	11–68
5	6,200	179	14–28
6	974	95	95–230
	(pg/cc)		
Glucagonomas			
1	24,000	2,900	1,320–2,400
2	10,000	800	600–1,750
3	10,650	?	856–2,213

*B-cell hyperplasia.

Glucagon (pg/cc)/Insulin (µU/cc)

1. v. lienal.	=	950/150
2. v. pancreatis (corpus)	=	1 200/300
3. v. pancreatis (corpus)	=	680/330
4. v. lienal. prox.	=	550/200
5. v. lienal. prox.	=	680/ 65
6. v. port.–mes. sup.–lienal. confluens	=	1 220/ 41
7. v. mes. sup. (below GCT)	=	600/ 5
8. v. PSPD	=	3 850/ 29
9. v. PSPD	=	5 750/ 60
10. v. lienal. dist. caudal	=	1 300/ 2
11. v. lienal. dist.	=	1 050/ 21
12. v. pancreat.	=	620/ 45
13. v. pancreat.	=	1 150/ 53
14. v. pancreat.	=	1 480/ 39
15. v. mes. inf.	=	1 490/ 3
16. v. ASPD	=	7 700/ 60
17. v. ASPD	=	10 000/ 69
18. v. GCT	=	800/ 7
19. v. pancreat. (cauda)	=	850/ 41
20. v. port. centr.	=	1 600/ 22
21. v. port. centr.	=	1 750/ 25
22. v. port. centr.	=	1 600/ 28

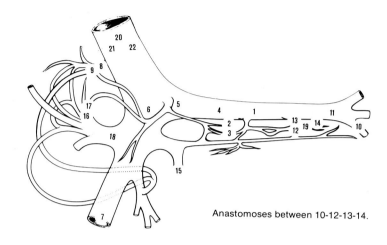

Anastomoses between 10-12-13-14.

Figure 63-12. Glucagon and insulin concentrations in different portal tributaries and pancreatic veins in a patient with glucagonoma of the head of the pancreas, mainly drained by the anterior superior pancreaticoduodenal vein (samples 16, 17).

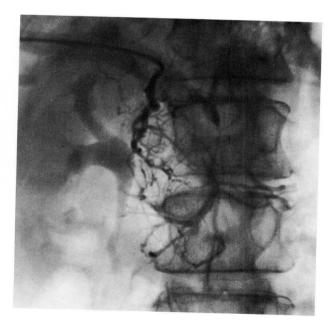

Figure 63-13. Chronic pancreatitis. Irregular intrapancreatic veins but patent collaterals between posterior superior and anterior superior pancreaticoduodenal vein. (From Reichardt [10].)

Pancreatitis

In patients with chronic relapsing pancreatitis, the pancreatic veins appear irregular, abruptly changing their course. If cystic lesions, edema, or abscess formation is present, the veins can be stretched and displaced. In general the veins are patent. When occlusion occurs, the discrepant finding of patent small veins adjacent to the occlusion may allow differentiation between chronic pancreatitis and a pancreatic carcinoma larger than 3 cm in size [10] (Fig. 63-13). This, however, means that the method is without clinical importance for detection of pancreatic carcinoma in patients with chronic pancreatitis because the majority of resectable tumors will be overlooked.

Peripancreatic Lesions

Selective phlebography has been performed in a few patients with peripancreatic disease when the indication for the examination was a possible pancreatic malignancy. The final diagnoses were multiple submucosal duodenal lipomas, retropancreatic malignant lymphoma, and common

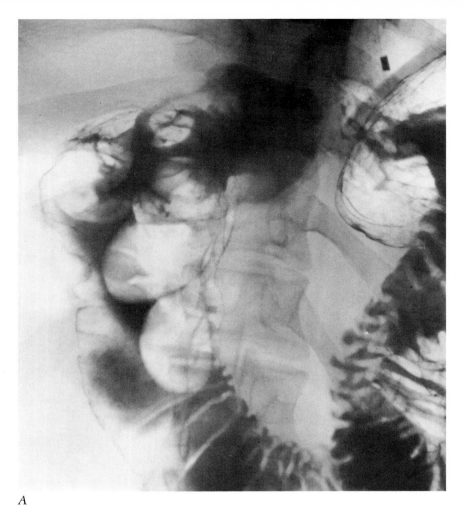

A

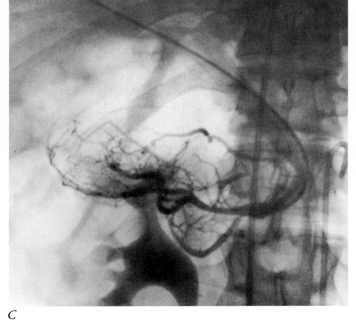

B   *C*

Figure 63-14. Submucosal duodenal lipomas. (A) Hypotonic duodenography. Injection into (B) posterior superior and (C) anterior superior pancreaticoduodenal veins demonstrates displaced and stretched veins without other abnormalities.

bile duct carcinoma. In lipomas and the retropancreatic lymphoma, pancreatic veins were not changed but adjacent veins including duodenal veins were displaced and stretched (Fig. 63-14).

References

1. Burcharth, F., Stage, J. G., Stadil, F., Jensen, L. I., and Fischermann, K.   Localization of gastrinomas by transhepatic portal catheterization and gastrin assay. *Gastroenterology* 77:444, 1979.
2. Douglass, B. E., Baggenstoss, A. H., and Hollinshead, W. H.   Anatomy of the portal vein and its tributaries. *Surg. Gynecol. Obstet.* 91:562, 1950.
3. Falconer, A., and Griffiths, E.   The anatomy of the blood vessels in the region of the pancreas. *Br. J. Surg.* 37:334, 1950.
4. Göthlin, J., Lunderquist, A., and Tylén, U.   Selective phlebography of the pancreas. *Acta Radiol.* [*Diagn.*] (Stockh.) 15:474, 1974.
5. Ingemansson, S., Holst, J., Larsson, L. I., and Lunderquist, A.   Localization of glucagonomas by catheterization of the pancreatic veins and with glucagon assay. *Surg. Gynecol. Obstet.* 145:509, 1977.
6. Ingemansson, S., Kühl, C., Larsson, L. I., Lunderquist, A., and Lundquist, I.   Localization of insulinomas and islet cell hyperplasia by pancreatic vein catheterization and insulin assay. *Surg. Gynecol. Obstet.* 146:725, 1978.
7. Ingemansson, S., Larsson, L. I., Lunderquist, A., and Stadil, F.   Pancreatic vein catheterization with gastrin assay in normal patients and in patients with the Zollinger-Ellison syndrome. *Am. J. Surg.* 134:558, 1977.
8. Lunderquist, A., Eriksson, M., Ingemansson, S., Larsson, L. I., and Reichardt, W.   Selective pancreatic vein catheterization for hormone assay in endocrine tumors of the pancreas. *Cardiovasc. Radiol.* 1:117, 1978.
9. Petrén, T.   Die Arterien und Venen des Duodenum und des Pankreaskopfes beim Menschen. *Z. Anat. Entwicklungsgesch.* 90:234, 1929.
10. Reichardt, W.   Selective phlebography in pancreatic and peripancreatic disease. *Acta Radiol.* [*Diagn.*] (Stockh.) 21:513, 1980.
11. Reichardt, W., and Cameron, R.   Anatomy of the pancreatic veins. A post mortem and clinical phlebographic investigation. *Acta Radiol.* [*Diagn.*] (Stockh.) 21:33, 1980.
12. Reichardt, W., Ihse, I.   Percutaneous transhepatic portography in pancreatic carcinoma. Diagnosis and evaluation of resectability. *Acta Radiol.* [*Diagn.*] (Stockh.) 21:579, 1980.
13. Reichardt, W., and Ingemansson, S.   Selective vein catheterization for hormone assay in endocrine tumors of the pancreas. Technique and results. *Acta Radiol.* [*Diagn.*] (Stockh.) 21:177, 1980.

Hepatic Arteriography

STANLEY BAUM

Although the in vivo arterial pattern of the liver had been demonstrated with percutaneous translumbar aortography, it remained for Bierman et al. in 1951 [1] first to describe the technique of selective hepatic arteriography. The examination was performed by injecting contrast material directly into the hepatic artery during intraarterial catheterization or laparotomy. This procedure, however, did not become widely accepted as a diagnostic aid because of the many technical problems involved in the surgical exposure of the brachial artery for the passage of the intraarterial catheters and the relatively toxic nature of the contrast material available at the time. The introduction in 1953 of the Seldinger catheter replacement technique [2], serial film changers, automatic injectors, and safe water-soluble contrast agents was essential for the development of hepatic arteriography.

In 1958 Ödman published a monograph on percutaneous selective arteriography of the celiac artery [3], which demonstrated the ease with which the celiac and superior mesenteric arteries could be selectively catheterized and injected. Since that time, selective hepatic arteriography has become a valuable tool in the diagnosis of liver disease; it has also provided insight into many pathophysiologic states [4–8].

Technique

Celiac arteriography is performed in most angiographic laboratories by the same technique described by Ödman. A preshaped radiopaque catheter is percutaneously inserted into either the femoral or the axillary artery, and, by means of image-intensification fluoroscopy preferably with television monitoring, the celiac axis is selectively catheterized. In most patients the celiac axis arises as an anterior branch of the aorta at the T12–L1 interspace. Orientation can usually be obtained by identifying the last rib and counting the vertebral bodies. The superior mesenteric artery generally arises from the anterior portion of the abdominal aorta at the bottom of the midportion of the first lumbar vertebral body. The renal arteries are generally posterolateral branches of the aorta at the level of L1–L2. At times it is helpful to turn the patient to a sharp left posterior oblique position during the catheter manipulation so as to identify clearly the anterior

1479

portion of the abdominal aorta. After the tip of the catheter is securely in place in the celiac trunk, approximately 0.5 to 0.75 cc per kilogram of body weight of a water-soluble diatrizoate contrast material is injected by automatic injector at a rate of 4 to 8 cc per second. Filming begins with the injection of the contrast material and continues during the arterial, capillary, and venous phases (spanning a total of 24 to 28 seconds after the start of the injection). During the arterial phase of the study, exposures are made every 0.5 second. Then films are taken every second, and finally one every third second. The hepatic arteriogram can be divided into an arterial phase, a capillary hepatogram phase, and a portal hepatogram phase.

In keeping with the current trend in vascular opacification studies of introducing the catheter as close as possible to the organ being studied, the hepatic artery is frequently catheterized directly by passing the catheter more peripherally after its insertion into the celiac trunk. This superselective injection technique provides excellent visualization of the intrahepatic arterial branches. The technique also avoids superimposition of extraneous vessels, such as the left gastric, gastroepiploic, and splenic arteries. It has the disadvantage that it does not afford evaluation of the portal hepatogram phase, since there is no contrast returning from the spleen. The performance of superselective arteriography of the hepatic artery requires more experience with catheter manipulation than does celiac arteriography. The techniques currently employed for superselective catheterization include the use of catheter manipulators, coaxial catheter methods, and specially shaped catheters and guidewires. Prior to superselective hepatic arteriography it is useful to have a celiac arteriogram, since this affords an arterial road map of the arterial blood flow to the liver. When the injection of contrast material is made directly into the hepatic artery, the volume used in the average adult is 20 to 40 cc (depending on the size of the liver) injected at a rate of 4 to 6 cc per second. This is generally accompanied by a sensation of warmth in the right upper quadrant.

The use of direct serial magnification techniques with fractional focal-spot x-ray tubes and air gap radiography has greatly increased the resolution obtained during arteriography. Vessels of approximately 100 μ in diameter can readily be seen.

Normal Anatomy

Because of the great frequency of anatomic variation in the arterial blood supply to the liver, only half the patients will have the entire hepatic arterial supply demonstrated after the injection into a common hepatic artery. The remaining 40 to 50 percent of patients have significant anatomic variations in the celiac and superior mesenteric arteries and, as Michels has pointed out [9], these variations occur most often in the origins of the hepatic artery. The most common of them are:

1. Right hepatic and middle hepatic arteries arising from the celiac axis with the left hepatic artery arising from the left gastric artery (approximately 10–12%) (Figs. 64-1, 64-2).
2. Left hepatic and middle hepatic arteries arising from the celiac common hepatic artery with the right hepatic artery arising from the superior mesenteric artery (approximately 14%) (Fig. 64-3).
3. Right, left, and middle hepatic arteries arising from the celiac common hepatic with an accessory left hepatic artery from the left gastric artery (8%).
4. Right, middle, and left hepatic arteries arising from the celiac common trunk with an accessory right hepatic artery arising from the superior mesenteric artery (6%).
5. The entire common hepatic artery arising from the superior mesenteric artery and no hepatic artery originating from the celiac axis (2.5%).

Additional, less frequent variations such as hepatic-lienal-mesenteric trunks have also been reported (Fig. 64-4). Almost all the major variations described by Michels in his dissection of the arterial trees of cadavers have also been noted in vivo during visceral angiography.

Corrosion casts of human livers by Healey and Schroy [10] have shown that it is the internal distribution of the arteries, bile ducts, and portal veins rather than the external morphology that determines the surgically significant divisions. The morphologic plane of division of the liver, therefore, is the lobar fissure and not the falciform ligament, left sagittal fossa, or ligamentum venosum. The lobar fissure is a parasagittal plane through the liver corresponding to a line extending from the gallbladder anteroinferiorly to the fossa of the inferior vena cava on the poste-

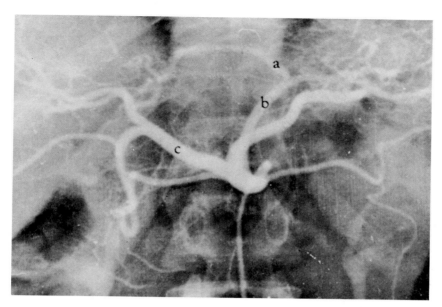

Figure 64-1. Left hepatic artery originating from a left gastric artery. *a* = left hepatic artery, *b* = left gastric artery, *c* = common hepatic artery.

Figure 64-2. Selective left gastric–left hepatic arteriogram. (A) Selective arteriography of a common left gastric–left hepatic trunk demonstrates site of bleeding stress ulcer in the stomach (*arrow*). (B) Infusion of vasopressin selectively into the common trunk demonstrates marked vasoconstriction of the left gas-tric portion of the vessel with little effect on the caliber of the left hepatic branches. The infusion of vasopressin continued for 2 days, and there was complete control of the patient's bleeding without any evidence of injury to the liver.

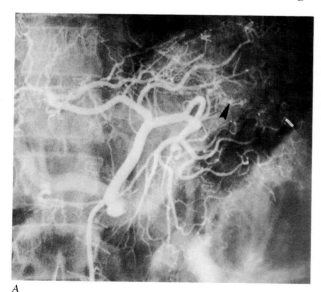

A

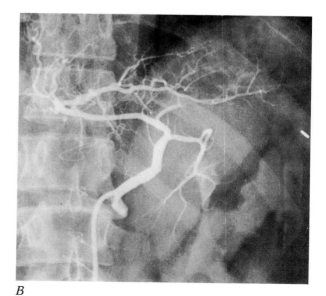

B

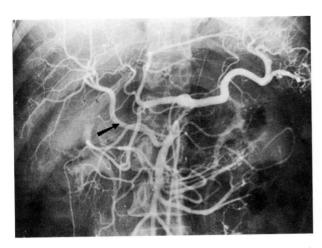

Figure 64-3. Selective celiac and superior mesenteric arteriography performed by injecting two catheters simultaneously, one positioned in the celiac axis and the other in the superior mesenteric artery. The right hepatic artery takes origin from the superior mesenteric artery (*arrow*). The celiac axis gives origin to the middle and left hepatic arteries, and the gastroduodenal artery is a branch of the left hepatic artery.

rior surface of the liver. This fissure is characterized by the absence of hepatic arteries, portal veins, and bile ducts. No significant branches of the bile ducts, hepatic arteries, or portal veins cross the main lobar fissure, and thus it is a surgically safe plane for hepatic incisions and partial or complete lobectomies.

Nebesar et al. [11] pointed out that the bifurcation of the common hepatic artery, even when it arises from the celiac axis itself, may be atypi-

Figure 64-4. Common hepatic-lienal-mesenteric trunk.

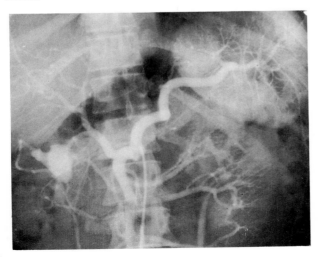

cal. Examples of a very proximal bifurcation of a common hepatic artery into a right hepatic and a middle hepaticogastroduodenal trunk have been seen. Other unusual bifurcations of the common hepatic artery are also encountered on occasion. All of these are important surgically because they may cause considerable confusion if they are not appreciated.

On account of the frequency of anatomic variations in the arterial supply of the liver, hepatic arteriography has proved to be a valuable procedure prior to major hepatic surgery. Since displacement and occasional thrombosis of the hepatic artery occur in the presence of neoplastic disease, arteriography is a prerequisite to hepatic arterial cannulation in cancer chemotherapeutic infusions [12].

Cirrhosis

The arteriographic appearance of the cirrhotic liver depends on the amount of volume loss of the liver itself. In the fibrotic, contracted, cirrhotic liver, the intrahepatic branches of the hepatic artery exhibit a characteristic corkscrew tortuosity (Fig. 64-5) [13, 14]. This correlates very well with the disorganization of the vascular tree as seen in corrosion studies of the hepatic artery of cirrhotic livers. Such tortuosity, however, is not present until substantial loss in liver parenchyma has occurred. In the early stages of cirrhosis, therefore, the arterial changes are not at all obvious.

There is considerable evidence to indicate that in cirrhosis an increased blood flow through the hepatic artery occurs, and this itself has caused intrahepatic vascular changes, including telangiectasis and aneurysms [15]. Hepatic arterial–portal venous shunting has long been postulated in cirrhotic patients, and on occasion it can be demonstrated duing hepatic arteriography (Fig. 64-6).

In the presence of portal hypertension, selective celiac and superior mesenteric arteriography has proved to be a valuable technique for the evaluation of the portal venous system and for the demonstration of venous collaterals.

In the normal patient, the hepatic artery accounts for only 20 to 25 percent of the total hepatic blood flow, with the remainder coming from the portal vein. There appears to be a sensitive reciprocal nature to the blood flow to the

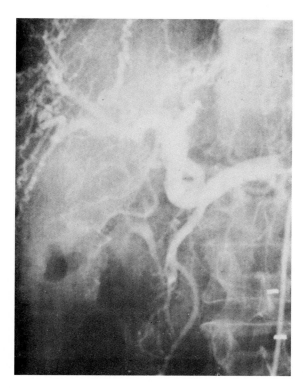

Figure 64-5. Cirrhosis. Selective hepatic arteriography demonstrates characteristic intrahepatic arterial tortuosity due to fibrosis in a contracted, cirrhotic liver.

liver so that a reduction of flow in one vessel causes an almost immediate increase in the other. Angiographically, this reciprocity can be readily demonstrated during the selective hepatic arterial infusion of vasopressin. Initially there is a decrease in the hepatic arterial blood flow. However, a rise in the systemic level of vasopressin causes a decrease in superior mesenteric blood flow and hence a decrease in the amount of portal venous return. The hepatic artery then appears to break free of the vasoconstricting effect of the vasopressin, and there is a reciprocal increase of hepatic arterial flow [16].

Around the periphery of the hepatic lobule there are portal spaces containing branches of the hepatic artery, portal vein, bile duct, and lymphatics. As pointed out by Reuter and Redman [17], the terminal arterioles of the hepatic artery and the terminal radicles of the portal vein empty into a common sinusoid. This mixed hepatic arterial and portal venous blood flows through the sinusoid, in contact with the hepatocytes, and finally drains via the central vein into the hepatic veins. Some of the angiographic features seen in cirrhosis are related to the drainage of the hepatic artery and portal venous radicles into a common sinusoidal space [18].

In early cirrhosis, when the amount of portal venous flow is normal, the hepatic arterial changes are minimal. If fatty infiltration exists within the liver, the small hepatic arterial branches appear stretched, and not infrequently there is a peculiar mottled appearance during the parenchymal phase of the study. When the cirrhosis is moderate to severe, there tends to be reduction in the portal venous return to the liver and therefore an increase in hepatic artery blood flow [19, 20]. The peripheral branches of the hepatic artery exhibit characteristic corkscrew appearance as fibrosis becomes a prominent feature of the disease.

One must always be alert to the possibility of a hepatoma superimposed on a cirrhotic liver. Because of the hepatic arterial changes that are present in cirrhosis, the diagnosis of a hepatoma can be difficult to make, especially since both cirrhosis and hepatomas tend to exhibit hepatic arterial–portal venous shunting. The presence of regenerating nodules in cirrhosis causes further confusion, since these may often be confused with hepatomas (Fig. 64-7). The regenerating nodule has fewer hepatic arterial branches than does the adjacent liver, but because of the mass effect of the nodule, the arteries appear stretched and on occasion distorted [21]. Regenerating nodules usually do not show the hypervascularity of hepatomas, nor does one see the hepatic arterial–portal venous shunting.

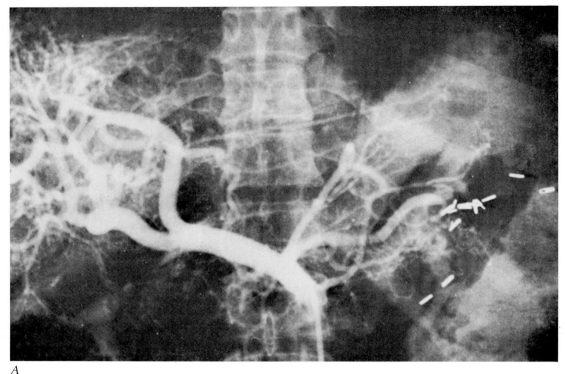

A

B

Figure 64-6. Hepatic arterial–portal venous shunt in a patient with portal hypertension and cirrhosis. (A) Selective celiac arteriography demonstrates large intrahepatic arterial branches and marked tortuosity of the smaller vessels due to a contracted, fibrotic liver. The splenic artery had been tied off as part of the patient's splenorenal shunt. (B) During the late arterial phase of the examination, prompt filling of the portal vein can be seen. (C) Several seconds later there is reversal of flow within the portal system with filling of gastric collaterals. The splenorenal shunt is nonfunctioning. (Courtesy of K. Kuroda, M.D.)

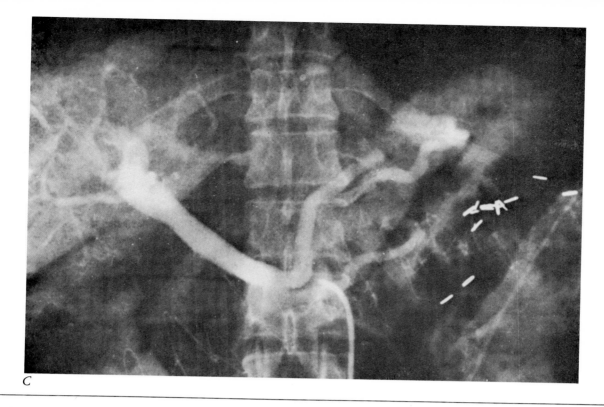

C

Figure 64-7. Large regenerating nodule in the right lobe of the liver in a patient with advanced cirrhosis. (A) Selective hepatic arteriography demonstrates a large mass extending down from the inferior portion of the right lobe of the liver. The vessel supplying the nodule appears stretched (*arrows*). The peripheral branches of the remaining portion of the hepatic artery exhibit the characteristic changes of advanced cirrhosis (*curved arrow*). (B) The venous phase of a superior mesenteric arteriogram demonstrates an elongated branch of the portal vein (*arrows*). (Courtesy of Josh Becker, M.D.)

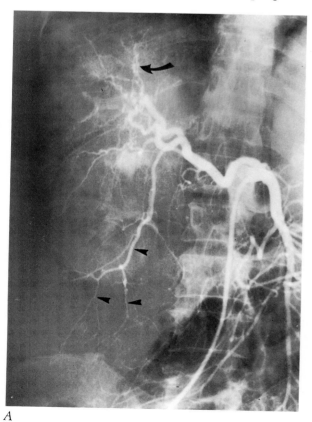

A

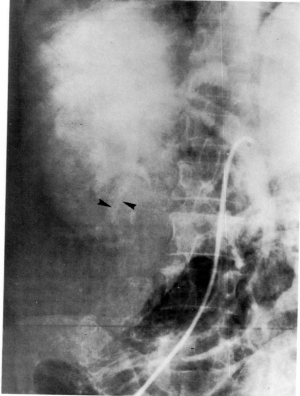

B

Inflammatory Disease

Inflammatory disease of the liver generally takes the form of either a diffuse process involving all of the organ (as in cholangitis, serum hepatitis, and infectious hepatitis) or hepatic abscesses, which may be solitary or multifocal.

CHOLANGITIS, SERUM HEPATITIS, AND INFECTIOUS HEPATITIS

The arteriographic findings in these diseases are not characteristic. In the few cases that have been reported, the findings have ranged from normal arteriograms to diffuse hypervascularity. Evans [14] has described an attenuated spastic appearance of the intrahepatic branches (Fig. 64-8). This

Figure 64-8. Viral hepatitis. Selective celiac arteriography demonstrates thin, spastic intrahepatic branches of the hepatic artery. The capillary hepatogram phase of the study was less dense than normal.

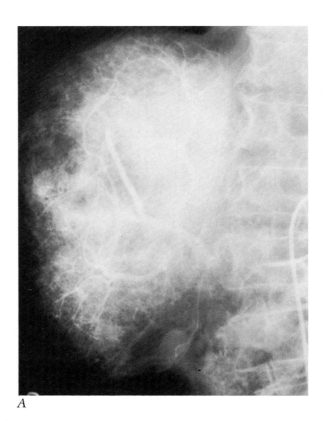

A

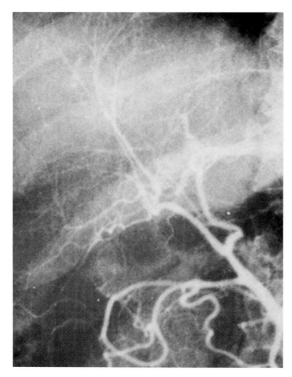

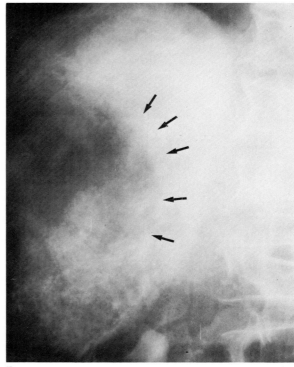

B

Figure 64-9. Hepatic abscess. (A) Arterial phase of ▶ the selective arteriogram shows displacement of peripheral branches of the hepatic artery. (B) Various-sized radiolucent defects are seen during the capillary phase of the study. In addition, the walls of the abscess cavity exhibit increased vascularity (*arrows*).

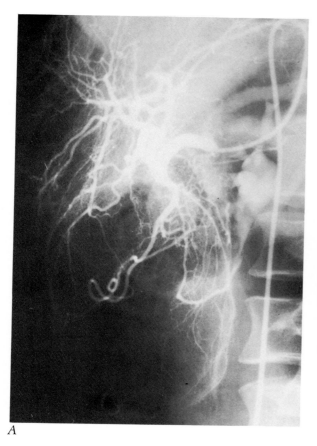

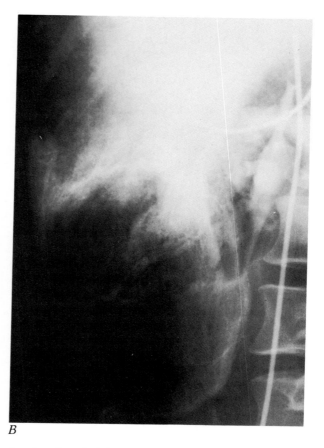

A

B

Figure 64-10. Echinococcus cyst. (A) The arterial phase of the study demonstrates a 10-cc avascular mass extending from the inferior margin of the right lobe of the liver. Because the patient was in a right posterior oblique position during the filming, the gastro-duodenal and right gastroepiploic arteries as well as the pancreatic arcades are superimposed on the superior portion of the cyst. (B) During the capillary phase of the study, the wall of the cyst appears hypervascular and thickened.

angiographic appearance is probably due to the stretching of the vessels in the swollen and inflamed liver. It certainly does not appear to be pathognomonic, and a similar arteriographic configuration is seen in cholangitis and the fatty infiltration that frequently accompanies cirrhosis.

HEPATIC ABSCESS

The arteriographic appearance of a hepatic abscess is very much like the appearance of abscess cavities anywhere in the body. If the abscess cavity is large, the arteriogram will reflect a relatively avascular mass with increased vascularity within the wall (Fig. 64-9). This is also the angiographic appearance of echinococcus (Fig. 64-10) [22, 23] and ameba cysts [24]. Obviously, the clinical history is of great importance in making the diagnosis and in differentiating wide-spread abscess cavities in the liver from metastatic disease.

Benign Hepatic Tumors

CAVERNOUS HEMANGIOMA

Cavernous hemangiomas are the most common of the benign hepatic tumors and are usually very characteristic in their angiographic features [25–27]. Some pathologists question whether they should be considered true neoplasms or hamartomatous malformations. These lesions are usually no larger than 3 cm in diameter (Figs. 64-11, 64-12), although occasionally they may be quite big and occupy large areas of the liver (Fig. 64-13). Histologically the vascular spaces are lined by endothelium and in most cases can be

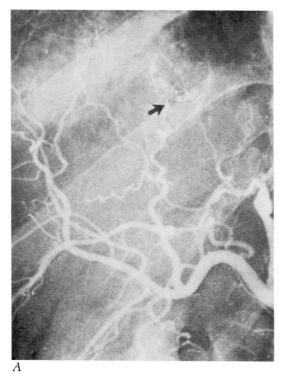

A

B

Figure 64-11. Cavernous hemangioma. (A) Selective hepatic arteriogram demonstrates a round vascular mass being fed by branches of the hepatic artery (*arrow*). (B) During the capillary phase of the study a spherical vascular stain is identified associated with pooling of contrast material without any evidence of arterial shunting (*arrows*).

Figure 64-12. Enhanced visualization of multiple hepatic hemangiomas. (A) Nonenhanced hepatic arteriogram showing multiple hemangioma. (B) Thirty seconds following the intraarterial injection of 10 μg of epinephrine.

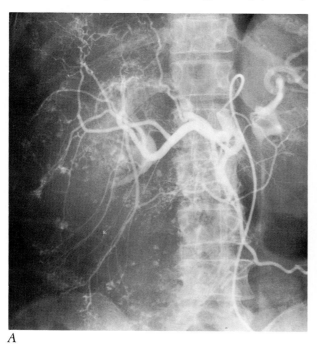

A

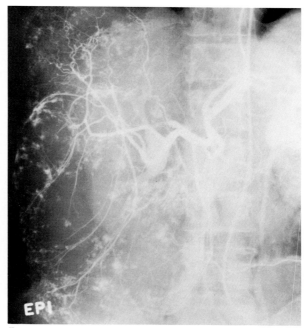

B

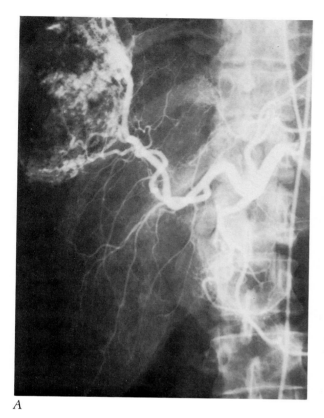

A

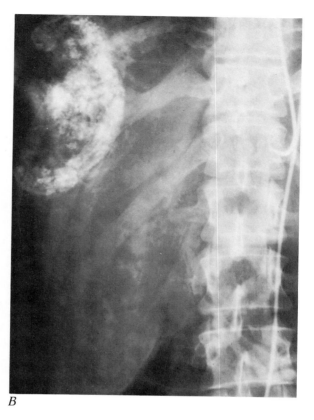

B

Figure 64-13. Cavernous hemangioma involving a large portion of the right lobe of the liver. (A) Selective hepatic arteriography demonstrates a large vascular mass deriving its blood supply from the right and middle hepatic arteries. (B) Contrast material persists within large vascular spaces of the cavernous hemangioma well into the venous phase of the examination.

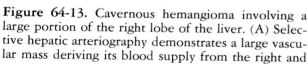

seen extending from one or more arterial branches. On the arteriogram, the contrast-containing vascular spaces are usually orderly in their configuration, and the opaque material persists well into the venous phase of the study because of the extremely slow blood flow. Often these contrast-filled spaces are curvilinear. Arteriovenous shunting, which is so typical of primary hepatocellular carcinoma, is not seen.

The vascular pattern of hemangioendothelioma [28], the other form of hepatic angioma, frequently mimics malignant disease and can be difficult to diagnose angiographically (Fig. 64-14).

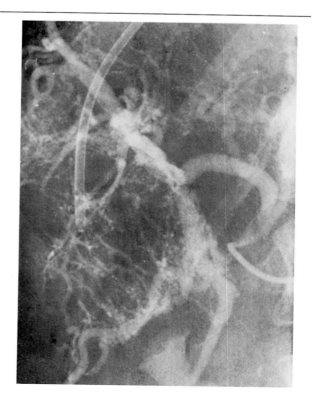

Figure 64-14. Hemangioendothelioma. Selective hepatic arteriogram demonstrates markedly increased vascularity in the right lobe of the liver associated with saccular dilatation of many intrahepatic arterial branches. During the capillary phase there was an intense tumor blush. No arteriovenous shunting was visible.

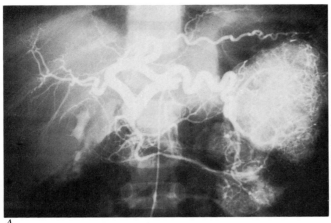
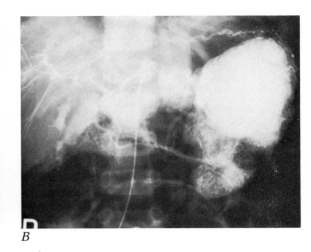

A

B

Figure 64-15. Focal nodular hyperplasia. (A) Hypervascular mass in the left lobe of the liver is supplied by a dilated left hepatic artery. As the artery penetrates the mass, it divides into small, fine branches. (B) During the capillary phase of the study, the tumor shows an intense, homogeneous, granular blush.

FOCAL NODULAR HYPERPLASIA

This lesion is benign, generally innocuous, and of uncertain pathogenesis [29]. Because of its multicellular nature, some pathologists have called it hepatic hamartoma [30], parenchymal hamartoma [31], focal nodular cirrhosis [32], and even minimal deviation hepatoma [33]. When possible, such lesions should be differentiated from hepatic adenomas, which have a different pathogenesis and prognosis.

Focal nodular hyperplasia tends to be well circumscribed, subcapsular, occasionally pedunculated, and, in approximately 20 percent of cases, multiple [34]. Pathologically the tumor is white and hard and has a central scar out of which radiate fibrous bands. Histologically these fibrous septa separate normal-appearing liver tissue. There are many blood vessels and bile ducts interspersed among the normal hepatocytes, and one can usually identify Kupffer cells. Angiographically focal nodular hyperplasia tends to be hypervascular and associated with dense capillary blushing. In large lesions, a dilated branch of the hepatic artery penetrates the mass and in the center of the lesion divides into small, fine branches that seem to radiate like spokes on a wheel (Fig. 64-15). There is an absence of arteriovenous shunting, and during the hepatographic phase the lesion looks granular or nodular. In smaller tumors, large penetrating arteries are not visible; however, there is a diffuse hypervascularity caused by small branches that penetrate the lesion, resulting in a reticular pattern during the hepatographic phase.

The pathogenesis of focal nodular hyperplasia remains obscure. It is probably not related to the ingestion of oral contraceptives, nor does it appear to be hormone-dependent. After an extensive literature review, Casarella et al. [35] concluded that there is no association between focal nodular hyperplasia and hepatocellular carcinoma. No deaths have been reported as being due to the natural history of the disease, but several deaths have occurred during attempted surgical resections. Although focal nodular hyperplasia has been seen in young children as well as in the elderly, in whom it is found as an incidental finding at autopsy, Knowles and Wolff [34] found 86 percent of patients with this lesion to be female with a mean age of 39 years. Because of the presence of Kupffer cells in focal nodular hyperplasia, some patients have normal uptake of labeled colloid on radionuclide scans.

HEPATIC ADENOMA

Liver cell adenomas tend to be solitary, encapsulated tumors that differ both macroscopically and microscopically from focal nodular hyperplasia [36]. Adenomas are likely to be larger than the lesions in focal nodular hyperplasia and when cut do not have the characteristic radiating scar of focal nodular hyperplasia. Also, areas of hemorrhage, necrosis, and bile stasis are often seen. Histologically adenomas are composed of atypical hepatocytes without any evidence of bile ducts or Kupffer cells. As pointed out by Phillips et al. [30], the hepatocytes are very uniform and show an abnormally simplified ultrastructure. In

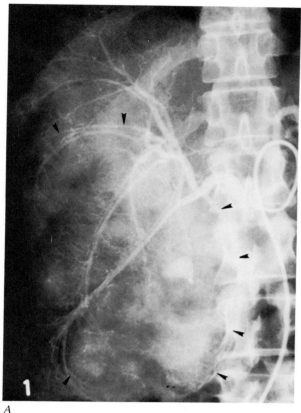

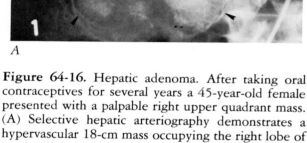

A

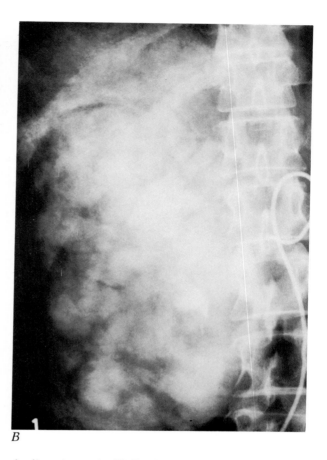

B

Figure 64-16. Hepatic adenoma. After taking oral contraceptives for several years a 45-year-old female presented with a palpable right upper quadrant mass. (A) Selective hepatic arteriography demonstrates a hypervascular 18-cm mass occupying the right lobe of the liver (*arrows*). (B) During the capillary phase of the examination the staining of the mass is not homogeneous but exhibits areas of radiolucency, due presumably either to necrosis or to small areas of hemorrhage. This hepatic adenoma was successfully resected.

1973 Baum et al. [37] reported an association between adenomas and the ingestion of oral contraceptives. Unlike focal nodular hyperplasia, with its innocuous natural history, hepatic adenomas have the potential for spontaneous intraabdominal hemorrhage. The exact frequency of these tumors is unknown, since they are asymptomatic and come to attention only incidentally during laparotomy or angiography or when they cause massive hemorrhage.

Angiographically adenomas have a wide spectrum of appearances. Although some may be as, or even more, vascular than focal nodular hyperplasia, cases are also seen in which the tumors appear hypovascular. The angiographic picture may be further complicated by areas of necrosis and hemorrhage. In general, the vascularity of adenomas is not as fine and orderly as the pattern seen in focal nodular hyperplasia (Fig. 64-16), nor does one usually see the septa within the tumor. The tumor staining also tends to be more homogeneous than in hyperplasia. At times, however, the arteriogram can be quite difficult to differentiate from that obtained in hyperplasia, and in these cases radionuclide scans can be helpful. Since adenomas do not have any Kupffer cells, they do not take up labeled colloid.

Whether adenomas have a malignant potential is not altogether clear, especially since histologically it can be difficult at times to differentiate an adenoma from a hepatocellular carcinoma. Because of the chance of malignancy plus the risk of life-threatening hemorrhage, many hepatic adenomas are surgically removed.

HAMARTOMAS AND OTHER RARE TUMORS

Hepatic hamartomas are rare, and their angiographic appearance varies greatly, depending on

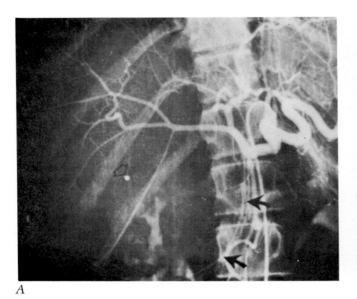

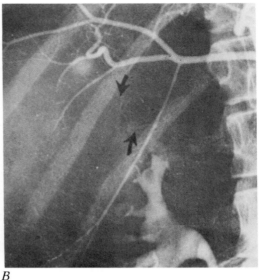

A   *B*

Figure 64-17. Cystic degeneration of a hamartoma. (A) A 15-year-old girl had selective celiac arteriography to investigate a right upper quadrant mass. A lead shot (*open arrow*) was placed on the palpable portion of the mass prior to the study. The intrahepatic branches of the hepatic artery are displaced medially and inferiorly (*arrows*) by a large cystic lesion arising from the liver. (B) Direct serial magnification study demonstrates small arterial branches coursing through the otherwise avascular cyst (*arrows*). At surgery this proved to be a hamartoma that had undergone cystic degeneration; the abnormal vasculature noted within the mass was due to vessels accompanying the remaining biliary ductal systems.

the primary cell type involved in the tumor mass [38]. These lesions frequently undergo cystic degeneration, and when this occurs, they may resemble benign cysts (Fig. 64-17). Other benign tumors of the liver are very rare, and although biliary adenomas, cystadenomas, and leiomyomas have been reported, characteristic arteriographic findings in these tumors have not been described.

Primary Malignant Tumors

HEPATOMA

Primary carcinoma of the liver, or hepatoma, is almost always seen arteriographically as a vascular tumor [39–41]. The hepatic artery feeding the tumor is usually wider than normal, and the intrahepatic branches are generally displaced. During the arterial phase of a selective hepatic arteriogram the abnormal neovasculature, unlike that of hemangiomas, exhibits a chaotic and disorganized pattern. During the capillary phase of the examination, there is generally an intense tumor blush (Figs. 64-18–64-20). Marked arteriovenous shunting is a common finding in hepatomas (Figs. 64-21, 64-22) and on occasion the shunting into the portal venous system may be so great as actually to delineate tumor thrombi within the portal vein (Fig. 64-23) [42]. Primary hepatic neoplasms derive almost all of their blood supply from the hepatic arteries. The portal venous system, which usually contributes approximately 75 percent of the blood supply to the normal liver, does not form the neovasculature of tumor masses [43]. As a result, splenoportography or arterial portography gives only indirect evidence of a mass, which is seen as a filling defect in an otherwise homogeneous portal hepatogram. Approximately 75 percent of patients with hepatomas have preexisting alcoholic or postnecrotic cirrhosis. The very distorted arterial pattern of advanced liver disease sometimes makes it difficult to detect a superposed carcinoma. A modification of the technique of hepatic arteriography for patients with suspected tumors has been the intrahepatic arterial administration of a vasoconstricting drug before the injection of contrast material (Fig. 64-24). This is based on the principle that tumor vessels, unlike normal vessels, do not react to vasoactive drugs. Small doses of epinephrine (5–10 μg) or vasopressin (1 pressor unit) injected into the hepatic artery immediately before injection of contrast

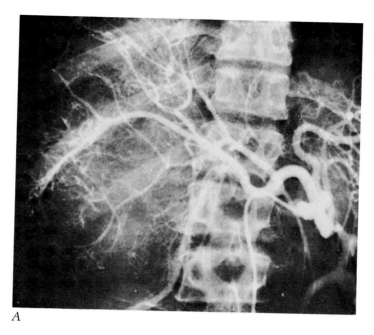

A

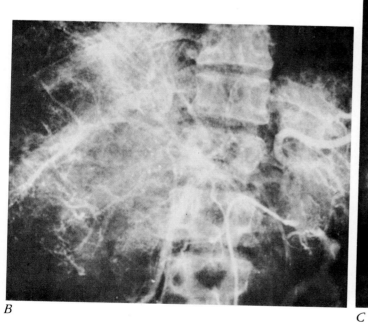

B

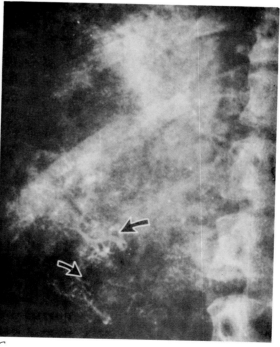

C

Figure 64-18. Hepatoma. (A) Arterial phase of a selective celiac arteriogram demonstrates marked displacement of the intrahepatic arterial branches involving primarily the right and middle lobes. (B) During the capillary phase, an intense tumor stain is seen associated with many abnormal tumor vessels. (C) During the late capillary phase, abnormal "laking" is seen within the tumors with persistence of contrast material within abnormally dilated veins (*arrows*).

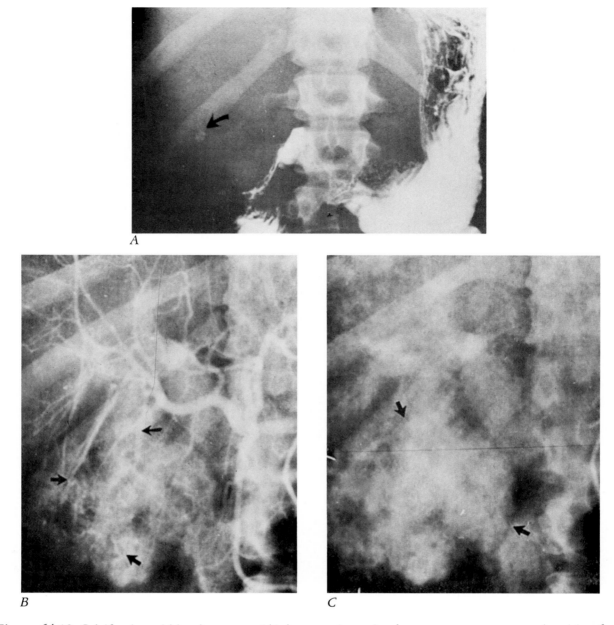

A

B   *C*

Figure 64-19. Calcification within a hepatoma. (A) An upper gastrointestinal study in a 22-year-old man demonstrates a large right upper quadrant mass displacing the first and second portions of the duodenum. Calcification is noted within the mass (*arrow*). Calcification within hepatomas is seen more often in children and young adults. (B) Selective hepatic arteriography demonstrates tumor vessels arising from the right hepatic artery (*arrows*) supplying this large, vascular tumor. (C) During the capillary phase of the study, an intense tumor blush is seen (*arrows*). The patient underwent successful resection of this lesion, which necessitated removal of the entire right lobe of the liver.

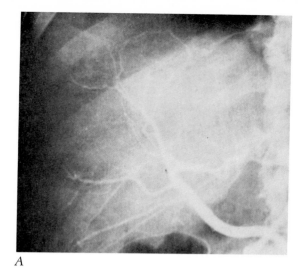

A

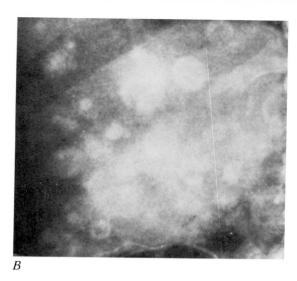

B

Figure 64-20. Multicentric hepatoma. (A) Selective hepatic arteriography fails to demonstrate tumor vessels or arteriovenous shunting. (B) During the capillary phase of the study, multiple tumor stains of various sizes can be identified. The arteriographic pictures resemble those of hepatic metastases. At surgery this was found to be a diffuse hepatoma. (Courtesy of Sidney Wallace, M.D.)

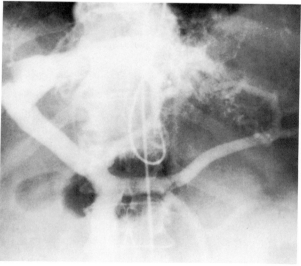

Figure 64-21. Hepatoma involving the left lobe of the liver. Selective injection into a common left hepatic–left gastric artery in a patient with cirrhosis and portal hypertension demonstrates marked arteriovenous shunting as a result of a hepatoma in the left lobe of the liver. The shunting into the portal venous system demonstrates hepatofugal flow.

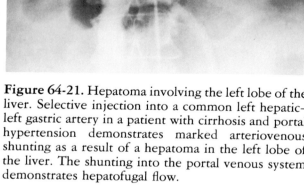

A

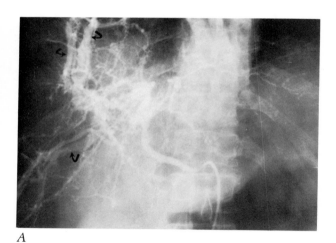

B

Figure 64-22. Hepatoma with marked hepatic ▶ arterial–portal venous shunting. (A) Selective hepatic arteriogram in a patient with cirrhosis and portal hypertension demonstrates hepatic arterial–portal venous shunting (*arrows*) secondary to a hepatoma. (B) During the hepatographic phase of the examination there is complete filling of the portal venous radicals with hepatofugal flow and filling of the coronary vein.

1495

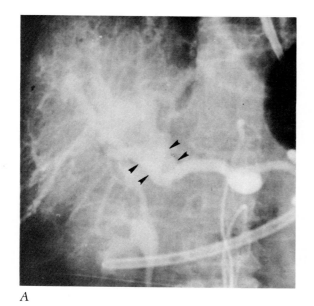

A

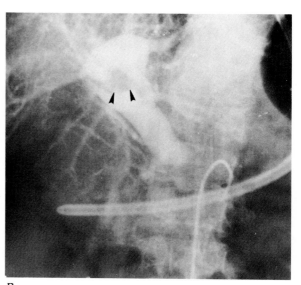

B

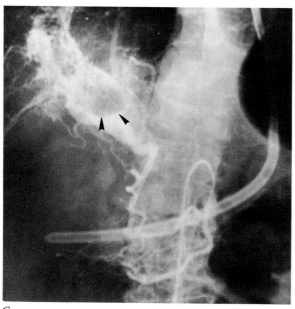

C

Figure 64-23. Hepatoma exhibiting marked arteriovenous shunting and a tumor thrombus in the portal vein. The patient presented with bleeding in the esophageal varices. (A) Selective celiac arteriography shows abundant tumor vascularity within the right lobe of the liver associated with arteriovenous shunting and opacification of the portal vein (*arrows*). (B) During the hepatographic phase of the injection a large filling defect can be seen within the main portal vein; this proved to be a tumor thrombus (*arrows*). (C) During the late phase of a selective inferior pancreaticoduodenal artery injection once again retrograde opacification of the portal vein can be seen due to arteriovenous shunting within the tumor. The tumor thrombus (*arrows*) is again identified extending upward into the liver.

material are often useful for the demonstration of tumor vessels [44].

Because of the trend in surgery to attempt hepatectomies in this disease, it is important for the arteriographer to assess the operability of these tumors and to determine the plane of the tumor in relation to the plane of division of the liver, the so-called lobar fissure. It is also important to delineate clearly which branches of the hepatic artery supply the tumor. Since as many as 35 percent of hepatomas have macroscopic invasion of the portal vein, percutaneous splenoportography is of value in determining the extent of portal venous invasion and hence the feasibility of surgical resection.

PRIMARY BILE DUCT CARCINOMA

Primary tumors of the biliary system are less vascular than hepatomas and do not exhibit the arteriovenous shunting that is so often seen in hepatomas [45, 46]. The arterial branches going to the primary tumor of the common duct or gallbladder exhibit displacement, margin irregularity, and on occasion complete obstruction (Fig. 64-25). During the capillary phase of the study, a

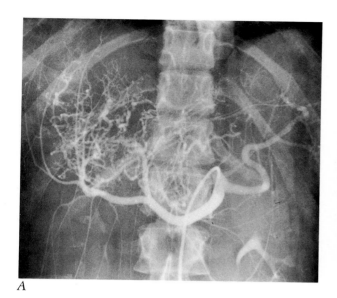

A

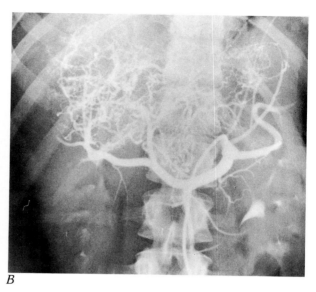

B

Figure 64-24. Hepatoma seen best after the injection of 1 unit of vasopressin. (A) Selective hepatic arteriography in a patient with cirrhosis of the liver and a superimposed hepatoma. Abnormal tumor vessels are seen within the liver as outlined by an irregular mass. (B) After injection of 1 unit of vasopressin into the hepatic artery there is vasoconstriction of the normal branches without any significant change of the tumor vessel diameter in the mass itself. Because of the vasoconstriction of the normal vessels more of the contrast is shunted to the mass, making it more clearly visible.

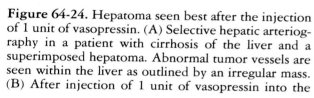

Figure 64-25. Carcinoma of the common duct. (A) The arterial phase of the selective celiac arteriogram demonstrates spreading of the common duct branches of the gastroduodenal artery (*solid black arrows*). Small, indistinct, irregular vessels are seen extending from the right hepatic artery (*open arrow*). (B) During the capillary phase of the study, a tumor stain can be identified in the area of the abnormal vasculature (*arrows*) that is irregular and extends into the liver parenchyma. This was an inoperable carcinoma of the common duct infiltrating deeply within the liver.

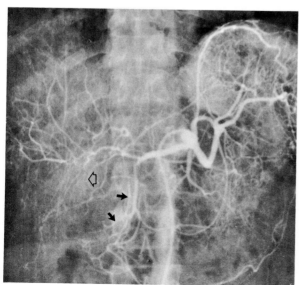

A

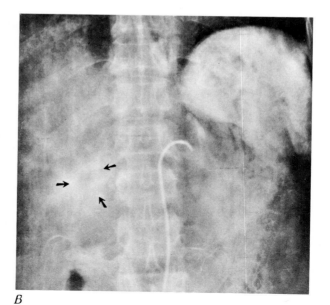

B

tumor stain can frequently be seen, but it tends not to be as dense as that seen in hepatomas.

The angiographic findings in hepatomas and cholangiomas correlate well with their histologic appearance. Hepatomas have extremely rich capillary stroma, while cholangiomas are hard tumors with a predominance of connective tissue overgrowth and few capillaries. Since cholangiocarcinomas can spread through the biliary ducts, large and extensive tumors may be present without angiographic evidence of a large mass.

ANGIOSARCOMA

Whelan et al. [47] have described the angiographic and radionuclide-uptake characteristics of hepatic angiosarcoma found following vinyl chloride exposure. The few cases described had a normal appearance of the hepatic artery associated with very small, fine tumor vessels around the periphery of the tumor. Contrast material persisting within the tumor extended very late into the venous phase of the examination. Areas of the tumor appeared hypovascular. The latter finding was probably a result of the central necrosis that frequently accompanies angiosarcomas.

Malignant Disease Metastatic to the Liver

Hepatic metastases, like primary tumors of the liver, are almost exclusively supplied by the hepatic artery. The metastatic lesion usually exhibits the same angiographic characteristics as the primary tumor. If the primary tumor is very vascular, as is renal cell carcinoma, carcinoid tumor (Fig. 64-26), or leiomyoma (Fig. 64-27) of the gastrointestinal tract, the metastatic deposits in the liver are also vascular. Poorly vascularized tumors, like adenocarcinoma of the gastrointestinal tract, when metastatic to the liver, may appear as either avascular masses or tumors exhibiting very small tumor vessels that stain sparsely during the capillary phase (Fig. 64-28). The latter changes are generally seen only when most of the hepatic parenchyma has been replaced by metastatic disease. The diagnosis of small scattered metastatic deposits within the liver is usually difficult to establish during arteriography. Rarely, as in carcinoma of the pancreas, the metastatic lesion to the liver is more vascular than the primary tumor.

Figure 64-26. Ileal carcinoid tumor metastatic to the liver. Hepatic arteriography demonstrates multiple vascular metastases to the liver from a carcinoid tumor of the small bowel.

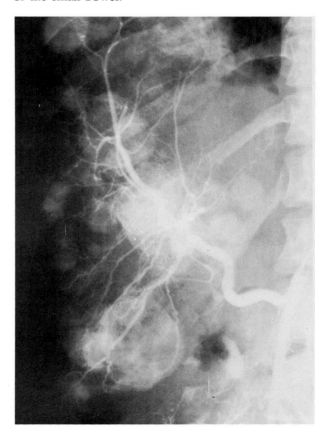

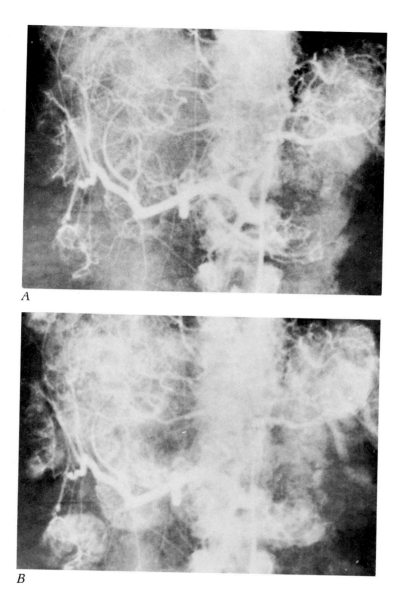

A

B

Figure 64-27. Leiomyosarcoma metastatic to the liver. (A) Selective hepatic arteriography demonstrates marked enlargement of the liver associated with displacement of intrahepatic arterial branches. Numerous irregular large tumor vessels can be identified. (B) During the late arterial phase of the examination, tumor stains of various sizes are seen. This patient had a primary leiomyosarcoma in the small intestine.

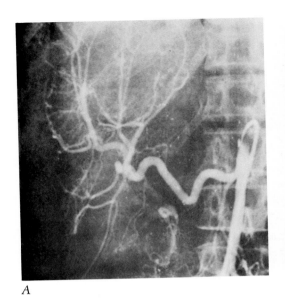
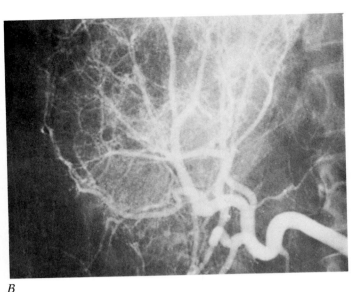

A *B*

Figure 64-28. Adenocarcinoma of the colon metastatic to the liver. (A) The hepatic artery arises from the superior mesenteric artery. Selective superior mesenteric arteriography demonstrates displaced intrahepatic branches associated with a mottled appearance of the finer intrahepatic radicles. (B) Direct serial magnification arteriography demonstrates small tumor vessels as well as displacement of the intrahepatic branches to much greater advantage. Vessels of approximately 100 μ in diameter can be visualized with direct radiographic magnification using a fractional focal-spot x-ray tube.

Hepatic Trauma

Although only 15 to 20 percent of abdominal injuries damage the liver, more than 50 percent of deaths from abdominal trauma are caused by hepatic rupture [48]. The mortality is even higher in blunt hepatic trauma than in perforating injury and may go as high as 70 percent. Because of this high mortality, emergency surgery is frequently indicated and often lifesaving in patients with hepatic rupture. Since it may well be impossible to evaluate the extent of the injury at surgery—in fact, sometimes it is not even possible to identify the lesion within the liver—emergency hepatic arteriography should be performed if at all feasible [49]. The indications for angiography are as follows:

1. To document the presence of liver damage and to evaluate and localize its extent.
2. To follow the natural course of an angiographically diagnosed lesion if surgery is not performed.
3. To evaluate for complications of trauma, whether they be aneurysms, subcapsular hematomas, or hemobilia, following either conservative or surgical management.
4. To control hepatic bleeding by the use of transcatheter embolization techniques (Fig. 64-29).

Any of the following angiographic findings may be seen in hepatic trauma:

1. Liver contusion.
   a. Elongation and straightening of arterial branches.
   b. Delay in hepatic blood flow to specific segments of the liver.
   c. Small areas of contrast accumulation in affected areas.
2. Liver laceration.
   a. Hepatic arterial occlusion.
   b. Contrast extravasation.
   c. Pseudoaneurysm formation (Fig. 64-30).
   d. Arterioportal fistula.
   e. Arteriobiliary fistula.
3. Subcapsular or intrahepatic hematoma (Fig. 64-31).
   a. Arterial displacement.
   b. Liver displacement.
   c. Contrast extravasation.

Small ruptures that are either subcapsular or central in location need no intervention if they

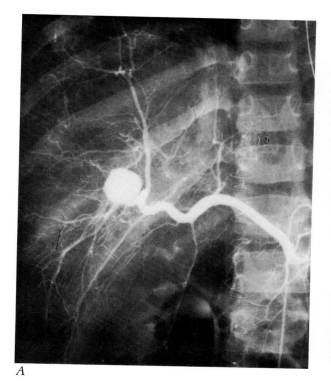

A

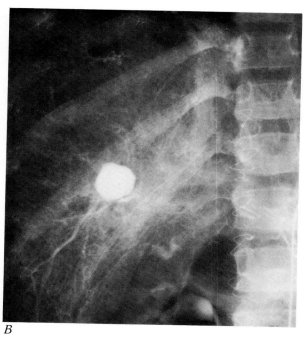

B

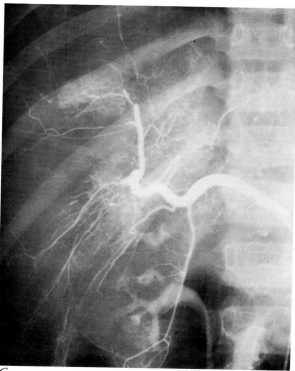

C

Figure 64-29. Bleeding false aneurysm of the hepatic artery treated by transcatheter arterial embolization. (A) Selective hepatic arteriogram demonstrates a large false aneurysm of the right hepatic artery. (B) Persistent contrast material in the false aneurysm can be seen 29 seconds after the start of the injection. (C) Repeat hepatic arteriogram after the injection of Gelfoam plugs fails to demonstrate any evidence of continued arterial extravasation. This child's hepatic bleeding was caused by blunt abdominal trauma sustained during a bicycle accident. The transcatheter embolization successfully controlled the bleeding.

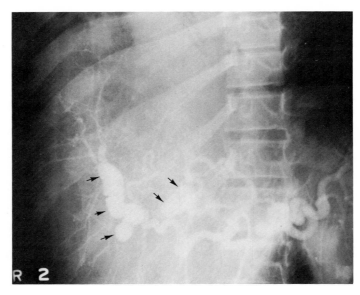

Figure 64-30. Traumatic false aneurysms of the right and middle hepatic arteries (*arrows*) in a patient who had sustained abdominal trauma several weeks earlier.

Figure 64-31. Traumatic subcapsular hepatic hematoma. (A) Arterial phase of a selective arteriogram demonstrates abrupt termination of the intrahepatic branches (*arrows*) before they reach the lateral body wall. (B) Capillary phase of the study shows the characteristic beaking due to compressed parenchyma and a radiolucent defect between the blush of the liver and the rib cage. The angiographic appearance of a subcapsular hepatic hematoma is identical to that of a subcapsular hematoma of the spleen.

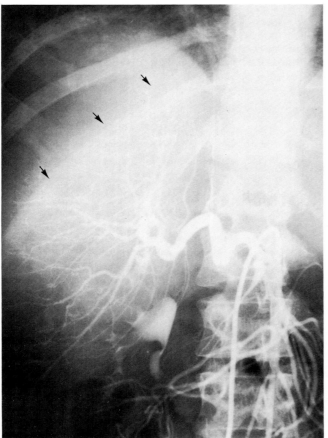

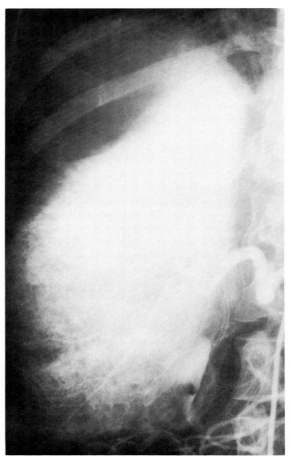

A

B

are clinically silent. Boijsen et al. [50] reported that 11 of 25 patients with unequivocal angiographic signs of liver damage were not operated on and did well. Because of the high association of renal and splenic injuries following either blunt or penetrating abdominal trauma, hepatic arteriography is often combined with splenic and renal arteriography.

References

1. Bierman, H. R., Byron, R. L., Jr., Kelly, K. H., and Grady, A. Studies on the blood supply of tumors in man: Vascular patterns of the liver by hepatic arteriography in vivo. *J. Natl. Cancer Inst.* 12:107, 1951.
2. Seldinger, S. L. Catheter replacement of needle in percutaneous arteriography; a new technique. *Acta Radiol.* (Stockh.) 39:368, 1953.
3. Ödman, P. Percutaneous selective angiography of the celiac artery. *Acta Radiol. [Suppl.]* (Stockh.) 159:1, 1958.
4. Tylén, U., Simert, G., and Vang, J. Hemodynamic changes after distal splenorenal shunt studied by sequential angiography. *Radiology* 121:585, 1976.
5. Viamonte, M., Jr., LePage, J. R., Russel, E., Roen, S. A., Pereiras, R., Zeppa, R., and Viamonte, M. The hemodynamics of diffuse liver disease. *Semin. Roentgenol.* 10:187, 1975.
6. Bookstein, J. J., Boijsen, E., Olin, T., and Vang, J. Angiography before and after end-to-side portacaval shunt. Clinical, laboratory, and pharmacoangiographic observations. *Invest. Radiol.* 6:101, 1971.
7. Kreel, L. Vascular radiology in liver disease. *Postgrad. Med. J.* 46:618, 1970.
8. Kim, D. K., McSweeney, J., Yeh, S. D. J., and Fortner, J. G. Tumors of the liver as demonstrated by angiography, scan, and laparotomy. *Surg. Gynecol. Obstet.* 141:409, 1975.
9. Michels, N. A. *Blood Supply and Anatomy of the Upper Abdominal Organs.* Philadelphia: Lippincott, 1955.
10. Healey, J. E., and Schroy, P. C. Anatomy of the biliary ducts within the human liver: Analysis of the prevailing pattern of branchings and the major variations of the biliary ducts. *Arch. Surg.* 66:599, 1953.
11. Nebesar, R. A., Kornblith, P. L., Pollard, J. J., and Michels, N. A. Anatomic Considerations. In R. A. Nebesar et al. (eds.), *Celiac and Superior Mesenteric Arteries: A Correlation of Angiograms and Dissections.* Boston: Little, Brown, 1969.
12. Wagner, D., and Baum, S. Preliminary arteriography in hepatic artery infusions for cancer. *Surg. Gynecol. Obstet.* 120:817, 1965.
13. Baum, S., Roy, R., Finkelstein, A. K., and Blakemore, W. S. Clinical application of selective celiac and superior mesenteric arteriography. *Radiology* 84:279, 1965.
14. Evans, J. A. Specialized roentgen diagnostic technics in the investigation of abdominal disease (Annual Oration in Memory of Clarence Elton Hufford). *Radiology* 82:579, 1964.
15. Boijsen, E., Ekman, C.-A., and Lundh, G. Selective splanchnic angiography. *Adv. Surg.* 3:13, 1968.
16. Simmons, J. T., Baum, S., Sheehan, B. A., Ring, E. J., Athanasoulis, C. A., Waltman, A. C., and Coggins, P. C. The effect of vasopressin on hepatic arterial blood flow. *Radiology* 124:637, 1977.
17. Reuter, S. R., and Redman, H. C. *Gastrointestinal Angiography* (2nd ed.). Philadelphia: Saunders, 1977.
18. Rosenberg, R. F., and Sprayregen, S. The hepatic artery in cirrhosis: An angiographic pathophysiologic correlation. *Angiology* 25:499, 1974.
19. Viamonte, M., Jr., Warren, W. D., Fomon, J. J., and Martinez, L. O. Angiographic investigations in portal hypertension. *Surg. Gynecol. Obstet.* 130:37, 1970.
20. Viamonte, M., Jr., and Viamonte, M. Liver circulation. *Crit. Rev. Clin. Radiol.* 27:214, 1974.
21. Rabinowitz, J. G., Kinkabwala, M., and Ulreich, S. Macroregenerating nodule in the cirrhotic liver. *AJR* 121:401, 1974.
22. McNulty, J. G. Angiographic manifestations of hydatid disease of the liver: A report of two cases. *AJR* 102:380, 1968.
23. Rizk, G. K., Tayyarah, K. A., and Ghandur-Mnaymneh, L. The angiographic changes in hydatid cysts of the liver and spleen. *Radiology* 99:303, 1971.
24. Lomba Viana, R. Selective arteriography in the diagnosis and evaluation of amebic abscess of the liver. *Am. J. Dig. Dis.* 20:632, 1975.
25. Abrams, R. M., Beranbaum, E. R., Santos, J. S., and Lipson, J. Angiographic features of cavernous hemangioma of liver. *Radiology* 92:308, 1969.
26. Alfidi, R. J., Rastogi, H., Buonocore, E., and Brown, C. H. Hepatic arteriography. *Radiology* 90:1136, 1968.
27. Pantoga, E. Angiography in liver hemangioma. *AJR* 104:874, 1968.
28. Curry, J. L., Johnson, W. G., Feinberg, D. H., and Updegrove, J. H. Thorium induced hepatic hemangioendothelioma: Roentgen-angiographic findings in two additional cases with clinical "informed consent" problems. *AJR* 125:671, 1975.
29. McLoughlin, M. J., Colapinto, R. F., Gilday, D. L., Hobbs, B. B., Korobkin, M. T., McDonald, P., and Phillips, M. J. Focal nodular hyperplasia of the liver: Angiography and radioisotope scanning. *Radiology* 107:257, 1973.

30. Philips, M. J., Langer, B., Stone, R., Fisher, M., and Ritchie, S. Benign liver cell tumors: Classification and ultrastructural pathology. *Cancer* 32:463, 1973.

31. Tate, R. C., Chacko, M. V., and Singh, S. Parenchymal hamartoma of the liver in infants and children. *Am. J. Surg.* 123:346, 1972.

32. Aronsen, K. F., Ericcson, B., Lunderquist, A., Malmborg, O., and Norden, J. G. A case of operated focal nodular cirrhosis of the liver. *Scand. J. Gastroenterol.* 3:58, 1968.

33. Galloway, S. J., Casarella, W. J., Lattes, R., and Seaman, W. B. Minimal deviation hepatoma: A new entity. *AJR* 125:184, 1975.

34. Knowles, D. M., and Wolff, M. Focal nodular hyperplasia of the liver: A clinicopathologic study and review of the literature. *Hum. Pathol.* 7:533, 1976.

35. Casarella, W. J., Knowles, D. M., Wolff, M., and Johnson, P. M. Focal nodular hyperplasia and liver cell adenoma: Radiologic and pathologic differentiation. *AJR* 131:393, 1978.

36. Sorensen, T. I., and Baden, H. Benign hepatocellular tumors. *Scand. J. Gastroenterol.* 10:113, 1975.

37. Baum, J. K., Holtz, F., Bookstein, J. J., and Klein, E. W. Possible association between benign hepatomas and oral contraceptives. *Lancet* 2:926, 1973.

38. McLoughlin, M. J., and Phillips, M. J. Angiographic findings in multiple bile duct hamartomas of the liver. *Radiology* 116:41, 1975.

39. Boijsen, E., and Abrams, H. L. Roentgenologic diagnosis of primary carcinoma of the liver. *Acta Radiol.* [*Diagn.*] (Stockh.) 3:257, 1965.

40. Reuter, S. R., Redman, H. C., and Siders, D. B. The spectrum of angiographic findings in hepatoma. *Radiology* 94:89, 1970.

41. Neiman, H. L., Goldstein, H. M., Silverman, P. J., and Bookstein, J. J. Angiographic features of peripancreatic malignant lymphoma. *Radiology* 115:589, 1975.

42. Okuda, K., Musha, H., Yoshida, T., Kanda, Y., Yamazaki, T., Jinnouchi, S., Moriyama, M., Kawaguchi, S., Kubo, Y., Shimokawa, Y., Kujiro, M., Kuratomi, S., Sakamotu, K., and Nakashima, T. Demonstration of growing casts of hepatocellular carcinoma in the portal vein by celiac angiography: The thread and streaks sign. *Radiology* 117:303, 1975.

43. Breedis, C., and Young, G. The blood supply of neoplasms in the liver. *Am. J. Pathol.* 30:969, 1954.

44. Kahn, P. C., Frates, W. J., and Paul, R. E., Jr. The epinephrine effect in angiography of gastrointestinal tract tumors. *Radiology* 88:686, 1967.

45. Abrams, R. M., Meng, C. H., Firooznia, H., Beranbaum, E. R., and Epstein, H. Y. Angiographic demonstration of carcinoma of the gallbladder. *Radiology* 94:277, 1970.

46. Reuter, S. R., Redman, H. C., and Bookstein, J. J. Angiography in carcinoma of the biliary tract. *Br. J. Radiol.* 44:636, 1971.

47. Whelan, J. G., Jr., Creech, J. L., and Tamburro, C. H. Angiographic and radionuclide characteristics of hepatic angiosarcoma found in vinyl chloride workers. *Radiology* 118:549, 1976.

48. Boijsen, E., Judkins, M. P., and Simay, A. Angiographic diagnosis of hepatic rupture. *Radiology* 86:66, 1966.

49. Aakhus, T., and Enge, L. Angiography in rupture of the liver. *Acta Radiol.* [*Diagn.*] (Stockh.) 11:353, 1971.

50. Boijsen, E., Kaude, J., and Tylén, U. Angiography in hepatic rupture. *Acta Radiol.* [*Diagn.*] (Stockh.) 11:363, 1971.

Transhepatic Portal Venography

ANDERS LUNDERQUIST
JÜRGEN HOEVELS
TORBEN OWMAN

Percutaneous transhepatic portography was described by Bierman et al. in 1952 [3]. Using a ventral approach they punctured the portal vein with a needle and injected contrast medium without any attempt at catheterization of the portal vein branches.

Wiechel [60] reported an improved puncture technique including the possibility of simultaneous catheterization of the portal vein and its branches. This technique has since been widely used at different centers [11, 20, 40, 59]. The puncture should not be performed in patients with severe coagulopathy. In elective studies we have regarded as contraindications a platelet count below 50,000 and a prolonged prothrombin time. In these cases, the prothrombin time has been measured with Normotest (Nyegaard & Co., Oslo, Norway), normal values being above 70 percent. Values below 40 percent have been considered a contraindication to transhepatic portography.

Technique

The puncture site is selected in the right midaxillary line. Fluoroscopically the liver hilus can be roughly localized, as can the costophrenic tip of the lung.

In the first series of patients who underwent this examination we asked the patient to take a deep breath so that the lowermost position of the costophrenic sinus of the pleura could be visualized, and the puncture was performed below this. However, in these cases the needle had to be directed too steeply upward and medially when it was aimed toward the liver hilus. Moreover, the angulation between the parenchymal part of the catheter and that in the portal vein made manipulation of the catheter difficult. Since then we have made the puncture in the midrespiratory position of the diaphragm, as straight as possible toward the liver hilus and through the obliterated costophrenic sinus of the pleura when this happened to be deep. A 25-cm-long needle sheathed by a radiopaque polyethylene catheter (ID/OD 1.1/1.6 mm) is used. The puncture is performed under local anesthesia and immediately above the rib to prevent damaging an intercostal artery. If the needle is introduced in the midaxillary line and moved horizontally toward the liver hilus up to 1 or 2 cm to the right of the spine, it will usually hit the

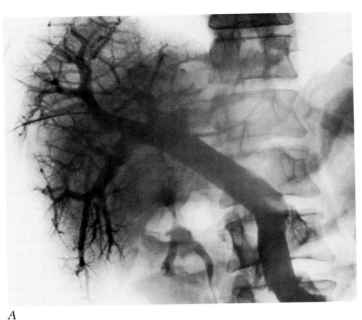
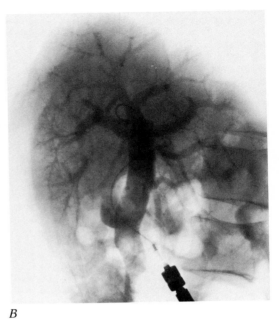

A   B

Figure 65-1. Transhepatic portography, normal anatomy. (A) Anteroposterior view. (B) Lateral view.

portal vein at its bifurcation (Fig. 65-1). The needle is removed, and the catheter is slowly pulled back under intermittent aspiration. When blood can be freely aspirated, a test injection of contrast medium will show whether the tip of the catheter is in a portal vein branch. If this is the case, a slightly curved guidewire is introduced and manipulated into the main stem of the portal vein. The catheter is then pushed over the guidewire until end to end with it and the guidewire is removed.

In patients with liver cirrhosis, ascites, and a hard fibrotic liver, it is sometimes difficult or impossible to advance the catheter over the guidewire all the way into the main stem of the portal vein. The guidewire and catheter often kink between the liver and the abdominal wall. In these cases a specially designed guidewire [29] with a soft tip will be of great help.

If the liver parenchyma is to be examined for primary or secondary tumors, 40 cc of 76 percent contrast medium is injected into the main stem of the portal vein at the rate of 8 cc per second, and films are exposed one per second for 5 seconds, two per second for 4 seconds, and one every other second for 6 seconds. The fast filming rate is chosen during the parenchymal phase of the portogram when filling defects can most easily be interpreted.

In patients with portal hypertension the catheter has to be introduced into the splenic vein and sometimes also into the superior mesenteric vein for injection of the contrast medium. Again 40 cc of contrast medium is injected at a rate of 8 cc per second. To cover the often slow flow of contrast through collateral vessels, eight films are exposed one per second followed by another eight films over 16 seconds.

At the end of the procedure, when the catheter is to be removed, a small piece of Gelfoam is injected into the puncture canal about 2 cm below the surface of the liver.

Complications

Complications accompanying percutaneous transhepatic catheterization of the portal vein are relatively few. Serious complications are most often seen in already severely ill patients such as those with liver cirrhosis, bleeding esophageal varices, or obstructive jaundice.

In 440 transhepatic catheterizations of the portal vein performed in 398 patients at the University Hospital, Lund, Sweden, three patients died later of complications from the procedure. One patient with liver cirrhosis and severe coagulopathy died of bleeding from the puncture site and generalized gastrointestinal hemorrhage, and two patients with malignant obstructive jaundice died because of intraabdominal bleeding. In the latter patients the examination had been performed in combination with percutaneous drainage of the bile ducts.

Laparotomy had to be performed in seven patients because of intraabdominal hemorrhage. Four of the patients had either liver cirrhosis or obstructive jaundice.

Portal Hypertension

INTRAHEPATIC FLOW PATTERN

In order to understand the intrahepatic flow pattern in the portal vein during portal hypertension, a short review of the blood flow through the normal liver is necessary.

Hepatic artery and portal vein branches follow each other within the liver on their way to the sinusoids. Presinusoidal anastomoses exist between the hepatic artery and the portal vein [10, 33]. These anastomoses are present directly between the hepatic artery and the portal vein and between the arterial plexus surrounding the bile duct and the adjacent portal vein.

The flow through the anastomoses and through the sinusoids is regulated by sphincters, which in fact are endothelial cells with the ability to increase and decrease in size [32]. Through the action of the sphincters, the sinusoids in one part of the liver can be perfused by a mixture of arterial and portal blood, pure portal blood, or pure arterial blood. The outflow from the sinusoids in each lobule is not restricted to its own hepatic vein. Sinusoids of all lobules are interconnected, and the drainage of one group of sinusoids can thus be through adjacent lobules and their central veins. From the sinusoids the blood is drained through the hepatic veins [27].

One of the first angiographic signs of portal hypertension is the development of extrahepatic portosystemic collaterals. When the liver parenchyma is damaged and replaced by fibrotic tissue, the flow through the sinusoids is impaired and portal venous pressure increases. When increased pressure is not enough to accomplish perfusion of all portal venous blood through the liver, the excess is first drained through collaterals with the least resistance, usually the left gastric vein and the inferior mesenteric vein. Still the intrahepatic vascular pattern shows very few changes from normal. The portal vein branches show more right-angled bifurcations and are less numerous than normal.

Later, portal flow resistance increases in areas of more severe parenchymal destruction. When arterial inflow through sinusoidal and presinusoidal anastomoses is in excess of hepatic venous

drainage, the portal flow in this part of the liver is reversed. The reversal is reflected in the portogram by lack of filling of portal vein branches and in the selective hepatic arteriogram by contrast filling of these portal vein branches (Figs. 65-2, 65-3). Certainly this can be the result not only of hepatofugal flow but also of thrombotic occlusion or external compression of the portal vein branch by a regenerative nodule or tumor. If, however, the lack of filling is due to segmental hepatofugal flow, oscillations of contrast medium are most often seen within a distance of a centimeter or so. The oscillations are produced by changes in portal venous pressure from injection of the contrast medium or by the patient's straining when holding his breath. Respiratory movements and straining can cause significant changes in portal venous pressure [35].

Hepatofugal flow of the portal venous blood can also be seen through a paraumbilical vein originating from the left portal vein branch (Fig. 65-4) or, less often, through an anomalous left gastric vein ending in the left portal vein branch [43].

If the arterial inflow to the whole liver is in excess of the capacity of hepatic vein drainage, the flow in the main stem of the portal vein becomes hepatofugal (Fig. 65-5). The part of the arterial flow to the liver that is not drained through the hepatic veins, together with venous blood from the splenic and superior mesenteric veins, is thus drained through the large number of portosystemic collaterals that usually develop [22, 50].

Under certain circumstances the flow in the main stem of the portal vein can be hepatopetal in spite of total hepatofugal flow within the liver. Hepatopetal flow can be seen when a wide paraumbilical vein has the capacity to drain not only the whole arterial inflow but also part of the flow from the splenic and the superior mesenteric veins (Fig. 65-6).

It has not been possible to show any correlation between the portal venous pressure and the degree of hepatofugal flow in the portal vein or the size or spectrum of portosystemic collaterals [22, 35, 50].

PORTOSYSTEMIC COLLATERALS

The obstruction of the hepatic veins because of fibrosis and formation of regeneration nodules in the cirrhotic liver appears to be the most important reason for the pressure rise in the portal vein and its tributaries [8, 14, 26, 34, 42]. Increasing

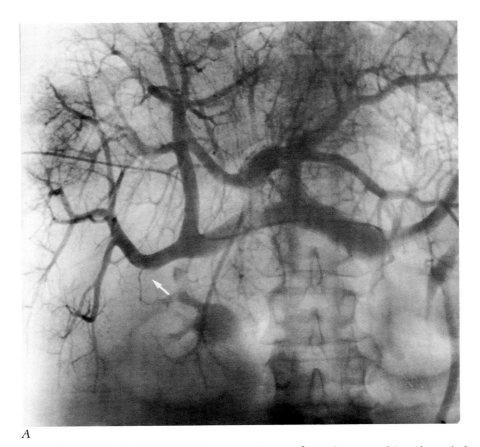

A

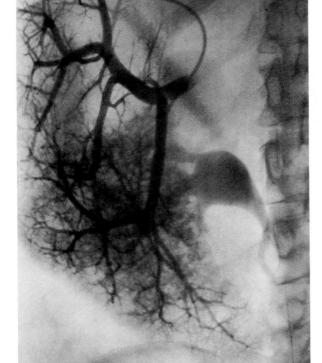

B

Figure 65-2. Segmental intrahepatic hepatofugal flow in patient with portal hypertension. (A) Hepatofugal flow is indicated by lack of filling of one portal vein branch (*arrow*). (B) Selective catheterization and injection of contrast into the branch with hepatofugal flow demonstrated in (A).

intrahepatic vascular resistance to the portal venous flow will finally result in spontaneous diversion of splanchnic blood through portosystemic collateral pathways into the systemic venous circulation.

Celiac, hepatic, splenic, superior mesenteric, and left gastric angiographic studies are the most important methods for the evaluation of the intrahepatic arterial and portal venous blood flow as well as for the study of the hemodynamics in the portal and splanchnic veins. Portosystemic collateral pathways may, however, escape detection at arteriography, when the concentration of the contrast medium in the venous phase is too low. Complementary morphologic and hemodynamic information can be provided by selective transhepatic catheterization of the portal vein and its tributaries.

Various authors [9, 45, 52] have demonstrated an abundance of normally patent portosystemic

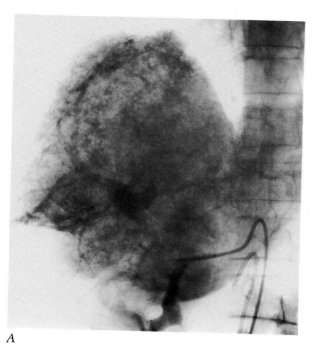

A

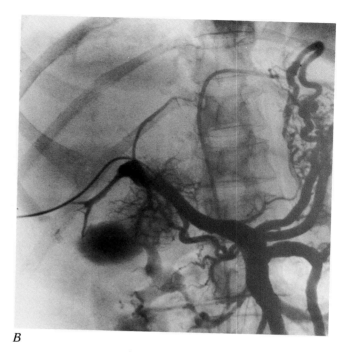

B

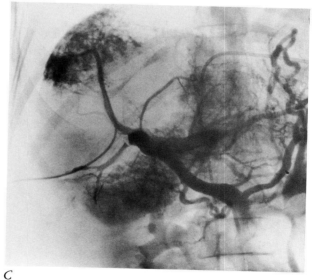

C

Figure 65-3. Portal hypertension with severe parenchymal damage. (A) Parenchymal phase after selective injection of contrast medium into common hepatic artery shows marked arterioportal shunting of contrast. (B) Transhepatic portography. Injection of contrast into main stem of portal vein demonstrates almost total hepatofugal flow and wide portosystemic collaterals. (C) Selective catheterization and injection of contrast into one portal vein branch with hepatofugal flow demonstrates patency of this branch.

communications in the pelvis, across the retroperitoneal surfaces of the abdominal viscera, and in the mediastinum, which are rarely shown intra vitam (Figs. 65-7, 65-8). The demonstration of portosystemic collateral blood flow depends primarily on the site of injection of the contrast medium at transhepatic portal venography. Collateral flow through the left gastric vein to esophageal varices may be demonstrated when the contrast medium is injected selectively into the superior mesenteric vein but may remain undetected when the contrast medium is injected into the splenic vein (Fig. 65-9). Consequently, the most important advantage of transhepatic portal venography as opposed to percutaneous splenoportography in the evaluation of portosystemic collateral flow is the selective access to the splanchnic veins.

The pattern of portosystemic collaterals varies widely among patients with portal hypertension due to liver cirrhosis. In three large series [7, 22, 36], using the percutaneous transhepatic access

to the portal and splanchnic veins, a wide variety and multiple combinations of portosystemic collaterals were observed. In the vast majority of the patients hepatofugal blood flow through left gastric and short gastric veins to gastroesophageal varices (Figs. 65-10, 65-11) seems to be present. Spontaneous reversal of blood flow in the inferior mesenteric vein is another common finding in patients with portal hypertension (Figs. 65-12, 65-13). The distribution of portosystemic collaterals in 93 cases of portal hypertension in patients with liver cirrhosis [22] is given in Table 65-1 (Figs. 65-14 to 65-19). In many of these

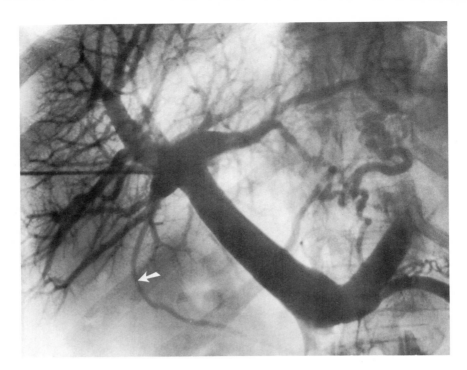

Figure 65-4. Transhepatic portography in patient with portal hypertension. There is hepatofugal flow through a tiny paraumbilical vein (*arrow*) and the left gastric and inferior mesenteric veins.

Figure 65-5. Transhepatic portography in a patient with portal hypertension. Hepatofugal flow is demonstrated in the main stem of the portal vein, and there are wide portosystemic collaterals over the left and short gastric veins and inferior mesenteric vein.

Figure 65-6. Transhepatic portography in a patient with portal hypertension. There is total hepatofugal intrahepatic portal vein flow in spite of hepatopetal flow in the main stem of portal vein. A wide paraumbilical vein serves as portosystemic collateral.

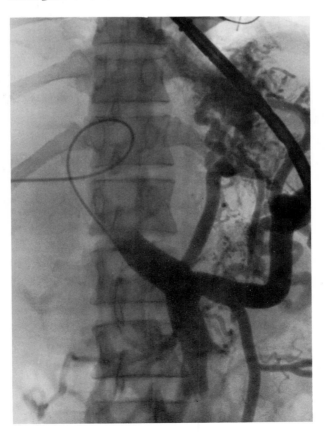

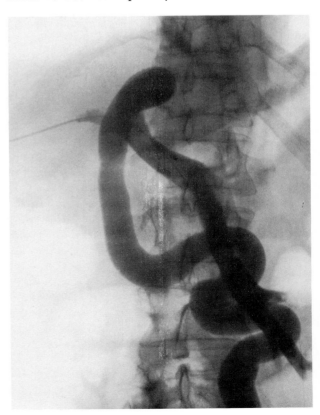

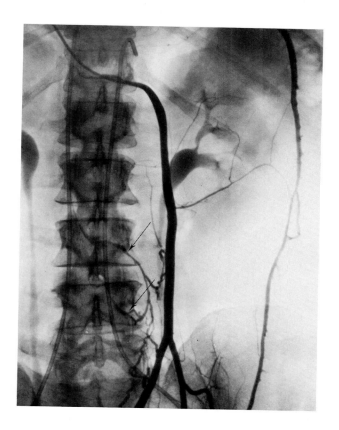

cases the collateral pathways, especially within the retroperitoneal space, were not shown or were insufficiently shown at the venous phase of arteriography.

Because esophageal varices are a potential source of bleeding, their frequency, morphology, and size in liver cirrhosis at various levels of increased portal pressure have been extensively discussed in the literature. Some authors [2, 22, 38, 53] have concluded that there is no correlation between a certain pressure level in the portal venous system and the severity of esophageal varices. Others [7, 48, 54] report a positive correlation between portal pressure and the degree of esophageal varices.

Esophageal varices of various degrees may exist whether or not large paraumbilical, splenorenal, gastrorenal, or mesentericocaval communications are present [22]. Contrary to the

Figure 65-7. Transhepatic portal venography in a patient with normal portal venous pressure. Selective injection of contrast medium into the inferior mesenteric vein demonstrates a connection with the inferior vena cava via small retroperitoneal veins (*arrows*).

Figure 65-8. Transhepatic portal venography in a patient with liver cirrhosis. The portal venous pressure was within normal limits. There is portosystemic flow from an intrahepatic portal vein branch (*arrows*) to a mediastinal vein.

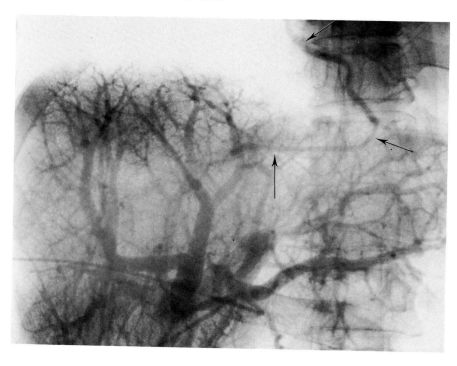

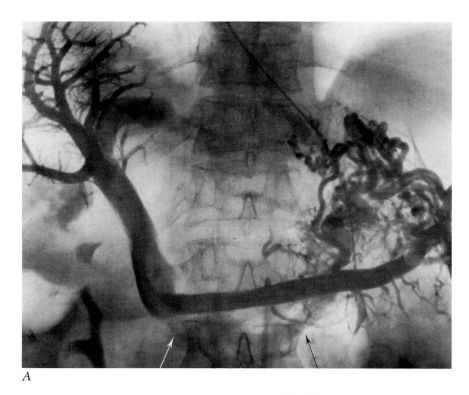

A

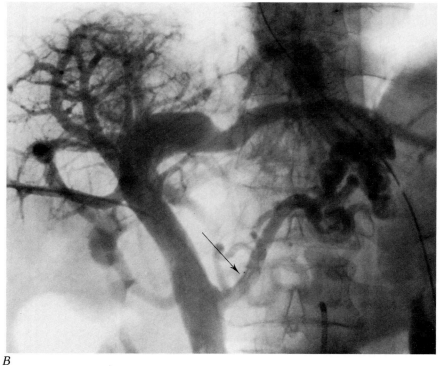

B

Figure 65-9. Transhepatic portal venography in a patient with portal hypertension. (A) Selective injection of contrast medium into the splenic vein shows partial drainage through short gastric and capsular veins of the spleen to a spontaneous splenorenal shunt (*arrows*). The left gastric vein and esophageal varices are not demonstrated. (B) Selective injection of contrast medium into the superior mesenteric vein. There is hepatofugal flow through left gastric vein (*arrow*) to esophageal varices and hepatofugal flow through a paraumbilical vein in ligamentum falciforme hepatis.

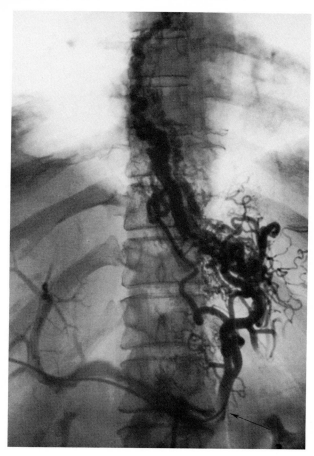

Figure 65-10. Transhepatic portal venography in a patient with portal hypertension. Selective catheterization and injection of contrast medium into left gastric vein (*arrow*) shows hepatofugal flow to gastric and esophageal veins. Endoscopy confirmed the presence of submucosal esophageal varices.

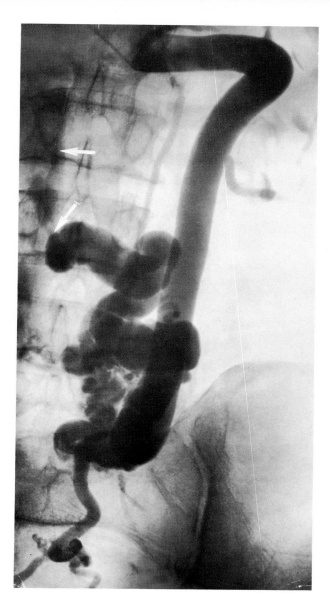

Figure 65-12. Transhepatic catheterization of markedly enlarged inferior mesenteric vein in a patient with portal hypertension. There is hepatofugal flow via retroperitoneal collaterals to the inferior vena cava (*upper arrow*). The portosystemic anastomosis (*lower arrow*) is very narrow in comparison to feeding collateral vein.

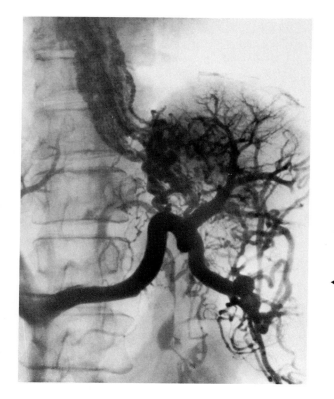

◄ **Figure 65-11.** Transhepatic portal venography in a patient with portal hypertension. Selective injection of contrast medium into the splenic vein near hilus of spleen. There is hepatofugal flow via short gastric and capsular veins of the spleen to esophageal varices. At endoscopy multiple submucosal veins in the region of the cardia and the distal segment of the esophagus were demonstrated.

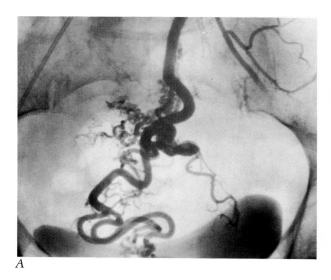

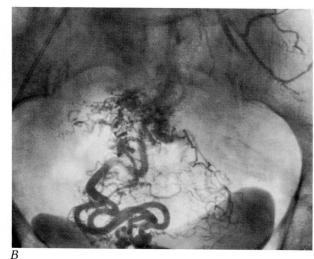

A

B

Figure 65-13. Selective catheterization of the inferior mesenteric vein in a patient with portal hypertension demonstrates hepatofugal flow to the venous plexus of the ampulla recti. (A) Early phase of phlebographic study. (B) Late phase of phlebographic study.

findings of other authors [57], large portosystemic collaterals in a recent series [22] did not reduce the portal pressure to normal values. When the portosystemic anastomosis itself is demonstrated (Figs. 65-15, 65-19), it is much narrower than the feeding collateral [22, 36], a feature that may contribute to its ineffectiveness in reducing the portal pressure. No correlation seems to exist between the portal pressure and the portosystemic collateral flow to the drainage region of the inferior or superior vena cava [22].

OBLITERATION OF VARICES

Many different treatments have been tried in patients with bleeding esophageal varices. The high operative mortality when an emergency portacaval shunt operation is performed [37] has led to the development of several methods to stop the bleeding and make an elective shunt procedure possible.

After endoscopy has verified the source of bleeding, intravenous vasopressin infusion and fresh blood transfusion are usually first tried [23, 51]. If the bleeding does not stop, a Sengstaken-Blakemore tube will in most cases control the bleeding. However, if it does not, a few nonsurgical alternatives remain. In some centers transesophageal sclerotherapy [39], in others percutaneous transhepatic obliteration of the esophageal varices [28, 30, 40, 55], is performed.

Table 65-1. Portosystemic Collaterals in 93 Cases of Portal Hypertension Caused by Liver Cirrhosis

Left gastric vein	80	Splenorenal/gastrorenal collaterals	24
Short gastric veins	54	Paraumbilical vein	27
Esophageal veins (varices)	82	Inferior mesenteric vein	55
Paraesophageal veins	27	Colon veins	22
Upper splenic hilus veins	11	Retroperitoneal veins	28
Lower splenic hilus veins	24	Inferior epigastric veins	8
Right intercostal veins	3	Posterior-superior pancreatico-duodenal vein	25
Left intercostal veins	21		
Right/left diaphragm veins	8	Anterior-superior pancreatico-duodenal vein	11
Mediastinal veins	15		
Left inferior phrenic vein	16	Azygos/hemiazygos veins	18

From Hoevels et al. [22].

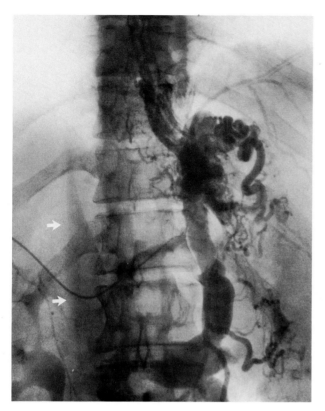

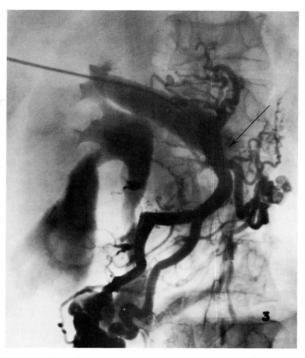

Figure 65-16. Selective catheterization of a dilated posterior superior pancreaticoduodenal (PSPD) vein (*arrow*) demonstrates hepatofugal flow via dilated pancreatic and tortuous retroperitoneal veins to the inferior vena cava.

Figure 65-14. Selective catheterization and injection of contrast medium into the left gastric vein demonstrating, in addition to esophageal varices, hepatofugal flow via a gastrorenal collateral to inferior vena cava (*arrows*).

Figure 65-15. Transhepatic catheterization of a spontaneous splenorenal shunt. The portosystemic anastomosis (*arrow*) is narrower than the feeding collateral.

Technique

The technique for obliterating the esophageal varices was first described in 1974 [31] and has since been modified and improved. Severe coagulopathy was first considered a contraindication, but it was often found that, for vital indications, the procedure had to be performed despite coagulopathy. The technique of portal vein catheterization was described earlier (pp. 1505 to 1506). We discuss here only the special technique for obliteration of the veins. The collaterals draining to the esophageal varices as demonstrated at a previous portographic examination (Fig. 65-20A) are catheterized with the aid of a slightly curved guidewire (Fig. 65-20B). The catheter is manipulated as far out in this vein as possible to prevent reflux of embolic material into the portal vein. A small catheter is introduced coaxially into the first catheter and advanced about 1 cm beyond the tip of the outer catheter. Through a three-way stopcock both catheters are filled with isotonic glucose. Glucose is then injected through the larger catheter when the embolic material (isobutyl 2-cyanoacrylate; bucrylate) is injected through the smaller one. After bucrylate injection the smaller catheter is

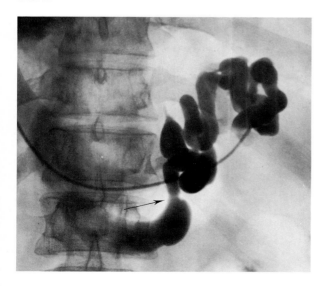

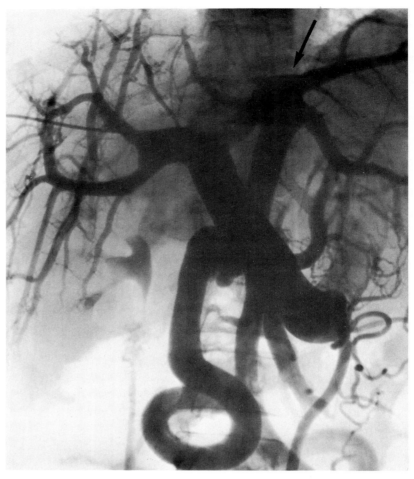

Figure 65-17. Transhepatic portal venography demonstrates hepatofugal flow via a markedly enlarged paraumbilical vein originating from the main left branch of the portal vein (*arrow*).

Figure 65-18. Selective transhepatic catheterization of a phrenic vein in the area of the attachment of the left liver lobe to the diaphragm (pars affixa) demonstrates hepatofugal flow via left pericardiacophrenic vein.

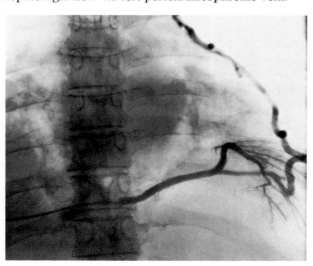

immediately flushed with glucose, and both catheters are withdrawn a few centimeters to prevent their becoming fixed to the vessel wall. To make bucrylate radiopaque we first tried tantalum powder, but this mixed poorly with the monomer. Lipiodol, on the other hand, homogeneously mixed with bucrylate in equal volumes, and the mixture had the advantage of slightly prolonged polymerization time. Depending on the size of the vein to be obliterated, 0.5 to 1.0 cc of the mixture is injected.

Control portography will reveal whether all venous connections to the esophageal varices are obliterated (Fig. 65-20C). If this is not the case, the remaining vein or veins are catheterized and occluded. Collateral veins from the lateral part of the splenic vein or from the splenic capsule are more difficult, or impossible, to catheterize.

If bucrylate is not available, other embolic materials can be used. Lunderquist et al. [28] used a mixture of thrombin, Gelfoam, and Eto-

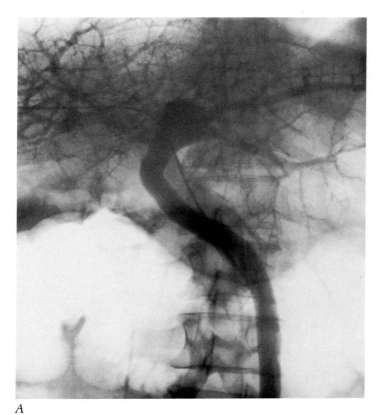

A

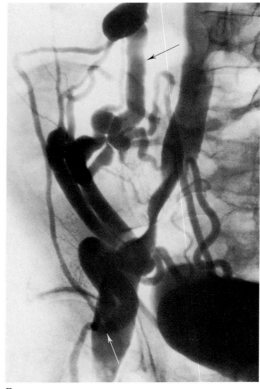

B

Figure 65-19. Transhepatic portal venography in a patient with portal hypertension demonstrates hepatofugal flow through large (A) paraumbilical and (B) inferior epigastric vein (*black arrow*) to femoral-iliac-inferior vena caval veins. The portosystemic anastomosis (*white arrow*) is narrower than feeding collaterals.

lein (monoethanolamine olease; Astra, Södertälje, Sweden). Viamonte et al. [55] and Pereiras et al. [40] used autogenous blood clots, Gelfoam, and Sotradecol. Funaro et al. [12] obliterated the veins with the steel coil. When these materials are injected, a coaxial system of catheters is not necessary.

At the end of the procedure, when the catheter is removed, and in order to prevent bleeding into the peritoneal cavity, a small piece of Gelfoam is injected into the puncture canal beneath the surface of the liver.

Results

Regardless of what kind of embolic material is used, rebleeding is frequent [1, 28, 30]. Using the combination of thrombin, Gelfoam, and Etolein, Lunderquist et al. [30] found a high degree of recanalization of occluded veins (Fig. 65-21). Follow-up on 10 patients treated by Viamonte et al. [55] did not, however, show any recanalization when autogenous blood clots, Gelfoam, and Sotradecol were used. When bucrylate

obliteration was performed, a few cases with recanalization of veins were found [28], but rebleeding often occurred in the absence of recanalization [1]. The main reason for rebleeding was most often that new collaterals opened up and drained the portal blood to the dangerous esophageal varices. These new veins most often originated from the lateral part of the splenic vein, or from the splenic capsular veins, which were difficult or impossible to catheterize.

Complications

Complications reported from the procedure are intraabdominal bleeding caused by the transhepatic puncture, intrapleural bleeding or effusion, and portal vein thrombosis.

Intraperitoneal bleeding may occur in spite of obliteration of the puncture canal with Gelfoam [1, 58]. Ordinarily this bleeding can be controlled with blood transfusion, but surgery may be necessary. If the puncture is performed through the costophrenic sinus, intrapleural bleeding can occur [1, 49, 58], or pleural effusion may be

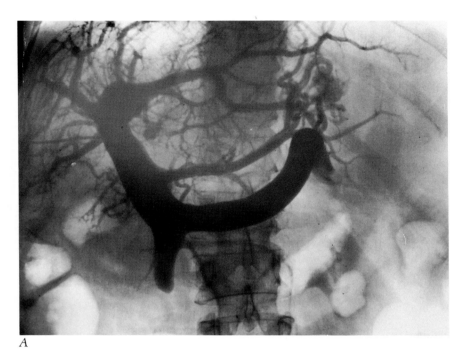

A

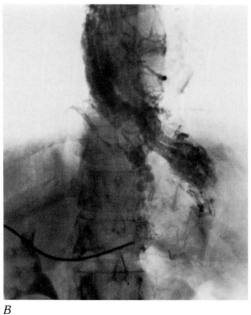

B

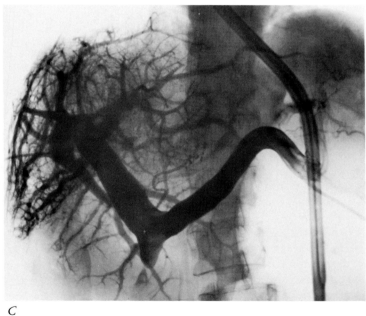

C

Figure 65-20. Percutaneous transhepatic portography in a patient with portal hypertension and bleeding esophageal varices. (A) Retrograde flow in the left gastric vein. (B) Selective catheterization of the left gastric vein demonstrating wide esophageal varices. (C) Transhepatic portography after obliteration of the left gastric vein with bucrylate. Flow is no longer seen to the esophageal varices.

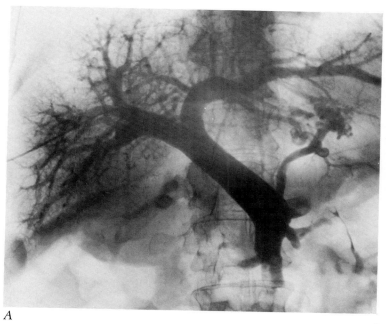

A

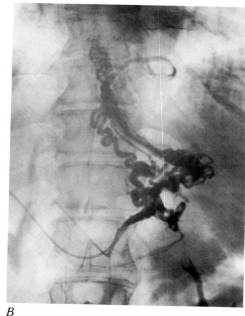

B

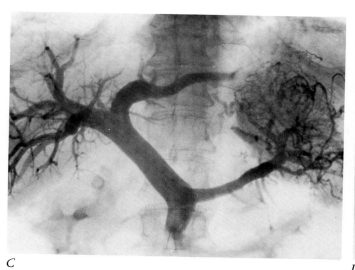

C

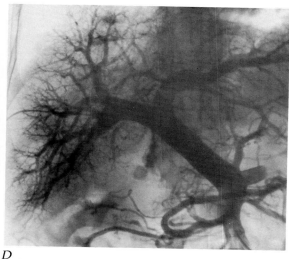

D

Figure 65-21. Transhepatic portography in a patient with portal hypertension and bleeding esophageal varices. (A) Retrograde flow in the left gastric vein. (B) Selective catheterization of the left gastric vein showing wide esophageal varices. (C) Transhepatic portography after obliteration of the left gastric vein with thrombin, Gelfoam, and Etolein. (D) Transhepatic portography 8 months after obliteration of left gastric vein showing recanalization of the previously obliterated vein.

caused by leaking of ascitic fluid. Portal vein thrombosis is another serious complication [1, 16, 58]. The cause of this thrombosis may be spilled embolic material or, more probably, stagnation of the portal blood flow. To prevent reflux of embolic material into the portal vein, balloon catheter obliteration may be useful [47].

The first expectation that percutaneous transhepatic obliteration of gastroesophageal varices could be a permanent way of treating patients with portal hypertension and esophageal varices has not been confirmed. It has, however, been possible to stop the acute bleeding in most cases where other nonsurgical methods have failed [1, 40]. We must stress the importance of a surgical portosystemic shunt operation as soon as this can be electively performed after the percutaneous transhepatic obliteration of the varices. Portal vein thrombosis may otherwise be an undesired complication.

Malignant Lesions

INTRAHEPATIC LESIONS

According to the results of postmortem injections, the blood supply of malignant tumors of the liver comes only from the hepatic arteries [5, 15, 41]. Visualization of the intrahepatic portal venous system will therefore demonstrate only indirect signs of expansive lesions (Fig. 65-22), making differentiation between malignant and benign masses impossible.

The diagnostic value of portography depends on the visualization of the complete intrahepatic portal venous system. Because of their ventral position, the portal vein branches of the left liver lobe in the majority of cases are insufficiently visualized when the patient is examined supine, regardless of which access to the portal venous system is used. In percutaneous splenoportography this problem may be overcome when the examination is performed with the patient in a prone position. However, the best demonstration of the portal venous system of the left lobe of the liver is obtained through selective catheterization of the left main branch of the portal vein via either the percutaneous transhepatic (Fig. 65-23) or the transumbilical access.

In cirrhosis of the liver, obstructive scarring affects predominantly the hepatic veins [8, 14, 25, 42]. Various degrees of hepatic vein obliteration may be present in different parts of the liver, resulting in diversion of portal venous blood from areas with high flow resistance to areas in which hepatic venous drainage is less obstructed (Fig. 65-24). Permanent or intermittent reversal of blood flow in intrahepatic portal vein branches [21] will result in nonvisualization of large areas of the liver at transhepatic portography. Furthermore, distortion and dislodgment of intrahepatic portal vein branches due to destruction and regeneration of the liver tissue make the identification of a neoplastic lesion by transhepatic portal venography impossible (Fig. 65-25).

In a comparative diagnostic study with transhepatic portal venography and infusion hepatic angiography [18], the detection of malignant tumors of the liver by transhepatic portal venography was found to be dependent on their size,

Figure 65-22. Transhepatic portal venography in a patient with malignant lymphoma demonstrates multiple expansive lesions in both liver lobes resulting in distortion and occlusion of intrahepatic portal vein branches. The main stem of the portal vein is compressed.

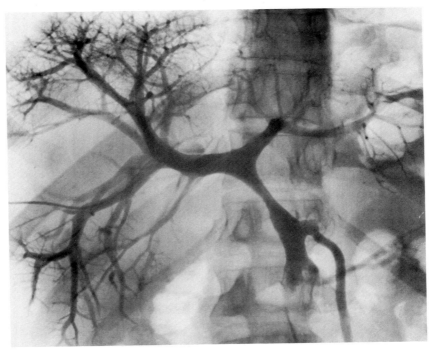

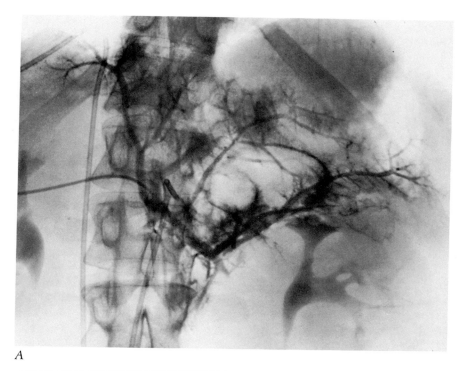

A

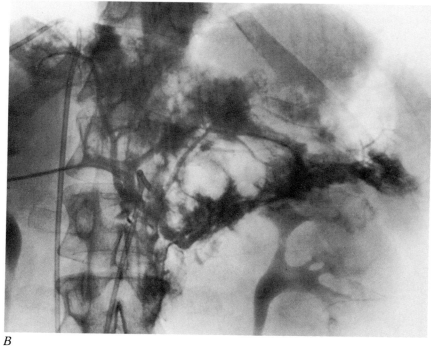

B

Figure 65-23. Transhepatic portal venography in a patient with multiple metastases to the liver secondary to a carcinoid tumor. Selective study of the portal vein branch to the left liver lobe. (A) Early phase. There is occlusion and displacement of portal vein branches by multiple expansive lesions. (B) Sinusoidal phase. The multiple areas without accumulation of contrast medium represent metastases in the left lobe.

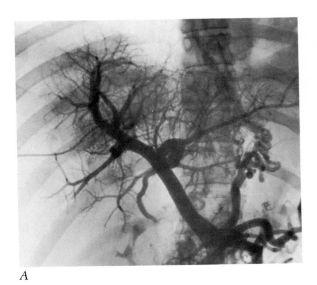

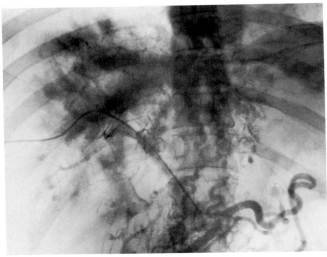

A

B

Figure 65-24. Transhepatic portal venography in a patient with liver cirrhosis, portal venous hypertension, and esophageal varices, but without suspicion of liver malignancy. (A) Portal venous phase. There is a marked flow disturbance, especially in caudal part of right lobe, resulting in incomplete demonstration of intrahepatic portal vein branches. (B) Sinusoidal phase. There is an irregular and sparse accumulation of contrast medium in multiple areas throughout the right and left liver lobes.

Figure 65-25. Liver cirrhosis and multinodular primary hepatic carcinoma involving both liver lobes. (A) Infusion hepatic angiography, early phase. Multiple hypervascular tumors, about 2 to 3 cm, are shown in both liver lobes. In addition, a 5-×-7-cm hypervascular tumor originates from the ventrolateral segment of left liver lobe. (B) Transhepatic portal venography. Selective study of left liver lobe, portal venous phase. The left lobe is enlarged with moderate distortion of intrahepatic portal vein branches in the medial segment. The tumor in the ventrolateral segment displaces minor portal vein branches (*arrows*). Differentiation from vessel displacement due to cirrhosis is not possible. No other space-occupying lesions are seen.

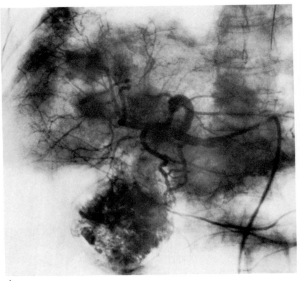

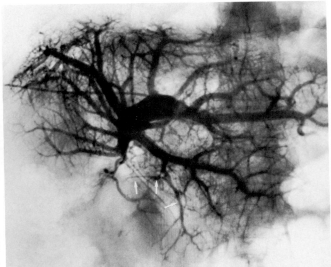

A

B

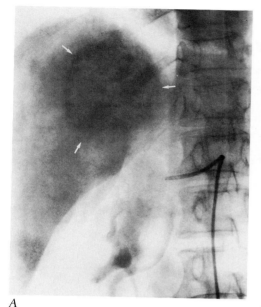

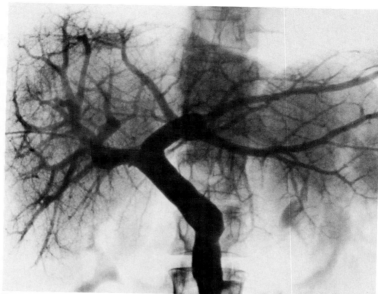

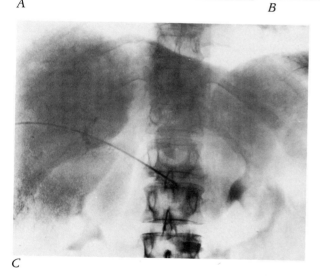

A

B

C

Figure 65-26. Solitary metastasis of carcinoma of the colon in central part of the liver, infiltrating both lobes. (A) Infusion hepatic angiography. Cranially, in midportion of the liver, there is an increased accumulation of contrast medium (*arrows*) representing an approximately 5-cm metastasis. (B) Transhepatic portal venography, portal venous phase. (C) Sinusoidal phase. No space-occupying lesion is demonstrated in either phase.

number, and location. All tumors larger than 7 cm were detected, and multiple 1- to 2-cm metastases were demonstrated in most cases. Solitary lesions smaller than 2 cm located in the central part of the liver were not detected. Metastases of 2 to 4 cm in the right liver lobe were visualized mainly in the sinusoidal phase of transhepatic portal venography. Overprojection of portal vein branches generally made the identification of space-occupying lesions of this size impossible in the portal venous phase. Tumors as large as 4 to 5 cm may remain undetected when they are located in the center of the liver and involve both lobes (Fig. 65-26). Selective catheterization of the left main branch

of the portal vein should theoretically overcome the diagnostic problems in lesions of the left lobe due to overprojection of the spine and the unfavorable hemodynamics involved when the patient is examined in supine position. However, comparison of the results of infusion hepatic angiography and transhepatic portal venography showed that portography is an unreliable method for detection of solitary lesions smaller than 5 cm in the left liver lobe. Multiple lesions and tumors larger than 6 cm in the left liver lobe were easily demonstrated during the portal venous and sinusoidal phases of transhepatic portal venography.

In conclusion: Transhepatic portal venography, like other methods of direct portography, is obsolete and far inferior in diagnostic effectiveness to infusion hepatic angiography, which better demonstrates the true degree of tumor spread in either or both liver lobes in the vast majority of cases.

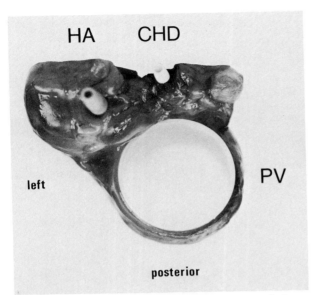

Figure 65-27. Cross-section specimen of hepatoduodenal ligament in porta hepatis. The topographic relation between the main vascular and ductal structures is clearly delineated. The hepatic artery (*HA*), which is anterior to the portal vein (*PV*), was cannulated with a gray catheter; the common hepatic duct (*CHD*) was cannulated with a white catheter.

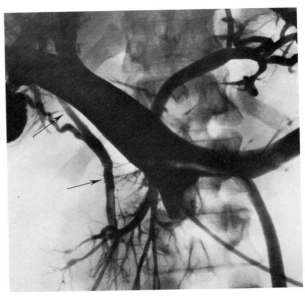

Figure 65-28. Combined portographic and cholangiographic postmortem study demonstrating relationship between main stem of portal vein and extrahepatic bile ducts (*arrows*).

EXTRAHEPATIC LESIONS

The portal vein and the extrahepatic part of the biliary duct system come into close contact with each other in the hilus of the liver and the hepatoduodenal ligament [17] (Figs. 65-27, 65-28). A tumor of the bile ducts in this region may spread to the portal vein (Figs. 65-29, 65-30). Lymphomas and metastases to the lymph nodes in the hepatoduodenal ligament and in the hilus of the liver may influence the portal vein and its main branches. A carcinoma of the pancreas may infiltrate both the main stem of the portal vein and its main tributaries, i.e., the superior mesenteric and splenic veins. Because of the relationship between the portal vein and the biliary ducts within their extrahepatic course and the adjacency of the pancreas to the confluence of the portal vein, involvement of the portal venous system by a malignant tumor in this region is likely to occur by the time surgical procedures are considered.

Various authors [4, 13, 24, 46, 56] have, however, reported a low incidence of portal vein involvement in carcinoma of the extrahepatic bile ducts. This conclusion was drawn from the findings of the venous phase of celiac and/or superior mesenteric angiography. However, correlation of the findings of transhepatic portal venography and angiography in patients with bile duct carcinoma [19] revealed that tumor involvement of the portal vein occurs in most cases, but its incidence is underestimated by the venous phase of celiac and superior mesenteric studies. Even pharmaco-enhanced arterial (i.e., indirect) mesentericoportography may result in an insufficient demonstration of morphologic abnormalities of the superior mesenteric and portal veins [19]. The portal vein is far better demonstrated by transhepatic portal venography because of higher concentration of contrast medium. Nevertheless, there is evidence that even transhepatic portal venography may fail to demonstrate existing tumor growth into the wall of the portal vein [19] (Fig. 65-31).

A high frequency of tumor involvement of the splenic, superior mesenteric, and portal veins demonstrated at angiography is on record, and the importance of the venous phases of celiac and superior mesenteric angiography in the evaluation of pancreatic carcinoma has been stressed [6].

In a recent investigation [44] the findings at

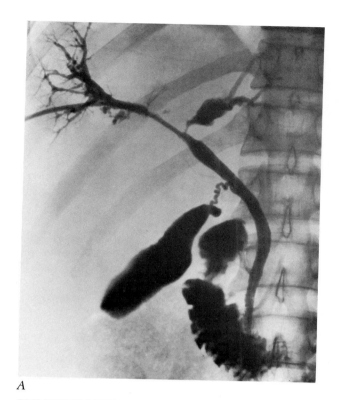

A

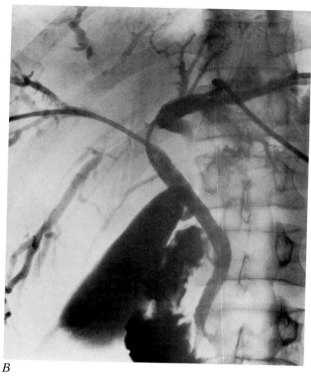

B

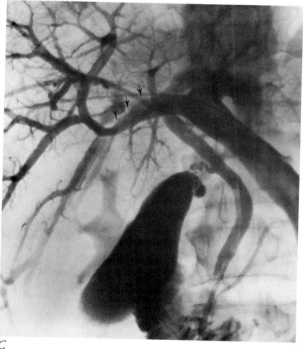

C

Figure 65-29. Cholangiocarcinoma at confluence of hepatic ducts. Infiltration of liver in porta hepatis. (A) Percutaneous transhepatic intubation of biliary duct system from right lateral approach. The tumor obstruction is passed by a catheter with its tip in the duodenum. Side holes proximal and distal to obstruction make possible internal decompression and drainage of the bile duct system of one segment of the right liver lobe. There is tumor stricture of left hepatic duct near hepatic confluence. (B) For decompression and drainage, a separate catheter is placed in the dilated bile duct of the left liver lobe from a ventral approach. The tip of the catheter is placed in the distal segment of the common bile duct, with the side holes positioned proximal and distal to the tumor stricture of the left hepatic duct for internal drainage. (C) Transhepatic portal venography with simultaneous contrast filling of extrahepatic bile ducts via drainage catheters. There is infiltration of the main stem of the portal vein to the right liver lobe about 3 cm distal to its origin (*arrows*).

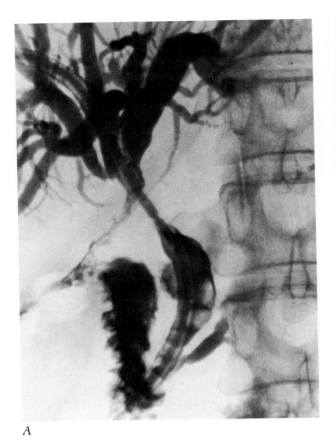

A

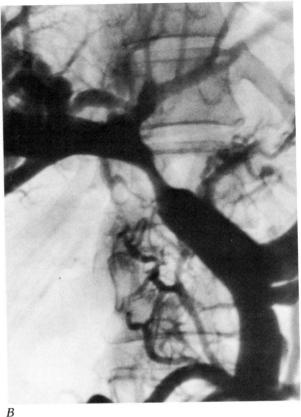

B

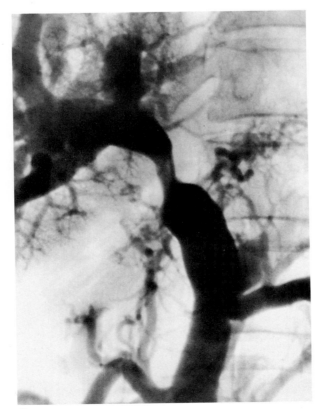

C

Figure 65-30. Cholangiocarcinoma involving the gallbladder and structures of the hepatoduodenal ligament. (A) Cholangiography via operatively placed transhepatic drainage tube. Stricture of the common hepatic duct and dilatation of intrahepatic bile ducts is shown. There are stones in the moderately dilated common bile duct, and the distal segment of the pancreatic duct is filled with contrast medium. (B and C) Transhepatic portal venography, anteroposterior projection (B) and slightly left anterior oblique projection (C). Circular stenosis of the main stem of portal vein near liver hilus is due to tumor infiltration.

transhepatic portal venography and selective pancreatic phlebography were compared with the findings at angiography in patients with pancreatic carcinoma. The results of this study indicate the usefulness of transhepatic portal venography in the evaluation of resectability of pancreatic carcinoma. It was concluded that the method should be used as a complement in patients in whom angiography does not give unequivocal information about nonresectability of the tumor.

It may be difficult to decide whether there is true infiltration of the portal venous system by a tumor when smooth compression and/or a dislocation of the mesenteric or portal veins is

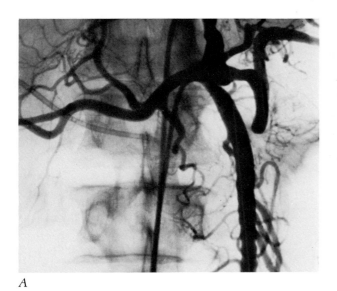

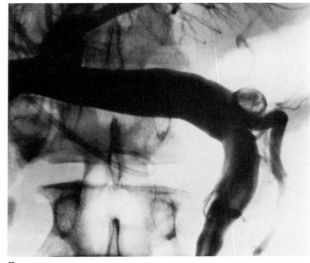

A

B

Figure 65-31. Cholangiocarcinoma originating from the distal (pancreatic) segment of the common bile duct. (A) Simultaneous angiography of the celiac and superior mesenteric arteries. The main stem of the splanchnic arteries is displaced to the left by a previous partial resection of the stomach. There are no findings to indicate a tumor. (B) Transhepatic portal venography shows confluence of portal vein displaced to left by previous partial resection of stomach. There are no signs of tumor infiltration. At operation, tumor was found adherent to proximal segment of portal vein.

observed at transhepatic portal venography or angiography. However, there is evidence that compression of the vein by a tumor may be equivalent to infiltration of the respective vein, making the patient an unsuitable candidate for radical surgery [19, 44].

In conclusion: Transhepatic portal venography as a complement to arteriography may provide information about tumor infiltration of the portal vein and its main tributaries in cases in which this is not demonstrated by the venous phases of celiac and mesenteric studies. Negative findings at transhepatic portal venography, however, do not exclude tumor growth along and in the wall of the portal and splanchnic veins and are therefore of little importance in the preoperative evaluation of tumor extirpability.

References

1. Bengmark, S., Börjesson, B., Hoevels, J., Joelsson, B., Lunderquist, A., and Owman, T. Obliteration of esophageal varices by PTP—a follow-up of 43 patients. *Ann. Surg.* 190:549, 1979.
2. Bergstrand, I., and Ekman, C. A. Portal circulation in portal hypertension. *Acta Radiol.* (Stockh.) 47:1, 1957.
3. Bierman, H. R., Steinbach, H. L., White, L. P., and Kelly, K. H. Portal venipuncture. Percutaneous transhepatic approach. *Proc. Soc. Exp. Biol. Med.* 79:550, 1952.
4. Boijsen, E., and Reuter, S. R. Combined percutaneous transhepatic cholangiography and angiography in the evaluation of obstructive jaundice. *AJR* 99:153, 1967.
5. Breedis, C., and Young, G. The blood supply of neoplasms of the liver. *Am. J. Pathol.* 30:969, 1954.
6. Buranasiri, S., and Baum, S. The significance of the venous phase of celiac and superior mesenteric arteriography in evaluating pancreatic carcinoma. *Radiology* 102:11, 1972.
7. Burcharth, F., Sörensen, T. J. A., and Andersen, B. Percutaneous transhepatic portography: III. Relationships between portosystemic collaterals and portal pressure in cirrhosis. *AJR* 133:1119, 1979.
8. Carter, J. H., Welch, C. S., and Barron, R. E. Changes in the hepatic blood vessels in cirrhosis of the liver. *Surg. Gynecol. Obstet.* 113:133, 1961.
9. Edwards, E. A. Functional anatomy of the porta-systemic communications. *Arch. Intern. Med.* 88:137, 1951.
10. Elias, H., and Petty, D. Terminal distribution of the hepatic artery. *Anat. Rec.* 116:9, 1953.
11. Freeny, P. C., and Kidd, R. Transhepatic portal venography and selective obliteration of gastroesophageal varices using isobutyl 2-cyano-

acrylate (bucrylate). *Am. J. Dig. Dis.* 24:321, 1979.

12. Funaro, A. H., Ring, E. J., Freiman, D. B., Oleaga, J. A., and Gordon, R. L. Transhepatic obliteration of esophageal varices using the stainless steel coil. *AJR* 133:1123, 1979.

13. Haertel, M., and Anderson, R. Die Angiographie bei biliären Neoplasien. *ROEFO* 124:314, 1976.

14. Hales, M. R., Allan, J. S., and Hall, E. M. Injection-corrosion studies of normal and cirrhotic livers. *Am. J. Pathol.* 35:909, 1959.

15. Healey, J. E., Jr. Vascular patterns in human metastatic liver tumors. *Surg. Gynecol. Obstet.* 120:1187, 1965.

16. Henderson, J. M., Buist, T. A. S., and MacPherson, A. I. S. Percutaneous transhepatic occlusion for bleeding esophageal varices. *Br. J. Surg.* 66:569, 1979.

17. Hoevels, J. Topographic relation of portal vein to extrahepatic bile ducts. A combined portographic-cholangiographic study in 25 cadavers. *ROEFO* 129:217, 1978.

18. Hoevels, J. A comparative diagnostic study of malignant lesions of the liver by infusion angiography and percutaneous transhepatic portography. *ROEFO* 130:676, 1979.

19. Hoevels, J., and Ihse, I. Percutaneous transhepatic portography in bile duct carcinoma. Correlation with percutaneous transhepatic cholangiography and angiography. *ROEFO* 131:140, 1979.

20. Hoevels, J., Lunderquist, A., and Tylén, U. Percutaneous transhepatic portography. *Acta Radiol.* [*Diagn.*] (Stockh.) 19:643, 1978.

21. Hoevels, J., Lunderquist, A., and Tylén, U. Spontaneous intermittent reversal of blood flow in intrahepatic portal vein branches in cirrhosis of the liver. *Cardiovasc. Radiol.* 2:267, 1979.

22. Hoevels, J., Lunderquist, A., Tylén, U., and Simert, G. Portosystemic collaterals in cirrhosis of the liver. Selective percutaneous transhepatic catheterization of the portal venous system in portal hypertension. *Acta Radiol.* [*Diagn.*] (Stockh.) 20:865, 1979.

23. Johnson, W. C., Widrich, W. C., Ansell, J. E., Robbins, A. H., and Nabseth, D. C. Control of bleeding varices by vasopressin. A prospective randomized study. *Ann. Surg.* 186:369, 1977.

24. Kaude, J., and Rian, R. Cholangiocarcinoma. *Radiology* 100:573, 1971.

25. Kelly, A. O. J. The nature and the lesions of cirrhosis of the liver, with special reference to the regeneration and rearrangement of the liver parenchyma. *Am. J. Med. Sci.* 130:951, 1950.

26. Kelty, R. H., Baggenstoss, A. H., and Butt, H. R. The relation of the regenerated liver nodule to the vascular bed in cirrhosis. *Gastroenterology* 15:285, 1950.

27. Lunderquist, A. Portal vein flow pattern in portal hypertension. *Clin. Radiol.* 31:395, 1980.

28. Lunderquist, A., Börjesson, B., Owman, T., and Bengmark, S. Isobutyl 2-cyanoacrylate (bucrylate) in obliteration of gastric coronary vein and esophageal varices. *AJR* 130:1, 1978.

29. Lunderquist, A., Lunderquist, M., and Owman, T. Guide wire for percutaneous transhepatic cholangiography. *Radiology* 132:228, 1979.

30. Lunderquist, A., Simert, G., Tylén, U., and Vang, J. Follow-up of patients with portal hypertension and esophageal varices treated with percutaneous obliteration of gastric coronary vein. *Radiology* 122:59, 1977.

31. Lunderquist, A., and Vang, J. Transhepatic catheterization and obliteration of the coronary vein in patients with portal hypertension and esophageal varices. *N. Engl. J. Med.* 291:646, 1974.

32. McCuskey, R. S. A dynamic and static study of hepatic arterioles and hepatic sphincters. *Am. J. Anat.* 119:455, 1966.

33. Mitra, S. K. The terminal distribution of the hepatic artery with special reference to arterioportal anastomosis. *J. Anat.* 100:651, 1966.

34. Mitra, S. K. Hepatic vascular changes in human and experimental cirrhosis. *J. Pathol. Bacteriol.* 92:405, 1966.

35. Moreno, A. H., Burchell, A. R., Rousselot, L. M., Panke, W., Slafsky, S. F., and Burke, J. H. Portal blood flow in cirrhosis of the liver. *J. Clin. Invest.* 46:436, 1967.

36. Nunez, D., Jr., Russell, E., Yrizarry, J., Pereiras, R., and Viamonte, M., Jr. Portosystemic communications studied by transhepatic portography. *Radiology* 127:75, 1978.

37. Orloff, M. J., Chartes, A. C., Chandler, J. G., Condon, J. K., Grambort, D. E., Modafferi, T. R., Levin, S. E., Brown, N. B., Sviokla, S. C., and Knox, D. G. Portacaval shunt as emergency procedure in unselected patients with alcoholic cirrhosis. *Surg. Gynecol. Obstet.* 141:59, 1975.

38. Palmer, E. D. On correlations between portal venous pressure and the size and extent of esophageal varices in portal cirrhosis. *Ann. Surg.* 138:741, 1953.

39. Paquet, K. J., and Oberhammer, E. Sclerotherapy of bleeding esophageal varices by means of endoscopy. *Endoscopy* 10:7, 1978.

40. Pereiras, R., Viamonte, M., Jr., Russell, E., LePage, J., White, P., and Hutson, D. New techniques for interruption of gastroesophageal venous blood flow. *Radiology* 124:313, 1977.

41. Pinet, F., Amiel, M., Bougoin, J. J., Clermont, A., Pierluca, P., and Dargent, M. Microangiographie des tumeurs malignes du foie. *Ann. Radiol.* (Paris) 15:437, 1972.

42. Piper, D. W. A radiographic study of the portal and hepatic venous systems in cirrhosis of the liver. *Am. J. Dig. Dis.* 6:499, 1961.

43. Reichardt, W., Bützow, G. H., and Erbe, W. Anomalous venous connections involving the portal system. *Cardiovasc. Radiol.* 2:41, 1979.

44. Reichardt, W., and Ihse, I.   Percutaneous transhepatic portography in pancreatic carcinoma. Diagnosis and evaluation of resectability. *Acta Radiol. [Diagn.]* (Stockh.) 21:579, 1980.

45. Retzius, A. A.   Bemerkungen über Anastomosen zwischen der Pfortader und der unteren Hohlader ausserhalb der Leber. *Z. Physiol.* 5:105, 1835.

46. Reuter, S. R., Redman, H. C., and Bookstein, J. J.   Angiography in carcinoma of the biliary tract. *Br. J. Radiol.* 44:636, 1971.

47. Roche, A., Kunstlinger, F., Curet, P., and Doyon, D.   Balloon catheter to control transhepatic obliteration of gastroesophageal varices. *AJR* 132:647, 1979.

48. Rousselot, L. M., Moreno, A. H., and Panke, W. F.   Studies on portal hypertension: IV. The clinical and physiopathologic significance of self-established (nonsurgical) portal systemic venous shunts. *Ann. Surg.* 150:384, 1959.

49. Scott, J., Dick, R., Long, R. G., and Sherlock, S.   Percutaneous transhepatic obliteration of gastroesophageal varices. *Lancet* 2:53, 1976.

50. Simert, G., Lunderquist, A., Tylén, U., and Vang, J.   Correlation between percutaneous transhepatic portography and clinical findings in 56 patients with portal hypertension. *Acta Chir. Scand.* 144:27, 1978.

51. Terblanche, J., Saunders, S. J., and Louw, J. H.   Surgical Forum. In R. Smith (ed.), *The Liver.* London: Butterworth, 1974.

52. Thamm, M.   Die portocavalen Venenverbindungen des Menschen. *Zentralbl. Chir.* 39:1828, 1940.

53. Turner, M. D., Sherlock, S., and Steiner, R. E.   Splenic venography and intrasplenic pressure measurement in the clinical investigation of the portal venous system. *Am. J. Med.* 23:846, 1957.

54. Viallet, A., Legare, A., and Lavoie, P.   Hepatic and umbilicoportal catheterization in portal hypertension. *Ann. N.Y. Acad. Sci.* 170:177, 1970.

55. Viamonte, M., Jr., Pereiras, R., Russell, E., LePage, J., and Hutson, D.   Transhepatic obliteration of gastro-esophageal varices: Results in acute and nonacute bleeders. *AJR* 129:237, 1977.

56. Walter, J. F., Bookstein, J. J., and Boufford, E. V.   Newer angiographic observations in cholangiocarcinoma. *Radiology* 118:19, 1976.

57. Wexler, M. J., and MacLean, L. D.   Massive spontaneous portal-systemic shunting without varices. *Arch. Surg.* 110:995, 1975.

58. Widrich, W. C., Robbins, A. H., Nabseth, D. C., Johnson, W. C., and Goldstein, S. A.   Pitfalls of transhepatic portal venography and therapeutic coronary vein occlusion. *AJR* 131:637, 1978.

59. Widrich, W. C., Robbins, A. H., Nabseth, D. C., O'Hara, E. T., Johnson, W. C., and Loughlin, K. V.   Portal hypertension changes following selective splenorenal shunt surgery. Evaluation by percutaneous transhepatic portal catheterization venography and cinefluorography. *Radiology* 121:295, 1978.

60. Wiechel, K. L.   Tekniken vid perkutan transhepatisk portapunktion (PTP). *Nord. Med.* 86:912, 1971. (In Swedish.)

Splenic Arteriography

HERBERT L. ABRAMS

The spleen is an organ that is considered a vital element in the reticuloendothelial system. Until recently, its removal was thought to be unaccompanied by signs that man misses it sorely. It is now clear, however, that asplenic patients may be subject to overwhelming sepsis and that the decreased immunologic competence that follows splenectomy cannot be ignored [24, 73]. In portal hypertension the spleen may become huge and unwieldy; it is frequently involved in lymphoma; and in congenital hemolytic anemia it plays a central role in the disease process itself. Although newer modalities, such as computed tomography, are valuable noninvasive methods of assessing splenic trauma [55, 66, 67] and of determining splenic volume and mass [42], angiography remains the definitive diagnostic method, and thus the vascular anatomy of the spleen is of special importance.

Some years ago, we studied the variations in the anatomy of the splenic artery, the frequency of visualization of its important branches, the variable sites of origin of the splenic artery branches, and the intrasplenic circulatory patterns recorded by serialographic filming [56]. By determining normal variations as visualized angiographically, it was hoped that a more precise background for judging significant alterations in the splenic arterial patterns and their relationship to gastric, pancreatic, and splenic disease would be afforded.

This chapter is based on that analysis, as well as on our accumulated experience and a review of the literature.

Anatomy of the Splenic Artery

The classic anatomic description of the splenic artery has been given by Michels on the basis of 100 human dissections [68, 69]. Michels' descriptions have generally been confirmed and amplified in vivo in our clinical studies. The basic anatomic observations must first be summarized.

ORIGIN

The splenic artery typically originates from the celiac artery via a hepatolienogastric trunk. This situation was found in 82 percent of the dissections. In the most common form, the left gastric artery is given off first and the splenic and hepatic arteries then form a common trunk. In about 25

1531

percent of cases the left gastric, splenic, and hepatic arteries arise from the same point to form a tripod celiac configuration. Less often the dorsal pancreatic or middle colic artery arises from the same point to form a tetrapod configuration; this phenomenon occurred in 5 percent of the dissections. Occasionally the splenic artery arises from the aorta or the superior mesenteric artery, and, rarely, a double splenic artery is formed when a smaller branch to a superior pole of the spleen originates from the celiac axis.

DISTRIBUTION

The arterial blood supply to the spleen is so varied that no two vascularization patterns were exactly alike in 100 dissections [68, 69]. There are, however, two basic types of splenic architecture associated with two different types of splenic arterial patterns.

1. A distributed type of spleen has a wide hilus, notches in the anterior and posterior borders, a thumblike lobe at the inferior pole, and a tubercle at the superior pole. This constitutes the *distributed* configuration, which occurred in approximately 70 percent of dissections. The splenic trunk is relatively short, with terminal branching at any point from the celiac axis to the hilus of the spleen. The branches are usually numerous and small in caliber and enter 75 percent of the medial surface of the spleen.
2. A compact type of spleen has smooth, even borders with a narrow hilus, giving rise to a *magistral* configuration (found in approximately 30 percent of dissections). The splenic trunk is long; terminal division occurs near the hilus; and the terminal branches are few and large and enter 25 to 33 percent of the spleen's medial surface.

Measurements of the splenic artery have revealed an average length of 13 cm (with a range of 8–32 cm) and an average width of 7.5 mm (with a range of 5–12 mm).

SEGMENTATION

The splenic artery can be divided into the following four main segments:

1. Suprapancreatic. This is the first 1 to 3 cm of the vessel.

2. Pancreatic. This portion of the vessel usually is found on the dorsal surface of the pancreas. It is the most tortuous of the segments, lies adjacent to the pancreas, and supplies the small pancreatic branches that enter the organ at frequent intervals.
3. Prepancreatic. This segment runs obliquely along the anterior surface of the tail of the pancreas. Terminal branching usually occurs in this segment and gives rise to a distributed pattern. In 80 percent of dissections the main trunk was divided into a superior terminal artery and an inferior terminal artery. In some cases an additional medial terminal artery was also present.
4. Prehilar. This segment is found between the tail of the pancreas and the spleen. If branching into a terminal division occurs at this point, the arterial pattern is magistral.

TORTUOSITY

One of the most pronounced characteristics of the splenic artery is its tortuosity, which is manifested in curves, loops, and spirals, primarily along the splenic trunk and secondarily in the terminal branches. Michels [69] feels that the tortuous appearance is correlated with age: it becomes progressively more marked in individuals over 50 years of age.

Branches of the Splenic Artery

PANCREATIC BRANCHES (FIG. 66-1)

Dorsal Pancreatic Branch (Superior Pancreatic Branch of Testut)

This vessel was described by Michels [69] as the "most varied of celiac-mesenteric vessels in its origin, branching and distribution." It measured 1 to 4 mm in width and originated from the splenic artery in 40 percent of dissections. Occasionally it arises from the celiac, hepatic, or superior mesenteric arteries. It supplies the dorsal and ventral surfaces of the pancreas in the region of the neck. Two right branches may originate from the dorsal pancreatic branch, one anastomosing with the superior pancreaticoduodenal artery and the other directly supplying the uncinate process. A left branch, the transverse pancreatic, runs along the inferior surface of the organ to its tail for an anastomosis with the arteria pancreatica

Table 66-6. Causes of Splenomegaly

Inflammation
    "Acute splenic tumor" (acute infections)
    Chronic infections (e.g., tuberculosis, malaria)
    Miscellaneous inflammations (e.g., sarcoidosis, lupus
      erythematosus)
Cysts and tumors
    True cysts (e.g., congenital echinococcus)
    False cysts (posttraumatic)
    Benign tumors
    Malignant tumors
      Primary tumors (e.g., leukemia, lymphoma)
      Metastatic tumors
Infiltrative diseases
    Gaucher's disease, Neimann-Pick disease
    Amyloidosis, hemosiderosis
Hyperplastic disorders
    Hemolytic anemias
    Myelofibrosis
    Polycythemia vera
    Thrombocytopenia purpura
    Other anemias (e.g., pernicious anemia)
Splenic vein hypertension
    Cirrhosis of the liver
    Portal or splenic vein thrombosis

tive disorders, including Gaucher's disease and amyloidosis, are relatively rare. The hyperplastic disorders are frequently associated with splenomegaly, including all the hemolytic anemias, except sickle cell disease, which in its most chronic form is generally associated with a small, infarcted spleen. Finally, splenic vein hypertension, such as that found in cirrhosis of the liver or in portal or splenic vein thrombosis, may be associated with splenic enlargement and hypersplenism.

The angiographic appearance of splenomegaly reflects to some degree the underlying cause of the disease. In all forms of splenomegaly, the most common appearance is of stretching and separation of the vessels, with a splenogram or capillary phase that is uniformly diminished in intensity. In the neoplastic or infiltrative disorders, there may be more or less uniform separation of the vessels, but, in addition, irregularity and encasement of arteries are visible at times. Inflammatory disorders, including arteritis, as well as cirrhosis of the liver, may be associated with aneurysmal change in the intrasplenic arteries, as well as with attenuation and wide separation of the vessels.

CONGENITAL ANOMALIES

Anomalies of Position
These may be divided into two categories: (1) anomalies that are variants of the normal spleen and (2) anomalies of the so-called wandering, or ectopic, spleen. In anomalies that are variants of the normal spleen, the spleen may be located transversely immediately below the diaphragm (Fig. 66-14), a finding of no pathologic significance. Similarly, the spleen may assume any level of obliquity (see Figs. 66-2, 66-3, 66-6), or it may approach a vertical orientation.

Radionuclide scanning with technetium Tc 99m sulfur colloid and ultrasonography can reliably establish the position of the spleen and assist in the diagnosis of such entities as situs inversus [19].

Wandering Spleen
The spleen may be located aberrantly in the left flank (Fig. 66-15) of the midabdomen or the left lower quadrant or pelvis (Fig. 66-16) [38]. Such instances of wandering spleen are rare, and they constitute a diagnostic challenge since the findings are relatively nonspecific. The discovery of a mass in the midabdomen or near the lower

Figure 66-14. Transverse position of the spleen. The spleen lies in the left upper quadrant beneath the diaphragm in horizontal position, rather than in its usual vertical or oblique orientation. This represents a normal variation, and has no pathologic significance.

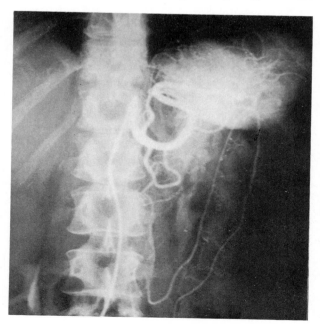

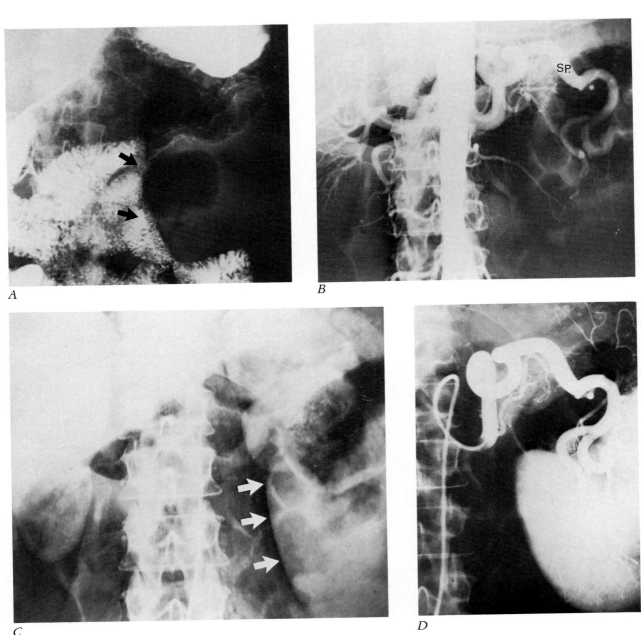

Figure 66-15. "Wandering," or ectopic, spleen. (A) Upper gastrointestinal series. The stomach fills the left upper quadrant in the area where the spleen normally is located. In addition, a mass is visible displacing small bowel loops (*arrows*) in the left midabdomen. (B) Aortogram. The coiled splenic artery (*SP*), instead of being directed laterally and cephalad, extends in a caudal direction. (C) Splenographic phase. The spleen is visible in the left midabdomen (*arrows*), in precisely the area where the mass was noted on the upper gastrointestinal series. (D) Selective splenic arteriogram. The position of the spleen, well out of the left upper quadrant, is now clearly delineated. (Courtesy of David Levin, M.D.)

pole of the left kidney on plain films, together with evidence of the splenic hump's absence on excretory urography and medial or anterior displacement of the spleen on barium examination, should prompt ultrasonography, radioisotope scanning with agents specific for the spleen, and/or angiography.

Patients with wandering spleen may be symptomatic or asymptomatic. Diagnosis is important in symptomatic cases since symptoms derive from torsion, which carries possible complications of infarction, gangrene, and abscess; the mortality is 50 percent in such cases [1]. In a case reported by Sorgen and Robbins [114], bleeding fundal varices were associated with a wandering spleen in a 14-year-old girl. It was theorized that the varices developed as a result of splenic vein occlusion caused by torsion with consequent retrograde filling of short gastric and left gastroepiploic veins.

Wandering spleen has been reported in 0 to 0.4 percent of splenectomies [29, 93, 102]. Various causes have been suggested, including congenital anomalies of the lienogastric and lienorenal ligaments [36]. In the case illustrated in Figure 66-15, a left flank mass was palpated, and the absence of the normal spleen shadow on upper gastrointestinal series led to a tentative diagnosis of wandering spleen. The patient whose films are shown in Figure 66-16 had a palpable pelvic mass and lower abdominal pain. Angiography and radionuclide studies finally established the diagnosis.

Anomalies of Number

Accessory Splenic Tissue. Accessory spleens may be present in as many as 16 percent of people [29] and may be more common in people with hematologic disorders [82]. The classic accessory spleen is single and is located in the hilus of the spleen or adjacent to the tail of the pancreas. As a consequence, at the time of splenic surgery, accessory spleens may be readily recognized. Angiographically, these spleens are seen as small nodules with an arterial and a capillary phase similar to that of splenic tissue, which may be separate from and/or immediately adjacent to the hilus of the spleen or may be embedded in the pancreas. Computed tomography has also been able to identify accessory spleens, particularly during contrast enhancement.

The classic accessory spleen must be differentiated from "splenosis." Although approximately 20 percent of patients who have had splenectomy for hematologic indications have Howell-Jolly bodies or have "pitted" red cells, suggesting persistence of splenic activity, over 50 percent of children who have had splenectomy for splenic trauma have demonstrated persistent splenic activity. The fact that such patients develop splenosis may explain the relatively low incidence of sepsis in patients who have had splenectomy for traumatic indications [89].

While the presence of more than one spleen normally is of no significance, the accessory splenic tissue can occasionally present a diagnostic or therapeutic challenge. In one case reported by Fitzer [33], a splenic hematoma could not be ruled out on radionuclide scans because of the presence of an accessory spleen, and arteriographic studies were necessary to arrive at a definitive diagnosis. Infarction of an accessory spleen, simulating acute appendicitis, has been reported [84], and accessory spleens may cause recurrence of hematologic disorders after surgical removal of the primary spleen [8]. In addition, an accessory spleen can be a source of problems in treatment planning in Hodgkin's disease [47].

Asplenia. Although asplenia may appear as an isolated anomaly [43], it most often occurs as part of the asplenia, or Ivemark, syndrome, in conjunction with complex, characteristic cardiovascular malformations and other anomalies [65]. The minimal incidence has been estimated as 1 in 40,000 live births [108]. The conjunction of anomalies in the asplenia syndrome has led some embryologists to postulate that it results from a teratogenic insult to the embryo between the thirty-first and thirty-sixth day of gestation [81]. It has also been suggested that the asplenia syndrome may represent an autosomal recessive trait [48]. Neither of these mechanisms can explain all cases of asplenia, however. In a case reported by Wilkinson et al. [123], one monozygotic twin suffered from the asplenia syndrome while the other twin was normal; genetic factors could not have played a part in this instance, nor is it likely that a teratogen could have affected one twin and not the other.

The diagnosis of asplenia is suggested by a complex of cardiac and extracardiac anomalies, including some anomalies that represent a bilateral right-sidedness [64]: mesocardia or dextrocardia, bilateral superior vena cava, a single ventricle or two ventricles with a ventricular septal defect, a large atrial septal defect, trans-

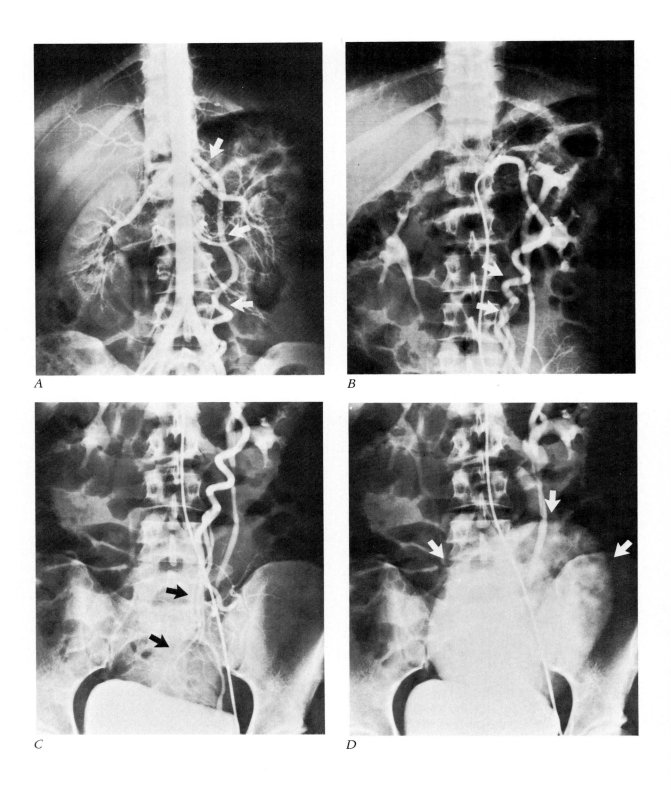

A

B

C

D

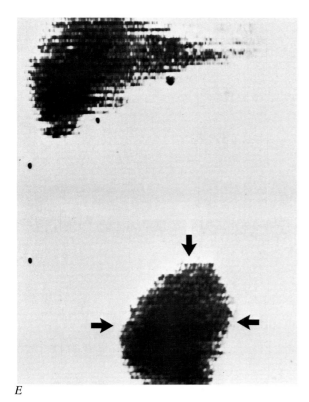

E

Figure 66-16. "Wandering," or ectopic, spleen. A mass was palpable in the pelvis. (A) Aortogram. A long, tortuous vessel extends toward the pelvis (*arrows*). (B) Selective arteriogram. The catheter is emplaced in the mouth of this vessel (*arrows*), which is a branch of the celiac axis. (C) Selective splenic arteriogram, view of lower abdomen and pelvis. The tortuous vessel visualized on the prior two films arborizes extensively (*arrows*) in the pelvis. (D) Selective arteriogram, capillary phase. A large homogeneously dense mass (*arrows*) is visible in the pelvis above the contrast-filled bladder. The diagnosis of a wandering spleen was made because the vessel selectively catheterized was thought to be the splenic artery. (E) Radionuclide scan. The liver is visualized in its normal position in the right upper quadrant. No spleen is seen in the left upper quadrant. Instead, the wandering spleen in the pelvis is well visualized (*arrows*). (Courtesy of Melvin Clouse, M.D.)

position of the great vessels, total anomalous pulmonary venous return, bilateral trilobed lungs with bilateral eparterial bronchi, a symmetric liver, a midline gallbladder, and malrotation of the gastrointestinal tract. Cyanosis and heart failure are often evident soon after birth. Chest films usually reveal mesocardia or dextrocardia, decreased pulmonary vasculature, and a central symmetric liver [60, 101].

Although there have been reports of prolonged survival after surgery to repair complex cardiac anomalies in asplenic infants [4, 6], most such infants die soon after birth. In a series reported by Majeski and Upshur, the lifespan of 14 live-born asplenic infants averaged 38 days [65]. The first-year mortality of such infants was estimated in 1972 as being greater than 95 percent [116].

In patients with isolated asplenia, the diagnosis may be more obscure. These patients have a high incidence of sepsis because of the absence of splenic tissue and the altered immunologic response early in life [118]. Honigman and Lanzkowsky [43] suggest that all infants and children with septicemia, especially of a pneumococcal or *Haemophilus influenzae* type, be assessed for the presence of Howell-Jolly bodies. Although isolated asplenia has been diagnosed in people as old as 69 [53], it can also predispose to early, sudden death [48].

Polysplenia. Polysplenia syndrome is also a complex congenital disorder in which multiple discrete spleens are coupled with cardiac and extracardiac abnormalities. With polysplenia there is a tendency toward bilateral left-sidedness, with bilateral bilobed lungs and hyparterial bronchi. Interruption of the inferior vena cava with azygos or hemiazygos continuation is common. The liver is generally located centrally, and there is frequently malrotation of the bowel.

While the cardiac disease is usually more benign in patients with polysplenia than in those with asplenia (because of the infrequent occurrence of transposition of the great arteries and total anomalous pulmonary venous return), the cardiac anomalies may lead to pulmonary vascular disease if they are not promptly corrected.

Radionuclide spleen scans will generally show abnormal results, but they usually do not suggest the diagnosis of polysplenia with any precision [102]. Arteriography may be necessary to establish the diagnosis (Fig. 66-17).

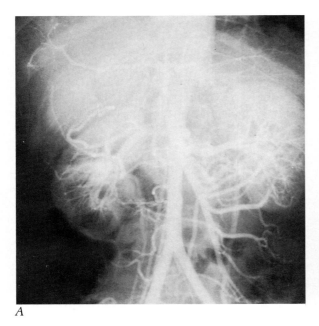

A

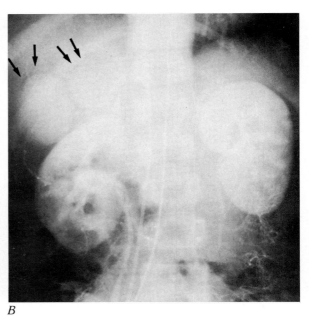

B

Figure 66-17. Polysplenia. This young patient had congenital heart disease associated with an absent hepatic portion of the inferior vena cava. (A) Aortogram. The splenic artery extends into the right upper quadrant instead of the left upper quadrant. (B) Capillary phase. Two separate splenic shadows (*arrows*) are visible in the right upper quadrant. There is no evidence of a spleen located on the left upper quadrant.

PRIMARY ABNORMALITIES OF THE SPLENIC VASCULAR BED

Arteriosclerosis

The splenic artery is commonly affected by arteriosclerosis, and visible calcification of the highly tortuous vessels may be observed as an incidental finding on conventional films of the abdomen (Fig. 66-18). The involvement is largely medial rather than intimal so that adequate lumen size is preserved in some of the most heavily calcified arteries. The splenic artery is particularly prone to elongation and tortuosity, which generally increase with age. Since the splenic artery is closely related to the stomach, tortuosity can produce an extrinsic impression on the barium-filled stomach that may simulate a neoplasm [20]. Plaques may form and produce wall irregularities on the splenic arteriogram. Severe stenosis is unusual but occurs. When it does, it need produce no symptoms as long as it is gradual. Splenic arteriosclerosis, therefore, is of little clinical significance by itself. Its major importance clinically is determined by the extent to which it predisposes to aneurysm formation or, occasionally, to complete thrombosis.

Dysplasia of the Splenic Artery

The corrugated or string-of-beads pattern frequently described in the renal vessels may be visualized in the splenic trunk on rare occasions, as noted by Palubinskas and Ripley [86]. Splenic artery fibroplasia has been reported as an incidental finding in a 9-year-old boy [36]. When the lesion is quite localized, it may be impossible to differentiate from atherosclerosis.

Arteritis

Although primary arteritis of the splenic artery is rare, the artery may be involved in arteritis affecting the aorta (e.g., giant cell arteritis) (Fig. 66-19) or other visceral branches. The inflammatory process involves the vessel wall to varying degrees, with destruction of media, areas of fibrosis and cicatrix, and at times aneurysm formation (Fig. 66-19).

Splenic Artery Aneurysm

Splenic artery aneurysm is the most common intraabdominal aneurysm aside from those of the abdominal aorta and the iliac arteries. Splenic artery aneurysms may be multiple [15] and may occur in association with other visceral artery aneurysms [13].

They are observed most often in the third and sixth decades of life, and they are two to three times more common in the female. Half the women of childbearing age in whom they are discovered are pregnant at the time of discovery.

Congenital splenic artery aneurysm ruptures more commonly than any other visceral artery aneurysm in women, especially those under 45 years of age, although it is rarely responsible for hemorrhage in men [90]. Splenic artery aneurysms may be largely congenital in women and atherosclerotic in men.

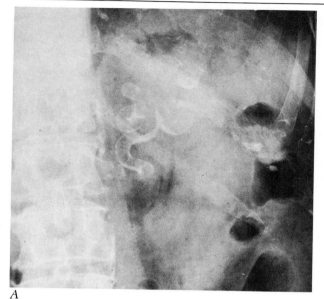

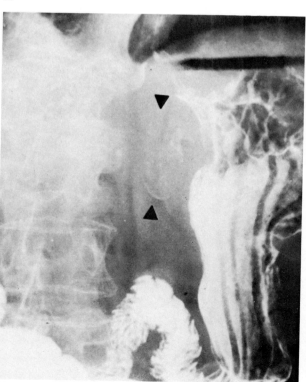

A

B

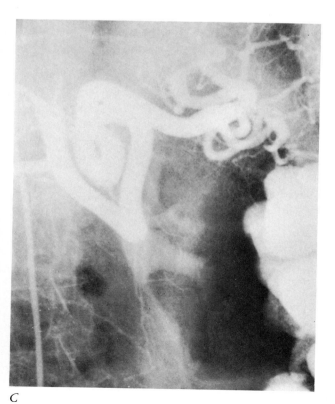

C

Figure 66-18. Arteriosclerosis of the splenic artery. (A) Calcified splenic artery. The splenic artery is grossly calcified throughout its course. Arteriosclerosis is manifested by both the tortuosity and the extensive calcium deposits in the wall. Note also the calcification of the abdominal aorta. See also Figure 66-9, in which carcinoma of the pancreas has invaded the wall of the splenic artery and resembles arteriosclerosis. (B) Calcified splenic artery (*arrowheads*). The tortuous vessel inserts at the lesser curvature of the stomach. (C) Arteriogram. Same patient as in (B). Note the great elongation but relative absence of intimal filling defects.

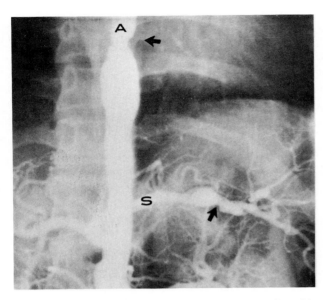

Figure 66-19. Splenic artery in arteritis. This 23-year-old hypertensive woman had a systolic bruit in the back. Aortography demonstrates marked irregularity in the lumen of the aorta (*A*), with a thickened wall (*arrow*). The splenic artery (*S*) is also irregular in appearance, with areas of aneurysmal dilatation (*arrow*) both along the course of the main trunk and in the peripheral branches. These changes were considered characteristic of an arteritis, a diagnosis consistent with the laboratory and biopsy data.

The diagnosis may be made on the plain film by demonstration of a ringlike calcific shadow in the region of the splenic artery (Fig. 66-20; see also Fig. 66-23C). It is important to visualize this shadow in two projections because a tortuous splenic artery may simulate the ring of a splenic aneurysm [85]. Rupture of a splenic aneurysm may be well demonstrated by celiac arteriography. In a case described by Baum et al., diagnosis led to prompt surgical intervention that was almost certainly lifesaving [9].

Splenic artery aneurysms have been reported as incidental findings in 0.78 percent of all selective celiac axis angiographic examinations and in 0.1 percent of all autopsy studies [99]. Pollak et al., noting the benign course of most splenic artery aneurysms, suggest that resection of small, asymptomatic aneurysms in older patients is unnecessary [90]. In women who are pregnant or of childbearing age, resection is necessary because of the danger of rupture during pregnancy [110].

Figure 66-19 shows an unusual aneurysm in association with arteritis. Figure 66-20 demonstrates a calcified splenic artery aneurysm in a 68-year-old patient with septicemia. The aneurysms shown in Figures 66-21 and 66-22 are large enough to warrant concern about rupture. Multiple aneurysms in a patient with celiac artery

Figure 66-20. Calcified splenic artery aneurysm. This 68-year-old woman had septicemia incidental to a renal abscess. (A) Film of the abdomen during an intravenous pyelogram shows a circumscribed area of calcification (*arrows*) in the left upper quadrant. (B) Abdominal aortogram to evaluate the renal arteries demonstrates filling of the calcified aneurysm (*arrows*) of the distal splenic artery.

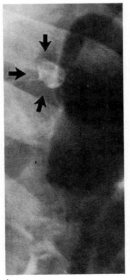

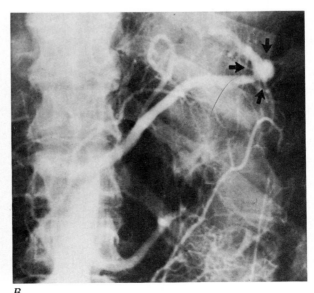

A

B

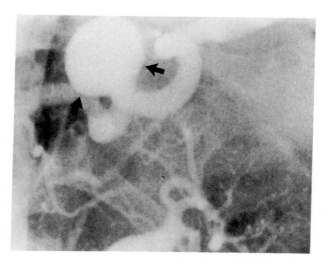

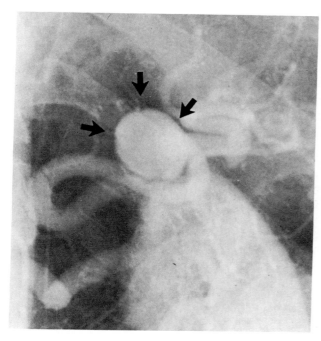

Figure 66-21. Splenic artery aneurysm. A large saccular aneurysm is visible (*arrows*) arising at the junction of the middle and distal thirds of the splenic artery. The caudal border of the aneurysm is irregular, suggesting the presence of thrombus within it.

Figure 66-22. Splenic artery aneurysm. A large, smooth-walled sac (*arrows*) arises from the splenic artery at the junction of the proximal and middle thirds. The remainder of the artery is smooth walled, strongly suggesting the congenital origin of this aneurysm.

occlusion are seen in Figure 66-23. Figure 66-24 demonstrates numerous aneurysmal dilatations of the peripheral intrasplenic branches without early filling of veins in a patient with hypersplenism, while Figure 66-25 shows similar findings in a patient with cirrhosis.

Splenic Arteriovenous Fistula

Splenic arteriovenous fistulas are said to cause cardiac failure rarely because the portal venous bed is much smaller than the systemic circulation and the return to the heart is delayed by the vascular resistance of the liver [115]. The fistulas may be congenital or acquired. The acquired lesions may be traumatic in origin, but they are also thought to result from rupture of splenic artery aneurysms. A bruit is usually heard in the left upper quadrant [111]. The spleen is commonly enlarged, and portal hypertension may be present [76].

Figure 66-26 shows an arteriovenous fistula in a lower part of the spleen in a 57-year-old woman. Acker et al. [3] described a traumatic fistula between the proximal splenic artery and the splenic vein through which a catheter was placed, which resulted in a transaortic portogram.

Percutaneous occlusion of a large splenic arteriovenous fistula exacerbating portal hypertension was performed in a patient bleeding from esophageal varices after both mesocaval shunting and transthoracic esophageal and gastric devascularization with splenectomy (the Sugiura procedure); transhepatic obliteration of the varices was carried out at the same time [49]. Although a transcatheter approach was chosen in this case because of the patient's poor clinical status, the procedure may also be advantageously applied to other, less critically ill, patients [98].

Splenic Infarction

Infarction of the spleen is relatively common in association with sickle-cell anemia or emboli from the left atrium in mitral stenosis. Radionuclide studies and computed tomography are useful screening methods (Fig. 66-27). Arteriographic studies demonstrate abrupt occlusion of intrasplenic branches associated with a localized ischemic zone, which is usually triangular (Fig. 66-28) [105].

Splenic Artery Thrombosis

Splenic artery thrombosis is relatively rare. Arteriography reveals obstruction with filling of intrasplenic vessels through collateral channels (Figs. 66-29, 66-30).

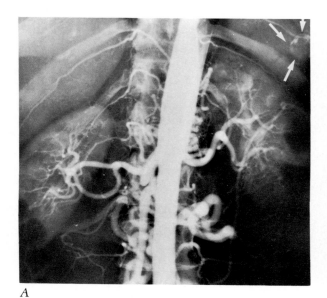

A

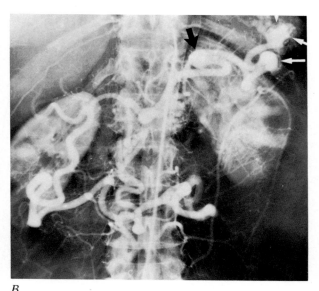

B

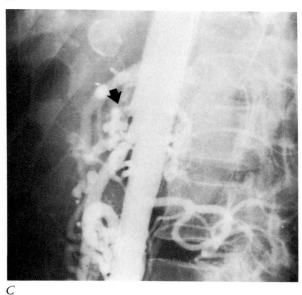

C

Figure 66-23. Multiple splenic artery aneurysms, associated with celiac artery occlusion. (A) Abdominal aotogram. The renal, superior mesenteric, and multiple lumbar arteries are visualized. No splenic artery is opacified following aortic injection. Note the ring-shaped calcification (*arrows*) in the left upper quadrant in the region of the spleen. (B) Aortogram, 3 seconds. Filling of the gastroduodenal artery has occurred from the common pancreaticoduodenal arteries arising from the superior mesenteric artery. There is retrograde flow into the common hepatic artery, with filling as well of the splenic artery, visualizing multiple aneurysms (*arrows*). (C) Lateral projection. Abdominal aortogram. The calcified splenic artery is visible ventral to the aorta. In addition, there is complete occlusion of the celiac artery (*arrow*).

Changes After Surgery

After splenorenal arterial shunts, the proximal intrapancreatic branches of the splenic artery may undergo remarkable enlargement and provide a collateral supply to the distal portion of the previously divided splenic trunk (Fig. 66-31). While immediate postoperative studies have shown little diversion of blood flow from the liver in patients with distal splenorenal venous (Warren) shunts [97], two-year follow-up studies have demonstrated reversal of portal venous flow from the liver to the low-pressure shunt [122]. In patients who had a Warren shunt performed that involved ligation of the left gastric and gas-

troepiploic veins, other collateral vessels formed postoperatively, while in patients who had a modified shunt without ligation of these branches, the left gastric and gastroepiploic veins enlarged and served as collateral vessels [122].

Portal Hypertension

The splenic artery may enlarge in the presence of cirrhosis and portal hypertension. Intrasplenic branch aneurysms may also develop (see Fig. 66-28).

Splenic Vein Occlusion

Pancreatic and retroperitoneal disease may cause splenic vein occlusion with a consequent increase in intrasplenic and peripheral splenic vein pressures and venous flow to gastric varices through the splenoportal collateral vessels (the short gas-

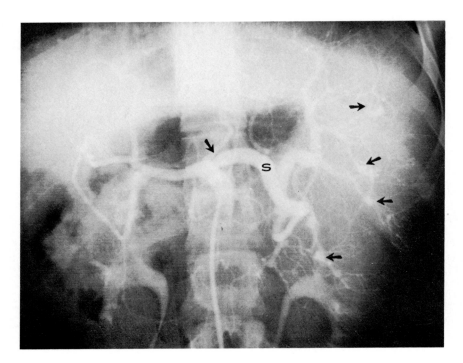

Figure 66-24. Intrasplenic arterial aneurysms. This 16-year-old girl had splenomegaly, leukopenia, thrombocytopenia, and a coagulation defect. The celiac arteriogram shows marked splenomegaly with slight stenosis (*single arrow at left*) at the origin of the splenic artery (*S*). There are numerous aneurysmal dilatations (*arrows*) of the peripheral intrasplenic branches. Early draining veins were not identified, but multiple arteriovenous fistulas could not be completely ruled out.

Figure 66-25. Intrasplenic branch artery aneurysms in cirrhosis of the liver. This 45-year-old chronic alcoholic had cirrhosis of the liver with chronic liver failure. He had had multiple bleeding episodes because of esophageal varices. Selective splenic arteriogram demonstrates multiple intrasplenic arterial aneurysms, with profound narrowing of the intrasplenic arterial branches. The appearance resembles that in periarteritis, but represents one of the findings sometimes associated with cirrhosis of the liver and portal hypertension.

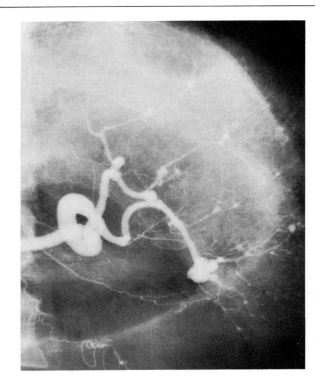

tric, coronary, and gastroepiploic veins) [21, 45, 75]. Gastric varices may give rise to massive acute or recurrent hemorrhaging [50], which can be forestalled by splenectomy.

Abdominal pain, weight loss, or iron-deficiency anemia is commonly associated with splenic vein occlusion [75]. Radiographic investigation may reveal a normal-size spleen [45, 75] or splenomegaly. The presence of gastric varices in the absence of esophageal varices is evidence of splenic vein occlusion, while the coexistence of varices of both venous systems rather suggests

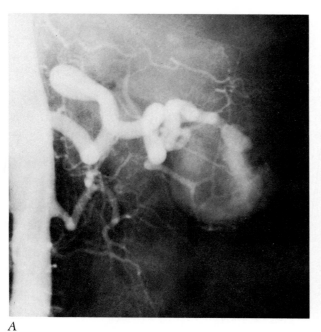

A

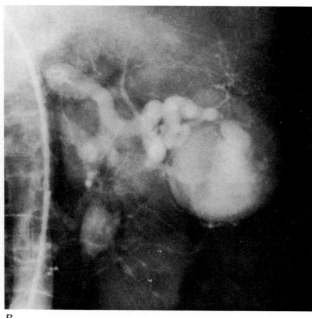

B

Figure 66-26. Splenic arteriovenous fistula in a 57-year-old woman complaining of weight loss, diarrhea, malaise, and an enlarging abdomen. Physical examination showed ascites without evidence of a mass and severe edema of both lower extremities. Angiography showed a large arteriovenous fistula. (A) Early phase. A tortuous splenic artery fills a large blood sac in the spleen. (B) Late phase. The sac retains contrast, and its true size is now clearly defined. (Courtesy of Arthur Pryde, M.D.)

Figure 66-27. Splenic infarction. Computed tomographic scan demonstrates two wedge-shaped areas of diminished absorption in the spleen (*arrows*). These represent areas of splenic infarction in a patient with multiple embolic episodes.

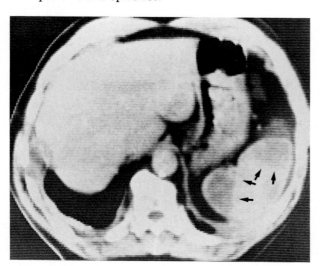

portal hypertension [21]. In a study of 19 patients with angiographically demonstrated splenic vein occlusion, gastric varices were evident on barium examination in 74 percent as "broad, serpentine, redundant filling defects or clusters of polypoid defects, simulating thickened rugal folds" [21]. Definitive diagnosis, however, requires angiographic studies.

Cysts
Splenic cysts are rare lesions; fewer than 700 cases have been reported in the literature [25]. Although large splenic cysts have been found in neonates [40], cysts in children are rare. Most cysts occur in people under 40 years of age [94], and there is a female predominance [34]. Of six cases reported by Doolas et al. [25], three were found in association with pregnancy.

Symptoms, including dyspnea, coughing, respiratory infections, nausea, vomiting, and urinary frequency, frequently arise as a result of visceral compression [94]. Twenty-five percent of splenic cysts rupture, and 45 percent are demonstrated as splenomegaly [94]. Although splenic cysts are usually diagnosed prior to surgery only

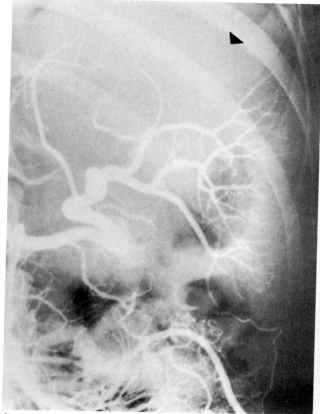

A

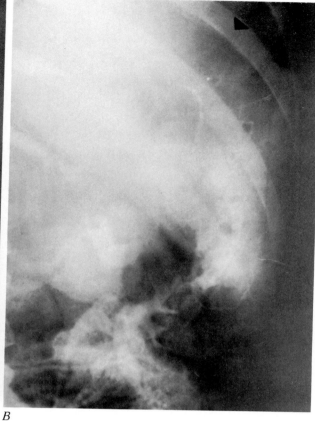

B

Figure 66-28. Splenic infarction. This 23-year-old woman had rheumatic heart disease with atrial fibrillation. She had a series of embolic episodes to the abdomen and then developed a bout of both left and right upper quadrant pain. (A) Splenic arteriography demonstrates complete occlusion of the superior splenic arterial branch. No evidence of filling of the small vessels is observed in this area (*arrowhead*). (B) In the capillary phase, a large radiolucent area representing the zone of ischemia is apparent (*arrowhead*).

Figure 66-29. Splenic artery thrombosis. Selective celiac arteriogram. (A) Early phase. There is complete occlusion of the splenic artery 2 cm distal to its origin from the celiac artery (*arrow*). Multiple collateral channels are filling. (B) Later phase at 1.5 seconds. The distal splenic artery (*arrows*) is densely opacified via collateral vessels, and arborizes normally into the terminal branches in the spleen.

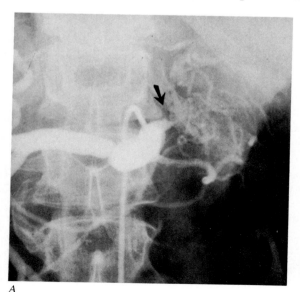

A

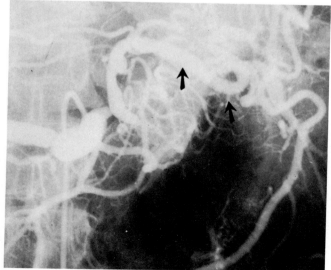

B

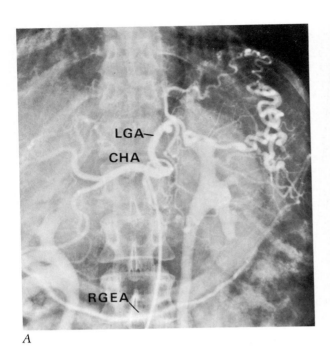

A

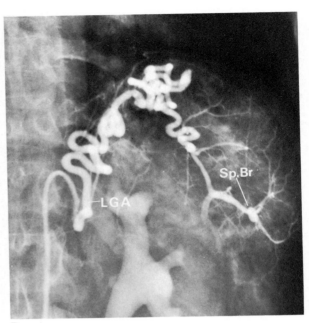

B

Figure 66-30. Splenic artery thrombosis. (A) Selective celiac arteriogram. There is complete occlusion of the splenic artery just beyond its origin. Collateral filling to the spleen via the left gastric artery (*LGA*) and the right gastroepiploic artery (*RGEA*) is apparent. (B) Selective left gastric arteriogram. Left posterior oblique projection. The left gastric artery is profoundly tortuous in its course, and communicates with branches to the spleen, filling the rather thin intrasplenic arterial branches. *LGA* = left gastric artery; *CHA* = left hepatic or common hepatic artery; *RGEA* = right gastroepiploic artery; *Sp. Br.* = intrasplenic branches.

when calcified, a high index of suspicion should be maintained because of the danger of cyst rupture. Excretory urography may demonstrate a splenic cyst as a suprarenal mass [14], and although nonspecific, the liver-spleen scan shows defects in 60 to 70 percent of cases of splenic cyst (Fig. 66-32) [27]. While ultrasonography plays a critical role in the evaluation of splenic cysts [92], computed tomography may also be of value if ultrasonography fails to determine adequately the location and characteristics of the cyst (Fig. 66-33) [31]. Cystic fluid may be obtained by percutaneous puncture, as has been demonstrated inadvertently during attempted splenoportography [28, 44]; however, cyst puncture is not recommended because of the possibility of cyst rupture, leading to abscess and peritonitis [113]. Angiography (Fig. 66-34) is valuable at times in excluding the diagnosis of abscess or neoplasm [31, 54].

Splenic cysts are divided into two large groups: (1) the true cysts, of either parasitic or nonpara-

sitic origin, which have an epithelial lining; and (2) the false cysts, which frequently arise secondary to trauma and which lack an epithelial lining. The most common cause of splenic cysts is echinococcus infection; in such cysts peripheral calcification may be present in the cyst wall. In countries in which echinococcus disease is not endemic, false cysts have been reported to constitute 80 percent of splenic cysts [31].

Characteristically, cysts cause compression and displacement of surrounding normal parenchyma. They are avascular [91, 103], and they may demonstrate large capsular vessels coursing over them. There is rarely any problem with the distinction from neoplasm because the intrasplenic vessels are smoothly compressed and displaced by the avascular cyst (Fig. 66-35) [91]. Frequently there may be only a densely opacified shell of parenchyma during the capillary phase as a reflection of the high degree of replacement by the cyst [52]. The edge is usually sharp and smooth.

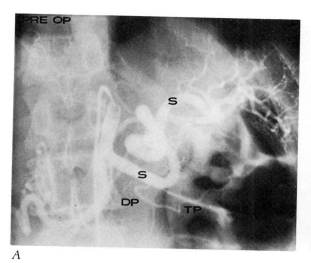

A

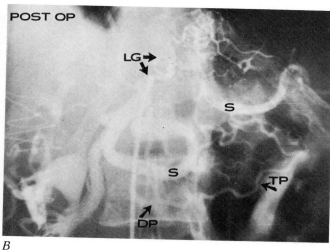

B

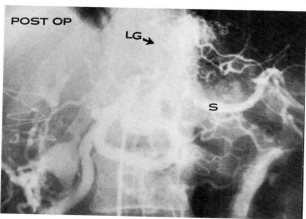

C

Figure 66-31. Postoperative changes in the splenic artery. This 46-year-old hypertensive man had severe left renal artery stenosis demonstrated by renal angiography. A splenorenal shunt was constructed at surgery. (A) Preoperative study. A normal, somewhat tortuous main splenic trunk (*S*) with dorsal pancreatic (*DP*) and transverse pancreatic (*TP*) branches is opacified. (B) Postoperative study 8 days after surgery. The splenic trunk (*S*) has been divided. The distal portion fills from the dorsal pancreatic (*DP*) and transverse pancreatic (*TP*) anastomosis, which has enlarged in the interval. *LG* = left gastric artery. (C) Later phase in the serialographic study. Additional collateral supply to the spleen via tortuous channels originating from the left gastric artery (*LG*) is evident.

Figure 66-32. Splenic cyst. Radionuclide scan demonstrates multiple round negative defects in the spleen, representing subcapsular cysts.

Figure 66-33. Calcified splenic cyst. Computed tomography. A large cyst of the spleen is visible (*arrows*) with a calcific wall. Although the appearance is compatible with an echinococcus cyst, this represented a congenital cyst of the kidney.

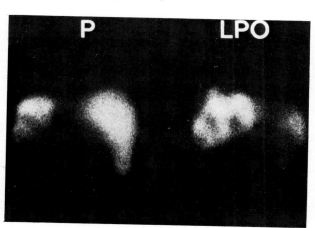

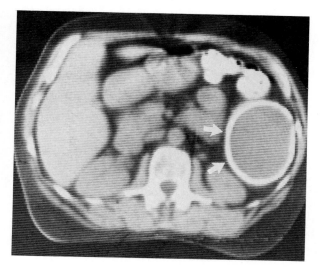

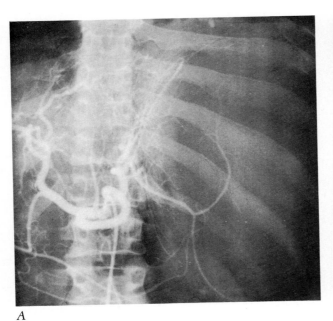

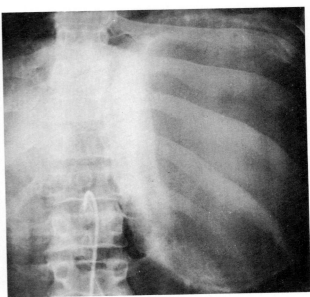

A

B

Figure 66-34. Cyst of the spleen. This 45-year-old man had left upper quadrant pain and a palpable mass. (A) Celiac arteriogram demonstrates a huge mass lesion, with distortion and compression of the peripheral splenic vessels. (B) A later phase of the same study shows a large, avascular area of mass compressing the remainder of the splenic parenchyma, which is filled with contrast medium. At laparotomy, the preoperative diagnosis of splenic cyst was confirmed.

Figure 66-35. Splenic cyst. Splenographic phase of a selective celiac arteriogram. A large lucent area is visible (*arrows*) in the hilus of the spleen, slightly compressing the visualized splenic vein (*Sp. V.*). Notice the thin rim of compressed splenic tissue around the congenital cyst.

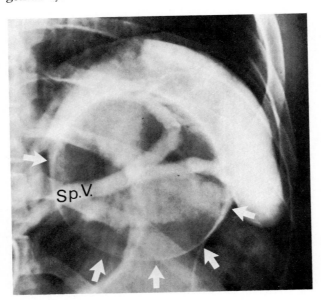

NEOPLASMS

Benign Tumors

The benign tumors of the spleen are of many varieties: fibromas, osteomas, chondromas, lymphangiomas, hemangiomas, and hamartomas. Most of these tumors are round or oval and displace surrounding arterial branches significantly. Atrophy of the adjacent parenchyma may also be observed. A relative lack of vascularity in the parenchal phase is generally apparent. The hamartomas, by contrast, may be richly vascular tumors with large, plexoid vessels that may simulate those of malignant neoplasms (Fig. 66-36). The vessels may be tortuous, with aneurysmal dilatations and multiple vascular lakes [54]: they ramify irregularly and may communicate directly with veins [119]. They resemble the neovasculature of malignant tumors of the kidney and other viscera.

Malignant Tumors

Malignant splenic neoplasms are characteristically those that involve the lymph nodes and the bone marrow (lymphosarcoma, Hodgkin's disease, reticulum cell sarcoma, and the leukemias). The

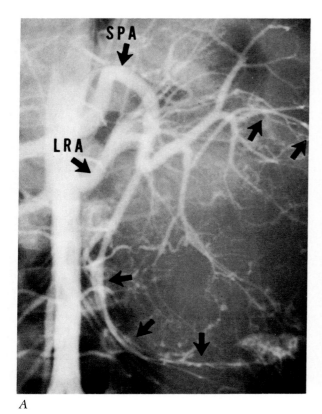

A

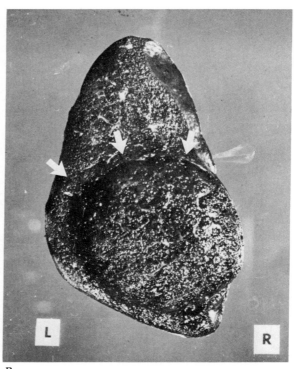

B

Figure 66-36. Hamartoma of the spleen. (A) Arteriogram. This 4-year-old boy had an abdominal mass and the nephrotic syndrome. A retrograde abdominal aortogram showed splaying of the branches (*arrows*) of the splenic artery (*SPA*) around a tumor occupying approximately 50 percent of the splenic substance. In the early arterial phase, numerous large, tortuous vessels were visualized within the tumor mass. Vascular lakes and early venous filling were demonstrated on later serial films. The left renal artery (*LRA*) was also displaced superiorly and medially with stretching of the lower pole branches. A diagnosis of congenital angiomatous malformation (hemangioma) or hemangiosarcoma was suggested. (B) Gross pathologic specimen. At laparotomy, the spleen weighed 300 gm and contained a well-delimited 7-cm mass (*arrows*). On microscopic section, the appearance was considered characteristic of a hamartoma. The splenic mass was causing compression and stretching of the left renal vein. After splenectomy, proteinuria and hypoproteinemia disappeared.

subject has been reviewed by Das Gupta et al. [23], Rösch [104], and Kishikawa et al. [53]. In addition, hemangiosarcomas and fibrosarcomas may also be observed. All of these neoplasms, with the exception of the hemangiosarcomas and the fibrosarcomas, cause a diffuse increase in the size of the spleen; the neoplastic tissue is distributed generally rather than localized.

Arteriography has not been commonly employed in the study of malignant neoplasms of the spleen because nonlymphomatous malignancies are unusual and because patients with metastases of epithelial neoplasms to the spleen generally have disseminated metastases. In 1954, Edsman [26] described the first case of malignant tumor of the spleen studied by angiography. The histology was that of a malignant splenic endothelioma.

As in malignant tumors elsewhere, the vessels may be irregularly narrowed, amputated, and displaced. By far the commonest finding is displacement: stretching and distortion of the vessels by diffuse tumor infiltration. The appearance demonstrated in Figure 66-12, splenomegaly with Hodgkin's disease, is typical. There is more or less stretching and distortion of the major branches of the splenic artery, with distinct separation of the distal small branches and, frequently, rather striking narrowing as well.

In a study of the angiographic findings in splenic neoplasms, Kishikawa et al. [54] noted similar angiographic appearances in five cases of reticulum cell sarcoma and one case of Hodgkin's disease. In these cases, the lesions were visualized as "multiple, poorly defined round defects in the splenic parenchymograms." Arterial encasement was shown in all cases, while fine tumor vessels and venous obstruction were evident in, respectively, three and two of the cases of reticulum cell sarcomas. Splayed intrasplenic branches, vascular lakes in the late arterial-to-venous phase, and no obvious tumor vessels or stains were found in two cases of hemangiosarcoma [53].

Vascular changes may also occur in the leukemias. In Figure 66-13, the stretching of the intrasplenic branches is obvious, and the capsular circulation is somewhat richer than is normally seen. The opacification of the spleen is relatively less than normal because of the replacement of a significant volume of tissue by the leukemic infiltrates.

Both computed tomography and ultrasonography yield valuable information in splenic lymphoma (Figs. 66-37, 66-38). As has been demonstrated in a case reported by Cunningham [22], ultrasonography cannot reliably distinguish lymphoma from abscess; however, when angiography shows typical neovascularity and irregular, en-

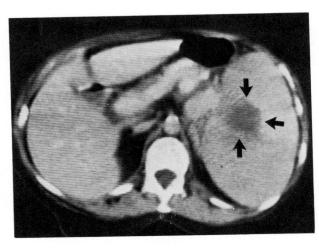

Figure 66-38. Hodgkin's disease of the spleen. Computed tomographic scan. The spleen is grossly enlarged. There is, thus, diffuse involvement of the spleen by Hodgkin's disease. In addition, there is an area of low attenuation (*arrows*), representing a localized implant of Hodgkin's tissue.

cased vessels, as in the reticulum cell sarcoma illustrated in Figure 66-39, an unequivocal diagnosis of malignancy can be made. Computed tomography has proved helpful in detecting moderate-size splenic metastases (Fig. 66-40), as has angiography (Fig. 66-41). On angiography metastases may displace vessels but more commonly are demonstrated as round, lucent areas in the capillary phase. With the development of new contrast agents, computed tomography may well have the capacity to detect smaller avascular splenic masses [117]. The concept that the spleen is immune to metastases from epithelial neoplasms and that such metastases are extremely rare has not been borne out by autopsy studies [2].

Trauma

The spleen is ruptured more often than any other intraabdominal organ in nonpenetrating abdominal injuries, and it is also frequently injured in penetrating trauma. In a review of 335 consecutively studied patients undergoing splenectomy for trauma [35], 57 percent of the patients had three or more associated injuries. While no patient with only a splenic injury died, the mortality was greater than 30 percent among patients with more than three associated injuries. In penetrating trauma, the chest is the commonest site of associated injury; in blunt trauma, the skeletal system is the commonest site (Table 66-7) [78]. In both blunt and penetrating splenic trauma,

Figure 66-37. Splenic lymphoma. Ultrasonogram. The spleen (*SP*) is grossly enlarged. A discrete echogenic tumor mass is visible within the splenic shadow (*arrows*). The kidney (*K*) is well visualized.

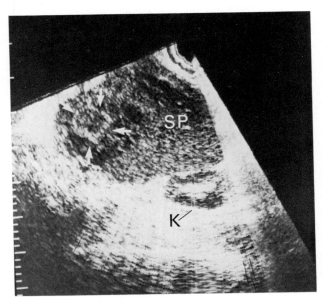

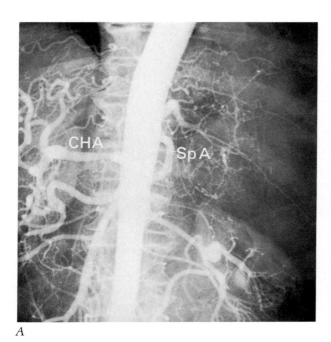

A

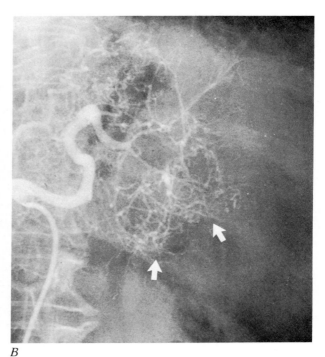

B

Figure 66-39. Reticulum cell sarcoma of the spleen and retroperitoneum. (A) Abdominal aortogram. The splenic artery (*SpA*) is visualized arising from the celiac axis and extending into the left upper quadrant. It then becomes obscured by a meshwork of malignant vessels extending into the spleen. Incidentally noted are extension of the tumor to involve the common hepatic artery (*CHA*) with encasement and an aneurysm of the left renal artery. (B) Selective splenic arteriogram. Magnification view. Encasement of the splenic artery is demonstrated, reflected in the areas of narrowing and irregularity. The tumor has completely surrounded the vessel, which gives rise to a large cluster of tumor vessels (*arrows*) extending into the spleen.

Figure 66-40. Metastasis to the spleen. Computed tomographic scan. The splenic shadow (*Sp*) is well visualized, with a round nodule (*arrows*) representing metastasis from an ovarian carcinoma. The negative filling defects in the spleen (*barred arrows*) also represent metastatic disease.

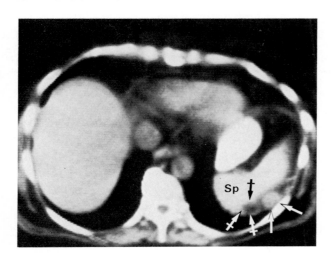

shock and pulmonary complications are the commonest causes of death (Table 66-8). It is likely that blunt trauma leads to splenic fractures in the areas between the intrasplenic arteries since the arteries serve as the major structural supports of the parenchyma [24]; if this is true, it would mean that the injuries themselves follow a natural segmental distribution.

Although diagnostic paracentesis may establish the presence of blood in the peritoneal cavity and permit a presumptive diagnosis of splenic rupture [35], imaging methods are frequently applied both for making the primary diagnosis and for defining the associated injuries. Indications of splenic trauma include depression of the splenic flexure of the colon, elevation of the diaphragm, obliteration of the splenic shadow, and prominent gastric rugae. Rib fractures, pleural fluid at the base of the left lung, and free peritoneal fluid may also be observed. These signs are not, however, always present.

Computed tomography has shown promise in

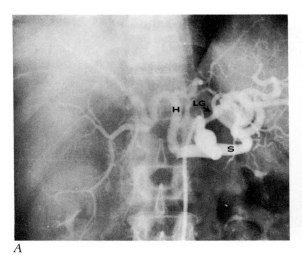

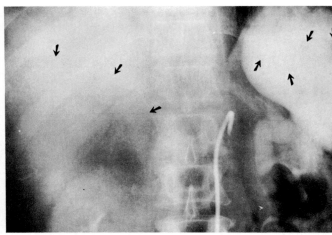

A   B

Figure 66-41. Metastases to the spleen and liver. This 50-year-old man had a diagnosis of malignant melanoma established on skin biopsy several years prior to the present study. He was admitted to the hospital complaining of malaise, anorexia, and abdominal pain. On physical examination, hepatosplenomegaly was found to be present, and the patient was subsequently found to have widespread metastatic disease. (A) Celiac arteriogram demonstrates enlargement of the liver and spleen. Hepatic branches (H) are stretched peripherally. The splenic trunk (S) is tortuous and compressed by the enlarged spleen. LG = left gastric artery. (B) Later phase of same study reveals filling defects (arrows) in the opacified parenchyma of both the liver and the spleen due to metastatic deposits.

the diagnosis of both splenic laceration [66] and subcapsular splenic hematoma [55]. Radioisotope studies lack specificity and cannot demonstrate very small subcapsular hematomas; nevertheless, positive studies in patients with a history of trauma may permit laparotomy to be performed without the necessity for angiographic confirmation. Displacement of the barium-filled stomach from the inner rib margin in the left lateral decubitus position may provide a simple means of diagnosing splenic rupture [77].

A positive angiographic diagnosis can best be made when extravasation is visualized. "Mottling," or apparent areas of subcapsular ischemia or fluid collection, is a less reliable sign [57] although Scatliff has pointed out that mottling is frequently present and probably represents stasis of contrast material and blood in the marginal sinuses of the traumatized spleen [109]. Splenic "notching," or lobulation, may be incorrectly considered as evidence of splenic rupture (Fig. 66-42) [57]. Extravasation is usually unmistakable (Fig. 66-43), but at times may be best demonstrated by intraarterial administration of epinephrine or vasopressin. By increasing resistance at the precapillary arteriolar level, contrast leakage

Table 66-7. Associated Injuries with Splenic Trauma

Blunt Injuries (150 patients)		Penetrating Injuries (186 patients)	
Orthopedic	79	Chest	104
Chest	64	Stomach	71
Central nervous system	48	Liver	52
Liver	31	Colon	46
Genitourinary	28	Genitourinary	36
Pancreas	19	Pancreas	32
Diaphragm (ruptured)	11	Extremity	26
Intestine	15	Small bowel	20

From Naylor et al. [78].

Table 66-8. Breakdown of Causes
of Death Following Splenic Trauma

| Cause of Death | Number of Deaths | | Total Number of Deaths |
	Blunt Trauma	Penetrating Trauma	
Shock	16	5	21
Pulmonary disorder	13	3	16
Central nervous system disorder	5	1	6
Sepsis	1	3	4
Unknown	1	1	2
Total	36	13	49

From Naylor et al. [78].

may be enhanced (Fig. 66-44). The site of bleeding may be demonstrated by the leakage of contrast medium into the splenic pulp (Fig. 66-45) [11, 41]. Characteristic findings also include (1) a large, avascular area with spreading of the intrasplenic branches (see Figs. 66-45, 66-47); (2) irregularities in the opacified spleen in the region of the hematoma (Fig. 66-46); (3) loss of the continuous splenic contour (see Fig. 66-43); (4) simultaneous visualization of the splenic artery and vein (see Fig. 66-45); (5) extravasation of contrast material in the spleen (see Figs. 66-43–66-45); (6) a clear break ("fracture") in the splenic contour (Fig. 66-47); and (7) an increased distance between the spleen and the left flank (see Figs. 66-43–66-46) [80]. The spleen may be displaced medially and the kidney inferiorly [59].

Figure 66-42. "Notching" of the spleen. This patient was in an automobile accident and was suspected of having splenic rupture. A splenic arteriogram was performed. (A) Early phase. There appears to be a defect in the contour of the spleen (*arrow*) located just below the diaphragm, and originally interpreted as possibly representing splenic hematoma consequent to trauma. (B) Splenographic phase. The spleen is densely but nonuniformly opacified, and a number of areas of lucency are visible at the edge of the spleen (*arrows*). Splenectomy was performed on this patient, and no evidence of splenic trauma was visible. Instead, congenital notching of the spleen was found.

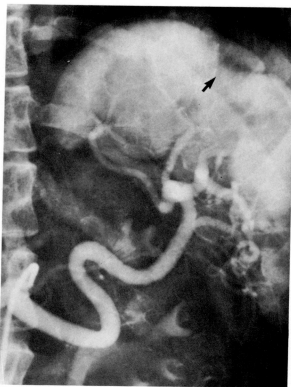

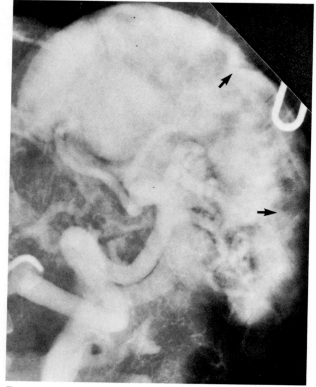

A   *B*

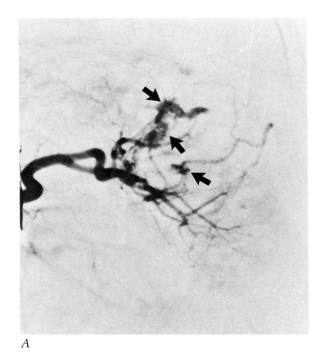

A

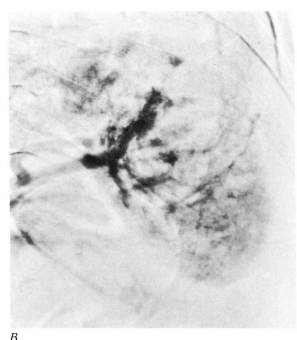

B

Figure 66-43. Splenic trauma. Selective splenic arteriography. (A) Early phase. Subtraction demonstrates unequivocal extravasation (*arrows*) of contrast agent outside the vascular bed into the splenic tissue. (B) Later phase. The contrast agent puddles within the splenic tissue, indicating the presence of gross splenic trauma. Notice that the lateral wall of the spleen is separated from the lateral abdominal wall by a subcapsular collection of blood.

Figure 66-44. Splenic trauma. (A) Selective splenic arteriogram. Although there is some spreading of the intrasplenic vessels, there is no definite evidence of extravasation or local collections of blood within the spleen. (B) Selective splenic arteriogram 15 seconds after the administration of 6 gm of epinephrine. With the increase in the intrasplenic arterial resistance, there is clear evidence of multiple areas of extravasation (*arrows*) throughout the spleen. The epinephrine, by raising the vascular resistance at the precapillary level, has helped establish an unequivocal diagnosis of splenic trauma. (Courtesy of Stanley Baum, M.D.)

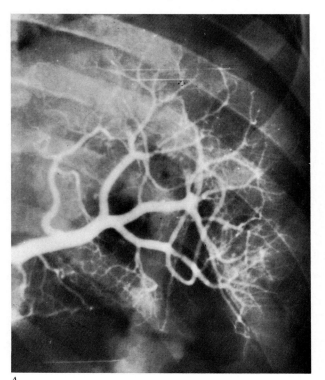

A

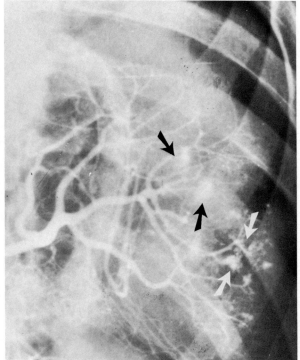

B

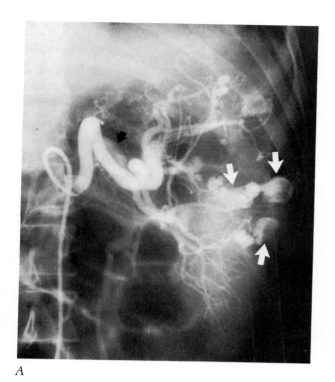

A

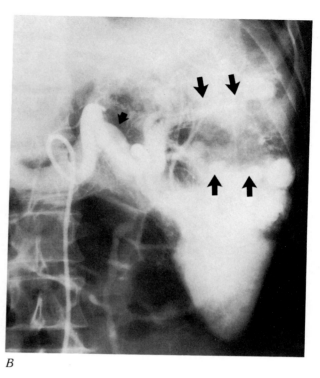

B

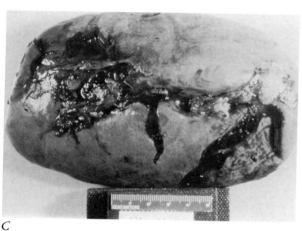

C

Figure 66-45. Splenic trauma. (A) Selective splenic arteriogram, early phase. Gross extravasation is visible within the splenic tissue (*white arrows*), as are profound separation of vessels and early filling of the splenic vein (*black arrow*). (B) Selective splenic arteriogram. Splenographic phase. In addition to the gross extravasation, there is a large area of nonfilling (*large arrows*), representing intrasplenic hemorrhage. The splenic vein is densely visualized (*small arrow*). (C) Specimen of ruptured spleen. Multiple rents are visible in the surface of the spleen, with gross intrasplenic hemorrhage also demonstrated.

In subacute or chronic trauma, intrasplenic "channels" may be visualized (Fig. 66-47).

In those patients in whom the diagnosis is suspected but uncertain, splenic arteriography should be performed. It is an accurate method of establishing the diagnosis and of assessing the degree of splenic injury (Fig. 66-48) [12, 59, 96].

A recent report by Morag and Rubenstein [72] on cases in which angiography was performed supports the feasibility of conservative management of some cases of trauma. In their two patients with definite angiographic evidence of serious splenic injury, repeat angiography two months later showed a normal splenic appear-

ance. Fischer et al. [32] have employed scintigraphy in the diagnosis and follow-up of splenic trauma in pediatric patients, and they have shown that splenic tissue, and therefore immunologic competence, may be preserved in this group [32].

Partial splenectomy, exploiting the segmental distribution of intrasplenic arteries, has come into increasing favor as a means of preserving immunologic competence and decreasing the chance of postoperative sepsis [24, 73]. Partial splenectomy offers promise in the treatment of cysts and hamartomas and, especially, in cases of trauma without coexisting multiple abdominal injuries [73].

In recent years, occult rupture of the spleen has been recognized as a diagnostic challenge. While splenic injury results in immediate rupture

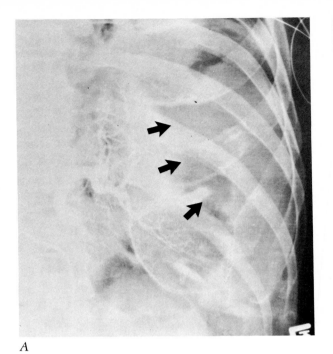

A

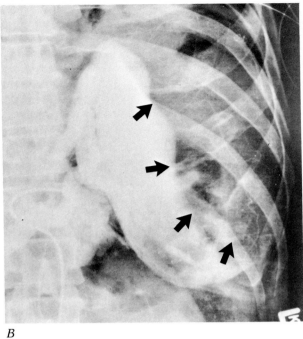

B

Figure 66-46. Splenic rupture with subcapsular hematoma. Selective splenic arteriogram. (A) Arterial phase. The splenic arterial branches are clumped together at the medial aspect of the kidney, and a large area of nonfilling is visible (*arrows*). (B) Splenographic phase. The splenic tissue is grossly compressed and very densely opacified. A large subcapsular hematoma is well visualized (*arrows*). It separates the opacified splenic tissue from the lateral abdominal wall to a striking degree.

Figure 66-47. Splenic trauma. This patient was in an automobile accident and had multiple fractures. Although there was a suspicion of splenic trauma, arteriographic studies were delayed until 3 weeks after the accident. (A) Selective splenic arteriogram. There is profound separation of intrasplenic arterial branches, with clumping and compression of splenic parenchyma. (B) Capillary phase. There is striking evidence of splenic trauma. A large laceration of the spleen is visible, with intrasplenic hemorrhage (*arrows*). The splenic edge is separated from the lateral abdominal wall because of a subcapsular collection of blood. Intrasplenic tracts of contrast agent representing channels in an otherwise hemorrhagic area are clearly visible (*barred arrows*).

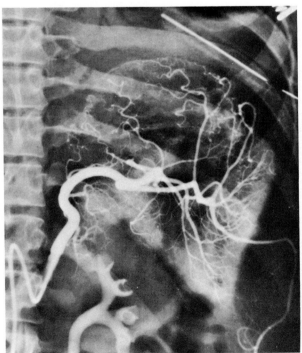

A

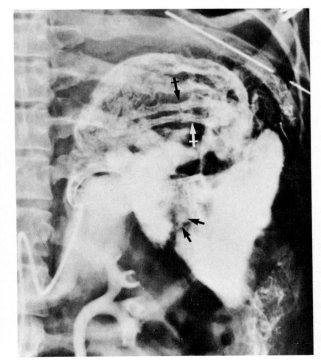

B

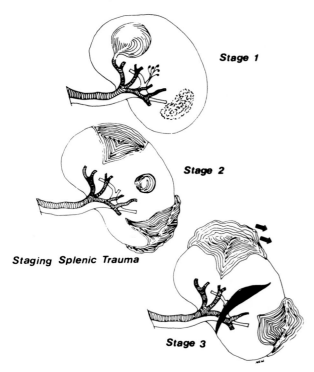

Figure 66-48. Diagrammatic representation of splenic trauma. (Courtesy of Mark Wholey, M.D.). Stage 1. Intrasplenic hemorrhage. Stage 2. Subcapsular and extracapsular hemorrhage. Stage 3. Splenic fraction with extracapsular bleeding.

in 85 percent of patients and in delayed rupture (some days or weeks later) in 14 percent of patients, in 1 percent of patients the splenic rupture may take place without immediate symptoms and become clinically evident months or years after the trauma in a confusing welter of symptoms. In such cases of occult rupture, the hemorrhage is contained by an intact capsule or adhesions to adjacent organs [16]. The characteristic angiographic pattern comprises a peripheral avascular splenic area, tortuosity of the splenic artery with hilar vessel compression, and a smooth filling defect between the diaphragm and the spleen [16].

Trauma is not necessarily implicated in all cases of splenic rupture [16]; in five cases collected by McMahon [62], infectious mononucleosis was the underlying cause in two patients, Hodgkin's disease in one, and amyloidosis in one, while in one patient no cause was ever determined. Preoperative diagnosis is important. In a case reported by Moskovitz [74] in which the diagnosis was not established preoperatively, extensive resection was carried out because the organized hematoma resembled infiltrating neoplasm.

Inflammation

Splenic abscess is a rare but serious lesion, and it is frequently difficult to diagnose. Two angiographic patterns have been described: (1) an avascular mass with tortuous peripheral arteries as well as collateral veins if the splenic vein is narrowed or obstructed [100] and (2) splenomegaly with an irregular mass lacking a vascular rim in association with normal veins and stretched arteries without encasement [46]. In some cases, the angiographic findings may be nonspecific or misleading, suggesting, for example, the presence of a subcapsular hematoma. Miller et al. [71], noting that a mycotic aneurysm has been associated with a splenic abscess in a number of cases, have suggested that abnormal splenic arteriographic findings in the presence of a mycotic aneurysm be interpreted as evidence of a splenic abscess. In one case studied by Grant et al. [39], arteriography, computed tomography, and ultrasonography successfully defined the nature of the mass, whereas a radioisotope liver-spleen scan suggested a lesion of the liver.

Interventional Techniques

Interventional techniques have been increasingly applied to the splenic circulation. Attempts at transcatheter splenic infarction have frequently been unsuccessful when this approach has been used alone [5, 18, 37, 63, 87]. In patients with hematologic disorders, sepsis may ensue; Wholey et al. have reported that splenic artery occlusion and embolization resulted in abscess formation in two such patients and in septicemia and spontaneous rupture in a third [121]. While splenectomy itself may cause infectious complications, bacterial contamination in the angiographic laboratory further increases the chance of infection. Skin and catheter cultures obtained after standard aseptic techniques were maintained revealed a 60 percent rate of bacterial contamination [121]. Although the organisms cultured are normally not pathogenic, they pose a risk to patients with compromised immunologic defenses.

Occlusion of the splenic artery has shown promise, however, as a preparatory measure before operative splenectomy [18]. In one case reported by Levy [58], a patient with myelofibrosis and severe pancytopenia underwent successful preoperative splenic artery occlusion with Gianturco coils to reduce the massive splenomegaly and to decrease the possibility of intraoperative hemorrhage. Catheter infusion of cytotoxic agents has also been successfully employed to decrease splenomegaly in patients with chronic granulocytic leukemia although the reduction in splenic size persisted only 4 to 6 weeks [17].

The applications of "medical splenectomy" require a careful weighing of the risks against the potential benefits. In disorders in which the surgical mortality is high (e.g., hypersplenism with thrombocytopenia and portal hypertension); in emergent situations, such as gastrointestinal bleeding with hypersplenism and portal hypertension; in idiopathic thrombocytopenia (to obviate platelet transfusion); and in splenic trauma (to decrease bleeding prior to definitive surgery), catheter occlusion of the splenic artery may afford substantial benefit in selected cases.

Diagnostic Decision Pathway

Radiologic methods play an important role in establishing the presence or absence of splenic disease, as well as in defining its character when present. Splenomegaly may be well depicted by plain abdominal films, the upper gastrointestinal series, the barium enema, and the intravenous urogram. In trauma, multiple associated injuries may be detected. The conventional examinations, however, shed little light on the *nature* of the splenic abnormality that is present, and they may show entirely normal findings in many types of splenic disease.

Radionuclide scintigraphy, ultrasonography, computed tomography, and angiography have all been considered *complementary* imaging approaches to the spleen; they are, in fact, *competitive* more often than not. The difficult problem is to determine a sequence and pattern of use of imaging methods that optimally clarifies the diagnostic problem while it avoids expensive, unnecessary, and invasive examinations.

A sequence that has proved useful is illustrated in Figure 66-49. It is a modification of the algorithm proposed by Shirkhoda et al. [112]. Except when there is a strong probability of trauma, this approach would utilize scintigraphy, ultrasonography, or computed tomography as a primary imaging method, accepting the concept that the sensitivity and specificity of these methods are approximately equal. If the results of the examinations employed are normal, the diagnostic triage is terminated. If the results are abnormal, but diffusely so and diagnostic only of splenomegaly (as in infiltrative, hyperplastic, or congestive disorders), no further examinations

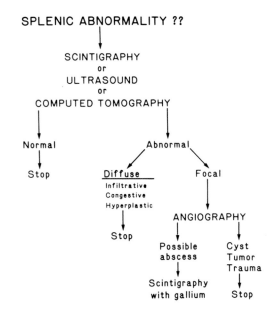

Figure 66-49. Diagnostic decision tree in splenic disease. (Modified from Shirkhoda et al. [112].)

are indicated. The congestive disorders are by far the most common, as in cirrhosis of the liver.

If a focal lesion or focal lesions are defined, and if they are well characterized, as in a classic simple cyst demonstrated by ultrasonography or computed tomography, or multiple metastases found in a patient with malignant disease, the diagnostic sequence is complete. If the nature of the splenic abnormality is undefined, angiography is employed as the definitive diagnostic method. The diagnosis of splenic abscess is difficult to make, and if the clinical and angiographic data suggest its presence, gallium scintigraphy may then be indicated.

This diagnostic decision pathway is short-circuited only when there is a high clinical suspicion of splenic trauma. Even in such patients, if they are in the pediatric age group, scintigraphy may prove to be adequate and permit follow-up as a part of the effort to avoid splenectomy. In patients with evidence of persistent bleeding, however, angiography should be initiated rapidly, and, depending on the clinical assessment, it may be followed by catheter occlusion as a means of controlling bleeding prior to surgery.

References

1. Abell, I.   Wandering spleen with torsion of the pedicle. *Ann. Surg.* 98:722, 1933.

2. Abrams, H. L. The incidence of splenic metastasis of carcinoma. *Calif. Med.* 76:281, 1952.
3. Acker, J. J., Galambos, J. T., and Weens, H. S. Selective celiac angiography. *Am. J. Med.* 37:417, 1964.
4. Albert, H. M., Fowler, R. L., Glass, B. A., and Yu, S-K. Cardiac anomalies and splenic agenesis. *Am. Surg.* 34:94, 1968.
5. Anderson, J. H., VuBan, A., Wallace, S., Hester, J. P., and Burke, J. S. Transcatheter splenic arterial occlusion: An experimental study in dogs. *Radiology* 125:95, 1977.
6. Ando, F., Shirotani, H., Kawai, J., Kanzaki, Y., Setsuie, N., Yamaguchi, K., Okamoto, F., Yokoyama, T., Makino, S., Tateishi, K., and Nishi, K. Successful total repair of complicated cardiac anomalies with asplenia syndrome. *J. Thorac. Cardiovasc. Surg.* 72:33, 1976.
7. Barnhart, M. I., Baechler, C. A., and Lusher, J. M. Arteriovenous shunts in the human spleen. *Am. J. Hematol.* 1:105, 1976.
8. Bart, B. B., and Appel, M. F. Recurrent hemolytic anemia secondary to accessory spleens. *South Med. J.* 71:608, 1978.
9. Baum, S., Greenstein, R. H., Nusbaum, M., and Blakemore, W. Diagnosis of ruptured, noncalcified splenic artery aneurysm by selective celiac arteriography. *Arch. Surg.* 91:1026, 1965.
10. Baum, S., Kuroda, K., and Roy, R. H. Value of special angiographic techniques in the management of patients with abdominal neoplasms. *Radiol. Clin. North Am.* 3:583, 1965.
11. Baum, S., Roy, R., Finkelstein, A. K., and Blakemore, W. S. Clinical application of selective celiac and superior mesenteric arteriography. *Radiology* 84:279, 1965.
12. Berk, R. N., and Wholey, M. H. The application of splenic arteriography in the diagnosis of rupture of the spleen. *AJR* 104:662, 1968.
13. Boontje, A. H. Multiple aneurysms of the visceral branches of the abdominal aorta. *Vasa* 8:42, 1979.
14. Breslin, J. A., Turner, B. I., Rhamy, R. K., and Faber, R. B. Splenic cysts in the differential diagnosis of suprarenal masses. *J. Urol.* 119:559, 1978.
15. Bücherl, E. S., and Rucker, G. Das Aneurysma der Arteria Coeliaca und ihre Äste. *Chirurg* 35:354, 1964.
16. Budd, D. C., Fouty, W. J., Jr., Johnson, R. B., and Lukash, W. M. Occult rupture of the spleen: A dilemma in diagnosis. *J.A.M.A.* 236:2884, 1976.
17. Canellos, G. P., Sutliffe, S. B., DeVita, V. T., and Lister, T. A. Treatment of refractory splenomegaly in myeloproliferative disease by splenic artery infusion. *Blood* 53:1014, 1979.
18. Castaneda-Zuniga, W. R., Hammerschmidt, D. E., Sanchez, R., and Amplatz, K. Nonsurgical splenectomy. *AJR* 129:805, 1977.
19. Chandramouly, B. S., Kihm, R. H., and Flesh, L. H. Dextrocardia with total situs inversus: Radionuclide imaging and ultrasonography of liver and spleen. *N.Y. State J. Med.* 80:655, 1980.
20. Childress, M. H., Cho, K. J., Newlin, N., and Martel, W. Arterial impression on the stomach. *AJR* 132:769, 1979.
21. Cho, K. J., and Martel, W. Recognition of splenic vein occlusion. *AJR* 131:439, 1978.
22. Cunningham, J. J. Ultrasonic findings in isolated lymphoma of the spleen simulating splenic abscess. *JCU* 6:412, 1978.
23. Das Gupta, T., Coombes, B., and Brasfield, R. D. Primary malignant neoplasms of the spleen. *Surg. Gynecol. Obstet.* 120:947, 1965.
24. Dixon, J. A., Miller, F., McCloskey, D., and Siddoway, J. Anatomy and techniques in segmental splenectomy. *Surg. Gynecol. Obstet.* 150:516, 1980.
25. Doolas, A., Nolte, M., McDonald, O. G., and Economou, S. G. Splenic cysts. *J. Surg. Oncol.* 10:369, 1978.
26. Edsman, G. Malignant tumor of the spleen diagnosed by lienal arteriography. *Acta Radiol.* (Stockh.) 42:461, 1954.
27. Eisenstat, T. E., Morris, D. M., and Mason, G. R. Cysts of the spleen: Report of a case and review of the literature. *Am. J. Surg.* 134:635, 1977.
28. Ellis, H. Splenic cysts diagnosed by splenography. *Br. J. Radiol.* 31:331, 1958.
29. Eraklis, A. J., and Filler, R. M. Splenectomy in childhood: A review of 1413 cases. *J. Pediatr. Surg.* 7:382, 1972.
30. Evans, J. Techniques in the detection and diagnosis of malignant lesions of the liver, spleen and pancreas. *Radiol. Clin. North Am.* 3:567, 1965.
31. Faer, M. J., Lynch, R. D., Lichtenstein, J. E., Madewell, J. E., and Feigin, D. S. Traumatic splenic cyst: RPC from the AFIP. *Radiology* 134:371, 1980.
32. Fischer, K. C., Eraklis, A., Rossello, P., and Treves, S. Scintigraphy in the follow-up of pediatric splenic trauma treated without surgery. *J. Nucl. Med.* 19:3, 1978.
33. Fitzer, P. M. Accessory spleen simulating splenic hematoma. *Va. Med.* 104:782, 1977.
34. Fowler, R. H. Nonparasitic benign cystic tumors of the spleen. *Intern. Abstr. Surg.* 96:209, 1953.
35. Fry, D. E., Garrison, R. N., and Williams, H. C. Patterns of morbidity and mortality in splenic trauma. *Ann. Surg.* 46:28, 1980.
36. Garti, L. J., and Meiraz, D. Fibromuscular

dysplasia of the splenic artery in a child; case report. *Vasa* 8:83, 1979.

37. Goldstein, H. M., Wallace, S., Anderson, J. H., Bree, R. L., and Gianturco, C. Transcatheter occlusion of abdominal tumors. *Radiology* 120:539, 1976.

38. Gordon, D. H., Burrell, M. I., Levin, D. C., Mueller, C. F., and Becker, J. A. Wandering spleen—the radiological and clinical spectrum. *Radiology* 125:39, 1977.

39. Grant, E., Mertens, M. A., and Mascatello, V. J. Splenic abscess: Comparison of four imaging methods. *AJR* 132:465, 1979.

40. Griscom, N. T., Hargreaves, H. K., Schwartz, M. Z., Reddish, J. M., and Colodny, A. H. Huge splenic cyst in a newborn: Comparison with 10 cases in later childhood and adolescence. *AJR* 129:889, 1977.

41. Haertel, M., and Ryder, D. Radiologic investigation of splenic trauma. *Cardiovasc. Radiol.* 2:27, 1979.

42. Heymsfield, S. B., Fulenwider, T., Nordlinger, B., Barlow, R., Sones, P., and Kutner, M. Accurate measurement of liver, kidney, and spleen volume and mass by computerized axial tomography. *Ann. Intern. Med.* 90:185, 1979.

43. Honigman, R., and Lanzkowsky, P. Isolated congenital asplenia: An occult case of overwhelming sepsis. *Am. J. Dis. Child.* 133:552, 1979.

44. Iban, R. E. Splenic cysts, with preoperative diagnosis. *Br. J. Radiol.* 32:821, 1959.

45. Itzchak, Y., and Glickman, M. G. Splenic vein thrombosis in patients with a normal size spleen. *Invest. Radiol.* 12:158, 1977.

46. Jacobs, R. P., Shanser, J. D., Lawson, D. L., and Palubinskas, A. J. Angiography of splenic abscesses. *AJR* 122:419, 1974.

47. Jacobson, J. M., and Reynolds, R. D. Accessory spleen in Hodgkin's disease. *J.A.M.A.* 240:2081, 1978.

48. Katcher, A. L. Familial asplenia, other malformations, and sudden death. *Pediatrics* 65:633, 1980.

49. Keller, F. S., Rösch, J., and Dotter, C. T. Bleeding from esophageal varices exacerbated by splenic arterial-venous fistula: Complete transcatheter obliterative therapy. *Cardiovasc. Intervent. Radiol.* 3:97, 1980.

50. Khan, A. H., O'Reilly, C. J., Avakian, V. A., and Lucina, P. A. Splenic vein thrombosis: An unusual case of gastric bleeding. *Angiology* 28:725, 1977.

51. Kim, E. E., and DeLand, F. H. Myelofibrosis presenting as hypermetabolic bone disease by radionuclide imaging in a patient with asplenia. *Clin. Nucl. Med.* 3:406, 1978.

52. King, M. C., Glick, B. W., and Freed, A. The diagnosis of splenic cysts. *Surg. Gynecol. Obstet.* 127:509, 1968.

53. Kishikawa, T., Numaguchi, Y., Tokunaga, M., and Matsuura, K. Hemangiosarcoma of the spleen with liver metastases: Angiographic manifestations. *Radiology* 123:31, 1977.

54. Kishikawa, T., Numaguchi, Y., Watanabe, K., and Matsuura, K. Angiographic diagnosis of benign and malignant splenic tumors. *AJR* 130:339, 1978.

55. Korobkin, M., Moss, A. A., Callen, P. W., De-Martini, W. J., and Kaiser, J. A. Computed tomography of subcapsular splenic hematoma: Clinical and experimental studies. *Radiology* 129:441, 1978.

56. Kupic, E. A., Marshall, W. H., and Abrams, H. L. Splenic arterial patterns: Angiographic analysis and review. *Invest. Radiol.* 2:70, 1967.

57. Lepasoon, J., and Olin, T. Angiographic diagnosis of splenic lesions following blunt abdominal trauma. *Acta Radiol.* [*Diagn.*] (Stockh.) 11:257, 1971.

58. Levy, J. M., Wasserman, P., and Pitha, N. Presplenectomy transcatheter occlusion of the splenic artery. *Arch. Surg.* 114:198, 1979.

59. Love, L., Greenfield, G. B., Braun, T. W., Moncada, R., Freeark, R. J., and Baker, R. J. Arteriography of splenic trauma. *Radiology* 91:96, 1968.

60. Lucas, R. V., Jr., Neufeld, H. N., Lester, R. G., and Edwards, J. E. The symmetrical liver as a roentgen sign of asplenia. *Circulation* 25:973, 1962.

61. Lunderquist, A. Angiography in carcinoma of the pancreas. *Acta Radiol.* [*Suppl.*] (Stockh.) 235:1, 1965.

62. McMahon, M. J., Lintott, J. D., Mair, W. S. J., Lee, P. W. R., and Duthie, J. S. Occult rupture of the spleen. *Br. J. Surg.* 64:641, 1977.

63. Maddison, F. E. Embolic therapy of hypersplenism. *Invest. Radiol.* 8:280, 1973.

64. Majeski, J. A. Asplenia associated with a congenital diaphragmatic defect and neurologic anomalies. *South. Med. J.* 71:1448, 1978.

65. Majeski, J. A., and Upshur, J. K. Asplenia syndrome: A study of congenital anomalies in 16 cases. *J.A.M.A.* 240:1508, 1978.

66. Mall, J. C., and Kaiser, J. A. CT diagnosis of splenic laceration. *AJR* 134:265, 1980.

67. Messina, S., Goodman, M., van der Schaaf, A., and Surveyor, I. The radioisotope spleen scan in the assessment of patients with suspected spleen trauma. *Med. J. Aust.* 1:144, 1979.

68. Michels, N. A. The variational anatomy of the spleen and splenic artery. *Am. J. Anat.* 70:21, 1942.

69. Michels, N. A. *Blood Supply and Anatomy of the Upper Abdominal Organs.* Philadelphia: Lippincott, 1955.

70. Mikhail, Y., Kamel, R., Nawar, N. N. Y., and Rafla, M. F. M. Observations on the mode of

termination and parenchymal distribution of the splenic artery with evidence of splenic lobulation and segmentation. *J. Anat.* 128:253, 1979.

71. Miller, F. J., Rothermel, F. J., O'Neill, M. J., and Shocat, S. J. Clinical and roentgenographic findings in splenic abscess. *Arch. Surg.* 111:1156, 1976.

72. Morag, B., and Rubinstein, Z. J. Conservative management of splenic trauma: Angiographic observations. *ROEFO* 129:517, 1978.

73. Morgenstern, L., and Shapiro, S. J. Techniques of splenic conservation. *Arch. Surg.* 114:449, 1979.

74. Moskovitz, M. Occult splenic rupture: Presentation as a gastric pseudotumor. *Conn. Med.* 42:498, 1978.

75. Muhletaler, C., Gerlock, A. J., Goncharenko, V., Avant, G. R., and Flexner, J. M. Gastric varices secondary to splenic vein occlusion: Radiographic diagnosis and clinical significance. *Radiology* 132:593, 1979.

76. Murray, M. J., Thol, A. J., and Greenspan, R. Splenic arteriovenous fistulas as a cause of portal hypertension. *Am. J. Med.* 29:849, 1960.

77. Myers, R. A. M., Andrew, W., and Wilkinson, A. E. Reappraisal of the left lateral decubitus x-ray in splenic rupture. *Br. J. Surg.* 64:482, 1977.

78. Naylor, R., Coln, D., and Shires, G. T. Morbidity and mortality from injuries to the spleen. *J. Trauma* 14:773, 1974.

79. Nebesar, R. A., Pollard, J. J., Edmunds, L. H., Jr., and McKhann, C. F. Indications for selective celiac and superior mesenteric angiography: Experience with 128 cases. *AJR* 92:1100, 1964.

80. Ödman, P. Percutaneous selective angiography of the coeliac artery. *Acta Radiol. [Suppl.]* (Stockh.) 159:1, 1958.

81. Okayasu, I., Mori, W., and Kajita, A. A study on so-called splenic agenesis syndrome—pathological examination of 27 autopsy cases. *Acta Pathol. Jpn.* 24:495, 1974.

82. Olsen, W. R., and Beaudoin, E. D. Increased incidence of accessory spleens in hematologic disease. *Arch. Surg.* 98:762, 1969.

83. Olsson, O. Angiographic diagnosis of an islet cell tumor of the pancreas. *Acta Chir. Scand.* 126:246, 1963.

84. Onuigbo, W. I. B., Ojukwu, J. O., and Eze, W. C. Infarction of accessory spleen. *J. Pediatr. Surg.* 13:129, 1978.

85. Otto, W. J. Calcification in the left upper quadrant, or "All that glisters . . ." *J.A.M.A.* 193:1406, 1965.

86. Palubinskas, A. J., and Ripley, H. R. Fibromuscular hyperplasia in extrarenal arteries. *Radiology* 82:451, 1964.

87. Papadimitriou, J., Tritakis, C., Karatzas, G., and Papaioannou, A. Treatment of hypersplenism by embolus placement in the splenic artery. *Lancet* 2:1268, 1976.

88. Paul, R. E., Jr., Miller, H. H., Kahn, P. C., Callow, A. D., Edwards, T. L., Jr., and Patterson, J. F. Pancreatic angiography, with application of subselective angiography of the celiac or superior mesenteric artery to the diagnosis of carcinoma of the pancreas. *N. Engl. J. Med.* 272:283, 1965.

89. Pearson, H. A., Johnston, D., Smith, K. A., and Touloukian, R. J. The born-again spleen: Return of splenic function after splenectomy for trauma. *N. Engl. J. Med.* 298:1389, 1978.

90. Pollak, E. W., and Michas, C. A. Massive spontaneous hemoperitoneum due to rupture of visceral branches of the abdominal aorta. *Am. Surg.* 45:621, 1979.

91. Poller, S., and Wholey, M. H. Splenic cysts: Confirmation by selective visceral angiography. *AJR* 96:418, 1966.

92. Propper, R. A., Weinstein, B. J., Skolnick, M. L., and Kisloff, B. Ultrasonography of hemorrhagic splenic cysts. *JCU* 7:18, 1979.

93. Pugh, H. L. Collective review, splenectomy with special reference to historical background; indications and rationale, and comparison of reported mortality. *Intern. Abstr. Surg.* 83:209, 1946.

94. Qureshi, M. A., and Hafner, C. D. Clinical manifestations of splenic cysts: A study of 75 cases. *Am. Surg.* 31:605, 1965.

95. Ranniger, K., and Saldino, R. M. Arteriographic diagnosis of pancreatic lesions. *Radiology* 86:470, 1966.

96. Redman, H. C., Reuter, S. R., and Bookstein, J. J. Angiography in abdominal trauma. *Ann. Surg.* 169:57, 1969.

97. Reichle, F. A., and Owen, O. E. Hemodynamic patterns in human hepatic cirrhosis: A prospective randomized study of the hemodynamic sequelae of distal splenorenal (Warren) and mesocaval shunts. *Ann. Surg.* 190:523, 1979.

98. Reuter, S. R. Embolization of gastrointestinal hemorrhage. *AJR* 133:557, 1979.

99. Reuter, S. R., Fry, W. J., and Bookstein, J. J. Mesenteric artery branch aneurysms. *Arch. Surg.* 97:497, 1968.

100. Reuter, S. R., and Redman, H. C. *Gastrointestinal Angiography.* Philadelphia: Saunders, 1972. P. 202.

101. Roguin, N., Auslaender, L., Zelter, M., Katzir, J., Sujov, P., and Riss, E. Asplenia syndrome: Report of two cases. *Isr. J. Med. Sci.* 15:451, 1979.

102. Roguin, N., Pelled, B., Amikam, S., Auslaender, L., and Riss, E. Polysplenia syndrome: A study of five new cases. *Isr. J. Med. Sci.* 14:948, 1978.

103. Rösch, J. Roentgenologic possibilities in spleen diagnosis. *AJR* 94:453, 1965.

104. Rösch, J. Tumors of the spleen: The value of selective arteriography. *Clin. Radiol.* 17:183, 1966.

105. Rösch, J. *Roentgenology of the Spleen and Pancreas.* Springfield, Ill.: Thomas, 1967.

106. Rösch, J., and Bret, J. Arteriography of the pancreas. *AJR* 94:182, 1965.

107. Rösch, J., and Herfort, K. Contribution of splenoportography to the diagnosis of diseases of the pancreas: Inflammatory diseases. *Acta Med. Scand.* 171:263, 1962.

108. Rose, V., Izukawa, T., and Moes, C. Syndrome of asplenia and polysplenia. *Br. Heart J.* 37:840, 1975.

109. Scatliff, J. H., Fisher, O. N., Guilford, W. B., and McLendon, W. W. The "starry night" splenic angiogram: Contrast material opacification of the malpighian body marginal sinus circulation in spleen trauma. *AJR* 125:91, 1975.

110. Schug, J., and Bankin, R. P. Rupture of the splenic artery aneurysm in pregnancy. *Obstet. Gynecol.* 25:717, 1965.

111. Shah, V. V., Mehtalia, S. D., Shah, K. D., and Hansoti, R. C. Splenic arteriovenous fistula. *Angiology* 18:23, 1967.

112. Shirkhoda, A., McCartney, W. H., Staab, E. V., and Mittelstaedt, C. A. Imaging of the spleen: A proposed algorithm. *AJR* 135:195, 1980.

113. Sirinek, K. R., and Evans, W. E. Nonparasitic, splenic cysts. Case report of epidermoid cyst with review of the literature. *Am. J. Surg.* 126:8, 1973.

114. Sorgen, R. A., and Robbins, D. I. Bleeding gastric varices secondary to wandering spleen. *Gastrointest. Radiol.* 5:25, 1980.

115. Stone, H. H., Jordan, W. D., Aker, J. J., and Martin, J. D. Portal arteriovenous fistulas, review and case report. *Am. J. Surg.* 109:191, 1965.

116. Van Mierop, L. H. S., Gessner, I., and Schiebler, G. Asplenia and polysplenia syndromes. *Birth Defects* 8:5, 1972.

117. Vermess, M., Chatterji, D. C., Doppman, J. L., Grimes, G., and Adamson, R. H. Development and experimental evaluation of a contrast medium for computed tomographic examination of the liver and spleen. *J. Comput. Assist. Tomogr.* 3:25, 1979.

118. Waldman, J. D., Rosenthal, A., Smith, A. L., Shurin, S., and Nadas, A. S. Sepsis and congenital asplenia. *J. Pediatr.* 90:555, 1977.

119. Wexler, L., and Abrams, H. L. Hamartoma of the spleen: Angiographic observations. *AJR* 92:1150, 1964.

120. Whipple, H. O. The medical-surgical splenopathies. *Bull. N.Y. Acad. Med.* 15:174, 1939.

121. Wholey, M. H., Chamorro, H. A., Rao, G., and Chapman, W. Splenic infarction and spontaneous rupture of the spleen after therapeutic embolization. *Cardiovasc. Radiol.* 1:249, 1978.

122. Widrich, W. C., Robbins, A. H., Johnson, W. C., and Nasbeth, D. C. Long-term follow-up of distal splenorenal shunts. *Radiology* 134:341, 1980.

123. Wilkinson, J. L., Holt, P. A., Dickinson, D. F., and Jivani, S. K. Asplenia syndrome in one of mono-zygotic twins. *Eur. J. Cardiol.* 10:301, 1979.

Splenoportography

INGEMAR BERGSTRAND

Radiography of the portal venous system in man with injection of contrast medium into a portal vein tributary during laparotomy was introduced in 1945 [14]. Injection of contrast medium percutaneously via the spleen was first described in 1951 [18, 39] after Abeatici and Campi [1] had shown in dogs that contrast medium injected into the spleen flows into the splenic and portal veins. This examination method is now widely used. Minor variations of the examination technique have been reported [48, 53]. Modifications intended to permit application of the method for studying portal hemodynamics have also been described by several authors [2, 5, 10–13, 19, 27, 30, 37, 40]. A number of monographs on the roentgenologic and clinical aspects of the portal system have been published [21, 22, 26, 33, 38, 42, 43, 46].

The method has been described under various names (for example, hepatic angiography, transparietal splenoportal roentgenography, splenic venography, percutaneous splenic portal venography). The term most widely used and generally accepted is *splenoportography*, introduced in 1952 [50]. The term *percutaneous lienoportal venography* [30] is the most descriptive, but it has proved too long for clinical use.

Technique

The technique described here is based on many years' experience in more than 500 examinations and a critical analysis of the results obtained.

(1) Precautions are taken against hypersensitivity to the contrast medium and renal failure.

(2) The patient is examined in the fasting state with the bowel cleared.

(3) One hour before the examination the patient receives pentobarbital sodium as premedication (morphine is contraindicated in liver disease).

(4) Preliminary films are taken for assessment of the size of the spleen. Lead markers are placed on the patient's skin to show the position of the spleen in the respiratory phase in which the puncture is to be made.

(5) Local anesthesia of the skin is sufficient. Only in children is general anesthesia necessary.

(6) Posture influences the distribution of contrast medium in the portal system because of its effect on portal hemodynamics and because the relatively high specific gravity of the contrast

medium promotes incomplete admixture with blood. The position of the patient during the examination must therefore be standardized—supine on a horizontal examination table. The prone position is not comfortable and is likely to cause wide respiratory excursions.

(7) The diameter of the cannula or catheter used should be just large enough to permit rapid manual injection of the relatively viscous contrast medium. An internal diameter of 1.2 mm and a length of 10 cm are suitable.

(8) The site of puncture in an intercostal space and the depth to which the needle is inserted are selected according to the size and position of the spleen as seen in the preliminary films. The spleen should be punctured in the area closest to the abdominal wall to diminish the risk of hemorrhage. The cannula should be directed somewhat cranially in the frontal plane in order to avoid neighboring organs such as the colon and pleural cavity. The tip of the cannula or catheter should be placed near the hilus of the spleen. In this way flow of the contrast medium from the parenchyma into the veins is facilitated and extrasplenic escape is decreased. Respiration should be as shallow as possible as long as the cannula is in the spleen. Excursions of the free end of the cannula should not be restricted. Strict observance of these two points will obviate splenic damage.

Puncture with a cannula is simple and is preferred in splenomegaly. By a three-way stopcock the cannula is connected to a 10-cc syringe filled with saline and to a 50-cc syringe filled with contrast medium. The cannula is introduced in the midaxillary line until its tip is felt to scrub the rough surface of the spleen (in the presence of splenic adhesions, however, this sign is absent). The patient is instructed to hold his breath in inspiration, and the cannula is quickly introduced toward the hilus (about 3–5 cm). In order to clear the passage through the cannula, 3 to 4 cc of saline is injected. Then the syringe with saline is disconnected from the stopcock, and a free blood flow is observed through the tubing as a sign of correct position. Not until this sign occurs is the stopcock switched to the other syringe and the contrast medium injected. The time for the described procedure is short enough to permit apnea.

Puncture with a catheter is preferred in patients with a normal-sized spleen. A suitable intercostal space is selected in the posterior axillary line. A small skin incision is made, and a catheter pro-

vided with a mandrin is introduced toward the hilus of the spleen (Longdwell Teflon catheter 15 G × 4 inches). A multiple side-hole catheter has been described that proved useful after animal experimentation and clinical trial [49]. The procedure is done by television fluoroscopy. The patient is not moved to the serial film changer until test injections of contrast medium have demonstrated the correct position of the tip of the catheter.

(9) Injection should be rapid (about 7–8 cc per second), and the contrast medium should be concentrated in order to secure satisfactory definition of the vessels. A dose of 30 to 50 cc of 60 percent Urografin is sufficient. The patient is instructed not to strain during the injection. The cannula is withdrawn immediately following the injection.

(10) Demonstration of the direction and velocity of flow in different parts of the portal system from the spleen to and through the liver requires exposure of one film per second for 13 seconds and then one every third second during about 20 seconds. An automatic film changer and an automatic program selector are therefore necessary. In this way films are obtained of all portal vessels while their filling is optimal; of the liver parenchyma during the densest stage of the hepatographic phase; and of the venae hepaticae. We take films in the frontal plane only because biplane examinations produce too much scattered radiation.

(11) A plain film is taken afterward to determine the site and amount of any contrast medium outside the spleen.

(12) The patient is instructed to lie on the left side for 4 to 5 hours immediately after the examination. In this way a certain degree of mechanical compression of the spleen at the site of the puncture may be attained.

Hazards

Intraabdominal hemorrhage is the most serious complication of splenoportography. Blood has been noted at surgery after splenoportography in quantities up to a few hundred cubic centimeters. Splenic arteriography performed in 14 patients immediately following splenoportography demonstrated splenic hematoma in 3 patients, while in the remaining 11 no arteriographic abnormalities were detected [36]. Hemorrhage producing clinical signs of intraperitoneal bleeding appears to be rare, however [30, 51]. The frequency of bleeding was not found to vary with the prothrombin index [12]. In a few small series, especially of splenic puncture at laparotomy, a high frequency of intraabdominal hemorrhage has been reported. A survey of the available literature reveals that abdominal hemorrhage after splenoportography has been fatal in 4 of about 1,200 examinations [3]. Probst et al. explored the use of both Ivalon and Gelfoam injected in the needle tract after splenoportography as a means of diminishing the risk of hemorrhage. They found that in dogs, complete cessation of bleeding occurred after plugging of the needle tract, even when the animals were fully heparinized [45]. Emboldened by their success, they undertook the procedure in five clinical subjects with decreased platelets and severe hypertension, without sequelae. At surgery, successful plugging of the needle tract was found [45].

Aneurysms of the splenic artery occur in almost 20 percent of patients with cirrhosis and portal hypertension. In three out of four the aneurysm is located in or near the splenic hilus [16]. Puncture of an aneurysm or an arterial branch involves an increased risk of hemorrhage. Selective celiac angiography prior to splenoportography has therefore been recommended [16]. Local intrasplenic arterial aneurysms secondary to splenoportography may be demonstrated by splenic arteriography in one-third of patients with portal hypertension [15]. These aneurysms are relatively small and have not been reported to have clinical consequences.

If the injection is successful, the patient will feel only a sensation of warmth or burning during the injection. The quantities and types of contrast medium under discussion do not cause vascular or hepatic damage; neither have they been known to produce damage in animal experiments conducted.

Extrasplenic deposition of contrast medium will cause pain varying in intensity and duration with the amount. In small quantities the discomfort lasts about 15 minutes. If the entire dose of contrast medium is injected intraperitoneally, the patient may have subsiding pain for 6 hours. No serious sequelae have been seen.

Indications

Splenoportography has been used mainly in the investigation of diseases interfering with hemodynamic conditions in the portal system. The method can, however, also be used for investigating the morphology of the portal system.

Obstruction to the drainage of splenic or portal blood is the commonest condition disturbing portal hemodynamics. The obstruction may be extrahepatic (usually thrombosis or malformations) or intrahepatic (usually cirrhosis). The blood in the congested vascular area bypasses the obstruction via collaterals to that part of the portal system behind the obstruction or to the caval veins, usually via the clinically important esophageal veins. The diagnosis and localization of such a disorder is important and may make possible lifesaving surgery such as the establishment of a portacaval or a splenorenal shunt. Splenoportography will show the hemodynamic changes and thereby clarify the presence and the approximate site of obstruction. This examination is therefore employed in the investigation of patients with symptoms or signs of obstruction in any segment of the portal system, such as esophageal varices, gastrointestinal hemorrhage of unknown cause, or splenomegaly. The method is far more accurate than the conventional upper gastrointestinal series in depicting gastric varices [29]. Splenoportography is also indicated for checking the patency of a surgically established portacaval shunt [26].

Vascular morphology is changed in many diseases of organs situated alongside the venous pathways (for example, the pancreas, the hepatoduodenal ligament, and the liver). The changes demonstrable by splenoportography are essentially the same in the extrahepatic and the intrahepatic part of the pathway. They consist in displacement, compression, or occlusion of vessels [7, 38, 47] according to the nature and extent of the pathologic process. Spenoportography may therefore be indicated in the investigation of known or suspected liver cirrhosis and of hepatomegaly or suspected tumors along the splenoportal pathway, such as pancreatic cysts, pancreatic cancer, liver cysts, and liver metastases. Recent progress in splanchnic arteriography has decreased the indications for splenoportography except in patients with portal hypertension [17]. Nevertheless, the value of splenoportography has recently been reemphasized [28, 34], and the simplicity of the method has been stressed [34]. Furthermore, some workers believe that both arterioportography and splenoportography are indicated in the presence of liver disease [35].

Contraindications

With the technique described, the risks involved in splenoportography are slight compared with the value of the information obtained. Because of the risk of hemorrhage, examination of patients with decreased clotting power should be restricted, and performed only after restorative treatment, such as blood transfusions and parenteral administration of vitamin K. Splenic puncture during laparotomy or in combination with pneumoperitoneum is not advisable. In infective splenomegaly the spleen is fragile. Examination of patients with long-standing infectious diseases should therefore be avoided.

Normal Hemodynamics

During the injection contrast medium flows continuously into those veins draining the punctured part of the spleen. The spleen does not actively expel contrast medium into the veins. After successful puncture only a very small portion of the amount injected persists in the splenic paren-

Figure 67-1. Vessels normally demonstrated by splenoportography (*red*); portal and splenic tributaries and systemic veins capable of forming important collateral pathways (*blue*). Arrows indicate normal direction of flow. In this drawing, as in other figures, the names of the vessels are abbreviated as follows:

> *sp.* = splenic vein
> *p.* = portal vein
> *i.m.* = inferior mesenteric vein
> *s.m.* = superior mesenteric vein
> *co.* = coronary vein
> *s.g.* = short gastric veins
> *g.e.* = gastroepiploic vein

> *cy.* = cystic vein
> *pu.* = parumbilical vein
> *sp. r.* = connections between the splenic vein and the left renal vein
> *sp. c.* = collateral veins connecting the spleen and hepatodistal part of the splenic vein to systemic veins in the lateral abdominal wall
> *I.V.C.* = inferior vena cava
> *haz.* = hemiazygos vein
> *e.* = esophageal veins
> *d.* = diaphragmatic veins
> *p.c.* = pericardial veins
> *r.* = left renal vein

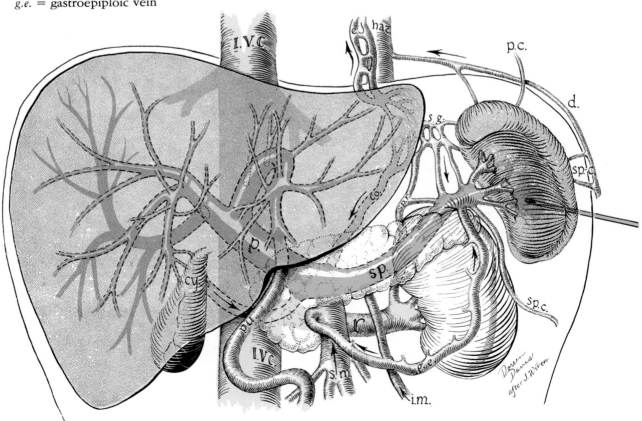

chyma, whence it disappears within half an hour. The velocity and direction of flow recorded are measures of the actual hemodynamic conditions. Judging from clinical experience as well as from experiments on dogs, intrasplenic injection by the technique described does not disturb portal hemodynamics [13]. Thus, in normal subjects the contrast medium never fills the vessels emptying into the splenoportal pathway, such as the coro-

nary vein and the mesenteric veins. On the contrary, on its way to the liver the contrast medium is diluted more and more by blood from these veins (Figs. 67-1–67-4).

The velocity of portal flow is sometimes changed, even in an early stage of portal obstruction. Normally the contrast medium reaches the porta hepatis 1 to 2 seconds after its passage through the splenic vein radicles (see Fig. 67-2A,

Figure 67-2. Normal splenoportogram. (A) Exposure made 1 second after beginning of injection. Contrast medium has filled the splenic vein. (Dorsocaudal branches are in solid black and ventrocaudal branches are striated in the diagrams of this chapter.) *sp.* = splenic vein. (B) Two seconds. Contrast medium has filled the splenic and portal veins and has entered the intrahepatic branches. *p.* = portal vein; *sp.* = splenic vein. (C) Four seconds. Contrast medium has filled the entire right intrahepatic ramification but only part of the left. Note filling defect in the portal vein caused by mesenteric blood. *p.* = portal vein; *s.m.* = superior mesenteric vein; *sp.* = splenic vein; *4* = left principal portal venous ramus. (D) Six seconds. Contrast medium begins to fill the liver parenchyma. Entire left intrahepatic ramification is filled. *p.* = portal vein; *9* = ventrolateral portal venous ramus. (E) Eight seconds (4 seconds after the end of injection). Contrast medium has left the intrahepatic portal branches and is accumulated evenly in the liver parenchyma. Note contrast defect corresponding to fossa venae cavae.

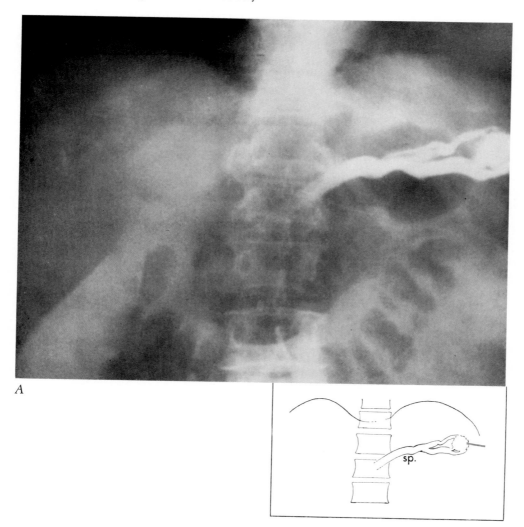

A

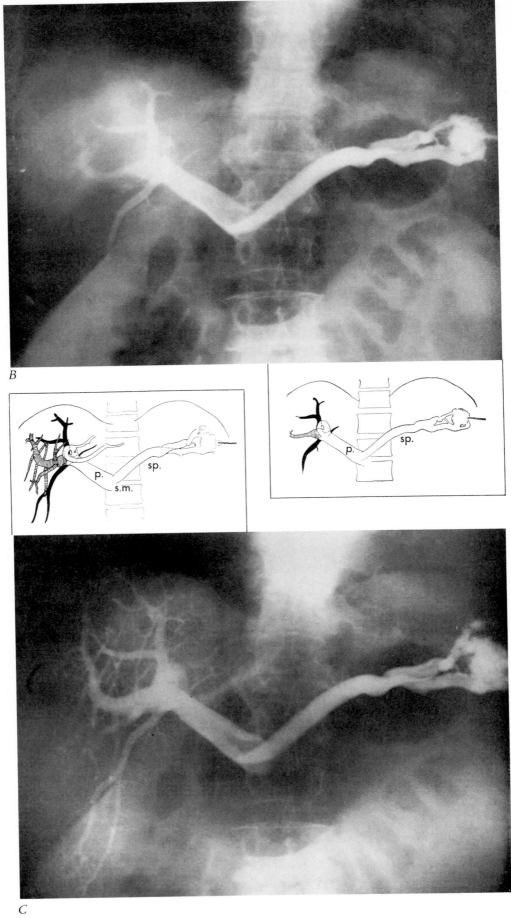

B

C

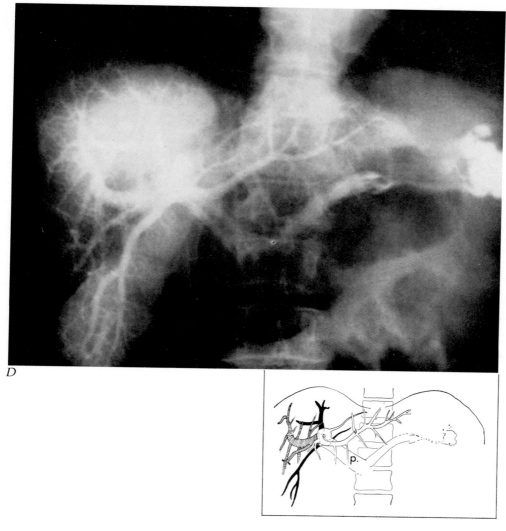

D

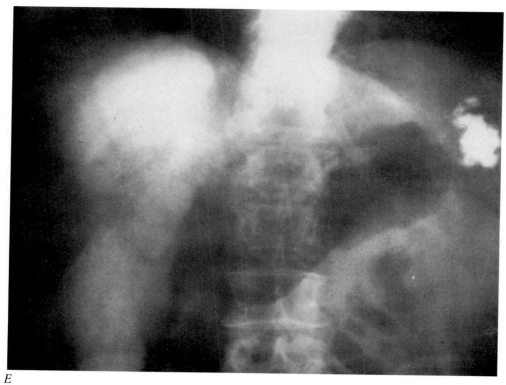

E

1579

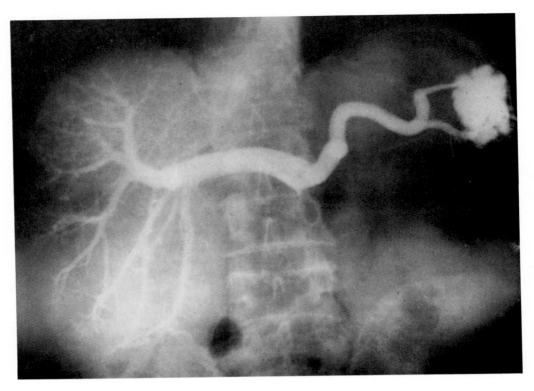

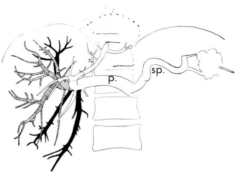

Figure 67-3. Normal splenoportogram. Slight cranially convex curve of portal vein. Note the straight vessel projected along the right margin of the spine and running to the liver, presumably a dorsal portal venous ramus (vpr). *sp.* = splenic vein; *p.* = portal vein; 7 = dorsal vpr.

B). This means a relatively high venous velocity (10–20 cm/second), which, like the relatively high oxygen tension of splenic venous blood, may be explained by the low resistance of the capillary splenic bed to arterial flow. Within 3 to 5 seconds after the beginning of the injection, the intrahepatic vessels of the right portion of the liver are optimally filled (see Fig. 67-2C). The branches to the left portion fill somewhat later, and the filling obtained there is often less dense (see Fig. 67-2D). After another 3 to 5 seconds (3 to 5 seconds after the *end* of the injection), the contrast medium has left the intrahepatic portal branches and fills the hepatic sinusoids. The liver is then opacified diffusely (see Fig. 67-2E). At the end of the hepatographic phase, the hepatic veins are faintly visible (about 20–30 seconds after the beginning of the injection). Opacification of the liver disappears completely about 30 to 40 seconds after the beginning of the injection. The velocity of flow may be influenced to some extent by straining during the injection of contrast medium.

The width of the splenic and portal veins is often influenced by conditions such as portal stasis and increased intraabdominal pressure (for

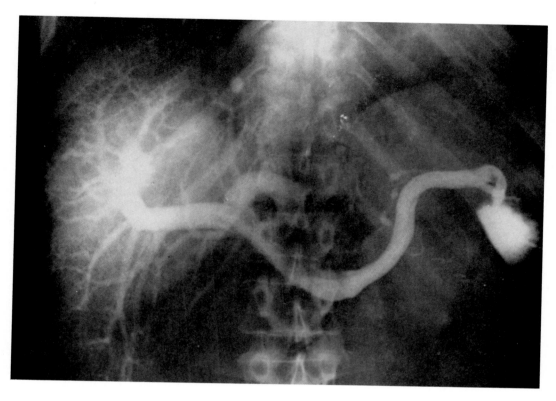

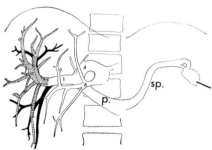

Figure 67-4. Normal splenoportogram. Note good filling of the ventral vpr. but no filling of the dorsolateral and ventrolateral vpr. Careful palpation of the left part of the liver at laparotomy and 1 year's follow-up revealed no signs of tumor. *sp.* = splenic vein; *p.* = portal vein; *1* = right principal vpr.; *4* = left principal vpr.; *6* = ventral vpr.

example, in patients with ascites). In normal studies we conducted, the width of the splenic vein, as measured in the films proximal to the liver, did not exceed 15 mm. The diameter of the portal vein, as measured distal to the liver, was 15 to 22 mm.

Normal Anatomy

The technique described demonstrates the vessels in frontal projection only. Because of incomplete intermixture between contrast-free blood from the mesenteric veins and opacified blood from the splenic vein, the portal vein and its ventrally situated intrahepatic branches are often less well opacified than the dorsal branches. This discrepancy, however, facilitates orientation in the ventrodorsal direction, as do differences in geometric enlargement and blur.

EXTRAHEPATIC VASCULAR ANATOMY

The normal variations of the splenic and portal veins, as well as of their tributaries, have been studied in living subjects and cadavers [25].

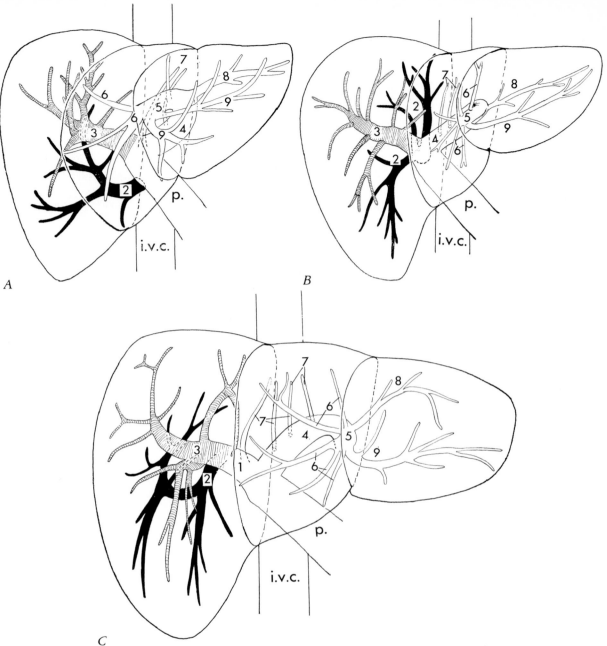

Figure 67-5. Schematic drawings showing normal intrahepatic portal vascular arrangement. The contours of the liver are roughly depicted with the two main fissures drawn in anatomic position. The drawings also show the intrahepatic portal nomenclature used by the author.

(A) Dorsocaudal vpr. is an arcuate vessel that leaves the portal vein before the origin of the left principal vpr. Thus the right principal vpr. is missing. The ventroflexed vpr. is visible cranial to the left principal vpr. (B) Three dorsocaudal vpr. leave the portal vein at the same level as the left principal vpr. The ventroflexed vpr. is projected over the left principal vpr. (C) The ventroflexed vpr. projects to the left of the left principal vpr.

<table>
<tr><td>p.</td><td>=</td><td>portal vein</td><td></td></tr>
<tr><td>i.v.c.</td><td>=</td><td>inferior vena cava</td><td></td></tr>
<tr><td>1</td><td>=</td><td>right principal portal venous ramus (vpr.)</td><td rowspan="3">} right main part of the liver</td></tr>
<tr><td>2</td><td>=</td><td>dorsocaudal vpr. (black)</td></tr>
<tr><td>3</td><td>=</td><td>ventrocranial vpr. (striated)</td></tr>
</table>

4 = left principal vpr.
5 = ventroflexed vpr.
6 = ventral vpr. } central portion
7 = dorsal vpr.
8 = dorsolateral vpr. } lateral portion
9 = ventrolateral vpr.

left main part of the liver

1582

Knowledge of these variations is a prerequisite for detecting the presence of any space-occupying lesion in the vicinity of these vessels.

The splenic vein is formed by convergence of the short splenic radicles. The course of the splenic vein varies; sometimes it is straight, sometimes tortuous (see Figs. 67-1–67-4). It regularly meets the termination of the mesenteric vein and forms a caudally convex curve. The diameter of the splenic vein increases only slightly during its course toward the portal vein.

The portal vein is formed by the convergence of the splenic vein and the superior mesenteric vein. The blood from the latter causes a filling defect in the splenoportogram that should not be confused with mural thrombosis (see Fig. 67-2C). This point, which marks the hepatodistal and widest end of the portal vein, is projected over the spine at the level of the first to second lumbar vertebrae. The portal vein, 6 to 8 cm in length, usually pursues a straight dextrocranial course to form an angle of 40 to 90 degrees with the vertebral spine. Sometimes the vein is slightly curved, with the convexity cranial and to the left (see Fig. 67-3).

INTRAHEPATIC VASCULAR ANATOMY

A brief outline of the basic features of human liver anatomy will facilitate the description of the intrahepatic vascular anatomy.

The intrahepatic vascular tree is divided into two main parts. The plane of division passes to the right of the left sagittal fissure and the insertion of the falciform ligament and passes through the bed of the gallbladder to the inferior vena cava. The portal ramification of the right main part is divided into two main segments, one situated dorsocaudally and the other ventrocranially. These segments are then subdivided in different ways by different anatomists [23, 31, 32]. The left main part consists of two portions divided by a fissure corresponding to the insertion of the falciform ligament and the left sagittal fissure. The lateral portion is that part generally called the left liver lobe, and the central portion consists mainly of the ventrally situated quadrate lobe and the dorsally situated caudate lobe. The main branches of the hepatic veins run in the fissures formed between the different portal parts and segments.

The intrahepatic vascular nomenclature used here is based on an anatomic investigation by Hjortsjö [32]. It has been somewhat simplified [6] to suit roentgen diagnostic requirements. Figure 67-5 illustrates the nomenclature used and shows some usual types of intrahepatic portal vascular arrangement.

The extent to which different parts of the liver are opacified during the hepatographic phase depends on the amount of contrast medium actually passing through the sinusoids in the various parts of the liver and on the varying thickness of the liver. The left part of the liver is thin and located ventrally, so that it receives a relatively small amount of contrast medium. It is therefore only slightly opacified compared with the right part (see Figs. 67-2E, 67-13D). In the right part the ordinarily deep fossa for the gallbladder and the fossa venae cavae will often appear as well-defined defects (see Figs. 67-2E, 67-13D).

Portal Hemodynamics in Vascular Obstruction

Venous stasis is roentgenographically manifested by a low velocity of flow, dilatation of the veins, and a filling of collateral vessels. Of these signs, filling of collaterals is the most important and reliable. In our own investigation of patients with venous stasis verified in other ways—for example, by pressure measurements—all showed filling of collaterals [11]. In another study, however, a few exceptions to this rule were found [52]. The direction of collateral flow is always such as to bypass the occluded part of the vascular pathway. This can be demonstrated by the way contrast medium fills and leaves the collaterals.

The velocity of flow is usually, although not

Figure 67-6. Diagram of a splenoportogram indicating intrahepatic obstruction. The main types of hepatofugal collateral vessels are delineated. K = kidney; L = liver; S = spleen. (From Bergstrand [9].)

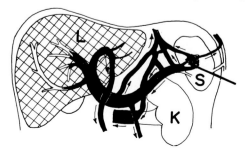

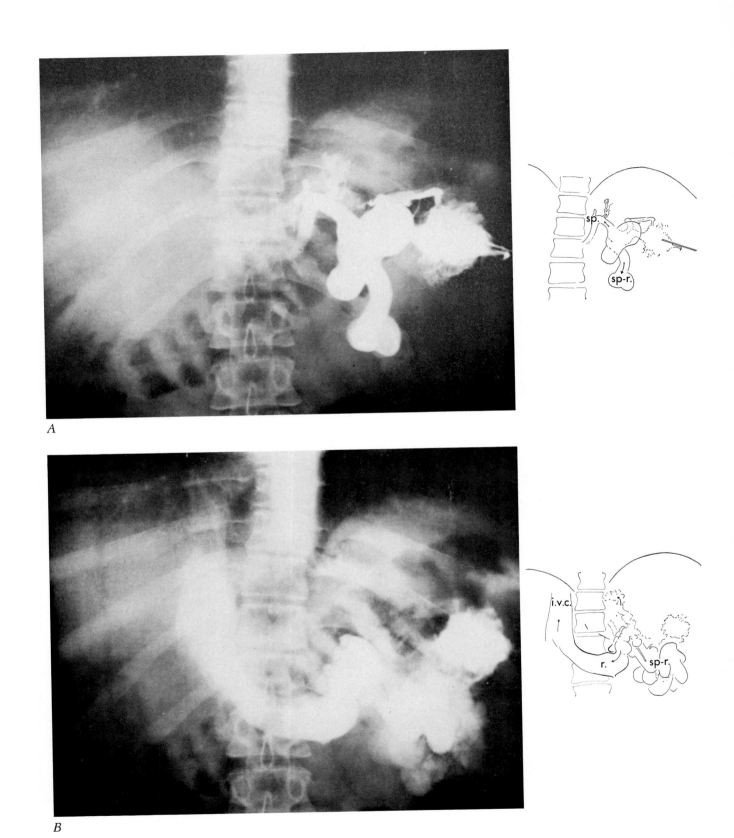

A

B

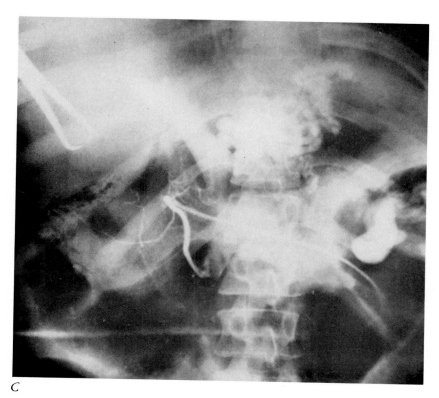

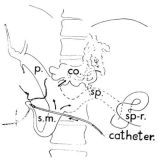

C

Figure 67-7. Cirrhosis of the liver (verified at laparotomy). (A) Splenoportogram shows filling of tortuous collateral veins draining the splenic vein. There is no filling of the portal vein. Only small, cranially directed collaterals are visible despite the presence of large esophageal varices. *sp.* = splenic vein; *sp-r.* = connections between splenic vein and left renal vein. (B) Eight seconds later. Contrast medium has reached the left renal vein and enters the inferior vena cava. *r.* = left renal vein; *i.v.c.* = inferior vena cava; *sp-r.* = connections between splenic vein and left renal vein. (C) Portography during laparotomy. (Contrast medium was injected in the superior mesenteric vein via catheter.) Filling of a patent portal vein and a large coronary vein running to the esophageal veins. Contrast medium has also reached the splenorenal connection demonstrated in the splenoportogram. *sp.* = splenic vein; *sp-r.* = connections between splenic vein and left renal vein; *p.* = portal vein; *co.* = coronary vein; *s.m.* = superior mesenteric vein.

always, abnormally low, and the vascular diameters are often abnormally large in vascular stasis with portal hypertension. In patients with ascites, however, the dilatation is usually slight at most.

The extent and capacity of the collateral circulation as judged by the number of the collaterals, vascular size, and velocity of flow are difficult to estimate. The large variations observed are apparently due mainly to differences in the duration and severity of the obstruction and to individual differences in the readiness with which a collateral circulation can be formed. Even in patients with a well-developed collateral circulation, its inability to drain the congested vascular bed adequately is apparent from a low velocity of flow and pathologically high pressures.

Figure 67-8. Diagram of a splenoportogram indicating extrahepatic portal vein obstruction. K = kidney; L = liver; S = spleen. (From Bergstrand [9].)

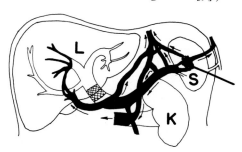

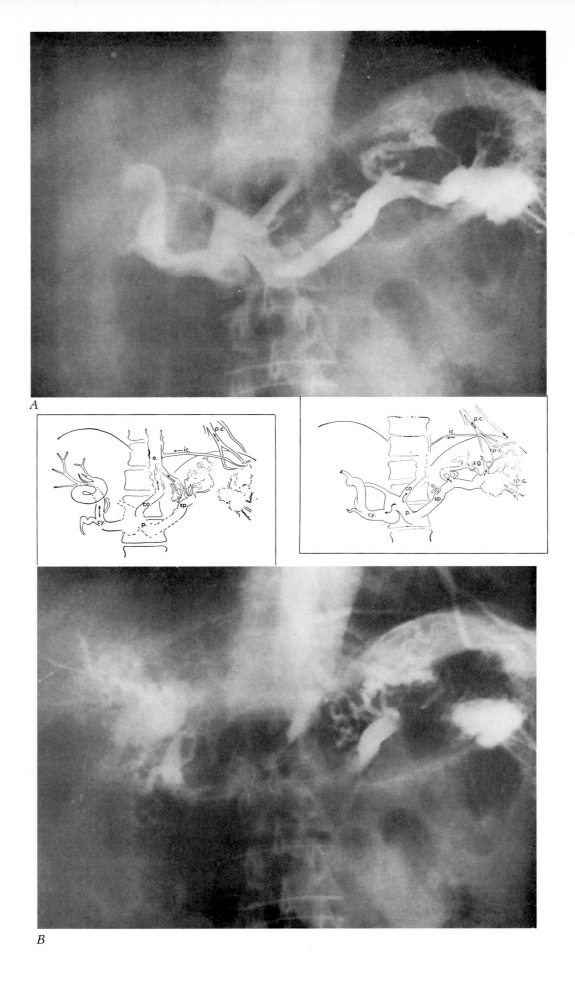

◀ **Figure 67-9.** Portal thrombosis (verified at autopsy). Filling of splenic vein and hepatodistal part of portal vein (A) from which contrast medium flows to the liver via dilated cystic veins (B). Note collateral circulation to the superior vena cava via the coronary vein, short gastric veins, intercostal veins, and pericardial veins. *sp.* = splenic vein; *p.* = portal vein; *cy.* = cystic vein; *co.* = coronary vein; *s.g.* = short gastric veins; *sp-c.* = collateral veins connecting spleen and hepatodistal part of splenic vein to systemic veins in the lateral abdominal wall; *p.c.* = pericardial veins; *ic.* = intercostal veins; *e.* = esophageal veins.

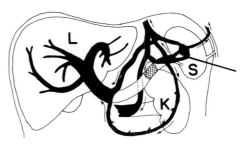

Figure 67-11. Diagram of a splenoportogram indicating extrahepatic splenic vein obstruction. *K* = kidney; *L* = liver; *S* = spleen. (From Bergstrand [9].)

INTRAHEPATIC OBSTRUCTION

In cirrhosis of the liver the portal intrahepatic ramifications are often involved to such a degree as to cause venous stasis and portal hypertension. Even widespread intrahepatic metastases cause only comparatively slight signs of vascular obstruction, probably because of the rapid and fatal course of the obstructing disease.

When the vascular obstruction is intrahepatic, the collateral vessels will drain the congested vascular area toward the low-pressure systemic veins and not to the liver. This is called a *hepatofugal* (away from the liver) collateral circulation. On the other hand, when the obstruction is extrahepatic, the collateral circulation will usually develop toward the portal system behind the obstruction and toward the liver where, in both locations, the portal pressure is normal. This is called a *hepatopetal* (toward the liver) collateral circulation [9].

In intrahepatic obstruction the commonest of the collateral connections demonstrable establish communication with the superior caval system via the coronary vein and short gastric veins on the one hand and the esophageal venous plexus on

the other (Fig. 67-6; see Figs. 67-17, 67-18A, 67-19A, and 67-20A). Some cases, however, despite large esophageal varices, show no cranially directed collaterals. The absence can almost always be ascribed to imperfect contrast filling [8]. Demonstrable communications with the inferior caval system via the inferior mesenteric vein and hemorrhoidal vein plexus or via retroperitoneal connections with the left renal vein are less common (see Figs. 67-17, 67-18A). In advanced intrahepatic obstruction, a collateral communication may be demonstrated between the portal venous ramus ventroflexus and the caval system via recanalized remnants of the umbilical vein and veins in the abdominal wall (see Fig. 67-20). Such a picture is suggestive of the Cruveilhier-Baumgarten syndrome [4]. Even in cases of advanced obstruction, filling may be obtained of at most a few centimeters of the superior mesenteric vein (see Fig. 67-18A). The contrast medium slowly returns by the same route, indicating the impossibility of significant collateral flow through that channel.

In complete intrahepatic obstruction the portal blood is entirely diverted to the caval system by the routes mentioned earlier without any filling

Figure 67-10. Diagram of a splenoportogram that does not indicate the site of obstruction (extrahepatic, intrahepatic, or both). *K* = kidney; *L* = liver; *S* = spleen. (From Bergstrand [9].)

Figure 67-12. Diagram of a splenoportogram indicating extrahepatic obstruction (splenic, portal, or both). *K* = kidney; *L* = liver; *S* = spleen. (From Bergstrand [9].)

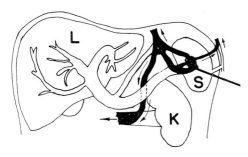

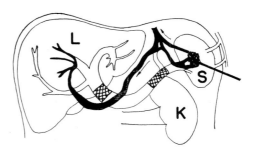

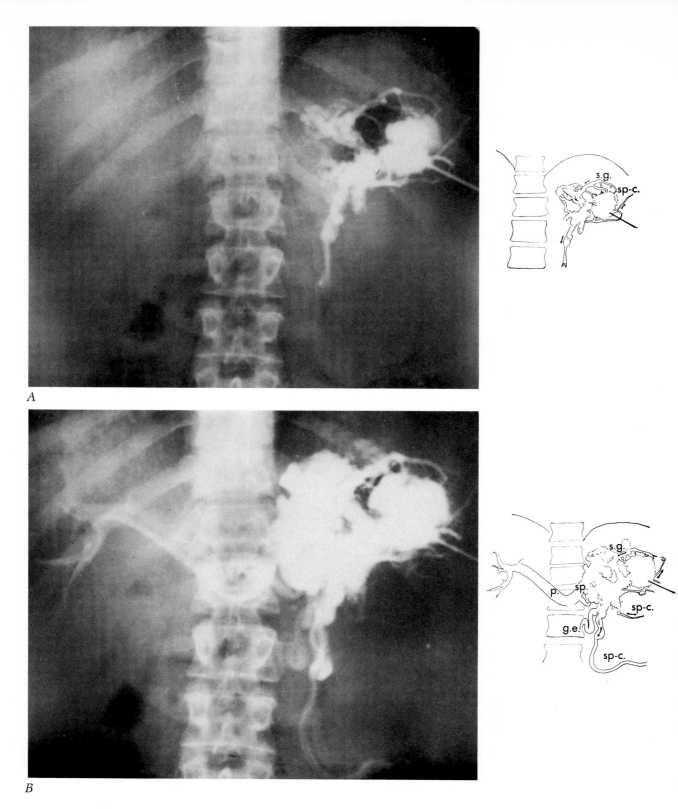

A

B

Figure 67-13. Thrombosis of splenic vein (verified at laparotomy). (A) Exposure made 2 seconds after beginning of injection. Filling of collaterals from hilus of the spleen. *s.g.* = short gastric veins; *sp-c.* = collateral veins connecting spleen and hepatodistal part of splenic vein to systemic veins in the lateral abdominal wall. (B) Five seconds. Collaterals empty into the hepatoproximal part of the splenic vein. *sp.* = splenic vein; *p.* = portal vein; *s.g.* = short gastric veins; *g.e.* = **1588** gastroepiploic vein; *sp-c.* = collateral veins connecting spleen and hepatodistal part of splenic vein to systemic veins in the lateral abdominal wall. (C) Nine seconds. Filling of the portal vein and of intrahepatic portal branches. Note filling of the gastroepiploic vein emptying into the superior mesenteric vein. *p.* = portal vein; *g.e.* = gastroepiploic vein; *s.m.* = superior mesenteric vein; *6* = ventral vpr. (D) Twelve seconds. Hepatogram showing intense and even contrast accumulation in normal liver parenchyma. Note fossa for the gallbladder.

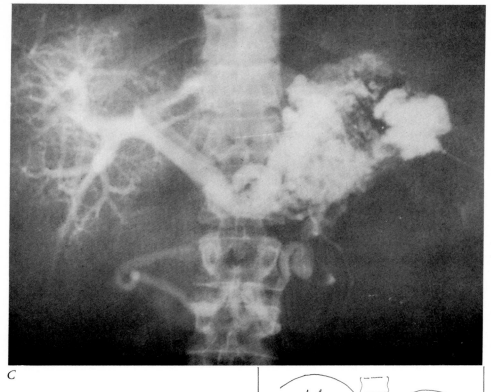

C

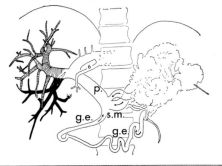

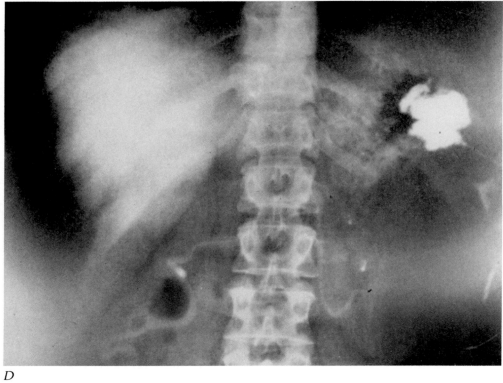

D

1589

of the occluded intrahepatic vessels. In the patent extrahepatic part of the pathway, blood flow is sometimes reversed toward the collaterals draining the splenic vein. Because contrast medium cannot fill a vessel against the blood flow, this patent part of the pathway is not demonstrated in the films and may falsely indicate extrahepatic obstruction (Figs. 67-7A, B; see 67-10). Clinical findings and portography with injection of contrast medium via the superior mesenteric vein during laparotomy reveal the true intrahepatic site of obstruction and other collaterals (Fig. 67-7C). This splenoportographic picture was found in 6 of 91 patients with verified intrahepatic portal obstruction [9].

EXTRAHEPATIC OBSTRUCTION

Extrahepatic obstruction is usually caused by thrombosis, malformations, or both, which are long-standing conditions with well-developed signs of stasis. But extrahepatic obstruction may also be caused by other diseases, such as malig-

nant tumors or pancreatic cysts, producing relatively slight signs of stasis. In partial vascular obstruction its exact site and extent are visible in the roentgenogram. In complete obstruction blood flow is sometimes reversed, so that its site may be deduced only from the type of the collateral circulation.

In most patients with complete obstruction of the portal vein, the correct diagnosis is made by demonstration of a hepatopetal circulation (Fig. 67-8) via paraportal tortuous collaterals (Fig. 67-9). In some of these patients, however, only a hepatofugal collateral circulation is demonstrated (Fig. 67-10).

In complete obstruction of the splenic vein or of the splenic and portal veins, the correct diagnosis is made by the demonstration of a hepatopetal collateral circulation and an absent filling of the obstructed part of the portal system (Figs. 67-11–67-13). Many times, however, the splenoportogram is not informative or is misleading in those patients in whom only hepatofugal collateral vessels are filled (Fig.

Figure 67-14. Thrombosis of splenic vein (verified at laparotomy). Filling of numerous collaterals to superior vena cava, such as the short gastric veins and connections to intercostal veins. There is no filling of the splenic vein. *s.g.* = short gastric veins; *sp-c.* = collateral veins connecting spleen and hepatodistal part of splenic vein to systemic veins in the lateral abdominal wall; *ic.* = intercostal veins.

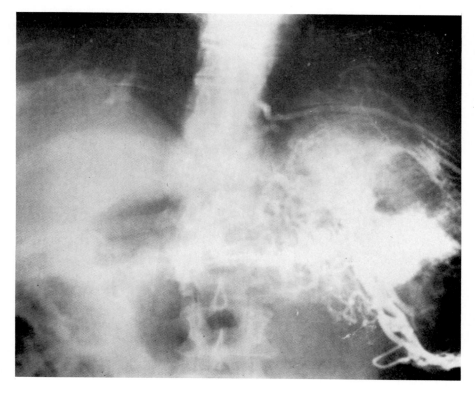
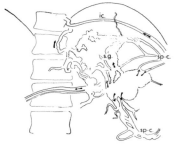

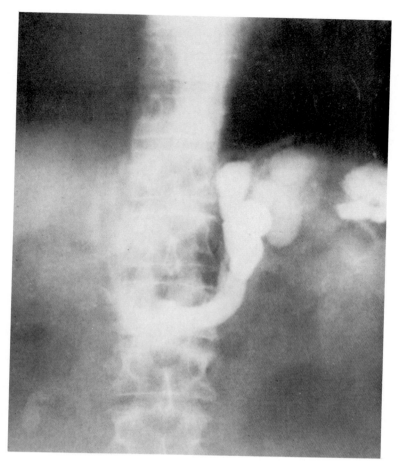

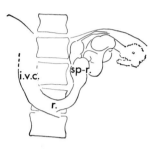

Figure 67-15. Thrombosis of splenic vein (verified during laparotomy). Contrast medium empties via dilated, tortuous retroperitoneal connections from hilus of the spleen into the left renal vein and inferior vena cava. There is no filling of splenic and portal veins. *sp-r.* = connections between splenic vein and left renal vein; *r.* = left renal vein; *i.v.c.* = inferior vena cava.

67-14; see also Figs. 67-7A, 67-10). Connections with the inferior vena cava via retroperitoneal veins and emptying into the left renal vein are not uncommon (Fig. 67-15).

In intrahepatic combined with extrahepatic obstruction (such as cirrhosis with complicating portal thrombosis), all collaterals run to the caval system (Fig. 67-16).

A surgically established shunt between the portal vein and the inferior vena cava is directly demonstrable in splenoportography. In adequately functioning shunts, no filling of collaterals is obtained (see Fig. 67-19B). If the portacaval shunt is inefficient, because of thrombosis or obstruction of flow in the inferior vena cava, collaterals are filled. The obstructing lesion is usually directly demonstrable (Fig. 67-16B; see also Fig. 67-20C).

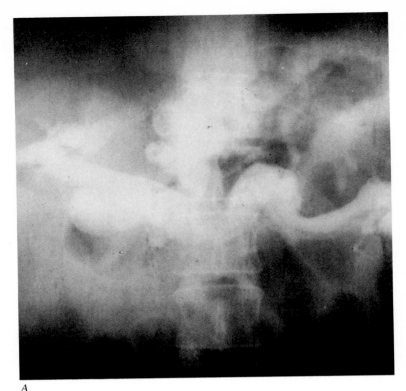

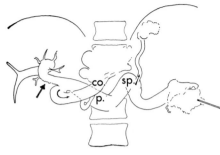

A

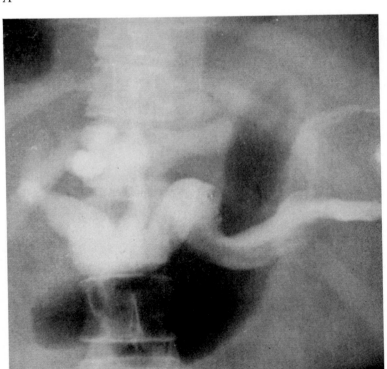

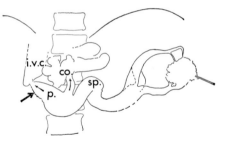

B

Figure 67-16. Liver cirrhosis and mural portal thrombosis (verified at laparotomy). (A) Splenoportogram before portacaval shunt shows mural thrombosis in the portal vein (*arrow*) and a thick, tortuous coronary vein emptying in a cranial direction. *sp.* = splenic vein; *p.* = portal vein; *co.* = coronary vein. (B) Splenoportogram after portacaval shunt shows the shunt partly obstructed by thrombosis (*arrow*), resulting in persistent filling of the coronary vein. *sp.* = splenic vein; *p.* = portal vein; *co.* = coronary vein; *i.v.c.* = inferior vena cava.

Intrahepatic Anatomic Changes

Diseases affecting the size of the liver can be diagnosed only to a limited degree by splenoportography. The normally wide variation in the size of the liver in the frontal plane, however, diminishes this possibility. In certain conditions with liver cell injury causing hepatic failure, neither the size of the liver nor its vascular tree is affected. On the other hand, liver-function tests may be normal in patients with severe vascular changes as seen by roentgenography.

There are two main groups of common diseases in which the actual intrahepatic vascular changes may be demonstrable by splenoportography: cirrhosis of the liver and intrahepatic malignant tumors.

CIRRHOSIS OF THE LIVER

The circulatory disturbances in advanced human cirrhosis have been described by McIndoe [36] on the basis of corrosion preparations and perfusion experiments. He stressed the noticeable

Figure 67-17. Cirrhosis of the liver. Splenoportogram shows narrow intrahepatic portal branches spread less than normally. Filling of collaterals toward superior vena cava (coronary vein, short gastric veins) and toward inferior vena cava (inferior mesenteric vein) indicates marked venous stasis. *sp.* = splenic vein; *p.* = portal vein; *co.* = coronary vein; *s.g.* = short gastric veins; *i.m.* = inferior mesenteric vein; *e.* = esophageal veins.

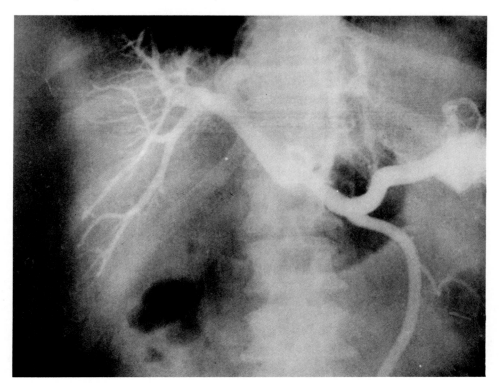

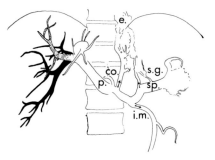

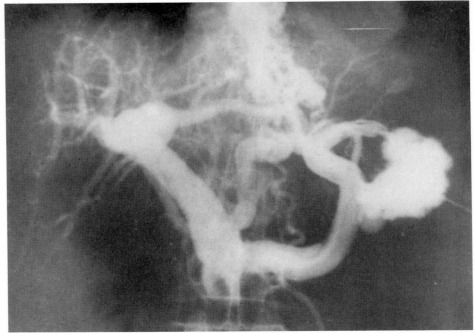

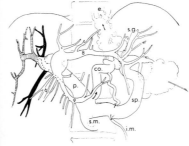

A

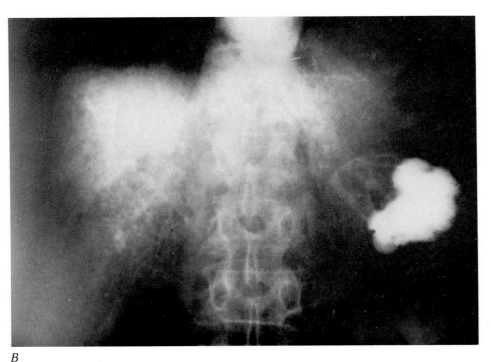

B

Figure 67-18. Cirrhosis of the liver. (A) Splenoportogram showing narrow and irregular intrahepatic portal branches. The left main part of the liver is abnormally large. There is filling of collateral vessels (coronary vein, short gastric veins, inferior mesenteric vein), indicating marked venous stasis. (B) Hepatogram of mottled appearance. *sp.* = splenic vein; *p.* = portal vein; *co.* = coronary vein; *s.g.* = short gastric veins; *i.m.* = inferior mesenteric vein; *s.m.* = superior mesenteric vein; *e.* = esophageal veins; *6* = ventral vpr.; *8* = dorsolateral vpr.; *9* = ventrolateral vpr.

Figure 67-19. Cirrhosis of the liver. (A) Splenoportogram. Filling is obtained of only a few intrahepatic branches, and there is no filling of the left principal vpr. Collateral circulation via the coronary vein and esophageal veins shows portal congestion. *sp.* = splenic vein; *p.* = portal vein; *co.* = coronary vein; *i.m.* = inferior mesenteric vein; *e.* = esophageal veins; *1* = right principal vpr. (B) Splenoportogram after portacaval shunt. There is no filling of collaterals. The contrast medium empties into the inferior vena cava. *sp.* = splenic vein; *p.* = portal vein; *i.v.c.* = inferior vena cava.

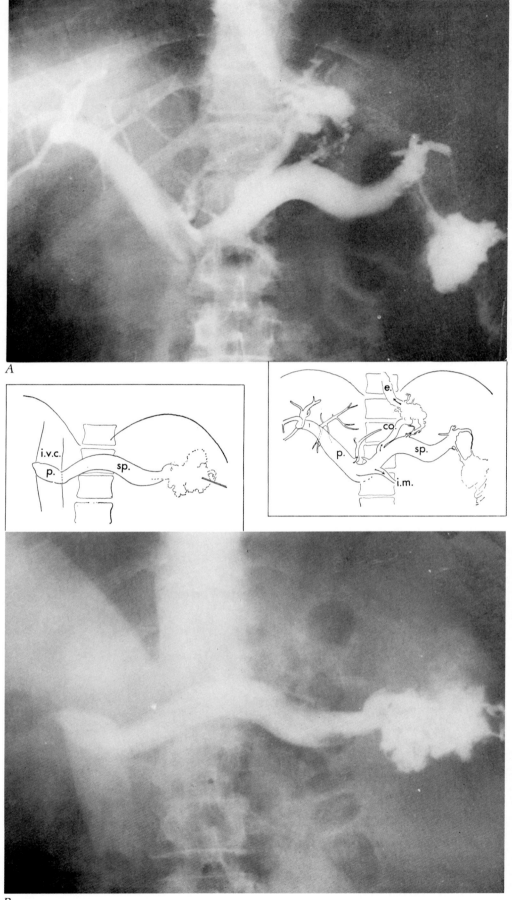

A

B

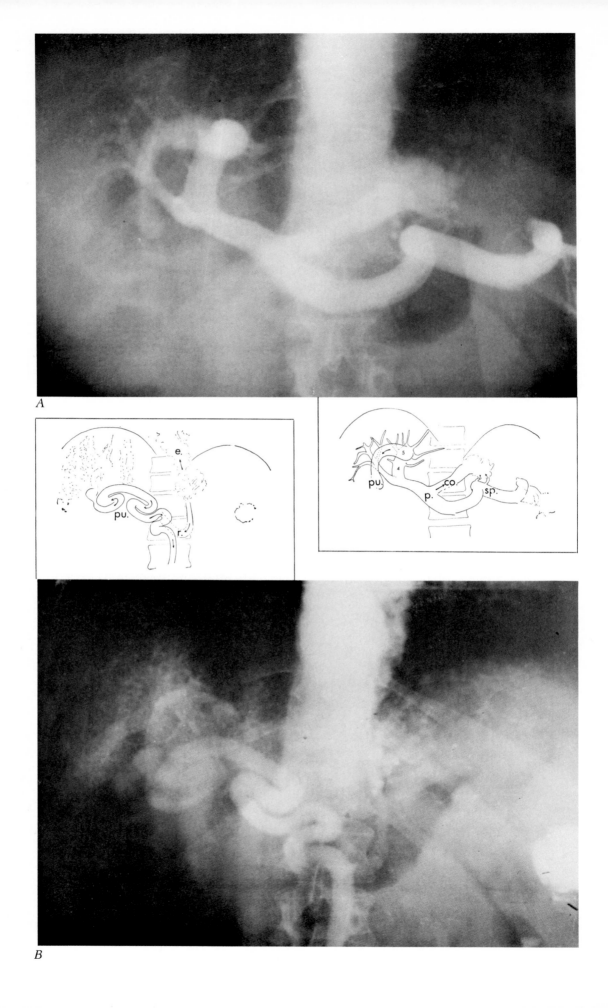

A

B

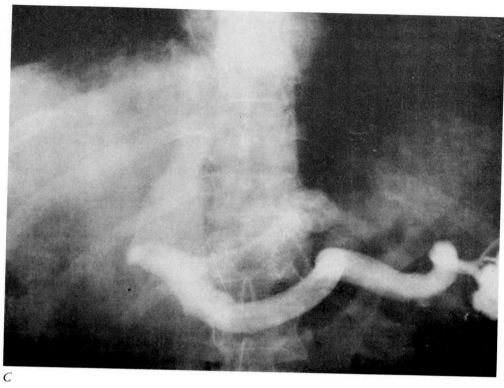

C

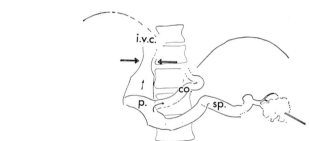

Figure 67-20. Cirrhosis of the liver. (A) Splenoportogram shows markedly changed intrahepatic ramification with few, narrow, and irregularly tapering vessels. Filling of a large coronary vein extending from the portal vein and a dilated parumbilical vein from ventroflexed vpr. indicate portal stasis. *sp.* = splenic vein; *p.* = portal vein; *co.* = coronary vein; *pu.* = parumbilical vein; *4* = left principal vpr.; *5* = ventroflexed vpr. (B) Six seconds later. Filling of the tortuous parumbilical vein is obtained. Contrast medium in the coronary vein plexus is emptying cranially into the esophageal veins and caudally via a retroperitoneal connection to the left renal vein. Note the mottled hepatographic appearance. *pu.* = parumbilical vein; *e.* = esophageal veins; *r.* = left renal vein. (C) Splenoportography after portacaval shunt still shows filling of the coronary vein despite a broad portacaval communication. This may be explained by the narrowing of the inferior vena cava on its passage behind the liver, probably caused by cirrhotic nodules (*arrows*). The incapacity of the inferior vena cava was also evidenced by a relatively small decrease in portal pressure after establishment of the portavacal shunt (from 37 to 30 mm H$_2$O) and by edema of the legs postoperatively. *sp.* = splenic vein; *p.* = portal vein; *co.* = coronary vein; *i.v.c.* = inferior vena cava.

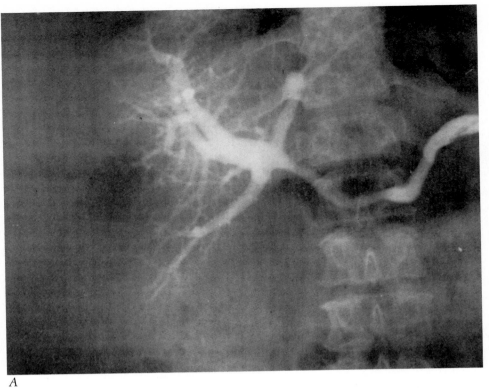
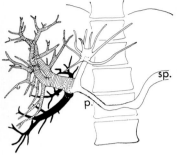

A

B

Figure 67-21. Tumor metastases. (A) Splenoporto-gram shows marked constriction of the portal vein. *sp.* = splenic vein; *p.* = portal vein. (B) Hepatogram shows one large filling defect corresponding to the lateral part of the ventrocranial segment.

Figure 67-22. Liver metastases. (A) Splenoporto-gram shows marked enlargement of the liver and displacement of the portal vein and intrahepatic branches. *sp.* = splenic vein; *p.* = portal vein; *1* = right principal vpr.; *8* = dorsolateral vpr.; *9* = ventrolateral ▶ vpr. (B) Hepatogram shows several filling defects corresponding approximately to displacement of the intrahepatic portal branches.

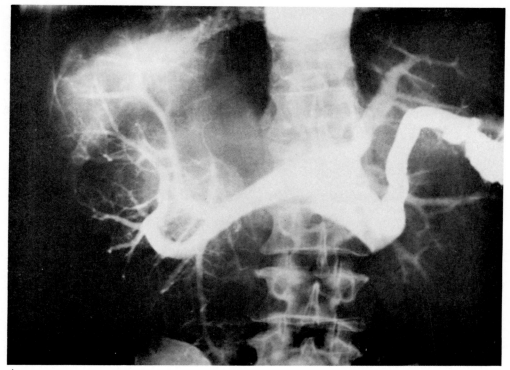

A

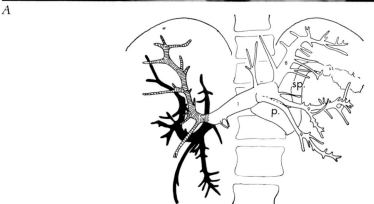

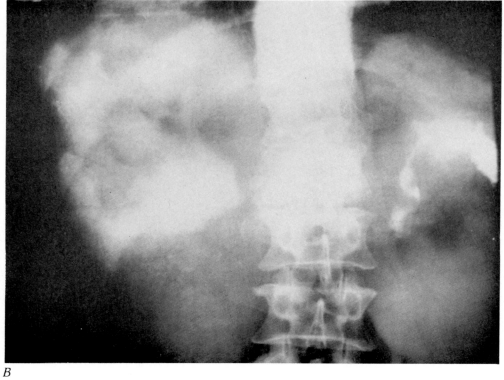

B

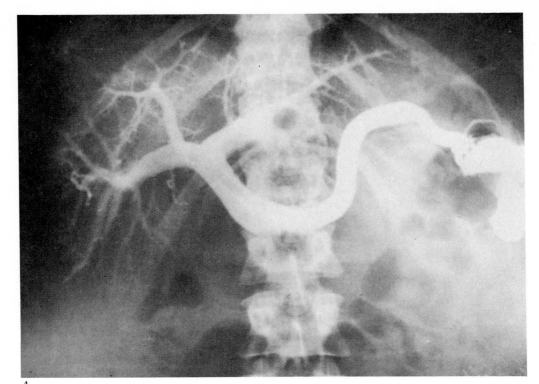

A

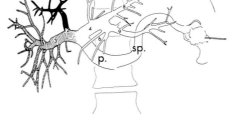

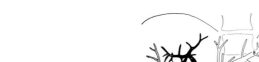

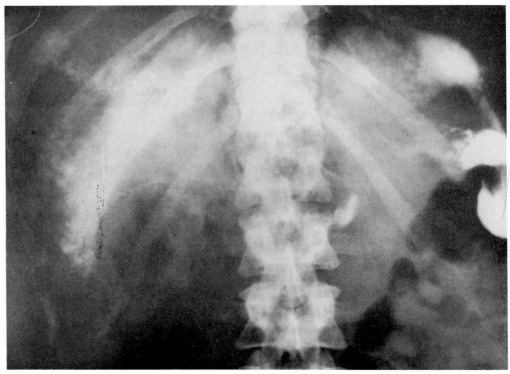

B

diminution in the hepatic vascular bed and the irregularity of the main branches. He also described the formation of direct intrahepatic connections between the portal and hepatic veins, which impaired the nutrition of the liver cells that were then dependent entirely on the arterial supply. Vascular intrahepatic obstruction may also be caused by compression of the smaller vessels by regenerating nodules or else by secondary thrombosis.

In the author's pathoanatomically verified material [7] derived from cirrhosis mainly combined with portal hypertension, two-thirds of the patients showed changes consisting of narrow branches (Fig. 67-17) or abruptly ending or irregularly tapering portal vessels whose course markedly deviated from the main direction (Fig. 67-18A). In several cases thrombi were directly visible or suggested by occlusion of branches (Fig. 67-19A). The left principal portal venous ramus and ventroflexed portal venous ramus were often wider than vessels of corresponding importance in the right main part and projected more dextrocranially than usual (Fig. 67-20A). The dilatation can often be attributed to a demonstrable collateral circulation from the ventroflexed portal venous ramus to the caval system via the parumbilical vein (Fig. 67-20B). About one-third of the patients with cirrhosis show no definite vascular changes intrahepatically.

Hepatographic changes in cirrhosis must be judged with caution. In many instances the appearance of the liver is mottled (see Fig. 67-18B). This should be regarded as a definite sign of cirrhosis. Less distinct differences in contrast density are, however, also observed in normal subjects. The hepatographic density is often poor in cirrhosis. It is most commonly explained by an extrahepatic collateral circulation so that the liver receives an abnormally small quantity of contrast medium. In several cases, however, a poor hepatographic density and an abnormally early appearance of hepatic veins are observed in patients with at most a small collateral circulation [7, 11]. These signs are probably the roentgenographic manifestation of the intrahepatic shunts from portal to hepatic veins, bypassing the sinusoids in cirrhosis [24, 41, 44].

INTRAHEPATIC MALIGNANT TUMORS

Liver metastases as well as primary intrahepatic malignant growths affect the intrahepatic venous ramification mainly by their tendency to invade and occlude veins rapidly. Since the supply to these tumors is almost entirely arterial [20], a contrast filling of tumor vessels in splenoportography is hardly to be expected.

The earliest change demonstrable by splenoportography usually consists of one or more clearly outlined, more or less irregular defects in the hepatogram (Figs. 67-21–67-23). This is a manifestation of invasion and occlusion of vessels too small to cause gross vascular changes. Sometimes tumor thrombi are seen in the vessels before obstruction is complete. A deficient filling of the left principal portal venous ramus or its branches should be interpreted with caution since this is also common in normal subjects (see Fig. 67-4). Sometimes a direct connection between portal and hepatic veins is demonstrable at the site of the tumor. Dislocation of vessels and signs of hepatomegaly are comparatively late signs (see Fig. 67-22A). In the absence of the above-mentioned signs of tumor invasion, any expansive process is probably not malignant. If the metastases are small and are evenly distributed, they do not appreciably change the roentgenogram.

Extrahepatic Anatomic Changes

The normally large variation in the course of the splenic vein makes it difficult to detect any dislocation.

Dislocation of or pressure on the portal vein, on the other hand, may be readily demonstrated because of the regularly straight or slightly curved normal course of this vessel. Such a change may, for example, be produced by tumor masses in the porta hepatis (Fig. 67-24; see also Fig. 67-21A) or in adjacent parts of the liver parenchyma.

◄ Figure 67-23. Liver metastases. (A) Splenoportogram shows occlusion of smaller intrahepatic branches. There is no dislocation. *sp.* = splenic vein; *p.* = portal vein; *2* = dorsocaudal vpr. (*black*); *3* = ventrocranial vpr. (*striated*); *4* = left principal vpr.; *6* = ventral vpr.; *8* = dorsolateral vpr.; *9* = ventrolateral vpr. (B) Hepatogram shows several major filling defects and numerous smaller ones.

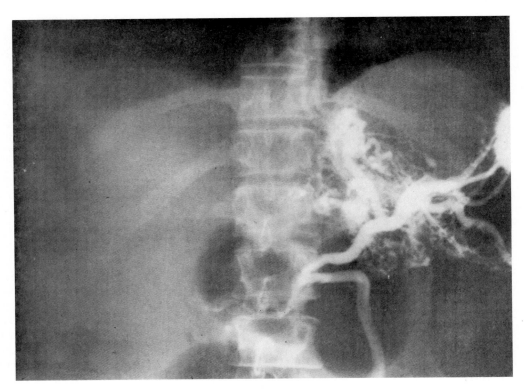

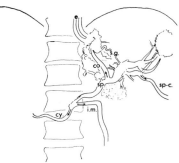

Figure 67-24. Portal occlusion owing to tumor metastases. Splenoportogram shows filling of collaterals (coronary vein, mesenteric vein, cystic vein). *sp.* = splenic vein; *s.g.* = short gastric veins; *co.* = coronary vein; *i.m.* = inferior mesenteric vein; *cy.* = cystic vein; *sp-c.* = collateral veins connecting spleen and hepatodistal part of splenic vein to systemic veins in the lateral abdominal wall; *e* = esophageal veins.

References

1. Abeatici, S., and Campi, L.   Sur les possibilités de l'angiographie hépatique: La visualisation du système portal. *Acta Radiol.* (Stockh.) 36:383, 1951.

2. Abeatici, S., Campi, L., and Ferrero, R.   Sulle curve di propagazione del circolo spleno-portale: Studio emodinamico del distretto lienoepatico mediante portografia seriata. *Minerva Chir.* 7:886, 1952.

3. Anacker, H., Devens, K., and Linden, G.   Leistungsfähigkeit und Grenzen der perkutanen Splenoportographie. *ROEFO* 86:411 1957.

4. Armstrong, E. L., Adams, W. L., Jr., Tragerman, L. J., and Townsend, E. W.   The Cruveilhier-Baumgarten syndrome; review of the literature and report of two additional cases. *Ann. Intern. Med.* 16:113, 1942.

5. Atkinson, M., Barnett, E., Sherlock, S., and Steiner, R. E.   The clinical investigation of the portal circulation with special reference to portal venography. *Q. J. Med.* 24:77, 1955.

6. Bergstrand, I.   Roentgen anatomy of the intrahepatic portal ramification: A study on autopsy material. *Kgl. Fysiograf. Sällskap. Lund Förh.* 27:85, 1957.

7. Bergstrand, I. Liver morphology in percutaneous lienoportal venography. *Kgl. Fysiograf. Sällskap. Lund Förh.* 27:105, 1957.

8. Bergstrand, I. Die portale Kollateralzirkulation und Ösophagusvarizen. In *Transactions of the Ninth International Congress of Radiology.* Stuttgart: Thieme, 1960.

9. Bergstrand, I. The localization of portal obstruction by splenoportography. *AJR* 85:1111, 1961.

10. Bergstrand, I., and Ekman, C.-A. Percutaneous lieno-portal venography. *Acta Radiol.* (Stockh.) 43:377, 1955.

11. Bergstrand, I., and Ekman, C.-A. Portal circulation in portal hypertension. *Acta Radiol.* (Stockh.) 47:1, 1957.

12. Bergstrand, I., and Ekman, C.-A. Percutaneous lieno-portal venography: Technique and complications. *Acta Radiol.* (Stockh.) 47:269, 1957.

13. Bergstrand, I., and Ekman, C.-A. Lieno-portal venography in the study of portal circulation in the dog. *Acta Radiol.* (Stockh.) 47:257, 1957.

14. Blakemore, A. H., and Lord, J. W., Jr. The technic of using vitallium tubes in establishing porta-caval shunts for portal hypertension. *Ann. Surg.* 122:476, 1945.

15. Boijsen, E., and Efsing, H.-O. Intrasplenic arterial aneurysms following splenoportal phlebography. *Acta Radiol.* [*Diagn.*] (Stockh.) 6:487, 1967.

16. Boijsen, E., and Efsing, H.-O. Aneurysm of the splenic artery. *Acta Radiol.* [*Diagn.*] (Stockh.) 8:29, 1969.

17. Boijsen, E., Ekman, C.-A., and Lundh, G. Selective Splanchnic Angiography. In C. E. Welch (ed.), *Advances in Surgery.* Chicago: Year Book, 1968.

18. Boulvin, R., Chevalier, M., Gallus, P., and Nagel, M. La portographie par voie splénique transpariétale. *Acta Chir. Belg.* 50:534, 1951.

19. Bourgeon, R., Dumazer, R., Pietri, H., and Guntz, M. Une forme nouvelle de l'hépatographie; son intérêt particulier dans l'étude des néoformations hépatiques. *Mem. Acad. Chir.* (Paris) 80:665, 1954.

20. Breedis, C., and Young, G. The blood supply of neoplasms in the liver. *Am. J. Pathol.* 30:969, 1954.

21. Cacciari, C., Pisi, E., and Cavalli, G. *Splenoportografia e Splenomanometria.* Bologna: Officina d'arte grafica Cacciari, 1957.

22. Child, C. G., III. *The Hepatic Circulation and Portal Hypertension.* Philadelphia: Saunders, 1954.

23. Couinaud, C. Étude de la veine porte intrahépatique. *Presse Med.* 61:1434, 1953.

24. Daniel, P. M., Prichard, M. L., and Reynell, P. C. The portal circulation in experimental cirrhosis of the liver. *J. Pathol.* 64:53, 1952.

25. Doehner, G. A., Ruzicka, F. F., Hoffman, G., and Rousselot, L. M. The portal venous system: Its roentgen anatomy. *Radiology* 64:675, 1955.

26. Eckman, C.-A. Portal hypertension; diagnosis and surgical treatment. *Acta Chir. Scand.* [Suppl.] 222:1, 1957.

27. Figley, M. M., Fry, W. J., Orebaugh, J. E., and Pollard, H. M. Percutaneous spleno-portography. *Gastroenterology* 28:153, 1955.

28. Foster, J. H., Conkle, D. M., Crane, J. M., and Burko. H. Splenoportography: An assessment of its value and risk. *Ann. Surg.* 179:773, 1974.

29. Gabrielsson, N. Diagnosis of gastric varices by conventional roentgenography as compared with splenoportal phlebography. *Acta Radiol.* [*Diagn.*] (Stockh.) 11:506, 1971.

30. Gvozdanović, V., and Hauptmann, E. Further experience with percutaneous lieno-portal venography. *Acta Radiol.* (Stockh.) 43:177, 1955.

31. Healey, J. E. Clinical anatomic aspects of radical hepatic surgery. *J. Int. Coll. Surg.* 22:542, 1954.

32. Hjortsjö, C.-H. Die Anatomie der intrahepatischen Gallengänge beim Menschen, mittels Röntgen- und Injektions-technik studiert. *Lunds Univ. Årsskr. N. F.* 44:3, 1948.

33. Hunt, A. H. *A Contribution to the Study of Portal Hypertension.* Edinburgh: Livingstone, 1958.

34. Kogutt, M. S., and Jander, P. Splenoportography—a valuable diagnostic technic, revisited. *South. Med. J.* 70:1210, 1977.

35. Korepanov, V. I., Zhuravlev, V. A., and Yung, E. P. Diagnostic value of hepatic arterial and portal angiography in focal liver diseases. *Cor Vasa* 15:178, 1973.

36. Lande, A., and Bard, R. Celiac arteriography following percutaneous splenoportography. *Radiology* 114:57, 1975.

37. Lebon, J., Fabregoule, M., and Le Go, R. Méthodes actuelles et données nouvelles en splénoportographie. Manométrie splénique. Seriographie portale. *Algerie Med.* 58:837, 1954.

38. Leger, L. *Spleno-Portographie.* Paris: Masson, 1955.

39. Leger, L., Albot, G., and Arvay, N. La phlébographie portale dans l'exploration des affections hépato-spléniques. *Presse Med.* 59:1230, 1951.

40. Leroux, G. F., and de Scoville, A. Contribution à la splénoportographie transpariétale: Étude de l'hépatogramme. *Acta Gastroenterol. Belg.* 19:697, 1956.

41. McIndoe, A. H. Vascular lesions of portal cirrhosis. *Arch. Pathol.* 5:23, 1928.

42. Ödman, P. Percutaneous selective angiography of the coeliac artery. *Acta Radiol.* [Suppl.] (Stockh.) 159:1, 1958.

43. Patrassi, G., d'Agnolo, B., dal Palù, C., and Ruol, A. *Il Circolo Epatoportale alla Luce della Moderne Techniche.* Padova: Tip. Editrice "La Garangola," 1957.

44. Popper, H., Elias, H., and Petty, D. E. Vascular pattern of the cirrhotic liver. *Am. J. Clin. Pathol.* 22:717, 1952.

45. Probst, P., Rysavy, J. A., and Amplatz, K. Improved safety of splenoportography by plugging of the needle tract. *AJR* 131:445, 1978.

46. Rösch, J., and Bret, J. *Roentgenology of the Spleen and the Pancreas.* Springfield, Ill.: Thomas, 1967.

47. Scoville, A. de, and Leroux, G. Déformations et thromboses de la veine splénique. *Acta Gastroenterol. Belg.* 19:629, 1956.

48. Seldinger, S. I. A simple method of catheterization of the spleen and liver. *Acta Radiol.* (Stockh.) 48:93, 1957.

49. Shin, M.-S. Splenoportography with multiple sidehole catheter. *AJR* 119:433, 1973.

50. Sotgiu, G., Cacciari, C., and Frassineti, A. Splénoportographie. *Presse Med.* 60:1295, 1952.

51. Steiner, R. E., Sherlock, S., and Turner, M. D. Percutaneous splenic portal venography. *J. Fac. Radiol.* 8:158, 1957.

52. Turner, M. D., Sherlock, S., and Steiner, R. E. Splenic venography and intrasplenic pressure measurement in the clinical investigation of the portal system. *Am. J. Med.* 23:846, 1957.

53. Wannagat, L. Das laparoskopische Splenoportogramm bei der hepatitischen Zirrhose. *Acta Hepatol.* 3:204, 1955.

Arterial Portography

KLAUS M. BRON

Evaluation of the portal venous system is essential in the management of patients with portal hypertension and its complications. Portal venography, although primarily useful for the investigation of portal hypertension, is also at times helpful in the assessment of pancreatic masses. The relative inaccessibility of the portal venous system has prompted the search for a variety of techniques, both intraoperative and nonsurgical, to explore this circulation. The objective of these procedures is to determine the anatomic patency of the splenoportal axis and the hemodynamic alterations due to the development of extrahepatic portosystemic collateral channels (a response to portal hypertension).

The earliest technique for portal vein visualization in man was devised by Blakemore and Lord [4] in 1945 (at the suggestion of Whipple [41]) and consisted of the direct injection of contrast material into the portal vein or one of its mesenteric tributaries at laparotomy. Further reports in the early 1950s [14, 29, 37] attested to the value of operative portal angiography at laparotomy, but it quickly became apparent that this method was cumbersome, time-consuming, and less than satisfactory. More important, it did not aid in the preoperative diagnosis of the patient and thus was of no use in planning the surgical approach.

During the 1950s, the nonoperative technique of percutaneous splenoportography was developed after Abeatici and Campi [1] in 1951 demonstrated this method in dogs. To Leger [26] goes the credit for the first successful percutaneous splenoportogram in man. Thereafter, this method became firmly entrenched as the preoperative diagnostic technique for investigating patients with portal hypertension. Numerous reviews have appraised the indications, hazards, and results of its use in large series of patients [3, 8, 18, 23, 33, 40].

Arterial portography, an alternative nonoperative technique, developed gradually after the observation in 1953 by Rigler et al. [36] that the portal venous system was occasionally visualized after injection of contrast material into the abdominal aorta. The technique was largely neglected because low concentration of contrast made visualization of the portal circulation by aortic injection poor. In 1958 Ödman [32] refined the technique by selective catheterization of the celiac axis and obtained excellent splenic and portal vein visualization. Two further modifications of the arterial technique have been

1605

suggested with the intent of improving visualization of the portal system: simultaneous selective contrast injection of the celiac and superior mesenteric arteries [5] and selective splenic artery injection [34].

Principles of Arterial Portography

The rationale inherent in arterial portography is that contrast material injected into the celiac or superior mesenteric arteries, individually or simultaneously, will remain sufficiently concentrated to demonstrate the venous portion of the circulation. This requires an amount of contrast and rate of injection sufficient to form a bolus that overcomes the diluting effect of the non-opacified blood.

The method is physiologically sound, for it takes advantage of the normal, patent circulatory pathways between the splanchnic arteries and the portal venous system. When the normal routes are altered by disease, creating venous obstruction and portosystemic collateral vessels, the angiogram will reflect and demonstrate these abnormalities. The technique of arterial portography utilizes the specific anatomy of the portal vein. This vessel, which is formed by the confluence of the splenic and superior mesenteric veins, receives blood from both the splenic and mesenteric circulations. Thus, the portal vein may be visualized after selective injection of either the celiac or the superior mesenteric arteries or both.

Selective injection of the celiac axis may be likened to remote percutaneous splenoportography because in both instances only the splenoportal axis is visualized. After arterial injection, however, additional information may be derived from the demonstration of the hepatic arteries and splenic size. In the patient with a previous splenectomy, neither selective celiac arteriography nor percutaneous splenoportography will effectively demonstrate the splenoportal axis. Selective injection of the superior mesenteric artery, however, demonstrates the portal vein via blood returning to the liver in the superior mesenteric vein and its tributaries. This is an advantage because the absence of a spleen does not preclude portal vein visualization by this technique. Therefore, the status of the portal circulation may still be investigated in patients who have had simple splenectomy or splenectomy in combination with an operative portosystemic shunt.

Technique

PATIENT PREPARATION

All patients, adults and children, are thoroughly familiarized with the procedure the day prior to the examination in order to allay unnecessary anxiety. A laxative is prescribed the evening prior to the examination, and all solid food is proscribed after the evening meal until conclusion of the study. Clear liquids are not restricted. Cleansing enemas may be ordered for constipated patients if barium has been administered within 48 hours prior to the scheduled portogram. A surgical preparation of both groin areas is performed; occasionally the left axilla is prepared if both femoral artery pulses are weak. The femoral artery is the site of choice from which to catheterize the various splanchnic aortic branches selectively, but these vessels may also be approached from the left axillary artery [9].

Preexamination analgesia is administered intramuscularly 30 to 45 minutes prior to the procedure. In adults this consists of Demerol (meperidine hydrochloride) and Seconal (sodium secobarbital) or Phenergan (promethazine hydrochloride) in amounts appropriate to the patient's age and weight. For children, morphine and Seconal are used.

Because patients with portal hypertension or retroperitoneal masses are frequently anemic from acute or chronic blood loss, the examination is postponed until the hemoglobin and hematocrit levels are in the range of 7 to 8 gm and 25 to 30 percent, respectively. This consideration, however, is waived in the critically ill, emergency patient, who may be examined in a state of clinical shock with blood replacement flowing in an effort to determine the bleeding source. Coagulopathies and bleeding tendencies are frequent in patients with cirrhosis and portal hypertension. These have not prevented successful arterial portography in patients with platelet counts as low as 30,000, and the procedure caused no untoward effects.

CATHETERS AND CATHETERIZATION

The percutaneous Seldinger technique [39] is used to puncture and catheterize the femoral artery. In adults a red Kifa (in the United States obtained from Universal Medical Instrument Corporation) catheter (60 cm long) with a tapered tip and a preformed curved end is used. In children the technique of introducing the catheter is slightly modified [12], and a Formocath RPX 045 (Becton, Dickinson and Co.) catheter (40 cm long and similarly precurved) is used. Under fluoroscopic control the catheter is selectively manipulated into the specific splanchnic artery.

Both the celiac and superior mesenteric arteries are catheterized and singly injected in most patients. In patients with splenectomy, only the superior mesenteric artery is catheterized because injection of the celiac axis will yield no information concerning the portal vein or portosystemic collaterals.

At conclusion of the examination, the catheter is withdrawn and manual pressure is exerted at the arterial puncture site to prevent bleeding and hematoma formation. In the majority of patients, to stop bleeding pressure need usually be maintained no longer than 10 to 15 minutes after catheter withdrawal. Once bleeding has stopped, a pressure dressing is applied to the puncture site and the patient is returned to bed. The vital signs are monitored regularly, and the puncture site must be examined for evidence of bleeding during the 4 hours of bed rest prescribed after the examination.

CONTRAST AND FILMING

The contrast material is injected by means of a pressure injector. In adults Renografin 76 percent (methylglucamine diatrizoate) is injected selectively into the celiac or superior mesenteric arteries at a rate of 9 to 13 cc per second in amounts ranging from 35 to 50 cc. The larger quantities are used in patients with splenomegaly or proved varices. Some investigators have reported routinely using doses in excess of 50 cc per injection, but I have not found this amount to be necessary. In children Renografin 60 percent is usually used and injected at a rate of 6 to 10 cc per second for a total of 25 to 30 cc per injection.

POSITION AND FILM PROGRAM

A scout film is obtained prior to any sequential filming to check exposure factors and position. The top of the film should include a least 2 to 3 inches of the distal esophagus in order to visualize any esophageal varices.

Routinely, an anteroposterior series of a selective injection into the celiac or splenic and superior mesenteric arteries is obtained. Another series of the superior mesenteric artery is exposed in the right posterior oblique position. The latter study permits better visualization of the junction of the superior mesenteric and portal veins because the vessels in this position are displaced from the vertebral bodies. An additional series of the celiac artery in the right posterior oblique view may be obtained because occasionally this position will better demonstrate esophagogastric varices that fill from the coronary vein.

Sequential films are obtained by means of a rapid serial changer and programmed to expose films through the arterial, capillary, and venous phases. Films are usually exposed for 22 to 25 seconds after the onset of contrast injection with filming of the arterial phase at two films per second for 3 seconds; the capillary phase at one film per second for 2 seconds; and the venous phase at one film per 2 seconds for the remainder. The film programming may have to be prolonged in extremely slow portal circulation. Unfortunately this condition is unpredictable but more frequently occurs in association with marked splenomegaly and is due to severe portal hypertension.

PHARMACOANGIOGRAPHY OF THE PORTAL SYSTEM

The degree of contrast visualization of the portal venous system and gastroesophageal varices, following selective celiac or superior mesenteric arteriography, is not always adequate to delineate the anatomic detail of these structures despite the selective injection of adequate amounts of radiopaque contrast material. This deficiency is particularly distressing in patients with previous splenectomy and/or a splenorenal shunt, which prevents the use of selective celiac or splenic arteriography for assessing the portal venous anatomy. From my own experience, inadequate contrast visualization of the portal venous anatomy following selective visceral arteriography occurs in an estimated 20 to 25 percent of cases. The use of various pharmacologic agents, mainly vasodilators, has been advocated in order to enhance mesenteric and portal vein visualization. In 1966 Boijsen and Redman [6] reported on the effects of infusing bradykinin into the celiac and superior mesenteric arteries prior to angiography to enhance portal vein visualization.

Subsequently, infusions of tolazoline [35], isoproterenol and phentolamine [15], glucagon [16], epinephrine [7], papaverine [42], and prostaglandin E_1 [22] prior to arteriography have been reported to improve contrast visualization of the portal venous system. Since 1972 I have used infusion of papaverine hydrochloride before selective superior mesenteric arteriography in order to improve the contrast visualization of the portal vein and gastroesophageal varices. This has proved to be extremely effective and safe in doses ranging from 0.6 to 0.9 mg per kilogram. My experience with this drug includes nearly 500 patients with portal hypertension, pancreatic carcinoma, hepatic tumors, gastrointestinal bleeding, and retroperitoneal tumors. The papaverine is infused with an automatic pump at the rate of 1.8 cc per minute for 1.5 minutes, for a total drug dose ranging from 50 to 65 mg. The papaverine may also be administered by hand injection over the same time period. Occasionally a very mild transient drop in systemic blood pressure has been observed with this dose. The papaverine causes a 40 percent increase in the superior mesenteric artery blood flow, but this effect is transient. Thus, there should be no delay between the papaverine infusion and the arteriography. If a repeat papaverine infusion is required, it can be safely done about 15 minutes after the first administration.

COMPLICATIONS

The complications of arterial portography are those caused by the technique of percutaneous catheterization and those produced by an allergic reaction to the contrast material. Among the minor hazards of the procedure are the formation of hematomas at the puncture site, intramural contrast deposition, inadvertent transmural passage of a guidewire, and arterial spasm. These are not generally associated with an increased morbidity, and their frequency is inversely proportional to the experience and skill of the attending angiographer.

One might anticipate that postcatheterization hematomas would be a more serious problem in portal hypertension patients with increased bleeding tendencies due to thrombocytopenia. In 52 percent of my patients with portal hypertension and thrombocytopenia with platelet counts of less than 100,000 and in 32 percent with thrombocytopenia with counts of less than 60,000, no significant increase in the rate or degree of hematoma formation was discerned.

A more serious complication is postcatheterization thrombosis at the puncture site, which occurs more often in elderly individuals with predisposing severe atherosclerosis. Because the majority of patients with portal hypertension usually do not fall into this category, this complication is infrequent. Generally, the complication rate from the technique of percutaneous catheterization ranges from 1 to 3 percent [19, 20, 25]. My own experience with percutaneous catheterization of more than 2,500 patients for a variety of indications agrees with this. Specifically, in selective visceral angiography of more than 500 patients, I have encountered no mortality and have had two patients who experienced symptoms of postcatheterization thrombosis (neither patient required thrombectomy).

Contraindications

A known sensitivity to contrast material probably constitutes the single contraindication to any type of elective contrast study. The hazard of an allergic reaction, however, must be weighed against the danger of ignorance concerning the portal circulation if a therapeutic operative procedure is being contemplated. The choice requires clinical judgment in each individual situation. In my own experience with arteriography, there was no mortality from an anaphylactic reaction even in patients with a known previous reaction to contrast material. Several patients who had previously experienced urticaria, itching, faintness, and transient, moderate hypotension during intravenous pyelography were premedicated with steroids and evidenced no similar symptoms during or after arterial portography.

Indications

The aim of arterial portography is to establish the etiology and to indicate a potential course of surgical management in patients with portal hypertension or retroperitoneal tumors. This is possible because the technique permits visualization of the component vessels of the portal circulation—the splenic, superior mesenteric, and portal veins—and the pathologic portosystemic collaterals.

One report [10] of the arterial technique in portal hypertension established specific indications; they are listed in Table 68-1. They have

Table 68-1. Indications for Arterial Portography

Portal hypertension
  Preoperative evaluation
    Differentiate intrahepatic and extrahepatic portal
      obstruction
    Demonstrate gastric and/or esophageal varices
    Evaluate technical failure of splenoportography
    Determine cause of nonvisualization of portal
      circulation by splenoportography
    Consider the relative contraindications for
      splenoportography (i.e., ascites, thrombocytopenia,
      and small spleen)
  Postoperative evaluation
    Demonstrate the function of shunts in
      nonsplenectomized patients
    Evaluate portal circulation after splenectomy
Extrahepatic tumors
  Pancreatic
    Carcinoma
    Pseudocyst

withstood the test of subsequent experience [21, 24, 28, 31, 38]. The arterial approach should be the method of choice in examining patients with portal hypertension, especially children with this disorder. Only if the desired information is not obtained by this technique should one resort to percutaneous splenoportography.

Normal Arterial Portogram

In arterial portography two different normal patterns must be distinguished because the vessels demonstrated will reflect which artery, the celiac or superior mesenteric, has been injected with contrast. Theoretically, all vessels between the point of arterial injection and venous outflow in the hepatic veins should be visualized, but in fact this is not the case. Only those vessels in the regional blood flow that receive a significant proportion of the injected contrast material will be visualized.

When the celiac axis is injected (celiac portography), the major branches (the common hepatic, left gastric, and splenic arteries) will be demonstrated during the arterial phase. Because the celiac axis is occasionally anomalous, only the splenic and left gastric arteries, or sometimes these two vessels and a hepatic artery branch, may be visualized. As the contrast proceeds peripherally, it enters the capillary phase and reveals a distinct, rather homogeneously dense outline of the spleen (splenogram) and a less dense outline of the liver (hepatogram). The car-

dia of the stomach, when not distended with air, may be visualized as a dense, rounded structure, sometimes with a very sharp and distinct margin, which should not be confused with a tumor mass. Infrequently, portions of the stomach wall in the fundus or portions of the pancreas may be densely outlined by contrast during the capillary phase.

Slightly later, in the venous phase of the celiac portogram (Fig. 68-1), the tributaries and then the main splenic and portal veins are visualized. The splenic and portal veins are noted in most instances almost simultaneously, so that separate splenic and portal vein transit times cannot be established. The contrast density usually increases to a maximum in these vessels, then gradually fades. The splenic vein normally follows a straight course between the spleen and extrahepatic portion of the portal vein. The portion of the splenic vein that overlies the vertebral body may be poorly seen. The degree of intrahepatic portal vein filling is usually poor. The main right and left lobe intrahepatic branches are noted at their origins, but the peripheral vessels are largely imperceptible. The right intrahepatic branch may be better filled with contrast than the left because in the supine position the right branch is more dependent and thus enhances the gravitational effect of the contrast material. The hepatic veins draining the liver lobules into the systemic venous circulation are usually not visualized. The coronary vein (left gastric), draining the lesser curvature and cardia of the stomach, is normally infrequently visualized. It may enter the splenic or portal vein. Another seldom noted vessel is the right gastroepiploic vein, which drains the greater curvature of the stomach. The pancreatic veins are never clearly visualized as distinct vessels. The inferior mesenteric vein, a tributary of the splenic vein, is not normally visualized.

Injection of contrast into the superior mesenteric artery (mesenteric portography) demonstrates a different group of regional vessels from that revealed by a celiac injection until the contrast reaches the portal vein. In the arterial phase the vessels to the duodenum and pancreas (the inferior pancreatic arcade arteries) are filled, and these in turn may demonstrate the gastroduodenal artery. The entire small bowel is supplied by jejunal and ileal branches that arise primarily along the left side of the main superior mesenteric artery. The colon from the cecum to the splenic flexure area receives its blood supply from vessels that generally arise from the right side

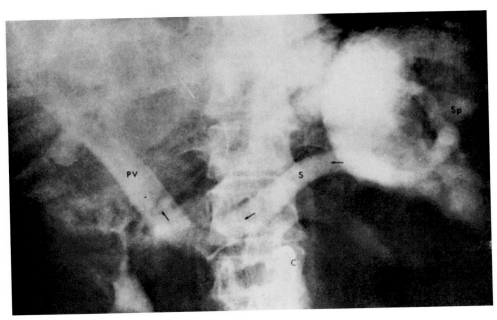

Figure 68-1. Celiac portogram. A normal venous phase after injection of the celiac artery (*C*). Arrows indicate the direction of blood flow from the spleen (*Sp*) into the splenic vein (*S*) and then into the extrahepatic portal vein (*PV*). The portion of splenic vein crossing the vertebrae may be indistinct, but note the caliber and straight course of the remainder of both vessels.

of the superior mesenteric artery. In the capillary phase the contrast is distributed in the wall of the various loops of bowel and when visualized *on end* may be mistaken for tumor staining.

As the contrast proceeds into the venous phase of the mesenteric portogram (Fig. 68-2), the different mesenteric tributaries draining the various portions of the small bowel and colon are visualized. These branches are named for the parts of the gut that they drain, and although a general pattern exists, there is marked variability in the individual patient. These regional veins coalesce into the main superior mesenteric vein, which joins with the splenic to form the portal vein.

There is usually no difference in the degree of frequency of visualization of the intrahepatic branches of the portal and hepatic veins after either celiac or superior mesenteric artery injection. The portal vein may demonstrate a stream-

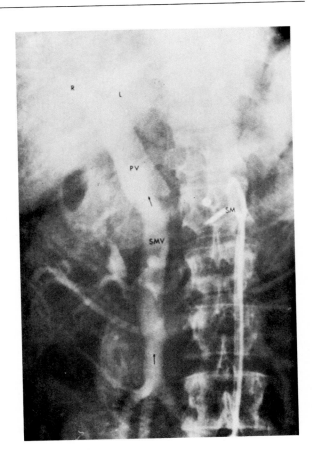

Figure 68-2. Superior mesenteric portogram. A normal venous phase after injection of the corresponding artery (*SM*). Arrows indicate the hepatopetal blood flow from the venous tributaries into the superior mesenteric vein (*SMV*), then into the extrahepatic portal vein (*PV*), and finally into the right (*R*) and left (*L*) intrahepatic branches.

ing effect caused by mixing of the two separate blood flows from the splenic and superior mesenteric veins when only one of these regional flows is opacified. This may render visible only a portion of the total diameter of the portal vein.

Abnormal Portograms

INTRAHEPATIC PORTAL OBSTRUCTION

The most frequent cause of portal hypertension is intrahepatic obstruction secondary to cirrhosis of the portal, biliary, or postnecrotic variety. The pathologic changes cause distortion of the hepatic parenchyma with intermingling of necrotic, fibrotic, and regenerating areas of liver tissue. This progressive process eventually results in impaired circulation through the liver with consequent portal hypertension. The normal direc-

tion of portal blood flow is toward the liver (hepatopetal), but as the intrahepatic circulation becomes progressively impaired, portosystemic collateral vessels develop and blood flows away from the liver (hepatofugal).

The major types of collateral channels are the esophagogastric, splenorenal, retroperitoneal, and umbilical varieties. These are formed by vessels normally present but unused in the absence of elevated portal pressure rather than from the growth of new vessels. The vessels that constitute the collateral circulation are generally dilated and markedly tortuous, and the blood flow through them is sluggish. Esophagogastric varices occur most frequently. More than one type of collateral circulation is often present (Fig. 68-3), and there seems to be no correlation between the degree of portal hypertension and the type of collateral developed. The esophagogastric varices (Fig. 68-4)

Figure 68-3. Collateral drainage. (A) Celiac portogram demonstrates two types of collaterals: gastric varices (*G*) and a dilated, tortuous umbilical vein (*C*). The gastric varices are supplied by vessels directly from the lower pole of the spleen (*arrows*). The splenic vein has emptied, and only the portal vein (*PV*) and the collateral vessel (*C*) remain visualized. The direction of blood flow is indicated by the arrows.

S = spleen. (B) The superior mesenteric portogram also shows the umbilical vein collateral (*C*), and its extent is better appreciated in the oblique view. This collateral vessel originates from left branch of the portal vein (*PV*). Arrows indicate the direction of blood flow from the superior mesenteric vein (*SM*) toward the umbilicus.

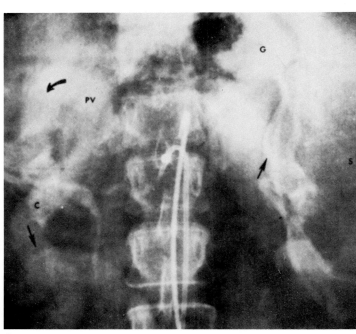

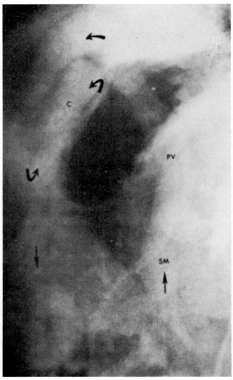

A   *B*

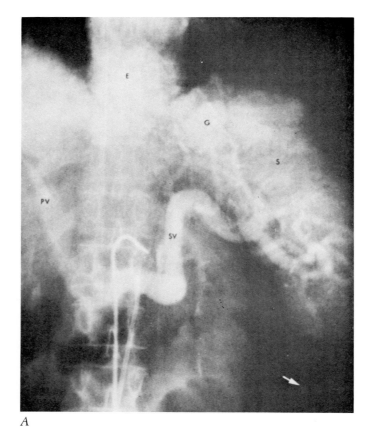

A

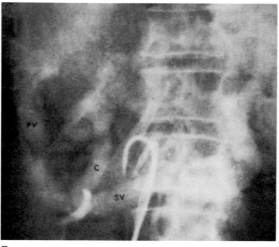

B

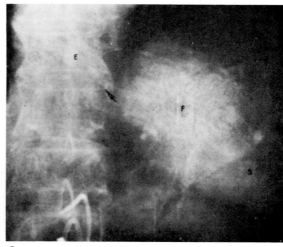

C

Figure 68-4. Esophagogastric varices. (A) A celiac portogram in the anteroposterior position demonstrates gastric (*G*) and esophageal (*E*) varices, supplied by the short gastric vessels from the spleen (*S*). The splenic vein (*SV*) is tortuous and dilated, reflecting the portal hypertension. The portal vein (*PV*) is patent. A dilated retroperitoneal vein (*arrow*) that functions as a collateral is visible at the caudal margin of the spleen.

(B) A celiac portogram in the right posterior oblique position demonstrates a dilated coronary vein (*C*) that feeds esophageal varices. This vessel and the varices were not evident in the anteroposterior view. The splenic (*SV*) and portal (*PV*) veins are dilated. (C) Esophageal varices (*E*) are supplied by a vessel (*arrow*) directly from the cardia (*F*) of the stomach; this latter structure overlies the medial portion of the spleen (*S*).

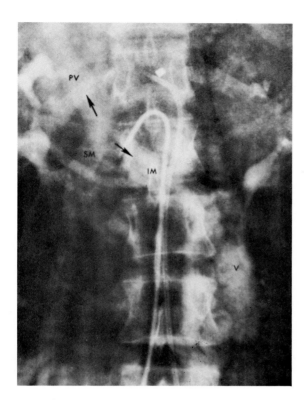

Figure 68-5. Intestinal varices. An intestinal varix (*V*) is present in the course of the inferior mesenteric vein (*IM*). This is a localized area of venous dilatation and tortuosity. The mesenteric portogram reveals that the blood flow from the superior mesenteric vein (*SM*) continues to be hepatopetal (*arrow*) in the portal vein (*PV*) but is hepatofugal (*arrow*) in the inferior mesenteric vein (*IM*).

are formed by either the coronary or short gastric veins or both. It is not unusual for either the esophageal or the gastric varices to appear more prominent than the other because both may not be developed to the same degree. The umbilical vein collateral arises from the left portal vein branch because during embryologic development this anatomic connection existed. Occasionally an intestinal varix (Fig. 68-5) occurs because of the development of collaterals.

The esophagogastric, splenorenal, and retroperitoneal collaterals are usually best demonstrated by a celiac axis injection because these abnormal vessels are formed by branches of the splenic vein. But when the coronary vein arises from the portal vein, the esophagogastric varices may be seen after a superior mesenteric artery injection. The umbilical vein collateral may be equally well demonstrated after a celiac or superior mesenteric artery injection because the

abnormal venous connection arises from the left intrahepatic branch of the portal vein.

These collaterals represent a natural mechanism that attempts to reduce the portal pressure by diverting the portal circulation away from the abnormal liver. That the attempt is usually unsuccessful is attested to by the development of hematemesis, melena, and ascites, the complications of portal hypertension.

EXTRAHEPATIC PORTAL OBSTRUCTION

The portal circulation can be obstructed by partial or complete occlusion of the extrahepatic portion of the portal and/or splenic veins. Obstruction of the hepatic veins is a less frequent cause, and rarely is the superior mesenteric vein directly included in the obstructive process. Unlike intrahepatic obstruction, which is secondary to hepatic tissue destruction, extrahepatic obstruction is the result of intrinsic vascular pathology in the form of thrombosis caused by infection, congenital malformation, or tumor compression and/or invasion.

The portal is more often affected than the splenic vein. Neonatal umbilical vein infection and congenital malformation are responsible for the high incidence of portal vein obstruction and are the leading causes of portal hypertension in children. In adults there is associated portal vein obstruction in about 10 percent of patients with portal cirrhosis of the liver. Extrahepatic portal obstruction is considerably less frequent than intrahepatic obstruction as the cause of portal hypertension. A biopsy of the liver in extrahepatic portal obstruction, unless associated with hepatic cirrhosis, will usually reveal normal liver architecture.

Recanalization may follow portal vein thrombosis and cause smaller than normal caliber, irregular contour, or replacement by multiple channels (Fig. 68-6). There may also be evidence of calcification reflecting the previous thrombosis (see Fig. 68-13A).

The collateral vessels reflect the site of venous occlusion. When the splenic vein is occluded but the portal vein remains patent, collaterals will attempt to bypass the occlusion in order to reconstitute the portal vein (Fig. 68-7). If both the portal and splenic veins are occluded (Fig. 68-8), drainage from the spleen may be via esophagogastric, retroperitoneal, or splenorenal collateral vessels. If the recanalized portal vein cannot accommodate the portal circulation, portal

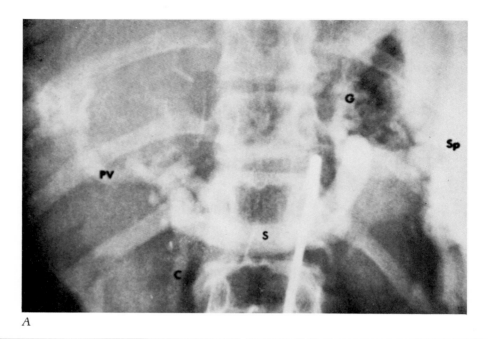

A

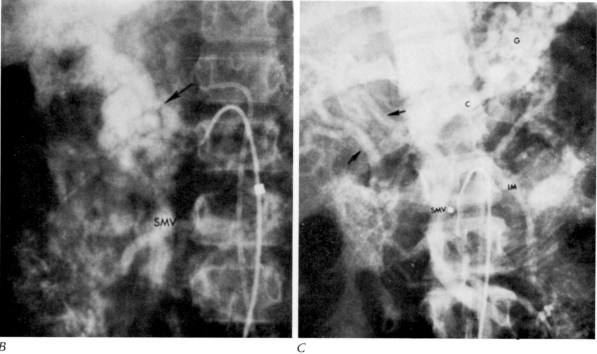

B   *C*

Figure 68-6. Extrahepatic portal obstruction. The vein displays a variety of changes reflecting the antecedent pathology. (A) The portal vein (*PV*) is reduced in caliber, and its junction with the splenic vein (*S*) is abnormal. A collateral vessel (*C*) and gastric varices (*G*) are present. The spleen (*Sp*) was enlarged. (B) The portal vein has been deformed into a tortuous tangle of vessels (*arrow*) at its origin from the superior mesenteric vein (*SMV*). (C) A previous splenec-tomy in this patient precluded any nonoperative evaluation of the status of the portal vessel other than superior mesenteric portography. The portal vein (*arrows*) consists of multiple channels which fill from the superior mesenteric vein (*SMV*). A dilated coronary vein (*C*) demonstrates gastric varices (*G*). The direction of blood flow in the inferior mesenteric vein (*IM*) is retrograde from the superior mesenteric vein.

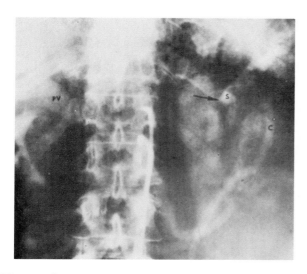

Figure 68-7. Splenic vein obstruction. The splenic vein (*S*) is occluded proximally (*arrow*). Dilated, tortuous collateral vessels (*C*) originate from the spleen and bypass the splenic vein obstruction to reconstitute the patent portal vein (*PV*).

Figure 68-8. Splenic and portal vein obstruction. The splenic and portal veins are occluded, with resultant splenomegaly (*Sp*) and venous drainage into esophageal varices (*E*) via the short gastric veins (*arrowhead*). The spleen is also decompressed by retroperitoneal collaterals (*C*). The metallic clips are from a partial gastrectomy and vagotomy that confirmed the venous occlusion.

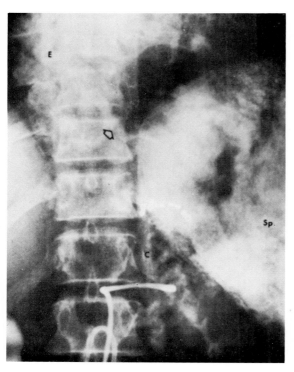

hypertension ensues with consequent collateral vessels and varices.

PRIOR SPLENECTOMY

The problem of evaluating the status of the portal circulation in the patient with a prior splenectomy is a serious challenge. This patient has usually had one or more surgical procedures in an attempt to alleviate the complications of portal hypertension. Splenectomy alone is a form of therapy for portal hypertension with hypersplenism, but more often a splenorenal shunt is performed or attempted in conjunction with splenectomy. Recurrence of hematemesis, melena, or ascites generally signals failure of the previous therapy, and before any further surgical intervention, the existing portal circulation must be carefully evaluated (Fig. 68-9).

When the spleen is absent, the splenoportal axis has been interrupted. Any attempt to visualize the portal vein from the celiac circulation is therefore unsuccessful, and percutaneous splenoportography is impossible. In this situation

Figure 68-9. Postsplenectomy status. The patient presented with recurrent hematemesis after failure of a previous portacaval shunt and a subsequent unsuccessful splenorenal shunt that resulted in splenectomy. A superior mesenteric portogram demonstrates the status of the portal venous system. The superior mesenteric (*SM*) and portal (*PV*) veins are patent, and no evidence of a functioning portacaval shunt is observed. Gastric varices (*G*) are supplied by the coronary vein (*arrow*).

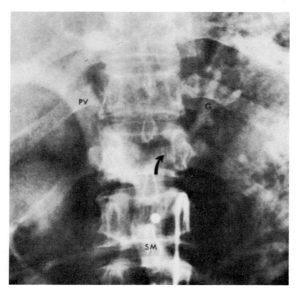

the value of arterial portography via the superior mesenteric artery has been pointed out by Boijsen et al. [5]. It is the only safe and effective nonoperative technique for demonstrating the portal vein, any varices, and patency of a splenorenal shunt that may be present after splenectomy (see Fig. 68-6C).

SURGICAL SHUNTS

Therapy aimed at relieving portal hypertension and its complications—gastrointestinal bleeding and ascites—is based on reducing the portal pressure by the creation of portosystemic shunts. These surgically formed shunts may be of the portacaval, splenorenal, or mesocaval variety. The operative shunts generally reduce portal pressure, whereas the natural shunts usually do not lower the pressure and result in varices. Unfortunately, shunt surgery is likely to afford relief only from the acute symptoms, which may be life-threatening; it does not provide a permanent cure. The recurrence of symptoms subsequent to surgery raises the question of shunt patency or adequacy to handle the portal circulation.

End-to-side portacaval shunts are usually the procedure of choice when technically feasible. A splenorenal shunt may be the primary procedure when splenectomy is contemplated because of severe hypersplenism, but it may be reserved for failure of a portacaval shunt. Mesocaval shunts

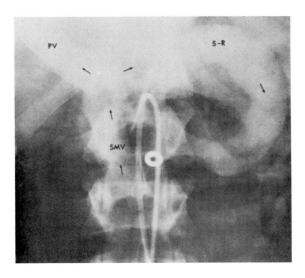

Figure 68-11. Splenorenal shunt. A superior mesenteric portogram is required to demonstrate patency of a splenorenal shunt. The arrows indicate the direction of blood flow from the superior mesenteric vein (SMV), which then continues into both the portal vein (PV) and splenorenal shunt (S–R). Dilution of the contrast by nonopacified renal vein blood causes poor visualization of the inferior vena cava. (Courtesy of Sam E. Morris, M.D.)

Figure 68-10. Portacaval shunt. A celiac portogram demonstrates the patent portacaval shunt. A dilated splenic vein (S) and the end-to-side anastomosis be- tween the portal vein and inferior vena cava (IVC) are noted.

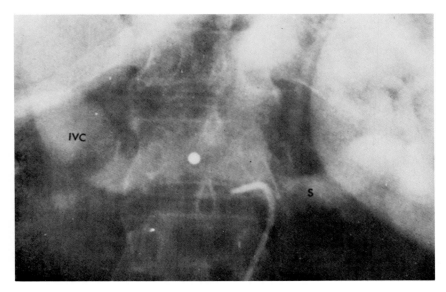

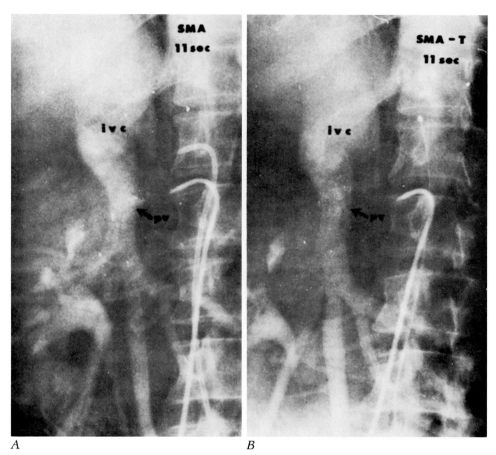

A   *B*

Figure 68-12. Portacaval shunt. (A) Patency of the portacaval shunt is demonstrated by the superior mesenteric portogram with filling of the inferior vena cava (*Ivc*) from the portal vein (*pv*). (B) Visualization of a patent portacaval shunt may be enhanced by reducing the dilution effect of nonopacified blood re-turning in the inferior vena cava. Tying tourniquets around both thighs accomplishes this by decreasing the venous return from the extremities. *SMA* = control superior mesenteric arteriogram; *SMA–T* = arteriogram with tourniquets around thighs. (From Bron and Fisher [10].)

are usually performed when both a portacaval and a splenorenal shunt have failed. Portacaval shunts may be demonstrated by either celiac (Fig. 68-10) or superior mesenteric arteriography (see Fig. 68-12A) when the spleen is intact, but, like splenorenal and mesocaval shunts, they are demonstrated only by the mesenteric artery route after splenectomy (Fig. 68-11).

The demonstration of shunt patency can be rendered difficult by the rapid return of non-opacified lower extremity blood in the inferior vena cava. To obviate this problem, one may attempt to reduce the rate of return by application of vein-occluding tourniquets to both thighs. This reduces the contrast dilution in the inferior vena cava and improves the visualization of shunt patency (Fig. 68-12). The injection of tolazoline, a vasodilator, into the superior

mesenteric artery just prior to angiography has been reported to accomplish the same result in the demonstration of portacaval shunts [35].

PATENT BUT NONVISUALIZED SPLENOPORTAL AXIS

When the splenic and portal veins are not vi-sualized by percutaneous splenoportography but the portosystemic collaterals are, it is generally assumed that the splenoportal axis is anatomically occluded. Shortly after the introduction of per-cutaneous splenoportography, however, it be-came apparent that, in a definite percentage of patients in whom splenic or portal vein occlusion had been suspected on the basis of nonvisualiza-tion by this technique, these vessels were anatomically patent at surgery or autopsy [27,

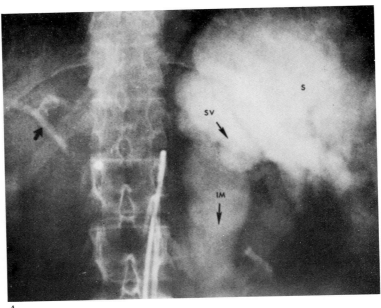

A

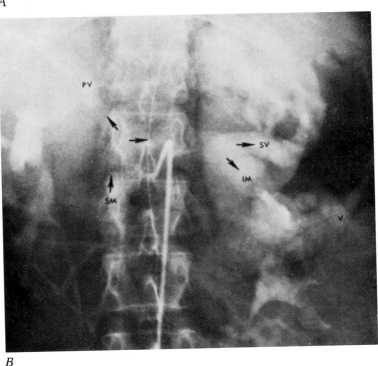

B

Figure 68-13. Splenic and/or portal vein thrombosis was suspected because a previous percutaneous splenoportogram had failed to demonstrate these vessels; calcification of the portal vein (*thick arrow*, A) was noted. (A) The celiac portogram demonstrates splenomegaly (*S*) and a dilated, tortuous splenic vein (*SV*) that empties into the inferior mesenteric vein (*IM*). Thin arrows indicate direction of blood flow. This study tends to confirm the conclusions of the percutaneous splenoportogram. (B) The superior mesenteric portogram, however, revealed that the splenic (*SV*) and portal (*PV*) veins were patent. The returning blood in the superior mesenteric vein (*SM*) flows antegrade in the portal vein but retrograde in the splenic and inferior mesenteric (*IM*) veins (*arrows*). Note the intestinal varix (*V*).

30]. The frequency of nonvisualization of the splenoportal axis by percutaneous splenoportography in the face of anatomic patency has been estimated at 17 percent [13] of such studies in patients who might benefit from a portacaval shunt. This serious limitation of percutaneous splenoportography must be recognized and cannot be lightly dismissed because the decision of whether to perform a portacaval shunt is usually based on the demonstration of a patent splenic and portal vein.

Several explanations have been advanced to account for this hemodynamic abnormality in portal hypertension. Ekman states that there is reversal of blood flow in the portal vein so that this vessel serves as a hepatic outflow tract rather than fulfills its normal function as an inflow tract [17]. Other investigators [2] claim that the bulk of the splenic blood flow is diverted into the portosystemic collaterals; thus, an insufficient quantity flows into the splenoportal axis to demonstrate these vessels. Burchell et al. [13], by measuring portal vein blood flows at surgery with an electromagnetic flowmeter, were unable to demonstrate any reversal in blood flow but found extremely low portal vein blood flows in patients with portal hypertension. Their observations tend to support the conclusion that the splenic and mesenteric venous blood flows were diverted through collaterals and thus caused nonvisualization of the splenic and portal veins.

In this situation of apparent splenoportal axis occlusion, arterial portography [11] can be very helpful in demonstrating that the vessels are patent. Because the superior mesenteric vein blood flow still maintains its hepatopetal direction despite severe elevation of portal pressure, arterial portography can demonstrate patency of these vessels in patients with portal hypertension and altered hemodynamics. In other words, the superior mesenteric vein, unlike the splenic and inferior mesenteric veins, does not generally function as a collateral channel to relieve portal hypertension. Thus, when the superior mesenteric artery is injected, the contrast returns in the vein and is distributed into the patent portal vessels and varices. Injection of contrast into the celiac axis or splenic artery in this situation will yield the same result as percutaneous splenoportography and will lead to a false conclusion of probable splenoportal vessel occlusion. The celiac injection (Fig. 68-13A) will demonstrate the marked portosystemic collaterals that accompany the hemodynamic alterations in the portal circulation. But injection of the superior mesenteric artery (Fig. 68-13B) will reveal the true nature of the alteration and will dispel any doubt concerning patency of the splenic and portal veins.

References

1. Abeatici, S., and Campi, L. Sur les possibilités de l'angiographie hépatique—la visualisation du système portal (recherches expérimentales). *Acta Radiol.* (Stockh.) 36:383, 1951.
2. Atkinson, M., Barnett, E., Sherlock, S., and Steiner, R. E. The clinical investigation of the portal circulation with special reference to portal venography. *Q. J. Med.* 24:77, 1955.
3. Bergstrand, I., and Ekman, C.-A. Percutaneous lieno-portal venography. *Acta Radiol.* (Stockh.) 47:269, 1957.
4. Blakemore, A. H., and Lord, J. W., Jr. Technique of using vitallium tubes in establishing portacaval shunts for portal hypertension. *Ann. Surg.* 122:476, 1945.
5. Boijsen, E., Ekman, C.-A., and Olin, T. Coeliac and superior mesenteric angiography in portal hypertension. *Acta Chir. Scand.* 126:315, 1963.
6. Boijsen, E., and Redman, H. C. Effect of bradykinin on celiac and superior mesenteric angiography. *Invest. Radiol.* 1:422, 1966.
7. Boijsen, E., and Redman, H. C. Effect of epinephrine on celiac and superior mesenteric angiography. *Invest. Radiol.* 2:184, 1967.
8. Bookstein, J. J., and Whitehouse, W. M. Splenoportography. *Radiol. Clin. North Am.* 2:447, 1964.
9. Bron, K. M. Selective visceral and total abdominal arteriography via the left axillary artery in the older age group. *AJR* 97:432, 1966.
10. Bron, K. M., and Fisher, B. Arterial portography: Indications and technique. *Surgery* 61:137, 1967.
11. Bron, K. M., Jackson, F. C., Haller, J., Perez-Stable, E., Eisen, H. B., and Poller, S. The value of selective arteriography in demonstrating portal and splenic vein patency following nonvisualization by splenoportography. *Radiology* 85:448, 1965.
12. Bron, K. M., Riley, R. R., and Girdany, B. R. Pediatric arteriography in abdominal and extremity lesions: Clinical experience, indications and technic. *Radiology* 92:1241, 1969.
13. Burchell, A. R., Moreno, A. H., Panke, W. F., and Rousselot, L. M. Some limitations of splenic portography. *Ann. Surg.* 162:981, 1965.
14. Child, C. G., III, O'Sullivan, W. D., Payne, M. A., and McClure, R. D., Jr. Portal venography: Preliminary report. *Radiology* 57:691, 1951.

15. Cioffi, C. M., Ruzicka, F. F., Jr., Carillo, F. J., and Gould, H. R. Enhanced visualization of the portal system using phentolamine and isoproterenol in combination. *Radiology* 108:43, 1973.

16. Danford, R. O., and Davidson, A. J. The use of glucagon as a vasodilator in visceral angiography. *Radiology* 93:173, 1969.

17. Ekman, C.-A. Portal hypertension, diagnosis and surgical treatment. *Acta Chir. Scand.* [Suppl.] 222, 1957.

18. Figley, M. M. Splenoportography: Some advantages and disadvantages. *AJR* 80:313, 1958.

19. Folin, J. Complications of percutaneous femoral catheterization for renal angiography. *Radiologe* 8:190, 1968.

20. Halpern, M. Percutaneous transfemoral arteriography. *AJR* 92:918, 1964.

21. Herlinger, H. Arterioportography. *Clin. Radiol.* 29:255, 1978.

22. Jonsson, K., Wallace, S., Jacobson, E. D., Anderson, J. H., Zornoza, J., and Granmayeh, M. The use of prostaglandin E₁ for enhanced visualization of the splanchnic circulation. *Radiology* 125:373, 1977.

23. Kogutt, M. S., and Jander, H. P. Splenoportography—a valuable diagnostic technic revisited. *South. Med. J.* 70:1210, 1977.

24. Kuroyangi, Y., Takagi, H., and Imanaga, H. Significance of selective arteriographic patterns in the celiac axis and superior mesenteric artery in portal hypertension. *Am. J. Surg.* 132:664, 1976.

25. Lang, E. K. A survey of the complications of percutaneous retrograde arteriography. *Radiology* 81:257, 1963.

26. Leger, L. Phlébographie portale par injection splénique intra-parenchymateuse. *Mem. Acad. Chir.* (Paris) 77:712, 1951.

27. Leger, L. L'inversion du courant portal—les fausses images d'obstacle à la circulation sur le tronc porte. *Presse Med.* 64:1189, 1956.

28. Levine, E. Preoperative angiographic assessment of portal venous hypertension. *S. Afr. Med. J.* 52:103, 1977.

29. Moore, G. E., and Bridenbaugh, R. B. Portal venography. *Surgery* 28:827, 1950.

30. Moreno, A. H., Burchell, A. R., Reddy, R. V., Steen, J. A., Panke, W. F., and Nealon, T. F. Spontaneous reversal of portal blood flow. *Ann. Surg.* 181:346, 1975.

31. Nebesar, R. A., and Pollard, J. J. Portal venography by selective arterial catheterization. *AJR* 97:477, 1966.

32. Ödman, P. Percutaneous selective angiography of the coeliac artery. *Acta Radiol. [Suppl.]* (Stockh.) 159, 1958.

33. Panke, W. F., Bradley, E. G., Moreno, A. H., Ruzicka, F. F., Jr., and Rousselot, L. M. Technique, hazards and usefulness of percutaneous splenic portography. *J.A.M.A.* 169:1032, 1959.

34. Pollard, J. J., and Nebesar, R. A. Catheterization of the splenic artery for portal venography. *N. Engl. J. Med.* 271:234, 1964.

35. Redman, H. C., Reuter, S. R., and Miller, W. J. Improvement of superior mesenteric and portal vein visualization with tolazoline. *Invest. Radiol.* 4:24, 1969.

36. Rigler, L. G., Olfelt, P. C., and Krumbach, R. W. Roentgen hepatography by injection of a contrast medium into the aorta. *Radiology* 60:363, 1953.

37. Rousselot, L. M., Ruzicka, F. F., Jr., and Doehmer, G. A. Portal venography via portal and percutaneous splenic routes: Anatomical and clinical studies. *Surgery* 34:557, 1953.

38. Ruzicka, F. F., Jr., and Rossi, P. Arterial portography: Patterns of venous flow. *Radiology* 92:777, 1969.

39. Seldinger, S. I. Catheter replacement of needle in percutaneous arteriography: New technique. *Acta Radiol.* (Stockh.) 39:368, 1953.

40. Weitzman, J. J., and Stanley, P. Splenoportography in the pediatric age group. *J. Pediatr. Surg.* 13:707, 1978.

41. Whipple, A. O. The problem of portal hypertension in relation to the hepatosplenopathies. *Ann. Surg.* 128:449, 1945.

42. Widrich, W. C., Nordahl, D. L., and Robbins, A. H. Contrast enhancement of the mesenteric and portal veins using intra-arterial papaverine. *AJR* 121:374, 1974.

5. Mesenteric Angiography

69

Superior Mesenteric Angiography

ERIK BOIJSEN

Modern, noninvasive methods, i.e., ultrasonography and computed tomography (CT), will not have the great impact on the diagnosis of bowel disease that they have had on the diagnosis of diseases of other abdominal organs. Similarly, while improvements in double-contrast techniques have certainly increased the accuracy with which intestinal lesions are diagnosed, these methods only rarely give clearcut evidence of extension of disease in the bowel wall or in the mesentery.

Angiography of the mesenteric arteries can supply important information in addition to that provided by the conventional methods. Angiography should therefore always be considered in patients in whom conventional methods have failed to explain symptoms referring to the bowel or when obscure findings are present in small and large bowel series. Vascular lesions as a cause or consequence of intestinal disease are not recognized as often as they should be. It is therefore the radiologist's responsibility to inform his clinical colleagues about the potential of angiography in a given situation.

During the decade that has passed since superior mesenteric angiography was discussed in the previous edition of *Angiography* [36] many important contributions to the field have been made. The results of extensive work on ischemic bowel disease, highlighted by Scott Boley and his co-workers in a 1971 book [56], have been followed by significant studies indicating a relationship between early angiography and intraarterial therapy and improved prognosis. Another area in which superior mesenteric angiography with intraarterial therapy has found application is in acute gastrointestinal hemorrhage; Stanley Baum and his collaborators [22, 23, 269] initiated an intense clinical research program that is still going on. This chapter is intended to show the central role superior mesenteric angiography has taken in the diagnosis of intestinal disease, with the exception of gastrointestinal hemorrhage.

Anatomy

Anatomic and topographic studies of the blood supply of the small and large bowel through dissection, corrosion, and arteriography of autopsy specimens have extensively demonstrated the normal variations of the superior mesenteric artery [18, 19, 94, 125, 168, 238, 246, 306, 325, 353]. However, the anatomic studies cannot re-

1623

place a well-documented analysis of a series of normal superior mesenteric angiograms, especially when correlations are made to dissection studies [12, 263].

ARTERIES

The extensive work of Michels et al. [246, 263] provides detailed information on the anatomy of the superior mesenteric artery. The following description is based mainly on their work.

The superior mesenteric artery originates from the anterior aspect of the aorta at the level of the twelfth thoracic to the second lumbar vertebral bodies [94]. It arises 1 to 20 mm below the origin of the celiac artery. Rarely, the superior mesenteric artery arises from the celiac artery as a celiomesenteric trunk. The first part of the superior mesenteric artery is immediately posterior to the body of the pancreas and can be surrounded by this organ when the uncinate process extends medially.

The width of the main stem varies from 6 to 16 mm [246] or from 8.0 to 15.5 mm [94]. At angiography the width of the artery has been observed to be 8 to 10 mm [274], 5 to 13 mm [373], and 6.7 to 12.3 mm (mean 9.5) [42]. The slightly lower figures found at angiography may depend on the fact that the measurements were made in the anteroposterior projection. In this view the first part of the superior mesenteric artery is not observed because the vessel runs more or less parallel to the central ray. Hearn [178] found in a small series of angiographic studies that the artery normally coursed in a 45- to 60-degree angle to the aorta. I have often observed a 90-degree angle. The course of the first part of the superior mesenteric artery depends mainly on the amount of adipose tissue in the abdomen.

Certain anatomic landmarks are seen at superior mesenteric angiography, and they should always be defined (Fig. 69-1). These are the inferior pancreaticoduodenal artery, the jejunal arteries, the ileal arteries, and the ileocolic artery. Less often found but usually present are the right and the middle colic arteries. Finally, the hepatic, pancreatic, and gastric arteries may occasionally arise from the superior mesenteric artery.

Inferior Pancreaticoduodenal Artery

This vessel arises either from the main stem or from the first jejunal artery. It may arise as a single artery or as one anterior and one posterior branch with separate origins. When arising from the first jejunal artery, it passes behind the superior mesenteric artery; when directly from the superior mesenteric artery, it passes from the right side directly to the duodenum and pancreas. An intercommunicating arterial arcade between the inferior pancreaticoduodenal artery and the first jejunal artery, according to Michels et al. [246], is present in approximately 60 percent of individuals. This arcade, which supplies the fourth part of the duodenum, represents an important anastomotic arcade in occlusive disease.

Jejunal and Ileal Arteries

These vessels vary in number and size. Because there is no distinct anatomic border between the jejunum and the ileum, there is no way to decide where the jejunal arteries end and the ileal arteries begin. As a general rule, it is simplest to regard those arteries that arise from the superior mesenteric artery before the origin of the ileocolic artery as jejunal arteries, and those distal to this origin as ileal arteries. The jejunal arteries number between 2 and 7, and the ileal arteries between 7 and 17, not including those supplying the terminal ileum. The latter is supplied by 3 to 15 branches originating from the ileal branch of the ileocolic artery. This ileal branch anastomoses directly with the distal part of the superior mesenteric artery forming a distal arcade (Fig. 69-1).

The presence of intraarterial arcades is characteristic of the mesenteric circulation. The number of arcades varies at different levels from

Figure 69-1. Angiomatous lesion of the cecum in a ▶ 55-year-old man with melena and anemia for 3 months. Gastrointestinal studies were normal. (A) At superior mesenteric arteriography a 10-×-10-mm area of the cecum showed an abnormal blood supply with wide, tortuous arteries and early shunting to the veins (lower arrows). Observe the anatomic landmarks: the posterior inferior pancreaticoduodenal artery (1a) arises from aberrant branch of the right hepatic artery. The anterior inferior pancreaticoduodenal artery (1b) arises from the first jejunal artery (2). Four jejunal (2) and eight ileal arteries (3) are observed. The ileocolic artery divides into ileal (4a) and colic (4b) branches. A short arcade (upper arrow) is present between the two arteries. The right colic artery (5) arises from the middle colic artery (6). (B and C) After injection of 5 μg of norepinephrine, a repeat angiogram demonstates a general decrease in width of all arteries, but the dysplastic lesion is not affected by the drug and is therefore better observed.

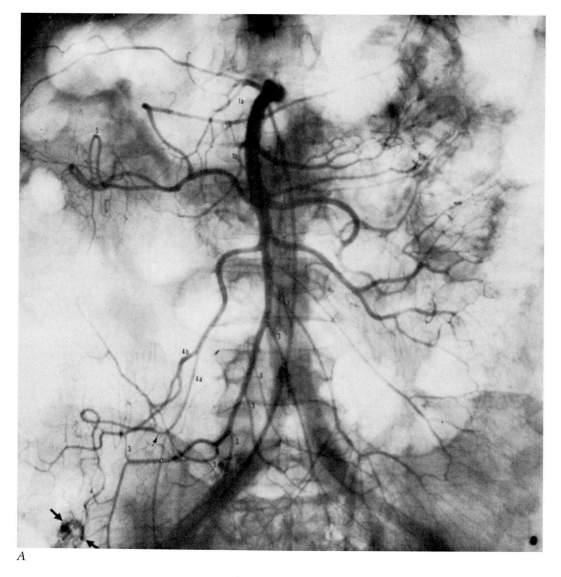

A

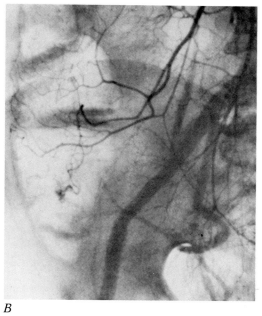

B

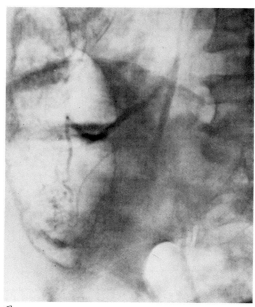

C

1625

one to five; the largest number is observed in the midportion of the small bowel, the smallest in the terminal ileum. The long vasa recta of the small bowel arise from the last arcades, which are close to the mesenteric border. These vasa recta pass to the anterior and posterior surface of the bowel wall, but in man they usually do not communicate at the antimesenteric border because they penetrate the bowel wall and enter the submucosal layer earlier. The short vasa recta arising from the last arcade directly or branching from the long vasa enter the submucosa of the intestinal wall at its mesenteric border. A rich interarterial anastomotic network among the vasa recta is present in the small bowel wall, but the connections in the large bowel are poor [325]. Angiographically the vasa recta of the jejunum appear wider and more tortuous than those of the ileum (Fig. 69-1). Usually the width of the ileal arteries decreases distally, and the smallest vessels are observed in the terminal ileum.

Because of the large number of intercommunicating arcades in the mesenteric circulation, there is, as in the large bowel, an arterial channel running parallel to the mesenteric border. The vasa recta take their origin from this channel. It was first described by Dwight [128] and has the same importance in maintaining the viability of the small intestine as the marginal artery of Drummond has for the large intestine. The two channels communicate via the arcades in the terminal ileum and thus form an uninterrupted pathway from the duodenum to the rectum. Because these channels can be demonstrated with angiography and represent important collateral pathways in vascular disease or after surgery, they should be identified at superior mesenteric angiography. Since there are few communications between the vasa recta of the large bowel, preservation of the marginal artery is essential in colonic resection [168].

Ileocolic Artery

This is the only constant artery from the right side of the superior mesenteric artery. It supplies the terminal ileum, the appendix, the cecum, and the proximal part of the ascending colon. Distal extension of supply may occur when the right colic artery is absent or originates from the ileocolic artery.

The ileocolic artery divides into one colic and one ileal artery. Usually there is an ileocolic arcade between them. The ileal artery communicates directly with the superior mesenteric ar-

tery. The terminal ileum has a precarious blood supply because the arcade at the mesenteric border, the recurrent ileal artery, is missing in 61 percent of individuals, and in 16 percent there is a 3- to 5-cm segment of distal ileum without vasa recta [246]. At arteriography of autopsy specimens this area is hard to fill adequately [306]. At superior mesenteric angiography the vasa recta of the terminal ileum are difficult or impossible to define, and the accumulation of contrast medium in the wall is often insignificant. With magnification techniques, however, more information is obtained about these small vessels [20].

Right Colic Artery

This vessel has a variable origin from the superior mesenteric, middle colic, or ileocolic artery. It supplies the ascending colon and hepatic flexure.

Middle Colic Artery

This vessel supplies the transverse colon. It usually arises from the first part of the superior mesenteric artery at the level of the first jejunal artery but may originate more distally or from the celiac artery. An accessory middle colic artery is occasionally present. The left branch of the middle colic artery is in direct communication with the left colic artery from the inferior mesenteric artery. This channel is the most important collateral in the mesenteric circulation. It proceeds in a proximal direction as the right branch of the middle colic artery, the right colic artery, and the ileocolic artery. A second collateral pathway is the marginal artery of Drummond, which represents the arcades along the mesenteric border of the colon. This marginal artery is usually not complete because the vasa recta of the transverse colon often arise directly from the middle colic artery. Riolan's artery is a third anastomosis between the superior and inferior mesenteric arteries. It is a short, direct connection running retroperitoneally from the root

Figure 69-2. Occlusion of celiac axis and marked concentric stenosis of the superior mesenteric artery in a 31-year-old woman with postprandial pain and malabsorption. (A and B) At lumbar aortography the arterial constrictions are observed, as well as collateral circulation from the inferior mesenteric artery (*lower arrow*). Retroperitoneal collaterals are present to the left of the aorta (*upper arrows*). (C) At superior mesenteric angiography the complete celiac arterial system is contrast-filled via wide pancreaticoduodenal arcades. The stenosis is not observed in this view.

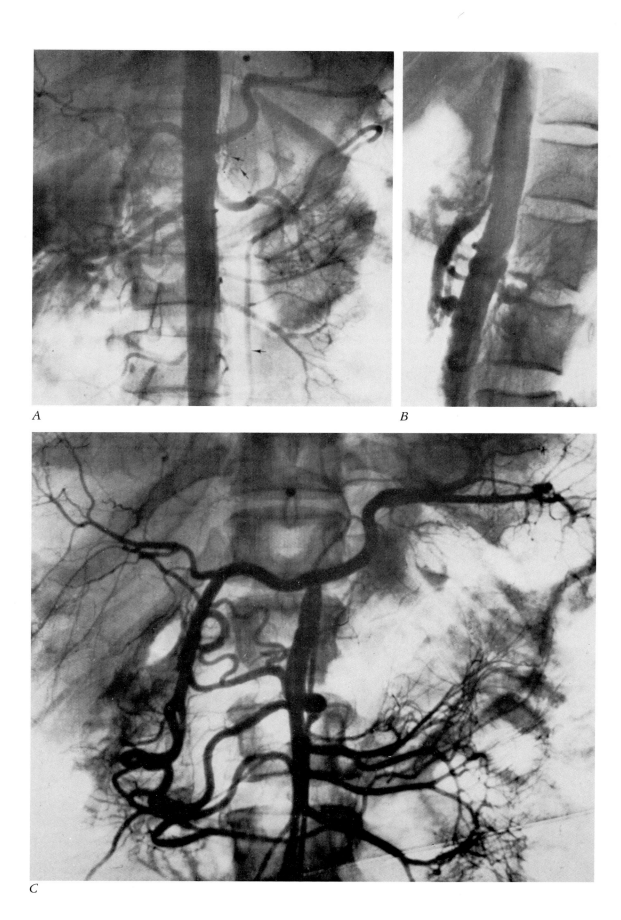

A

B

C

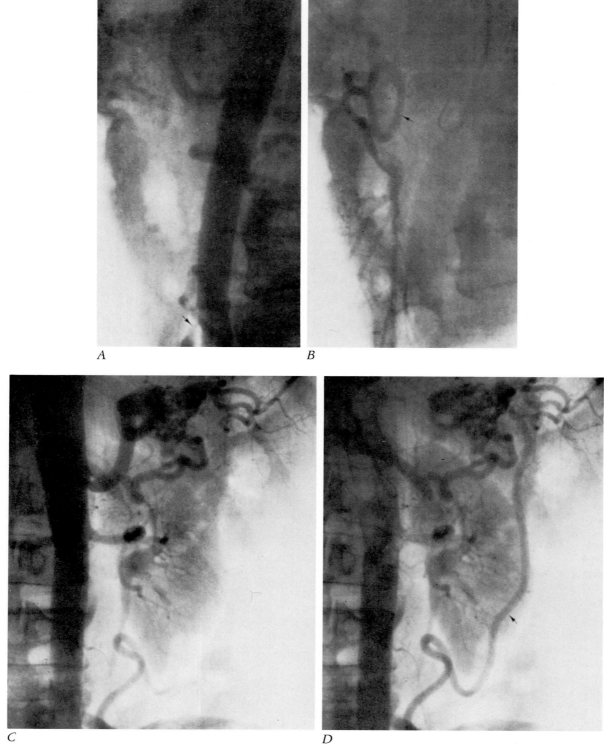

A   *B*

C   *D*

Figure 69-3. Complete occlusion of the superior mesenteric artery and of the common hepatic artery at its origin from the celiac artery and marked stenosis of the celiac and inferior mesenteric arteries in a 58-year-old man who had no gastrointestinal symptoms. Aortography in lateral (A and B) and left posterior oblique (C, D, and E) projections was performed after percutaneous puncture of the left axillary artery in order to demonstrate patency of previous operation for occlusion at the aortic bifurcation. Wide pancreatic arterial collaterals from the splenic artery supply the hepatic artery. The wide left and middle colic arteries (*arrows* in B, D, and E) supply the superior mesenteric artery from the stenotic inferior mesenteric artery (*arrow* in A).

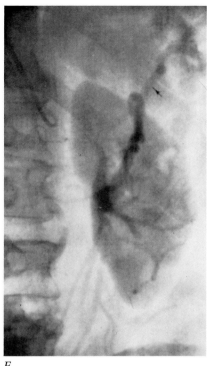

E

of the superior mesenteric artery or one of its primary branches to the inferior mesenteric artery or one of its branches [19].

The common hepatic or, more often, the right hepatic artery may originate from the superior mesenteric artery. According to Michels et al. [246] this occurs in 16 percent of individuals, which finding is in agreement with angiographic observations [221, 222, 358, 373]. Not uncommonly seen are the dorsal pancreatic, transverse pancreatic, and gastroduodenal arteries with their origin from the first part of the superior mesenteric artery.

Collateral Arteries

"A knowledge of collateral circulation is of fundamental importance in surgical interference with the intestinal blood supply" [246]. The same is true for the proper understanding of the angiographic study. More than 50 collateral pathways are listed by Michels et al. in the small and large bowels, and for complete information the reader is referred to their work [246]. In addition to those arcades in the mesenteric circulation mentioned previously, the pancreatic and pancreaticoduodenal arteries serve as collaterals in stenosis or occlusion of the main stem of the superior mesenteric artery (Figs. 69-2, 69-3). The

collateral arteries from the inferior mesenteric artery are also important in this type of lesion. Further connections are the epiploic arteries, at least in more distal occlusion of the superior mesenteric artery. Retroperitoneal parietal arteries, including renal capsular arteries, inferior phrenic arteries, and arteries supplying the adipose tissue of the mesentery, are also collateral vessels that may take part in the bowel supply in vascular occlusion [306, 328, 364] (see Fig. 69-2).

VEINS

The superior mesenteric vein follows the course of the superior mesenteric artery. The veins following the vasa recta are usually duplicated. At superior mesenteric angiography the mesenteric veins are seldom well demonstrated unless a lesion is present or special techniques are used to delineate them.

Physiologic Considerations

Superior mesenteric blood flow is two to three times greater than blood flow to one renal artery [362]. The total capacity of the splanchnic circulation, of which the superior mesenteric artery conveys the main part, is as great as the entire blood volume [185]. The regulation of the mesenteric circulation is complex. While humoral, neurogenic, and cardiovascular factors play the dominant roles, autoregulation and arteriovenous shunting are also important components of this control process that must be recognized in order to understand the variations in splanchnic blood flow in normal and pathologic situations [185, 188, 396].

In vascular shock the size of the vascular bed is markedly reduced [106, 153, 219]. Vasoactive substances administered by intravenous or intraarterial injection cause a complex response in the superior mesenteric vascular bed that depends on autoregulatory escape and on the tone of the intestinal wall [167, 185]. The effects of such substances have in part been confirmed by intraarterial injections in combination with superior mesenteric angiography [38, 44, 45, 98, 268, 270, 297, 300, 322, 350, 384]. Bowel distention and increased intraluminal pressure have a profound influence on intestinal blood flow [51, 266]; at angiography a decreased flow and arteriovenous shunting are observed [20].

Technique and Complications

Originally, selective angiography was performed with antegrade technique after cutdown of the brachial artery [32, 253]. The retrograde technique with percutaneous puncture of the femoral artery, as recommended by Ödman [273], has replaced the antegrade method. Only in selected cases, when the femoral technique has failed because of advanced atherosclerosis, is the antegrade method used today; percutaneous puncture of the axillary artery is then employed [34, 175, 326] (Fig. 69-3). A thin-walled red Ödman-Ledin catheter (inner diameter, 1.4 mm; outer diameter, 2.2 mm) is used irrespective of the percutaneous route taken [37]. Ödman [273] originally recommended a larger, thick-walled catheter, but with the development of image amplification and television there is no longer any need for this type of catheter.

The optimal type and amount of contrast media have been extensively considered because serious complications in terms of bowel necrosis have been observed both clinically and experimentally [104, 147, 163, 166, 239, 336]. Initially, out of concern for possible bowel injury, small amounts of dilute contrast media were commonly used, although the information provided was incomplete. Because no complications were observed, larger doses and more concentrated contrast media were used. A reevaluation of previous complications suggested that they were largely caused by the technique employed and the effects of the earlier, more toxic contrast agents. The experimentally produced bowel necroses seemed to be the result of temporary vascular occlusion that permitted prolonged contact of the toxic contrast medium with the intima. A repeat experimental study could not reproduce the toxic effects when the superior mesenteric artery was not occluded by the catheter, even when larger contrast doses were used [299]. Temporary occlusion of the superior mesenteric artery with a balloon catheter during contrast-medium injection did not damage the bowel [283]. However, electron microscopic analysis has shown mitochondrial changes caused by contrast media injected into the superior mesenteric artery of the rabbit, suggesting damage to the intracellular enzyme production [259]. The significant elevation of SGOT and alkaline phosphatase observed in dogs following contrast injection suggests possible liver damage in these animals [61].

The present clinical use of 40 to 50 cc of a 76 percent solution of methylglucamine salts of metrizoate, diatrizoate, or iothalamate has not caused any complications, even when the dose is repeated. It should be delivered at a rate of 7 to 10 cc per second. The transit of the contrast medium to the veins is followed by a series of exposures in the anteroposterior projection for at least 20 seconds. For complete evaluation of the superior mesenteric artery, a short series with approximately 15 cc of contrast medium in the lateral view is necessary. Before the full dose of contrast medium is delivered, a test injection with 10 cc should be performed under fluoroscopic control in order to avoid subintimal injection. Despite this precaution subintimal deposition of contrast medium may occur, but in my experience it has not had any severe sequelae. After translumbar aortography, however, several serious accidents with bowel necrosis or paralytic ileus have been reported [164, 243, 293, 294, 372, 374].

When there is simultaneous injection into the celiac and superior mesenteric arteries, the flow of the contrast medium is commonly observed to be slower through the superior mesenteric artery than through the splenic or hepatic arteries [35]. The reason is not clear, and the variance is contradictory to the physiologic findings of superior mesenteric flow. The contrast medium may cause an initial vasoconstriction in the superior mesenteric arterioles, which may also explain the usually poor opacification of the superior mesenteric vein. Or it may be that the deformed red blood cells have greater difficulty in passing through the mesenteric vascular bed as compared with that of the splenic or hepatic. The prolonged contact of the hypertonic contrast medium with the capillaries results in an increase in intravascular fluid with consequent dilution of the medium. The response to selective injection will within 20 seconds be vasodilation with increased mesenteric flow lasting for 15 minutes [343]. Thus, when a larger amount of contrast medium is used and the injection period is markedly extended, the vasodilating effect will be dominant. The contrast medium will be less diluted and the venous information consequently enhanced [226, 349].

There is no objection to single doses of larger amounts of contrast medium than were just recommended, but a complete angiographic study usually includes repeated injections into the superior mesenteric artery and also into the celiac axis. The total dose of contrast medium may then be too high. There is no defined upper limit to the total amounts of contrast medium that can be given to a patient over a period of 1 hour. My present policy is not to exceed a single dose of 1 cc per kilogram of body weight and to keep the total amount given to less than 3 cc per kilogram of body weight.

Pharmacoangiography

Pharmacoangiography is now a well-established method and should be used in the mesenteric circulation whenever increased information about the mesenteric vein is required.

Vasodilation has been employed to improve the visualization of, for example, angiodysplastic lesions of the bowel [344]. Various vasodilating drugs have been utilized. The best and most consistent results are obtained with bradykinin and tolazoline [44, 298, 300], but prostaglandin E_1 and F_2-alpha, isoproterenol, secretin, glucagon, cholecystokinin, and extended epinephrine infusion have been used with good results [96, 98, 111, 112, 116, 193, 297, 298, 349, 365, 366, 384]. Injection of 20 to 30 cc of normal saline containing 5 cc of 2 percent Xylocaine immediately prior to the injection of contrast medium is said to cause good opacification of the superior mesenteric vein [182].

Improved venous opacification may also be achieved when superior mesenteric angiography is performed during digestion [227]. The most reliable technique, not yet fully tested in humans, is to inject contrast medium after balloon occlusion of the superior mesenteric artery with release of the occlusion at the end of the contrast medium injection [283, 379]. Higher venous concentrations of contrast have also been achieved experimentally by balloon occlusion of the celiac axis and contrast injection into the superior mesenteric artery [187].

Injection of 5 to 10 μg of bradykinin into the superior mesenteric artery within 30 seconds prior to angiography has been, in my experience with more than 1,000 patients, a reliable and safe method for demonstrating the superior mesenteric and portal veins. While the bradykinin produces such an increased flow that arterial detail is lost, it usually causes a marked accumulation of contrast medium in the bowel wall, giving an "intestinogram," which can aid in demonstrating local abnormalities of the gut.

Because bradykinin is not widely available, tolazoline is sometimes substituted. Tolazoline will enhance the venous opacification to approximately the same extent as bradykinin. My present technique for obtaining maximum information about the venous system is to inject 25 mg tolazoline followed by 70 to 80 cc of the contrast medium, beginning at a slow rate of 2 to 3 cc per second and then increasing slowly to a rate of 10 cc per second. With this technique, advantage is taken of the dilating effect of both tolazoline and the contrast medium (Fig. 69-4). Tolazoline, however, may also be difficult to obtain. In the future, it is likely that prostaglandins will be available for use in this technique.

In order to enhance arterial detail and to differentiate an inflammatory lesion from a tumor, *vasoconstrictive substances* may be helpful [36, 38, 45, 46, 133, 157, 192, 197, 250, 350] (Fig. 69-5). Although no consistent advantage of this method has been demonstrated, it appears that the vessels of an active inflammatory lesion are more susceptible to constriction than are normal or tumor vessels.

Other methods of superior mesenteric angiography have also been used, including operative mesenteric angiography [230, 240, 329]. Because of the complicated procedures required during operation and the lack of serial films, the information afforded is less than that of conventional superior mesenteric angiography despite the better arterial detail of operative angiography.

Routine superior mesenteric angiography does not always necessitate administration of drugs prior to contrast-medium injection. On the contrary, in a routine study a small amount of contrast medium (20–30 cc) injected at a rate of 8 to 10 cc per second without any previous injection of drugs will often give the required information. A series of films covering about 20 seconds should be taken with a film speed of two frames per second for 5 seconds, one frame per second for 5 seconds, and one frame every other second for 10 seconds.

The arteriogram contains morphologic as well as functional information about the splanchnic vasculature; therefore, the emptying time of the arteries as well as the appearance time of the veins should be recorded. There is a sequential arterial emptying of contrast medium from the proximal jejunal to the distal ileal and colic arteries [40, 44, 45, 334]. The appearance times for the veins are approximately in the same sequence. The contrast medium of the jejunal, ileal, and colic arteries disappears within 2 seconds after the end of injection, and the veins of

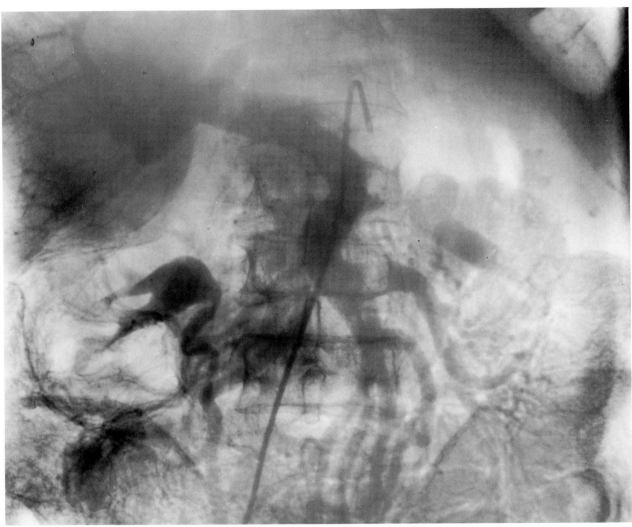

A

Figure 69-4. Venous phase of superior mesenteric angiogram after 25 mg tolazoline and 60 cc contrast medium were injected into the artery. (A) Normal venogram. (B) Portal hypertension with dilatation and reversal of flow in inferior mesenteric vein (*arrows*) in a patient with cholangiocarcinoma infiltrating the portal vein in the hilus of the liver.

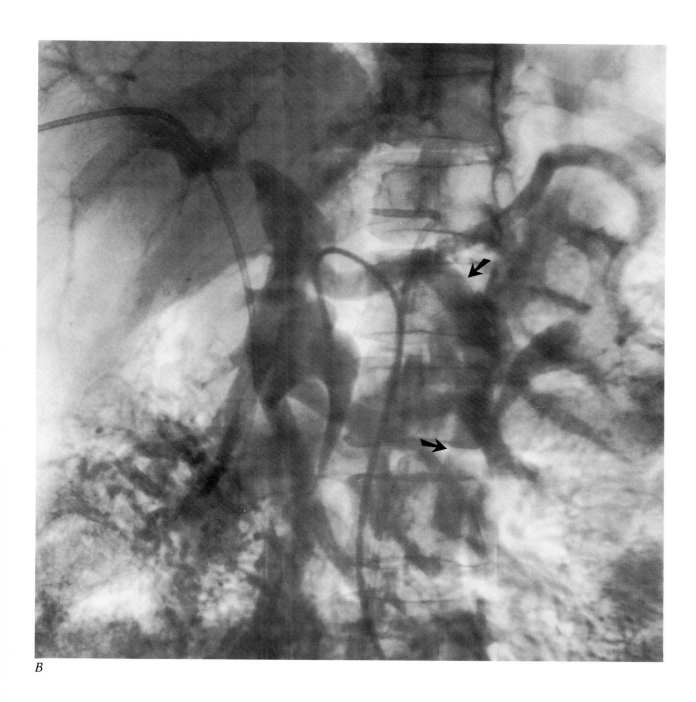

B

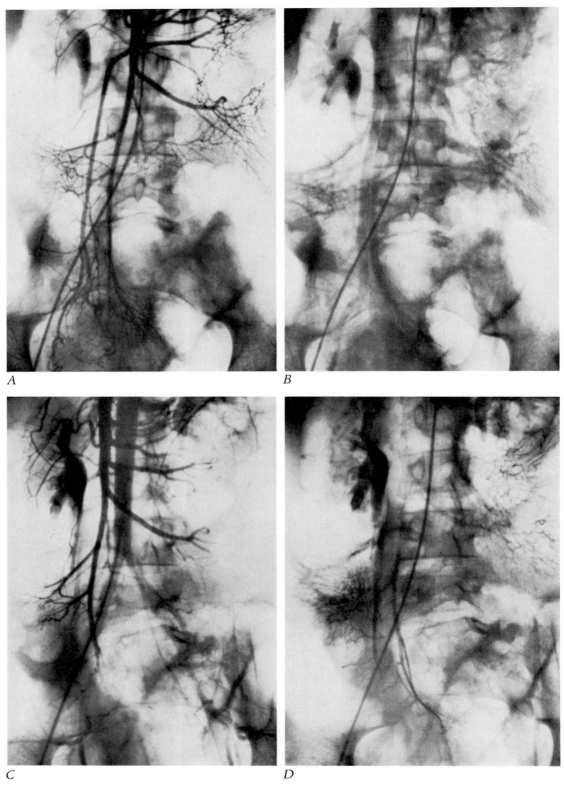

A

B

C

D

Figure 69-5. Granulomatous enterocolitis of terminal ileum and cecum in a 17-year-old boy. (A and B) At conventional superior mesenteric angiography, irregular, stenosed arteries are present within the field of supply of the ileocolic and distal superior mesenteric arteries. There is marked hypervascularization with early transit of contrast medium to the veins, especially in the terminal ileum but also in the remaining part of the small bowel. (C and D) After injection of 1 IU of vasopressin into the superior mesenteric artery, angiography reveals marked constriction of all peripheral branches, but it is most pronounced in the region of the terminal ileum.

the small bowel usually appear within 8 to 10 seconds after the start of the injection. Abnormalities in the sequence of filling and emptying of mesenteric arteries and veins can be a guide to the diagnosis of a variety of bowel disorders [40, 46, 47, 60, 334].

Mesenteric Vascular Insufficiency

Stenosis or occlusion of the main stem or branches of the superior mesenteric artery produces symptoms of various types and severity. The results of surgical correction have been improving, in large part because angiography is being employed with greater frequency. The main clinical problem is to know when the patient has a vascular insufficiency and, if it is acute, to suspect a lesion early enough for adequate diagnosis and treatment. Angiography is today the only method by which a reliable diagnosis can be made and is therefore an important part in the understanding of the morphologic and functional events that occur.

ACUTE OCCLUSION

Acute obstruction of the superior mesenteric artery or its branches causes symptoms that are difficult to interpret clinically. Diagnosis is therefore likely to be delayed, with serious consequences [235, 375].

Bowel ischemia may be due to acute arterial occlusion (thrombosis or embolization), venous obstruction, and "nonocclusive ischemia." The clinical symptomatology is basically the same for all three causes and depends mainly on the duration of the ischemia. Since the therapeutic approach is contingent on whether or not an occlusion is present, the specific cause should be defined as precisely as possible. Even if plain films and barium studies may suggest a vascular catastrophe, angiography is the only method that will provide information of importance for therapeutic activity. Although the patients are usually in poor general condition, angiography will not cause any additional risks to the patient or any essential delay in the therapy [3, 4, 386, 389, 392].

Mortality is extremely high in this disease. Abnormalities are observed in the mucosa within minutes of the occlusion, followed by extensive necrosis with submucosal edema and hemorrhage. In the literature the maximum time delay between onset of occlusion and operation for successful result varies. While it appears that irreversible damage to the bowel may occur within 12 hours of the occlusion [59], good results have been obtained in patients who had angiography and operation within 24 hours of the occlusion [201]. In the world literature there are few cases of successful removal of emboli or thrombi; in 1974 there were 49 out of 69 patients surviving this type of operation [28]. An aggressive clinical approach will, however, reveal more operable cases, consequently yielding a better outcome [201, 341, 342].

The *angiographic examination* should start with a lumbar aortogram in lateral and frontal projections in order to define the degree of aortic atherosclerosis and occlusions of the main stems and first branches of the splanchnic arteries. If the main stem of the superior mesenteric artery is patent, a superior mesenteric angiogram should be performed in frontal projection (Fig. 69-6).

The incidence of various causes of bowel ischemia varies in different series. The incidence of nonocclusive mesenteric infarction is recognized in 50 to 75 percent of patients with acute bowel ischemia, while venous thrombosis is rarely seen [29, 72, 276, 284, 386].

Acute arterial occlusion is caused by either an embolus or a thrombus (Fig. 69-6). The site of the occlusion observed at angiography may give some information about the cause, but in most cases angiography alone will not achieve a firm diagnosis [392]. As a rule, moderate to severe aortic atherosclerosis is associated with thrombotic occlusion, while minimal atherosclerosis strongly suggests embolic disease. Thrombosis is usually situated at the origin of the superior mesenteric artery, but branch thrombosis is frequently encountered in autopsy series [305].

Occlusion of multiple splanchnic and renal arteries speaks in favor of embolic disease. Embolic occlusion of the superior mesenteric artery is angiographically observed at the level of the middle colic artery or within the first 10 cm of the main stem [1, 3, 4, 82, 296, 392], but single or multiple emboli can occur in branches of the superior mesenteric artery [296]. Arteries proximal and distal to an embolic occlusion show marked constriction, and collateral flow may not be present [1, 3, 4, 286, 392]. Consequently, there is increased resistance to flow with delayed arterial visualization and decreased vascularity [60]. Ap-

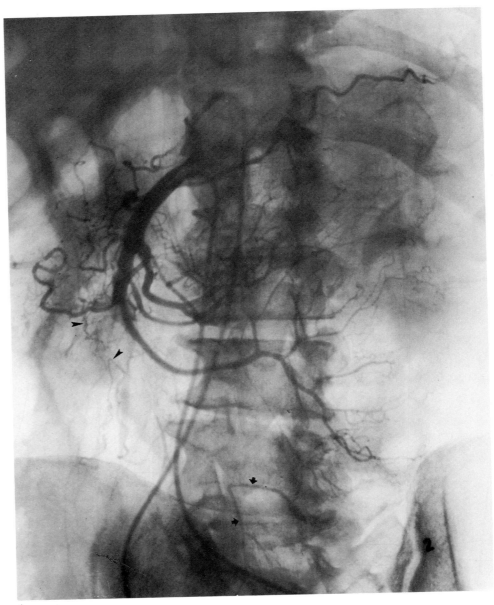

A

Figure 69-6. Short thrombosis of the superior mesenteric artery at the level of the third jejunal artery in a 77-year-old man with progressive abdominal pain during the last week. Marked atheromatosis was observed at lumbar aortography, but the first part of the superior mesenteric artery was patent. (A) At superior mesenteric angiography, collateral circulation to the distal jejunal and ileal arteries is shown to be incomplete and insufficient via arcades (*arrows*) or vessels in the mesentery (*arrowheads*). (B) At inferior mesenteric angiography, the right colon and distal small bowel are found to be supplied via the left colic–middle colic–right colic artery. At operation 50 cm of jejunum had to be removed because of partial necrosis in the wall.

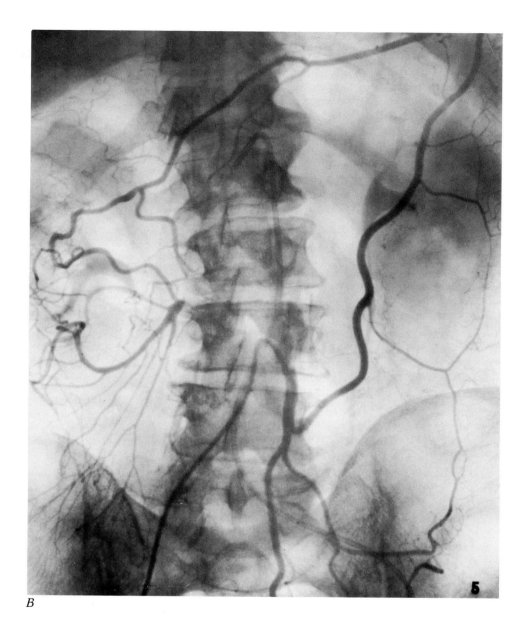

B

parently spasm does not occur immediately following embolization; in iatrogenic embolization it was never observed when angiography was performed soon after occlusion [211].

When present, the angiographic characteristics of the collateral circulation are the same as in chronic obliterative disease of the splanchnic arteries [25, 73, 74, 83, 103, 121, 159, 258, 261, 311, 328, 351]. If adequate collateral circulation is established in an acute occlusion, operation appears to be unnecessary.

Extensive experimental and clinical research has shown that the degree and extent of bowel damage depends largely on the duration of the occlusion and its site and extent [52, 62, 64, 65,

82, 195, 201, 211, 267, 292, 301, 304, 332]. An acute occlusion proximal to the origin of the middle colic artery may not cause any necrosis, and the result of surgery is good also in cases of ischemia [201]. The incidence of emboli is probably higher than reported, because large emboli may pass unnoticed and without symptoms in iatrogenic embolism [211] and in therapeutic embolism in patients with intestinal hemorrhage [63, 198, 375]. This is particularly the case for the small bowel when segmental arteries are occluded, and intentional occlusions of the large bowel arteries have caused necrosis [375]. Occlusion of arteries close to the bowel wall may thus not cause alarming symptoms but, nevertheless,

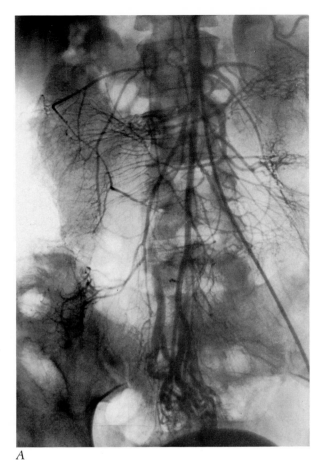

A

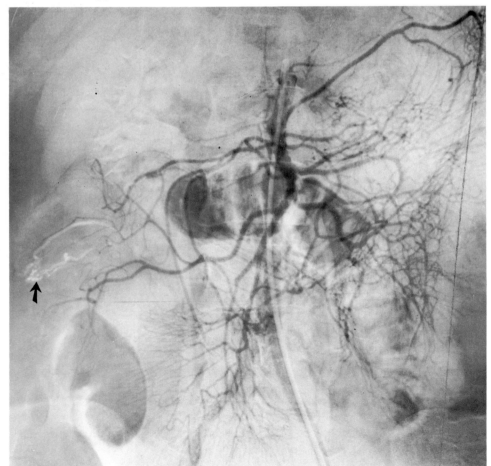

B

result in serious complications such as perforation, ulceration, stenosis, or hemorrhage depending on the extent of the vascular compromise (Fig. 69-7) [40, 301, 316, 331, 361, 363, 368, 394]. Stenosis of the bowel may later cause malabsorption or small bowel obstruction [52, 60, 177, 324, 333]. It is essential to realize that a patient with "intestinal angina" may be subject to acute occlusion of the superior mesenteric artery, be it by thrombosis or embolism [280]. About 50 percent of patients who have an acute infarction secondary to a thrombus had had previous symptoms of abdominal angina [27, 79]. The poor correlation between the incidence of stenosis of splanchnic arteries and intestinal angina is well known, but any patient with abdominal symptoms and arteriographic evidence of significant arterial obstruction should be considered a candidate for reconstructive surgery in order to prevent a later catastrophe [79, 386].

In patients with atrial fibrillation or myocardial infarction, the emboli usually originate from the heart. It has been suggested that the primary heart disease may favor a complicating spasm in the mesenteric circulation, thus decreasing the bowel perfusion, with a consequently greater risk of bowel necrosis [201, 211]. Paradoxical embolism to the superior mesenteric artery from venous thrombosis has also been observed [201]. Cholesterol embolism is another, perhaps too often overlooked, cause of occlusion of the mesenteric artery [279, 333].

Thrombosis of the superior mesenteric artery is most often secondary to the atheromatosis, but recent increased activity in vasopressin therapy has caused thrombosis of both arteries and veins in the mesenteric circulation [26, 307, 318].

In addition to embolus and thrombosis secondary to atherosclerosis, a wide variety of other disorders may cause acute occlusion of small mesenteric arteries. Mesenteric angiography can provide information about abnormalities due to lupus erythematosus, polyarteritis nodosa, rheumatoid disease, and other types of vasculitis [6, 75, 97, 108, 110, 139, 141, 282, 288, 289, 316, 332]. Intimal arterial hyperplasia and thrombus formation in small mesenteric arteries may also cause infarction [5, 81]. Bowel ischemia due to operation [316], catheterization [211], and trauma [216, 237] are other causes of vascular occlusions that can be defined by angiography.

It should be realized that occlusion of branches of the superior mesenteric artery can occur without causing any symptoms at all (Fig. 69-8) [36, 303].

Occlusion of the superior mesenteric vein may be secondary to hematologic or intraabdominal disease or to vasopressin infusion. In primary occlusion no obvious cause is found. The angiographic findings are constriction of superior mesenteric artery branches, delayed emptying, and absence of the venous phase [144, 158, 230, 234, 285, 291]. Preoperative phlebography will demonstrate the extension of a thrombus [30]. Vascular compromise—particularly venous, but also arterial—is noted in bowel intussusception, strangulated bowel obstruction, intestinal volvulus, and midgut malrotation. Clinical and experimental angiographic work has demonstrated the abnormal circulation [2, 86, 95, 191, 212, 242, 334]. Clinical as well as angiographic symptomatology may mimic occlusive or nonocclusive ischemia, leading to a wrong preoperative diagnosis. However, typical findings with an abnormal course of mesenteric vessels should direct the radiologist's attention to the lesions [86, 101, 191, 212, 335].

Nonocclusive mesenteric ischemia usually occurs in patients with low-flow syndromes due to myocardial insufficiency, hypotension, and low cardiac output [15, 31, 57, 106, 124, 134, 154, 160, 170, 184, 251, 390]. It is probably the commonest cause of bowel necrosis today. Damage to the bowel occurs despite patency of the major intestinal arteries and veins. The pathologic lesions are similar to those found in dogs dying of shock [124, 214, 219]. Enteritis gravis is another entity probably caused by shock and spasm in the peripheral branches of the superior mesenteric artery [84, 278, 391]. A severe pancreatitis may display features like those of nonocclusive ischemia [49, 392]. A persistent vasoconstriction is regarded as being responsible for bowel necrosis [342, 387], but a shunt mechanism in the bowel wall has also been claimed as the cause of nonocclusive ischemia [376]. Dig-

◀**Figure 69-7.** (A) Superior mesenteric angiography in a 24-year-old woman with repeated episodes of intestinal hemorrhage. An angiomatous lesion is present in the distal small bowel with early venous filling. At operation and histopathologic examination, an ischemic stricture with ulceration and thrombosed arteries in the wall of the bowel was found but no malformation. There were no further hemorrhages from the bowel, but reevaluation was made 4 years later because of hypertension. (B) At renal angiography an aneurysm was found on the renal artery, and repeated mesenteric angiography showed a dysplastic lesion in the right colon (subtraction film, *arrow*).

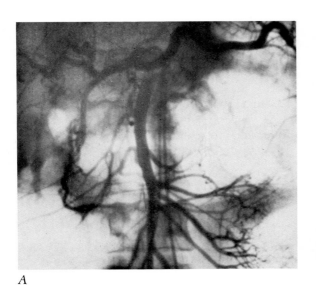

A

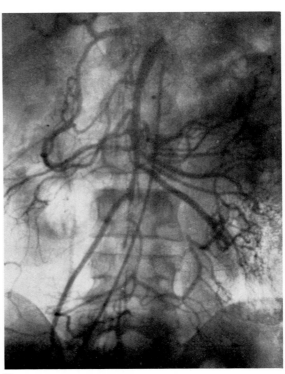

B

Figure 69-8. Thrombosis of the superior mesenteric artery in a man who at the age of 25, after an upper respiratory infection and recurrent fever, had arthritis in multiple joints. Weight loss and an elevated sedimentation rate indicated the need for celiac and superior mesenteric angiography. (A) Except for some irregular pancreatic arteries and moderately widened pancreaticoduodenal arcades, nothing abnormal was observed. After a period of improvement, hypertension and multiple pulmonary lesions appeared. With medical treatment the pulmonary lesions disappeared. At the age of 29 the patient was in good health, but he was continuously treated for hypertension. (B) Repeat superior mesenteric angiography was performed. The main stem was reduced in width and was occluded distal to the origin of the ileocolic artery. The ileum was supplied from peripheral arterial collaterals via jejunal and ileocolic arteries. Similar changes were present in the renal arteries. The patient had no symptoms from the gastrointestinal tract.

italis has a definite constrictive effect on the mesenteric circulation [356]. Since it is a common prescription, it may produce bowel necrosis, especially when given in too high a dose [370].

The angiographic findings vary. Usually, a generalized narrowing of the superior mesenteric tree is present with smooth tapering of jejunal and ileal branches. These arteries may also show a pattern of repetitive narrowings producing a beaded appearance (Fig. 69-9) [1, 3, 4, 11, 15, 36, 57, 228, 341, 342, 370, 392]. Such findings are, however, not present in all cases [392].

Early operation should not be performed because there is no vascular occlusion to correct and the degree and extent of bowel lesion are difficult to determine at an early stage [390]. Since the prognosis is extremely poor, many suggestions have been made for improving the circulation by intraarterial injection of vasodilating drugs [11, 36, 57, 169, 228, 276, 341, 342, 367]. The most successful therapy reported so far was achieved by the infusion of 30 to 60 mg of papaverine per hour for 16 to 24 hours [341, 342].

Ischemic colitis is a specific vascular disorder of the large bowel, usually present within the supply of the inferior mesenteric artery but often observed in the splenic flexure and sometimes more proximally [54, 55, 393]. Plain film and barium enema examination provide important information on its site and extent [55, 135, 233, 331, 340, 377]. Angiography is of less importance because it does not provide a therapeutic implication [393]. The pathoanatomic abnormalities are mucosal necrosis and submucosal edema and hemorrhage [257]. Compared with other types of ischemic disease, ischemic colitis has a relatively

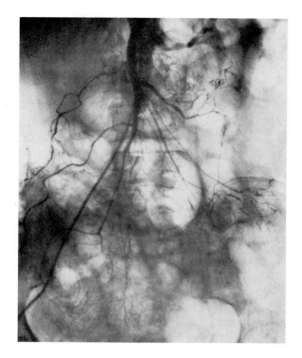

Figure 69-9. Hemorrhagic infarction of the small bowel in a 77-year-old woman who had had severe abdominal pain for the previous 24 hours. Superior mesenteric angiography showed that the main stem was patent but reduced in width. Marked constriction of all arteries to the small bowel is noted as well as signs of increased peripheral resistance. Multiple small branches and arcades are occluded, and there is insufficient collateral supply. Ileocolic and right colic arteries are less constricted, while blood supply of the transverse colon is missing. The angiographic findings were almost the same after injection of 10 μg of bradykinin into the superior mesenteric artery with only slight improvement of blood flow. At autopsy no occlusion was observed. Hemorrhagic necrosis was present in the small bowel and transverse colon. An old myocardial infarction was also found.

good outcome, with recovery in about two-thirds of the cases without acute resection. The lesion may heal completely or cause a fibrous narrowing later requiring resection. The etiology may be an arterial occlusion brought about by atherosclerosis, vasculitis, aortic surgery, or catheterization for angiography [9, 55, 126, 138, 310]. Often, however, no vascular occlusion is observed but instead increased blood flow with dilated arteries and early venous filling (Fig. 69-10) [46, 115, 180, 310, 331, 388, 393]. This type of ischemic colitis thus should not be confused with the very serious forms of colitis that occur in nonocclusive ischemia, which usually include the

small bowel as well as the right part of the large bowel.

CHRONIC OBSTRUCTION

Congenital lesions such as prenatal occlusion of the superior mesenteric artery [330] are not observed at angiography because collateral supply to the duodenum and proximal jejunum is absent; the child will therefore not survive. Abdominal coarctation with marked stenosis or occlusion of the large trunks arising from the proximal lumbar aorta is a congenital lesion diagnosed by lumbar aortography [42, 186]. The celiac and mesenteric lesions are usually accidental findings, the main symptom being hypertension. A well-developed collateral circulation to the abdominal viscera eliminates bowel ischemia and the typical symptoms following it.

Chronic obstruction of the superior mesenteric artery is ordinarily of arteriosclerotic origin and is most often located in the first 1 to 2 cm of the artery [93, 118, 155, 218]. The stenosis is best observed at angiography in the lateral projection (see Fig. 69-2). Contrast medium should therefore be injected in the lumbar aorta at the origin of the superior mesenteric artery [76, 142, 143, 254–256, 287, 315, 316, 368].

Autopsy studies of arteriosclerotic changes in the mesenteric circulation have shown that they are less pronounced and less common than in the coronary arteries or the aorta [93, 213, 305]. Various opinions are on record concerning the frequency of arteriosclerotic narrowing of the celiac and superior mesenteric arteries. Derrick et al. [118] found approximately the same frequency in both vessels in a consecutive series of patients (44% and 37%, respectively). In patients above 50 years of age, on the other hand, Goertler [155] found moderate and severe stenosis in more than 25 percent in the superior mesenteric artery and in only 6 percent in the celiac axis.

These findings are at variance with angiographic studies, in which celiac stenoses are much more frequently seen than stenoses of the superior mesenteric artery. Thus, in a series of 713 patients Bron and Redman [76] found celiac stenoses in 12.3 percent and stenoses of the superior mesenteric artery in only 3.4 percent. This report may be explained by the observations of Dunbar et al. [127] and Rob [316] that the celiac stenosis is usually not arteriosclerotic but rather is caused by a compression of the crura of

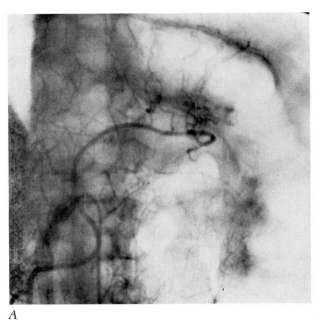
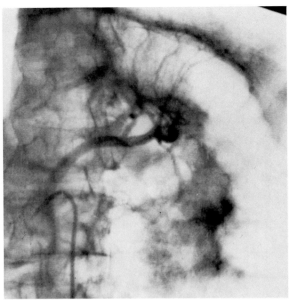

A

B

Figure 69-10. Reversible infarction of the splenic flexure of the colon in a 64-year-old man with acute rectal bleeding and abdominal pain. Two years previously he had had a myocardial infarction. At barium study typical findings of bowel infarction of the splenic flexure were observed. (A and B) At superior mesenteric angiography 10 days after onset of symptoms, no vascular occlusion is present but there is marked hypervascularization of the diseased area. Later examination with barium enema showed a complete regression.

the diaphragm or of the celiac ganglion. On the other hand, the high frequency of superior mesenteric stenosis found at autopsy cannot be verified by angiography, perhaps because small plaques at the orifice are not angiographically demonstrable. Although the commonest angiographic finding due to atherosclerosis is a concentric constriction at or near the origin (see Fig. 69-2), the earliest morphologic appearance is an eccentric, degenerative lesion [155].

Arteriosclerotic stenosis or occlusion in the branches of the superior mesenteric artery has been considered rare by some observers [93, 316]. Reiner et al. [305, 306], using arteriography of autopsy specimens, frequently found peripheral arteriosclerotic disease of the mesenteric circulation but mentioned that dissection studies alone did not give adequate information.

A stenosis or occlusion of the main stem of the superior mesenteric artery is not an uncommon finding at autopsy in patients who have had no symptoms related to the gastrointestinal tract [189, 215, 305]. In fact, occlusion of two or three main stems does not necessarily cause symptoms of ischemic bowel disease [76, 80, 209, 258]. Stenosis of the superior mesenteric artery alone

may, on the other hand, cause abdominal symptoms—most commonly postprandial pain and malabsorption with fatty stools and weight loss. Some authors believe that at least two main stems must be occluded for these symptoms to be produced [71, 146, 247, 254–256, 303]. The first reports on malabsorption in connection with vascular disease showed, however, occlusion of only the superior mesenteric artery [236, 237]. This finding has been verified by others [88, 103, 316, 332, 368]. Partial ligation of the superior mesenteric artery produced intestinal malabsorption in dogs with partial villous atrophy [277]. Improvement of mucosal changes and symptoms of malabsorption after 3 weeks agrees with the clinical observations by Connolly et al. [103] that these symptoms depend on the potentialities of the collateral supply. The varying ability of each individual to develop a collateral circulation may be the most important factor in determining whether or not the syndrome of abdominal angina will appear [312].

Obstruction of peripheral branches of the superior mesenteric artery may also cause intestinal ischemia with malabsorption [92, 177, 316, 332]. Reiner [303], on the other hand, found peripheral occlusion due to local arteriosclerosis and thrombosis that were often silent during life. Joske et al. [190] reported two patients who developed malabsorption after temporary occlusion of the superior mesenteric artery. Aortography in one of the patients revealed a widely patent superior mesenteric artery, but peripheral branches could not be observed in detail. The importance of using aortography to demonstrate the stenosis in abdominal angina or malabsorption has been stressed by all authors, but in order to evaluate the malabsorption syndrome fully, selective angiography is required, especially when the main stem of the superior mesenteric artery is patent.

Experimental experience suggests that malabsorption may appear also when the superior mesenteric artery is patent, i.e., when a relative insufficiency is present or there is mesenteric steal due to stenosis of the celiac and inferior mesenteric arteries [277]. Mesenteric steal causing relative ischemia of the villi may likewise be due to aortoiliac steal [148, 258], to stenosis of the celiac and inferior mesenteric arteries, or to arteriovenous shunting in the mesenteric circulation [36].

Celiac and superior mesenteric angiography was performed in patients with signs of malabsorption [48]. In these patients, all of whom had steatorrhea, there were different types of alterations in the mesenteric circulation that could cause relative anoxia of the villi. In one group shunting of blood was due to Crohn's disease (see Fig. 69-5), ileocecal carcinoma, colitis, or arteriovenous fistula (Fig. 69-11). Because of the shunting, a form of mesenteric steal was present with relative anoxia to the otherwise normal bowel. In another group of patients with gluten-induced steatorrhea, the superior mesenteric artery was wider than normal but there was no evidence of shunting because the veins were not observed early and were poorly opacified (Fig. 69-12). An explanation for the dilated artery may be the special anatomic and physiologic arrangements in the bowel wall [153, 326, 396]. Gluten-induced steatorrhea is probably a form of allergy [359]. It is postulated that because of this allergic reaction vasospasm occurs in the villi and blood is short-circuited to the veins. Anoxia and villous atrophy, which are characteristic for sprue, result. The contrast medium may be pooled in the mesenteric blood reservoir and therefore diluted so that early filling of veins cannot be observed during angiography. General in-

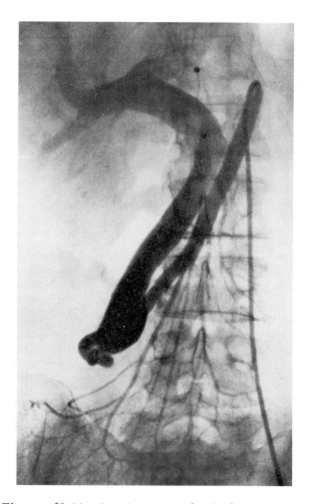

Figure 69-11. Arteriovenous fistula between the superior mesenteric artery and vein in a 61-year-old woman with gluten-induced steatorrhea who had a normal gastrointestinal barium study. The fistula was secondary to a previous bowel resection for intussusception due to a lipoma of the ileum with gangrene.

creased width of the superior mesenteric artery and the marked general venous shunting have been reported in a few cases of nontropical sprue [109] and in patients with *Strongyloides stercoralis* enteritis [220]. Patients with reticulum cell sarcoma of the bowel, a disease related to idiopathic sprue, may also have a wide superior mesenteric artery [225].

Another common finding in the ischemic syndrome is occult blood in the feces [202, 229, 255]. Angiography of the superior mesenteric artery should therefore be performed in every patient with unexplained bleeding from the gastrointestinal tract. Boijsen and Reuter [47] found a high percentage of vascular stenosis in patients with this symptom, which later was verified by

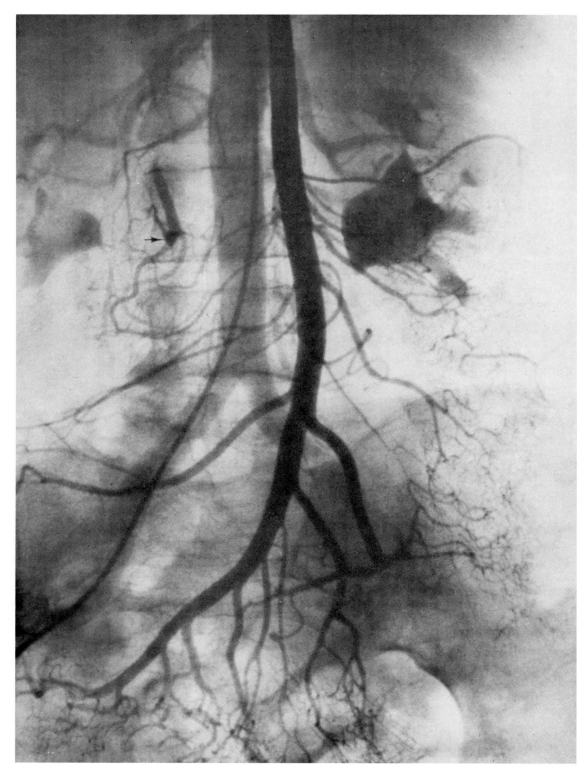

Figure 69-12. Idiopathic sprue in a 63-year-old woman. At angiography the superior mesenteric as well as the ileal arteries are seen to be unusually wide, while the jejunal arteries are small. No shunting is observed, but there is an aneurysm of the gastroduodenal artery (*arrow*).

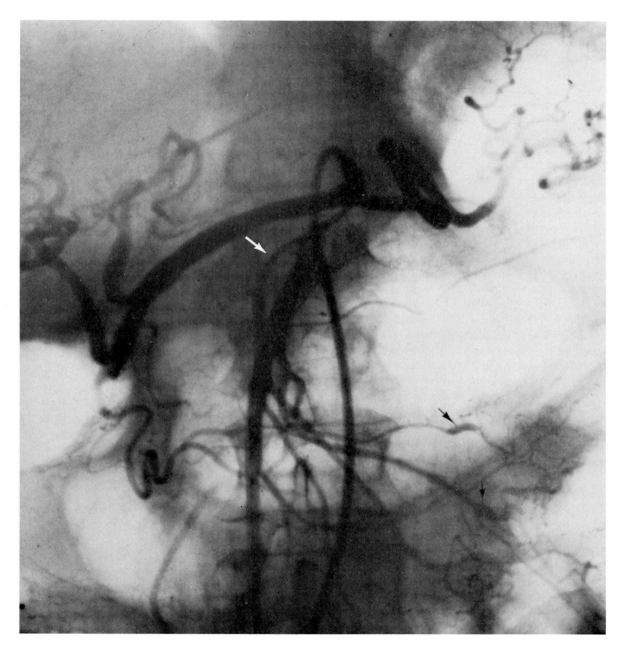

Figure 69-13. Chronic pancreatitis in a 66-year-old woman with abdominal pain. At celiac angiography the superior mesenteric artery is filled in a retrograde direction from a dilated dorsal pancreatic artery, also called the anastomosis of Bühler (*upper arrow*). Irregular arterial walls are present within the splenic, common hepatic, dorsal pancreatic, superior mesenteric, and first jejunal arteries. Peripheral aneurysms are visible in the jejunal arteries (*lower arrows*).

others [205, 338, 385]. Since collateral circulation is often observed at angiography, this observation in patients with hemorrhage to the gastrointestinal tract is difficult to evaluate.

Although narrowing of the superior mesenteric artery is ordinarily atherosclerotic in origin, other causes are known. The commonest are tumor encasement, usually due to pancreatic carcinoma, and stenosis secondary to chronic pancreatitis. Splanchnic angiography is the best preoperative method for diagnosis of these lesions (Fig. 69-13). Although aortography may demonstrate the local constriction, for detailed analysis selective angiography is necessary. The malabsorption syndrome often seen in pancreatic disease may be related not only to a reduction of pancreatic exocrine function but also to a stenosis of the superior mesenteric artery itself.

Distal stenoses of the superior mesenteric artery or its branches are common in carcinoma infiltrating the mesentery. The stenosis is different from that caused by arteriosclerosis because the vessels are irregularly infiltrated by the tumor [46]. Fibromuscular hyperplasia [132, 312, 314, 395], pseudoxanthoma elasticum [14], thromboangiitis obliterans [323], and other types of arteritis [162] (see Fig. 69-8) cause narrowing or occlusion of the main stem or branches of the superior mesenteric artery, sometimes with abdominal angina. More peripheral arteries are stenosed or occluded in systemic amyloidosis [330], polyarteritis nodosa [122], necrotizing angiitis due to drug abuse [99], carcinoid tumors [41, 308], and peritoneal carcinomatosis [46]. In granulomatous enterocolitis, irregular stenosis of the vasa recta may be observed at angiography [46, 66, 199, 226, 249], an observation that is not verified by microangiography [68, 194].

With the development of modern therapeutic dilatation technique in diagnostic radiology, it appears that some of the central stenoses of the superior mesenteric artery can be treated percutaneously [148].

Aneurysms

Aneurysms of the superior mesenteric artery or its branches are seldom observed at autopsy or operation. In a review of the literature Rob [316] found that approximately 20 percent of aneurysms in the splanchnic viscera were located in the superior mesenteric artery. The aneurysms reported were mycotic and located in the main stem. Previous experience gave the impression that most aneurysms of the main stem were syphilitic or necrotic [241, 380], but with the increasing use of angiography, these lesions seem to be arteriosclerotic. Furthermore, with today's high frequency of mesenteric angiography, particularly performed in patients with gastrointestinal hemorrhage, few aneurysms are reported [39, 309, 338, 348]. One reason is that most aneurysms are silent; another is that angiography of the superior mesenteric artery is not performed as often as it should be in patients with disease entities complicated with aneurysms,

i.e., polyarteritis nodosa [85, 89, 97, 122, 174, 183], necrotizing angiitis [98], and pancreatitis [50] (Fig. 69-13). Destruction of the arterial wall by pancreatic enzymes [49] or by neoplasms [232] may cause large pseudoaneurysms of the mesentery or pancreas, or the aneurysms may rupture into the peritoneal cavity. The small arteriosclerotic aneurysms of the superior mesenteric artery and its branches rarely cause any symptoms, but rupture may occur without previous symptoms (Fig. 69-14). They may also cause thrombotic occlusion of branches of the superior mesenteric artery, which may or may not elicit abdominal symptoms.

The aneurysms of polyarteritis nodosa have a varying appearance at angiography. They are usually small (1–5 mm) and situated in peripheral branches close to the mesenteric border, but secondary or tertiary branches may also be engaged, with extensive, irregular destruction of the arterial wall and thrombotic occlusion of branches [85, 122, 174] (Fig. 69-15).

Figure 69-14. Aneurysm of the left branch of the middle colic artery in a 56-year-old man with hypertension and sudden bleeding into the abdominal cavity. At superior mesenteric angiography a 7-×-7-mm aneurysm is visible surrounded by a hematoma displacing the marginal artery. Collateral circulation was demonstrated in the area at angiography. The aneurysm could therefore be extirpated without compromising the bowel circulation.

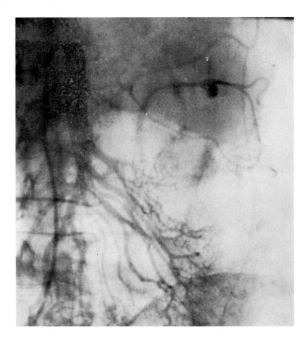

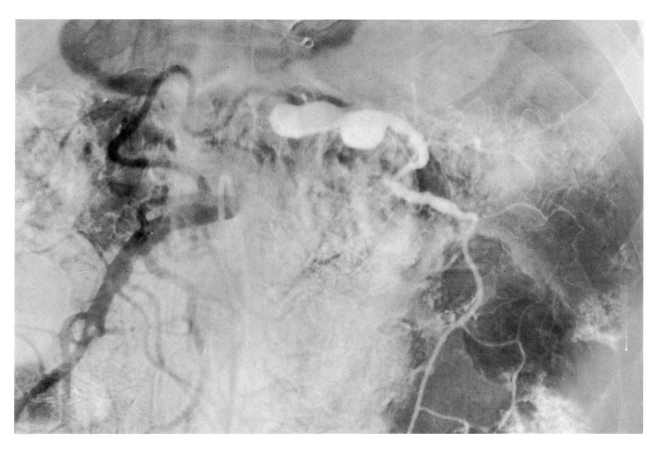

Figure 69-15. Aneurysm formation in the middle colic artery in a 56-year-old man, previously operated on for a lumbar aortic aneurysm. The complicated operation involved the left renal artery, and reoperation was necessary because of insufficiency in graft anastomosis. Four months later, he rebled to the gastroin-testinal tract, and a long irregular aneurysm of the type found in polyarteritis nodosa was observed in the middle colic artery at superior mesenteric angiography. The aneurysm was resected. It was probably the result of the complicated operation.

Arteriovenous Communications

ANGIOMATOUS LESIONS

A large variety of benign vascular lesions with abnormal arteriovenous connections may be recognized at selective superior mesenteric angiography: angioma, hemangioma, hamartoma, angiodysplasia, phlebectasia, and telangiectasia. Some of them (e.g., angiodysplasia and phlebectasia) are thus benign vascular tumors that have a different histologic appearance in which widened mucosal or submucosal veins are the most characteristic finding. These lesions are often called vascular malformations. *Angiomatous lesions* would be a better name because some of the lesions are hereditary (hereditary hemorrhagic telangiectasia), others are congenital (blue rubber bleb nevus, Klippel-Trenaunay syndrome), and

still others are acquired (old age, congestive heart failure, aortic stenosis). The latter are usually called angiodysplasia. A distinction between these lesions based on angiography alone is usually not possible.

The angiomatous lesions have other characteristics in common. They usually cause gastrointestinal hemorrhage and they are difficult or impossible to find at exploratory laparotomy. Since the first description in 1960 by Margulis et al. [231], based on operative angiography, a large number of reports have shown that selective splanchnic angiography, particularly superior mesenteric angiography, is a useful method to demonstrate these lesions [8, 12, 21, 40, 47, 58, 70, 105, 149, 152, 171–173, 196, 210, 248, 252, 269, 271, 272, 338, 354, 381, 383].

The characteristic and most frequent angiographic observation of the *angiodysplastic lesion* is that of a small (less than 1 cm) vascular lesion of the cecum or ascending colon. It is fed by a slightly enlarged vasa recta, and early filling of a widened draining vein is seen (see Fig. 69-1) [21, 58, 248, 252, 272]. Delayed emptying of the early filled draining vein is also noted [58, 272]. This has been believed to be an indication of venous stasis, presumably induced by increased luminal bowel pressure, and a cause of the phlebectasia observed [53]. Another hypothesis is that the lesion is secondary to mucosal ischemia [21], since most lesions occur in elderly patients and shunting has been found in cases in which arteries in the region were thrombosed (see Fig. 69-7) [40]. This hypothesis is also in line with the observation that some of the lesions occur in patients with aortic stenosis [149, 378] or in patients with cardiac, vascular, or pulmonary insufficiency [320].

The diagnosis of the angiodysplastic lesions is thus made by angiography of the superior mesenteric artery. In many patients repeated gastrointestinal barium studies and colonoscopy have failed to demonstrate the lesions [21, 149, 252, 272, 354]. On the other hand, it is known that angiography may be falsely negative and that colonoscopy may reveal the lesion [171]. Magnification angiography or pharmacoangiography may improve the diagnostic accuracy (see Fig. 69-1) [36, 171, 272, 344]. With increasing experience the angiodysplastic lesions have also been observed at angiography in the small bowel and in the left colon and rectosigmoid area [40, 105, 248, 272, 378, 382], and new lesions are seen to appear after resection of the primary lesion [21, 272] (see Fig. 69-7). Of particular interest is the fact that angiodysplastic lesions also occur in the upper gastrointestinal tract, as has been observed at endoscopy in patients with aortic stenoses [378]. Certainly, some of the unexplained recurrent gastrointestinal hemorrhages with negative angiography could be referred to these lesions. Perhaps the local hypervascularization of the stomach or duodenum sometimes observed in otherwise unexplained hemorrhage [47] could be accounted for by similar lesions.

The angiomatous lesions discovered at angiography in patients with *hereditary hemorrhagic telangiectasia* occur in all abdominal organs including the gastrointestinal tract [173, 210, 252, 271, 272]. At superior mesenteric angiography multiple punctate lesions may be observed but usually only single lesions are noted, looking much like angiodysplasia of the colon. Often the vascular tufts are too small to be observed. Angiography may then show a localized early filling of the vein, or the angiogram may appear normal.

A *diffuse angiomatous lesion* of the small bowel in infants is a particular entity that appears angiographically as a general shunting from the widened superior mesenteric artery [252, 272].

In *Klippel-Trenaunay syndrome* [152, 272], *blue rubber bleb nevus* [13] and other congenital angiomatous lesions of the small or large bowel, the angiographic findings are not similar to those of angiodysplasia. Usually there is no arteriovenous shunting, and the feeding arteries are not dilated.

In localized lesions such as angiodysplasia of the large bowel, resection has been the method of choice. During the last few years, however, embolization [345] or electrocoagulation via the endoscope [320, 378] has been successful.

ARTERIOVENOUS FISTULA

Whereas the angiomatous lesion rarely grows to be a shunt of hemodynamic import, the arteriovenous fistula may very well shunt significant amounts of blood. This fistula represents a direct communication between the main stem or branches and their respective veins and is of traumatic origin. The main-stem fistulas are secondary to direct violence [70, 357, 360], while those of the peripheral branches are secondary to previous complicated operations [260, 262, 295, 352]. Congenital arteriovenous fistula of the mesentery has also been described [10]. Because of a markedly increased flow, the superior mesenteric artery becomes wider and a shunt can be observed even at lumbar aortography [262, 295, 357, 360]. The exact site of the fistula, however, may be difficult to define by aortography [357] but selective angiography readily delineates the exact position of the lesion [352] (see Fig. 69-11).

Although malabsorption has been reported in patients with arteriovenous fistula [260, 262], it is not a constant finding. One patient with the disorder had a gluten-induced steatorrhea, which disappeared after ligation of the fistula. Biopsy showed that the villi were normal, but the enzymes in the villi were reduced. Thus decreased peripheral resistance due to the fistula can reduce perfusion pressure in the bowel wall, resulting in reduction of the enzymes [48].

Tumor and Inflammatory Disease

Inflammatory and neoplastic disease of the intestine has been studied by microangiography, and differences in the vascular pattern of the lesions have been observed [68, 194, 346, 347]. Even though it does not achieve the same detailed vascular anatomy as microangiography, conventional selective angiography adds more information about the pathophysiologic changes within these lesions (Fig. 69-16). Changes in the vascular patterns are seen during selective angiography in most neoplastic [24, 43, 113, 114, 120, 131, 196, 200, 207, 208, 245, 265, 275, 308, 312] and inflammatory lesions within the bowel [46, 66, 67, 123, 136, 179, 199, 223, 226, 249]. The differential diagnosis of a specific neoplastic or inflammatory origin, however, may be difficult. From the present collected experience it seems that certain angiographic findings are characteristic, but at times it is impossible to make a definite diagnosis.

INFLAMMATION

The two main types of inflammatory disease, regional enterocolitis and ulcerative colitis, have distinct angiographic patterns when they are fully developed. The pathologic and microangiographic changes explain the angiographic findings. In Crohn's disease degenerative vascular changes are observed, with granulomatous reaction and diffuse fibrosis of all layers of the bowel as well as the mesentery [194, 206]. Inflammatory vascular changes are relatively few in the early stages of the disease, when there is a nonspecific inflammatory reaction. Conversely, in ulcerative colitis the inflammatory vascular reaction dominates, and degenerative vascular changes are nonexistent. Thus, at angiography in advanced stages of Crohn's disease with stenosis the long vasa recta and the arteries near the mesenteric border appear irregularly stenosed or occluded, and collateral circulation with tortuous arteries in the gut wall is found [46, 66, 123, 226, 249]. These observations are not in agreement with other reports [67]. Microangiography and histoangiography have definitely shown that there is no occlusion of the vasa recta even in advanced stages of Crohn's disease [68, 194]. Since they are crowded, tortuous, and reduced in width, they will not be seen on routine angio-

grams. Other findings in Crohn's disease are wide-angle branching between the long vasa recta [179] and small vascular tufts in the bowel wall and mesentery [123]. The arterial changes in idiopathic ulcerative colitis [179, 223] are wide vasa recta and signs of hypervascularization. In cases of "zoning" [67, 179] (i.e., hypervascular areas present in the submucosa and serosa), the diagnosis of Crohn's disease can be made. Otherwise it is rarely possible to make a distinction between the two disease entities. Hypervascularization with shunting to densely opacified veins is observed in both types when activity is present (Fig. 69-17; see Fig. 69-5). This phenomenon may also be noted where there is delayed transit of contrast medium through the arteries of the diseased bowel [40]. Absence of early venous filling is frequently observed in the advanced stage of Crohn's disease.

To summarize, the interesting and somewhat controversial angiographic changes observed in inflammatory bowel disease are usually not specific [67, 194]. The extension of disease can be defined quite well as a rule, but the rather complicated procedure and the radiation risks of the method have made the indications for angiography obsolete in the young patients. To be sure, there is a certain risk of malignant change in the bowel of these patients. It occurs, however, late in the disease, and then other diagnostic methods will usually give the diagnosis.

TUMORS

Tumors of the small bowel are rare and often overlooked or misinterpreted at barium examination. Superior mesenteric angiography plays an important role in diagnosis, in preoperative evaluation of local extent, and in locating the exact site of the tumor in the small bowel wall [120, 131, 200].

The commonest primary tumor of the small bowel is the *carcinoid,* usually present in the ileum. Because of a marked desmoplastic reaction of the mesentery, the tumor has a typical angiographic pattern when it extends outside the bowel wall [33, 41, 100, 102, 157, 181, 203, 308, 339, 355, 369] (Fig. 69-18). Ileal mesenteric arteries and veins are stenosed or occluded. Often the ileocolic artery is narrowed in its entire length. Because of a mesenteric retraction the distal arcades and the vasa recta are arranged in a stellate pattern. Tumor vessels have been ob-

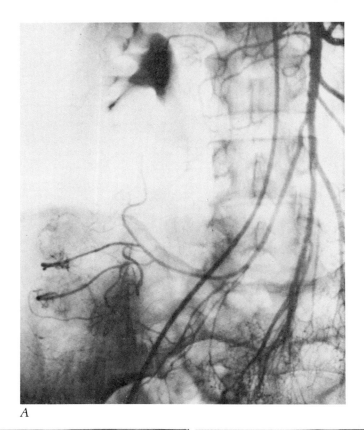

A

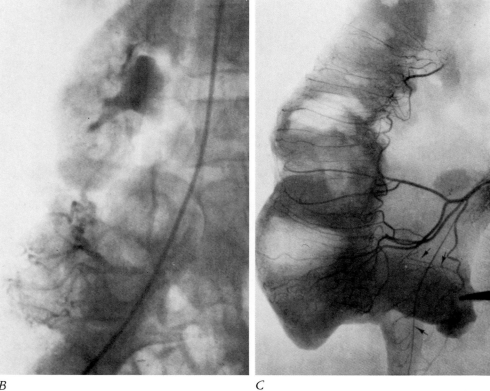

B   *C*

Figure 69-16. Carcinoma of the cecum in a 52-year-old woman. (A and B) At superior mesenteric angiography tumor vessels and early venous filling are observed in a 5-×-5-cm area of the cecum. (C) Arteriography of the operative specimen demonstrates that the slight arterial changes can hardly be seen with this method and that the pathophysiologic changes due to the tumor are far better observed with serial angiography. Note in the specimen the recurrent ileal artery supplying the terminal ileum (*upper arrows*) and the artery supplying the appendix (*lower arrow*).

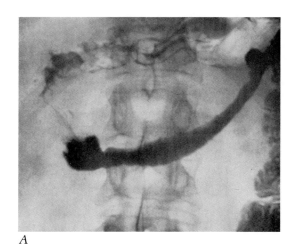

A

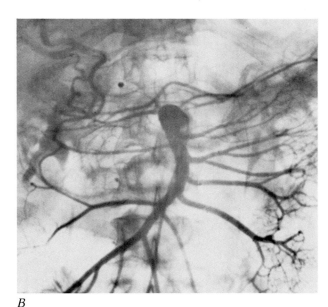

B

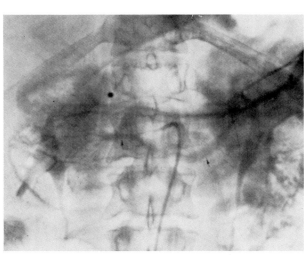

C

served, but they are probably collateral channels opened up because of occlusion of arterial arcades. Tumor stain is usually not discerned but may occur [102, 157, 203, 339]. Pharmacoangiography may enhance the information [36, 38, 157]. Although in small tumors without the desmoplastic change of the mesentery, the primary lesion will not be seen [41, 102, 203, 302], local metastases in the mesentery as well as hepatic metastases will nevertheless be shown [203, 302]. The angiographic findings are thus, as a rule, typical, but similar findings in mesenteric fibrosis have been noted [156]. It appears, however, that vascular displacement and distortion are more typical for this lesion than is incasement [91, 120, 327].

Carcinoid tumors of the large bowel within the superior mesenteric territory are rarely examined by angiography despite the fact that the most frequent site is in the appendix. Only two cases are reported [203], with the same findings as in small bowel tumors.

Leiomyoma or neurinoma of the small bowel has a characteristic appearance [46, 90, 113, 114, 196, 200, 245, 290, 381]. The tumor has well-circumscribed margins. Prominent feeding arteries and draining veins are observed, and many irregular tumor vessels give rise to a dense stain (Fig. 69-19). Malignancy can rarely be ruled out, but if the tumor is small (3–4 cm) it is probably benign. Angiography appears to be extremely reliable and is not infrequently used in the diagnosis of chronic, otherwise unexplained, melena [47, 131, 200, 205, 338]. Only one case of angiography of a leiomyoma of the large bowel has been reported [200].

The *hamartoma* in patients with Peutz-Jegher's disease is a vascular tumor, but at angiography it is usually noted as a hypovascular mass with lack of venous drainage [140, 150, 317].

Adenocarcinoma of the small bowel is a rare lesion, and angiography is therefore seldom reported [130]. The large bowel adenocarcinoma

---

Figure 69-17. Regional enteritis of the duodenum in a 31-year-old man. (A) Typical changes observed at upper gastrointestinal barium study. (B and C) At superior mesenteric angiography slightly irregular changes are observed in the peripheral branches of the pancreaticoduodenal arteries and gastroduodenal artery. Hypervascularization with early shunting to the veins is visible (*arrows*).

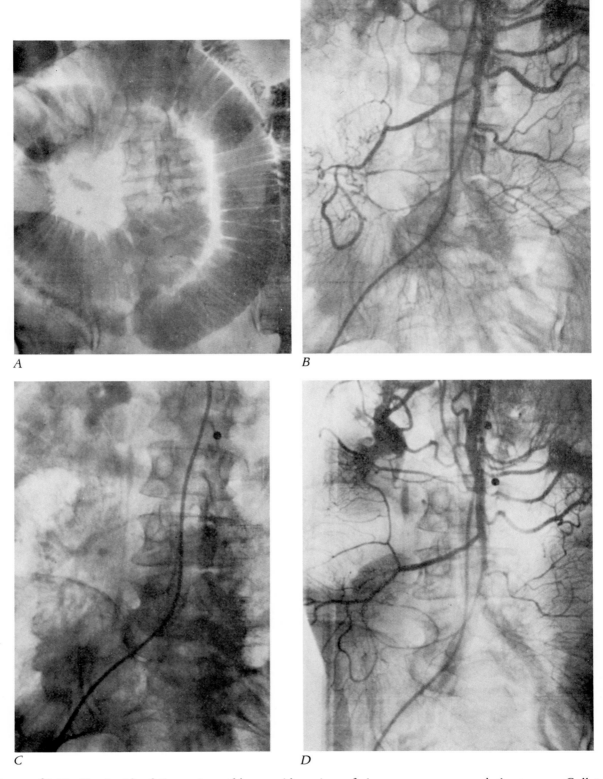

A

B

C

D

Figure 69-18. Carcinoid of ileum in a 64-year-old woman with malabsorption and a palpable mass to the right in the abdomen. (A) Small bowel study demonstrates dilated ileal loops surrounding a tumor. (B and C) At superior mesenteric angiography the terminal part of the artery as well as peripheral branches and arcades are found to be irregularly infiltrated. The mesentery is infiltrated with consequent typical radia-

tion of the vasa recta toward the tumor. Collateral supply is present from the infiltrated ileocolic artery. Ileal and ileocolic veins are occluded by tumor (C). (D) At pharmacoangiography using 0.5 IU of vaso-pressin, the irregular arterial infiltrations of larger branches are somewhat better observed but fewer tumor vessels are seen.

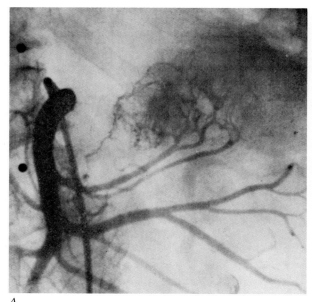

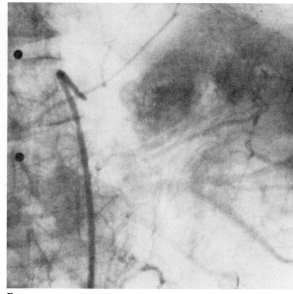

A

B

Figure 69-19. Leiomyoma of the jejunum in a 67-year-old man with repeated bleeding from the bowel. Previous operation for diverticula of the colon did not stop the bleeding. Repeated small bowel studies were reported negative. (A and B) At superior mesenteric angiography a 3.5-×-2.5-cm richly vascularized tumor was found to be supplied by the first jejunal artery.

has been frequently observed at superior mesenteric angiography [46, 205, 250, 338]. The angiographic appearance varies with the type of growth. Thus, the infiltrating, scirrhous tumor is avascular or hypovascular and infiltrates the vasa recta with no tumor stain and no early venous filling. This is most often seen in the small bowel adenocarcinoma (Fig. 69-20). Tumors of the large bowel supplied from the superior mesenteric artery are, on the other hand, usually hypervascular and show tumor stain as well as dense and early venous drainage (see Fig. 69-16). Infiltration of arteries of the mesentery signifies extension of tumor outside the bowel wall.

Villous tumor of the ascending colon may have a slightly different appearance from that of carcinoma [313].

Lymphoma, lymphosarcoma and *reticular cell sarcoma* of the bowel are rarely examined by mesenteric angiography. Findings in the few cases reported are noncharacteristic [7, 46, 119, 120, 225, 338]. Vascular displacement and incasement are reported as well as early shunting, but occasionally no abnormality is observed despite the extensive involvement of the mesentery [225].

Cystic lesions of the mesentery cause vascular displacement, and sometimes accumulation of contrast medium in the wall may be noted [120, 161].

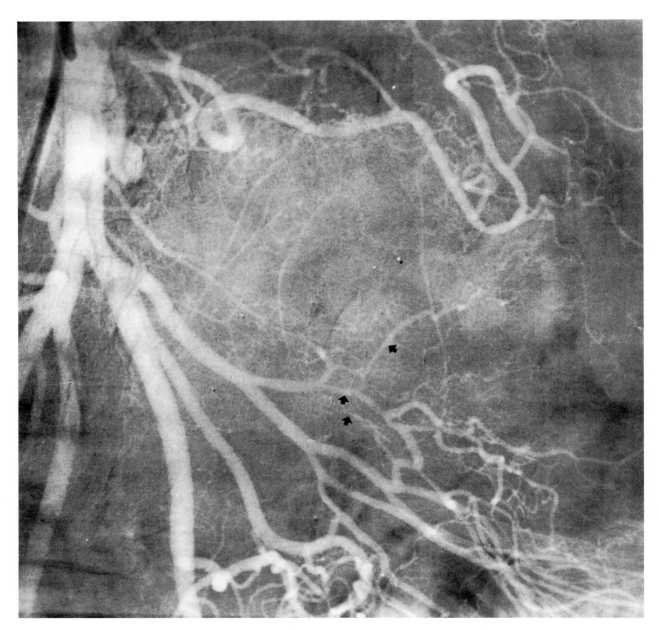

Figure 69-20. Adenocarcinoma of the jejunum with marked infiltration of jejunal arteries (*arrows*). Few tumor vessels are observed, but there is a slight accumulation in the tumor. (×2.5 magnification, subtraction film.)

Miscellaneous Conditions

Besides primary vascular lesions, tumors, and inflammatory disease, angiography may reveal the presence of *internal herniation, intussusception, volvulus, malrotation,* or *adhesions.* These are of particular importance to define when there is a vascular compromise [2, 86, 95, 101, 130, 191, 205, 212, 224, 242, 244, 334, 335] that may cause acute bowel ischemia, symptoms of gastrointestinal hemorrhage, or abdominal pain.

Meckel's diverticulum may also be revealed by angiography, particularly in acute bleeding when extravasation or accumulation of contrast medium in the ectopic gastric mucosa is observed [69, 107, 129, 137, 145, 151, 205, 281, 338].

Radiation enteritis is another lesion of the bowel that appears angiographically as irregular stenosis or occlusion of superior mesenteric artery branches including the vasa recta. The latter are often tortuous and crowded [117, 321]. The bowel wall appears hypovascular, and the veins are often stenosed.

Ileal varicosities may be seen at angiography in patients with portal hypertension. In the venous phase of the superior mesenteric angiogram large venous varicosities are observed in the bowel wall [17, 120, 165, 204].

Superior mesenteric angiography is thus a useful method for detecting a variety of gastrointestinal lesions. It should be taken advantage of particularly in situations in which other approaches, including CT and ultrasonography, have failed.

References

1. Aakhus, T. The value of angiography in superior mesenteric artery embolism. *Br. J. Radiol.* 39:928, 1966.
2. Aakhus, T. Angiography in experimental strangulating obstruction of the small intestine in dogs. *Acta Radiol. [Diagn.]* (Stockh.) 6:337, 1967.
3. Aakhus, T., and Brabrand, G. Angiography in acute superior mesenteric arterial insufficiency. *Acta Radiol. [Diagn.]* (Stockh.) 6:1, 1967.
4. Aakhus, T., and Evensen, A. Angiography in acute mesenteric arterial insufficiency. *Acta Radiol. [Diagn.]* (Stockh.) 19:945, 1978.
5. Aboumrad, M. H., Fine, G., and Horn, R. C., Jr. Intimal hyperplasia of small mesenteric arteries. *Arch. Pathol.* 75:196, 1963.
6. Adler, R. H., Norcross, B. M., and Lockie, L. M. Arteritis and infarction of the intestine in rheumatoid arthritis. *J.A.M.A.* 180:922, 1962.
7. Albrechtsson, U., and Tylén, U. Angiography in reticulum cell sarcoma. *Acta Radiol. [Diagn.]* (Stockh.) 18:210, 1977.
8. Alfidi, R. D., Esselstyn, C. D., Tarar, R., Klein, H. J., Hermann, R. E., Weakley, F. L., and Turnbull, R. B., Jr. Recognition and angiosurgical detection of arteriovenous malformations of the bowel. *Ann. Surg.* 174:573, 1971.
9. Andersen, P. E. Ischemic colitis caused by angiography. *Clin. Radiol.* 20:414, 1969.
10. Anderson, R. D., Liebeskind, A., and Lowman, R. M. Arteriovenous fistula of the mesentery. *Am. J. Gastroenterol.* 57:453, 1972.
11. Athanasoulis, C. A., Wittenberg, J., Bernstein, R., and Williams, L. F. Vasodilatory drugs in the management of nonocclusive bowel ischemia. *Gastroenterology* 69:146, 1975.
12. Baer, J. W., and Ryan, S. Analysis of cecal vasculature in the search for vascular malformations. *AJR* 126:394, 1976.
13. Baker, A. L., Kahn, P. C., Binder, S. C., and Patterson, J. F. Gastrointestinal bleeding due to blue rubber bleb nevus syndrome. A case diagnosed by angiography. *Gastroenterology* 61:530, 1971.
14. Bardsley, J. L., and Koehler, P. R. Pseudoxanthoma elasticum: Angiographic manifestations in abdominal vessels. *Radiology* 93:559, 1969.
15. Barth, K., Strecker, E. P., Schmidt-Hieber, M., Brobmann, G. F., and Schmidt, H. A. Klinische und experimentelle Beiträge zum Krankheitsbild der non-occlusive mesenteric Ischemia. *Radiologe* 14:431, 1974.
16. Barth, K. H., Scott, W. W., Jr., Harrington, D. P., and Siegelman, S. S. Abnormalities in the sequence of filling and emptying of mesenteric arteries and veins. A guide to ischemic disease of the bowel. *Gastrointest. Radiol.* 3:85, 1978.
17. Barth, V., and Kölmel, B. Blutende Dunndarmvarizen bei portaler Hypertension als seltene Komplikation nach abdominellen Operationen. *ROEFO* 132:219, 1980.
18. Basmajian, J. V. The marginal anastomoses of the arteries to the large intestine. *Surg. Gynecol. Obstet.* 99:614, 1954.
19. Basmajian, J. V. The main arteries of the large intestine. *Surg. Gynecol. Obstet.* 101:585, 1955.
20. Baum, S. Magnification Arteriography in Intestinal Vascular Disease. In S. J. Boley, S. S. Schwartz, and L. F. Williams, Jr. (eds.), *Vascular Disorders of the Intestine.* New York: Appleton-Century-Crofts, 1971.
21. Baum, S., Athanasoulis, C. A., Waltman, A. C., Galdabini, J., Schapiro, R. H., Warshaw, A. L., and Ottinger, L. W. Angiodysplasia of the right colon: A cause of gastrointestinal bleeding. *AJR* 129:789, 1977.
22. Baum, S., and Nusbaum, M. The control of gastrointestinal hemorrhage by selective mesenteric arterial infusion of vasopressin. *Radiology* 98:497, 1971.
23. Baum, S., Nusbaum, M., Clearfield, H. R., Kuroda, K., and Tumen, H. J. Angiography in the diagnosis of gastrointestinal bleeding. *Arch. Intern. Med.* 119:16, 1967.
24. Baum, S., Roy, R., Finkelstein, A. K., and Blakemore, W. S. Clinical application of selective celiac and superior mesenteric arteriography. *Radiology* 84:279, 1965.
25. Baum, S., Stein, G. N., and Baue, A. Extrinsic pressure defects on the duodenal loop in mesenteric occlusive disease. *Radiology* 85:866, 1965.
26. Berardi, R. S. Vascular complications of superior mesenteric artery infusion with Pitressin in treatment of bleeding oesophageal varices. *Am. J. Surg.* 127:757, 1974.

27. Bergan, J. J.   Recognition and treatment of intestinal ischemia. *Surg. Clin. North Am.* 47:109, 1967.

28. Bergan, J. J., Dean, R. H., Conn, J., and Yao, J. S. T.   Revascularisation in treatment of mesenteric infarction. *Ann. Surg.* 182:430, 1975.

29. Bergan, J. J., Dry, L., Conn, J., and Trippel, O. H.   Intestinal ischemic syndromes. *Ann. Surg.* 169:120, 1969.

30. Bergentz, S. E., Ericsson, B., Hedner, U., Leandoer, L., and Nilsson, J. M.   Thrombosis in the superior mesenteric and portal veins: Report of a case treated with thrombectomy. *Surgery* 76:286, 1974.

31. Berger, L., and Bryne, J. J.   Intestinal gangrene associated with heart disease. *Surg. Gynecol. Obstet.* 112:529, 1961.

32. Bierman, H. R., Miller, E. R., Bryon, R. L., Jr., Dod, K. S., Kelly, K. H., and Black, D. H.   Intra-arterial catheterization of viscera in man. *AJR* 66:555, 1951.

33. Bjørn-Hansen, R., and Aakhus, T.   Angiography in intestinal carcinoid. *Acta Radiol.* [*Diagn.*] (Stockh.) 14:721, 1973.

34. Boijsen, E.   Selective visceral angiography using a percutaneous axillary technique. *Br. J. Radiol.* 39:414, 1966.

35. Boijsen, E.   Selective visceral angiography with Isopaque B. *Acta Radiol.* [*Suppl.*] (Stockh.) 270:121, 1967.

36. Boijsen, E.   Superior Mesenteric Angiography. In H. L. Abrams (ed.), *Angiography* (2nd ed.). Boston: Little, Brown, 1971.

37. Boijsen, E., and Bron, K. M.   Visceral arteriography. *Ann. Rev. Med.* 15:273, 1964.

38. Boijsen, E., and Göthlin, J.   Effect of vasopressin on celiac and superior mesenteric angiography. *Acta Radiol.* [*Diagn.*] (Stockh.) 21:523, 1980.

39. Boijsen, E., Göthlin, J., Hallböök, T., and Sandblom, P.   Preoperative angiographic diagnosis of bleeding aneurysms of abdominal visceral arteries. *Radiology* 93:781, 1969.

40. Boijsen, E., and Härtel, M.   Kontrastmittelpassagezeiten im Versorgungsgebiet der Arteria mesenterica superior. *ROEFO* 118:491, 1972.

41. Boijsen, E., Kaude, J., and Tylén, U.   Radiologic diagnosis of ileal carcinoid tumors. *Acta Radiol.* [*Diagn.*] (Stockh.) 15:65, 1974.

42. Boijsen, E., and Larini, G. P.   Aortic hypoplasia combined with coarctation of the thoracic and lumbar aorta. *J. Can. Assoc. Radiol.* 17:81, 1966.

43. Boijsen, E., and Olin, T.   Zöliakographie und Angiographie der Arteria mesenterica superior. *Ergeb. Med. Strahlenforsch.* 1:112, 1964.

44. Boijsen, E., and Redman, H. C.   Effect of bradykinin on celiac and superior mesenteric angiography. *Invest. Radiol.* 1:422, 1966.

45. Boijsen, E., and Redman, H. C.   Effect of epinephrine on celiac and superior mesenteric angiography. *Invest. Radiol.* 2:184, 1967.

46. Boijsen, E., and Reuter, S. R.   Mesenteric angiography in the evaluation of inflammatory and neoplastic disease of the intestine. *Radiology* 87:1028, 1966.

47. Boijsen, E., and Reuter, S. R.   Angiography in diagnosis of chronic unexplained melena. *Radiology* 89:413, 1967.

48. Boijsen, E., and Tylén, U.   Angiographic findings in malabsorption. Unpublished results, 1969.

49. Boijsen, E., and Tylén, U.   Angiography in diagnosis in the exocrine pancreas. *Clin. Gastroenterol.* 1:85, 1972.

50. Boijsen, E., and Tylén, U.   Vascular changes in chronic pancreatitis. *Acta Radiol.* [*Diagn.*] (Stockh.) 12:34, 1972.

51. Boley, S. J., Agrawal, G. P., Warren, A. R., Veith, F. J., Levowitz, B. S., Treiber, W. F., Dougherty, J., Schwartz, S. S., and Gliedman, M. L.   Pathophysiologic effects of bowel distension on intestinal blood flow. *Am. J. Surg.* 117:228, 1969.

52. Boley, S. J., Krieger, H., Schultz, L., Robinson, K., Siew, F. P., Allen, A. C., and Schwartz, S.   Experimental aspects of peripheral vascular occlusion of the intestine. *Surg. Gynecol. Obstet.* 121:789, 1965.

53. Boley, S. J., Sammartano, R., Adams, A., Dibiase, A., Kleinhaus, S., and Sprayregen, S.   On the nature and etiology of vascular ectasias of the colon. Degenerative lesions of aging. *Gastroenterology* 72:650, 1977.

54. Boley, S. J., and Schwartz, S. S.   Colonic Ischemia: Reversible Ischemic Lesions. In S. J. Boley, S. S. Schwartz, and L. F. Williams, Jr. (eds.), *Vascular Disorders of the Intestine.* New York: Appleton-Century-Crofts, 1971.

55. Boley, S. J., Schwartz, S., Lash, J., and Sternhill, V.   Reversible vascular occlusion of the colon. *Surg. Gynecol. Obstet.* 116:53, 1963.

56. Boley, S. J., Schwartz, S. S., and Williams, L. F., Jr. (eds.).   *Vascular Disorders of the Intestine.* New York: Appleton-Century-Crofts, 1971.

57. Boley, S. J., and Siegelman, S. S.   Experimental and Clinical Non-occlusive Mesenteric Ischemia: Pathogenesis, diagnosis, and management. In S. Hilal (ed.), *Symposium on Small Vessel Angiography.* St. Louis: Mosby, 1973.

58. Boley, S. J., Sprayregen, S., Sammartano, R. J., Adams, A., and Kleinhaus, S.   The pathophysiologic basis for the angiographic signs of vascular ectasias of the colon. *Radiology* 125:615, 1977.

59. Boley, S. J., Sprayregen, S., Veith, F. J., and Siegelman, S. S.   An Aggressive Roentgenologic and Surgical Approach to Acute Mesenteric Ischemia. In L. M. Nyhus (ed.), *Surgery*

Annual. New York: Appleton-Century-Crofts, 1973. Vol. 5, pp. 355–378.

60. Bonakdarpour, A. Angiography of mesenteric arterial occlusion. *Invest. Radiol.* 5:316, 1970.

61. Bonakdarpour, A., Shea, F. J., Esterhai, J. L., and Siplet, H. Serum enzyme changes following selective superior mesenteric arteriography in dogs. *Radiology* 104:427, 1972.

62. Bonte, F. J., Curry, G. C., and Parkey, R. W. Experimental studies of the splanchnic circulation of the rabbit after ligation of the superior mesenteric artery: Angiographic and physiologic studies. *AJR* 106:691, 1969.

63. Bookstein, J. J., Naderi, M. J., and Walter, J. F. Transcatheter embolization for lower gastrointestinal bleeding. *Radiology* 127:345, 1978.

64. Bosniak, M. A. Experimental In-Vivo Magnification Intestinal Angiography Utilizing Photographic Enlargement Techniques. In S. J. Boley, S. S. Schwartz, and L. F. Williams, Jr. (eds.), *Vascular Disorders of the Intestine.* New York: Appleton-Century-Crofts, 1971. Pp. 257–271.

65. Bosniak, M. A., Farmelant, M. H., Bakos, C., Hasiotis, C. A., and Williams, L. F., Jr. Experimental in vivo photographic magnification angiography of the canine kidney and bowel. *Invest. Radiol.* 3:120, 1968.

66. Brahme, F. Mesenteric angiography in regional enterocolitis. *Radiology* 87:1037, 1966.

67. Brahme, F., and Hildell, J. Angiography in Crohn's disease revisited. *AJR* 126:941, 1976.

68. Brahme, F., and Lindström, C. A comparative radiographic and pathological study on intestinal vaso-architecture in Crohn's disease and in ulcerative colitis. *Gut* 11:928, 1970.

69. Bree, R. L., and Reuter, S. R. Angiographic demonstration of a bleeding Meckel's diverticulum. *Radiology* 108:287, 1973.

70. Brehm, H., Hoeffken, W., and Gehl, H. Präoperative angiographische Darstellung eines blutenden Dünndarmskavernoms. *Fortschr. Med.* 85:233, 1967.

71. Brette, R., Descotes, J., and Lambert, R. A propos d'un cas d'insuffisance artérielle mésentérique traitée par ré-implantation de l'artère mésentérique supérieure. *Arch. Fr. Mal. App. Dig.* 51:1425, 1962.

72. Britt, L. G., and Cheek, R. C. Non-occlusive mesenteric vascular disease. Clinical and experimental observations. *Ann. Surg.* 169:704, 1969.

73. Brolin, I., and Paulin, S. Abdominal communications between splanchnic vesels. *Acta Radiol. [Diagn.]* (Stockh.) 2:460, 1964.

74. Bron, K. M. Thrombotic occlusion of the abdominal aorta: Associated visceral artery lesions and collateral circulation. *AJR* 96:887, 1966.

75. Bron, H. W., and Ghosh, S. Polyarteritis nodosa presenting as an acute abdomen. *Int. Surg.* 51:30, 1969.

76. Bron, K. M., and Redman, H. C. Splanchnic artery stenosis and occlusion: Incidence; arteriographic and clinical manifestations. *Radiology* 92:323, 1969.

77. Brown, C. H., Rankin, G. B., Meaney, R. R., and Turnbull, R. B., Jr. Normal mesenteric arteriograms in a case of senile ulcerative colitis. *J. Am. Geriatr. Soc.* 12:215, 1964.

78. Brunner, J. H., and Stanley, R. J. Superior mesenteric arteriovenous fistula. Report of a case with increased systemic flow. *J.A.M.A.* 223:316, 1973.

79. Buchardt Hansen, H. J., and Christoffersen, J. K. Occlusive mesenteric infarction. *Acta Chir. Scand. [Suppl.]* 472:102, 1976.

80. Buchardt Hansen, H. J., and Efsen, F. Occlusive disease of the mesenteric arteries. *Dan. Med. Bull.* 24:117, 1977.

81. Buchardt Hansen, H. J., Jørgensen, S. J., and Engell, H. C. Acute mesenteric infarction caused by small vessel disease. *Acta Chir. Scand. [Suppl.]* 472:109, 1976.

82. Buchardt Hansen, H. J., and Øigaard, A. Embolization to the superior mesenteric artery. *Acta Chir. Scand.* 142:451, 1976.

83. Bücheler, E., Düx, A., and Rohr, H. Mesenteric-Steal-Syndrom. *ROEFO* 106:313, 1967.

84. Buckley, J. J., Seiden, S. P., Jimenes, F. A., and Kaufman, G. Enteritis gravis: Report of three cases. *Gastroenterology* 42:330, 1962.

85. Buranasiri, S. I., Baum, S., Nusbaum, M., and Finkelstein, D. Periarteritis of the middle colic artery. *Am. J. Gastroenterol.* 59:73, 1973.

86. Buranasiri, S. I., Baum, S., Nusbaum, M., and Tumen, H. The angiographic diagnosis of mid-gut malrotation with volvulus in adults. *Radiology* 109:555, 1973.

87. Busson, A., and Hernandez, C. L'artériographie séléctive mésentérique dans la rectocolite hémorrhagique et la colite ulcéreuse d'emblée: Résultats; déductions cliniques et pathogéniques. *Arch. Fr. Mal. App. Dig.* 54:441, 1965.

88. Busson, A., Natali, J., Charleux, H., and Davezac, J.-F. Syndrome douloureux hyperalgique péri-ombilical par sténose de l'origine du tronc de l'artère mésentérique supérieure, traité par pontage entre l'aorte et la mésentérique supérieure. *Arch. Fr. Mal. App. Dig.* 53:1089, 1964.

89. Cabal, E., and Holtz, S. Polyarteritis as a cause of intestinal hemorrhage. *Gastroenterology* 61:99, 1971.

90. Capdeville, R., Bennet, J., Dubois, F., and Toulet, J. L'artériographie des tumeurs du grêle. A propos de 3 cas de schwannomes. *Arch. Fr. Mal. App. Dig.* 59:453, 1970.

91. Carillo, F. J., Ruzicka, F. F., Jr., and Clemett, A.

R.   Value of angiography in the diagnosis of retractile mesenteritis. *AJR* 115:396, 1972.

92. Carron, D. B., and Douglas, A. P.   Steatorrhoea in vascular insufficiency of the small intestine. *Q. J. Med.* 34:331, 1965.

93. Carucci, J. J.   Mesenteric vascular occlusion. *Am. J. Surg.* 85:47, 1953.

94. Cauldwell, E. W., and Anson, B. J.   The visceral branches of the abdominal aorta: Topographical relationships. *Am. J. Anat.* 73:27, 1943.

95. Chang, T., and Huang, T.   Arteriographic diagnosis of intussusception: Three case reports. *AJR* 117:317, 1973.

96. Cho, K. J., Chuang, V. P., and Reuter, S. R.   Prostaglandin E$_1$ as a pharmacoangiographic agent for arterial portography. *Radiology* 116:207, 1975.

97. Chudacek, Z.   Angiographic diagnosis of polyarteritis nodosa of the liver, kidney, and mesentery. *Br. J. Radiol.* 40:864, 1967.

98. Cioffi, C. M., Ruzicka, F. F., Jr., Carillo F. J., and Gould, H. R.   Enhanced visualization of portal venous system using phentolamine and isoproterenol in combination. *Radiology* 108:43, 1973.

99. Citron, B. P., Halpern, M., McCarron, M., Lundberg, G. D., McCormick, R., Pincus, I. J., Tatter, D., and Haverback, B. J.   Necrotizing angiitis associated with drug abuse. *N. Engl. J. Med.* 283:1003, 1970.

100. Claps, R. J., Lande, A., Lilienfeld, R., and Mieza, M.   Angiographic demonstration of an ileal carcinoid. *Radiology* 103:87, 1972.

101. Cohen, A. M., and Patel, S.   Arteriographic findings in congenital transmesenteric internal hernia. *AJR* 133:541, 1979.

102. Collatz Christensen, S., Stage, J. G., and Henriksen, F. W.   Angiography in the diagnosis of carcinoid syndrome. *Scand. J. Gastroenterol.* [Suppl.] 14:111, 1979.

103. Connolly, J. E., Abrams, H. L., and Kieraldo, J. H.   Observations on the diagnosis and treatment of obliterative disease of the visceral branches of the abdominal aorta. *Arch. Surg.* 90:596, 1965.

104. Cooley, R. N., Schreiber, M. H., and Brown, R. W.   Effects of transaortic catheter injection of Renografin, Urokon, Hypaque and Miokon into the superior mesenteric arteries of dogs. *Angiology* 15:107, 1964.

105. Cooperman, A. M., Kelly, K. A., Bernatz, Ph. E., and Huizenga, K. A.   Arteriovenous malformation of the intestine. *Arch. Surg.* 104:284, 1972.

106. Corday, E., Irving, D. W., Gold, H., Bernstein, H., and Skelton, R. B. T.   Mesenteric vascular insufficiency. *Am. J. Med.* 33:365, 1962.

107. Cornet, A., Abelent, R., Chaumont, P., Debesse, P., Terris, G., Dadoune, J. P., Epois, A.,
and Reboul, R.   Diverticule de Meckel à form hémorrhagique.   Dépistage artériographique. *Sem. Hop. Paris* 43:3441, 1967.

108. Craig, R. D. P.   Multiple perforations of small intestine in polyarteritis nodosa. *Gastroenterology* 44:355, 1963.

109. Cynn, W.-S., Herasme, V. M., Levin, B. L., Gureghian, P. A., and Schreiber, M. N.   Mesenteric angiography of non-tropical sprue. *AJR* 125:442, 1975.

110. Czembirek, L., Garbsch, H., Thurnher, B., and Zandanell, E.   Dickdarmstenose bei Periarteriitis nodosa. *Radiol. Austria.* 18:307, 1968.

111. Danford, R. O., and Davidson, A. J.   The use of glucagon as a vasodilator in visceral angiography. *Radiology* 93:173, 1969.

112. Davis, L. J., Anderson, J. H., Wallace, S., Gianturco, C., and Jacobson, E. D.   The use of prostaglandin E$_1$ to enhance the angiographic visualization of the splanchnic circulation. *Radiology* 114:281, 1975.

113. Debray, C., Leymarios, J., Hernandez, C., Marche, C., Hardouin, J.-P., and Pironneau, A.   Tumeur bénigne de l'intestine grêle (léiomyome) diagnostiquée par artériographie mésentérique supérieure. *Presse Med.* 72:3005, 1964.

114. Debray, C., Morin, G., Leymarios, J., Hernandez, C., Pironneau, A., Validire, J., Marche, C., and Hass, R.-M.   Tumeurs de l'intestine grêle diagnostiquées exclusivement par l'artériographie sélective de la mésentérique supérieure: A propos de 2 cas. *Arch. Fr. Mal. App. Dig.* 54:593, 1965.

115. DeDombal, F. T., Fletcher, D. M., and Harris, R. S.   Early diagnosis of ischemic colitis. *Gut* 10:131, 1969.

116. Dencker, H., Göthlin, J., Hedner, P., Lunderquist, A., Norryd, C., and Tylén, U.   Superior mesenteric angiography and blood flow following intra-arterial injection of Prostaglandin F$_2\alpha$. *AJR* 125:111, 1975.

117. Dencker, H., H:Son Holmdahl, K., Lunderquist, A., Olivecrona, H., and Tylén, U.   Mesenteric angiography in patients with radiation injury of the bowel after pelvis irradiation. *AJR* 114:476, 1972.

118. Derrick, J. R., Pollard, H. S., and Moore, R. M.   The pattern of arteriosclerotic narrowing of the celiac and superior mesenteric arteries. *Ann. Surg.* 149:684, 1959.

119. DeScheffer, A., Hubens, A., Van Vooren, W., and Verbraken, H.   Angiography in diagnosis of small bowel tumors. *Radiologe* 14:425, 1974.

120. Diamond, A. B., Meng, C.-H., and Goldin, R. R.   Arteriography of unusual mass lesions of the mesentery. *Radiology* 110:547, 1974.

121. Diemel, H., Rau, G., and Schmitz-Dräger, H.-G.   Die Riolansche Kollaterale: Ihre diagnostische Bedeutung für die Angiographie bei

Verschlusskrankheiten der Mesenterialarterien. *ROEFO* 101:253, 1964.

122. D'Izarn, J. J., Boulet, C. P., Convard, J. P., Bonnin, A., and Ledoux-Lebard, G. L'artériographie dans la périartérite noueuse. A propos de 15 cas. *J. Radiol. Electrol. Med. Nucl.* 57:505, 1976.

123. Dombrowski, H., and Korb, G. Das Gefässbild bei Enteritis regionalis (Morbus Crohn) und sein diagnostische Bedeutung. *Radiologe* 10:17, 1970.

124. Drucker, W. R., Davis, J. H., Holden, W. D., and Reagan, J. R. Hemorrhagic necrosis of the intestine: A clinical syndrome present without organic vascular occlusion. *Arch. Surg.* 89:42, 1964.

125. Drummond, H. Some points relating to the surgical anatomy of the arterial supply of the large intestine. *Proc. R. Soc. Med.* 7:185, 1913.

126. Dunbar, J. D. Reversible cecal infarction. *Am. J. Surg.* 112:447, 1966.

127. Dunbar, J. D., Molnar, W., Beman, F. F., and Marable, S. A. Compression of the celiac trunk and abdominal angina: Preliminary report of 15 cases. *AJR* 95:731, 1965.

128. Dwight, T. Cited by Michels et al. [246].

129. Eisenberg, D., and Sherwood, C. E. Bleeding Meckel's diverticulum diagnosed by arteriography and radioisotope imaging. *Am. J. Dig. Dis.* 20:573, 1975.

130. Ekberg, O., and Ekholm, S. Radiology in primary small bowel adenocarcinoma. *Gastrointest. Radiol.* 5:49, 1980.

131. Ekberg, O., and Ekholm, S. Radiography in primary tumors of the small bowel. *Acta Radiol. [Diagn.]* (Stockh.) 21:79, 1980.

132. Ekelund, L., Gerlock, J., Molin, J., and Smith, C. Roentgenologic appearance of fibromuscular dysplasia. *Acta Radiol. [Diagn.]* (Stockh.) 19:433, 1978.

133. Ekelund, L., and Lunderquist, A. Pharmacoangiography with angiotensin. *Radiology* 110:533, 1974.

134. Ende, N. Infarction of the bowel in cardiac failure. *N. Engl. J. Med.* 258:879, 1958.

135. Engelhardt, J. E., and Jacobson, G. Infarction of the colon, demonstrated by barium enema. *Radiology* 67:573, 1956.

136. Eriksson, U., Fagerberg, S., Krause, U., and Olding, L. Angiographic studies in Crohn's disease and ulcerative colitis. *AJR* 110:385, 1970.

137. Faris, J. C., and Whitley, J. E. Angiographic demonstration of Meckel's diverticulum: Case report and review of the literature. *Radiology* 108:285, 1973.

138. Farman, J. Vascular lesions of the colon. *Br. J. Radiol.* 39:575, 1966.

139. Feller, E., Rickert, R., and Spiro, H. M. Small Vessel Disease of the Gut. In S. J. Boley, S. S.

Schwartz, and L. F. Williams, Jr. (eds.), *Vascular Disorders of the Intestine.* New York: Appleton-Century-Crofts, 1971.

140. Fenlon, J. W., and Schackelford, G. D. Peutz-Jeghers syndrome. Case report with angiographic evaluation. *Radiology* 103:595, 1972.

141. Finkbine, R. B., and Decker, J. P. Ulceration and perforation of the intestine due to necrotizing arteriolitis. *N. Engl. J. Med.* 268:14, 1963.

142. Fontaine, R., Kieny, R., Japy, C., and Warter, P. Etude angiographique des oblitérations de l'artère mésentérique supérieure. *J. Radiol. Electrol. Med. Nucl.* 47:1, 1966.

143. Fontaine, R., Kim, M., and Kiney, R. Le traitement chirurgical des oblitérations des artères mésentériques: Aspect clinique, artériographique et indications chirurgicales. *Lyon Chir.* 58:641, 1962.

144. Friedenberg, M. J., Polk, H. C., Jr., McAlister, W. H., and Shochat, S. J. Superior mesenteric arteriography in experimental mesenteric venous thrombosis. *Radiology* 85:38, 1965.

145. Friedmann, G., Bützler, H. O., and Wehrle, J. Angiographische Befunde bei zwei rezidivierend blutenden Meckelschen Divertikeln (MD). *ROEFO* 120:446, 1974.

146. Fry, W. J., and Kraft, R. O. Visceral angina. *Surg. Gynecol. Obstet.* 117:417, 1963.

147. Fujii, K., Grayson, T., Margulis, A. R., and Saltzstein, S. L. The effects of intra-arterial injection of contrast media on canine intestine. *AJR* 89:730, 1963.

148. Furrer, J., Grüntzig, A., Kugelmeier, J., and Goebel, N. Treatment of abdominal angina with percutaneous dilatation of an arteria mesenterica superior stenosis. Preliminary communication. *Cardiovasc. Intervent. Radiol.* 3:43, 1980.

149. Galloway, S. J., Casarella, W. J., and Shimkin, P. M. Vascular malformations of the right colon as a cause of bleeding in patients with aortic stenosis. *Radiology* 113:11, 1974.

150. Gasquet, C., and Barbier, J. L'artériographie sélective mésentérique supérieure dans le syndrome de Peutz-Jeghers. *Sem. Hop. Paris* 44:1953, 1968.

151. Gershater, R. Enterolith causing bleeding in a patient with Meckel's diverticulum. Angiographic demonstration. *Radiology* 120:327, 1976.

152. Ghahremani, G. G., Kangarloo, H., Volberg, F., and Meyers, M. A. Diffuse cavernous hemangioma of the colon in the Klippel-Trenaunay syndrome. *Radiology* 118:673, 1976.

153. Gilbert, R. P. Mechanisms of the hemodynamic effects of endotoxin. *Physiol. Rev.* 40:245, 1960.

154. Glotzer, D. J., and Shaw, R. S. Massive bowel infarction: An autopsy study assessing the

potentialities of reconstructive vascular surgery. *N. Engl. J. Med.* 260:162, 1959.

155. Goertler, K. Das Gefässystem in Bauchraum aus der Sicht des Pathologen. In H. Bertelheimer and N. Heisig (eds.), *Aktuelle Gastroenterologie.* Stuttgart: Thieme, 1968.

156. Gold, R. E., and Redman, H. C. Mesenteric fibrosis simulating the angiographic appearance of ileal carcinoid tumor. *Radiology* 103:85, 1972.

157. Goldstein, H. M., and Miller, M. Angiographic evaluation of carcinoid tumors of the small intestine: The value of epinephrine. *Radiology* 115:23, 1975.

158. Goldstone, J., More, W. S., and Hall, A. P. Chronic occlusion of the superior and inferior mesenteric veins. *Ann. Surg.* 36:235, 1970.

159. Gonzales, L. L., and Jaffe, M. S. Mesenteric arterial insufficiency following abdominal aortic resection. *Arch. Surg.* 93:10, 1966.

160. Gooding, R. A., and Couch, R. D. Mesenteric ischemia without vascular occlusion. *Arch. Surg.* 85:186, 1962.

161. Gordon, R. B., Capetillo, A., and Principato, D. J. Angiographic demonstration of a lymphatic cyst of the mesentery: A case report. *AJR* 104:870, 1968.

162. Gotsman, M. S., Beck, W., and Schrire, V. Selective angiography in arteritis of the aorta and its major branches. *Radiology* 88:232, 1967.

163. Gottlob, R. *Angiographie und Klinik.* Wien-Bonn: Maudrich, 1956.

164. Grainger, K., and Aber, C. Dissection of the superior mesenteric artery during aortography with recovery—report of a case. *Br. J. Radiol.* 34:265, 1961.

165. Gray, R. K., and Grollman, J. H., Jr. Acute lower gastrointestinal bleeding secondary to varices of the superior mesenteric venous system. Angiographic demonstration. *Radiology* 111:559, 1974.

166. Grayson, T., Margulis, A. R., Heinbecker, P., and Saltzstein, S. L. Effects of intra-arterial injection of Miokon, Hypaque, and Renografin in the small intestine of the dog. *Radiology* 77:776, 1961.

167. Green, H. D., and Kepchar, J. H. Control of peripheral resistance in major systemic vascular beds. *Physiol. Rev.* 39:617,1959.

168. Griffiths, J. D. Extramural and intramural blood supply of colon. *Br. Med. J.* 1:323, 1961.

169. Guy, J. M., Davies, R. L., McLachlan, M. S. F., and Evans, K. T. Effects of intra-arterial phentolamine in experimental intestinal ischemia in the rabbit. *Br. J. Radiol.* 46:440, 1973.

170. Habboushe, F., Wallace, H. W., and Nusbaum, M. Nonocclusive mesenteric vascular insufficiency. *Ann. Surg.* 180:819, 1974.

171. Hagihara, P. F., Chuang, V. P., and Griffen, W. O. Arteriovenous malformation of the colon. *Am. J. Surg.* 133:681, 1977.

172. Halpern, M., Turner, A. F., and Citron, B. P. Angiodysplasia of the abdominal viscera associated with hereditary hemorrhagic telangiectasia. *AJR* 102:783, 1968.

173. Halpern, M., Turner, A. F., and Citron, B. P. Hereditary hemorrhagic telangiectasia. An angiographic study of abdominal visual angiodysplasia associated with gastrointestinal hemorrhage. *Radiology* 90:1143, 1968.

174. Han, S. Y., Jander, H. P., and Laws, H. L. Polyarteritis nodosa causing severe intestinal bleeding. *Gastrointest. Radiol.* 1:285, 1976.

175. Hanafee, W. Axillary artery approach to carotid, vertebral, abdominal aorta, and coronary angiography. *Radiology* 81:559, 1963.

176. Harris, P. L., and Charlesworth, D. Chronic intestinal ischemia due to aortoiliac steal. *J. Cardiovasc. Surg.* (Torino) 15:122, 1974.

177. Hawkins, C. F. Jejunal stenosis following mesenteric artery occlusion. *Lancet* 2:121, 1957.

178. Hearn, J. B. Duodenal ileus with special reference to superior mesenteric artery compression. *Radiology* 86:305, 1966.

179. Herlinger, H. Angiography in Crohn's disease. *Clin. Gastroenterol.* 1:383, 1972.

180. Herlinger, H. Angiography of visceral arteries. *Clin. Gastroenterol.* 1:547, 1972.

181. Hermanutz, K. D., Bücheler, E., and Biersack, H. J. Zur Röntgendiagnose des Karzinoids. *ROEFO* 121:186, 1974.

182. Hernandez, C., Morin, G., and Ecarlat, B. L'émbol pulsé en artériographie sélective digestive. *Presse Med.* 73:2889, 1965.

183. Herschman, A., Blum, R., and Lee, Y. C. Angiographic findings in polyarteritis nodosa. Report of a case. *Radiology* 94:147, 1970.

184. Hoffman, F. G., Zimmerman, S. L., and Cardwell, E. S., Jr. Massive intestinal infarction without vascular occlusion associated with aortic insufficiency. *N. Engl. J. Med.* 263:436, 1960.

185. Jacobson, E. D. Physiologic Aspects of the Intestinal Circulation. In S. J. Boley, S. S. Schwartz, and L. F. Williams, Jr. (eds.), *Vascular Disorders of the Intestine.* New York: Appleton-Century-Crofts, 1971.

186. Janson, R., and Beltz, L. Abdominelle Aortakoarktation, kombiniert mit Abgangsstenosen des Truncus coeliacus, der Arteria mesenterica superior und der Arteria renalis beidseits. *ROEFO* 118:690, 1973.

187. Jensen, R., and Olin, T. Balloon catheters in angiography. An experimental investigation in rabbits. *Acta Radiol.* [*Diagn.*] (Stockh.) 12:721, 1972.

188. Johnson, P. C. Autoregulation in the Intestine and Mesentery. In S. J. Boley, S. S. Schwartz, and L. F. Williams, Jr. (eds.), *Vascular Disorders of the Intestine.* New York: Appleton-Century-Crofts, 1971.

189. Johnsson, C. C., and Baggenstoss, A. H.

Mesenteric vascular occlusion: II. Study of 60 cases of occlusion of arteries and of 12 cases of occlusion of both arteries and veins. *Mayo Clin. Proc.* 24:649, 1949.

190. Joske, R. A., Shamma'a, M. H., and Drummey, G. D. Intestinal malabsorption following temporary occlusion of the superior mesenteric artery. *Am. J. Med.* 25:449, 1958.

191. Kadir, S., Athanasoulis, C. A., and Greenfield, A. J. Intestinal volvulus: Angiographic findings. *Radiology* 128:595, 1978.

192. Kahn, P. C., Frates, W. J., and Paul, R. E., Jr. The epinephrine effect in angiography of gastrointestinal tract tumors. *Radiology* 88:686, 1967.

193. Kahn, P. C., O'Halloran, J. F., Jr., and Paul, R. E., Jr. Improved portography by delayed postepinephrine celiac and mesenteric arteriography. *Radiology* 92:86, 1969.

194. Kalima, T. V., Peltokallio, P., and Myllärniemi, H. Vascular pattern in ileal Crohn's disease. *Ann. Clin. Res.* 7:23, 1975.

195. Kameron, G. R., and Khanna, S. D. Regeneration of the intestinal villi after extensive mucosal infarction. *J. Pathol.* 77:505, 1959.

196. Kanter, I. E., Schwartz, A. J., and Fleming, R. J. Localization of bleeding point in chronic and acute gastrointestinal hemorrhage by means of selective visceral arteriography. *AJR* 103:386, 1968.

197. Kaplan, J. H., and Bookstein, J. J. Abdominal visceral pharmacoangiography with angiotensin. *Radiology* 103:79, 1972.

198. Katzen, B. T., Rossi, P., Passariello, R., and Simonetti, G. Transcatheter therapeutic arterial embolization. *Radiology* 120:523, 1976.

199. Katzen, B. T., Sprayregen, S., Chisolm, A., and Rossi, P. Angiographic manifestations of regional enteritis. *Gastrointest. Radiol.* 1:271, 1976.

200. Kaude, J., Silseth, Ch., and Tylén, U. Angiography in myomas of the gastrointestinal tract. *Acta Radiol. [Diagn.]* (Stockh.) 12:691, 1972.

201. Kaufman, S. L., Harrington, D. P., and Siegelman, S. S. Superior mesenteric artery embolization: An angiographic emergency. *Radiology* 124:625, 1977.

202. Keeley, F. X., Misanik, L. F., and Wirts, C. W. Abdominal angina syndrome. *Gastroenterology* 37:480, 1959.

203. Kinkhabwala, M., and Balthazar, E. J. Carcinoid tumors of the alimentary tract: II. Angiographic diagnosis of small intestinal and colonic lesions. *Gastrointest. Radiol.* 3:57, 1978.

204. Kinkhabwala, M., Mousavi, A., Iyer, S., and Adamsons, R. Bleeding ilear varicosity demonstrated by transhepatic portography. *AJR* 129:514, 1977.

205. Klein, H. J., Alfidi, R. J., Meaney, T. F., and Poirier, V. C. Angiography in the diagnosis of chronic gastrointestinal bleeding. *Radiology* 98:83, 1971.

206. Knutson, H., Lunderquist, A., and Lunderquist, A. Vascular changes in Crohn's disease. *AJR* 103:380, 1968.

207. Koehler, P. R. Dir Darstellung von massiven akuten Blutungen des Magen-Darm-Kanals durch Arteriographie. *ROEFO* 110:1, 1969.

208. Koehler, P. R., and Salmon, R. B. Angiographic localization of unknown acute gastrointestinal bleeding sites. *Radiology* 89:244, 1967.

209. Koikkalainen, K., and Köhler, R. Stenosis and occlusion in the celiac and mesenteric arteries. *Ann. Chir. Gynaecol.* 60:9, 1971.

210. Lande, A., Bedford, A., and Schechter, L. S. The spectrum of arteriographic finding in Osler-Weber-Rendu's disease. *Angiology* 27:223, 1976.

211. Lande, A., and Meyers, M. A. Iatrogenic embolization of the superior mesenteric artery: Arteriographic observations and clinical implications. *AJR* 126:822, 1976.

212. Lande, A., Schechter, L. S., and Bole, P. V. Angiographic diagnosis of small intestinal intussusception. *Radiology* 122:691, 1977.

213. Lapicirella, V., and Weber, G. La claudicazione mesenterica sindroma di allarme della malattia coronarica. *Arch. De Vecchi Anat. Pathol.* 19:1123, 1953.

214. Laufman, H., Nora, P. F., and Mittelpunkt, A. I. Mesenteric blood vessels: Advances in surgery and physiology. *Arch. Surg.* 88:1021, 1964.

215. Laufman, H., and Scheinberg, S. Arterial and venous mesenteric occlusion. Analysis of 44 cases. *Am. J. Surg.* 58:84, 1942.

216. Ledgerwood, A., and Lucas, C. E. Survival following proximal superior mesenteric artery occlusion from trauma. *J. Trauma* 14:622, 1974.

217. Leonidas, J. C., Amoury, R. A., Aschcraft, K. W., and Fellows, R. A. Duodenojejunal atresia with "apple-peel" small bowel: A distinct form of intestinal ischemia. *Radiology* 118:661, 1976.

218. Leymarios, J. Contribution à l'Étude de la Pathologie de l'Artère Mésentérique Supérieure: l'Ischémie Intestinale Non Nécrosante. Thèse Médicine, Paris, 1960.

219. Lillehei, R. C. The intestinal factor in irreversible hemorrhagic shock. *Surgery* 42:1043, 1957.

220. Louisy, C. L., and Barton, C. J. The radiological diagnosis of *strongyloides stercoralis* enteritis. *Radiology* 98:535, 1971.

221. Lunderquist, A. Angiography in carcinoma of the pancreas. *Acta Radiol. [Suppl.]* (Stockh.) 235:1, 1965.

222. Lunderquist, A. Arterial segmental supply of the liver: An angiographic study. *Acta Radiol. [Suppl.]* (Stockh.) 272:1, 1967.

223. Lunderquist, A., and Lunderquist, A. Angiography in ulcerative colitis. *AJR* 99:18, 1967.

224. Lunderquist, A., and Lunderquist, A. Arterio-

graphic appearance of intestinal adhesions. *AJR* 103:354, 1968.

225. Lunderquist, A., Lunderquist, A., H:Son Holmdahl, K., and Clemens, F. Selective superior mesenteric arteriography in reticulum cell sarcoma of the small bowel. *Radiology* 98:113, 1971.

226. Lunderquist, A., Lunderquist, A., and Knutsson, H. Angiography in Crohn's disease of the small bowel and colon. *AJR* 101:338, 1967.

227. Lunderquist, A., Lunderquist, A., and Nommesen, N. Angiographic changes during digestion. *AJR* 107:191, 1969.

228. MacGregor, A. M. C., Abney, H. T., and Morris, L. Pharmacodynamic response in nonocclusive mesenteric ischemia. *Am. Surg.* 40:381, 1974.

229. Mandell, H. N. Abdominal angina: Report of a case and review of the literature. *N. Engl. J. Med.* 257:1035, 1957.

230. Margulis, A. R., and Heinbecker, P. Mesenteric arteriography. *AJR* 86:103, 1961.

231. Margulis, A. R., Heinbecker, P., and Bernard, H. R. Operative mesenteric arteriography in the search for the site of bleeding in unexplained gastrointestinal hemorrhage: A preliminary report. *Surgery* 48:534, 1960.

232. Marks, W. M., Jacobs, R. P., and Clark, R. E. Neoplastic pseudoaneurysm of the superior mesenteric artery. *Radiology* 126:622, 1978.

233. Marshak, R. H., Maklansky, D., and Calem, S. H. Segmental infarction of the colon. *Am. J. Dig. Dis.* 10:86, 1965.

234. Matthews, A. E., and White, R. R. Primary mesenteric venous occlusive disease. *Am. J. Surg.* 122:579, 1971.

235. Mavor, G. E., and Chrystal, K. M. R. Problems in mesenteric infarction. *J. Cardiovasc. Surg. (Torino)* 3:250, 1962.

236. Mavor, G. E., and Michie, W. Chronic midgut ischaemia. *Br. Med. J.* 2:534, 1958.

237. May, A. G., Lipchik, E. O., and Deweese, J. A. Repair of injured visceral arteries. *Ann. Surg.* 162:869, 1965.

238. Mayo, C. W. Blood supply of the colon: Surgical considerations. *Surg. Clin. North Am.* 35:1117, 1955.

239. McAfee, J. G. A survey of complications of abdominal aortography. *Radiology* 68:825, 1957.

240. McAlister, W. H., Margulis, A. R., Heinbecker, P., and Spjut, H. Arteriography and microangiography of gastric and colonic lesions. *Radiology* 79:769, 1962.

241. McClelland, R. N., and Duke, J. H. Successful resection of an idiopathic aneurysm of the superior mesenteric artery. *Ann. Surg.* 164:167, 1966.

242. McPhedran, N. T., Holliday, R., and Colapinto, R. F. Angiographic diagnosis of strangulated bowel obstruction. *Can. J. Surg.* 13:90, 1970.

243. Melick, W. F., Byrne, J. E., and Boler, T. D. The experimental and clinical investigation of various media used in translumbar aortography. *J. Urol.* 67:1019, 1952.

244. Meyers, M. A. Arteriographic diagnosis of internal (left paraduodenal) hernia. *Radiology* 92:1035, 1969.

245. Meyers, M. A., and King, M. C. Leiomyosarcoma of the duodenum: Angiographic findings and report of a case. *Radiology* 91:788, 1968.

246. Michels, N. A., Siddarth, P., Kornblith, P. L., and Parke, W. W. The variant blood supply to the small and large intestines: Its import in regional resections. *J. Int. Coll. Surg.* 39:127, 1963.

247. Mikkelsen, W. P., and Zaro, J. A., Jr. Intestinal angina: Report of a case with preoperative diagnosis and surgical relief. *N. Engl. J. Med.* 260:912, 1959.

248. Miller, K. D., Jr., Tutton, R. H., Bell, K. A., and Simon, R. K. Angiodysplasia of the colon. *Radiology* 132:309, 1979.

249. Miller, M. H., Lunderquist, A., and Tylén, U. Angiographic spectrum in Crohn's disease of the small intestine and colon. *Surg. Gynecol. Obstet.* 141:907, 1975.

250. Miller, W. J., Reuter, S. R., and Redman, H. C. Epinephrine effect in angiography of colonic carcinoma: An inconsistent aid in diagnosis. *Invest. Radiol.* 4:246, 1969.

251. Ming, S.-C., and Levitan, R. Acute hemorrhagic necrosis of the gastrointestinal tract. *N. Engl. J. Med.* 263:59, 1960.

252. Moore, J. D., Thompson, N. W., Appelman, H. D., and Foley, D. Arteriovenous malformations of the gastrointestinal tract. *Arch. Surg.* 111:381, 1976.

253. Morino, F., Tarquini, A., and Olivero, S. Artériographie abdominale sélective par le cathétérisme de l'artère humérale. *Presse Med.* 64:1944, 1956.

254. Morris, G. C., Jr. Abdominal angina. *Heart Bull.* 10:5, 1961.

255. Morris, G. C., Jr., Crawford, E. S., Cooley, D. A., and DeBakey, M. E. Revascularization of the celiac and superior mesenteric arteries. *Arch. Surg.* 84:95, 1962.

256. Morris, G. C., Jr., and DeBakey, M. E. Abdominal angina—diagnosis and surgical treatment. *J.A.M.A.* 176:89, 1961.

257. Morson, B. C. Pathology of ischemic colitis. *Clin. Gastroenterol.* 1:765, 1972.

258. Moskowitz, M., Zimmerman, H., and Felson, B. The meandering mesenteric artery of the colon. *AJR* 92:1088, 1964.

259. Moss, A. A., Margulis, A. R., Lee, J. C., and Youker, J. E. The effect of intra-arterial contrast media on the small intestine of rabbit: An electron microscopic study. *Radiology* 108:279, 1973.

260. Mowitz, D., and Finne, B. Postoperative arteriovenous aneurysm in mesentery after small bowel resection. *J.A.M.A.* 173:42, 1960.

261. Muller, R. F., and Figley, M. M. The arteries of the abdomen, pelvis, and thigh: I. Normal roentgenographic anatomy. II. Collateral circulation in obstructive arterial disease. *AJR* 77:296, 1957.

262. Munnell, E. R., Mota, C. R., and Thompson, W. B. Iatrogenic arteriovenous fistula: Report of a case involving the superior mesenteric vessels. *Am. Surg.* 26:738, 1960.

263. Nebesar, R. A., Kornblith, P. L., Pollard, J. J., and Michels, N. A. *Celiac and Superior Mesenteric Arteries: A Correlation of Angiograms and Dissections.* Boston: Little, Brown, 1969.

264. Nebesar, R. A., and Pollard, J. J. Portal venography by selective arterial catheterization. *AJR* 97:477, 1966.

265. Nebesar, R. A., Pollard, J. J., Edmunds, L. H., Jr., and McKhann, C. F. Indications for selective celiac and superior mesenteric angiography: Experience with 128 cases. *AJR* 92:1100, 1964.

266. Noer, R. J., Derr, J. W., and Johnston, C. G. The circulation of the small intestine: An evaluation of its revascularizing potential. *Ann. Surg.* 130:608, 1949.

267. Noonan, C. D., Rambo, O. N., and Margulis, A. R. Effect of timed occlusions at various levels of mesenteric arteries and veins: Correlative study of arteriographic and histologic patterns of rat gut. *Radiology* 90:99, 1968.

268. Norryd, C., Dencker, H., Lunderquist, A., and Olin, T. Superior mesenteric blood flow in man following injection of bradykinin and vasopressin into the superior mesenteric artery. *Acta Chir. Scand.* 141:119, 1975.

269. Nusbaum, M., and Baum, S. Radiographic demonstration of unknown sites of gastrointestinal bleeding. *Surg. Forum* 14:374, 1963.

270. Nusbaum, M., Baum, S., Kuroda, K., and Blakemore, W. S. Control of portal hypertension by selective mesenteric arterial drug infusion. *Arch. Surg.* 97:1005, 1968.

271. Nyman, U. Angiography in hereditary hemorrhagic telangiectasia. *Acta Radiol.* [*Diagn.*] (Stockh.) 18:581, 1977.

272. Nyman, U., Boijsen, E., Lindström, C., and Rosengren, J.-E. Angiography in angiomatous lesions of the gastrointestinal tract. *Acta Radiol.* [*Diagn.*] (Stockh.) 21:21, 1980.

273. Ödman, P. Percutaneous selective angiography of the superior mesenteric artery. *Acta Radiol.* (Stockh.) 51:25, 1959.

274. Olivero, S. Angiografia selettiva dell'arteria mesenterica superiore. *Minerva Cardioangiol.* 8:55, 1960.

275. Olsson, O. Viszerale angiographie. *Bibl. Gastroenterol.* 8:127, 1965.

276. Ottinger, L. W., and Austen, W. G. A study of 136 patients with mesenteric infarction. *Surg. Gynecol. Obstet.* 124:251, 1967.

277. Passi, R. B., and Lansing, A. M. Experimental intestinal malabsorption produced by vascular insufficiency. *Can. J. Surg.* 7:332, 1964.

278. Penner, A., and Bernheim, A. I. Acute postoperative enterocolitis: A study on the pathologic nature of shock. *Arch. Pathol.* 27:966, 1939.

279. Perdue, G. D., Jr., and Smith, R. B. Atheromatous microemboli. *Ann. Surg.* 169:954, 1969.

280. Perdue, G. D., Jr., and Smith, R. B. Intestinal ischemia due to mesenteric arterial disease. *Am. Surg.* 36:152, 1970.

281. Perlberger, R. R. Demonstration of bleeding from Meckel's diverticulum by means of selective arteriography of the superior mesenteric artery. *Radiol. Clin.* (Basel) 44:397, 1975.

282. Philips, J. C., and Howland, W. J. Mesenteric arteritis in systemic lupus erythematosus. *J.A.M.A.* 206:1569, 1968.

283. Phillips, D. A., Adams, D. F., Beckmann, C. F., and Abrams, H. L. Balloon-occlusion superior mesenteric arteriography for improved visualization of the mesenteric and portal venous anatomy of dogs. *Invest. Radiol.* 15:129, 1980.

284. Pierce, G. E., and Brockenbrough, E. C. The spectrum of mesenteric infarction. *Am. J. Surg.* 119:233, 1970.

285. Polk, H. C. Experimental mesenteric venous occlusion. *Ann. Surg.* 163:432, 1966.

286. Pollard, J. J., and Nebesar, R. A. Abdominal angiography. *N. Engl. J. Med.* 279:1148, 1968.

287. Porcher, P., Chérigié, E., Chalut, J., Bennet, J., and Prot, D. Les syndromes douloureux abdominaux d'origine vasculaire. *Ann. Radiol.* (Paris) 7:483, 1964.

288. Pugh, J. I., and Stringer, P. Abdominal periarteritis nodosa. *Br. J. Surg.* 44:302, 1956–57.

289. Rabinovitch, J., and Rabinovitch, S. Infarction of the small intestine sequent to polyarteritis nodosa of the mesenteric vessels. *Am. J. Surg.* 88:896, 1954.

290. Ramer, M., Mitty, H. A., and Baron, M. G. Angiography in leiomyomatous neoplasms of the small bowel. *AJR* 113:263, 1971.

291. Rankin, R. S., and Hussey, J. L. Idiopathic inferior mesenteric venous thrombosis demonstrated by angiography. *Gastrointest. Radiol.* 1:275, 1976.

292. Ranniger, K., and Scheiner, D. L. Experimental bowel ischemia. *Arch. Surg.* 95:768, 1967.

293. Ratschow, M., and Hasse, H. M. Angiologie. *Munch. Med. Wochenschr.* 95:1040, 1953.

294. Read, R. C., and Meyer, M. The role of red cell agglutination in arteriographic complications. *Surg. Forum* 10:472, 1959.

295. Reams, G. B. A middle colic arteriovenous

fistula developing as a postgastrectomy complication. *Arch. Surg.* 81:757, 1960.

296. Recek, C., Kren, V., Fixa, B., and Steinhart, L. Selective mesentericography as a guide to diagnosis and treatment of acute superior mesenteric artery occlusion. *J. Cardiovasc. Surg.* (Torino) 9:184, 1968.

297. Redman, H. C. Mesenteric arterial and venous blood flow changes following selective arterial injection of vasodilators. *Invest. Radiol.* 9:193, 1974.

298. Redman, H. C. Demonstration of portocaval shunts and superior mesenteric venous collateral channels following selective intra-arterial injection of vasodilators. *Invest. Radiol.* 9:199, 1974.

299. Redman, H. C., Berg, N. O., and Boijsen, E. Absence of toxicity of contrast media in the superior mesenteric artery: A pathologic study in rabbits. *Invest. Radiol.* 2:123, 1967.

300. Redman, H. C., Reuter, S. R., and Miller, W. J. Improvement of superior mesenteric and portal vein visualization with tolazoline. *Invest. Radiol.* 4:24, 1969.

301. Reeves, J. D., and Wang, C. C. The stages of mesenteric artery disease. *South. Med. J.* 54:541, 1961.

302. Reichardt, W. Angiographischer Befund bei Karzinoidmetastasen im Mesenterium. *ROEFO* 129:185, 1978.

303. Reiner, L. Mesenteric arterial insufficiency and abdominal angina. *Arch. Intern. Med.* 114:765, 1964.

304. Reiner, L., Platt, R., Rodriguez, F. L., and Jimenez, F. A. Injection studies on the mesenteric arterial circulation: II. Intestinal infarction. *Gastroenterology* 39:747, 1960.

305. Reiner, L., Rodriguez, F. L., Jimenez, F. A., and Platt, R. Injection studies on mesenteric arterial circulation: III. Occlusions without intestinal infarction. *Arch. Pathol.* 73:461, 1962.

306. Reiner, L., Rodriguez, F. L., Platt, R., and Schlesinger, M. J. Injection studies on mesenteric arterial circulation: I. Technique and observations on collaterals. *Surgery* 45:820, 1959.

307. Renert, W. A., Button, K. F., Fuld, S. L., and Casarella, W. J. Mesenteric venous thrombosis and small-bowel infarction following infusion of vasopressin into the superior mesenteric artery. *Radiology* 102:299, 1972.

308. Reuter, S. R., and Boijsen, E. Angiographic findings in two ileal carcinoid tumors. *Radiology* 87:836, 1966.

309. Reuter, S. R., Fry, W. J., and Bookstein, J. J. Mesenteric artery branch aneurysms. *Arch. Surg.* 97:497, 1968.

310. Reuter, S. R., Kanter, J. E., and Redman, H. C. Angiography in reversible colonic ischemia. *Radiology* 97:371, 1971.

311. Reuter, S. R., and Olin, T. Stenosis of the celiac artery. *Radiology* 85:617, 1965.

312. Reuter, S. R., and Redman, H. C. *Gastrointestinal Angiography.* Philadelphia: Saunders, 1977.

313. Riba, P. O., and Lunderquist, A. Angiographic findings in villous tumors of the colon. *AJR* 117:287, 1973.

314. Ripley, H. R., and Levin, S. M. Abdominal angina associated with fibromuscular hyperplasia of the celiac and superior mesenteric arteries. *Angiology* 17:297, 1966.

315. Rob, C. Symposium on obliteration of visceral arteries: The indications for operation in occlusive disease of the visceral arteries. *J. Cardiovasc. Surg.* (Torino) 3:223, 1962.

316. Rob, C. Surgical diseases of the celiac and mesenteric arteries. *Arch. Surg.* 93:21, 1966.

317. Robert, P. E., Pradel, E., Hernandez, C., and Chemali, A. Utilisation et enseignement de l'artériographie sélective dans un syndrome de Peutz-Jeghers. *Sem. Hop. Paris* 42:1975. 1966.

318. Roberts, C., and Maddison, F. E. Partial mesenteric arterial occlusion with subsequent ischemic bowel damage due to pitressin infusion. *AJR* 126:829, 1976.

319. Robins, J. M., and Bookstein, J. J. Regressing aneurysms in periarteritis nodosa: A report of three cases. *Radiology* 104:39, 1972.

320. Rogers, B. H. A newly recognized syndrome: (1) Lower intestinal blood loss of obscure cause, (2) hemangiomas of the right large bowel and (3) cardiac vascular or pulmonary insufficiency. *Gastrointest. Endosc.* 25:47, 1979.

321. Rogers, L. F., and Goldstein, H. M. Roentgen manifestations of radiation injury to the gastrointestinal tract. *Gastrointest. Radiol.* 2:281, 1977.

322. Rösch, J., Dotter, C. T., and Rose, R. W. Selective arterial infusions of vasoconstrictors in acute gastrointestinal bleeding. *Radiology* 99:27, 1971.

323. Rosenberger, A., Munk, J., Schramek, A., and Arieh, J. B. The angiographic appearance of thromboangiitis obliterans (Buerger's disease) in the abdominal visceral vessels. *Br. J. Radiol.* 46:337, 1973.

324. Rosenman, L. D., and Gropper, A. N. Small intestine stenosis caused by infarction: An unusual sequel of mesenteric artery embolism. *Ann. Surg.* 141:254, 1955.

325. Ross, A. J. Vascular patterns of small and large intestine compared. *Br. J. Surg.* 39:330, 1952.

326. Roy, P. Percutaneous catheterization via the axillary artery: A new approach to some technical roadblocks in selective arteriography. *AJR* 94:1, 1965.

327. Sacks, B., Joffe, N., and Harris, N. Isolated mesenteric dermoids (mesenteric fibromatosis). *Clin. Radiol.* 29:95, 1978.

328. Sacks, R. P., Sheft, D. J., and Freeman, J. H. The demonstration of the mesenteric collateral circulation in young patients. *AJR* 102:401, 1968.

329. Schobinger, R., Blackman, G., and Kan Lin, R. Operative intestinal arteriography. *Acta Radiol.* (Stockh.) 48:330, 1957.
330. Schroeder, F. M., Miller, F. J., Nelson, J. A., and Rankin, R. S. Gastrointestinal angiographic findings in systemic amyloidosis. *AJR* 131:143, 1978.
331. Schwartz, S., Boley, S., Lash, J., and Sternhill, V. Roentgenologic aspects of reversible vascular occlusion of the colon and its relationship to ulcerative colitis. *Radiology* 80:625, 1963.
332. Schwartz, S., Boley, S., Schultz, L., and Allen, A. A survey of vascular diseases of the small intestine. *Semin. Roentgenol.* 1:178, 1966.
333. Schwartz, S., and Waters, L. Cholesterol embolization. *Radiology* 106:37, 1973.
334. Scott, W. W., Jr., Harrington, D. P., and Siegelman, S. S. Functional abnormalities of mesenteric blood flow. A guide to organic disease of the bowel. *Gastrointest. Radiol.* 1:367, 1977.
335. Seo, K. W., Bookstein, J. J., and Brown, H. S. Angiography of intussusception of the small bowel. *Radiology* 132:603, 1979.
336. Sewell, R. A. Small bowel injury by angiographic contrast media. *Surgery* 64:459, 1968.
337. Shaw, R. S., and Maynard, E. P., III. Acute and chronic thrombosis of the mesenteric arteries associated with malabsorption: A report of two cases successfully treated by thromboendarterectomy. *N. Engl. J. Med.* 258:874, 1958.
338. Sheedy, P. F., II, Fulton, R. E., and Atwell, D. T. Angiographic evaluation of patients with chronic gastrointestinal bleeding. *AJR* 123:338, 1975.
339. Shimkin, P. M., Devita, V. T., and Doppman, J. L. Arteriography of an ileal carcinoid tumor. *J. Can. Assoc. Radiol.* 23:259, 1971.
340. Shippey, S. H., Jr., and Acker, J. J. Segmental infarction of the colon demonstrated by selective inferior mesenteric angiography. *Am. J. Surg.* 109:671, 1965.
341. Siegelman, S. S. An Aggressive Approach to Acute Small Bowel Ischemia. In A. R. Margulis and C. H. Gooding (eds.), *Diagnostic Radiology.* San Francisco: University of California Printing Department, 1977. Pp. 85–97.
342. Siegelman, S. S., Sprayregen, S., and Boley, S. J. Angiographic diagnosis of mesenteric arterial vasoconstriction. *Radiology* 12:533, 1974.
343. Siegelman, S. S., Warren, A., Veith, F. J., and Boley, S. J. The physiologic response to superior mesenteric angiography. *Radiology* 96:101, 1970.
344. Sniderman, K. W., Baxi, R. K., Saddekni, S., and Sos, T. A. Use of tolazoline enhanced superior mesenteric arteriography to improve opacification of a cecal vascular ectasia: A case report. *Gastrointest. Radiol.* 4:339, 1979.
345. Sniderman, K. W., Franklin, J., Jr., and Sos, T. A. Successful transcatheter Gelfoam emboli-

zation of a a bleeding cecal vascular ectasia. *AJR* 131:157, 1978.
346. Spjut, H. J., and Margulis, A. R. Microangiographic patterns of chronic ulcerative colitis. *Dis. Colon Rectum* 8:215, 1965.
347. Spjut, H. J., Margulis, A. R., and McAlister, W. H. Microangiographic study of gastrointestinal lesions. *AJR* 92:1173, 1964.
348. Stanley, J. C., Thompson, N. W., and Fry, W. J. Splanchnic artery aneurysms. *Arch. Surg.* 101:689, 1970.
349. Steckel, R. J., Rösch, J., Ross, G., and Grollman, J. H., Jr. New developments in pharmacoangiography (and arterial pharmacotherapy) of the gastrointestinal tract. *Invest. Radiol.* 6:199, 1971.
350. Steckel, R. J., Ross, G., and Grollman, J. H., Jr. A potent drug combination for producing constriction of the superior mesenteric artery and its branches. *Radiology* 91:579, 1968.
351. Steger, C., and Cresti, M. Über das Verhalten und die Bedeutung der Arteria mesenterica caudalis in dem nach Verschluss der Bauchaorta und der Beckenarterien sich ausbildenden Kollateralkreislauf. *Z. Kreislaufforsch.* 53:404, 1964.
352. Steinberg, I., Tillotson, P. M., and Halpern, M. Roengenography of systemic (congenital and traumatic) arteriovenous fistulas. *AJR* 89:343, 1963.
353. Steward, J. A., and Rankin, F. W. Blood supply of the large intestine: Its surgical considerations. *Arch. Surg.* 26:843, 1933.
354. Stewart, B. W., Gathright, J. B., and Ray, J. E. Vascular ectasia of the colon. *Surg. Gynecol. Obstet.* 148:670, 1979.
355. Strasberg, Z., Hyland, J., Salem, S., Wilderspin, K., and Tuttle, R. J. The role of angiography in the management of intestinal carcinoid. *Angiology* 26:573, 1975.
356. Strecker, E.-P., Schmidt-Hieber, M., Barth, K., Brobmann, G. F., Birg, W., and Schmidt, H. A. Strophantineffekt auf die Mesenterialarterien (zur Pathogenese der non-occlusive-disease). *Vasa* 4:391, 1975.
357. Sumner, R. G., Kistler, P. C., Barry, W. F., Jr., and McIntosh, H. D. Recognition and surgical repair of superior mesenteric arteriovenous fistula. *Circulation* 27:943, 1963.
358. Suzuki, T., Imamura, M., Kawabe, K., and Honjo, J. Selective demonstration of the variant hepatic artery. *Surg. Gynecol. Obstet.* 135:209, 1972.
359. Taylor, K. B., and Truelove, S. C. Immunological reactions in gastrointestinal disease: A review. *Gut* 3:277, 1962.
360. Taylor, R. M. R., Douglas, A. P., Hacking, P., and Walker, F. C. Traumatic fistula between a main branch of the superior mesenteric artery and vein. *Am. J. Med.* 38:641, 1965.
361. Teicher, I., Arlen, M., Muehlbauer, M., and Allen, A. C. The clinical-pathological spectrum

of primary ulcers of the small intestine. *Surg. Gynecol. Obstet.* 116:196, 1963.

362. Texter, E. C.   Small intestinal blood flow. *Am. J. Dig. Dis.* 8:587, 1963.

363. Touloukian, R. J., Zikria, B. A., and Ferrer, J. M.   Segmental small bowel infarction associated with abdominal angina. *Am. J. Gastroenterol.* 46:347, 1966.

364. Turner, W.   On the existence of a system of anastomosing arteries between and connecting the visceral and parietal branches of the abdominal aorta. *Br. Foreign Med. Chir. Rev.* 32:222, 1963.

365. Udén, R.   Effect of secretin in celiac and superior mesenteric angiography. *Acta Radiol. [Diagn.]* (Stockh.) 8:497, 1969.

366. Udén, R.   Cholecystokinin-pancreozymin in celiac and superior mesenteric angiography. *Acta Radiol. [Diagn.]* (Stockh.) 12:363, 1972.

367. Ulano, H. B., Treat, E., Shanbour, L. L., and Jacobson, E. D.   Selective dilatation of the constricted superior mesenteric artery. *Gastroenterology* 62:39, 1972.

368. Varay, A., Orcel, L., Périer, E., Blondon, J., Durand, F., and Roland, J.   La malabsorption d'origine vasculaire: Contribution à l'étude des artériopathies ostiales mésentériques supérieures et des ulcères primitifs du grêle. *Arch. Fr. Mal. App. Dig.* 53:937, 1964.

369. Vesin, S., and Ochova, A.   Das angiographische Bild des Karzinoids des Verdauungstraktes. *ROEFO* 120:23, 1974.

370. Voegeli, E., and Binswanger, R.   Angiographie bei akuten Dunndarmischämien. *Schweiz. Med. Wochenschr.* 105:1258, 1975.

371. Vollmar, J.   Störungen der arteriellen Durchblutung im Bauchraum. In H. Bertelheimer and N. Heisig (eds.), *Aktuelle Gastroenterologie.* Stuttgart: Thieme, 1968.

372. Völpel, H. W.   Zur Indikation der Aortographie. *Verh. Dtsch. Ges. Kreislaufforsch.* 17:305, 1951.

373. Voorthuisen, A. E. van.   *Ervaringern met selectieve arteriografie van de arteria coeliaca en de arteria mesenterica superior.* Leiden: Staflen's Wetenschappelijke Uitgeversmaatschappij N.V., 1967.

374. Wagner, F. B., Jr., and Price, A. H.   Fatality after abdominal arteriography: Prevention by new modification of technique. *Surgery* 27:621, 1950.

375. Walker, W. J., Goldin, A. R., Shaff, M. I., and Allibone, G. W.   Per catheter control of a haemorrhage from the superior and inferior mesenteric arteries. *Clin. Radiol.* 31:71, 1980.

376. Waltman, A. C., Jang, G. C., Athanasoulis, C. A., Ring, E. J., and Baum, S.   Emergency gastrointestinal angiography. *Geriatrics* 29:48, 1974.

377. Wang, C. C., and Reeves, J. D.   Mesenteric vascular disease. *AJR* 83:895, 1960.

378. Weaver, G. A., Alpern, H. D., Davis, J. S., Ramsey, W. H., and Reichelderfer, M.   Gastrointestinal angiodysplasia associated with aortic valve disease: Part of a spectrum of angiodysplasia of the gut. *Gastroenterology* 77:1, 1979.

379. Weber, J., and Novak, D.   Occlusion arteriography: Diagnostic and therapeutic applicability of balloon catheters. *Cardiovasc. Intervent. Radiol.* 3:97, 1980.

380. Weidner, W., Fox, P., Brooks, J. W., and Vinik, M.   The roentgenographic diagnosis of aneurysms of the superior mesenteric artery. *AJR* 109:138, 1970.

381. Wenz, W., Roth, F.-J., and Brückner, U.   Die Angiographie bei der akuten Gastrointestinalblutung: Experimentelle Voraussetzung und klinische Ergenbnisse. *ROEFO* 110:616, 1969.

382. Whitehouse, G. H.   Solitary angiodysplastic lesions in the ileocecal region diagnosed by angiography. *Gut* 14:977, 1973.

383. Wholey, M. H., Bron, K. M., and Haller, J. D.   Selective angiography of the colon. *Surg. Clin. North Am.* 45:1283, 1965.

384. Widrich, W. C., Nordahl, D. L., and Robbins, A. H.   Contrast enhancement of the mesenteric and portal veins using intraarterial papaverine. *AJR* 121:375, 1974.

385. Williams, L. F., Jr.   Chronic Intestinal Ischemia. In S. J. Boley, S. S. Schwartz, and L. F. Williams, Jr. (eds.), *Vascular Disorders of the Intestine.* New York: Appleton-Century-Crofts, 1971.

386. Williams, L. F., Jr.   Vascular insufficiency of the intestines. *Gastroenterology* 61:757, 1971.

387. Williams, L. F., Jr., Anastasia, L. F., Hasiotis, C. A., Bosniak, M. A., and Byrne, J. J.   Experimental nonocclusive mesenteric ischemia. *Arch. Surg.* 96:987, 1968.

388. Williams, L. F., Jr., Bosniak, M. A., and Wittenberg, J.   Ischemic colitis. *Am. J. Surg.* 117:254, 1969.

389. Williams, L. F., Jr., and Grindlinger, G.   Hemodynamic Effects of Mesenteric Ischemia. In S. J. Boley, S. S. Schwartz, and L. F. Williams, Jr. (eds.), *Vascular Disorders of the Intestine.* New York: Appleton-Century-Crofts, 1971.

390. Williams, L. F., Jr., and Kim, J.-P.   Nonocclusive Mesenteric Ischemia. In S. J. Boley, S. S. Schwartz, and L. F. Williams, Jr. (eds.), *Vascular Disorders of the Intestine.* New York: Appleton-Century-Crofts, 1971.

391. Wilson, R., and Qualheim, R. E.   A form of acute hemorrhagic enterocolitis afflicting chronically ill individuals: A description of twenty cases. *Gastroenterology* 27:431, 1954.

392. Wittenberg, J., Athanasoulis, C. A., Shapiro, J. H., and Williams, L. F., Jr.   A radiological ap-

proach to the patient with acute extensive bowel ischemia. *Radiology* 106:13, 1973.

393. Wittenberg, J., Athanasoulis, C. A., Williams, L. F., Jr., Paredes, S., O'Sullivan, P., and Brown, B. Ischemic colitis: Radiology and pathophysiology. *AJR* 123:287, 1975.

394. Wolf, B. S., and Marshak, R. H. Segmental in-farction of the small bowel. *Radiology* 66:701, 1956.

395. Wylie, E. J., Binkley, F. M., and Palubinskas, A. J. Extrarenal fibromuscular hyperplasia. *Am. J. Surg.* 112:149, 1966.

396. Sweifach, B. W. *Functional Behavior of the Microcirculation.* Springfield, Ill.: Thomas, 1961.

Arteriographic Diagnosis and Treatment of Gastrointestinal Bleeding

STANLEY BAUM

Since its introduction in 1963, selective arteriography has become established as an accurate, safe, and important technique for the diagnosis and treatment of gastrointestinal bleeding [1–3]. When this procedure was initially introduced, it was used exclusively for diagnosis. The selective arterial infusion of vasoconstricting drugs through the same catheter used to identify the bleeding site was a natural outgrowth of diagnostic arteriography. This progression from a diagnostic to a therapeutic application of the angiographic catheter was in many ways the beginning of interventional radiology [4].

In order to utilize angiography effectively in the emergency management of gastrointestinal bleeding, one must perform it rapidly and efficiently. Well-trained personnel must be available on short notice, 24 hours a day. The indications as well as the limitations of angiography must be well understood by both the radiologist and the attending clinician. About 75 percent of patients requiring hospitalization for gastrointestinal bleeding can be managed conservatively with sedation, bed rest, and replacement of blood volume [5]. These patients are obviously not candidates for emergency angiography. Transcatheter therapy is most useful in patients in whom bleeding does not respond to conservative treatment or those who are poor surgical risks.

Bleeding Site Localization

Although angiography is only one of several methods available for locating sources of gastrointestinal bleeding, it has become a very important and commonly used clinical tool [6–9]. The procedure may be performed on severely ill patients and requires little patient cooperation. The angiographic criteria of bleeding are straightforward, and the examination requires little special preparation and can be performed despite the presence of large amounts of blood in the gastrointestinal tract.

For successful visualization, however, the patient must be bleeding at a rate of at least 0.5 cc per minute. The major limitation of the technique relates to the intermittent nature of gastrointestinal bleeding, which can result in a negative study if the bleeding has temporarily stopped at the time of the injection [10]. Another serious limitation has been the inability of a selective arteriogram to demonstrate venous bleeding. This is also a problem if the patients studied are bleeding massively from esophageal varices.

Prior endoscopy can be of great help to the angiographer. Even if the endoscopist cannot be certain exactly where the bleeding is coming from, the identification of the region of bleeding, such as the duodenum or stomach, is of value in guiding catheterization of the appropriate vessel. If the bleeding is observed coming from esophageal varices, initial therapy is directed toward intravenous vasopressin infusion rather than early angiography. Unfortunately, an accurate endoscopic diagnosis is not always possible since direct visualization is made difficult by active bleeding and blood in the gastrointestinal tract.

Recently, a radioisotopic examination was developed for demonstrating active bleeding as a preliminary to angiography. This technique is totally noninvasive, simple, and capable of visualizing both arterial and venous bleeding at

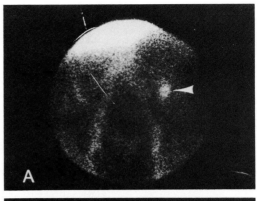

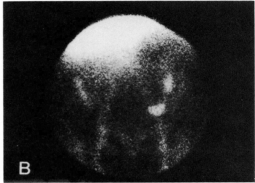

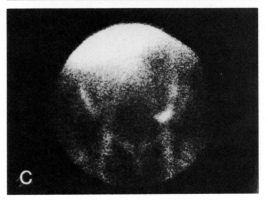

Figure 70-1. ^{99m}Tc sulfur colloid scan for the detection of gastrointestinal bleeding. Following the injection of ^{99m}Tc sulfur colloid into a patient who is actively bleeding, the radioactive agent is cleared by the liver and only a fraction of the injected material will extravasate at the bleeding site. This process is repeated each time the blood circulates, adding another, but smaller, fraction to the material already at the site of the hemorrhage. Immediately after the intravenous administration of the radioactive agent, the background activity decreases exponentially, while the activity at the bleeding site increases exponentially.

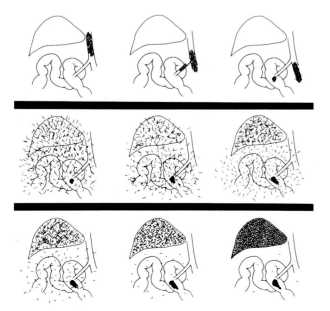

Figure 70-2. Bleeding diverticulum demonstrated with a ^{99m}Tc sulfur colloid scan. (A) Ten minutes after the injection of 10 mCi intravenously, an area of abnormal activity is seen in the left iliac fossa (*arrow*). (B and C) Scans obtained 15 and 30 minutes later demonstrate movement of activity in the lumen of the bowel. The activity outlines a configuration of the descending and proximal sigmoid colons. (D) Twenty minutes after the isotope scan, an inferior mesenteric arteriogram was obtained that demonstrates an area of extravasation (*arrow*) in the descending colon superimposed on the iliac fossa. (E) A late film obtained during inferior mesenteric arteriography shows persistence of extravasated contrast material in the descending colon (*arrow*). The patient was successfully treated by a vasopressin infusion. Prior to discharge, a barium examination showed the arteriographic abnormality to correspond to a colonic diverticulum.

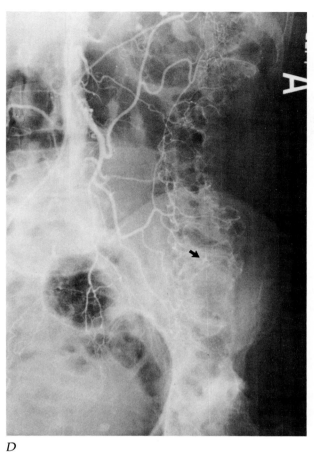

D

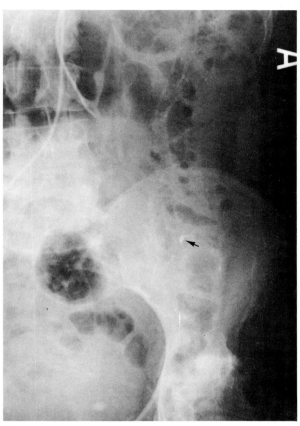

E

rates as low as 0.1 cc per minute. The isotope procedure is performed with an intravenous injection of technetium 99m sulfur colloid, a liver-scanning agent [11]. As the isotope reaches the bleeding site, a small amount extravasates. With each additional circulation, more of the isotope leaks into the gut. As activity in the vascular system is removed by the liver and spleen, a difference is quickly reached between the bleeding site and the background (Figs. 70-1, 70-2). The extravasated isotope within the gut can usually be demonstrated in the first 5 to 10 minutes after the injection. If sites of bleeding cannot be identified on the early scan, the examination is continued so as to identify activity that moves away from the hepatic or splenic flexure. Such an area may be obscured at first by the activity in the overlying spleen and liver, but as continued peristalsis moves the isotope along the gastrointestinal tract it becomes visible. The

technique is frequently used as a screening procedure and enables better selection of patients to be studied by angiography.

The value of emergency barium examinations in patients with severe gastrointestinal bleeding is limited. Large amounts of blood in the gut make upper gastrointestinal barium studies difficult to interpret except in the presence of very large and obvious lesions. Barium enemas are even more limited because of fecal material in the unprepared bowel. If the barium examination is positive, there is no assurance that the detected pathologic processes (e.g., duodenal ulcers, esophageal varices, or colonic diverticular disease) are responsible for the current bleeding episode [12, 13]. In addition, the presence of barium in the gastrointestinal tract precludes the possibility of a subsequent angiographic examination and also interferes with direct endoscopic visualization.

Angiographic Appearance of Bleeding

When bleeding is first detected during the arterial phase of a selective arteriogram, it typically appears as a localized puddle of contrast material. As the filming continues, the bleeding becomes increasingly obvious and persists after all the intravascular contrast has washed out. In the presence of very brisk bleeding one may see excellent opacification of the mucosa of the gastrointestinal tract. Small amounts of extravasation appear as

Figure 70-3. Bleeding gastric ulcer. (A) Selective left gastric arteriography demonstrates a common left hepatic–left gastric trunk and active bleeding (*arrow*) from a fundal branch of the left gastric artery. (B) Repeat left gastric arteriography during the infusion of vasopressin demonstrates marked vasoconstriction of the left gastric artery without any evidence of continued bleeding. The left hepatic artery branch appears unaffected by the vasopressin. This impression is in keeping with experimental evidence that, although vasopressin causes initial vasoconstriction of the hepatic artery, it does not maintain the vasoconstriction during an infusion. It is generally assumed, therefore, that it is safe to infuse the hepatic artery selectively in patients with normal liver function.

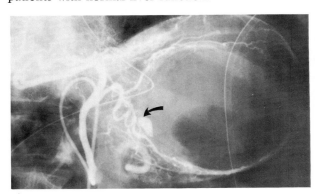

A

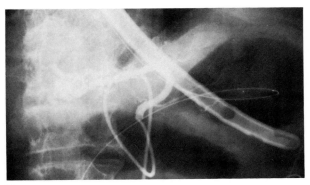

B

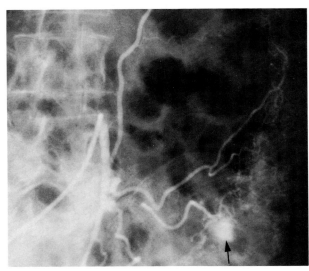

A

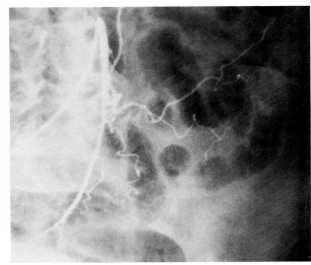

B

Figure 70-4. Bleeding diverticulum in the descending colon outlined with extravasated contrast material. (A) Arterial phase of a selective inferior mesenteric arteriogram shows extravasation of contrast material (*arrow*) in the midportion of the descending colon. The extravasated contrast appears to outline the diverticulum itself. (B) During the infusion of vasopressin at 0.2 unit per minute into the inferior mesenteric artery, a repeat arteriogram demonstrates peripheral vasoconstriction of the arterial branches and cessation of the bleeding. After the patient was weaned from the vasopressin, the bleeding did not recur and the patient was discharged without surgery.

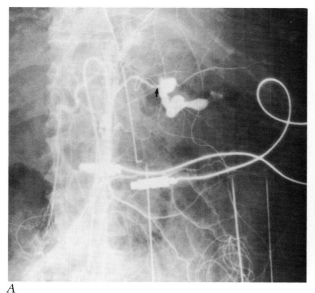

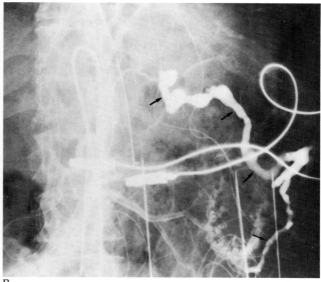

A   *B*

Figure 70-5. Pseudovein appearance of extravasated contrast material. (A) Selective left gastric arteriography performed on a patient with an actively bleeding stress ulcer in the fundus of the stomach demonstrates extravasation from a branch of the left gastric artery (*arrow*). (B) A film obtained during the capillary phase of the study demonstrates the extravasated contrast material (*arrows*) puddled between clots within a dilated, blood-filled stomach. Although the appearance of the contrast material is that of a vascular structure, this should not be confused with either an arterial or a venous malformation.

localized flecks, which occasionally outline either an ulcer crater (Fig. 70-3) or a colonic diverticulum (Fig. 70-4). If the lumen of the gastrointestinal tract is filled with blood clots, extravasated contrast material will occasionally appear tubular in configuration and resemble a venous structure [14]. This "pseudovein" (Fig. 70-5) is easily distinguished from a vascular malformation since the extravasated contrast persists well beyond the venous phase of the arteriogram.

Pitfalls in the Angiographic Diagnosis of Bleeding

The intermittent nature of bleeding in some patients can result in a negative angiographic study if during the injection the bleeding has ceased. Some angiographers have attempted to provoke bleeding in these cases; however, my own experience with both heparin and vasodilators such as Priscoline has not been successful. I have found the isotope technique very helpful in selecting those patients who are actively bleeding, and its use has reduced the number of negative arteriograms.

Venous bleeding is almost never demonstrated angiographically, and the diagnosis of esophageal bleeding is made on angiography only indirectly by demonstrating portal hypertension and excluding all other potential arterial and/or mucosal sites of bleeding.

FALSE-NEGATIVE EXAMINATION

Occasionally in a patient actively bleeding from an arterial and/or a capillary site, the arteriogram will not demonstrate an area of extravasation. This is usually the result of injecting the wrong vessel. If there is clinical or endoscopic evidence of upper gastrointestinal bleeding, a complete examination must include opacification of the left gastric, gastroduodenal, pancreaticoduodenal, and splenic arteries. In the absence of a gastrojejunostomy the history of having vomited blood generally indicates that the bleeding is coming from some portion of the gastrointestinal tract proximal to the ligament of Treitz. The history of having passed bright red blood per rectum, however, does not preclude the patient's having a bleeding site in the upper gastrointestinal tract. Examination of the vasculature of the stomach and duodenum should also be carried

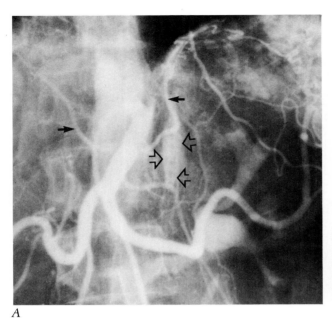

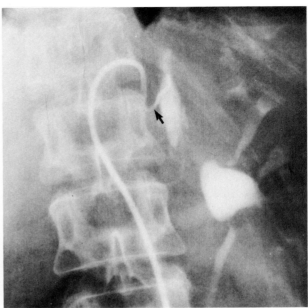

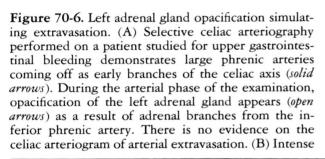

A   *B*

Figure 70-6. Left adrenal gland opacification simulating extravasation. (A) Selective celiac arteriography performed on a patient studied for upper gastrointestinal bleeding demonstrates large phrenic arteries coming off as early branches of the celiac axis (*solid arrows*). During the arterial phase of the examination, opacification of the left adrenal gland appears (*open arrows*) as a result of adrenal branches from the inferior phrenic artery. There is no evidence on the celiac arteriogram of arterial extravasation. (B) Intense opacification of the left adrenal gland persists well after the venous phase of the examination and is superimposed on the lesser curvature aspect of the fundus of the stomach. The fact that the tip of the catheter is partially wedged in the left inferior phrenic artery probably accounts for the intense opacification of the adrenal gland and the poor washout of the phrenic artery (*arrow*). The patient did not have any angiographic evidence of arterial or mucosal bleeding.

out if a negative superior and inferior mesenteric arteriogram is obtained in a patient presenting with lower gastrointestinal hemorrhage.

FALSE-POSITIVE EXAMINATION

False-positive diagnoses will occasionally be made when normal parenchymal blushes are confused with extravasation. One of the most commonly made errors is the superimposition of a densely opacified left adrenal gland on the gastric fundus (Fig. 70-6). This often occurs when the inferior phrenic arteries originate either as branches of or adjacent to the left gastric artery or celiac axis. The arteriographic parenchymal blush of the adrenal gland resembles a railroad track, being linear in appearance with a radiolucency in the center.

Another instance of a false-positive examination can occur in some patients in whom selective left gastric arteriography demonstrates a marked increase in the size and number of vessels supplying the gastric fundus accompanied by an intense mucosal stain. Although this appearance is similar to that seen in hemorrhagic gastritis, unless one can identify actual points of extravasation the diagnosis of bleeding gastritis should not be made. The hyperemic appearance can be caused by vigorous lavaging of the stomach prior to arteriography in an attempt to stop the bleeding. It must also be remembered that patients bleeding from other causes such as duodenal ulcers or Mallory-Weiss tears of the stomach will frequently have gastritis (Fig. 70-7).

Even after a site of extravasation is identified on the arteriogram, errors can occur in knowing exactly where the bleeding site is within the gastrointestinal tract. In the anteroposterior projection of a superior mesenteric arteriogram, extravasation from a bleeding duodenal ulcer that is being supplied from the inferior pancreaticoduodenal artery may seem to originate in

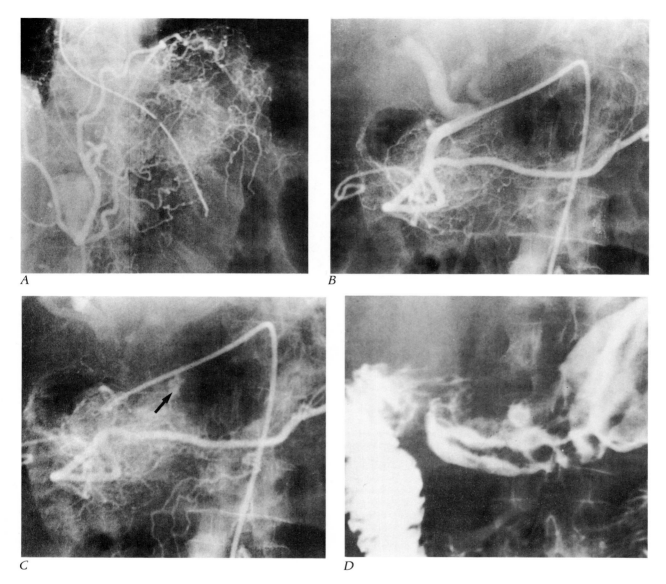

Figure 70-7. Fundal gastritis and actively bleeding lesser curvature peptic ulcer in a patient presenting with massive upper gastrointestinal bleeding. (A) Selective left gastric arteriography demonstrates marked hypervascularity in the gastric fundus without any evidence of discrete extravasation. The angiographic appearance is that of gastritis. (B) Early phase of a selective gastroduodenal arteriogram. (C) Late arterial phase of the gastroduodenal arteriogram demonstrates extravasation of contrast material (*arrow*) at the site of an antral ulcer that was seen on a prior upper gastrointestinal series. This bleeding was controlled by infusing vasopressin into the gastroduodenal artery. (D) Upper gastrointestinal series performed 2 weeks earlier demonstrates a lesser curvature ulcer.

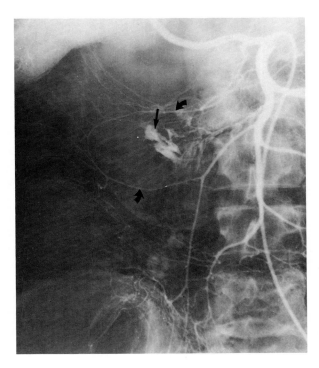

Figure 70-8. Bleeding duodenal ulcer that can be easily confused with bleeding in the proximal transverse colon. In an elderly man who presented with bright red rectal bleeding without any history of having vomited blood, superior mesenteric arteriography demonstrates right-upper-quadrant extravasation (*straight arrow*) surrounded by the right colic (*lower curved arrow*) and the middle colic (*upper curved arrow*) arteries. In view of the clinical history and the proximity of the colic vessels, this duodenal bleed, which actually derived its blood supply from the inferior pancreaticoduodenal artery, could very easily be taken for a bleeding lesion in the proximal transverse colon.

the transverse colon (Fig. 70-8). The surgeon will therefore be misled unless the angiographer is certain as to the site of extravasation. All doubt can be resolved by repeating the superior mesenteric arteriography with the patient in a right posterior oblique position. Another common error is confusing a prepyloric ulcer that is actively bleeding with a duodenal ulcer. This can also be resolved by repeating the injection with the patient in a left posterior oblique position.

THE PRECISE LOCALIZATION OF SMALL BOWEL BLEEDING

With superior mesenteric arteriography it is usually very difficult to be sure which loop of small bowel is bleeding. Athanasoulis has successfully demonstrated the pathologic segment of bleeding in the small bowel by subselectively catheterizing the specific superior mesenteric arterial branch involved immediately prior to the laparatomy [15]. After the small bowel has been surgically exposed, methylene blue or Evans blue is injected into the catheter, resulting in a transient staining of the abnormal bowel. If the patient is actively bleeding at the time of the surgery, the isotopic scanning technique developed by Alavi [11] can be used intraoperatively to localize the bleeding site in the small bowel.

Angiographic Techniques for the Control of Gastrointestinal Bleeding

Following the angiographic demonstration of a bleeding site the catheter can be used to diminish flow and thereby control bleeding. This can be accomplished pharmacologically, by selectively infusing a vasoconstrictor such as vasopressin into the vessel supplying the bleeding point, or the flow in the vessel can be mechanically obstructed by occluding the lumen with embolic materials.

PHARMACOLOGIC INFUSION

Vasopressin has had the greatest clinical acceptance as a safe and reliable vasoconstrictor for the angiographic control of gastrointestinal bleeding. The vasopressin used for this purpose is an aqueous solution of the pressor principle of the posterior pituitary gland and is relatively free of oxytocic principle. It causes contraction of the smooth muscles of the gastrointestinal tract as well as the vascular bed. These effects are not antagonized by adrenergic blocking agents or prevented by vascular denervation. The antidiuretic properties of vasopressin are important and well known [16].

Since its introduction, vasopressin has been the preferred drug for transcatheter infusion therapy of gastrointestinal bleeding because of its significant and sustained reduction in splanchnic blood flow [6–9]. More recently the prostaglandins have been investigated but to date have been untried in any large clinical series. Other vasoconstrictors such as norepinephrine were previously evaluated, but since they do not have sustained actions they have never become popular for this form of therapy.

Vasopressin's action is direct and immediate. A repeat arteriogram obtained 20 minutes after the infusion is begun will accurately determine the effectiveness of the therapy. Also, the dose of vasopressin can be modified so as to produce various degrees of vasoconstriction and thereby cause a more controlled and reversible ischemia than that of mechanical embolic therapy.

The selective infusion of vasopressin into a bleeding splanchnic vessel at the dose of 0.2 unit per minute is generally sufficient to stop gastrointestinal arterial or mucosal bleeding. Extensive experimental and clinical experience with this method has shown it to be safe when used in the gastrointestinal tract with little danger of significant organ ischemia. Even direct infusions into the hepatic [17, 18] or splenic artery are well tolerated, so that infusion of the celiac axis is a viable alternative when more subselective catheterization of the left gastric artery is not technically possible.

The use of vasopressin is particularly successful in gastric mucosal bleeding when the left gastric artery is selectively infused. If the bleeding is coming from the small or large bowel, the selective infusion of the main superior or inferior mesenteric artery is generally sufficient, obviating the need for subselective catheterization of the specific branch supplying the diseased segment.

Vasopressin diluted in saline or 5 percent dextrose and water is usually infused at a constant rate of 0.2 unit per minute for 20 minutes. Then a repeat arteriogram is obtained to evaluate the success of the therapy. If no further bleeding is demonstrated on the subsequent arteriogram, the infusion is continued at 0.2 unit per minute. If bleeding persists, however, the infusion can be increased to 0.4 unit per minute for another 20 minutes, followed by a repeat arteriogram. Failure to control the bleeding using 0.4 unit per minute indicates that the bleeding is unlikely to be controlled by vasopressin and that alternative methods of therapy should be considered. The angiogram obtained 20 minutes after the start of the infusion is analyzed to be sure that (1) moderate reduction in caliber of the infused vessels has occurred with preservation of good forward flow into the capillary and venous phases, (2) there is still filling of branches in the area of the bleeding point, and (3) there is no further extravasation.

If all these criteria are met, a pressure dressing is applied around the catheter entry site and the patient can be sent back to the intensive care unit for careful monitoring. If there is no clinical evidence of recurrent bleeding, the initial infusion rate is continued for 24 to 36 hours and then reduced by 50 percent for an additional 24 hours. The vasopressin infusion can then be stopped, but the catheter is generally kept in place and its patency maintained by the infusion of either normal saline or dextrose and water for another 12 hours. If the patient remains clinically stable, the catheter can then be removed. If there is recurrent bleeding as the vasoconstrictor dose is being tapered, a return to the initial dose rate usually controls it.

Role of Angiography in the Management of Esophageal Variceal Bleeding

Prior to its intraarterial use for gastrointestinal bleeding, vasopressin was injected intravenously in fairly large doses (20 units over 20 minutes) in an attempt to reduce portal pressure during the treatment of variceal bleeding [19]. Although bleeding esophageal varices cannot be constricted by direct infusion of pharmacologic agents, vasopressin is a potent splanchnic vasoconstrictor that causes significant reduction in mesenteric blood flow and consequently portal pressure. Since a relatively large dose of vasopressin given intravenously can be associated with side effects including decreased cardiac output and coronary artery vasoconstriction, the selective mesenteric artery infusion of vasopressin appeared to be an attractive alternative when it was first introduced in 1971 [20]. This technique of continuously infusing the superior mesenteric artery with doses of vasopressin at 0.2 unit per minute was highly effective in controlling variceal bleeding and could be maintained for long periods of time without the development of tachyphylaxis. It was less efficacious in controlling bleeding in patients with advanced cirrhosis [21], probably because of the increased arterialization of the portal system from the hepatic artery in patients with severe liver disease. In 1973 Barr et al. [22] showed that vasopressin, infused intravenously at the same low dose rates used in the superior mesenteric artery, reduces portal pressure by 40 to 50 percent. The systemic side effects with the low-dose intravenous infusions are about the same as those with the intraarterial infusion. Johnson and his associates [23] reported a randomized clinical study confirming that the systemic infusions of vasopressin at low dose

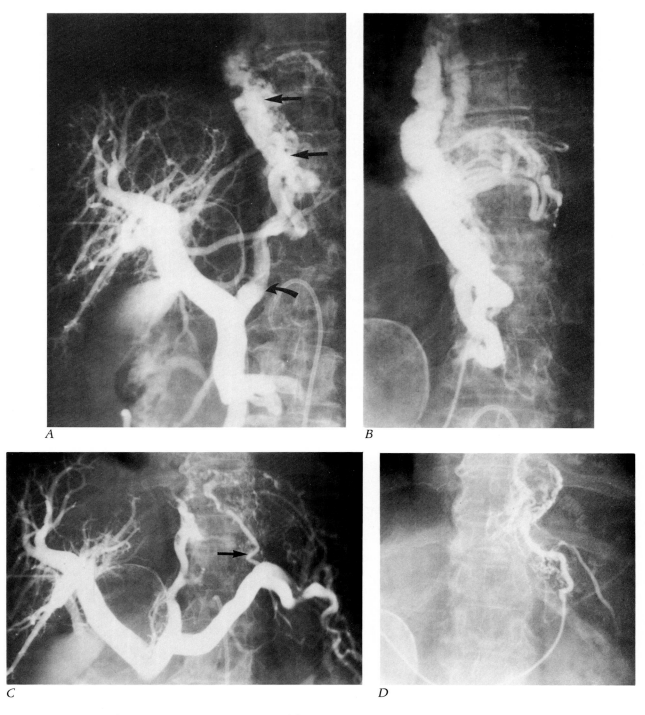

A

B

C

D

Figure 70-9. Bleeding esophageal varices treated by percutaneous transhepatic catheterization of the portal vein and embolization of the coronary veins. (A) Direct portography following percutaneous catheterization of the portal vein demonstrates a large coronary vein (*curved arrow*) supplying large gastric and esophageal varices (*straight arrows*). (B) Selective catheterization of the coronary vein defines with greater clarity the very large gastric and esophageal varices. (C) Following embolization of the coronary vein with Gelfoam, repeat direct portography demonstrates occlusion of the coronary vein. However, there is now filling of a short gastric vein (*arrow*) that appears to be supplying the gastric varices. (D) Selective catheterization of the short gastric vein demonstrates that it is indeed feeding the gastric and esophageal

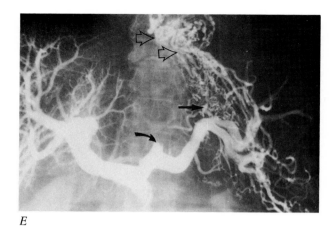

E

varices. This vessel was embolized with Gelfoam. After embolization of the coronary and short gastric veins, the patient stopped bleeding. (E) Repeat direct portography performed several days later when the patient's bleeding recurred demonstrates that the coronary vein (*curved arrow*) has remained occluded, as has the short gastric vein (*straight arrow*). Large gastric and esophageal varices (*open arrows*) are now being supplied by multiple gastric veins originating from the splenic vein in the area of the hilus of the spleen.

rates were as effective as intraarterial infusions at the same rate in controlling variceal bleeding. Therefore, there appears to be no advantage to the selective intraarterial infusion of vasopressin in the treatment of bleeding esophageal varices.

The percutaneous transhepatic approach to the portal vein was popularized in 1974 by Lunderquist [24, 25]. This technique gives direct access to the portal vein and its tributaries. In the absence of marked ascites the procedure is not technically difficult, and the risk of bleeding from the point of entry is negligible. The more common complication involved in this study is the formation of thrombi in the portal vein as a result of the introduction of the catheter [26]. After the catheter has been introduced into the portal vein, the coronary vein can generally be selectively catheterized without too much difficulty. Various embolic materials can then be introduced into the coronary gastric veins to interrupt flow to the varices rapidly, thereby, it would be hoped, controlling the bleeding [27] (Fig. 70-9).

Unfortunately, follow-up studies have shown that varices become patent within 1 to 4 weeks, and permanent occlusion seldom results [28]. Control of the bleeding by this technique is generally temporary and allows the patient to be stabilized and prepared for elective surgery.

Various materials have been used for occlusion of the coronary veins including Gelfoam, steel coils, balloons, and even bucrylate.

Bleeding Mesenteric Varices

On the parietal surface of the gut, very small, delicate venous communications join the portal branches of the mesenteric vein to the systemic venous channels in the retroperitoneum and abdominal wall. Most varices from portal hypertension occur in the esophagus, rectum, and umbilicus. Some patients, however, have intestinal varices as a result of dilatation of these preexisting intestinal branches—particularly patients who have had previous surgery and have developed adhesions between loops of bowel and the abdominal wall. In patients with portal hypertension the varices may become exceedingly large and capable of bleeding in a manner similar to that of esophageal varices [29].

Varicosities may also grow across adhesions in the pelvis, allowing for decompression of the portal vein by the gonadal systemic veins. The pelvic adhesions may be the result of either inflammatory disease or previous surgery (Fig. 70-10). Localized varicosities involving the superior mesenteric vein and its branches can occur secondary to pancreatitis or neoplasms of the pancreas that invade the superior mesenteric vein or to neoplasms of the gastrointestinal tract that secondarily occlude mesenteric veins (Fig. 70-11). Intestinal varices have been seen as a result of the extensive desmoplastic reaction that occurs in the root of the mesentery secondary to carcinoid tumors [30].

ARTERIAL EMBOLIZATION

Where arterial or capillary bleeding cannot be stopped pharmacologically with the infusion of vasopressin, an alternative approach is to attempt to occlude the supplying artery selectively. The catheter is positioned as close as possible to the site of extravasation, and embolic material is carefully injected through the catheter to block the artery. The very rich collateral arterial supply to the stomach and duodenum usually protects these organs from significant ischemia and infarction after embolization of the bleeding vessel (Fig. 70-12).

Although this method is frequently successful in stopping the bleeding, therapeutic failures may arise when bleeding takes place in an area that has a dual arterial blood supply [31]. The occlusion of

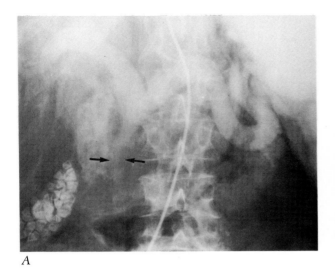

A

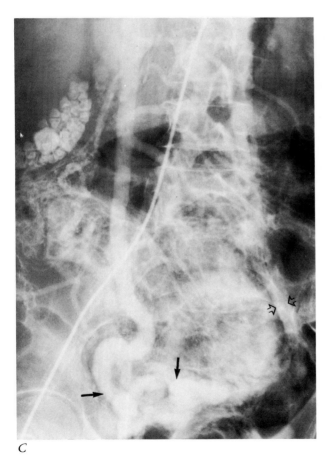

C

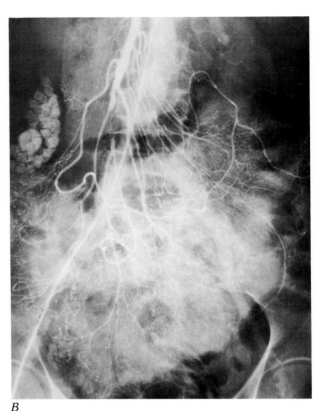

B

Figure 70-10. Bleeding mesenteric varices in a 68-year-old woman with cirrhosis referred for mesenteric arteriography because of lower gastrointestinal bleeding. (A) The venous phase of the selective splenic arteriogram demonstrates patency of the splenic and portal veins. There is retrograde filling of the superior mesenteric vein (*arrows*). (B) A selective superior mesenteric arteriogram fails to demonstrate evidence of an arterial or mucosal bleeding site. (C) During the venous phase of the superior mesenteric arteriogram, retrograde flow is seen in the superior mesenteric vein draining into large pelvic varicosities (*solid arrows*). The pelvic varices decompress the mesenteric vein by the left gonadal vein (*open arrows*). The patient had had pelvic surgery many years earlier. Following this examination, the patient was re-explored, and at surgery adhesions containing large varicosities were seen extending between the pelvic organs and the ileal loops of the small bowel. In the resected specimen of the ileum, one of the large mucosal veins was bleeding as a result of an overlying area of mucosal ulceration.

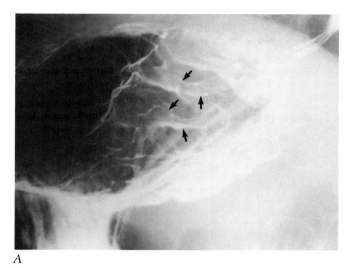

A

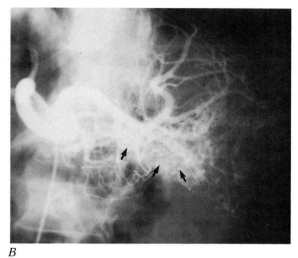

B

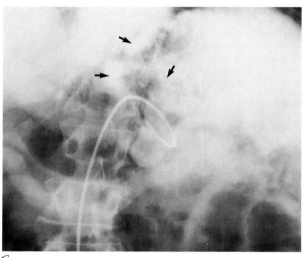

C

Figure 70-11. A 66-year-old man presented with a history of hematemesis. (A) An upper gastrointestinal series with the patient in a steep right posterior oblique position demonstrates gastric varices (*arrows*) without any evidence of esophageal varices. This picture suggested splenic vein obstruction; the patient was referred for angiography. (B) Selective splenic arteriography demonstrates tumor vessels in the distal portion of the pancreas extending into the hilus of the spleen (*arrows*). (C) In the venous phase of the splenic arteriogram, multiple gastric varices (*arrows*) are seen draining into a patent portal vein. The patient had had a left nephrectomy 15 years earlier for a renal cell carcinoma, and the tumor disclosed in the tail of the pancreas on the present examination was renal cell carcinoma metastatic to the pancreas, causing splenic vein occlusion and gastric varices.

only one limb of such a vascular arcade may result in failure to control bleeding because the abnormal segment continues to be supplied by a second arterial limb (Fig. 70-13). Successful control, therefore, may require individual treatment of each limb, whether by vasopressin infusion or occlusion (Fig. 70-14). A control arteriogram is essential to confirm cessation of previously demonstrated bleeding. If a dual blood supply exists, it may be necessary to embolize both sides of an arcade. Examples of vascular arcades that may be significant in the angiographic management of bleeding include (1) middle colic–left colic artery anastomosis at the splenic flexure of the colon, (2) superior pancreaticoduodenal–inferior pancreaticoduodenal arterial arcades in the duodenum, (3) left gastric–right gastric arcade along the lesser curvature of the stomach, and (4) right gastroepiploic–left gastroepiploic arterial communications along the greater curvature of the stomach.

Various embolic materials have been tried in a search for a safe, effective, and simple agent [32]. Gelfoam, a slowly absorbed gelatin sponge, is the most widely used embolic material in the treatment of gastrointestinal bleeding [33]. Although autologous blood clot has the advantage of providing very small emboli that lodge peripherally and thereby lessen the chance of collateral bleeding, this form of control tends to be only temporary because of lysis of the clot, generally within 12 to 14 hours [34, 35]. Clots that are pretreated with thrombin, aminocaproic acid, or oxidized cellulose (Oxycel) persist for a longer time. Ivalon particles provide even longer-lasting occlusions but are more difficult to use [36, 37].

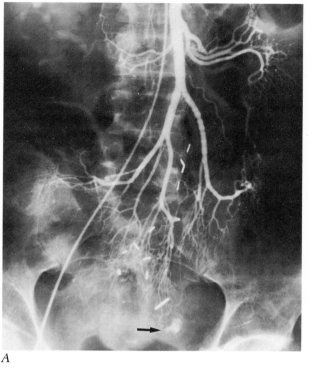

A

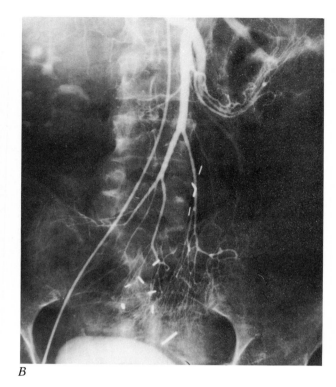

B

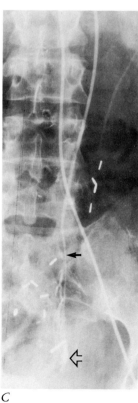

C

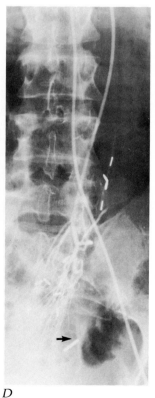

D

Figure 70-12. Bleeding ileitis in a patient with a long-standing history of ileitis and multiple surgical procedures, referred to angiography because of lower gastrointestinal bleeding. Since the pelvic ileal loops were bound together by multiple adhesions, the patient was a very poor surgical candidate. (A) Selective superior mesenteric arteriography demonstrates extravasation of contrast material (*arrow*) from one of the pelvic ileal branches. (B) Bleeding was controlled by the infusion of 0.2 unit of vasopressin per minute into the superior mesenteric artery. There was, however, great difficulty in weaning the patient from the vasopressin, and each time the dose was reduced, the bleeding recurred. (C) Because of the desire of the clinicians to avoid surgery, selective embolization of the bleeding vessel was attempted. The catheter was advanced into the small jejunal artery (*solid arrow*) supplying the bleeding site, and a small hand injection of contrast material once again shows extravasation (*open arrow*). (D) Following embolization with a small Gelfoam plug, the bleeding was controlled and repeat arteriography with the catheter partially withdrawn shows very selective occlusion of the small ileal branch (*arrow*). The patient did not rebleed and was discharged from the hospital without having to be operated on.

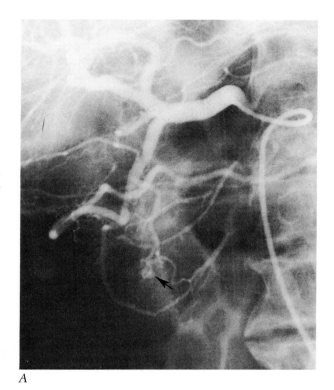

A

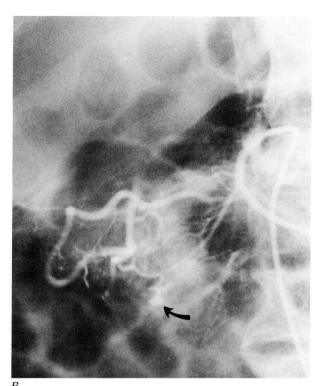

B

Figure 70-13. Dual blood supply of a bleeding duodenal ulcer. (A) Following selective hepatic arteriography, extravasation in the duodenum (*arrow*) can be identified as coming from a small branch of the superior pancreaticoduodenal artery. (B) Selective inferior pancreaticoduodenal arteriography demonstrates the same point of extravasation (*arrow*). In cases like these, infusions into both superior and inferior pancreaticoduodenal arteries may be necessary if angiographic control is attempted.

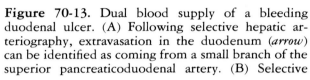

Figure 70-14. Bleeding duodenal ulcer controlled by angiographically treating both limbs of an arcade. (A) Selective gastroduodenal arteriogram demonstrates massive extravasation of contrast material (*arrows*) into the duodenum from a branch of the superior pancreaticoduodenal artery. (B) A balloon catheter (*curved arrow*) was placed through the angiographic catheter and is occluding the gastroduodenal artery. A second catheter was placed in the inferior pancreaticoduodenal branch of the superior mesenteric artery (*straight arrow*), and on injection of this vessel, bleeding is once again demonstrated in the duodenal ulcer (*open arrow*). (C) Embolization of the inferior pancreaticoduodenal artery with small Gelfoam plugs successfully interrupts the inferior pancreaticoduodenal arcade, and the bleeding is controlled.

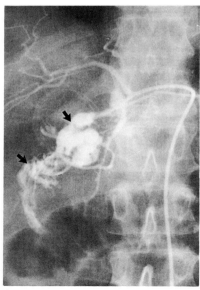

A

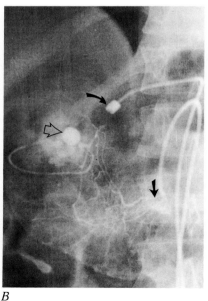

B

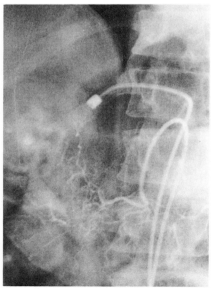

C

Rapidly setting tissue adhesives such as isobutyl 2-cyanoacrylate (bucrylate) produce long-term occlusion [38, 39] and are currently being evaluated in controlled trials but are not available for general use. These rapidly setting glues are liquid monomers that undergo rapid polymerization and solidification when they come in contact with charged ions in the blood. They are difficult to use and must be administered through a coaxial catheter system.

Double-lumen balloon-tipped catheters can be used for the temporary control of gastrointestinal bleeding [40, 41]. They can also be of great value with injection of embolic material, preventing possible reflux of emboli to more distant sites [42]. Small detachable balloons are at present under clinical trial [43]. These devices have some advantage in that they are flow-directed and can be retrieved and their position altered if they are not producing the desired effect. They give the angiographer much more control in occluding a vessel, and the danger of inadvertent occlusion, always associated with emboli, is thereby eliminated. One disadvantage of balloon-tipped catheters is that they occlude bleeding vessels much more proximally than do injected embolic materials. Because of the hemodynamics of bleeding in the presence of a rich collateral blood flow, distal occlusion is a desirable feature.

Wool- or nylon-tufted stainless steel coils have been successful in permanently occluding large vessels where Gelfoam emboli are not suitable. Although the original Gianturco coils [44] had to be delivered through a relatively large Teflon catheter, smaller coils are now available that can be delivered through smaller, more versatile catheters (Fig. 70-15); thus their field of application is extended.

A technique of producing occlusion of an artery by damaging the arterial wall electrically has been described [45], but there is still too little clinical experience available for evaluation.

In general, mechanical embolization techniques should be used only in patients in whom pharmacologic control has failed or in whom prolonged catheter infusions are not practical. Experience has shown that embolization is much more likely than vasopressin to control duodenal bleeding ulcer disease. However, embolization of the superior or inferior mesenteric arteries is still

---

Figure 70-15. Hemorrhagic gastritis treated with Gelfoam embolization and proximal occlusion of the left gastric artery with a nylon-tufted steel coil. (A) The patient was referred for angiography because of upper gastrointestinal bleeding following pancreatic surgery. Selective left gastric arteriography demonstrates a marked hyperemia involving the entire upper portion of the stomach consistent with the diagnosis of hemorrhagic gastritis. Oozing around the catheter site in the groin made it impossible to maintain a continuous infusion of vasopressin, and embolization techniques were therefore resorted to. (B) Gelfoam pellets were embolized into the left gastric artery, and the proximal portion of the left gastric artery was occluded by inserting a nylon-tufted Gianturco coil (*arrows*).

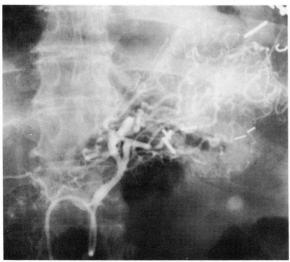

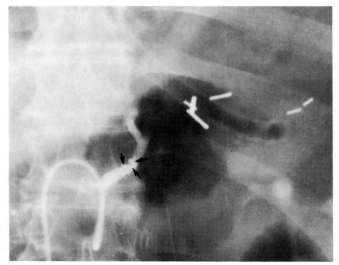

A

B

controversial and should probably be avoided if at all possible because of the danger of bowel infarction.

Angiographic Control of Gastrointestinal Hemorrhage from Specific Arterial Sites

ESOPHAGEAL BLEEDING

Esophageal tumors, esophagitis, and hiatus hernia rarely cause massive bleeding. When this does occur, however, angiography is able to demonstrate the bleeding site if the bleeding segment of the esophagus derives its blood supply from branches of the left gastric artery (Fig. 70-16). Bleeding of the upper and middle portions of the esophagus generally cannot be angiographically demonstrated because of the difficulty associated with catheterizing the appropriate vessels. If the bleeding site can be identified angiographically, the selective arterial infusion of vasopressin almost always controls the bleeding. Mallory-Weiss tears at the cardioesophageal junction as well as bleeding esophagitis are readily responsive to vasopressin infusions (Fig. 70-17).

GASTRIC MUCOSAL HEMORRHAGE

Acute ulcerations of the stomach and duodenum are frequently the cause of significant gastrointestinal bleeding. These ulcerations may be part of any of the following conditions: (1) stress ulcerations, (2) drug- or alcohol-induced gastritis, (3) idiopathic gastritis, (4) Curling's ulcers seen in burn patients, and (5) uremia.

Recent reports indicate that these conditions are being recognized more and more as a cause of massive gastrointestinal bleeding. In all of them the ulcers tend to be acute, are frequently multiple, and are capable of massive bleeding.

Patients who develop ulcerations of the gastrointestinal tract following severe physiologic stress usually have ulcers in the stomach, but in some cases they extend up to the esophagus or into the duodenum. The second and third portions of the duodenum may be another site of mucosal ulcerations, and in some patients these may be the only ulcers that are actively bleeding (Fig. 70-18). For reasons that are not completely understood, the ulcers in the second and third portions of the duodenum are seen more often in patients who have had recent cardiac surgery and who are receiving digitalis [46].

Figure 70-16. A 91-year-old man with a long history of a hiatus hernia was referred for arteriography because of massive hematemesis. (A) A selective left gastric arteriogram demonstrates arterial extravasation in the distal esophagus (*arrows*). In addition, there is marked hyperemia of the entire stomach, consistent with a gastritis. (B) Selective left gastric arteriography during infusion of 0.2 unit per minute of vasopressin shows vasoconstriction of the peripheral branches of the left gastric artery and cessation of the bleeding in the distal esophagus. The bleeding was controlled in this patient, and surgery was not required.

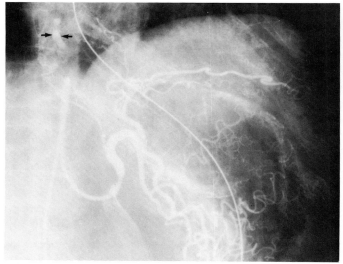

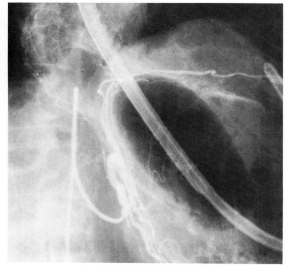

A

B

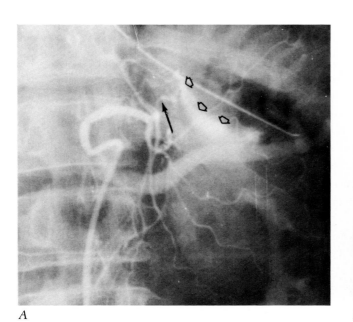

A

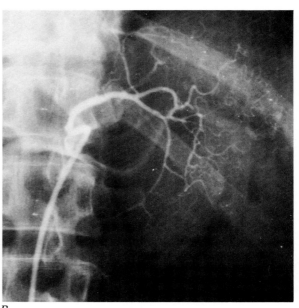

B

Figure 70-17. Bleeding Mallory-Weiss tear at the cardioesophageal junction controlled by the infusion of vasopressin into the left gastric artery. (A) Selective left gastric arteriography demonstrates extravasation of contrast material from a branch of the left gastric artery (*solid arrow*) into the stomach (*open arrows*). (B) During the infusion of 0.2 unit per minute of vaso- pressin, repeat arteriogram shows opacification of the left gastric artery and its branches without any further evidence of extravasation. The patient had an uneventful recovery with no recurrences of hemorrhage. (From Baum and Nusbaum [20]. Reproduced with permission from *Radiology*.)

The angiographic appearance of bleeding stress ulceration may be that of massive extravasation in an otherwise normal-appearing stomach (see Fig. 70-3) or duodenum. The bleeding of gastritis, on the other hand, may appear as multiple areas of extravasation in a vascular bed that is diffusely hyperemic [6] (Fig. 70-19).

Since the therapy in all these lesions is directed toward achieving hemostasis, the intraarterial infusion of vasopressin is a very attractive alternative to surgery when patients do not stop bleeding on medical therapy. Despite the theory that stress ulceration is ischemic in origin, experience has been that stress ulcers as well as ulcerations associated with gastritis heal during the infusion of vasopressin, and rebleeding usually does not occur. The selective infusion of vasopressin into the left gastric artery has been reported to control bleeding of this sort in more than 80 percent of cases [47]. Of this group about 15 percent of patients have recurrent bleeding after the initial control, and these patients are suitable candidates for repeat treatment.

PEPTIC ULCERATION OF THE STOMACH AND DUODENUM

Bleeding that is due to an erosion into a small branch vessel can generally be controlled by infusing the left gastric, gastroduodenal, or superior pancreaticoduodenal arteries. If there is erosion into a main vessel such as a gastroduodenal artery, vasopressin infusion has usually been unsuccessful [48, 49], and in this setting embolization of the bleeding vessel may be necessary to achieve hemostasis [34] (Fig. 70-20).

In most peptic ulcer patients angiography is only a temporary measure to control bleeding and is clearly not the definitive form of therapy. Surgery is still required to deal with the basic problem and prevent recurrence of the disease. Excessive time should not, therefore, be spent on the angiographic procedure unless the patient is unsuitable for surgery. The introduction of histamine antagonists such as cimetidine for the treatment of peptic ulcer disease has caused a reevaluation of the indications for surgery [50]. The angiographic control of bleeding coupled

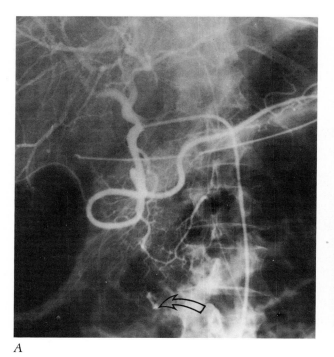

A

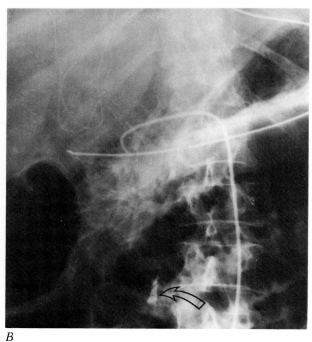

B

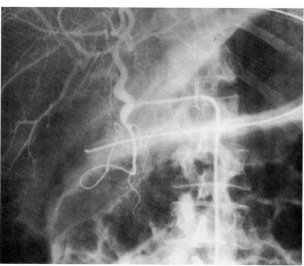

C

Figure 70-18. Bleeding stress ulcer at the junction of the second and third portions of the duodenum. (A) Selective gastroduodenal arteriogram of a patient presenting with massive upper gastrointestinal bleeding 4 days after aortic valve replacement demonstrates arterial bleeding at the junction of the second and third portions of the duodenum (*arrow*). (B) During the late capillary phase of the study, persistent contrast material remains (*arrow*), outlining mucosal folds. (C) Control of the bleeding stress ulcer was obtained by the infusion of 0.2 unit of vasopressin per minute into the gastroduodenal artery. Repeat arteriography shows peripheral vasoconstriction without any evidence of extravasation. The patient had no further clinical evidence of bleeding from this site.

with cimetidine therapy may in fact provide the definitive answer in some patients.

ANASTOMOTIC ULCERS

Selective mesenteric arteriography can be used to demonstrate bleeding from an anastomotic ulcer at the site of gastrojejunostomy [51]. The bleeding site is usually supplied by a jejunal branch of the superior mesenteric artery (Fig. 70-21) and can frequently be controlled by infusing vasopressin into the superior mesenteric artery. After

gastric surgery many collateral vessels are ligated, possibly making embolic therapy dangerous. In addition, embolization requires subselective catheterization of the appropriate feeding vessel, which is difficult to accomplish in this particular group of patients.

POSTOPERATIVE HEMORRHAGE

Bleeding caused by indwelling tubes or slipped ligatures can often be definitively controlled by vasopressin, thus avoiding the inconvenience and

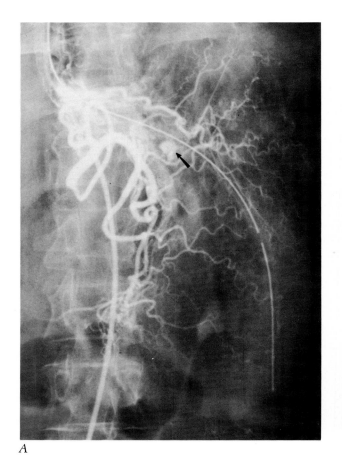

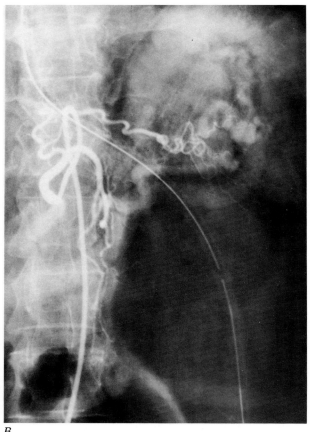

A

B

Figure 70-19. Bleeding hemorrhagic gastritis in a 60-year-old woman who had had multiple surgical procedures for regional enteritis. Postoperatively the patient began to bleed massively from the gastrointestinal tract. Endoscopy showed several ulcers in the gastric fundus. (A) Selective left gastric arteriography demonstrates extravasation from a branch of the left gastric artery (*arrow*). (B) Repeat left gastric arteriography during the infusion of 0.2 unit per minute of vasopressin shows constriction of peripheral arterial branches without further evidence of extravasation. The infusion was continued for 2 days, and the bleeding was clinically controlled.

hazard of reexploration and major abdominal surgery [52]. Further, since most of the patients do not have an underlying disease responsible for the bleeding, the therapy is directed only at the control of the hemorrhage. This method of treatment has also proved helpful following hemorrhage from endoscopic biopsies during colonoscopy (Fig. 70-22).

DIVERTICULAR BLEEDING

The complication of bleeding has been reported to occur in about 10 to 30 percent of patients with colonic diverticulosis [53, 54]. In most patients the blood loss is small and the bleeding stops when the patient is put at rest. Persistent severe diverticular bleeding, however, may re-

quire emergency operative treatment. Since this is a disease of the elderly, emergency colectomy carries an extremely high morbidity and mortality [55].

Establishing the diagnosis of hemorrhage from colonic diverticula by nonarteriographic techniques is difficult and is usually done by exclusion. Emergency mesenteric arteriography during the time of the actual bleeding episode is by far the best method for accurate localization of the bleeding site. The only other nonangiographic technique that has proved of significant value is radionuclide scanning with ^{99m}Tc sulfur colloid [11] (see Fig. 70-1).

Mesenteric arteriography can localize the site of bleeding to the right or left colon (Figs. 70-23, 70-24). Bleeding demonstrated angiographically

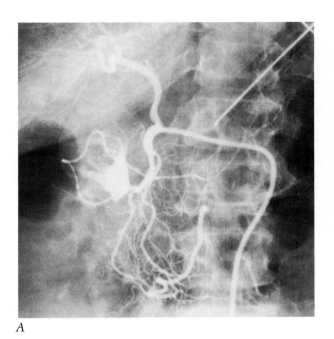

A

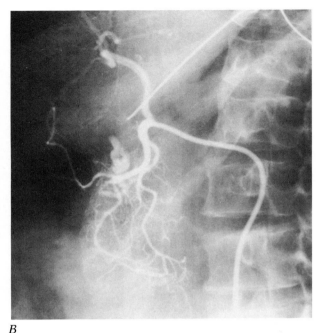

B

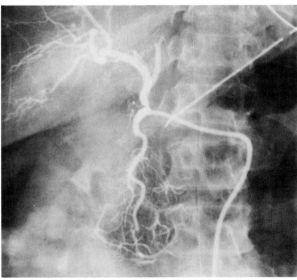

C

Figure 70-20. Actively bleeding duodenal ulcer controlled by the selective embolization of a small amount of autologous blood clot. (A) Arterial phase of a selective gastroduodenal arteriogram shows massive extravasation from a branch of the superior pancreaticoduodenal artery. (B) Infusion of 0.4 unit per minute of vasopressin was unable to stop the bleeding clinically, and on the repeat arteriogram continued extravasation can be seen. (C) Several strands of autologous clot were embolized into both the anterior and the posterior pancreaticoduodenal arcades, thereby disrupting the normal collateralization from the inferior pancreaticoduodenal artery. In addition, the superior pancreaticoduodenal artery was occluded. The bleeding stopped clinically, and a repeat arteriogram failed to show any evidence of extravasation.

is found more commonly in the ascending and transverse colon. In one series 75 percent of patients with massive diverticular bleeding had the bleeding site localized to the right of the splenic flexure [56, 57].

Once the extravasation of contrast material has been demonstrated, infusion of vasopressin into the artery supplying the bleeding point is successful in controlling the bleeding in approxi-

mately 90 percent of the patients treated [57, 58]. After the bleeding is controlled and the catheter removed, management of the patients remains controversial. If bleeding recurs, it usually does so within the first week following the angiographic treatment. The long-term follow-up of patients treated by vasopressin infusion suggests that after the first week these patients are probably no more likely to experience recur-

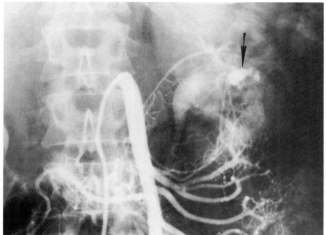

A

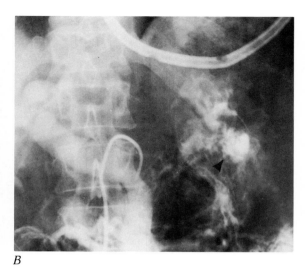

B

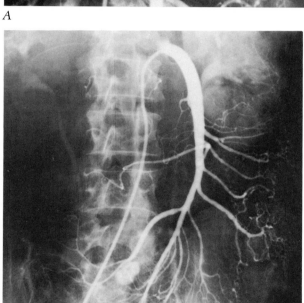

C

Figure 70-21. Bleeding anastomotic ulcer at the site of a Billroth II anastomosis. (A) Selective superior mesenteric arteriography demonstrates extravasation of contrast material (*arrow*) from a jejunal branch at the site of the gastrojejunostomy. (B) Venous phase of the examination shows persistence of contrast material within the jejunum (*arrowhead*). (C) Control of the bleeding was achieved by infusion of 0.2 unit per minute of vasopressin into the superior mesenteric artery.

rent bleeding than those with diverticular bleeding that resolves spontaneously. If, however, it is decided to operate on a patient either because of rebleeding or as prophylaxis, a segmental colonic resection based on the precise localization of the bleeding point can be performed rather than a subtotal colectomy or "blind" hemicolectomy. The initial control of the bleeding episode with vasopressin makes high-risk emergency surgical intervention unnecessary. It allows for prepara-

tion of the patient and elective surgery under more favorable circumstances.

INFLAMMATORY BOWEL DISEASE

Rectal bleeding may at times be the first manifestation of colitis. Some patients are therefore referred for emergency arteriography, and the diagnosis of bleeding colitis is first made by the angiographer (Fig. 70-25). The infusion of vasopressin in cases of actively bleeding colitis can quickly arrest the bleeding, thereby converting an emergency colectomy to an elective one that allows for much better patient preparation.

ANGIODYSPLASIA

Vascular ectasia or angiodysplasia of the colon is being demonstrated with increasing frequency as the cause of bleeding in elderly patients who have either chronic low-grade or intermittent acute lower gastrointestinal bleeding. The lesions tend to be very small and localized in the cecum, ascending colon, and proximal transverse

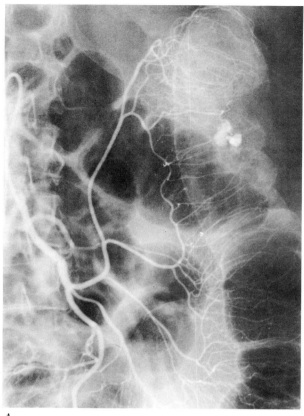

A

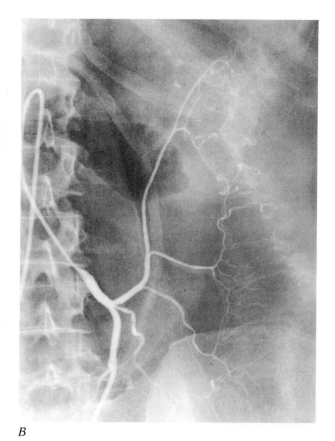

B

Figure 70-22. Lower gastrointestinal bleeding following the colonoscopic removal of a polyp from the descending colon. (A) Arterial phase of a selective inferior mesenteric arteriogram demonstrates bleeding from a branch of the left colic artery at the site of the previous polypectomy. (B) Repeat inferior mesenteric arteriogram 20 minutes after the beginning of an infusion of vasopressin at 0.2 unit per minute. Bleeding can no longer be identified and did not recur. The infusion was continued at the same rate for 12 hours and decreased to 0.1 unit per minute for another 12 hours. The patient was discharged from the hospital without surgery.

colon. They generally cannot be detected by barium studies and are only rarely seen on colonoscopy. The surgeon almost never finds these lesions at laparotomy, and the pathologist has difficulty demonstrating them unless guided by preliminary specimen injections.

The clinical manifestation of colonic vascular ectasia or angiodysplasia is usually assumed to be intermittent low-grade lower gastrointestinal bleeding. Nevertheless, in at least one series of 34 patients half the cases presented with acute episodes of massive rectal bleeding [59]. In most of these patients the stool became guaiac-negative between episodes of hemorrhage.

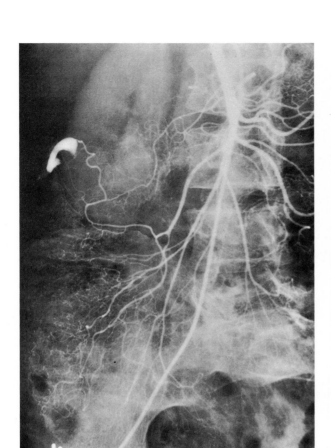

A

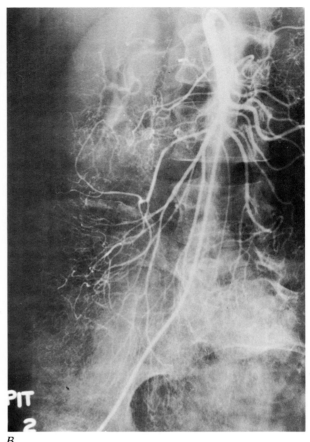

B

Figure 70-23. Bleeding diverticulum in the hepatic flexure in an 80-year-old man presenting with massive lower gastrointestinal bleeding. (A) Selective superior mesenteric arteriogram shows extravasation of contrast material from a branch of the right colic artery in the area of the hepatic flexure. (B) Repeat selective superior mesenteric arteriogram during infusion of 0.2 unit per minute of vasopressin shows complete cessation of the bleeding. The patient was infused with vasopressin for 72 hours at decreasing dosages, and the catheter was removed at the end of the third day. Bleeding did not recur, and he was discharged from the hospital without surgery.

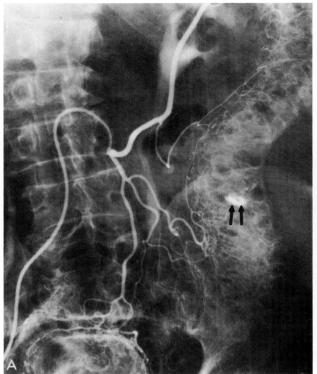
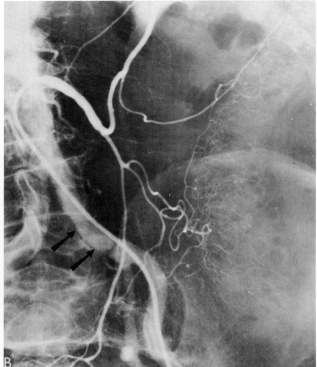

Figure 70-24. Bleeding diverticulum in the descending colon in a 73-year-old man with lower gastrointestinal hemorrhage. (A) Selective inferior mesenteric arteriography shows extravasation of contrast material in the sigmoid colon (*arrows*). (B) Repeat arteriogram during infusion of 0.2 unit per minute of vasopressin into the inferior mesenteric artery shows no further extravasation. Note the constriction of the peripheral vessels and reflux into the aorta and iliac vessels (*arrows*) confirming the increase in peripheral resistance. (From Baum et al. [58]. Reproduced with permission from *N. Engl. J. Med.*)

Figure 70-25. Chronic ulcerative colitis with massive lower gastrointestinal bleeding. (A) Selective superior mesenteric arteriogram shows extravasation from a cecal branch of the ileocecal artery. (B) The extravasated contrast material persists well into the venous phase of the arteriogram. (C) Bleeding stopped during the infusion into the superior mesenteric artery of 0.2 unit per minute of vasopressin. Control of the acute bleeding episode allowed the patient to be adequately prepared and to have a successful elective right colectomy several weeks later.

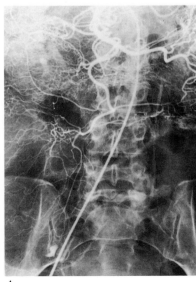
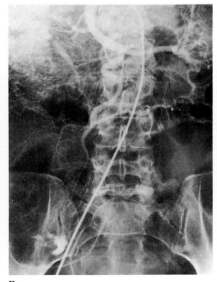
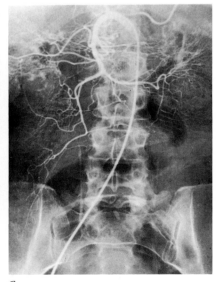

A   *B*   *C*   1693

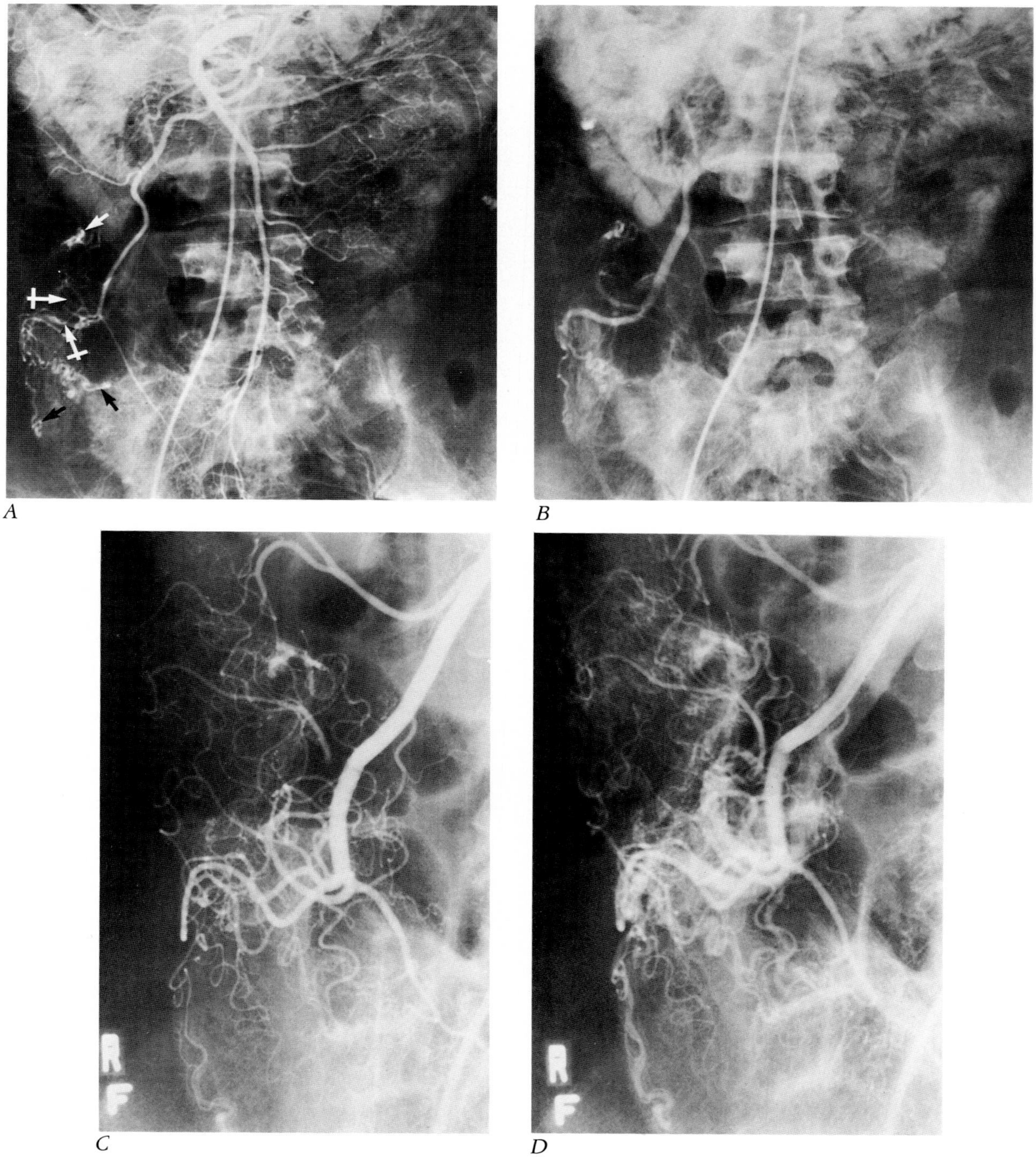

Figure 70-26. Angiodysplasia of the cecum and ascending colon. (A) During the arterial phase of a selective superior mesenteric arteriogram, abnormal clusters of small arteries can be identified in the cecum and ascending colon (*solid arrows*) associated with early-draining veins (*barred arrows*). (B) During the capillary phase of the examination, densely opacified colonic veins are seen draining the right colon. (C, D, and E) Direct serial magnification studies of the cecum and ascending colon with a catheter positioned in the ileocecal artery. The changes of angiodysplasia are clearly identified, with most of the increased vascularity and early-draining veins appearing on the antemesenteric border of the colon. The patient underwent a right colectomy, which extended from the cecum to the distal transverse colon. Pathologically, multiple areas of angiodysplasia were identified with large, thin-walled vascular channels in the colonic wall, predominantly in the submucosa and associated with ulceration and thinning of the overlying mucosa.

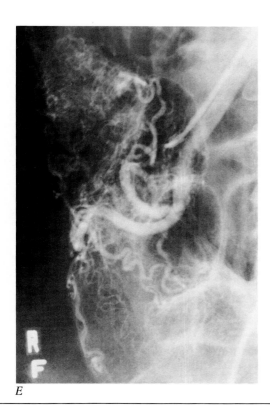

E

conventional x-ray barium examinations and colonoscopy assume great diagnostic importance. Other pathologic conditions must be excluded before a right colectomy is undertaken. Most patients with angiodysplasia are not studied during periods of active bleeding since the hemorrhage from this condition tends to be more episodic than continuous. Therefore, specific localization of a bleeding site, shown by the extravasation of contrast material, is the exception rather than the rule. Because the surgeon can neither see nor palpate the colonic angiodysplasia, the decision to resect the ascending and proximal transverse colon is generally made on the basis of preoperative angiographic findings. Pathologic identification of the lesions in the resected specimen is difficult; lesions are small and focal, and serial sections of the entire specimen are not practical. Hence injection of the right colic artery with silicone rubber is helpful, since this material causes the vessels to remain distended during the tissue fixation. Pathologically angiodysplasia appears as a conglomeration of vascular spaces, often multiple and often coalescent, with adjacent arteries and veins standing out against the homogeneous surface of the normal colonic mucosa. Histologically, the dilated vascular spaces correspond to thin-walled clusters of veins in the submucosa and mucosa.

Angiographically, an increased number of small arteries is seen during the arterial phase of the arteriogram. In the capillary phase of the study an accumulation of contrast material appears in the vascular spaces associated with a very intense opacification of the bowel wall. The veins draining the lesion are identified early in the examination and paradoxically seem to persist late into the venous phase (Figs. 70-26, 70-27).

The etiology of these angiodysplasias is obscure. It is generally assumed that they are acquired, since they are not seen in children. Some investigators consider the lesions related to a chronic form of ischemic bowel disease that results in poor mucosal perfusion associated with submucosal arterial venous shunting [59]. Other authors have compared them to localized varicosities within the submucosa [65].

NEOPLASMS

When bleeding occurs from a neoplasm of the gastrointestinal tract or from an invading contiguous tumor, the bleeding site may be demonstrated angiographically [66]. Vasopressin infu-

It is difficult to assess the incidence of colonic angiodysplasia among various age groups. The first description of the entity was probably recorded in 1839 [60]. In 1976 Bently collected 234 cases from the literature and added 110 cases from the Mayo Clinic files [61]. These reports, however, include a variety of vascular abnormalities of the intestines, such as congenital arteriovenous malformations and/or vascular neoplasms. Since 1960, when Margulis et al. [62] introduced operative angiography as a tool in the search for gastrointestinal bleeding sites, and 1965, when Baum et al. [63] introduced selective angiography for the preoperative localization of bleeding sites, the unusual character of colonic angiodysplasia has been recognized. These lesions have been reported in many patients with otherwise unexplained gastrointestinal hemorrhage. In one study on autopsy specimens colonic angiodysplasia was demonstrated in 2 percent of asymptomatic elderly patients [64].

Because colonic angiodysplasia may coexist with other lesions of the gastrointestinal tract,

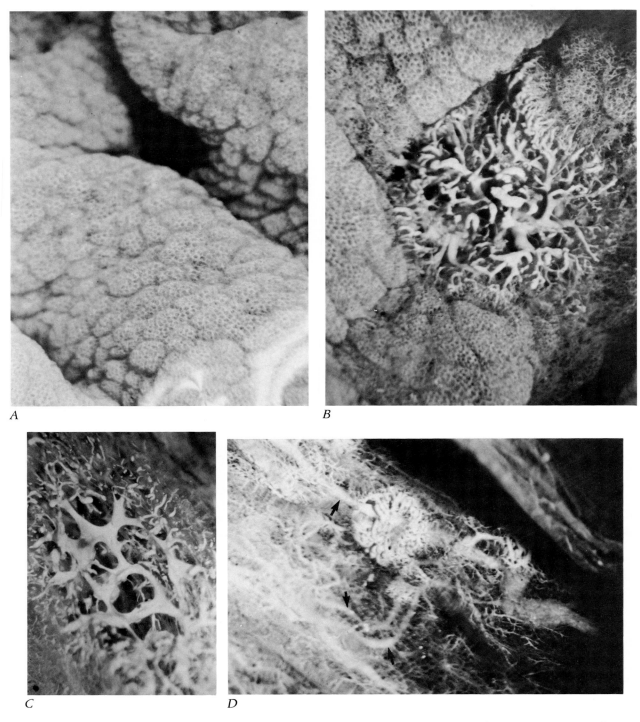

A

B

C

D

Figure 70-27. Microvascular anatomy of angio-dysplasia of the cecum and ascending colon on pathologic specimens. (A) Photograph (×40) of normal colonic mucosa viewed with a dissecting microscope after silicone rubber injection into right colic and ileocolic arteries and tissue clearing using absolute alcohol followed by methyl salicylate. (B, C, and D) Specimens of colonic angiodysplasia as viewed under the dissecting microscope following the tissue-clearing technique. The angiodysplasias appear as clusters of tortuous and dilated vessels against a homogeneous background of normal colonic mucosa. Histologically, these vessels are primarily venules extending from the submucosa into the mucosa. Occasionally, as in (D) (*arrows*), the draining arteries and veins can be identified.

sions have not been successful in controlling such bleeding because the tumor vessels themselves do not appear to respond to vasoconstrictors. If the bleeding is life-threatening and surgical intervention is contraindicated, embolization techniques may be employed. Wallace and Goldstein have reported a series of patients with gastrointestinal bleeding secondary to tumors who were successfully handled in this manner [67].

Complications

CATHETER-RELATED PROBLEMS

The risks involved in arteriography are low and well documented [68]. Thrombosis at the puncture site is clearly the most common complication and occurs in about 0.1 percent of studies. Patients studied on account of bleeding seem to have altered coagulability and are less likely to form thrombus around the catheter. Although many studies have shown that a catheter in the vascular system rapidly becomes coated with a fibrin sheath, catheters have been left in place during vasopressin infusion therapy for as long as 7 to 10 days without evidence of thromboembolic disease. Mild oozing in the groin and around the catheter may occur. When the catheter is removed, care should be taken not to press on it because this may cause the fibrin sheath that is almost always around the catheter itself to be stripped or to be milked from it and left behind in the femoral artery. Manual compression of the artery after removal of the catheter nearly always stops the bleeding although it may have to be applied for up to 2 hours.

PROBLEMS RELATED TO THE VASOPRESSIN INFUSION

Almost all patients complain of abdominal cramps when vasopressin is initially infused into the celiac or superior or inferior mesenteric arteries. The pain generally subsides within the first 10 to 15 minutes of the infusion and should not recur. It usually has been assumed that the discomfort experienced at first is due to contraction of the bowel itself and the increased peristalsis. Very often patients will evacuate as a sequel to the abdominal cramping. If the catheter tip changes position during the time of infusion and becomes lodged in a small jejunal or colic branch, localized bowel ischemia may result. Persistent severe abdominal cramps suggest ischemia, and the position of the catheter should be checked by repeat arteriography.

Although the dose of vasopressin that is infused intraarterially is quite small, the systemic antidiuretic effect almost always occurs after several hours of continuous infusion. Urinary output and electrolytes must be monitored carefully. Water retention and electrolyte imbalance should be treated by diuretics and suitable electrolyte infusions and not by alteration of the rate or dose of infusion of vasopressin.

Rarely, idiosyncratic reactions to the vasopressin are encountered, and the drug has to be discontinued. Sometimes patients exhibit a marked peripheral vasoconstriction in their extremities, which may have a mottled appearance. Occasionally this is troublesome enough so that the drug has to be discontinued. At the recommended dose rates, reduction in cardiac output is not a frequent problem, but this may depend on the individual cardiac status of the patient.

PROBLEMS RELATED TO EMBOLIZATION TECHNIQUES

After embolic material is discharged from the catheter tip, the emboli cannot be retrieved. The final position of an embolus cannot be precisely determined prior to its being injected, and therefore balance between hemostasis and end-organ ischemia is difficult to control. Embolic therapy is much less controllable than are pharmacologic infusions, which can be stopped, slowed, or increased, or balloons, which can be retrieved if they are not in the correct position. Complications that have occurred with the use of particulate emboli include end-organ necrosis [39] and reflux of embolic material from the selected artery with final embolization to unwanted sites. Embolic reflux can be prevented by using a balloon catheter; this is inflated proximally in the artery, and emboli are delivered distally through the lumen [42].

Following Gelfoam embolization, patients may experience a transient rise in temperature to about 39° C (102° F), which may persist for 24 to 36 hours before subsiding spontaneously. Blood cultures in these patients are sterile, and white cell counts tend to be normal.

References

1. Nusbaum, M., and Baum, S. Radiographic demonstration of unknown sites of gastrointestinal bleeding. *Surg. Forum* 13:374, 1963.
2. Baum, S., Stein, G. N., Nusbaum, M., and Chait, A. Selective arteriography in the diagnosis of hemorrhage in the gastrointestinal tract. *Radiol. Clin. North Am.* 7:131, 1969.
3. Baum, S., Nusbaum, M., Clearfield, H. R., Kuroda, K., and Tumen, H. J. Angiography in the diagnosis of gastrointestinal bleeding. *Arch. Intern. Med.* 119:16, 1967.
4. Baum, S. The radiologist intervenes. *N. Engl. J. Med.* 302:1141, 1980.
5. Welch, C. E., and Hedberg, S. Gastrointestinal hemorrhage: I. General considerations of diagnosis and therapy. *Adv. Surg.* 7:95, 1973.
6. Athanasoulis, C. A., Waltman, A. C., Novelline, R. A., Krudy, A. G., and Sniderman, K. W. Angiography, its contribution to the emergency management of gastrointestinal hemorrhage. *Radiol. Clin. North Am.* 14:265, 1976.
7. Conn, H. O., Ramsby, G. R., and Storer, E. H. Selective intraarterial vasopressin in the treatment of upper gastrointestinal hemorrhage. *Gastroenterology* 63:634, 1972.
8. Rösch, J., Gray, R. K., Grollman, J. H., Ross, G., Steckel, R. J., and Weiner, M. Selective arterial drug infusions in the treatment of acute gastrointestinal bleeding. *Gastroenterology* 59:341, 1970.
9. Baum, S., Athanasoulis, C. A., Waltman, A. C., and Ring, E. J. Angiographic Diagnosis and Control of Gastrointestinal Bleeding. In J. D. Hardy and R. M. Zollinger (eds.), *Advances in Surgery.* Chicago: Year Book, 1973. P. 149.
10. Sos, T. A., Lee, J. G., Wixson, D., and Sniderman, K. W. Intermittent bleeding from minute to minute in acute massive gastrointestinal hemorrhage: Arteriographic demonstration. *AJR* 131: 1015, 1978.
11. Alavi, A., Dann, R. W., Baum, S., and Biery, D. N. Scintigraphic detection of acute gastrointestinal bleeding. *Radiology* 124:753, 1977.
12. Conn, H. O., and Brodoff, M. Emergency esophagoscopy in the diagnosis of upper gastrointestinal hemorrhage. *Gastroenterology* 47:505, 1964.
13. McCray, R. S., Martin, F., Amir-Ahmadi, H., Sheahan, D. G., and Zamcheck, N. Erroneous diagnosis of hemorrhage from esophageal varices. *Am. J. Dig. Dis.* 14:755, 1969.
14. Ring, E. J., Athanasoulis, C. A., Waltman, A. C., and Baum, S. The pseudovein: An angiographic appearance of arterial hemorrhage. *J. Can. Assoc. Radiol.* 24:242, 1973.
15. Athanasoulis, C. A. Therapeutic applications of angiography. *N. Engl. J. Med.* 302:1117, 1980.
16. Goodman, L. S., and Gilman, A. *The Pharmacological Basis of Therapeutics* (5th ed.). New York: Macmillan, 1975. P. 855.
17. Barr, J. W., Lakin, R. C., and Rösch, J. Vasopressin and hepatic artery. Effect of selective celiac infusion of vasopressin on the hepatic artery flow. *Invest. Radiol.* 10:200, 1975.
18. Simmons, J. T., Baum, S., Sheehan, B. A., Ring, E. J., Athanasoulis, C. A., Waltman, A. C. and Coggins, P. C. The effects of vasopressin on hepatic artery blood flow. *Radiology* 124:637, 1977.
19. Shaldon, S., and Sherlock, S. The use of vasopressin (Pitressin) in the control of bleeding of oesophageal varices. *Lancet* 2:222, 1960.
20. Baum, S., and Nusbaum, M. The control of gastrointestinal hemorrhage by selective mesenteric arterial infusion of vasopressin. *Radiology* 98:497, 1971.
21. Conn, H. O., Ramsby, G. R., Stover, E. H., Mutchnick, M. G., Joshi, P. H., Phillips, M. M., Cohen, G. A., Fields, G. N., and Petrosk, D. Intraarterial vasopressin in the treatment of upper gastrointestinal hemorrhage: Prospective controlled clinical trial. *Gastroenterology* 68:211, 1975.
22. Barr, J. W., Lakin, R. C., and Rösch, J. Similarity of arterial and intravenous vasopressin on portal and systemic hemodynamics. *Gastroenterology* 69:13, 1975.
23. Johnson, W. C., Widrich, W. C., Ansell, J. E., Robbins, A. H., and Nabseth, D. C. Control of bleeding varices by vasopressin: A prospective radiological study. *Ann. Surg.* 186:369, 1977.
24. Lunderquist, A., and Vang, J. Transhepatic catheterization and obliteration of the coronary vein in patients with portal hypertension and esophageal varices. *N. Engl. J. Med.* 291:646, 1974.
25. Lunderquist, A., and Vang, J. Sclerosing injection of esophageal varices through transhepatic selective catheterization of the gastric coronary vein: A preliminary report. *Acta Radiol. [Diagn.]* (Stockh.) 15:546, 1974.
26. Lunderquist, A., Börjesson, B., Owman, T., and Bengmark, S. Isobutyl 2-cyanoacrylate (bucrylate) in obliteration of gastric coronary vein and esophageal varices. *AJR* 130:1, 1978.
27. Pereiras, R., Viamonte, M., Jr., Russell, E., Le-Page, J., White, P., and Hutson, D. New techniques for interruption of gastroesophageal venous blood flow. *Radiology* 124:313, 1977.
28. Lunderquist, A., Simert, G., Tylén, U., and Vang, J. Follow-up of patients with portal hypertension and esophageal varices treated with percutaneous obliteration of gastric coronary vein. *Radiology* 122:59, 1977.
29. Moncure, A. C., Waltman, A. C., Vander Salm,

T. J., Linton, R. R., Levine, F. H. and Abbott, W. M. Gastrointestinal hemorrhage from adhesion-related mesenteric varices. *Ann. Surg.* 183:24, 1976.

30. Case Records of the Massachusetts General Hospital (Case 1-1973). *N. Engl. J. Med.* 288:36, 1973.

31. Ring, E. J., Oleaga, J. A., Freiman, D., Husted, J. W., Waltman, A. C., Jr., and Baum, S. Pitfalls in the angiographic management of hemorrhage: Hemodynamic considerations. *AJR* 129:1007, 1977.

32. White, R. I., Jr., Strandberg, J. V., Gross, G. S., and Barth, K. H. Therapeutic embolization with long-term occluding agents and their effect on embolized tissues. *Radiology* 125:677, 1977.

33. Reuter, R. S., Chuang, V. P., and Bree, R. L. Selective arterial embolization for control of massive upper gastrointestinal bleeding. *AJR* 125:119, 1975.

34. Eisenberg, H., and Steer, M. L. The nonoperative treatment of massive pyloroduodenal hemorrhage by retracted autologous clot embolization. *Surgery* 79:414, 1976.

35. Bookstein, J. J., Closta, E. M., Foley, D., and Walter, J. F. Transcatheter hemostasis of gastrointestinal bleeding using modified autogenous clot. *Radiology* 113:277, 1974.

36. Tadavarthy, S. M., Moller, J. H., and Amplatz, K. Polyvinyl alcohol (Ivalon)—a new embolic material. *AJR* 125:609, 1975.

37. Castaneda-Zuniga, W. R., Sanchez, R., and Amplatz, K. Experimental observations on short- and long-term effects of arterial occlusion with Ivalon. *Radiology* 126:783, 1978.

38. Dotter, C. T., Goldman, M. L., and Rösch, J. Instant selective arterial occlusion with isobutyl 2-cyanoacrylate. *Radiology* 114:227, 1975.

39. Goldman, M. L., Freeney, P. C., Tallman, J. M., Galambos, J. T., Bradley, E. L., III, Salam, A., Oenk, T., Gordon, I. J., and Mennemeyer, R. Transcatheter vascular occlusion therapy with isobutyl 2-cyanoacrylate (bucrylate) for control of massive upper-gastrointestinal bleeding. *Radiology* 129:41, 1978.

40. Wholey, M. H. The technology of balloon catheters in interventional angiography. *Radiology* 125:671, 1977.

41. Dotter, C. T., Rösch, J., Lakin, P. C., Lakin, R. C., and Pegg, J. E. Injectable flow-guided coaxial catheters for selective angiography and controlled vascular occlusion. *Radiology* 104:421, 1972.

42. Greenfield, A. J., Athanasoulis, C. A., Waltman, A. C., and Le Moure, E. R. Prevention of embolic reflux using balloon catheters. *AJR* 131:651, 1978.

43. White, R. I., Jr., Ursic, T. A., Kaufman, S. L., Barth, K. H., Kim, W., and Gross, G. S. Therapeutic embolization with detachable balloons: Physical factors influencing permanent occlusion. *Radiology* 126:521, 1978.

44. Gianturco, C., Anderson, J. H., and Wallace, S. Mechanical devices for arterial occlusion. *AJR* 124:428, 1975.

45. Phillips, J. F. Transcatheter electrocoagulation of blood vessels. *Invest. Radiol.* 8:295, 1973.

46. Baum, S., Ward, S., and Nusbaum, M. Stress bleeding from the mid-duodenum: An often unrecognized source of gastrointestinal hemorrhage. *Radiology* 95:595, 1970.

47. Athanasoulis, C. A., Baum, S., Waltman, A. C., Ring, E. J., Imbembo, A., Vander Salm, T. J. Control of acute gastric mucosal hemorrhage: Intra-arterial infusion of posterior pituitary extract. *N. Engl. J. Med.* 290:597, 1974.

48. Waltman, A. C., Greenfield, A. J., Novelline, R. A., and Athanasoulis, C. A. Pyloroduodenal bleeding and intraarterial vasopressin: Clinical results. *AJR* 133:643, 1979.

49. Sherman, L. M., Shenoy, S. S., and Cerra, F. B. Selective intraarterial vasopressin: Clinical efficacy and complications. *Ann. Surg.* 189:298, 1979.

50. Fordtran, J. S., and Grossman, M. I. Third symposium on histamine H_2-receptor antagonists: Clinical results with cimetidine. *Gastroenterology* 74:339, 1978.

51. Rosenbaum, A., Siegelman, S., and Sprayregen, S. The bleeding marginal ulcer: Catheterization diagnosis and therapy. *AJR* 125:812, 1975.

52. Athanasoulis, C. A., Waltman, A. C., Ring, E. J., Smith, J. C., Jr., and Baum, S. Angiographic management of post-operative bleeding. *Radiology* 113:37, 1974.

53. Behringer, G. E., and Albright, N. L. Diverticular disease of the colon: A frequent cause of rectal bleeding. *Am. J. Surg.* 125:419, 1973.

54. Welch, C. E., and Hedberg, S. Gastrointestinal Hemorrhage. In J. D. Hardy and R. M. Zollinger (eds.), *Advances in Surgery*, Vol. 7. Chicago: Year Book, 1973. P. 95.

55. Rigg, M., and Ewing, M. R. Current attitudes on diverticulitis with particular reference to colonic bleeding. *Arch. Surg.* 92:321, 1966.

56. Casarella, W. J., Kanter, I. E., and Seaman, W. B. Right-sided colonic diverticula as a cause of acute rectal hemorrhage. *N. Engl. J. Med.* 286:450, 1972.

57. Athanasoulis, C. A., Baum, S., Rösch, J., Waltman, A. C., Ring, E. J., Smith, J. C., Jr., Sugarbaker, E., and Wood, W. Mesenteric arterial infusions of vasopressin for hemorrhage from colonic diverticulosis. *Am. J. Surg.* 129:212, 1975.

58. Baum, S., Rösch, J., Dotter, C. T., Ring, E. J., Athanasoulis, C. A., Waltman, A. C., and Courey, W. R. Selective mesenteric arterial infusions in

the management of massive diverticular hemorrhage. *N. Engl. J. Med.* 288:1269, 1973.

59. Baum, S., Athanasoulis, C. A., Waltman, A. C., Galdabini, J., Shapiro, R. H., Warshaw, A. L., and Ottinger, L. W.   Angiodysplasia of the right colon: A cause of gastrointestinal bleeding. *AJR* 129:789, 1977.

60. Phillips, B.   Letter to the editor. *London Med. Gaz.* 1:514, 1839.

61. Bently, P. G.   The bleeding caecal angioma: A diagnostic problem. *Br. J. Surg.* 63:455, 1976.

62. Margulis, A. R., Heinbecker, P., and Bernard, H. R.   Operative mesenteric arteriography in the search for the site in unexplained gastrointestinal hemorrhage. *Surgery* 48:534, 1960.

63. Baum, S., Nusbaum, M. H., and Blakemore, S. W.   The preoperative radiographic demonstration of intra-abdominal bleeding from undetermined sites by percutaneous selective celiac and superior mesenteric arteriography. *Surgery* 58:797, 1965.

64. Baer, J. W., and Ryan, S.   Analysis of cecal vasculature in the search for vascular malformations. *AJR* 126:394, 1976.

65. Boley, S. J., Sammartano, R. S., Adams, A., DiBiase, A., Kleinhaus, S., and Sprayregen, S.   On the nature and etiology of vascular ectasis of the colon: Degenerative lesions of aging. *Gastroenterology* 72:650, 1977.

66. Rösch, J., and Steckel, R. J.   Selective Angiography of the Abdominal Viscera. In W. N. Hanafee (ed.), *Selective Angiography*. Baltimore: Williams & Wilkins, 1972. P. 17.

67. Wallace, S., and Goldstein, H. M.   Intra-vascular occlusive therapy. *Postgrad. Med.* 59:141, 1976.

68. Sigstedt, B., and Lunderquist, A.   Complications of angiographic examinations. *AJR* 130:455, 1978.

Inferior Mesenteric Arteriography

HERBERT L. ABRAMS

Within recent years, mesenteric vascular disease has emerged as an important and difficult medical problem [11, 45, 46, 48, 61, 63, 67, 72, 90]. While the need for clinical recognition of abdominal angina has been emphasized, the capacity to define obstructive disease of the mesenteric arterial branches has simultaneously been enhanced [19, 50]. The frequency of occlusive disease has become apparent [21, 46], and the inferior mesenteric artery has become recognized as a major collateral channel. Nonocclusive ischemic colitis has also been clearly documented as a syndrome with multiple inciting factors [48]. Interest has also grown in the study of the tumor vascular bed and inflammatory disease of the colon. In 1962, Ström and Winberg demonstrated that selective mesenteric arteriography was technically feasible, and they devised a preshaped catheter for easy entrance into the vessel. They summarized their experience with carcinoma of the colon and diverticulitis [79]. Halpern indicated his enthusiasm for the method in a report of a limited series of cases [44]. Kahn and Abrams later discussed in detail the normal inferior mesenteric artery and the changes found in occlusive disease of the mesenteric vessels [50]. Wholey et al. noted the indications [92], and Boijsen and Reuter attempted to distinguish inflammatory disease and neoplastic disease [14]. Brahme has studied the changes in regional enterocolitis [18]. Perhaps of greatest importance, the detection and treatment of left colic bleeding via the angiographic catheter has now become a central aspect of the management of such disorders [5, 12, 74, 85].

This chapter summarizes the technique, normal anatomy, indications, and value of inferior mesenteric arteriography.

Technique

Percutaneous transfemoral catheter insertion is preferred, except when there is femoral artery occlusive disease. The transaxillary approach may then be employed. The inferior mesenteric circulation can be readily shown by intraaortic injection below the level of the renal arteries. If this method is used when selective studies are not feasible, 35 cc of 76 percent Renografin should be injected over a 2-second period. If the orifice of the inferior mesenteric vessel is to be seen dependably, an intraaortic injection must be obtained. By far the best projection is the lateral one. In cases in which vascular disease is suspected, it is often essential to place the catheter at the level of the celiac artery and to define the orifices of the celiac, superior mesenteric, and inferior mesenteric arteries simultaneously.

The preferable approach to selective arteriography is to employ a preshaped catheter so designed as to permit ready entry into the inferior mesenteric artery. The orifice is usually located on the left anterolateral wall of the aorta at the level of the third lumbar vertebra. The shape of the catheter that we use is similar to that described by Ström and Winberg [79] (it is illustrated in Fig. 71-2). During the introduction of the catheter into the femoral artery, the catheter tip is straightened by the metallic guidewire over which it is passed; the original shape returns with removal of the guidewire. The size of the catheter arch must not exceed the internal diameter of the aorta; if it does, the catheter tip will not regain its original shape.

Once localization has been accomplished under the image amplifier and satisfactory preliminary filming has been obtained, the study can proceed. After the injection of 18 cc of 76 percent Renografin at a rate of 6 cc per second (some investigators recommend a 60% concentration), serial filming is accomplished at two films per second for 5 seconds and one film per second for 7 seconds. The field of interest must be carefully collimated to obtain maximal detail, and the kilovoltage should be kept appropriately low to obtain good contrast. Frequently it will be desirable to perform a second study with the patient in a left posterior oblique projection to refine to a greater degree the analysis of the vessels and their distribution.

After the initial examination, it may be desirable to use a vasodilating drug to visualize the small vascular bed more effectively.

Normal Anatomy

Although the anatomy of the inferior mesenteric artery in cadavers has been well described [38, 42, 77, 81], there have been few serious, systematic attempts to analyze the angiographic anatomy and its variations. Some years ago, therefore, we undertook a review of 142 consecutive angiographic studies of the abdominal aorta and its branches. Such a study seemed warranted not only because there was considerable interest in inferior mesenteric artery insufficiency but also because the potential application of chemotherapeutic agents to bowel tumors by direct perfusion depends on a precise knowledge of the anatomy of the vascular bed. Furthermore, there was reason to believe that angiographic studies in vivo might yield information not attainable from postmortem studies and not necessarily in concord with conventional anatomic data [13]. In all except 6 of our 142 cases, analysis of the inferior mesenteric circulation was feasible. The material that follows on normal anatomy is drawn from that review [50].

The inferior mesenteric artery originates from the left anterior wall of the abdominal aorta at about the level of the third lumbar vertebra. After descending parallel to the aorta for 3 to 4 cm, it gives off an ascending branch. This branch may consist of the left colic artery alone or one or more sigmoid branches as well. In 60 percent of the cases studied, the left colic artery and one or more sigmoid branches arose jointly as a single major trunk; in about 40 percent of cases, the left colic artery arose as a separate and distinct vessel (Figs. 71-1, 71-2). The descending branch is the continuation of the inferior mesenteric artery and gives off the sigmoid branches not originating from the left colic artery. As it courses over the common iliac vessels, it becomes the superior hemorrhoidal artery. Branches of the left colic and sigmoid arteries participate in the large anastomosing channel of the mesocolon known as the marginal artery. This vessel, probably first described by Von Haller in 1786 [88] and subsequently reemphasized by Drummond in his classic paper in 1914 [32], is almost invariably visualized with good opacification of the inferior mesenteric artery. From it, as well as from the other arcades of the mesocolon, originate the vasa recta that supply the bowel wall. They are best demonstrated by selective arteriography (Fig. 71-2), but they may also be well seen after intraaortic injection.

The so-called marginal artery has been the source of much confusion in the literature. As Drummond described it, it represented a system of arcades to which the ileocolic, right colic, middle colic, left colic, and upper sigmoid arteries contributed. Although the colic arteries parallel the marginal artery at times, they also represent integral components of the marginal system. Thus, in injected specimens and in vivo, the colic arteries or their branches may give rise to the vasa recta of the colon directly and hence act as a

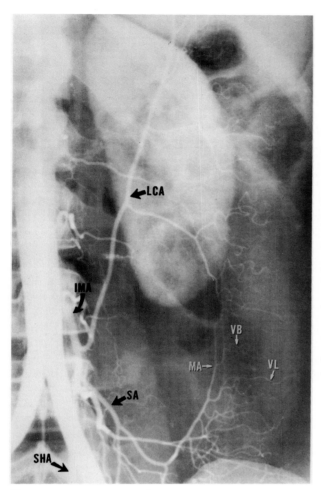

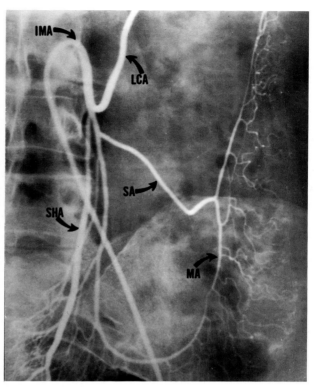

Figure 71-1. Normal inferior mesenteric arteriogram, aortic injection. The inferior mesenteric artery (*IMA*) gives off the left colic (*LCA*) and sigmoid branches (*SA*) and becomes the superior hemorrhoidal artery (*SHA*) after passing over the iliac vessels. The first branch of the left colic artery is the marginal artery (*MA*), which is continuous with the marginal branch of the sigmoid artery. The vasa brevia (*VB*) and vasa longa (*VL*) arise from the marginal artery and supply the wall of the colon.

Figure 71-2. Normal inferior mesenteric arteriogram, selective injection. The left colic artery (*LCA*) originates as a single branch. Immediately thereafter, a sigmoid trunk arises, which subsequently divides into three sigmoid arteries (*SA*). The marginal artery (*MA*) follows the course of the sigmoid colon and the descending colon. The inferior mesenteric artery (*IMA*) continues into the pelvis as the superior hemorrhoidal artery (*SHA*).

marginal artery. In such instances it is impossible to define where the colic arteries and their branches end and the marginal artery begins. We have therefore chosen to speak of the marginal artery as the total complex of arcades from which the nutrient vessels of the colon derive (particularly because the marginal artery itself connects the colon branches and merges imperceptibly with them). When the marginal system functions as a major collateral pathway in man between the superior and inferior mesenteric arteries, we

have designated the large major trunk as the marginal artery although elements of the left colic and middle colic arteries clearly may independently play an important role.

The inferior mesenteric vein is a continuation of the superior hemorrhoidal vein; it receives the drainage from the left colon through the left colic and sigmoid veins (into which the marginal vein empties) (Fig. 71-3). It lies in the retroperitoneal space to the left of the spine and empties into the splenic vein after passing behind the pancreas.

The circulation time through the inferior mesenteric system has been studied both by cine and large-film techniques. The time required for the development of threshold density in the inferior mesenteric vein after contrast injection into the inferior mesenteric artery is about 6 to 7 seconds in the normal individual.

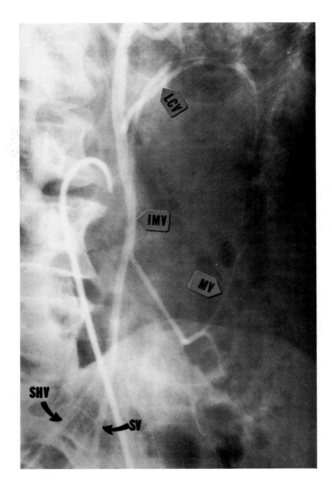

Figure 71-3. Normal inferior mesenteric venogram, selective injection. The venous phase demonstrates the superior hemorrhoidal vein (*SHV*), sigmoid veins (*SV*), left colic branches (*LCV*), and marginal vein (*MV*) draining into the inferior mesenteric vein (*IMV*). The inferior mesenteric vein empties into the splenic vein.

LEVEL OF ORIGIN OF THE INFERIOR MESENTERIC ARTERY

The inferior mesenteric artery may arise at any level from the second to the fourth lumbar vertebra. In 66 percent of all cases, it arose at the level of the third lumbar vertebra, and in 87 percent, between the lower border of the second and the upper border of the fourth lumbar vertebra (Fig. 71-4). Thus, it can be seen that in most instances its origin is sufficiently above the aortic bifurcation that thrombobliterative disease at the bifurcation need not involve the inferior mesenteric circulation.

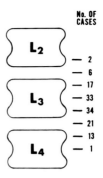

Figure 71-4. Level of aortic origin of the inferior mesenteric artery. The number of cases in which the artery arose at the level of the second, third, and fourth lumbar vertebrae (L2, L3, L4) is indicated.

SEGMENTS OF COLON SUPPLIED BY THE INFERIOR MESENTERIC ARTERY

In about 20 percent of the cases analyzed, the inferior mesenteric artery supplied the distal colon up to the middle or the lower descending colon. In 25 percent of cases, the area of supply reached but did not include the splenic flexure. In 44 percent of cases, the splenic flexure was included in the area of supply, and in an additional 10 percent the branches extended proximal to the splenic flexure. In only 3 percent of cases was the middle portion of the transverse colon supplied by the inferior mesenteric artery; the overwhelming bulk of cases demonstrated supply by the middle colic branch of the superior mesenteric artery.

SIZE OF THE INFERIOR MESENTERIC ARTERY AND ITS BRANCHES

There is great variability in the size of the inferior mesenteric artery in adults (1.2–5.5 mm in diameter) (Table 71-1). The same is true for the branches of the inferior mesenteric artery. The size bears no relationship to the degree of atheromatous disease of the aorta or of the inferior mesenteric artery itself. There is a rough correlation between the size of the left colic artery and the length of the colic segment supplied: the smaller diameters are found in patients in whom only the middle or the low descending colon is supplied by the left colic artery, whereas the larger diameters are found in those patients in whom the left colic branches are distributed to the splenic flexure and the transverse colon.

Table 71-1. Size of Inferior Mesenteric
Artery Branches in Normal Subjects*

Mesenteric Branch	Number of Patients	Range (mm)	Mean (mm)
Inferior mesenteric artery	110	1.2–5.5	3.34
Ascending branch (LC & S)	57	1.2–4.0	2.60
Ascending branch (LC)	35	1.0–3.1	2.07
Ascending branch (overall)	97	1.0–4.0	2.39
Left colic	106	1.0–2.8	1.70
Descending branch (part S)	53	1.0–4.0	2.47
Descending branch (all S)	36	1.2–4.4	2.58
Descending branch (overall)	95	1.0–4.4	2.54
Superior hemorrhoidal	37	1.0–3.0	2.02

*Patients under the age of 16 and those with occlusion have been
excluded.
LC = left colic artery; S = sigmoid artery.

Indications for Arteriography

MESENTERIC VASCULAR DISEASE

In those cases in which intestinal ischemia is
thought to be present, the demonstration of the
mesenteric vessels by arteriography is the only
method other than surgery to define the site and
degree of luminal compromise. In acute postoperative ischemia, arteriography may establish
the presence or absence of occlusion of the inferior mesenteric artery and the extent of the
collateral circulation. It may corroborate or rule
out embolic occlusion.

DIFFERENTIAL DIAGNOSIS OF
NEOPLASTIC MASSES FROM
INFLAMMATORY MASSES

At times the barium enema examination is
equivocal in the distinction of inflammatory masses from neoplastic ones. Inflammatory masses
may require conservative therapy, neoplastic
masses immediate surgery. Angiography offers
the opportunity to distinguish the two.

ASSESSMENT OF RESECTABILITY AND
EXTENT OF TUMORS

In the presence of large tumors, the extent of
tumor spread through and beyond the bowel wall
may be determined.

DETECTION OF RECURRENT TUMOR

At times recurrence is difficult to distinguish
from narrowing at the site of bowel anastomosis.
The angiogram will usually show tumor vessels.

ADEQUACY OF BLOOD SUPPLY OF
BOWEL SEGMENT TO BE
TRANSPLANTED FOR ESOPHAGEAL
PROSTHESIS

If there is significant atherosclerotic narrowing of
the vessels supplying the bowel segment to be
used, the chances of a successful operation are
significantly poorer.

COLIC BLEEDING OF UNDETERMINED
ETIOLOGY

Mesenteric arteriography may demonstrate the
site of bleeding or the presence of an angiomatous malformation in the bowel wall.

DEFINING SITE FOR
CHEMOTHERAPEUTIC INFUSION

Although chemotherapy is not widely used for
bowel neoplasms, in the presence of an inoperable tumor that may require regional chemotherapy the definition of the precise vascular
route of infusion and of the extent of the lesion
may be desirable.

Primary Vascular Abnormalities

INTESTINAL ISCHEMIA

The classic clinical picture of chronic intestinal ischemia includes postprandial pain, weight loss,
and bowel dysfunction. A history of cramping
upper abdominal pain that is worse after a large
meal is helpful if present. But the symptoms may
be relatively nondescript, and the character of the
pain is not always specific. Even in cases display-

ing classic symptoms, the diagnosis has frequently been missed until acute vascular insufficiency supervened [48]. Since the mortality is far higher for emergency than for elective surgical procedures [45], a high index of suspicion must be maintained for ischemic bowel disease, and symptoms suggestive of acute bowel ischemia should prompt immediate angiographic studies.

In the analysis of visceral ischemic syndromes, and of bowel infarction as well, emphasis traditionally has been on the superior mesenteric artery [78, 86], partly because it supplies such a large segment of the intestine. Nevertheless, it is clear that the inferior mesenteric artery is also a frequent site of atheromatous change and, at times, of occlusion. Perhaps a major factor in the persistent viability of the gut associated with significant disease of the inferior mesenteric artery is the richness of the collateral system.

The syndrome of mesenteric artery insufficiency of the colon or the rectum has been described with increasing frequency as a spontaneous occurrence [9, 22, 45] or as a result of aortic surgery [10, 24, 26, 36, 66, 76] or translumbar aortography [8, 55, 56, 65, 80]. Characteristically, the patient complains of left lower quadrant pain, melena, and, often, diarrhea [73]. Sigmoidoscopy may be diagnostic (showing bluish-black areas of ischemia, most often at the rectosigmoid junction) [23]. Because the surgical approach to mesenteric vascular disease is becoming more sophisticated [4, 9, 25, 27, 29, 35, 78, 91], the role of arteriography has been significantly amplified as a means of defining the site and the degree of major vessel narrowing. When arterial surgery is contemplated, an arteriographic map is essential. Once the presence of stenosis or occlusion of one of the mesenteric arteries has been established, the question still remains as to its relationship to the patient's symptoms. It is now clear that significant degrees of stenosis and occlusion of the mesenteric arteries may be present without symptoms [31, 35, 46, 50, 59]. A major determinant of the sufficiency of the blood supply is the extent of the collateral circulation.

COLLATERAL CIRCULATION TO LEFT COLON

The collateral circulation utilized after inferior mesenteric artery occlusion comprises primarily the marginal artery, which, adjacent to the splenic flexure, communicates with the middle colic branch of the superior mesenteric artery [7]. In addition, a short retroperitoneal loop connecting the superior and inferior mesenteric arteries or their major branches may be an important collateral element. Below the termination of the marginal artery and the lower sigmoid colon, collateral channels are more limited, but connections with the middle and inferior hemorrhoidal branches of the hypogastric artery and the middle sacral artery are present.

Among the 136 cases in which satisfactory inferior mesenteric arteriograms were obtained, there were 93 normal studies, 6 of which showed filling of potential collateral channels [50]. Such filling was best demonstrated by selective inferior mesenteric arteriography. After opacification of the inferior mesenteric and the left colic arteries, the middle colic artery filled from the marginal vessel, a continuation of the left colic artery (Fig. 71-5). Conversely, retrograde filling of an apparently normal left colic artery was seen on selec-

Figure 71-5. Retrograde filling of the middle colic artery from the inferior mesenteric artery. After selective injection into the inferior mesenteric artery (*IMA*), the left colic artery (*LCA*) and the marginal branches opacify, with retrograde flow into the middle colic artery (*MCA*). There is no evidence of mesenteric vascular disease. The inferior mesenteric artery trunk, after the origin of the left colic, divides into the sigmoidal artery (*SA*) and the superior hemorrhoidal artery.

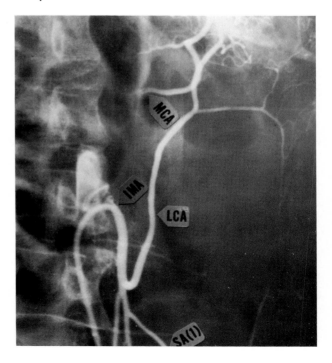

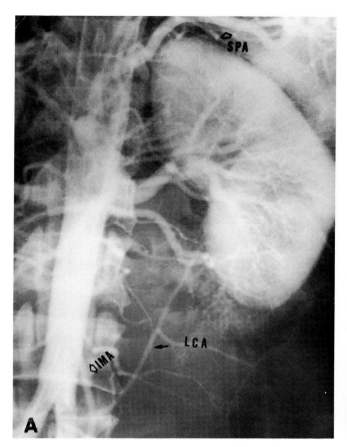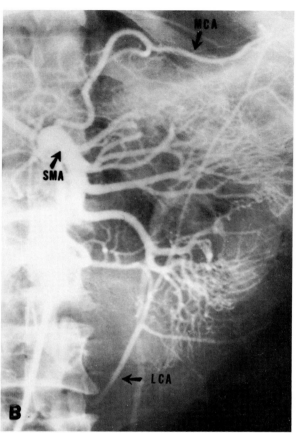

Figure 71-6. Retrograde filling of the left colic artery from the superior mesenteric artery. (A) Aortic injection. There is normal prograde filling of the inferior mesenteric (*IMA*) and left colic (*LCA*) arteries. Other branches of the aorta, such as the splenic artery (*SPA*) and the superior mesenteric and renal arteries are also filled. (B) Selective superior mesenteric arteriogram. After injection into the superior mesenteric artery (*SMA*), the middle colic artery (*MCA*) opacifies in continuity with the marginal loop, from which the left colic branch (*LCA*) of the inferior mesenteric artery fills.

tive superior mesenteric arteriography (Fig. 71-6). In addition, connections between the inferior mesenteric artery and the celiac axis were sometimes visible in the presence of otherwise normal mesenteric vessels (Fig. 71-7).

With occlusive disease of one or more of the major mesenteric arteries, the marginal loop may become strikingly prominent. In this way, the inferior mesenteric artery may supply the superior mesenteric channels (Fig. 71-8) or both the superior mesenteric and the celiac circulations (Fig. 71-9). By the same token, occlusive disease of the inferior mesenteric artery permits flow from the middle colic artery into the marginal artery and hence an adequate supply to the branches of the inferior mesenteric artery (Fig. 71-10). Under these circumstances, the enlargement of the marginal artery is not as great as it is

when a patent inferior mesenteric artery functions as a major avenue of supply to the proximal large bowel.

The degree to which the mesenteric arteries may function as an effective collateral network either prograde or retrograde has been emphasized in several articles [19, 50, 64]. The number of collateral vessels demonstrated by angiography was found by Hansen and Efsen to serve as a crude index of the significance of mesenteric vascular disease. In their study, patients with symptomatic disease had, on the average, twice as many collateral vessels as did asymptomatic patients. The relationship was not consistent, however; just as some symptomless patients exhibited collateral vessels, so some patients with symptomatic disease had none identified. Presumably, the intestinal blood sup-

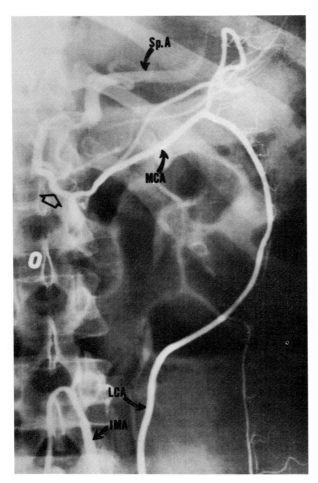

Figure 71-7. Retrograde filling of the splenic artery from the inferior mesenteric artery as shown by a selective inferior mesenteric arteriogram. After injection of the inferior mesenteric artery (*IMA*), good filling of the left colic artery (*LCA*) and the middle colic artery (*MCA*) is demonstrated. Through a retroperitoneal connection (*open arrow*), the splenic artery (*Sp. A*) is filled with contrast material and can be outlined throughout most of its course.

ply was maintained through collateral vessels that were not angiographically evident. The major cause of a developed collateral circulation is arteriosclerotic narrowing or occlusion, but congenital lesions, vasculitis, emboli, neoplastic disease, and inflammatory lesions may all alter regional flow to the bowel [69]. Even with acute occlusion of the superior mesenteric artery, the inferior mesenteric artery may function as a collateral channel [1]. Collateral flow from the inferior mesenteric and celiac arteries is of vital importance, because the superior mesenteric ar-

tery receives no extramesenteric collateral flow [46].

The inferior mesenteric artery also participates as a collateral channel in occlusive disease of the aorta and the iliac arteries. If the abdominal aorta is obstructed below the level of the superior mesenteric artery, the marginal loop may form one of the major pathways for blood to the lower aorta and the lower extremities (Fig. 71-11). When the obstruction in the aorta is below the origin of the inferior mesenteric artery, the superior hemorrhoidal anastomoses to the hypogastric artery become prominent and serve as important collateral vessels to the lower extremities (Fig. 71-12). The major supply to the rectum is through the middle and inferior hemorrhoidal arteries arising from the hypogastric artery. If the anastomoses between the superior and the middle hemorrhoidal arteries are inadequate, ischemia of the rectum may develop after distal aortic surgery or iliac artery ligation, even when the marginal artery supplies the remainder of the left colon.

ARTERIOSCLEROSIS, STENOSIS, AND OCCLUSION

The angiographic findings in arteriosclerosis of the inferior mesenteric arteries may be summarized as follows: (1) eccentric plaques; (2) eccentric filling defects, probably incorporating both plaque and thrombus; (3) concentric narrowing; (4) occlusion; and (5) segmental ste-

---

Figure 71-8. The intestinal collateral circulation in occlusive disease. Superior mesenteric artery stenosis. This 50-year-old woman had intermittent claudication of both lower extremities. Femoral arteriography demonstrated marked arteriosclerotic disease in both superficial femoral arteries. No symptoms referable to the abdomen were present. Aortography demonstrated a huge marginal artery as an important collateral system. (A) At 1 second after injection. Moderate atheromatous changes are visible in the aortic wall. The inferior mesenteric artery (*IMA*) is dilated and may be seen in continuity with an enlarged left colic (*LCA*) and marginal artery (*MA*). Notice that in spite of the excellent filling of the abdominal aortic branches, the superior mesenteric artery is not visualized. (B) At 2.5 seconds. The marginal artery is in continuity with the middle colic artery and follows the transverse mesocolon to the right. (C) At 4.5 seconds. The marginal artery (*MA*) can now be seen to anastomose with the superior mesenteric artery (*SMA*), which fills quite densely only after a long interval. (D)

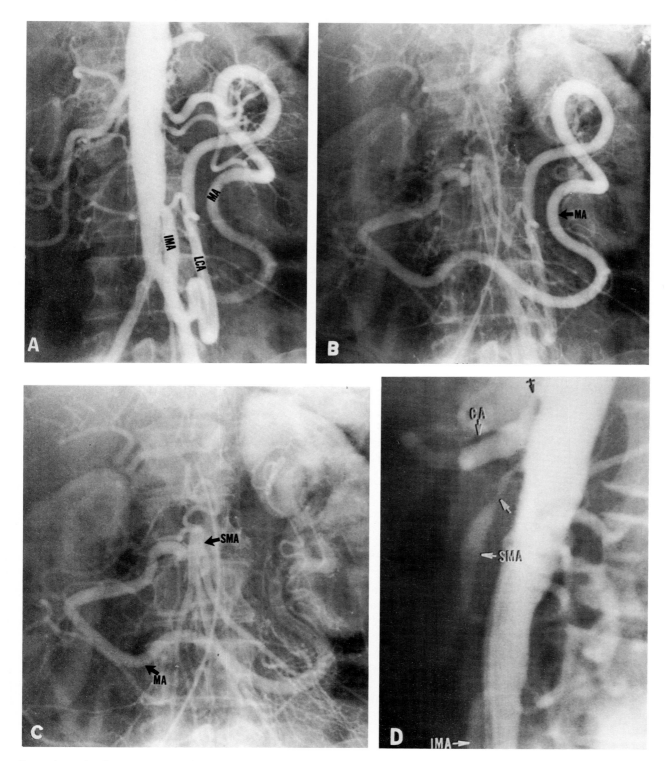

Lateral projection at 1 second. Stenosis of both the celiac artery (*CA*) and the superior mesenteric artery is clearly defined. The flow through the celiac artery seems adequate in spite of stenosis (*upper barred arrow*). The flow distally in the superior mesenteric artery, however, is significantly diminished, and, as can be seen from A, B, and C, most blood reaches the superior mesenteric circulation through the marginal artery. The proximal segment of the superior mesenteric artery is significantly narrowed (*arrow*). The inferior mesenteric artery (*IMA*) is not the site of stenosing lesions.

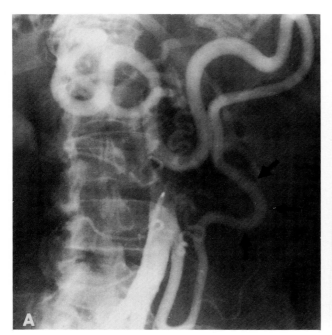

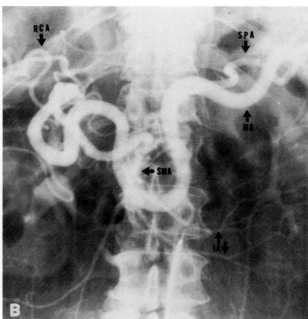

Figure 71-9. The intestinal collateral circulation in occlusive disease: stenosis of the celiac and superior mesenteric arteries. This 52-year-old woman had a 25-year history of hypertension and had noted the onset of intermittent claudication of both lower extremities a few months before admission. Femoral arteriography demonstrated arteriosclerotic disease with stenosis of the left external iliac and the left common femoral arteries and both hypogastric arteries. Aortography revealed the marginal artery as the source of blood to both the celiac and the superior mesenteric circulations. (A) Abdominal aortogram, right posterior oblique projection. The catheter has deliberately been placed below the renal arteries near the mouth of the inferior mesenteric artery. From the inferior mesenteric artery, a grossly dilated marginal artery (*arrows*) is visible. It pursues a circuitous course following the distribution of the left colic and the middle colic arteries. (B) Abdominal aortogram, anteroposterior projection, 2.5 seconds. The large marginal artery (*MA*) is seen to fill the branches both of the superior mesenteric artery (*SMA*) and the celiac artery. Filling of the splenic artery (*SPA*), the right colic artery (*RCA*), and the intestinal branches (*IA*) of the superior mesenteric artery is clearly demonstrated. A subsequent aortogram in the lateral projection demonstrated virtually complete occlusion of both the celiac and superior mesenteric arteries just distal to their origin.

nosis. Dysplasia involving the mesenteric arteries is rare. In two cases of nonocclusive intestinal infarction, histologic examination of distal branches of the superior mesenteric artery revealed ultrastructural changes similar to those that have been experimentally produced in the renal arteries by hypertension [57]. It is likely that such lesions may also occur in the inferior mesenteric artery in some hypertensive individuals. Thrombotic occlusion of the abdominal aorta may be associated with inferior mesenteric artery occlusion [20].

One of the major questions with regard to mesenteric artery insufficiency is the degree to which arterial lesions are found in asymptomatic patients as well as in symptomatic patients. In recent years, a significant amount of information has been accumulated on this subject. In our series, total occlusion of the inferior mesenteric artery was present in 9 (6.6%) of 136 patients with satisfactory studies (see Fig. 71-10) [50]. In an additional 23 patients (17%), stenosis or atheromatous change of a significant degree was visible in the inferior mesenteric artery (Fig. 71-13), but none of these patients had symptoms of intestinal ischemia. In association with arteriosclerosis of the inferior mesenteric artery, a characteristic plaque at the origin of this vessel was often seen. This plaque was usually best defined in the left posterior oblique projection (Fig. 71-13B). Arteriosclerotic change in the inferior mesenteric artery was unusual in the absence of significant atheromata in the aortic wall at other levels. In a review of 2,029 abdominal

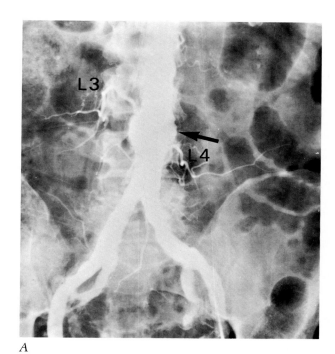

A

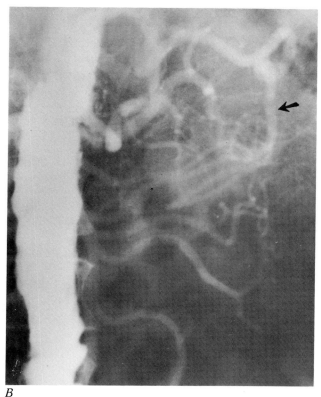

B

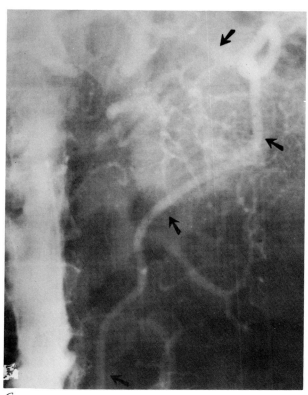

C

Figure 71-10. The collateral circulation in occlusive disease: inferior mesenteric artery occlusion. (A) Abdominal aortogram. There is extensive atheromatous disease of the abdominal aorta. The left third lumbar and the right fourth lumbar arteries are obstructed, together with the inferior mesenteric artery origin (*arrow*). (B and C) Collateral filling from the superior mesenteric artery. (B) At 1 second, gross atheromatous disease in the abdominal aorta, together with complete occlusion of the inferior mesenteric artery, is visible. A large marginal artery (*arrow*) may be seen filling during this phase of the study. (C) At 2 seconds, the left colic artery is now defined (*multiple arrows*), in continuity with the middle colic artery and the inferior mesenteric artery below. (D to G) Obstruction of the inferior mesenteric artery and the left common iliac artery. (D) The right common iliac (*RCI*) artery is opacified, but the left common iliac artery is not visualized because it was obstructed at its origin (*arrow*). A large plaque is seen on the left side of the aorta in the region of the origin of the inferior mesenteric artery, which is occluded (*barred arrow*). Filling of the superior mesenteric artery (*SMA*) and the celiac artery

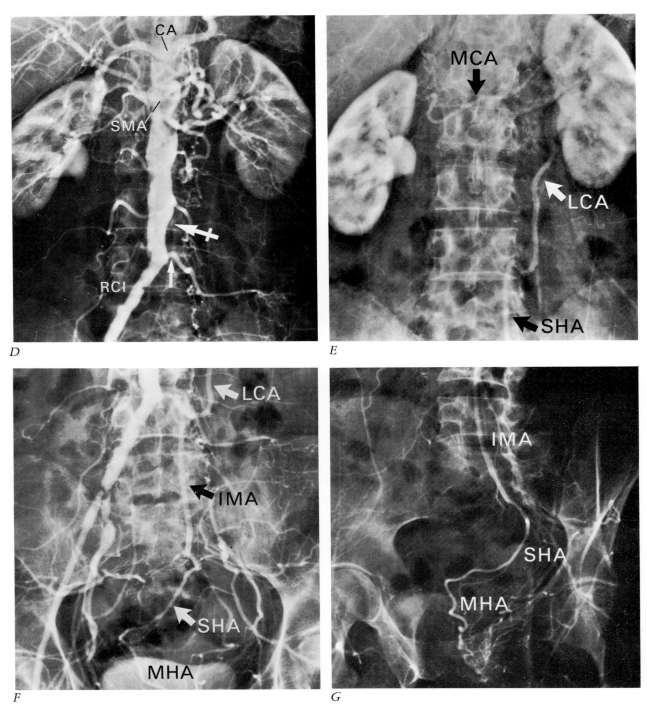

D

E

F

G

(*CA*) is well demonstrated. (E) At 3 seconds, the middle colic artery (*MCA, black arrow*) is opacified and may be seen extending to fill the left colic artery (*LCA, white arrow*). The left colic artery in turn is clearly in continuity with the superior hemorrhoidal artery below (*SHA, black arrow*). (F) The left colic (*LCA, white arrow*) and the inferior mesenteric (*IMA, black arrow*) arteries represent the channel whereby blood reaches the superior hemorrhoidal artery (*SHA, white arrow*) and the middle hemorrhoidal artery (*MHA*) below. (G) With opacification of the middle hemorrhoidal artery (*MHA*), the left obturator artery is the channel whereby the internal iliac and the common femoral arteries are filled and opacified. Thus, with complete obstruction of the common iliac artery, the circulation to the left limb is maintained largely via the inferior mesenteric and the superior hemorrhoidal arteries.

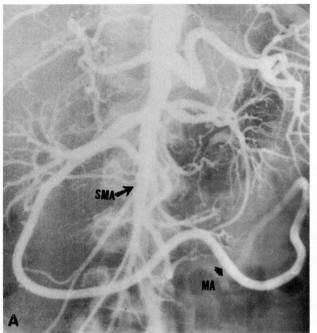

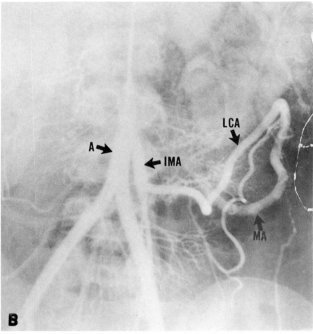

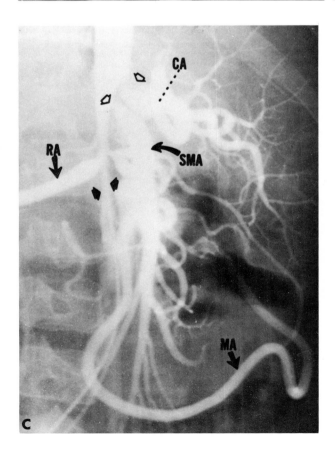

Figure 71-11. The intestinal collateral circulation in occlusive disease: stenosis of the upper abdominal aorta. This 6-year-old girl had a blood pressure of 180/110 mm Hg in the upper extremities and diminished femoral pulses. (A) Abdominal aortogram, anteroposterior projection, 1 second. The superior mesenteric artery (SMA) is large and is in continuity with a dilated marginal loop (MA). Notice the prominence of the intercostal arteries above, adjacent to the ribs. (B) Abdominal aortogram, anteroposterior projection, 2.5 seconds. Contrast has moved from the marginal artery (MA) into the left colic and inferior mesenteric arteries and retrograde to fill the distal abdominal aorta and the common iliac arteries. (C) Abdominal aortogram, left posterior oblique projection. In the oblique projection it can be seen that there is gross narrowing of the abdominal aorta (*solid arrows*), with stenosis as well of the origin of the celiac artery and the superior mesenteric arteries (*open arrows*). Both renal arteries (RA) are also narrowed at their origin. The dilated marginal artery in continuity with the superior mesenteric artery (SMA) is clearly seen in the oblique projection. In this case of abdominal coarctation, the origins of virtually all the great visceral vessels from the abdominal aorta were also involved. The marginal artery provided an avenue of distal aortic filling.

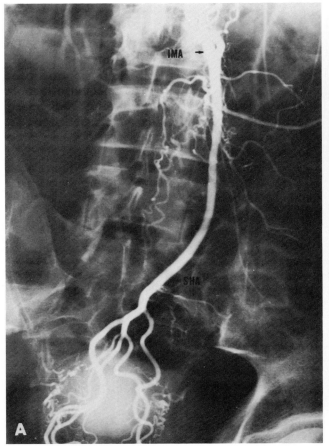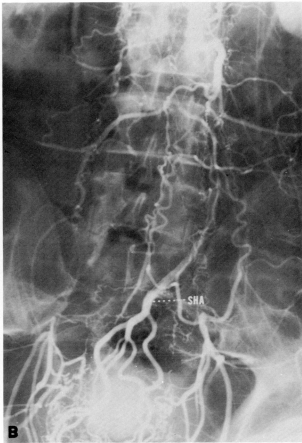

Figure 71-12. The intestinal collateral circulation in occlusive disease: occlusion of the distal abdominal aorta. This 40-year-old man had claudication of both legs and absent femoral pulses. Abdominal aortography was performed with percutaneous transaxillary catheterization of the distal aorta. (A) Intraaortic injection demonstrated complete occlusion of the distal aorta with a large inferior mesenteric artery (*IMA*) and superior hemorrhoidal artery (*SHA*). (B) At 2 seconds, the superior hemorrhoidal artery (*SHA*) and its branches are well delineated. There is retrograde filling of branches of the hypogastric arteries, and subsequent studies demonstrated that the inferior mesenteric artery was an important channel of blood flow to the lower extremities.

aortograms by Hansen and Efsen, 118 (5.6%) were found to show stenoses or occlusions in one or more of the three major visceral arteries [46]. Only 32 (27%) of the patients with arteriographically demonstrated abdominal vascular disease had symptoms of intestinal ischemia.

In contrast to the above patients without symptoms is a significant group in which mesenteric vascular disease is clearly associated with symptoms and in which the disease may be catastrophic if allowed to go unchecked. Some years ago we reported a group of such cases [25]. In one patient, celiac artery stenosis and superior mesenteric artery occlusion were associated with absence of the inferior mesenteric artery, which

had been sacrificed during a previous aortic resection. The basis for this patient's symptoms was not recognized until an acute exacerbation of signs and symptoms led to exploration and the discovery of gangrene. Earlier recognition might have avoided this sequence. In another patient, the presence of profound stenosis of the superior mesenteric artery as a cause of the patient's symptoms was not recognized even at surgery. Subsequently the patient developed infarction of the bowel and died. A more satisfying course was exemplified by a third patient. This woman had the classic symptoms of pain, diarrhea, and weight loss. Careful study led to a precise diagnosis. Surgical correction of a stenosis of the

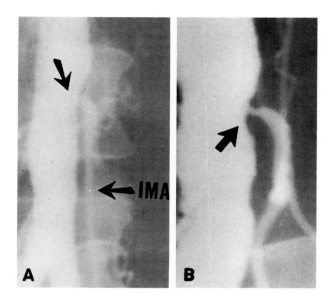

Figure 71-13. Stenosis of the inferior mesenteric artery. (A) Anteroposterior projection. A typical plaque is seen at the origin of the inferior mesenteric artery (*IMA*), with resulting stenosis of the vessel (*arrow*). (B) Left posterior oblique projection. In another case the plaque is again well defined (*arrow*). The stenosis of the origin of the inferior mesenteric artery is associated with slight poststenotic dilatation.

superior mesenteric artery was followed by cure [25].

Nevertheless, our own data support the concept that inferior mesenteric artery insufficiency rarely accompanies chronic, sustained, luminal compromise. Among the 32 individuals who had either occlusion or gross atheromatous change in the inferior mesenteric artery, none had the clinical signs of vascular insufficiency of the colon or rectum. While three patients in a surgical series reviewed by Hansen and Christofferson had intestinal angina as a result of occlusion of the inferior mesenteric artery alone [45], isolated inferior mesenteric artery disease was not associated with symptoms in any of the patients in Hansen's and Efsen's angiographic series. The relative rarity of symptomatic inferior mesenteric artery disease is explained by the rich collateral circulation available to the left colon. With slow diminution of the blood supply through the inferior mesenteric artery, the marginal artery may receive the bulk of its flow from the middle colic branch of the superior mesenteric artery and therefore continue to supply the small vessels of the colon with adequate oxygen and nutrients. Almost certainly an acute insult, such as surgical

trauma, acute thrombosis, or embolism, must be superimposed on an already compromised vascular bed to produce significant ischemia.

Several reports indicate that all three major arteries can be occluded without accompanying symptoms. In one patient described [59], the celiac and mesenteric circulations were filled by large retroperitoneal collateral vessels arising from the aorta. Although it has been clear that splanchnic vessel stenosis or occlusion may be asymptomatic, it has been assumed that occlusion of two major vessels is usually accompanied by symptoms. Apparently if time permits the development of an adequate collateral circulation, ischemia can be avoided.

The work of Hansen and Efsen also demonstrates that triple-vessel disease is not necessarily associated with symptoms of intestinal angina [46]. In 14 percent of their asymptomatic patients, all three vessels were diseased. Similarly, in a case reported by Hildebrand, an extensive collateral network from the internal iliac and the superior hemorrhoidal arteries supplied the visceral vessels retrogradely through their branches, preserving intestinal viability despite complete occlusion of the celiac artery, superior mesenteric artery, and inferior mesenteric artery. The patient, who also had marked aortoiliac stenosis that diminished the collateral flow, was symptomatic. In another reported case, the patient had occlusion of all three visceral arteries as well as of the right common iliac artery [48]. The entire gastrointestinal tract was supplied through a stenotic left iliac artery and through an artery of Drummond.

Bron and Redman have reported on 730 patients studied by aortography [21]. In 123 patients (17.3%), there was stenosis or occlusion of one or more vessels: the celiac artery was involved in 90 patients (12.5%), the superior mesenteric artery in 24 patients (3.4%), and the inferior mesenteric artery in 36 patients (5.5%). Of the last group, 25 patients showed stenosis, and 11 patients had occlusion. Hypertension or peripheral vascular disease were the major indications for aortography; abdominal pain was the indication in 18 percent of the patients. Among those with vessel obstruction, abdominal pain was present in 39 percent. The authors drew the inference that this pain was attributable to the vessel involvement although no patients had typical abdominal angina.

In the 118 patients found by Hansen and Efsen to have occlusive disease of the visceral arteries, lesions were found in 210 vessels: 90 in the celiac axis, 65 in the superior mesenteric artery, and 55 in the inferior mesenteric artery. While stenoses were frequent in the celiac axis and the superior mesenteric artery, occlusions occurred four times as frequently as stenoses in the inferior mesenteric artery.

An interesting quantitative approach to abdominal angina was described by Dick et al. [31]. They studied the splanchnic vessels by lateral lumbar aortography and attempted to estimate the sum of the cross-sectional areas of the celiac, superior mesenteric, and inferior mesenteric arteries. A significant difference was found in the cross-sectional areas of the group with ischemic gut disease as compared to a control group (27 patients with no evidence of arterial disease, 56 hypertensive patients, and 12 patients with known arteriosclerosis but without evidence of intestinal ischemia). A normal cross-sectional area was established, and, in cases of intestinal is-chemia, the cross-sectional area of the main arterial trunks was less than two-thirds of this normal level.

The patterns of involvement of the inferior mesenteric artery by arteriosclerosis must be kept in mind in the surgical management of the elderly patient [30]. The marginal artery may be a vital source of collateral supply in such a patient; it cannot be sacrificed without careful consideration [47]. Conversely, the inferior mesenteric artery itself may be a major source of blood to the viscera or even the lower extremities [34, 53], and the availability of other collateral channels should be assured before it is ligated. It is possible to compromise the collateral circulation of the left lower extremity by left colectomy when the inferior mesenteric artery is a major source of blood supply to this area. At least one case is on record in which gangrene followed such a procedure [70]. In addition, in those instances in which stenosis of the celiac and

Figure 71-14. Early aneurysm formation near the origin of the inferior mesenteric artery. A localized dilatation opposite the origin of the inferior mesenteric artery was visible in six cases. (A) The upper arrow points to the local bulge; the inferior mesenteric artery (IMA) is patent. (B) Similar local dilatation (*upper arrow*) in another subject. Notice that beyond the origin of the inferior mesenteric artery (IMA) there is a large plaque.

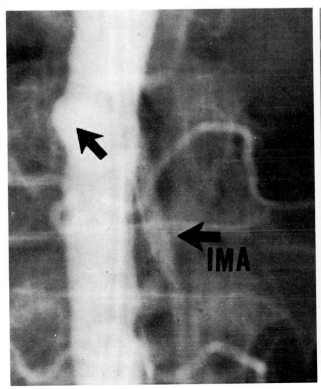

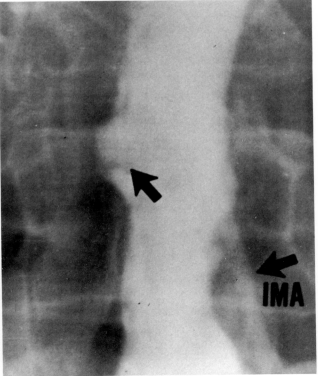

A

B

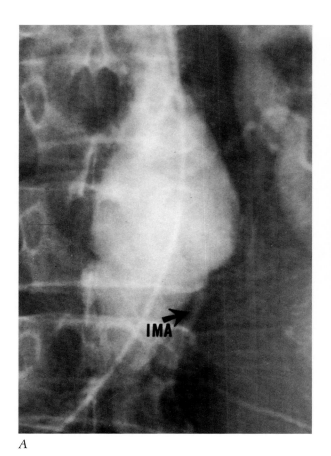

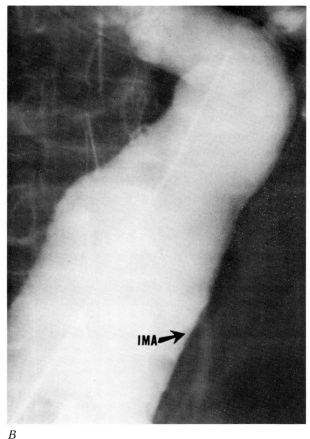

A   *B*

Figure 71-15. The inferior mesenteric artery in the presence of abdominal aortic aneurysm. (A) The inferior mesenteric artery (*IMA*) arises directly from the aneurysm and is clearly patent. (B) With a long, fusiform aneurysm of the abdominal aorta, the inferior mesenteric artery (*IMA*) arises from the midportion of the aneurysm. Contrast filling directly from the aorta indicates that it is patent.

superior mesenteric arteries is accompanied by a large mesenteric collateral system, surgery on the common iliac or femoral arteries may permit blood to be shunted away from the mesenteric circulation and into the periphery and thus create the so-called aortoiliac syndrome. In patients with complete occlusion of the infrarenal aorta and flow to the lower extremities through a central anastomotic artery connecting with the superior mesenteric artery, walking after meals may elicit symptoms of intestinal angina [26].

In six of the patients studied, a local dilatation of the abdominal aorta was visible directly opposite the origin of the inferior mesenteric artery (Fig. 71-14) [50]. This had the appearance of a small saccular aneurysm. In the presence of a large fusiform aneurysm, the inferior mesenteric artery origin was frequently within the wall of the aneurysm. Nevertheless, in six of seven patients

with large aneurysms, the inferior mesenteric artery filled directly from the aorta and was, therefore, not occluded (Fig. 71-15).

ACUTE VASCULAR OCCLUSION

The incidence of acute embolic occlusion of the inferior mesenteric artery is much lower than occlusion of the superior mesenteric artery. Not only is the latter a much larger vessel, but it runs parallel to the aorta and is ideally located for collecting emboli. Acute occlusion of the inferior mesenteric artery is well tolerated if the occlusion is limited to its proximal portion and if collateral vessels to the superior mesenteric artery are functional [27].

Acute occlusion may occur, however, as a consequence of arterial thrombosis. When it does, infarction of variable segments of the left colon may develop, with subsequent gangrene and death unless successful surgical intervention is possible. In some patients, occlusion may follow surgery; in others it may be associated with atheromatous plaques, blood dyscrasias, saccular aortic aneurysm, and sepsis [22]. Clinically, the course of such patients is characterized by the onset of sudden, severe, lower abdominal pain, tenderness, rigidity, and bloody rectal discharge. The mortality is high [45, 48], and an aggressive surgical approach is called for when the diagnosis is recognized. Arteriography is the only means of defining the precise lesion and the degree of collateral development.

Acute ischemia has been noted, particularly after resection of abdominal aortic aneurysms [10, 66, 70]. It has been treated by reattachment of the inferior mesenteric artery with a button of the aorta [27]. Although ligation of the inferior mesenteric artery alone need not be catastrophic if the marginal system is intact, ligation of the hypogastric arteries may be disastrous if the channels between the superior and the inferior hemorrhoidal arteries are not well established. Even temporary clamping of the hypogastric arteries after sacrifice of the inferior mesenteric artery for aortic aneurysm surgery may produce severe ischemia in about 10 percent of cases [76]. Asymptomatic patients with two- or three-vessel obstruction can develop gangrene after periods of hypotension, as may occur during intraabdominal surgery [27].

In the presence of acute embolic obstruction of the superior mesenteric artery, the inferior mesenteric artery may maintain a blood supply to the intestine via the marginal artery, but the blood supply is unlikely to be adequate in most cases [1].

Boley has pointed out that the course of the ischemic episode cannot be predicted from the initial clinical or radiographic findings [15, 16]. The patient should be observed carefully, the bowel placed at rest, and antibiotics and intravenous fluids administered. Steroids, which increase the chance of perforation, should not be given. The damage is considered irreversible if the patient's clinical state deteriorates or if symptoms persist for more than 2 weeks. In such cases, surgical treatment, involving resection of the involved intestinal segment with primary anastomosis of the remaining bowel, should be carried out. In Boley's series of 150 cases of colonic ischemia, 44.7 percent had reversible disease, 18.7 percent had persistent colitis, 12.7 percent had ischemic stricture, and 18.7 percent suffered gangrene or perforation. In 5.3 percent the follow-up was incomplete [15].

Carcinoma of the Colon

The importance of lesions of the segment of the gut supplied by the inferior mesenteric artery is hardly reflected by the volume of literature on this vascular bed. Over 75 percent of all polyps and cancers of the colon occur in the distribution area of the inferior mesenteric artery. Recent studies suggest the possibility of identifying these lesions by arteriographic techniques [14, 44, 79, 92].

Figure 71-16. Carcinoma of the colon. This 65-year-old woman was admitted to the hospital because of rectal bleeding. Barium enema examination revealed a short, stenotic segment of sigmoid colon (*arrowheads*), and the differentiation between carcinoma and diverticulitis was not clear. Inferior mesenteric angiography demonstrated unequivocal tumor vessels in the neoplasm, displacement of large branches, and profuse staining of the neoplastic mass. (Courtesy of Stewart Reuter, M.D.)

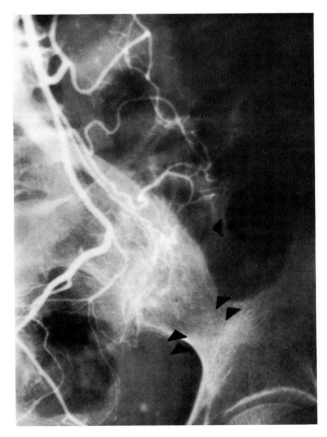

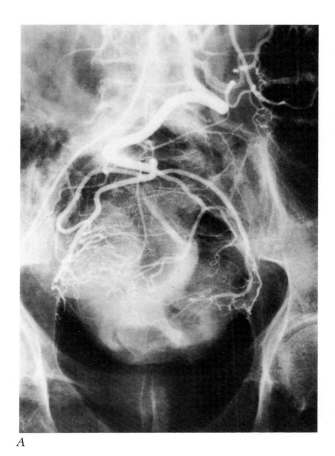

A

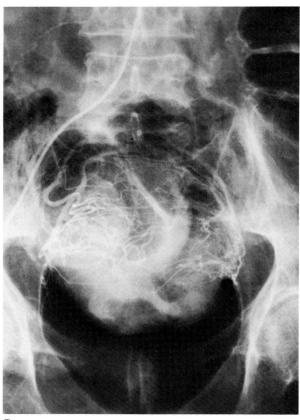

B

Figure 71-17. Villous adenoma of the colon. This 68-year-old man entered the hospital because of mucoid, watery diarrhea, persistent weakness, and occasional nausea and vomiting. Bowel movements varied from 10 to 50 a day, most of them watery. There was no history of rectal bleeding. Sigmoidoscopy revealed a lesion in the right lateral rectal wall about 15 to 18 cm from the mucocutaneous junction. Biopsy showed a villous adenoma. Angiography demonstrated a profusion of blood vessels to the tumor and gross displacement of the adjacent supplying vessels, indicating the size and extent of the tumor. There was contrast staining of the neoplastic mass. (A) Early phase. The hypervascularity of the tumor is clearly demonstrated, as are the tortuous vessels, their irregularity, and the displacement of adjacent large vascular trunks. (B) Later phase. There is persistent filling of many of the large branches and contrast accumulation in the tumor, somewhat difficult to define because of the opacified bladder. (Courtesy of Stewart Reuter, M.D.)

In all cases studied by Boijsen and Reuter [14], tumor vessels were observed. The tumors varied in vascularity and consequently in the number of abnormal vessels visualized. The vessels were tortuous in course, random in distribution, irregular in appearance, and abnormally tapered (Fig. 71-16). These findings are a requisite for the diagnosis of carcinoma. The contrast agent accumulates in the tumor, and many carcinomas also demonstrate premature venous filling [79]. Nevertheless, the density of the venous phase is significantly less than that seen in inflammatory disease.

Extension of the tumor through the bowel wall may be diagnosed by demonstrating irregularity of the arterial branches and marginal artery. Depending on the size of the tumor, there may be varying degrees of large-vessel displacement.

The distinction of recurrent tumor from scar formation at the site of the previous anastomosis may be difficult [21, 92]. Tumor vessels will usually be observed if there is a recurrence [14].

Figure 71-16 demonstrates the local vascular pattern in a 65-year-old woman in whom the clinical distinction between diverticulitis and carcinoma was not clear. Arteriography demon-

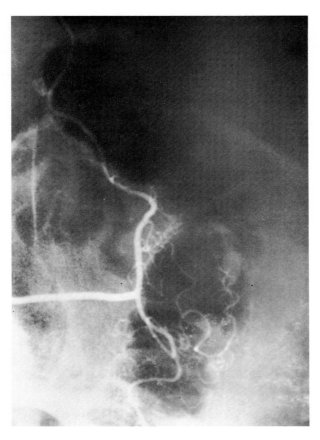

Figure 71-18. Malignant polyps of the colon. This 76-year-old man had polyps in the descending colon. Angiography demonstrated tortuous, abnormal vessels subserving these polyps. At resection the polyps were found to be adenocarcinomatous. (Courtesy of Stewart Reuter, M.D.)

strated unequivocal tumor vessels and a profound tumor stain.

Figure 71-17 shows the angiograms of a 68-year-old man admitted to the hospital because of mucoid, watery diarrhea, persistent weakness, and occasional nausea and vomiting. Angiography demonstrated a profusion of blood vessels—some of them tortuous and abnormal in their course. The extent of the tumor and the displacement of the adjacent vessels were clearly indicated. Biopsy showed a villous adenoma.

Figure 71-18 is an angiographic study of a 76-year-old man in whom polyps were noted in the descending colon on barium enema study. Selective inferior mesenteric angiography demonstrated abnormal vessels to the polyps. At surgery this area was resected, and the polyps were found to be adenocarcinomatous.

It is clear, then, that inferior mesenteric ar-

teriography may present unequivocal evidence of malignancy in certain instances in which the differential diagnosis from diverticulitis is difficult. The relative lack of an extensive vascular supply in diverticulitis is also helpful in the differentiation. More experience is required, however, before the accuracy of the arteriographic differentiation of inflammatory disease from malignant disease can be assessed adequately. Halpern [44] has emphasized that angiography may be particularly useful when carcinoma and diverticulitis coexist. In one of the cases that he reported, the arteriograms demonstrated unequivocally that malignancy was present in addition to diverticulitis. Brahme has reported a case in which chronic inflammatory disease was shown by barium enema examination to be a significant possibility. Arteriography demonstrated abundant abnormal vessels [18].

Inflammatory Disease of the Colon

Schobinger, on the basis of operative intestinal arteriography in diverticulitis, pointed out that mild degrees of inflammation had a vascular pattern similar to that of the surrounding normal bowel [71]. With acute inflammation, local hyperemia was visible but not the altered characteristics of the vascular bed seen with malignancy. No pooling of contrast agent was observed, nor were there arteriovenous shunts. Ström and Winberg also noted the absence of early venous filling in diverticulitis.

Boijsen and Reuter demonstrated that in regional enterocolitis the arteries and veins filled more rapidly than those in the surrounding normal bowel, increased vascularity was present, and there was slight dilatation of the supplying arteries and some dilatation and tortuosity of the

Figure 71-19. Ulcerative colitis. This 24-year-old ▶ woman had long-standing ulcerative colitis. (A) Selective inferior mesenteric arteriogram. There is good visualization of the major vessels to the left colon and the sigmoid. (B) Magnified view of A. (C) Later phase. (D) Magnified view of C. The vasa recta are prominent, and there is increased vascularity. The wall is slightly thickened, and the capillary phase is more intense than normal. The findings are nonspecific and less striking than in the acute phase. (Courtesy of Stanley Baum, M.D.)

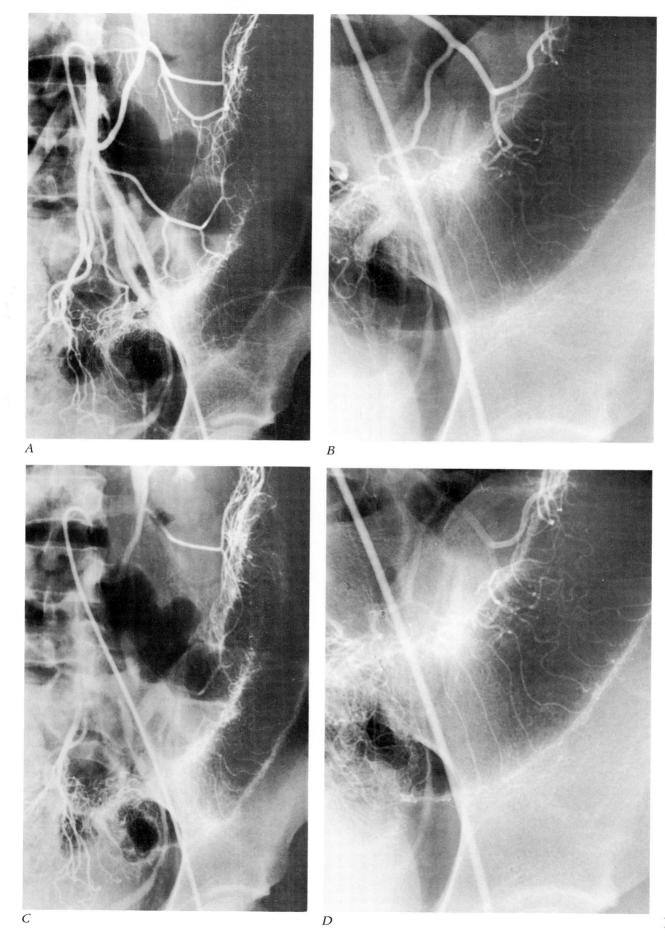

A

B

C

D

1721

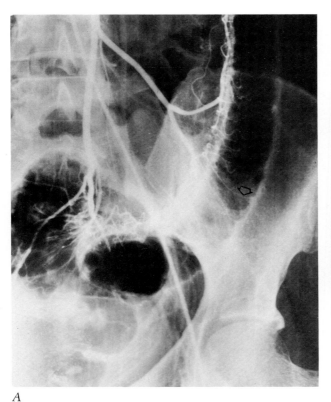

A

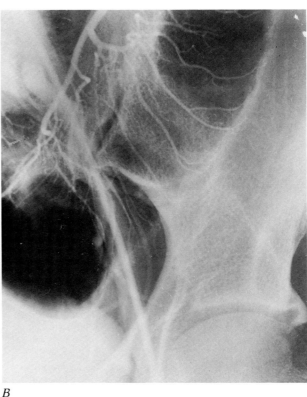

B

Figure 71-20. Ulcerative colitis. (A) Selective inferior mesenteric arteriogram. Augmented vascularity is apparent, and the capillary phase is increased. Loss of normal tapering is apparent (*arrowhead*). (B) Magnified view. Later films showed an early, intense venous phase. (Courtesy of Stanley Baum, M.D.)

veins draining the diseased segments [14]. During the capillary phase, thickened bowel could be seen in the presence of active disease. In ulcerative colitis there was also increased vascularity of the involved segment, but the vasa recta were smooth and regular (Figs. 71-19–17-21). In contrast to those in the normal bowel, there was relatively little tapering in the width of these vessels. In diverticulitis there was only a slight increase in vascularity of the diseased segment, and irregularity and distortion of the vasa recta were apparent.

Brahme, in describing the findings in regional enterocolitis, distinguished between (1) the changes in the ileum, in which the arteries of the bowel wall were reduced in number and the capillary phase was fainter than normal, and (2) inflammation in the colon, in which hypovascularization was not evident [18]. He pointed out that hypervascularization was also not seen (in contrast to the appearance in ulcerative colitis). The major changes were in the number of vessels and in the distorted course of those remaining. Relatively little accumulation of contrast medium

in the intestinal wall was observed. In the colon the vasa longa and the vasa brevia were tortuous and irregular in caliber (Fig. 71-22). Venous return appeared within a normal time.

Lunderquist and Lunderquist have reported detailed studies of angiography in ulcerative colitis [54]. In symptomatic cases, the inferior mesenteric artery and the vasa recta were widened. The vasa recta failed to taper toward the periphery, as they do in the normal colon. In some instances they terminated abruptly. A moderate increase in the thickness of the bowel wall was noted during the capillary phase. The veins were dilated, and their course was irregular. The large veins were abnormally wide and the contrast filling was unusually dense. These changes have been thought to be related to increased blood flow to the colon in ulcerative colitis [87]. In two symptom-free patients with ulcerative colitis, the angiographic studies were not dissimilar from the normal. The authors pointed out that the absence of tapering of the vasa recta might be useful in distinguishing ulcerative from

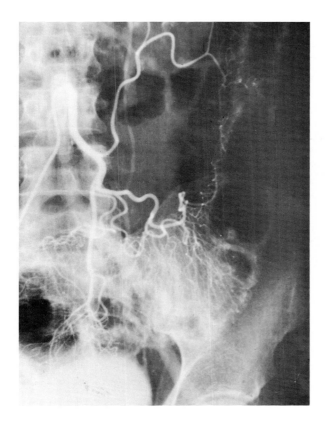

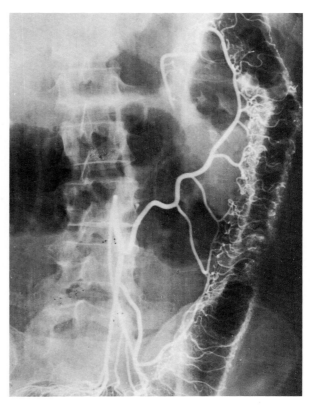

Figure 71-21. Ulcerative colitis in a 53-year-old man, selective inferior mesenteric arteriogram. There is a marked increase in vascularity, particularly to the sigmoid colon. The capillary blush is intense and the wall slightly thick. The vessels are relatively straight and do not taper normally. A small inflammatory polyp is visible in the descending colon. (Courtesy of Stanley Baum, M.D.)

Figure 71-22. Granulomatous colitis, selective inferior mesenteric arteriography. The inflammatory changes are not as marked as they are in ulcerative colitis. There is marked tortuosity of the vasa recta, with some loss of the normal smooth appearance of the walls. The vessels are somewhat stretched to the affected area of the bowel. The smaller mesenteric vessels may be narrowed in regional enteritis, and as the disease becomes chronic, irregularity and beading may be seen in some of the narrowed vessels. Note the marked thickening of the wall in the involved area and compare the tortuous vessels with those in the adjacent normal colon. (Courtesy of Stanley Baum, M.D.)

granulomatous colitis, in which the peripheral arteries in the intestinal wall are abnormally narrow and tortuous and have an irregular lumen. Tsuchiya et al. studied 25 patients with ulcerative colitis and found that the angiographic changes were correlated with the severity and activity of the disease, rather than with the duration or extent of involvement [87].

In summary, ulcerative colitis is distinguished by the findings of inflammation: dilated vessels, increased blood flow, augmented capillary phase, and large draining veins. In the chronic phase, the appearance may be normal. Granulomatous colitis reflects the involvement of the entire wall with tortuous vessels, narrowing and sometimes stretching of smaller branches, and irregularity of the vessel wall. The arteriogram may at times show a longer segment of involvement than does the barium enema examination.

Ischemic colitis, an unusual vascular disease that may cause occult bleeding and that may represent a phase of segmental ulcerative colitis, may also be distinguished angiographically [84].

Bleeding in the Left Colon

The subject of gastrointestinal bleeding is treated in Chapter 70, to which the reader is referred for a detailed discussion. Bleeding in the left colon is associated most commonly with diverticular disease and angiodysplasia [85]. Other important causes include neoplasms, ulcerative colitis, Crohn's disease, radiation proctitis, ischemic colitis, and infectious or inflammatory ulceration [37]. In idiopathic bleeding, associated factors include immunosuppression, chemotherapy, and anticoagulation for various disorders [37].

DIVERTICULAR BLEEDING

This is the commonest cause of bleeding in the large bowel, occurring generally in individuals over the age of 60. Although diverticula are more common in the left colon, bleeding from diverticula occurs three times more often in the right colon than in the left colon [85]. The cause of diverticular bleeding is thought to be erosion of a peridiverticular arteriole by fecal material within the diverticulum. Contrast extravasation is the only certain means of defining the precise site; when seen in the left colon in the absence of angiodysplasia or neoplasm, the cause is most likely diverticular. Vasopressin infusion may control diverticular bleeding [74, 89], but it is not always successful (Fig. 71-23) [89], presumably because of age and arteriosclerotic changes in the vessels.

ANGIODYSPLASIA

Angiodysplasia is a vascular malformation of the bowel wall in which dilated vascular channels—arterial, capillary, or venous—are present. These may be either gross or microscopic. Many terms, including vascular ectasia, dysplasia, or malformation, telangiectasia, and arteriovenous fistula or malformation, have been applied to these unique lesions, which are frequently a cause of chronic or recurrent gastrointestinal bleeding [12]. Most lesions have been found in the right side of the colon [17, 51, 62], but in some series left colic vascular malformations have represented an important group (Fig. 71–24), emphasizing the need for inferior mesenteric arteriography [12].

The most important angiographic features of angiodysplasia are: an early filling vein; a slowly emptying, tortuous intramural vein; a dilated feeding artery or arteries; a local wall stain; a vascular tuft; and prolonged venous opacification [17].

In chronic gastrointestinal bleeding with normal barium enema studies, angiodysplasia is a potentially correctable cause of bleeding if it can

be correctly diagnosed. It is essential, in such patients, that the inferior mesenteric artery as well as the superior mesenteric and celiac arteries be investigated angiographically.

ISCHEMIC COLITIS

Although there is good evidence that ischemic colitis may cause occult or massive bleeding [85], it must be considered an unusual cause of severe gastrointestinal hemorrhage. Occlusive mesenteric vascular disease has been thoroughly investigated, but nonocclusive mesenteric vascular insufficiency is not as well understood [48]. Particularly in the presence of central shock and low cardiac output, shunting of blood away from the mucosa may be associated with mucosal necrosis and, ultimately, erosion of vessels to the intestinal wall, with resultant bleeding into the bowel.

One type of ischemic colitis is illustrated in Figure 71-25. The woman whose case is illustrated had acute leukemia and was under treatment with cytotoxic drugs when she began to pass bright-red blood per rectum. She was hospitalized, and the bleeding increased 2 days after admission. Superior mesenteric arteriography was normal, but the inferior mesenteric arteriogram (Fig. 71-25) demonstrated the bleeding site in the sigmoid colon. Vasopressin infusion was initiated, and the bleeding was controlled. The infusion was tapered over 4 days; with the removal of the catheter, however, bleeding began anew, and the patient was taken to surgery. A segment of the sigmoid colon was resected. It demonstrated vasculitis and thrombosis of multiple small vessels, with ischemic sigmoiditis and ulcer formation (Fig. 71-25C). Thus, thrombosis of the small arteries was associated with mucosal ischemia and necrosis, ulcer formation, and, ultimately, with bleeding from a small and eroded artery.

Among the causes of nonocclusive ischemic colitis, the use of digitalis, certain vasopressors that constrict the splenic bed, antihypertensive medication, congestive heart failure and low blood volume have been identified. Other factors may be related to small vessel disease, with inflammation of small arteries producing mucosal damage, as in diabetes, lupus erythematosus, rheumatoid arthritis, polyarteritis nodosa, and radiation colitis. In these disorders, angiography frequently will not yield distinctive or diagnostic features. Barium enema studies may show the classic thumb printing, ulcerations, and strictures

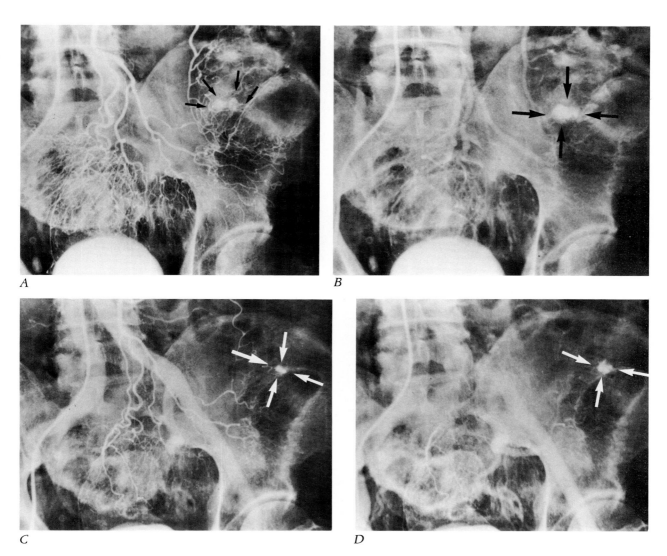

A

B

C

D

Figure 71-23. Left colic bleeding and diverticulosis. This 60-year-old man had massive bleeding into his lower gastrointestinal tract, and he required transfusion to maintain his blood volume. Superior mesenteric arteriography failed to disclose a bleeding site. Inferior mesenteric arteriography was then performed. (A) Inferior mesenteric arteriogram, 1 second. A discrete area of accumulation of contrast material in the lower descending colon is clearly visible (*arrows*). (B) At 3 seconds, during the venous phase, the accumulation of contrast material has become somewhat more dense (*arrows*). (C) Arteriogram. Following the administration of 0.2 unit of vasopressin per minute for 45 min- utes directly into the inferior mesenteric artery. Note the diminished caliber of the branch arteries. In spite of the response of the arteries to vasopressin infusion, evidence of bleeding is still visible in the descending colon (*arrows*). (D) Arteriogram during the venous phase. There is dense extravasation (*arrows*) in the descending colon, clearly less than on the initial examination but without cessation of bleeding. The patient was taken to surgery. Resection of the descending colon in the area of the bleeding demonstrated multiple diverticula, one of which had eroded at its base and destroyed the arterial wall.

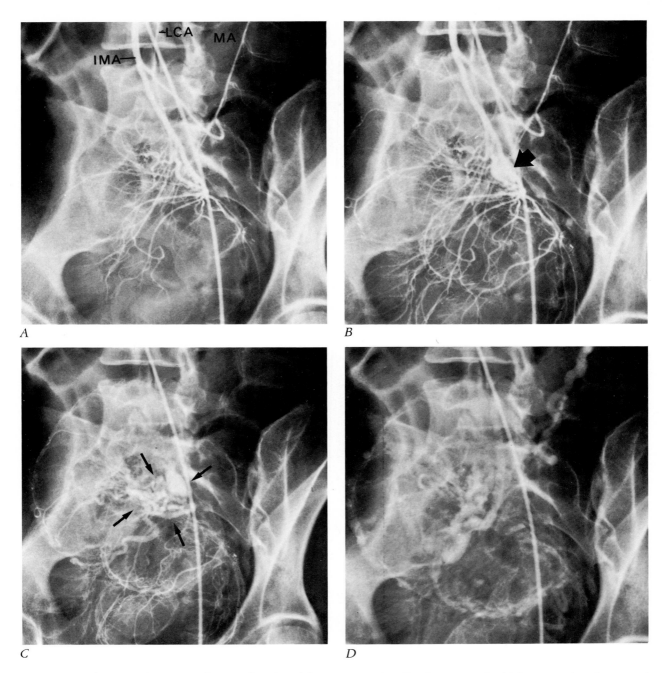

A

B

C

D

Figure 71-24. Angiodysplasia of the left colon. The patient had a history of recurrent bleeding. Superior mesenteric arteriography demonstrated no abnormalities. Inferior mesenteric arteriography was therefore performed. (A) Arteriogram, 0.5 second. No definite abnormalities are visible. (B) At 1 second. An area of contrast material accumulation (*arrow*) within a vascular wall is well demonstrated. (C) At 2 seconds. Multiple tortuous vessels are opacified, with premature venous drainage at the site of the angiodysplastic lesion (*arrows*). (D) At five seconds. Draining veins are now visualized, some of which are rather large and tortuous. These are particularly prominent in the region of the angiodysplasia. Thus this lesion demonstrates many of the classic features of colon angiodysplasia. Dilated feeding arteries are visible, together with an intense local wall stain, an early filling vein, dilated intramural veins, prolonged venous opacification, and a large vascular tuft. Identification of this lesion permitted a direct surgical approach to controlling chronic gastrointestinal bleeding in this patient.

Figure 71-25. Ischemic colitis. This 60-year-old woman with acute leukemia was placed on cytotoxic agents for her blood dyscrasia. She began to pass bright red blood per rectum, so she was hospitalized. Two days later, there was a sudden increase in bleeding, and arteriography was performed. The superior mesenteric arteriogram was normal. The inferior mesenteric arteriogram demonstrated a bleeding site and was followed by vasopressin infusion for 4 days, with cessation of bleeding. At the time of cathe- ▶

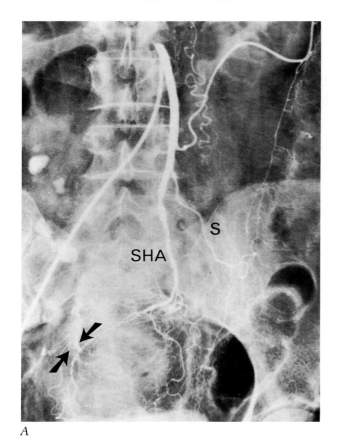

A

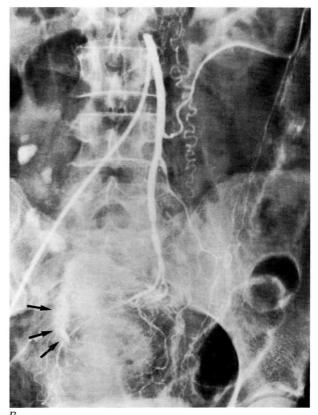

B

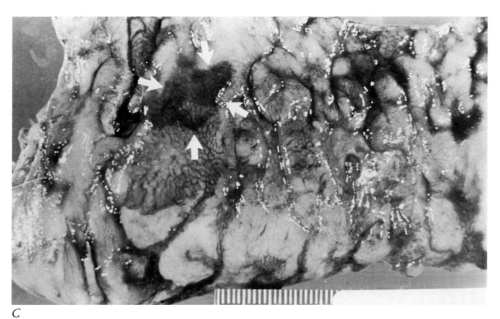

C

ter removal, however, the bleeding was reinitiated, and the patient was taken to surgery. Sigmoid resection was performed, and the involved segment demonstrated multiple thrombosed small vessels, with ischemic sigmoiditis and ulcer formation. (A) Inferior mesenteric arteriogram, 1 second. The inferior mesenteric artery and its left colic, sigmoid (*S*), and superior hemorrhoidal (*SHA*) arterial branches are well demonstrated. A branch of the superior hemorrhoidal artery to the sigmoid colon demonstrates a discrete area of intraluminal extravasation (*arrows*). (B) Inferior mesenteric arteriogram, 1.5 seconds. The contrast extravasation has increased (*arrows*). Note that in both A and B there are segments of irregular narrowing of the inferior mesenteric and superior hemorrhoidal branches, reflecting spasm in these branches. (C) Specimen of resected sigmoid colon. The mucosa is grossly inflamed, and an area of ulceration is visible (*arrows*). Beneath the area of ulceration, multiple thrombosed arteries were found, producing an ischemic sigmoiditis.

at the end stage, but the precise source of bleeding is frequently not well defined by angiography [6, 39].

ANGIOGRAPHIC DETECTION RATES IN COLONIC BLEEDING

In a study of 30 patients with massive gastrointestinal bleeding, Giacchino et al. were able to localize a site of bleeding in 23 patients (77%). Angiography was successful in 11 patients, barium enema study in 5 patients, and proctoscopy in 7 patients [37]. Bar et al., in an analysis of 24 patients with acute massive lower gastrointestinal bleeding, found that arteriography demonstrated a definite bleeding site in only 10 patients (about 40%) [5]. Best et al. analyzed angiographically 60 patients' studies for chronic gastrointestinal bleeding and noted a detection rate of 38 percent [12].

Thus, there is clearly a range of detection rates, but a minimum of one-third of all cases of occult chronic bleeding or of massive hemorrhage into the colon should be amenable to angiographic investigation. These figures are important because barium enema studies and colonoscopy may fail to define the bleeding site in many of these patients.

ACKNOWLEDGMENT

Many of the illustrations in this chapter were reproduced with permission from P. Kahn and H. L. Abrams, Inferior mesenteric arterial patterns: An angiographic study. *Radiology* 82:429, 1964.

References

1. Aakhus, T. The value of angiography in superior mesenteric artery embolism. *Br. J. Radiol.* 39:928, 1966.
2. Aakhus, T., and Evensen, A. Angiography in acute mesenteric arterial insufficiency. *Acta Radiol. [Diagn].* (Stockh.) 51:945, 1977.
3. Armstrong, B. G., Hunt, T. H., Price, C. W., and Resnick, M. I. Common origin of inferior mesenteric and accessory renal artery. *Urology* 14:298, 1979.
4. Atwell, R. B. Superior mesenteric artery embolectomy. *Surg. Gynecol. Obstet.* 112:257, 1961.
5. Bar, A. H., DeLaurentis, D. A., Parry, C. E., and Keohane, R. B. Angiography in the management of massive lower gastrointestinal tract hemorrhage. *Surg. Gynecol. Obstet.* 150:226, 1980.
6. Bartram, C. I. Obliteration of thumbprinting with double-contrast enemas in acute ischemic colitis. *Gastrointest. Radiol.* 4:85, 1979.
7. Basmajian, J. V. The marginal anastomoses of the arteries to the large intestines. *Surg. Gynecol. Obstet.* 99:614, 1954.
8. Baum, V., and Eufrate, S. A. Inferior mesenteric artery injury: A complication of translumbar aortography. *N.Y. State J. Med.* 62:3931, 1962.
9. Bergan, J. J., Dean, R. H., Conn, J., Jr., and Yao, J. S. T. Revascularization in treatment of mesenteric infarction. *Ann. Surg.* 182:430, 1975.
10. Bernatz, P. E. Necrosis of the colon following resection for abdominal aortic aneurysm. *Arch. Surg.* 81:373, 1960.
11. Bernstein, W. C., and Bernstein, E. F. Ischemic ulcerative colitis following inferior mesenteric arterial ligation. *Dis. Colon Rectum* 6:54, 1963.
12. Best, E. B., Teaford, A. K., and Rader, F. H. Angiography in chronic/recurrent gastrointestinal bleeding: A nine year study. *Surg. Clin. North Am.* 59:811, 1979.
13. Boijsen, E. Angiographic studies of the anatomy of single and multiple renal arteries. *Acta Radiol. [Suppl.]* (Stockh.) 183:1028, 1966.
14. Boijsen, E., and Reuter, S. R. Mesenteric arteriography in the evaluation of inflammatory and neoplastic disease of the intestine. *Radiology* 87:1028, 1966.
15. Boley, S. J., Brandt, L. J., and Veith, F. J. Ischemic disorders of the intestines. *Curr. Probl. Surg.* 15:1, 1978.
16. Boley, S. J., Schwartz, S., Krieger, H., Schultz, L., Siew, F. P., and Allen, A. C. Further observations on reversible vascular occlusion of the colon. *Am. J. Gastroenterol.* 44:260, 1965.
17. Boley, S. J., Sprayregen, S., Sammartano, R. J., Adams, A., and Kleinhaus, S. The pathophysiologic basis for the angiographic signs of vascular ectasias of the colon. *Radiology* 125:615, 1977.
18. Brahme, F. Mesenteric angiography in regional enterocolitis. *Radiology* 87:1037, 1966.
19. Brolin, I., and Paulin, S. Abnormal communications between splanchnic vessels. *Acta Radiol. [Diagn.]* (Stockh.) 2:460, 1964.
20. Bron, K. M. Thrombotic occlusion of the abdominal aorta: Associated visceral artery lesions and collateral circulation. *AJR* 96:887, 1966.
21. Bron, K. M., and Redman, H. C. Splenic artery stenosis and occlusion: Incidence; arteriographic and clinical manifestations. *Radiology* 92:323, 1969.
22. Carter, R., Vannix, R., Hinshaw, D. B., and Stafford, C. E. Acute inferior mesenteric vascular occlusion, a surgical syndrome. *Am. J. Surg.* 98:271, 1959.
23. Carter, R., Vannix, R., Hinshaw, D. B., and Stafford C. E. Inferior mesenteric vascular occlusion: Sigmoidoscopic diagnosis. *Surgery* 46:845, 1959.

24. Cole, F. H., Jr., and Richardson, R. L. Mesenteric thrombosis after penetrating cardiac trauma. *South. Med. J.* 69:1517, 1976.

25. Connolly, J. E., Abrams, H. L., and Kieraldo, J. H. Observations on obliterative disease of the visceral branches of the abdominal aorta. *Arch. Surg.* 90:596, 1965.

26. Connolly, J. E., and Kwaan, J. H. M. Prophylactic revascularization of the gut. *Ann. Surg.* 190:514, 1979.

27. Crawford, E. S., Morris, G. C., Jr., Myhre, H. O., and Roehm, J. O. F., Jr. Celiac axis, superior mesenteric artery, and inferior mesenteric artery occlusion: Surgical considerations. *Surgery* 82:856, 1977.

28. Cutler, D., Hernandex, B., Quintero, R., and Meza, E. Ten years' experience with artery thrombosis. *Am. J. Proctol.* 27:43, 1976.

29. Danesh, S. Abdominal angina and mesenteric insufficiency. *Angiography* 30:281, 1979.

30. Demos, N. J., Bahuth, J. J., and Urnes, P. D. Comparative study of arteriosclerosis in the inferior and superior mesenteric arteries: With a case report of gangrene of the colon. *Ann. Surg.* 155:599, 1962.

31. Dick, A. P., Graff, R., Gregg, D. M., Peters, N., and Sarner, N. An arteriographic study of mesenteric arterial disease: I. Large vessel changes. *Gut* 8:206, 1967.

32. Drummond, H. The arterial supply of the rectum and pelvic colon. *Br. J. Surg.* 1:677, 1914.

33. Duke, L. J., Lamberth, W. C., Jr., and Wright, C. B. Inferior mesenteric artery aneurysm: Case report and discussion. *Surgery* 85:385, 1979.

34. Edwards, E. A., and LeMay, M. Occlusion patterns and collaterals in arteriosclerosis of the lower aorta and iliac arteries. *Surgery* 38:950, 1955.

35. Eidemiller, L. R., Nelson, J. C., and Porter, J. M. Surgical treatment of chronic visceral ischemia. *Am. J. Surg.* 138:264, 1979.

36. Ernst, C. B., Hagihara, P. F., Daugherty, M. E., and Griffen, W. O., Jr. Inferior mesenteric artery stump pressure: A reliable index for safe IMA ligation during abdominal aortic aneurysmectomy. *Ann. Surg.* 187:641, 1978.

37. Giacchino, J. L., Geis, W. P., Pickleman, J. R., Dado, D. V., Hadcock, W. E., and Freeark, R. J. Changing perspectives in massive lower intestinal hemorrhage. *Surgery* 86:368, 1979.

38. Goligher, J. C. The blood supply to the sigmoid colon and rectum. *Br. J. Surg.* 37:157, 1949.

39. Gore, R. M., Calenoff, L., and Rogers, L. F. Roentgenographic manifestations of ischemic colitis. *J.A.M.A.* 241:1171, 1979.

40. Goswami, A., Chandnani, P., and Bansal, N. Parasitic blood supply from the inferior mesenteric arteries to the hypernephromas. *J. Urol.* 117:367, 1977.

41. Graham, J. M., Mattox, K. L., Beall, A. C., Jr., and DeBakey, M. E. Injuries to the visceral arteries. *Surgery* 84:835, 1978.

42. Griffiths, J. D. Surgical anatomy of the blood supply of the distal colon. *Ann. R. Coll. Surg. Engl.* 19:214, 1956.

43. Hagihara, P. F., Ernst, C. B., and Griffin, W. O., Jr. Incidence of ischemic colitis following abdominal aortic reconstruction. *Surgery* 149:571, 1979.

44. Halpern, N. Selective inferior mesenteric arteriography. *Vasc. Dis.* 1:294, 1964.

45. Hansen, H. J. B., and Christoffersen, J. K. Occlusive mesenteric infarction: A retrospective study of 83 cases. *Acta Chir. Scand.* [Suppl.] 472:103, 1976.

46. Hansen, H. J. B., and Efsen, F. Occlusive disease of the mesenteric arteries: A clinical and radiological study. *Dan. Med. Bull.* 24:117, 1977.

47. Harrison, A. W., and Croal, A. E. Left colon ischemia following occlusion or ligation of the inferior mesenteric artery. *Can. J. Surg.* 5:293, 1962.

48. Hildebrand, H. D., and Zierler, R. E. Mesenteric vascular disease. *Am. J. Surg.* 139:188, 1980.

49. Johnsrude, I. S., and Jackson, D. C. The role of the radiologist in acute gastrointestinal bleeding. *Gastrointest. Radiol.* 3:357, 1978.

50. Kahn, P., and Abrams, H. L. Inferior mesenteric arterial patterns: An angiographic study. *Radiology* 82:429, 1964.

51. Klein, H. J., Alfidi, R. J., Meaney, T. J., and Poirier, V. C. Angiography in the diagnosis of chronic gastrointestinal bleeding. *Radiology* 98:83, 1971.

52. Lau, J., Mattox, K. L., and DeBakey, M. E. Mycotic aneurysm of the inferior mesenteric artery. *Am. J. Surg.* 138:443, 1979.

53. Lindström, B. L. The value of the collateral circulation from the inferior mesenteric artery in obliteration of the lower abdominal aorta. *Acta Chir. Scand.* 100:367, 1950.

54. Lunderquist, A., and Lunderquist, A. Angiography and ulcerative colitis. *AJR* 99:18, 1967.

55. McAfee, J. C. A survey of complications of abdominal aortography. *Radiology* 68:825, 1957.

56. McDowell, R. F. C., and Thompson, I. D. Inferior mesenteric artery occlusion following lumbar aortography. *Br. J. Radiol.* 32:344, 1959.

57. McGregor, D. H., Pierce, G. E., Thomas, J. H., and Tilzer, L. L. Obstructive lesions of distal mesenteric arteries. *Arch. Pathol. Lab. Med.* 104:79, 1980.

58. McKain, J., and Shumacker, H. B., Jr. Ischemia of the colon associated with abdominal aortic aneurysms and their treatment. *Arch. Surg.* 76:355, 1958.

59. Matz, E. M., and Kahn, P. C. Occlusion of the

celiac, superior mesenteric and inferior mesenteric arteries: Angiographic demonstration in an asymptomatic patient. *Vasc. Dis.* 5:130, 1968.

60. Mayo, C. Blood supply of the colon: Surgical considerations. *Surg. Clin. North Am.* 35:117, 1955.

61. Miller, W. H., Maioriello, J. J., and Stein, D. B., Jr. Mesenteric vascular occlusion in infancy and childhood: Review of literature and report of an additional case. *J. Pediatr.* 59:567, 1961.

62. Moore, J. D., Thompson, N. W., Appleman, H. D., and Foley, D. Arteriovenous malformation of the gastrointestinal tract. *Arch. Surg.* 111:381, 1976.

63. Morris, G. C., Jr., DeBakey, M. E., and Bernhard, V. Abdominal angina. *Surg. Clin. North Am.* 46:919, 1966.

64. Moskowitz, M., Zimmerman, H., and Felson, B. Meandering mesenteric artery of colon. *AJR* 92:1088, 1964.

65. Padhi, R. K. Fatal infarction of the descending colon after lumbar aortography. *Can. Med. Assoc. J.* 82:199, 1960.

66. Perdue, G. D., and Lowry, K. Arterial insufficiency to the colon following resection of abdominal aortic aneurysms. *Surg. Gynecol. Obstet.* 115:39, 1962.

67. Ratner, I. A., and Swenson, O. Mesenteric vascular occlusion in infancy and childhood. *N. Engl. J. Med.* 263:1122, 1960.

68. Rosenberg, I. Left-sided colonoscopy in the office: A practical procedure. *Dis. Colon Rectum* 22:396, 1979.

69. Sacks, R. P., Sheft, D. J., and Freeman, J. H. The demonstration of the mesenteric collateral circulation in young patients. *AJR* 102:401, 1968.

70. Schobinger, R. Personal communication, 1964.

71. Schobinger, R. Operative intestinal arteriography in the diagnosis of diverticulitis of the colon. *Acta Radiol.* (Stockh.) 5:28, 1959.

72. Schwartz, S., Boley, S. J., Robinson, K., Krieger, H., Schultz, L., and Allen, A. C. Roentgenoologic features of vascular disorders of intestines. *Radiol. Clin. North Am.* 2:71, 1964.

73. Selby, D. K., and Bergan, J. J. Colonic infarction due to inferior mesenteric artery occlusion. *Q. Bull. Northw. Univ. Med. Sch.* 34:244, 1960.

74. Shaff, M. E., and Becker, H. Diagnosis and control of diverticular bleeding by arteriography and vasopressin infusion. *S. Afr. Med. J.* 56:72, 1979.

75. Siegel, B., and Pajewski, M. Selective embolization of the inferior mesenteric artery in massive colonic bleeding. *Isr. J. Med. Sci.* 14:481, 1978.

76. Smith, R. F., and Szilagyi, D. E. Ischemia of the colon as a complication in surgery of the abdominal aorta. *Arch. Surg.* 80:806, 1960.

77. Steward, J. A., and Rankin, F. W. Blood supply of the intestine: Its surgical considerations. *Arch. Surg.* 26:843, 1933.

78. Stoney, R. J., and Wylie, E. J. Recognition and surgical management of visceral ischemic syndromes. *Ann. Surg.* 164:714, 1966.

79. Ström, B. G., and Winberg, T. Percutaneous selective arteriography of the inferior mesenteric artery. *Acta Radiol.* (Stockh.) 57:401, 1962.

80. Sumner, D. S. Successful revascularization of mesenteric infarction following aortography. *Ann. Surg.* 43:743, 1977.

81. Sunderland, S. Blood supply of the distal colon. *Aust. N.Z. J. Surg.* 11:253, 1942.

82. Tarin, D., Allison, D. J., Modlin, I. M., and Neale, G. Diagnosis and management of obscure gastrointestinal bleeding. *Br. Med. J.* 2:751, 1978.

83. Tisnado, J., Amendola, M. A., and Beachley, M. C. Renal artery originating from the inferior mesenteric artery. *Br. J. Radiol.* 52:752, 1979.

84. Todd, G. J., and Forde, K. A. Lower gastrointestinal bleeding with negative or inconclusive radiographic studies: The role of colonoscopy. *Am. J. Surg.* 138:627, 1979.

85. Todd, M. C. Selective mesenteric angiography and colon bleeding. *Int. Surg.* 63:35, 1978.

86. Trotter, L. B. C. *Embolism and Thrombosis of the Mesenteric Vessels.* London: Cambridge University Press, 1913.

87. Tsuchiya, M., Miura, S., Asakura, H., Hibi, T., Tanaka, T., Aiso, S., and Hiramatsu, K. Angiographic evaluation of vascular changes in ulcerative colitis. *Angiology* 31:147, 1980.

88. Von Haller, A. Cited by Steward and Rankin [77].

89. Walker, W. J., Goldin, A. R., Shaff, M. I., and Allibone, G. W. Per catheter control of haemorrhage from the superior and inferior mesenteric arteries. *Clin. Radiol.* 31:71, 1980.

90. Wang, C. C., and Reeves, J. D. Mesenteric vascular disease. *AJR* 83:895, 1960.

91. Webb, W. R., and Hardy, J. D. Relief of abdominal angina by vascular graft. *Ann. Intern. Med.* 57:289, 1962.

92. Wholey, N. H., Bron, K. M., and Haller, J. B. Selective angiography of the colon. *Surg. Clin. North Am.* 45:1283, 1965.

Mesenteric Ischemia

SCOTT J. BOLEY
LAWRENCE J. BRANDT
SEYMOUR SPRAYREGEN

During the past two decades ischemic disorders of the intestine have been diagnosed with increasing frequency. In part this is due to a real increase in their incidence; more importantly, it is the result of the belated recognition of the many clinical manifestations that have as their common etiology interference with intestinal blood flow.

Although chronic intestinal ischemia was the subject of many articles in the 1960s, it has become evident that relatively few patients suffer from this problem. Far more common are episodes of acute mesenteric ischemia with either immediate or delayed effects of the circulatory insult. Angiography plays a major role in both the diagnosis and the management of mesenteric ischemia, especially in its acute forms.

Pathophysiologic Changes Accompanying Intestinal Ischemia

Reduction in blood flow to the intestine may be a reflection of generalized poor perfusion, as in shock or with a failing heart, or it may result from either local morphologic or functional changes. Narrowings of the major mesenteric vessels, focal atheromatous emboli, vasculitis as part of a systemic disease, and mesenteric vasoconstriction can all lead to inadequate circulation. However, whatever the cause, intestinal ischemia has the same end results—a spectrum ranging from completely reversible functional alterations to total hemorrhagic necrosis of portions of the bowel or all of it.

The intestines are protected from ischemia to a great extent by their abundant collateral circulation, which has been discussed in detail in Chapter 69, Superior Mesenteric Angiography.

Communications between the celiac and the superior and inferior mesenteric beds are numerous, and a general rule that has proved valid is that in gradual occlusion at least two of these vessels must be compromised to produce symptomatic intestinal ischemia. Moreover, occlusion of two of the three vessels occurs frequently without evidence of ischemia, and total occlusion of all three vessels in asymptomatic patients has been observed.

Collateral pathways around occlusions of smaller arterial branches in the mesentery are provided by the primary, secondary, and tertiary arcades in the small bowel and the marginal arterial complex of Drummond in the colon. Within the bowel wall itself, there is a network of communicating submucosal vessels that can maintain the viability of short segments of the intestine where the extramural arterial supply has been lost.

When a major vessel is occluded, collateral pathways open immediately in response to the fall in arterial pressure distal to the obstruction. Increased blood flow through this collateral circulation continues as long as the pressure in the vascular bed distal to the obstruction remains below the systemic pressure. If vasoconstriction develops in the distal bed, the arterial pressure there rises and causes diminution of collateral flow. If normal blood flow is reestablished, the flow through collateral channels ceases.

In the resting state, the splanchnic circulation receives 28 percent of the cardiac output. This may increase modestly after eating or may decrease during exercise, but major changes are usually related to increased sympathetic activity. Vasomotor control of the mesenteric circulation is mediated primarily through the sympathetic nervous system. Although beta-adrenergic receptors are present in the splanchnic vascular bed, alpha-adrenergic receptors predominate, and increased sympathetic activity produces vasoconstriction, which increases resistance and decreases blood flow. Folkow et al. [17] have shown that vasoconstriction induced by sympathetic nervous stimulation can virtually stop blood flow for brief intervals. Although vasoconstriction occurs in both the arterioles and venules, the increase in precapillary resistance is relatively greater than the increase in postcapillary resistance, and thus hydrostatic pressure within the capillary bed falls during prolonged vasoconstriction. This decrease in capillary pressure usually results in loss of plasma volume into the mesenteric bed.

In vascular disorders of the intestines, there is a frequently changing interrelationship between blood flow, the mesenteric vessels, and intestinal cellular viability. Mesenteric vasoconstriction may be present and cause a reduction in blood flow but not produce a fall to inadequate levels (ischemia). Similarly the lumen of a short segment of the superior mesenteric artery (SMA) may be reduced by 80 percent with no diminution in blood flow. Moreover, intestinal ischemia can be present without intestinal necrosis, and intestinal necrosis may be present with normal blood flow if blood flow is determined after a transient episode of ischemia has been relieved.

Intestinal ischemia may result from a reduction in blood flow, from redistribution of blood flow, or from a combination of both. With hypotension, there is decreased splanchnic blood flow due to vasoconstriction and also arteriovenous shunting within the bowel wall [10]. A similar situation occurs with intestinal distention [4]. In both the small and the large bowels, after an intraluminal pressure of 30 mm Hg is reached, further stepwise increases in pressure result in parallel decreases in intestinal blood flow. However, 20 to 35 percent of control blood flow remains even at a pressure of 210 mm Hg. Bowel injected with silicone rubber during distention and cleared to permit visualization of blood vessels reveals almost complete shunting away from the mucosa and muscularis propria, with filling of only the submucosal and serosal arteries. Thus, the remaining blood flow is redistributed away from the oxygen-consuming components of the intestine. This redistribution is reflected in a decreasing arteriovenous oxygen difference that parallels this fall in blood flow. The highly oxygenated blood flowing through the serosal arteries and veins results in a normal pink external appearance of the bowel, even when the total blood flow is only 20 percent of control. This phenomenon explains the frequent clinical observation of bowel that appears normal externally but in which there is pronounced hemorrhagic infarction of the mucosa.

The effects of intermittent distention on both a distended segment of small bowel and the rest of the small intestine are profound [35]. Intermittent increases in intraluminal pressure significantly reduce blood flow not only to the distended segment but also to the entire small bowel, and this diminution in flow persists for hours after relief of the distention.

Episodes of mesenteric ischemia may have delayed or protracted effects. Clinically, these effects are demonstrated by the occurrence of nonocclusive intestinal ischemia hours to days after the cardiovascular problem has been alleviated and by the well-documented progression of bowel infarction after an arterial occlusion has been corrected. In extensive animal experiments, *persistent mesenteric vasoconstriction* has been shown to be one explanation for these phenomena [6, 9, 16].

These investigations showed that when the SMA blood flow is decreased 50 percent with a hydraulic occluder, the mesenteric arterial pressure in the peripheral bed immediately falls proportionately, and blood flow through the sources of collateral blood supply (i.e., the celiac and the inferior mesenteric arteries) rises. However, a decreased SMA flow of several hours' duration results in mesenteric vasoconstriction, the pressure in the mesenteric bed rises to the level of the systemic arterial pressure, and blood flow through the arteries supplying collateral flow returns to normal. Initially, the mesenteric vasoconstriction is reversible with release of the SMA occlusion, but after it has been present for several hours the vasoconstriction persists even after the occlusion is removed. Thus, a low SMA flow initially produces mesenteric vascular responses that tend to maintain adequate intestinal blood flow, but if the diminished flow is prolonged, active vasoconstriction develops and may persist even after the primary cause of mesenteric ischemia is corrected.

Further studies showed that this persistent mesenteric vasoconstriction can be reversed by the selective injection of papaverine, a vasodilator, into the SMA. Such papaverine injections, therefore, could interrupt the vicious cycle that might result in persistent mesenteric ischemia following a transient fall in cardiac output or other temporary local or systemic causes of decreased mesenteric blood flow. This active and often persistent vasoconstriction can be identified angiographically and is the basis for the diagnosis of nonocclusive mesenteric ischemia [1, 2, 33].

Acute Mesenteric Ischemia

ANGIOGRAPHY

Emergency angiography is the keystone of our approach to acute mesenteric ischemia (AMI) [8]. Emboli, thromboses, and mesenteric vasoconstriction can be diagnosed and the adequacy of the splanchnic circulation evaluated. The angiographic catheter also provides a route for the intraarterial administration of vasodilators.

The angiographic technique used for diagnosing AMI is similar to that used for routine SMA arteriography, with the exception of the volume of contrast material employed. Since the initial angiographic examination and follow-up studies include multiple injections, and because most of the patients already have reduced renal blood flow, one-half the usual volume of contrast material is used in all selective studies to reduce renal damage. An initial flush aortogram with biplane filming is obtained to evaluate the aorta and the origin of the major aortic branches. The aorto-

gram is important since renal or splenic arterial emboli can also appear with abdominal pain of sudden onset. Such pain may reflect renal or splenic infarction or intestinal ischemia due to reflex mesenteric vasoconstriction (Fig. 72-1). Aortography is also used to evaluate the collateral circulation between the superior mesenteric, celiac, and inferior mesenteric arteries. Because mesenteric vasoconstriction may accompany hypotension, angiography is performed only in patients who are normotensive. A selective SMA angiogram is performed to identify emboli, thromboses, or mesenteric vasoconstriction and to assess the perfusion of the vascular bed distal to any obstruction. If an occlusion or a vasoconstriction is found, the angiogram is repeated after a single bolus of 25 mg of tolazoline is administered into the SMA catheter. This bolus of vasodilator permits better visualization of the peripheral circulation and indicates the potential effectiveness of a papaverine infusion. The response to tolazoline does not affect the decision to use a papaverine infusion in patients with nonocclusive mesenteric ischemia, but it may indicate the possibility of employing nonoperative therapy for patients with embolic obstructions. Previously, papaverine (60 mg) was used as the bolus, but tolazoline has been substituted because of its more rapid effect. Tolazoline is not used for continuous infusions because it is neither as effective nor as safe as papaverine by this method of administration.

In two of our patients with nonocclusive ischemia, the abdominal pain and marked peritoneal signs resulting from mesenteric vasoconstriction disappeared within 20 minutes after the tolazoline injection. The relief of pain and physical signs led to cancellation of scheduled laparotomies, and both patients survived without operation.

NONOCCLUSIVE MESENTERIC ISCHEMIA

Since Ende first described nonocclusive mesenteric ischemia in 1978 [15], the proportion of mesenteric vascular accidents resulting from this entity has risen from 12 percent [23] to over 50 percent in our series and other recently reported series [7, 27]. The pathogenesis of this entity is presently believed to be splanchnic vasoconstriction occurring in response to a decrease in cardiac output, hypovolemia, dehydration, vasopressor agents, or hypotension. This vasoconstriction may persist even after the initiating cause has

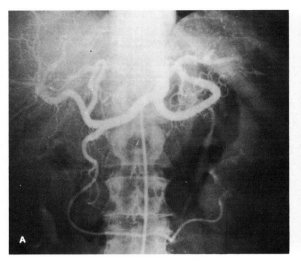
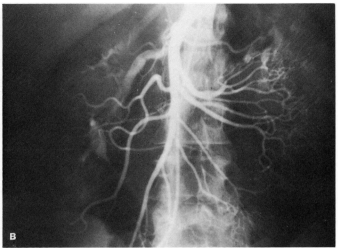
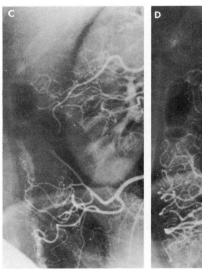
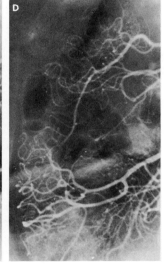

Figure 72-1. (A) Celiac angiogram from a 51-year-old woman with rheumatic heart disease, atrial fibrillation, and right lower quadrant pain of sudden onset. The embolus in the distal splenic artery was suspected on the flush aortogram. (B) Initial selective superior mesenteric arteriogram from the same patient, midarterial phase. The jejunal and ileal arcades are filled, but there is no filling of the arcades of the right colon. (C) Repeat angiogram after a bolus injection of papaverine shows a marked improvement in the circulation to the right colon. (D) Repeat angiogram after papaverine infusion for 20 hours shows excellent circulation with good visualization of the arcades and the intramural vessels. By this time, the abdominal pain had disappeared. (From Siegelman et al. [33]. Reproduced with permission from *Radiology.*)

been corrected. Predisposing conditions include myocardial infarction, congestive heart failure, aortic insufficiency, renal and hepatic disease, and major abdominal or cardiac operations. In addition, a more immediate precipitating cause, such as pulmonary edema, cardiac arrhythmia, or shock, is usually present, although the intestinal ischemic episode may not become manifest until hours to days later.

Treatment of nonocclusive mesenteric ischemia has been ineffective in reducing its 90 percent mortality. The patients are generally elderly and extremely ill, and in the majority of cases the underlying cause of the inadequate blood flow is not amenable to surgical correction. Since many of the patients are in coronary or intensive care units, there has been an understand-

able reluctance in the past to subject such patients to aggressive invasive diagnostic studies and therapy. However, despite their critical condition, a significant number of these patients survive the major cardiac insult only to succumb to intestinal infarction.

Angiographically, nonocclusive mesenteric ischemia is diagnosed when the signs of mesenteric vasoconstriction are seen in a patient who has a clinical picture suggestive of intestinal ischemia but who is neither in shock nor receiving vasopressors. Reliable angiographic criteria for the diagnosis of mesenteric vasoconstriction include: (1) narrowings at the origins of multiple branches of the SMA, (2) irregularities in intestinal branches, (3) spasms of arcades, and (4) impaired filling of intramural vessels [1, 2, 33]. The

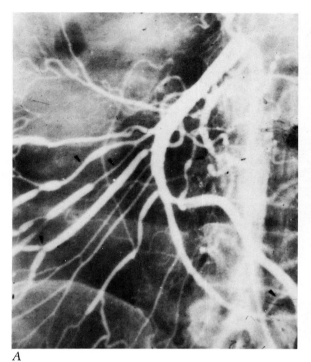

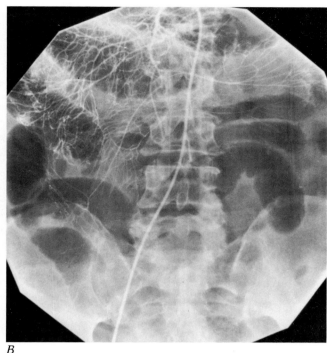

A   B

Figure 72-2. Angiographic appearance of mesenteric vasoconstriction. (A) Spasm at the origins of the major superior mesenteric artery (SMA) branches and multiple areas of intermittent spasm (*arrowheads*) and di-

latation ("string of sausages"). (Courtesy of S. S. Siegelman, M.D.) (B) Typical appearance of marked constriction of the entire SMA and its major branches.

angiographic findings may vary from localized spasm to a "pruned" appearance of the entire mesenteric tree (Fig. 72-2). Mesenteric vasoconstriction does occur with other conditions, such as hemorrhage (Fig. 72-3) and pancreatitis, but when it is present in patients without these disorders in whom intestinal ischemia is suspected, it is strong evidence of nonocclusive mesenteric ischemia. Thus, if angiography is performed sufficiently early in the course of their illnesses, patients with AMI of a nonocclusive origin, as well as patients with surgically correctable lesions, can be identified before bowel infarction occurs.

SUPERIOR MESENTERIC ARTERY EMBOLUS

Today, superior mesenteric artery emboli (SMAE) are responsible for 40 to 50 percent of episodes of acute mesenteric ischemia; they usually originate from a mural or an atrial thrombus [5, 26]. In the past, such thrombi were most commonly associated with rheumatic valvular disease, but in a review of our recent experience

with 47 patients with SMAE, arteriosclerotic heart disease was the cause in all but one case [5]. Many patients have a previous history of peripheral arterial embolism, and 20 percent or more have synchronous emboli in other arteries.

In a normal angiographic study, the major branches of the SMA, the intestinal arcades, the intramural arteries, and the mesenteric veins are all visualized. Emboli typically appear as sharp, rounded defects, but the duration of symptoms can influence this angiographic appearance. When angiography is performed immediately after the onset of abdominal pain, the emboli are apt to be sharply defined (Figs. 72-4A, 72-5B), but if the study is delayed for several days, secondary thrombus may build up proximally and distally and obscure the typical configuration (Figs. 72-4B, 72-5A). The artery may be completely occluded (Fig. 72-4A, B), but more often the embolus only partially obstructs blood flow (Fig. 72-4C). Mild-to-marked vasoconstriction is often present in arteries both proximal and distal to the embolus [1, 2]. The degree of vasoconstriction affects the retrograde filling of the SMA and its branches distal to the embolus,

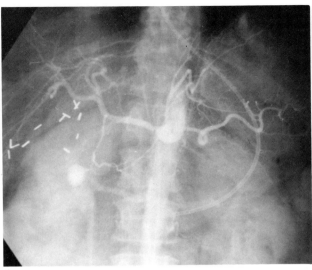

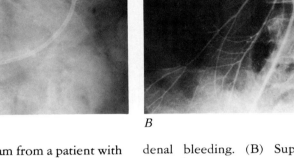

A

B

Figure 72-3. (A) Celiac angiogram from a patient with upper gastrointestinal tract bleeding and hypertension. Extravasation of contrast material from a branch of the gastroduodenal artery indicates the site of the duo- denal bleeding. (B) Superior mesenteric arterio- gram from the same patient showing mesenteric vasoconstriction in response to the hypotension.

which, together with the adequacy of the perfusion of the intestinal mural branches, should be evaluated before and after the injection of the tolazoline bolus.

Arterial emboli tend to lodge at points of normal anatomic narrowings, usually just distal to the origin of a major branch. In our series, the most frequent sites were just above the origin of the inferior pancreaticoduodenal artery, occluding all the main branches of the SMA, at or just above the origin of the middle colic artery, and just above or including the origin of the ileocolic artery. Approximately 10 percent of patients had more peripheral emboli, and in two patients the emboli were multiple (Fig. 72-5C).

ACUTE SUPERIOR MESENTERIC ARTERY THROMBOSIS

The incidence of acute superior mesenteric artery thrombosis (SMAT) varies in different reports. For example, Ottinger [27] and Jackson [23] found thromboses to be almost as common as emboli, whereas we found emboli to be three to four times more frequent. SMAT almost always is superimposed on severe atherosclerotic narrowing, most commonly in the region of the origin of the main artery. Since the acute episode represents the end stage of a chronic problem, it is not surprising that 30 to 50 percent of patients have had abdominal pain during the preceding weeks or months. Most patients have severe diffuse arteriosclerosis, and a prior history of coronary, cerebral, or peripheral arterial ischemia is frequent.

Identification of SMAT is usually made from the flush aortogram, which most often shows total occlusion of the SMA within 1 to 2 cm of its origin. Some filling of the artery distal to the obstruction is almost always present because of collateral circulation. Branches both proximal and distal to the occlusion may show local spasm or diffuse constriction. Angiographic differentiation between a thrombosis and an old embolus may be difficult; in such instances, the patients are treated initially as if they had emboli. A more difficult problem arises when a total occlusion of the SMA is demonstrated by angiography in a patient with abdominal pain but no abdominal findings. In such an instance, it is important to be able to differentiate an acute occlusion from a long-standing one since the long-standing one may be coincidental to the present illness. The presence or absence of prominent collateral vessels between the superior mesenteric and the celiac and/or the inferior mesenteric circulation is the decisive factor. If large collateral vessels are demonstrated on the angiogram, a chronic occlusion is presumed, and, in the absence of any peritoneal signs, the patient is treated expectantly (Fig. 72-6A). The absence of collateral vessels indicates an acute occlusion, and prompt interven-

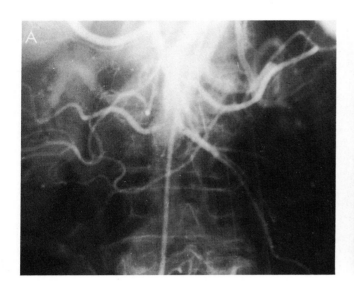
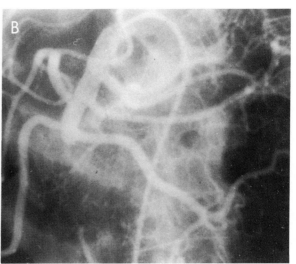
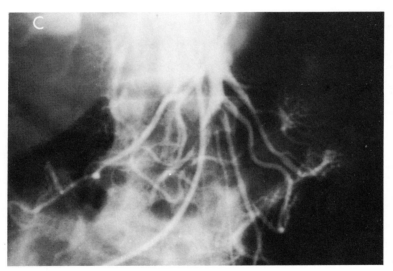

Figure 72-4. Angiographic appearance of superior mesenteric artery emboli. (A) Recent embolus lodged at the level of origin of the middle colic artery shows a well-defined round contour and a complete occlusion of the main artery. (B) Older embolus just below the origin of the right colic artery shows a complete obstruction, but the sharp contour seen in (A) is absent. (C) Recent embolus at the level of the ileocolic artery and extending into it. Well-defined round edges can be seen at the top and bottom of the embolus. The artery is only partially obstructed. (Reproduced with permission from S. J. Boley, L. J. Brandt, and F. J. Veith, Ischemic disorders of the intestines. In M. M. Ravitch et al. (eds.), *Curr. Probl. Surg.* 15:1, 1978. Courtesy of Year Book Medical Publishers, Inc., Chicago.)

tion is indicated whether or not peritoneal signs are present (Fig. 72-6B).

ACUTE MESENTERIC VENOUS THROMBOSIS

Acute mesenteric venous thrombosis, cited as the most frequent cause of intestinal infarction 50 years ago [11], is responsible for only a few cases today. Much of this decline is due to the fact that in the past, infarction in the absence of arterial occlusion was interpreted as being the result of venous thrombosis, whereas today nonocclusive mesenteric ischemia is recognized as the cause in most instances.

Mesenteric venous thrombosis can be primary (agnogenic) or secondary to a variety of conditions, including hematologic disorders, hypercoagulable states, intraabdominal sepsis, local venous stasis, and abdominal trauma. Recently

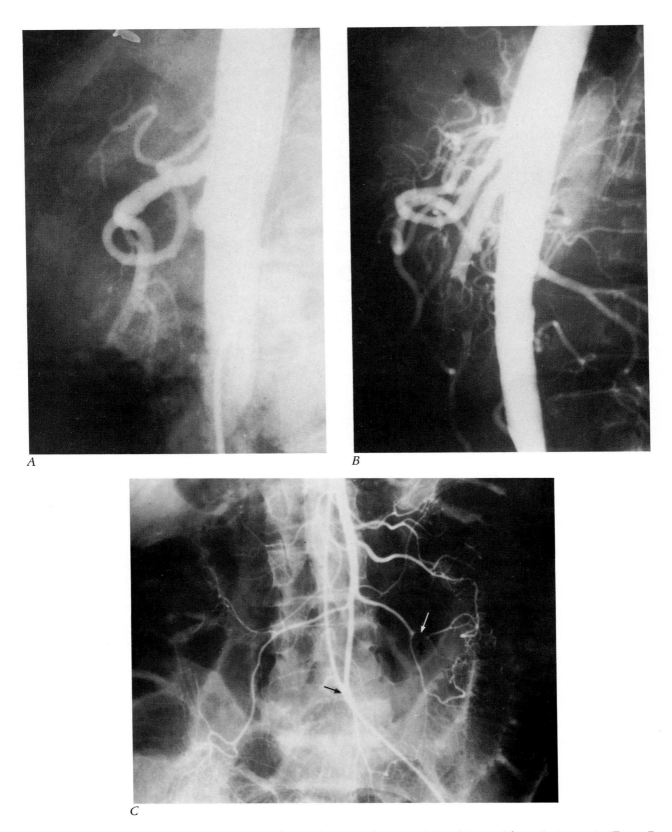

Figure 72-5. Angiographic appearance of superior mesenteric emboli. (A) Totally occluding embolus just distal to the origin of the SMA. (B) Embolus more distal in the main SMA with a well-defined round contour. (C) Multiple emboli to the ileocolic artery and the peripheral jejunal branch (*arrows*). (From R. Kieny and J. Cinqualbre, *Les Ischemies Intestinales Signes*. Paris: Expansion Scientifique Française, 1979. By permission of the authors and publishers.)

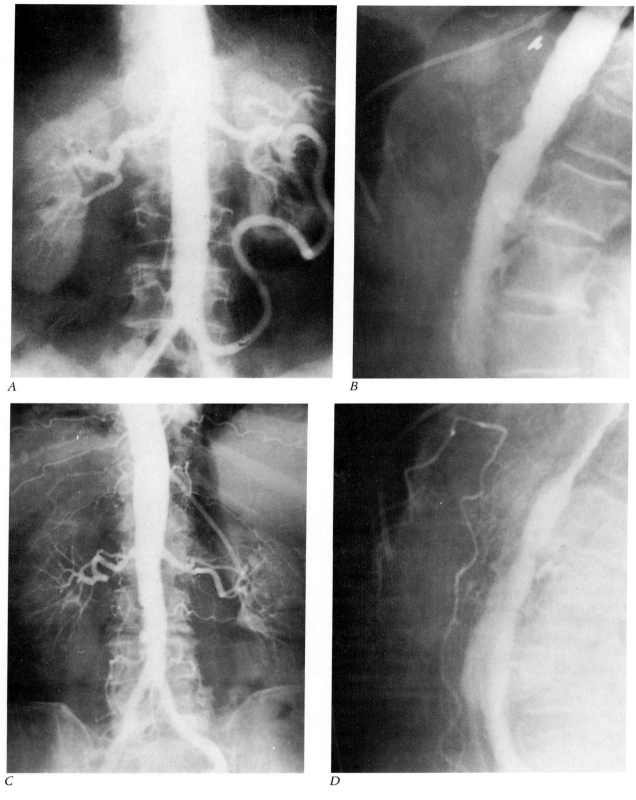

A

B

C

D

Figure 72-6. (A) Angiogram from a patient with a superior mesenteric artery occlusion. The prominent "meandering artery" shows that collateral channels have been present for some time and that the occlusion is not acute. (Reproduced with permission from S. J. Boley, L. J. Brandt, and F. J. Veith, Ischemic disorders of the intestines. In M. M. Ravitch et al. (eds.), *Curr. Probl. Surg.* 15:1, 1978. Courtesy of Year Book Medical Publishers, Inc., Chicago.) (B) Flush aortogram (lateral view) from another patient showing an occlusion of both celiac and superior mesenteric arteries. (C) Anteroposterior view shows no apparent prominent collateral vessels. (D) Late phase lateral view shows a small-caliber "meandering artery." The absence of large collateral vessels indicates an acute rather than a chronic occlusion.

1739

there have been a spate of reports of minor and major mesenteric venous thromboses in patients taking oral contraceptives. Angiographic studies in patients with mesenteric venous thrombosis may be normal, especially if only segmental veins are involved. While the angiographic diagnosis of mesenteric venous thrombosis has not been made in the clinical setting, based on experimental studies [28] the angiographic findings may include (1) spasm of the SMA and its major branches, (2) prolongation of the arterial phase, (3) intense opacification of the bowel wall, and (4) failure to opacify the mesenteric and portal veins.

PLAN FOR DIAGNOSIS AND THERAPY

All patients suspected of having AMI are promptly treated for associated cardiovascular problems and are sent for plain radiographic studies of the abdomen. Subsequent abdominal angiography is routinely performed unless some other intraabdominal condition is diagnosed on the plain film examination. Based on the angiographic findings and the presence or absence of signs of peritoneal irritation on physical examination, the individual patient is then treated according to the proposed plan of Figure 72-7.

Selection of Patients

AMI is most likely to develop in patients over 50 years of age with (1) valvular or arteriosclerotic heart disease; (2) long-standing congestive heart failure, especially with unsatisfactory control of digitalis therapy or prolonged use of diuretics; (3) cardiac arrhythmias of any cause; (4) hypovolemia or hypotension of any origin, such as burns, pancreatitis, or gastrointestinal or postoperative hemorrhage; or (5) recent myocardial infarctions.

Patients in any of these high-risk categories who have abdominal pain that started suddenly and has lasted more than 2 or 3 hours are started on the management protocol. Less absolute indications for an aggressive investigation are unexplained abdominal distention or gastrointestinal bleeding. These broad selection criteria are essential if early diagnosis and treatment are to be achieved, because the presence of more extensive and specific signs and symptoms usually signifies irreversible intestinal damage.

Even when the decision to operate has been made, an angiogram must be obtained to manage the patient properly at operation. Moreover, the relief of mesenteric vasoconstriction is an integral part of the therapy for emboli and thromboses, as well as for low-flow states, and can best be achieved by intraarterial infusion of papaverine through the angiography catheter.

Initial Preparation and Resuscitation

The initial treatment is directed toward correcting the predisposing or precipitating causes of the mesenteric ischemia. Relief of acute congestive heart failure, correction of cardiac arrhythmias, and replacement of blood volume precede any diagnostic studies. In general, efforts at increasing intestinal blood flow will be futile if low cardiac output, hypotension, or hypovolemia persists. On rare occasions, we have combined dopamine administered intravenously into a peripheral vein with papaverine administered intraarterially into the SMA, and we have been able to improve both systemic and mesenteric blood flow. Patients in shock should not undergo angiography, because mesenteric vasoconstriction will always be evident, even without intestinal ischemia. Such patients should not receive papaverine intraarterially since it will increase the size of the vascular bed and aggravate the hypovolemia (Fig. 72-8). The management of congestive heart failure or shock that is complicated by mesenteric ischemia is especially difficult, because the use of digitalis or vasopressors may further aggravate the diminished intestinal blood flow. Digitalis preparations all have a direct vasoconstrictor action on SMA smooth muscle, especially with the blood levels observed during rapid digitalization or with digitalis intoxication. The decision to discontinue digitalis is often a difficult one to make because the drug may be required to control rapid ventricular rates associated with atrial fibrillation or to manage severe congestive heart failure. Vasopressors are contraindicated in the treatment of shock if mesenteric ischemia is suspected.

When intestinal ischemia has progressed to the extent that systemic alterations associated with bowel infarction are present, appropriate correction of plasma volume deficits and fluid loss, gastrointestinal decompression, and parenteral antibiotics are included in the preparation prior to roentgenologic studies.

After the initial corrective and supportive measures have been completed, roentgenographic studies are undertaken irrespective of the abdominal physical findings or the surgeon's decision whether or not to operate.

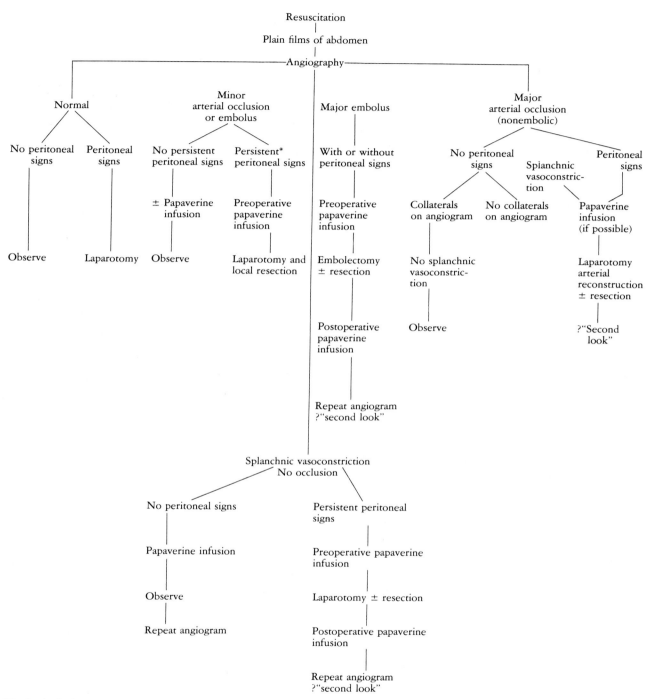

*Peritoneal signs are considered persistent if they are not relieved within 30 minutes following the bolus injection of tolazoline.

Figure 72-7. Proposed plan for the diagnosis and treatment of acute mesenteric ischemia.

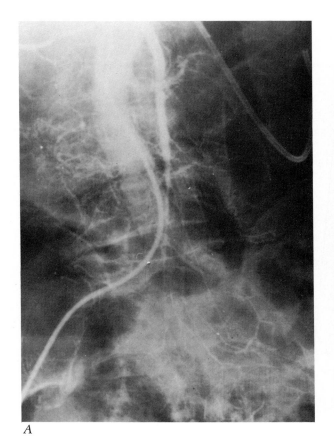

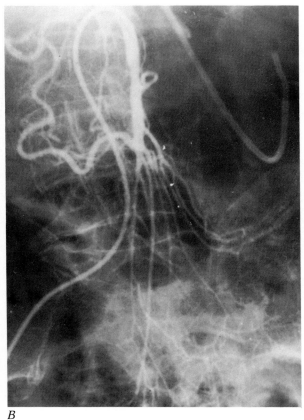

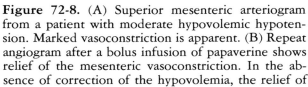

A

B

Figure 72-8. (A) Superior mesenteric arteriogram from a patient with moderate hypovolemic hypotension. Marked vasoconstriction is apparent. (B) Repeat angiogram after a bolus infusion of papaverine shows relief of the mesenteric vasoconstriction. In the absence of correction of the hypovolemia, the relief of the vasoconstriction was accompanied by a further fall in blood pressure. This sequence of events emphasizes the importance of adequate resuscitation before angiography is performed for suspected mesenteric ischemia.

Plain Film Studies

The initial examination includes a chest roentgenogram and roentgenograms of the abdomen with the patient in the supine, erect, and both lateral decubitus positions. Signs of intestinal ischemia on plain film studies occur late and usually indicate bowel infarction. In series of cases in which a significant portion of the patients have had such signs, the mortality has been dismaying [18, 22, 34].

A normal plain film of the abdomen does not exclude AMI, and, ideally, all patients should be studied before roentgenographic signs of ischemia develop. Thus, *the primary purpose of these plain film studies is not to help in the diagnosis of AMI, but to exclude other radiographically diagnosable causes of abdominal pain* (e.g., a perforated viscus or an intestinal obstruction). If no other acute abdominal condition is detected, angiography is performed.

Therapeutic Papaverine Infusion

When the therapeutic regimen includes the use of papaverine, the drug is infused through the angiography catheter, which is left in the SMA. To prevent dislodgment, the catheter is sutured to the skin at its point of entry in the thigh. The papaverine is administered at a constant rate of 30 to 60 mg per hour using an infusion pump. The drug is usually diluted in saline to a concentration of 1 mg per cc, but the concentration may vary according to the patient's fluid limitations or requirements. Continuous monitoring of systemic arterial pressure and cardiac rate and rhythm is indicated because these amounts of papaverine theoretically could have systemic effects. We have not observed such problems in either our experimental or clinical studies, probably because the drug is metabolized in the liver before it reaches the general circulation. Infusion at these rates has been used clinically for as long as 5 days without untoward systemic changes.

Heparin is not added to the infusion, because it is not compatible with papaverine hydrochloride and we have not found it necessary to prevent thrombus formation within the SMA. No other medications or fluids should be administered through the arterial catheter, and the patient must be observed carefully for evidence of dislodgment of the catheter.

The duration of the papaverine infusion varies with both the purpose for its use and the response of the patient. In conjunction with the embolectomy or arterial reconstruction, the infusion is continued for 12 to 24 hours if a "second-look" operation is not planned. After 12 to 24 hours, the angiogram is repeated, and, unless some specific indication for more prolonged vasodilator therapy is demonstrated, the infusion is discontinued. When a second-look operation is to be performed, the papaverine is continued until the abdomen is reopened, but a repeat angiogram is obtained prior to operation. The need for an additional period of infusion is determined intraoperatively, depending on the state of the bowel and the results of the preoperative angiogram.

When papaverine infusion is used as the primary treatment for nonocclusive mesenteric ischemia, it is continued for approximately 24 hours. Then the infusion is changed to isotonic saline without papaverine, and, 30 minutes after the change, a repeat angiogram is performed. Based on the clinical course of the patient (i.e., abdominal distention, bowel functioning, abdominal findings, and evidence of blood in the stools) and the response of the vasoconstriction to therapy as indicated by the angiogram, the infusion is discontinued or maintained for another 24 hours; the patient's condition is then reevaluated (Figs. 72-9, 72-10). Infusions have been continued for up to 5 days, but usually they can be stopped after 24 hours. When papaverine is used in conjunction with laparotomy for nonocclusive disease, a second-look operation is frequently necessary. In such cases, the infusion is continued as described previously for second-look operations following embolectomy. The papaverine infusion is discontinued when no signs of vasoconstriction are present on an an-

giogram that is obtained 30 minutes after the vasodilator infusion is temporarily replaced by saline alone. The SMA catheter is removed promptly when the intraarterial infusion is stopped.

Supportive Therapy

An essential aspect of the supportive therapy of patients with AMI is the maintenance of an adequate plasma volume. Just as massive losses of protein-rich fluids occur with early bowel infarction, so they may occur following revascularization of ischemic bowel. Hence it is important to correct continually for losses before undertaking treatment during papaverine infusions and following surgical relief of arterial occlusions. The use of low-molecular-weight dextran may serve a dual purpose because of its effect as a plasma expander and because of its potential value in decreasing sludging in the microcirculation.

The value of both systemic and locally administered antibiotics in improving the viability of compromised bowel is well accepted. For this reason, and because of the high incidence of positive blood cultures with AMI, systemic antibiotics are started as soon as the diagnosis is established.

Intestinal decompression by nasogastric suction, the use of furosemide and mannitol to maintain urinary output, and specific therapy for the cardiac problems all play a role in the management of most patients. Digitalis, as previously mentioned, must be used cautiously, and vasopressors should be avoided. Anticoagulant therapy during and immediately after operation is specifically avoided (except in venous thrombosis) because of the danger of intestinal hemorrhage. Early in our experience we had two patients who bled massively as a result of heparin therapy after successful embolectomy. Anticoagulant therapy is begun after 48 hours when a revascularization operation has been performed.

PROGNOSIS

The outlook for patients with AMI is improving. Although mortalities of 70 to 90 percent have been reported through 1979 with the use of traditional methods of diagnosis and therapy, the aggressive approach just described can reduce these catastrophic figures [7]. Of the first 50 patients managed by this approach, 35 (70%) proved to have AMI. Thirty-three had angio-

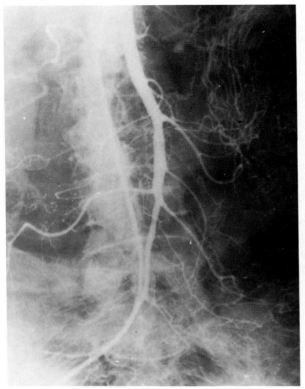
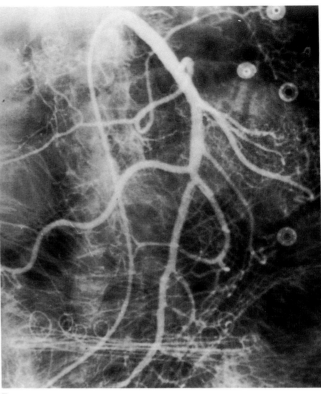

A   B

Figure 72-9. Patient with nonocclusive mesenteric is-chemia managed with papaverine infusion for 3 days. (A) Initial angiogram showing a spasm of the main superior mesenteric artery, origins of branches, and intestinal arcades. (B) Angiogram after 36 hours of papaverine infusion. The study was obtained 30 minutes after papaverine was replaced with saline. At this time, the patient's abdominal symptoms and signs were gone. (Reproduced with permission from S. J. Boley, L. J. Brandt, and F. J. Veith, Ischemic disorders of the intestines. In M. M. Ravitch et al. (eds.), *Curr. Probl. Surg.* 15:1, 1978. Courtesy of Year Book Medical Publishers, Inc., Chicago.)

---

graphic signs of nonocclusive or occlusive is-chemia. The other two patients had normal angiograms. Fifteen patients (30%) did not have mesenteric ischemia, but in 8 of these 15 the correct diagnosis was made from the angiographic study. Nineteen (54%) of the 35 patients with AMI survived, including 9 of 15 patients with nonocclusive mesenteric ischemia, 7 of 16 with SMA embolus, 2 of 3 patients with SMA thrombosis, and 1 patient with mesenteric venous thrombosis. Seventeen of the 19 survivors lost no bowel or had excision of less than 3 feet of small intestine [7].

Of special interest were the three patients with emboli managed initially with papaverine infusions for 24, 36, and 54 hours, respectively. Two were subsequently operated on, and the bowel was found to be normal. The third survived without operation. Future studies may justify wider use of this nonoperative management of SMA emboli.

The complications of the angiographic studies and prolonged infusions of vasodilator drugs have not been excessive. Of the first 50 patients, 3 developed transient acute tubular necrosis following angiography and treatment of their mesenteric ischemia. One patient developed arterial occlusions in both lower extremities during a papaverine infusion for an SMA embolus. These probably represented other emboli from the patient's primary source of embolization, but the SMA catheter could not be excluded as a factor. There were several instances of local hematomas at the arterial puncture site, but no other major problems were encountered with blood flow to the lower extremities.

Problems with prolonged papaverine infusions have been minimal. Infusions for more than 5

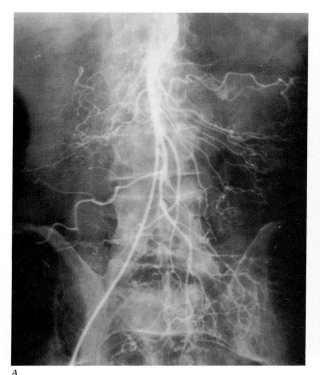

A

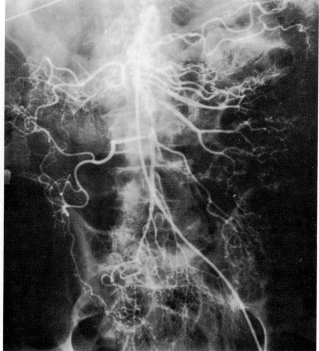

B

Figure 72-10. Patient with nonocclusive mesenteric ischemia following an episode of gastrointestinal hemorrhage and shock. (A) Initial superior mesenteric arteriogram showing diffuse vasoconstriction. (B) Repeat angiogram after papaverine infusion for 24 hours shows partial but not complete relief of the vasoconstriction. (C) Angiogram performed after 48 hours of papaverine infusion shows dilatation of all vessels. The patient was asymptomatic by that time. (Courtesy of Leon Schultz, M.D.)

days have been used without significant systemic effects. More than 90 percent of the drug is inactivated with each circulation through the liver, and so large doses can be given safely into the mesenteric circulation. Fibrin clots on the arterial catheter have been observed commonly, but have not caused any difficulty. Three catheters clotted and had to be removed, but this complication can be avoided if a continuous infusion pump is used. Catheter dislodgment occurred several times and required replacement under fluoroscopy.

C

The 54 percent survival in the present series is encouraging when it is compared with the 20 to 30 percent survival previously reported. Equally gratifying is the preservation of the normally functioning gastrointestinal tract in 85 percent of the surviving patients.

The survival of 9 of the 10 patients with acute

mesenteric ischemia who had angiography in the absence of physical signs of peritonitis demonstrates the potential value of early diagnosis. Ideally, all patients with AMI should be studied before physical signs develop, at a time when the plain films of the abdomen are normal. Physical signs and plain film abnormalities usually indicate the presence of bowel necrosis. Therefore, to wait for these signs to develop is to wait for ischemia to progress to infarction and to accept the high mortality that accompanies this progression.

Chronic Intestinal Ischemia (Abdominal Angina, Intestinal Angina, Recurrent Mesenteric Ischemia)

The term *chronic intestinal ischemia* (CMI) includes a host of conditions in which there is insufficient blood flow to satisfy the demands of increased motility, secretion, and absorption that develop after meals. These disorders manifest themselves either by ischemic visceral pain or by abnormalities in gastrointestinal absorption or motility. Patients with CMI are actually experiencing recurrent acute episodes of insufficient blood flow during periods of maximum intestinal work load. Therefore, the pain is similar to that arising in the myocardium with angina pectoris or that in the calf muscles with intermittent claudication.

Angiography plays a less important role in the diagnosis of CMI than it does in the diagnosis of AMI, because the demonstration of narrowed or occluded visceral vessels is not proof of chronic intestinal ischemia. Angiographic evaluation includes flush aortography in frontal and lateral views and selective injections of the SMA, the celiac axis (CA), and, if possible, the inferior mesenteric artery (IMA). The degree of occlusive involvement of the three major arteries can be best assessed on the lateral projections, and the collateral circulation and pattern of flow are best seen on the frontal views. The presence of prominent collateral vessels indicates a significant stenosis of a major vessel, but it also denotes a chronic process.

Although partial or complete occlusions of the SMA, CA, and IMA have been identified frequently in autopsy and angiographic studies, there have been relatively few patients with documented chronic intestinal ischemia. More-

over, there are many patients with occlusion of two or even all three of these vessels who remain asymptomatic (Fig. 72-11). Hence, the clinical significance of the angiographic demonstration of occlusion of one or more of these vessels remains controversial. The lack of any objective means of determining the inadequacy of intestinal blood flow before the morphologic changes of ischemia occur is the major obstacle to identifying patients with CMI.

Dick et al. [13] attempted to establish objective guidelines for the presence of CMI by angiographic measurements of the total cross-sectional area of the SMA, CA, and IMA in control patients, in hypertensive and arteriopathic patients, and in patients with chronic intestinal ischemia. These authors found that all patients with intestinal ischemia had total cross-sectional areas reduced to below two-thirds of normal. However, patients without ischemia had similar reductions. The inexact nature of such measurements is obvious. Moreover, the length of the stenosis, which is also an important factor, was not considered. A major shortcoming of estimating intestinal blood flow from the patency of the individual major vessels is the equal importance and variability of the collateral blood supply. The significance of stenoses of the major arteries is reduced in the presence of prominent collateral anastomosis but is of great importance in their absence. Determination of the presence or absence of these collateral circuits is an integral part of the angiographic evaluation of possible chronic intestinal ischemia. The absence of collateral vessels with occlusion of the SMA or CA is an ominous sign and suggests an acute rather than a chronic process.

A recent method of assessing the adequacy of splanchnic blood flow in which the angiographer plays a role is that described by Hansen et al. [21]. *Splanchnic blood flow* is defined as the total blood flow through the three splanchnic arteries and extrasplanchnic collateral vessels, and it is determined by measuring hepatic blood flow with indocyanine-green, both in the fasting state and after a standard meal. Oxygen consumption in the splanchnic bed is also measured. This technique involves catheterization of the radial artery, an arm vein, and a hepatic vein. In their study of 15 patients with abdominal pain, there was a significant failure of patients with abdominal angina to increase their splanchnic blood flow after the test meal. After arterial reconstruction, the postprandial increase in flow was similar to that in

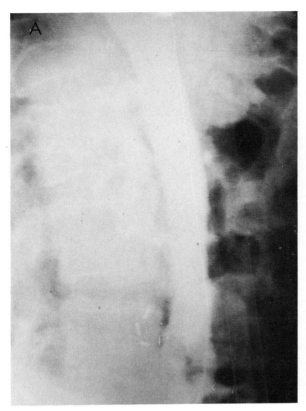

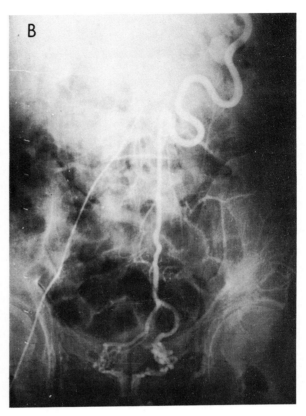

Figure 72-11. Angiogram from a patient with no abdominal symptoms. (A) Flush aortogram in lateral position shows an occlusion of the celiac axis, superior mesenteric artery (SMA), and inferior mesenteric artery. (B) Anteroposterior flush aortogram demonstrates filling from the middle hemorrhoidal arteries up to a large "meandering artery," with ultimate filling of the SMA and celiac axis through these collateral channels. (Reproduced with permission from S. J. Boley, L. J. Brandt, and F. J. Veith, Ischemic disorders of the intestines. In M. M. Ravitch et al. (eds.), *Curr. Probl. Surg.* 15:1, 1978. Courtesy of Year Book Medical Publishers, Inc., Chicago.)

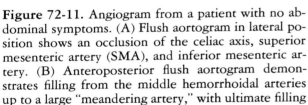

the control group. If these observations are corroborated, this method will provide an objective means of determining the need for treatment.

CMI has been reported with aneurysms of the aorta, CA, and SMA, with congenital and traumatic arteriovenous fistulas involving the SMA and the hepatic arteries, with coarctation of the aorta, and with congenital anomalies of the splanchnic vessels. Such cases are rare, however, and atherosclerotic involvement of the mesenteric vessels is the usual cause of this form of intestinal ischemia.

Atherosclerosis commonly involves the splanchnic arteries in individuals over 45 years of age. Of 88 adult patients studied by Reiner, Jiminez, and Rodriguez, 77 percent had evidence of atherosclerosis of the splanchnic vessels [29]. Some degree of luminal stenosis was observed in 72 percent of those with atherosclerosis, and in 65 percent the SMA, CA, or IMA was involved. Narrowing of the major vessels was almost always due to a plaque at the aortic ostium or in the proximal 1 to 2 cm of the artery. Severe stenoses were uniformly associated with marked aortic atherosclerosis, and, as expected, patients with severe mesenteric involvement had a higher incidence of coronary artery disease and diabetes mellitus. There was little correlation between the degree of mesenteric atherosclerosis and the clinical course.

DIAGNOSIS AND TREATMENT

There is no specific reliable diagnostic test for abdominal angina at this time. The diagnosis must be based on the clinical symptoms, the arteriographic demonstration of an occlusive process of the splanchnic arteries, and, to a great measure,

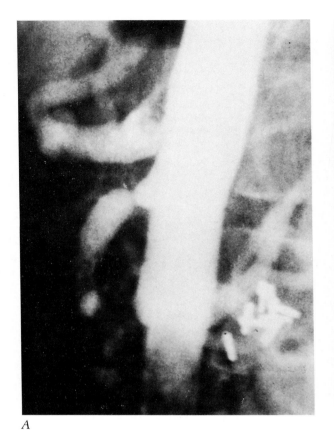

A

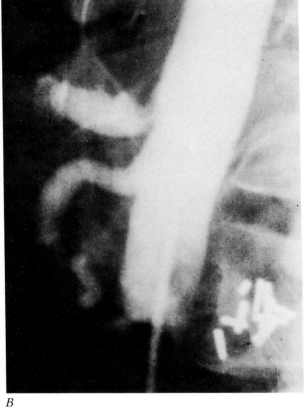

B

Figure 72-12. Transluminal angioplasty performed on a patient with symptoms of chronic intestinal ischemia. (A) Aortogram prior to dilatation shows stenosis and poststenotic dilatation of both celiac and superior mesenteric arteries. (B) Aortogram performed after dilatation of the SMA shows correction of the SMA stenosis. The patient was relieved of her symptoms. (Courtesy of Christos Athanasoulis, M.D.)

on the exclusion of other gastrointestinal disease. The one essential clinical symptom of CMI is abdominal pain, which is usually postprandial, progressive, and associated with weight loss. Physical findings are limited and nonspecific. A systolic bruit is heard in the upper abdomen in approximately one-half the patients although even when present its diagnostic significance must be questioned since similar bruits have been reported in 6.5 to 15.9 percent of healthy patients [14].

Conventional roentgenologic examinations of the gastrointestinal tract are usually unremarkable or are nonspecifically abnormal. Demonstration of extrinsic pressure defects along the medial border of the descending duodenum may indicate the presence of large collateral vessels between the SMA and the CA. Abnormalities in absorption studies or in small bowel biopsies may be present, but they are not specific for disease due to ischemia.

In the past, the only treatment for CMI was some form of operative arterial reconstruction. Today, transluminal angioplasty may afford an alternative approach of lesser magnitude and risk. Several patients have already been managed by transluminal dilatations, with good short-term responses (Fig. 72-12) [3, 19, 31]. In the absence of a method for measuring intestinal blood flow, precise criteria to define the need for operative arterial reconstruction have been lacking. There is agreement that a patient who has classic abdominal angina and unexplained weight loss, whose diagnostic evaluation has excluded other gastrointestinal disease, and whose angiogram shows occlusive involvement of at least two of the three major arteries should be treated. The issue has been much less clear if only one major vessel has been involved or if the nature of the clinical presentation has been atypical. With the availability of transluminal angioplasty, dilatation of stenoses of the SMA and the CA at the time of the original angiography is possible, and thus the indications for treatment may be liberalized. Further experience and follow-up will reveal whether this method will be as helpful in the management of patients with CMI as it has been in those with angina pectoris and renovascular hypertension.

There is one special situation in which reconstruction or dilatation of obstructed splanchnic arteries is indicated in the absence of abdominal complaints. This indication arises in a patient who is undergoing an aortic operation for peripheral vascular disease and in whom aortography has demonstrated occlusive involvement of the SMA and/or the CA and the presence of a large "meandering artery." In such a patient, the latter artery is supplying most of the blood flow to the splanchnic circulation from the IMA. Since the IMA may be compromised during the aortic procedure, it is advisable to provide another source of blood flow as part of this operation. The occurrence of acute intestinal ischemia resulting from "aortoiliac steal syndromes" has also been described in this situation after successful restoration of blood flow to the legs, but when no reconstructive procedure has been performed on the visceral vessels. Although we question whether or not the acute intestinal ischemia in these reports [24] represents a true "steal," the occurrence of this complication indicates the need for prophylactic revascularization.

Total occlusions or long stenoses of the SMA not amenable to transluminal angioplasty require operative revascularization of the splanchnic bed. Endarterectomy, reimplantation, and bypass procedures have all been successfully employed. Many surgeons believe that in the presence of CA and SMA occlusion, adequate management must include restoration of normal arterial pressures in both vessels and their branches [25].

RESULTS

Long-term follow-up information after operative revascularization is limited. In three recently reported series comprising 70 patients, the combined operative mortality was 7 percent, and 70 percent of patients were relieved of their symptoms [20, 24, 30]. Late deaths occurred in 21 percent of patients and are a reflection of the generalized arteriosclerotic disease in these patients. In McCollum et al.'s series of 33 patients, 83 percent were alive 5 years after operation, and 62 percent were alive after 10 years [24].

Properly selected patients with intestinal angina can be operated on successfully with a reasonable operative risk and a good long-term prognosis. Most will be relieved of their pain and malabsorption although complete relief of the latter may take months [12, 32]. While it has not been shown definitively that revascularization will protect against a fatal acute mesenteric infarction, the infrequency of these catastrophes after a successful operation suggests that that may be so.

References

1. Aakhus, T., and Brabrand, G. Angiography in acute superior mesenteric arterial insufficiency. *Acta Radiol. [Diagn.]* (Stockh.) 6:1, 1967.
2. Aakhus, T., and Evensen, A. Angiography in acute mesenteric arterial insufficiency. *Acta Radiol. [Diagn.]* (Stockh.) 19:945, 1978.
3. Athanasoulis, C. Personal communication, 1980.
4. Boley, S. J., Agrawal, G. P., Warren, A. R., Veith, F. J., Levowitz, B. S., Treiber, W. F., Dougherty, J. C., Schwartz, S., and Gliedman, M. L. Pathophysiologic effect of bowel distention on intestinal blood flow. *Am. J. Surg.* 117:228, 1969.
5. Boley, S. J., Feinstein, R., and Sammartano, R. J. Superior Mesenteric Artery Embolus. Presented at the American College of Surgeons, Atlanta, Georgia, Oct., 1980.
6. Boley, S. J., Regan, J. A., Tunick, P. A., Everhard, M. E., Winslow, P. R., and Veith, F. J. Persistent vasoconstriction—a major factor in nonocclusive mesenteric ischemia. *Curr. Top. Surg. Res.* 3:425, 1971.
7. Boley, S. J., Sprayregen, S., Siegelman, S. S., and Veith, F. J. Initial results from an aggressive approach to acute mesenteric ischemia. *Surgery* 82:848, 1977.
8. Boley, S. J., Sprayregen, S., Veith, F. J., and Siegelman, S. An Aggressive Roentgenologic and Surgical Approach to Acute Mesenteric Ischemia. In L. M. Nyhus (ed.), *Surgery Annual.* New York: Appleton-Century-Crofts, 1973.
9. Boley, S. J., Trieber, W., Winslow, P. R., Gliedman, M. L., and Veith, F. J. Circulatory response to acute reduction of superior mesenteric arterial blood flow. *Physiologist* 12:180, 1969.
10. Chou, C. C., Yu, L. C., and Yu, L. M. Effects of Acute Hemorrhage (H) and Carotid Artery Occlusion (CAO) on Compartmental Microcirculation in the G-I Tract. Presented at the First World Congress for Microcirculation, Toronto, Canada, 1975.

11. Cokkinis, A. J. *Mesenteric Vascular Occlusion.* London: Baillière, Tindall and Cox, 1926.
12. Dardik, H., Seidenberg, B., Parker, J. G., and Hurwitt, E. S. Intestinal angina malabsorption treated with elective revascularization. *J.A.M.A.* 194:1206, 1965.
13. Dick, A. P., Graff, R., Gregg, D. McC., Peters, N., and Sarner, M. An arteriographic study of mesenteric arterial disease. *Gut* 8:206, 1967.
14. Edwards, A. J., Hamilton, J. D., Nichol, W. D., Taylor, G. W., and Dawson, A. M. Experience with coeliac axis compression syndrome: A phonoarteriographic study. *Ann. Intern. Med.* 79:211, 1973.
15. Ende, N. Infarction of the bowel in cardiac failure. *N. Engl. J. Med.* 258:879, 1958.
16. Everhard, M. E., Regan, J. A., Veith, F. J., and Boley, S. J. Mesenteric vasomotor response to reduced mesenteric blood flow. *Physiologist* 13:191, 1970.
17. Folkow, B., Lewis, D., Lundgren, O., Mellander, S., and Wallentin, J. The effect of the sympathetic vasoconstrictor fibers on the distribution of the capillary blood flow in the intestine. *Acta Physiol. Scand.* 61:458, 1964.
18. Frimman-Dahl, J. Roentgen examination in mesenteric thrombosis. *AJR* 64:610, 1950.
19. Furrer, J., Grüntzig, A., Kugelmeier, J., and Goebel, N. Treatment of abdominal angina with percutaneous dilatation of an arteria mesenterica superior stenosis. *Cardiovasc. Intervent. Radiol.* 3:43, 1980.
20. Hansen, H. J. B. Abdominal angina. *Acta Chir. Scand.* 142:319, 1976.
21. Hansen, H. J. B., Engell, H. C., Ring-Larsen, H., and Raneck, L. Splanchnic blood flow in patients with abdominal angina before and after arterial reconstruction. *Ann. Surg.* 186:215, 1977.
22. Hessen, I. Roentgen examination in cases of occlusion of the mesenteric vessels. *Acta Radiol.* 44:293, 1955.
23. Jackson, B. B. Occlusion of the Superior Mesenteric Artery. In *American Lectures in Surgery.* Springfield, Ill.: Thomas, 1963.
24. McCollum, C. H., Graham, J. M., and DeBakey, M. E. Chronic mesenteric arterial insufficiency: Results of revascularization in 33 cases. *South. Med. J.* 69:1266, 1976.
25. Morris, G., DeBakey, M., and Bernhard, V. Abdominal angina. *Surg. Clin. North Am.* 46:919, 1966.
26. Ottinger, L. W. The surgical management of acute occlusion of the superior mesenteric artery. *Ann. Surg.* 188:721, 1978.
27. Ottinger, L. W., and Austen, W. G. A study of 136 patients with mesenteric infarction. *Surg. Gynecol. Obstet.* 121:789, 1965.
28. Polk, H. Experimental mesenteric venous occlusion. *Ann. Surg.* 163:432, 1966.
29. Reiner, L., Jiminez, F. A., and Rodriguez, F. L. Atherosclerosis in the mesenteric circulation: Observations and correlations with aortic and coronary atherosclerosis. *Am. Heart J.* 66:200, 1963.
30. Reul, G. J. Jr., Wukasc, D. C., Sandiford, F. M., Chiarillo, L., Hallman, G. L., and Cooley, D. A. Surgical treatment of abdominal angina: Review of 25 patients. *Surgery* 75:682, 1974.
31. Ring, E. Personal communication, 1980.
32. Rob, C. Surgical diseases of the celiac and mesenteric arteries. *Arch. Surg.* 93:21, 1966.
33. Siegelman, S. S., Sprayregen, S., and Boley, S. J. Angiographic diagnosis of mesenteric arterial vasoconstriction. *Radiology* 112:553, 1974.
34. Tomchik, F. S., Wittenberg, J., and Ottinger, L. W. The roentgenographic spectrum of bowel infarction. *Radiology* 96:249, 1970.
35. Tunick, P. A., Treiber, W. F., Frank, M., Veith, F. J., Gliedman, M. L., and Boley, S. J. Pathophysiologic effects of bowel distention on intestinal blood flow: II. *Curr. Top. Surg. Res.* 2:59, 1970.

6. Bladder and Pelvic Arteriography

Pelvic Angiography

ERICH K. LANG

The applications of pelvic angiography have been expanded and diversified in the last decade. In particular, the advent of interventional angiography has increased the demand for superselective arteriographic techniques, first to identify the precise location of traumatic or neoplastic lesions and then to limit therapeutic intervention to the vascular bed of the lesion, sparing adjacent normal tissues [3, 4, 17, 20, 40].

Improved techniques of microvascular surgery have made possible surgical correction of impotence. Such surgery, however, depends on precise angiographic identification of restrictive or occlusive vascular lesions afflicting tertiary vessels of the internal pudendal group [38, 62, 86].

The clinical challenge has been met with the refinement of superselective angiographic techniques for diagnostic and therapeutic purposes. The arteriographic array of resources has been enriched by sophisticated guidance systems aiding superselective catheterization of branch vessels, catheters equipped with balloons to isolate a vascular system (and hence selectively deliver embolic material), catheters equipped with detachable balloons or implantable umbrellas for occlusion of vessels, and catheters equipped with balloons for transluminal angioplasty [32, 33, 36, 42–44, 93, 124].

Technique

Percutaneous introduction of the arterial catheter (Seldinger technique) is favored.

The examination is best performed under local anesthesia. After the anesthetic agent infiltrates the subcutaneous tissues and periarterial space, a small skin incision is made and subcutaneous tissues are dissected with a straight hemostat to facilitate passage of catheters, particularly those equipped with inflatable balloons.

The artery should be entered via a single entry puncture. The arterial puncture site should be dilated by introduction of a vessel dilator over the guidewire, particularly if a balloon catheter is to be used [93].

Approach via a transaxillary or transfemoral route is determined by the etiology of the underlying disease, conditions of the vascular tree to be negotiated, and possible need to extend the procedure to one of intervention. The axillary route is favored in patients who have sustained massive pelvic trauma causing hematomas that complicate the percutaneous approach to the femoral arteries or in those treated by pneumatic compression suit, which makes the groin area inaccessible [3, 5, 31, 73, 100, 101].

To aid passage of the catheter into the desired segmental arterial branch, catheters are equipped with a variety of precurved tips. Guidance systems altering the curvature of the catheter tip by means of a tip deflector can also be used to help engage the desired vessel group.

To isolate a segment of the vascular bed or prevent regurgitation of embolic material into the main arterial branches, a catheter equipped with an inflatable balloon cuff can be used [93]. Catheters featuring detachable balloons or umbrellas are available for transcatheter embolization [73, 124].

The amount of contrast medium necessary for optimal opacification of the vascular system varies with the flow rate prevailing in a given region and the information sought by the study. Similarly, speed and duration as well as projections of the roentgenographic recordings are governed by the information sought, which varies for different pathologic entities.

Pharmacologic manipulation of blood flow may be useful for the study and management of certain pathologic entities. For example, normal tissues in the pelvis can be protected against inadvertent transcatheter embolization by temporarily constricting their vascular bed by intraarterial administration of epinephrine hydrochloride before attempting transcatheter embolization with inert embolic material or autologous blood clots [72].

To prevent clotting of blood in the catheter, periodic flushing with physiologic saline solution or saline solution containing 1,000 units of heparin per liter is advocated. After removal of the catheter, hemostasis is achieved by manually compressing the puncture site and applying a pressure dressing for 8 to 24 hours.

Applications

ARTERIOSCLEROTIC DISEASE OF PELVIC ARTERIES

The widespread acceptance and increased use of aortofemoral bypass grafts, endarterectomy, microsurgical techniques, and, most recently, transluminal angioplasty for correction of major artery

and small vessel occlusive disease have intensified the need for diagnostic studies capable of assessing physiologic and anatomic manifestions of such lesions as well as the existence and effectiveness of collateral vascular supply [62, 119].

Radionuclide studies are the best source for physiologic data. Flow and perfusion rates can be accurately calculated for resting and measured stress conditions, such as after treadmill exercise (Fig. 73-1). Moreover, this technique allows for assessment of flow via both natural and collateral pathways (Fig. 73-1). The effect of pharmacologic manipulation also can be measured.

Doppler ultrasound offers a noninvasive technique for evaluating the patency of major vessels [1].

Gray-scale and real-time ultrasonography can map the anatomy of the vascular tree and offer some information on the condition of or encroachment on the lumina of arteries [23].

For detailed assessment and mapping of arteriosclerotic disease of pelvic vessels, however, angiography is needed to determine management and to select the proper corrective surgical procedure. For this purpose the arteriogram must document conditions of the abdominal aorta, the aortic bifurcation, and the runoff vessels [119].

Injections of about 30 to 40 cc of contrast medium at a flow rate of 20 cc per second are suggested for the study of the distal abdominal

Figure 73-1. The computer-processed radionuclide flow curves demonstrate a near normal flow curve over the left femoral artery (*broken line*). Over the right femoral artery (*solid line*), the flow curve is abnormal (delayed ascent, lowered peak, delayed washout) reflecting blockage of the primary vessel and reconstitution via antegrade collaterals. *R FE* = right femoral artery; *L FE* = left femoral artery.

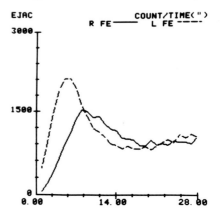

aorta, aortic bifurcation, and common, external, and internal iliac vessels. The flow rate may be modified according to the magnitude of arteriosclerotic disease present. Selective study of the common iliac arteries calls for a total volume of 20 to 25 cc of contrast medium injected at a flow rate of 15 cc per second; that of the hypogastric artery, for a total volume of 20 cc at a flow rate of about 10 cc per second.

To demonstrate the magnitude of arteriosclerotic plaques, biplane recording in anteroposterior and cross-table lateral projection is favored (Fig. 73-2).

The severity of arteriosclerotic disease and the presence of collateral flow—particularly reconstitution of flow distal to areas of total obstruction—determine the duration of roentgenographic recording. Reconstitution via collateral flow distal to sites of total obstruction may occur with delays of up to 40 seconds, and late documentation is necessary.

The connection between the superior, mid, and inferior hemorrhoidal arteries is the base for collateral flow from the inferior mesenteric artery via the hemorrhoidal arteries to the hypogastric artery and common iliac arteries and vice versa. The status of the inferior mesenteric artery supply should be determined before any bypass surgery, to identify dependence on collateral flow

and prevent inadvertent severance of such supply with attendant anoxic damage to the rectum, sigmoid, or descending colon [18, 115] (Figs. 73-3, 73-4).

TRANSLUMINAL ANGIOPLASTY OF PELVIC ARTERIES

Transluminal angioplasty with a Grüntzig balloon catheter has been found advantageous in the treatment of arteriosclerotic lesions involving the common, external, and internal iliac arteries [33] (Fig. 73-5). The method can be combined with microsurgical techniques, making feasible a concomitant treatment of multiple lesions impeding flow in proximal and distal vessels. The necessity of simultaneous correction of proximal and distal lesions to prevent thrombosis at peripheral endarterectomy sites or microvascular anastomoses makes transluminal angioplasty the procedure of choice for management of the proximal lesion.

PUDENDAL ARTERIOGRAPHY

Arterial insufficiency is one of the established causes of erectile impotence. After psychologic and psychiatric causes of erectile failure have been eliminated, vascular flow to the corpora cavernosa should be assessed and the site or sites

Figure 73-2. (A and B) Biplane arteriograms in anteroposterior and cross-table lateral projections optimally demonstrate arteriosclerotic plaques encroaching upon the lumen of vessels (*arrows*). Elevation of one leg and bolstering with water bags assure homogeneous density and facilitate differentiation of the vessels of the right and left side on cross-table lateral arteriograms.

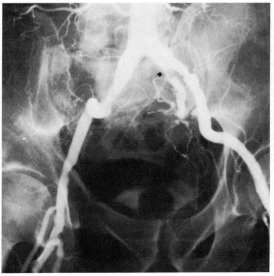

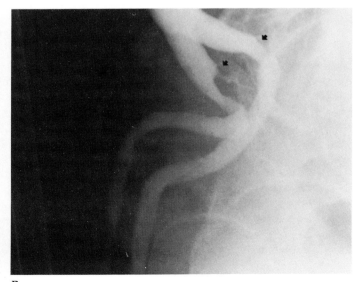

A   B

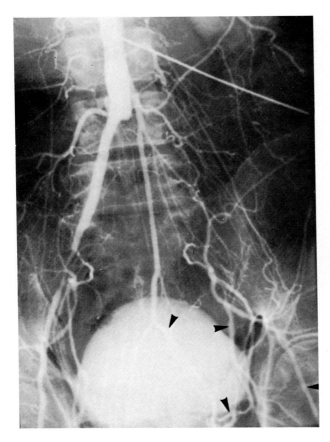

Figure 73-3. The late-phase inferior mesenteric arteriogram demonstrates huge collaterals between the superior, mid, and inferior hemorrhoidal arteries and retrograde opacification of the hypogastric arteries and external iliac and femoral arteries (*arrowheads*). The left lower extremity depends entirely on collateral circulation, the aorta being occluded at the level of the bifurcation.

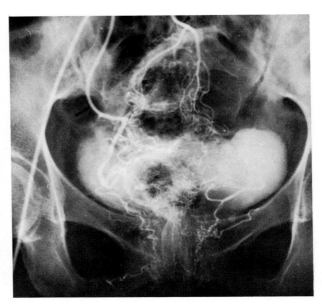

Figure 73-4. Selective injection of the right superior vesical artery demonstrates extensive tumor neovascularity involving the bladder, cervix, uterus, cul de sac, and rectum. Note retrograde opacification of the branches of the inferior mesenteric artery (*arrow, arrowhead*) via this collateral system. It suggests obstruction of the proximal inferior mesenteric artery and dependence of rectum and sigmoid upon collateral vascular supply via this pathway. (From Lang [72].)

of obstruction pinpointed to determine whether the condition can be corrected by one of the arterial circulatory augmentation procedures [1, 30, 37, 38, 48, 62]. Selective arteriography of the internal pudendal artery and its radicles (the superficial dorsal penile, deep cavernosal, and corpus spongeosal arteries) offers the most detailed information as to the condition of the vessels, the precise site of obstruction, and the magnitude of residual flow and runoff (Figs. 73-6, 73-7). In the presence of arteriosclerotic disease and particularly in diabetic patients, detailed study of the proximal vessels is mandatory [48]. Plaques at the proximal site could reduce the

peripheral flow rate and, unless corrected, would jeopardize the patency of the microvascular anastomosis [119]. Arteriographic findings determine which microvascular technique to choose—anastomosis of the inferior epigastric artery to the corpus cavernosum or anastomosis of the inferior epigastric artery to the superficial dorsal artery of the penis—or whether the patient's condition should be corrected by implantation of a Small-Kerion prosthesis (abandoning primary correction of the vascular insufficiency) [37, 38, 48, 62, 86].

Lesions afflicting the proximal segment of the internal pudendal artery are amenable to management by anastomosis of an inferior epigastric artery to a superficial dorsal artery of the penis, whereas lesions afflicting the terminal branches of the cavernosal or corpus spongeosal branches are best treated by a microvascular anastomosis between the inferior epigastric artery and the corpus cavernosum or by implanta-

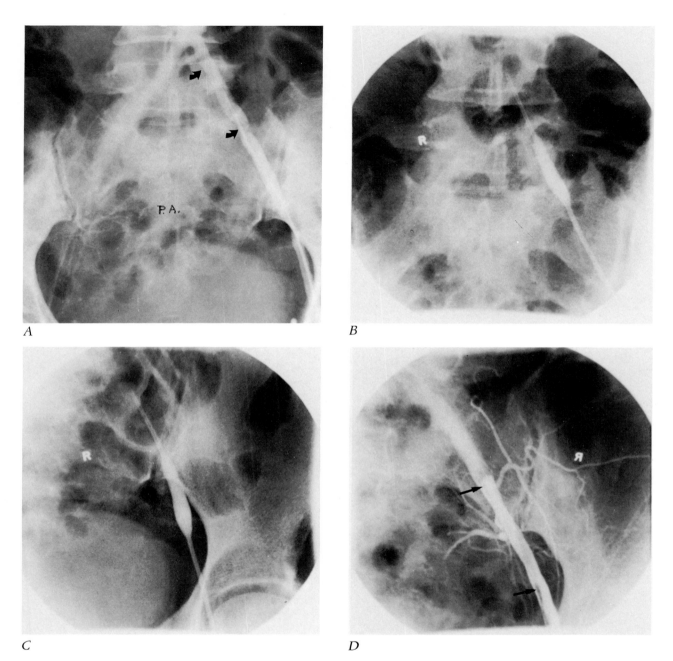

Figure 73-5. (A) Extensive arteriosclerotic disease is demonstrated in the area of aortic bifurcation and involves common and external iliac arteries (*arrows*). (B) Transluminal dilatation is carried out with a 1½-cc Grüntzig balloon, at multiple levels. At this point, the area of arteriosclerotic narrowing of the junction segment of common and external iliac arteries is being dilated. (C) The Grüntzig balloon has been withdrawn to a lower position, dilating an arteriosclerotic segment of the external iliac artery. Note the waistlike compression of the balloon, reflecting the location of the arteriosclerotic narrowing. (D) The postdilatation control arteriogram demonstrates improvement of the lumen of the artery, though a small intimal flap may have been created (*arrows*). Miniheparinization was instituted to prevent thrombosis. The computer-processed radionuclide angiograms confirmed marked improvement of perfusion of the extremity. A microsurgical approach to treating additional arteriosclerotic lesions at the level of the trifurcation was now considered feasible.

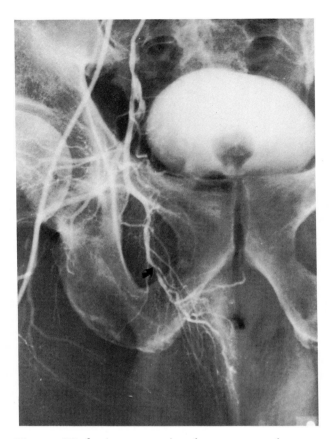

Figure 73-6. An eccentric plaque encroaches on the lumen of the distal segment of the internal pudendal artery (*arrow*). Hemodynamic significance is suggested by poststenotic dilatation.

tion of a Small-Kerion prosthesis [37, 38, 62, 86] (Figs. 73-8, 73-9).

Concentric narrowing in the pudendal artery must be differentiated from spasm induced by passage of the guidewire. Angiographic documentation after intraarterial administration of 3 to 5 mg of tolazoline (Priscoline) should show unabated concentric narrowing in the presence of organic stenosis or stricture, whereas "lesions" attributable to vascular spasm will disappear (see Fig. 73-7).

Transluminal angioplasty attacking proximal lesions in the common and internal iliac arteries can be combined with microvascular arterial augmentation techniques bypassing distal lesions.

ARTERIOGRAPHY OF THE BLADDER

Bladder Neoplasms

The stage of a bladder neoplasm largely determines the type of treatment and is the best prognostic indicator [118]. Clinical staging—by bimanual examination under anesthesia and deep-muscle biopsy—is unfortunately inaccurate [71, 90, 126, 127]. Some investigators have reported an accuracy rate as low as 34 percent for clinical staging [90]. Imaging examinations such as fractional cystography, arteriography, triple cystography, lymphangiography, ultrasonography, and computed tomography have been advocated to improve staging accuracy [14, 67, 71, 76, 78, 85, 90, 91, 109–112].

Staging of bladder tumors on computed tomograms rests on demonstration of the relationship of the lesion to the bladder wall, perivesical fat, and adjacent structures [109]. A stage B2 lesion (invasion through the entire muscularis) is indicated by localized thickening of a segment of the bladder wall but an intact and well-defined perivesical fat plane. Conversely, a stage C lesion (tumor extension into the perivesical fat) shows loss of definition of the perivesical fat plane [118] (Fig. 73-10). The diagnosis of a stage D lesion (tumor extension or metastases to other organs) depends on identification of contiguous tumor extension into adjacent structures or lymph node or distant metastases [78, 109–112, 118] (Fig. 73-11). To confirm permeation of the fat plane by the neoplasm or its contiguous extension into adjacent structures, patients are best scanned in decubitus and supine positions to encourage separation by gravity of adjacent structures from the bladder wall [109]. Distention of the bladder with gas creates favorable conditions for dependent gravity pull by the tumor and demonstration of its base and/or permeation of the muscularis and extension into the perivesical fat or adjacent structures [111]. Under optimal technical conditions, staging of bladder neoplasms by computed tomography should achieve an accuracy rate of about 80 percent [111].

Arteriograpic diagnosis and assessment of tumor extension are based on identification of highly specific tumor neovascularity. An abnormal development of the muscularis of tumor vessels occasions the characteristic erratic caliber and lack of normal tapering [67, 76, 91, 126] (Fig. 73-12). Arteriovenous shunts within the tumor result in increased flow and cause enlargement and marked tortuosity of the vesical artery [67,

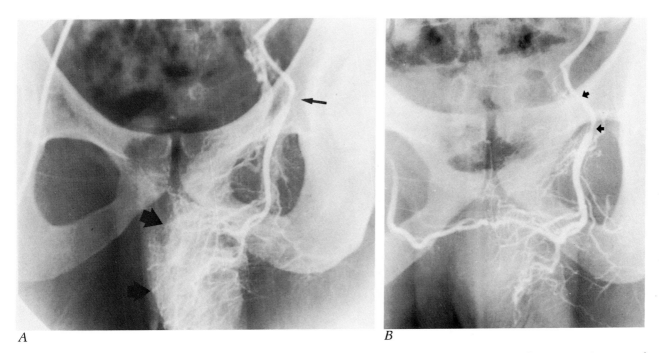

A   *B*

Figure 73-7. (A and B) Arteriogram obtained after intraarterial administration of 3 mg of Priscoline documents unabated concentric narrowing of the internal pudendal artery (*arrows*). The pharmacoan- giogram confirms the diagnosis of organic stricture and eliminates vascular spasm induced by passage of the guidewire as possible cause.

Figure 73-8. Selective internal pudendal arteriogram demonstrates arteriosclerotic lesions involving the distal segment of this vessel (*arrows*). There is, how- ever, excellent runoff into the deep cavernosal and corpus spongeosal arteries. This type of obstructive lesion can be corrected by flow augmentation via a microvascular anastomosis between the inferior epi- gastric and the superficial dorsal arteries of the penis.

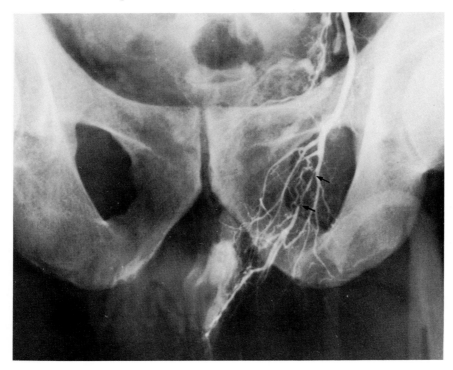

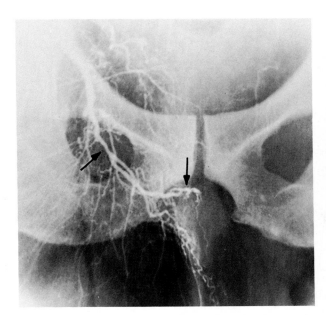

Figure 73-9. Only minor arteriosclerotic plaques involve the main internal pudendal artery (*left arrow*). However, there is a lack of runoff into the deep cavernosal and corpus spongeosal branches, indicating severe endarterial disease (*right arrow*). This finding militates against a microanastomotic procedure to the dorsal artery of the penis. Only a direct anastomosis of the inferior epigastric artery to the corpus cavernosum or implantation of the Small-Kerion prosthesis can improve function under this condition.

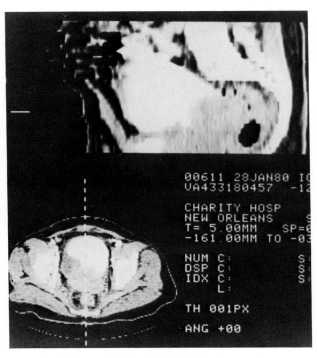

Figure 73-10. Computed tomogram suggests contiguous extension of a bladder tumor into the perivesical fat along the right lateral and posterior circumference. A sagittal reconstruction demonstrates the posterior extension of the tumor particularly well.

91] (Fig. 73-12). Puddling of contrast medium is a sign of tumor necrosis [67, 76, 91, 126].

Arteriographic staging is based on documentation of the characteristic tumor neovascularity in the muscularis, extending into the perivesical fat or contiguously into adjacent structures [67, 76, 91, 127]. To demonstrate such extension of the neoplasm, the tumor-bearing area must be projected tangentially [67, 76, 91] (Fig. 73-13). Distention of the bladder with gas and dissection of the perivesical fat plane by gas further improve the delineation of the tumor extension [67, 91] (Fig. 73-14). For optimal visualization of the neoplasm, selective injections of the anterior division of the hypogastric arteries or, if identified as the source of supply, of the respective superior or inferior vesical arteries are favored (Fig. 73-15).

About 90 percent of bladder carcinomas exhibit prominent tumor neovascularity, which makes possible staging by arteriography [91].

The remainder may appear as hypovascular masses on arteriograms [91]. Encasement and/or amputation of vessels is the salient arteriographic feature of this type of bladder neoplasm. These arteriographic findings are similar to the features of endarteritis obliterans of chronic inflammatory lesions and hence do not permit diagnosis or staging with acceptable confidence [61].

Arteriographic staging of bladder neoplasms is most accurate for advanced lesions [71, 128]. For early neoplasms, staging by clinical examination is more accurate; however, arteriography is still useful because it tends to eliminate some of the false-positives of clinical staging [71, 90, 127]. Overstaging is the most common error incurred with arteriography and is most often attributable to coexistent unrecognized inflammatory disease. Nonetheless, the 80 to 90 percent accuracy rate achieved when staging advanced bladder neoplasms by arteriography compares favorably with

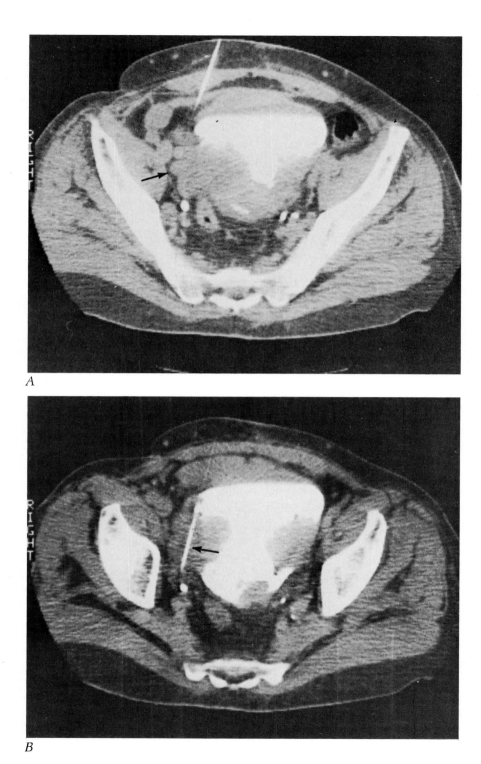

A

B

Figure 73-11. (A) Computed tomogram at a level 0.5 cm lower demonstrates nodular masses that could represent metastatic tumor to hypogastric nodes (*arrow*). The cut level localizer of the computed tomogram clearly establishes an appropriate point of entry for thin-needle biopsy. (B) The precise biopsy site, as confirmed on control computed tomograms, in this case yielded neoplastic deposits to the hypogastric nodes (*arrow*). The diagnosis of a stage D lesion was thus established.

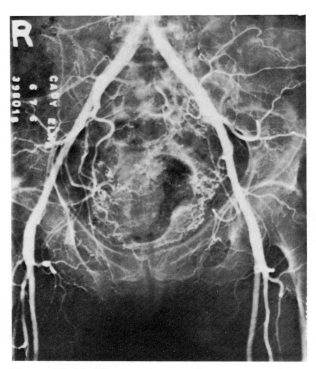

Figure 73-12. The arteriogram demonstrates characteristic tumor neovascularity (vessels of erratic caliber) in a huge tumor involving the right and left lateral bladder walls and replacing the entire posterior bladder wall. Note the size of the right superior vesical artery, reflecting the increased flow caused by arteriovenous shunts within the tumor. Puddling of contrast medium is a sign of tumor necrosis. (From E. K. Lang, *Roentgenographic Diagnosis of Bladder Tumors.* Springfield, Ill.: Thomas, 1968.)

that obtained by computed tomography, ultrasonography, or, particularly, clinical examination.

As might be expected, lymphangiography, involving as it does different diagnostic criteria, can further improve the accuracy for staging of advanced bladder neoplasms [56, 121, 127, 128]. Even though pedal lymphangiography does not normally opacify hypogastric nodes, the nodes surrounding the obturator nerve may be demonstrated [85]. The capability of lymphangiography to identify architectural changes in normal-sized nodes advances detection of metastatic disease to lymph nodes beyond the capabilities of computed tomography or ultrasonography, which depend solely on the criterion of lymph node enlargement. Though the observation of architectural changes is more specific for the diagnosis of neoplasms than is that of mere enlarge-

ment, it is subject to the same source of error as the arteriographic demonstration of a sustained stain in nodes, namely, inflammatory disease of lymph nodes. The addition of thin-needle biopsy under fluoroscopic control can improve diagnostic accuracy by eliminating false-positives attributable to inflammatory diseases that may appear on lymphangiograms with architectural changes in lymph nodes [83] (Fig. 73-16).

Since the criteria used for staging of bladder neoplasms by arteriography, computed tomography, and lymphangiography are based on different observations, the three techniques complement one another, and their combination improves the accuracy of staging [127, 128].

A variety of benign lesions involving the bladder, such as chronic nonspecific cystitis, tuberculosis, pheochromocytoma, hemangiopericytoma, hemangioma, arteriovenous malformation, primary amyloidosis, and pelvic lipomatosis, have been reported to be manifested as hypervascular lesions involving the bladder or perivesical tissues [21, 24, 25, 34, 50–52, 55, 57, 60, 61, 63, 73, 79].

A clinical history of hypertensive crisis precipitated by micturition should raise suspicion of a biochemically active tumor such as a pheochromocytoma involving the bladder. Documentation of elevated urine vanillylmandelic acid levels, elevated blood and urine catecholamine levels, and characteristic arteriographic findings are considered diagnostic for a functioning chromaffin tumor involving the bladder.

A spoke-wheel appearance is the arteriographic hallmark of pheochromocytoma of the bladder. Large feeding arteries enveloping the periphery of this tumor and dispatching branches toward its center cause this appearance [21, 24, 25, 35, 52, 55, 79]. The capillary phase is characterized by an intense and homogeneous stain. Visualization of dilated and tortuous veins during the early capillary phase attests to the rapid circulation within the tumor (Fig. 73-17). The intensity and homogeneity of the capillary stain have been advocated as differential diagnostic criteria against other malignant bladder neoplasms. The injection of contrast medium may provoke a hypertensive crisis, and treatment with Dibenzyline and phentolamine, alpha- and beta-adrenergic blocking agents, has been recommended in preparation for arteriography [53].

The arteriographic appearance of hemangiopericytomas of the bladder is similar to that of

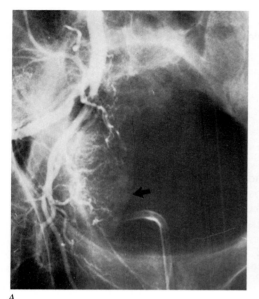

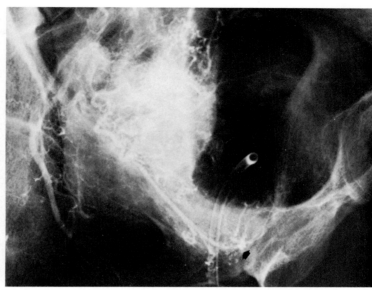

A   B

Figure 73-13. (A) Arteriogram in anteroposterior projection demonstrates tumor neovascularity involving the right lateral bladder wall (*arrow*). (B) The arteriogram is repeated in oblique projection to demonstrate the tumor tangentially (*arrow*) and allow assessment of the precise depth of tumor penetration.

Figure 73-14. A triple cystogram—showing distention of the bladder with nitrous oxide and dissection of the perivesical fat plane by insufflation of nitrous oxide into the perivesical space, and including an arteriogram—optimally demonstrates the large extra-vesical tumor component (iceberg tumor, *arrows*). (From E. K. Lang, *Professional Self-evaluation and Continuing Education Programs, Set #10.* Chicago: American College of Radiology, 1976).

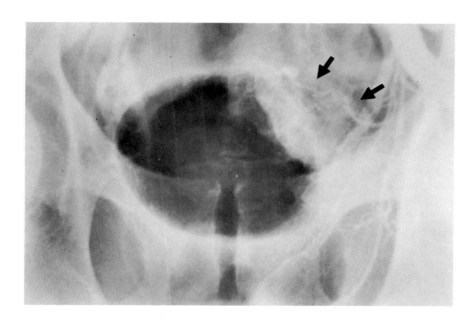

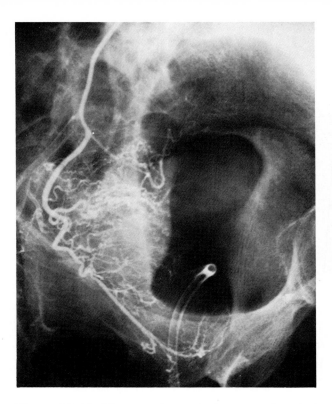

Figure 73-15. The superior vesical artery, identified on prior survey arteriograms as the principal vascular supply of the tumor, is selectively injected. This technique best demonstrates invasion into the perivesical fat on appropriate tangential projections.

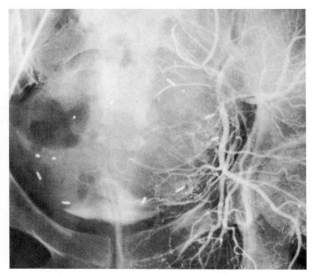

Figure 73-17. A fine neovascular pattern is identified in a mass indenting the dome of the bladder. Late capillary phase films demonstrated increase of the patchy staining observed on this early arterial phase roentgenogram. The appearance is quite characteristic for a pheochromocytoma.

Figure 73-16. (A and B) Percutaneous transperitoneal thin-needle biopsy of an external inguinal lymph node demonstrating architectural changes in its upper half on lymphangiograms is carried out under biplane fluoroscopic control. Since only a portion of the node exhibits architectural changes suggestive of neoplastic involvement, precise localization of the biopsy needle is mandatory to assure a representative sample.

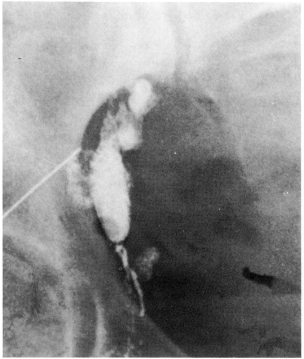

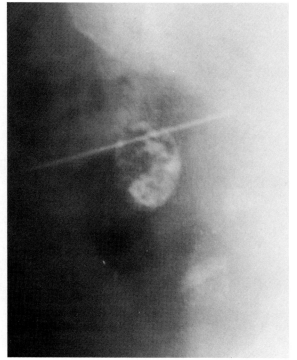

A

B

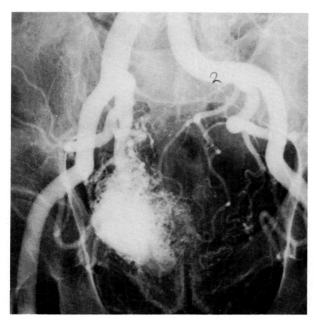

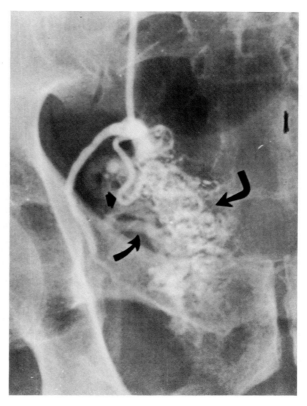

Figure 73-18. A flush aortogram demonstrates a huge arteriovenous malformation involving the right bladder wall. (From Lang et al. [73].)

Figure 73-20. A later phase arteriogram best demonstrates hemangiomatous elements (*long arrows*) arising from the feeding vessel (*short arrow at left*) and congenital phlebectasia in this tumefactive arteriovenous malformation. (From Lang et al. [73].)

Figure 73-19. Superselective arteriogram of the superior vesical artery (*arrows*) proves this vessel to be the principal feeder of the arteriovenous malformation.

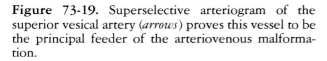

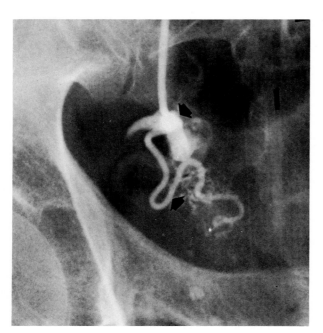

pheochromocytomas. Small corkscrew vessels penetrate into the tumor in a spoke-wheel fashion, feeding from prominent circumferential feeder arteries. A dense tumor stain is once again observed during the capillary phase. The characteristically sustained opacification of dilated draining veins has been advocated as a principal differential diagnostic criterion against pheochromocytoma [52].

Hemangiomas of the bladder occurring as part of the Klippel-Trenaunay syndrome may not be demonstrable on arteriograms [34, 63]. However, another variety of hemangioma associated with congenital phlebectasias and arteriovenous fistulas is readily demonstrable by arteriography [63, 73] (Figs. 73-18–73-21). These lesions are noted for an extensive collateral supply from

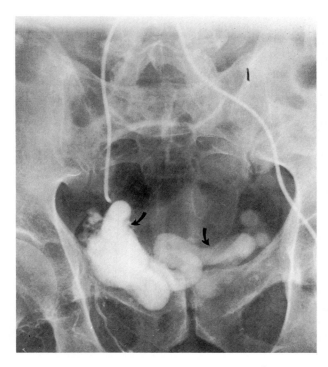

Figure 73-21. Premature opacification of an enormously dilated draining vein (*arrows*) is the consequence of multiple arteriovenous shunts. The size of the draining vein attests to the hemodynamic significance of the lesion. (From Lang et al. [73].)

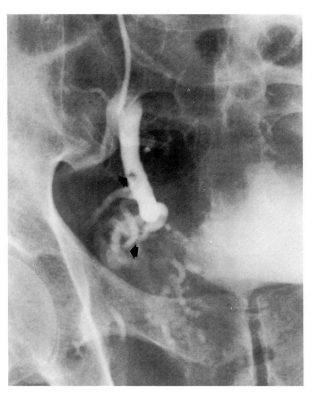

Figure 73-22. Following transcatheter embolization with Gelfoam particles of 2 × 2 × 2-mm size (*arrows*) there appears to be salutary obliteration of the hemangiomatous elements of the large arteriovenous malformation. Unfortunately, the arteriovenous malformation recurred, developing new collaterals to such remote branches as the circumflex femoral artery. (From Lang et al. [73].)

practically all pelvic vessels and even branches originating from the circumflex femoral artery, which explains the difficulty encountered when one attempts to eradicate such malformations by surgical ligation or transcatheter embolization of feeder vessels with inert embolic material (Fig. 73-22).

Cystitis generally produces arteriographic features consistent with inflammatory hyperemia. However, sometimes conglomerates of tortuous vessels mimic a neoplastic lesion [52, 61]. The variable appearance of tubercular bladder lesions on arteriograms probably reflects different stages of activity of the tubercular process. At one point, the number of arteries seems to be increased, the individual vessels look dilated and

tortuous, and even vessels of variable caliber may be observed [50] (Fig. 73-23). The inflammatory process may cause thickening of the bladder wall and mimic tumefaction. Once the lesion becomes fibrotic, the hypervascularity attributable to dilated vessels disappears [50]. Differentiation of tubercular from nonspecific cystitis is not possible on the basis of the arteriogram.

Tumefactive primary amyloidosis of the bladder may, likewise, appear as a hypervascular lesion [52].

Pelvic lipomatosis can present as an avascular or a markedly hypervascular lesion involving preponderantly the perivesical tissues [51, 57, 60] (Fig. 73-24). The diagnosis of pelvic lipomatosis is suggested on plain films by a strik-

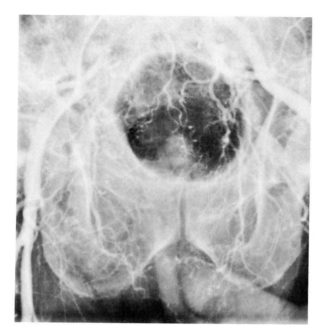

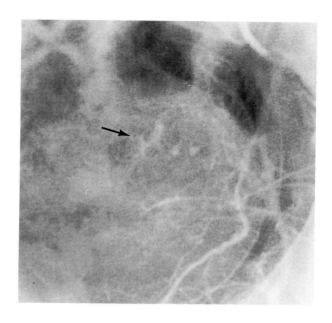

Figure 73-23. A 2-second arteriogram shows an increase in number as well as dilatation of small arteries in the perivesical fat and muscularis of the bladder. This nonspecific hypervascularity occurs with cystitis or particularly following radiation therapy.

Figure 73-25. A highly vascular tumor is demonstrated on an early-phase roentgenogram of a selective arteriogram of the anterior division of the left hypogastric artery. Numerous corkscrew intramural arteries (*arrow*) distinguish the tumor. The appearance is characteristic for an intramural chorioepithelioma.

Figure 73-24. (A) An increased number of small arteries and segmental dilatation of individual vessels in the perivesical space (*arrows*) suggest pelvic lipomatosis. The arteriographic manifestations are indistinguishable from those seen with cystitis or attendant radiation therapy. (B) The cystogram demonstrates a characteristic pear-shaped deformity of the floor of the bladder. Inordinate radiolucency of a mass enveloping the bladder and filling the pelvis affirms the diagnosis of pelvic lipomatosis.

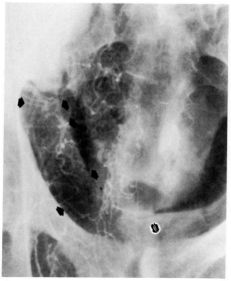

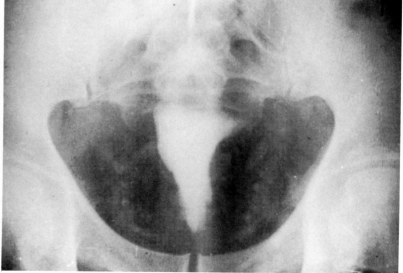

A   *B*

ing radiolucency in the pelvis, on cystograms by a characteristic pear-shaped deformity of the urinary bladder, and on barium enemas by a typical tubular narrowing afflicting the rectum and rectosigmoid. A low attenuation coefficient of the pelvic mass on computed tomograms and marked echogenicity on ultrasonograms are dependable criteria to affirm the diagnosis of pelvic lipomatosis and eliminate such misdiagnoses as cystitis or bladder neoplasm, which might have been entertained because of the hypervascular appearance on the arteriogram [51, 57, 60, 61, 113].

Arteriographic assessment of mass lesions of the prostate may be useful for differentiation of inflammatory masses and sarcoma of the prostate. The fleeting heterogeneous stain throughout the mass indicates a prostatic sarcoma, whereas a late-appearing and sustained rim stain around a lucent center is commonly associated with prostatic abscess (Fig. 73-25).

Pelvic Angiography in Obstetrics

Although today ultrasonography has largely replaced pelvic arteriography for the diagnosis of abnormal conditions of pregnancy, the latter technique is still favored for the follow-up of chorioepithelioma and hydatidiform mole treated by chemotherapeutic agents [8, 10, 12, 13, 22, 47, 59, 64, 82]. Though titers of human gonadotropin are generally obtained for diagnosis and follow-up of treated hydatidiform mole and chorioepithelioma, arteriograms are sometimes credited with identifying trophoblastic elements before the titer of chorionic gonadotropins has reached a diagnostic level or while production of the hormone is still suppressed by chemotherapy [20, 47].

The arteriographic diagnosis of hydatidiform mole is based on the demonstration of avascular spaces within the uterine content. Arteriograms obtained 5 to 10 seconds after completion of contrast-medium injection demonstrate filling of the intervillous spaces, which in patients with hydatidiform moles appear to be unduly widely separated because of the large hydropic vesicles of the mole (Fig. 73-25). The discrepancy between enlarged spiral myometrial vessels and the relatively avascular uterine content is another arteriographic observation suggesting hydatidiform

mole [8, 12, 22, 47]. Perseverance of cavities within the uterine wall and arteriographic demonstration of persistent arteriovenous communications suggest incomplete evacuation of the mole or malignant degeneration [8].

Chorioepithelioma and chorioadenoma destruens are characterized by an excessive pathologic vascularization of the myometrium. Hugely enlarged spiral myometrial arteries feed directly into vascular pools, which in turn communicate with prominent veins. The magnitude of the shunt across the arteriovenous fistulas is suggested by premature opacification of the ovarian veins [47, 53, 54, 64] (see Fig. 73-27). In hydatidiform mole the spiral arteries are uniformly dilated and stretched apart, but in malignant trophoblastic disease the spiral arteries are enormously hypertrophied around areas of localized growth [47]. In patients with hydatidiform mole the uterine content is strikingly avascular, whereas in those with malignant trophoblastic disease a highly vascularized space in the uterus or parametrium is characteristic. Arteriography is, therefore, particularly useful for differentiation of hydatidiform mole and malignant trophoblastic tumors that may not be differentiable by gonadotropin titer.

Today the diagnosis of placenta previa is made on ultrasonography, which offers a noninvasive and more accurate method than arteriography [11, 13].

Pelvic Arteriography in Gynecology

Computed tomography and ultrasonography in particular have proved more sensitive than arteriography for the detection of gynecologic masses. They are as accurate in indicating the diagnosis and assessing the extent of most gynecologic masses and are therefore favored for initial triage examination [19, 65, 71, 80, 98, 123].

However, arteriography offers criteria useful for differentiation of some entities such as pedunculated subserous uterine fibromyomas and ovarian tumors difficult to distinguish by ultrasonography or computed tomography [80, 98, 123].

Fibromyomas are generally hypervascular and derive their blood supply from intramural branches of the uterine artery [9, 29, 102, 106] (Fig. 73-26). Conversely, ovarian tumors have a

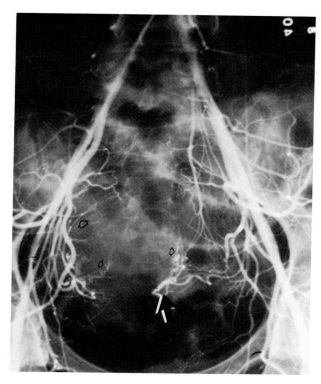

Figure 73-26. A hypervascular tumor featuring corkscrew arteries (*small open arrows*) is demonstrated eccentric to the corpus of the uterus, its size reflected by stretching and splaying of arteries (*large open arrow*). The blood supply is derived from intramural branches of the uterine artery (*black arrow*). These features are characteristic for a uterine fibromyoma. (From E. K. Lang, Arteriography in Gynecology. *Radiol. Clin. North Am.* 5:133, 1967.)

sparse vasculature and derive their supply from the adnexal branches of the uterine or ovarian arteries. The arteriographic diagnosis of an ovarian tumor, however, must rest on demonstrable neovascularity, since mere stretching of the adnexal branches of the uterine artery indicates solely the presence of an adnexal mass but offers no specific indication of the etiology. A predominant vascular supply to uterus and adnexa from the ovarian arteries requires aortography in addition to pelvic arteriography to ensure complete documentation of the vascular supply [6, 7, 13, 29].

The diagnostic criteria of ultrasonography and computed tomography on the one hand and arteriography on the other are dissimilar for ovarian and uterine tumors, and so the examinations complement each other [123] (Fig. 73-27). Ultrasonography offers rapid viewing of the pelvis in multiple planes, which facilitates demonstration of ovarian neoplasms and differentiation from masses originating from the uterus and adnexa [123]. However, criteria that serve to differentiate tissues—such as a low attenuation coefficient or low echogenicity—can be mimicked by necrotic uterine fibroids, and differentiation of an ovarian tumor from pedunculated necrotic fibromyomas of the uterus then depends on arteriographic criteria [102, 123].

Pelvic angiography has also been advocated for staging of carcinoma of the cervix. The propensity of carcinoma of the cervix to demonstrate tumor neovascularity and a dense stain in about 80 percent of patients can be used for positive localization of the neoplastic mass [71, 74, 75, 92, 95, 102, 106] (Fig. 73-28).

The cervicovaginal branch of the uterine artery is the predominant vascular supply for a carcinoma of the cervix. A marked hypertrophy of the cervicovaginal branch reflects increased flow associated with carcinoma of the cervix. Frank tumor neovascularity—that is, vessels of erratic caliber in the normally avascular cervical segment of the uterus—identifies the neoplasm [6, 29, 71, 74, 75] (Fig. 73-29). A sharp and curvilinear demarcation of the neovascularity suggests that the neoplasm is confined within the vaginal fornix (Fig. 73-30). Stretching and splaying of the parametrial segment of the uterine artery indicates the presence of a mass, whereas demonstration of neovascularity in the normally avascular parametrium confirms its neoplastic etiology [6, 71, 74, 75] (see Fig. 73-28).

Differentiation of coexistent inflammatory and neoplastic disease on arteriograms may be difficult [71, 74, 102, 106]. In general, neoplastic tumor stain appears within 2 seconds and is sustained for about 4 seconds; conversely, stain attributable to inflammatory hyperemia appears after 5 to 6 seconds' delay but may persevere for 5 to 6 seconds thereafter [74]. Though the arteriographic criterion for diagnosing coexistent inflammatory and neoplastic disease is of limited reliability, competitive examinations, such as computed tomography and ultrasonography, offer no criteria for the differentiation. Definitive diagnosis is therefore possible only by thin-needle biopsy [65, 78, 123] (Fig. 73-31).

The identification of lymph node metastases of carcinoma of the cervix presents vexing problems. Clinical staging has been found extremely inaccurate. Morton et al. in a review of the literature established an incidence of lymph node

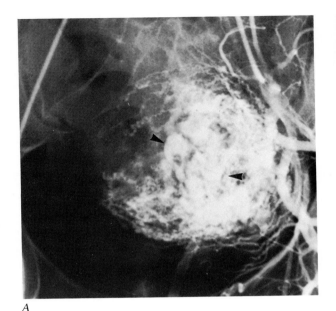

A

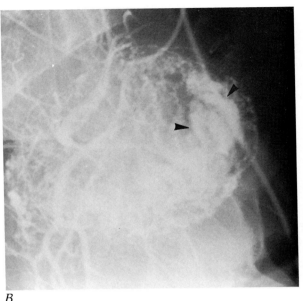

B

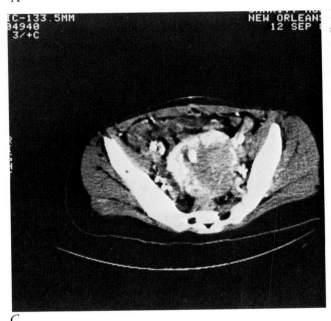

C

Figure 73-27. (A) A highly vascularized tumor (*arrowheads*) is demonstrated on an early-phase selective arteriogram of the anterior division of the left hypogastric artery. (B) A cross-table lateral projection of this same selective arteriogram demonstrates numerous intramural corkscrew arteries that appear to traverse the tumor (*arrowheads*). This appearance is characteristic for an intramural chorioepithelioma. (C) A dynamic computed tomogram demonstrates the densely opacified intramural elements of a chorioepithelioma destruens on an appropriate section.

metastases based on histologic examination: 16.6 percent in patients staged clinically as having a stage 1 carcinoma of the cervix, 32.5 percent in those in stage 2, and 45.6 percent in those in stage 3 [89]. While arteriographic demonstration of tumor neovascularity in a lymph node is a reliable criterion for the diagnosis of lymph node metastases, an unacceptably high rate of false-negative results limits the usefulness of this technique [71, 74] (Fig. 73-32). Unfortunately, other imaging modalities such as lymphangiography, computed tomography, and ultrasonography are beset by similar difficulties. The diagnosis of metastatic disease to pelvic lymph nodes often hinges on demonstrable changes of internal architecture in normal-sized lymph nodes and on identification of abnormal collateral lymphatic channels [78]. This is possible only on lymphangiograms. However, lymphangiograms offer no criteria for differentiation between inflammatory and malignant causes of such architectural changes, thus increasing the rate of false-positive findings [78]. A combination of computed tomography (for enlarged nodes) and lymphangiography with guided thin-needle biopsy has been advocated to establish a histologic diagnosis and reduce the rate of false-positives (see Fig. 73-16).

Neither ultrasonography nor computed tomography provides criteria for differentiating recurrent carcinoma of the cervix and radiation-induced fibrosis. Arteriography is the only modality short of guided thin-needle biopsy that can establish the diagnosis of tumor recurrence on the basis of characteristic tumor neovascularity

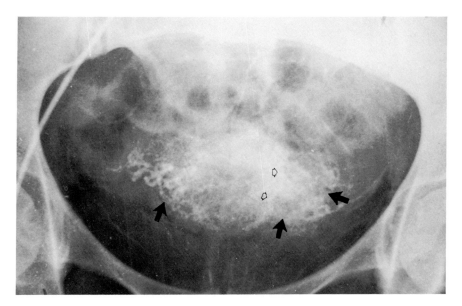

Figure 73-28. The late-phase films of an aortogram demonstrate a dense stain extending from the uterus laterally into the medial parametrium (*black arrows*). The findings are more marked in the left medial parametrium than on the right side. Tumor neovascularity is identifiable. The cleavage plane of the uterus is clearly defined by the marginal artery (*open arrows*). The arteriogram establishes extension of the carcinoma of the cervix to the medial parametrium, hence a stage 2A lesion. (From Lang and Greer [74].)

Figure 73-29. Selective arteriogram of the anterior division of the hypogastric artery demonstrates typical tumor vessels (erratic caliber) in the normally avascular cervical segment of the uterus (*long arrows*). The plane of the parametrium is defined by the parametrial segment of the uterine artery (*short black arrow*). The corpus and fundus of the uterus are located cephalad to the point of deflection of the parametrial and marginal arteries (*open arrow*). The magnitude of flow to the neoplasm is reflected by simultaneous opacification of tumor vessels in the cervix and myometrial branches of the uterus.

Figure 73-30. Extensive tumor neovascularity is seen in the normally avascular cervical segment of the uterus (*small arrowheads*). The tumor neovascularity is characterized by encasement of vessels, presenting a distinctly different pattern from that of the corkscrew vessels found in normal uterine myometrium (*arrows*). Despite contribution to the blood supply of the neoplasm from the internal pudendal group (*large arrowhead*), tumor stain and neovascularity are sharply confined, suggesting that the tumor is contained within the vaginal fornix.

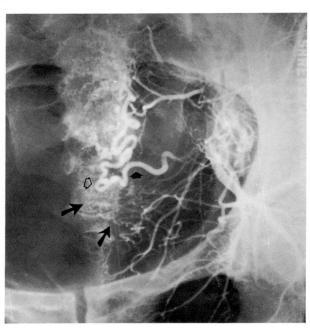

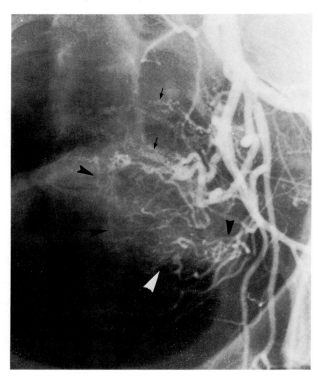

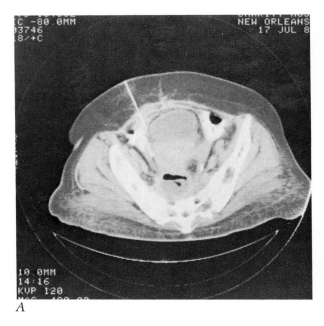

A

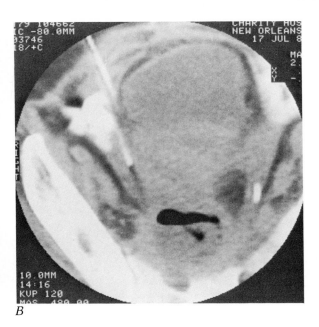

B

Figure 73-31. (A and B) A transperitoneal percutaneous thin-needle biopsy obtains material from a mass contiguously extending from the cervix uteri into the parametrium. The biopsy was performed under CT control. Documentation of the precise site from which the biopsy has been obtained is of paramount importance to validate the histopathologic diagnosis and particularly to authenticate a negative biopsy.

Figure 73-32. (A) An early stain is seen in two nodes of the obturator group (*small arrows*). A dense tumor stain and neovascularity supplied from the internal pudendal artery help identify a tumor implant at the vaginal introitus (*large arrows*). (B) Delayed roentgenograms recording the venous phase demonstrate several more staining nodes along the path of the veins draining the metastatic implant to the vaginal introitus (*arrows*). Dissemination of the neoplasm via these draining veins is suggested.

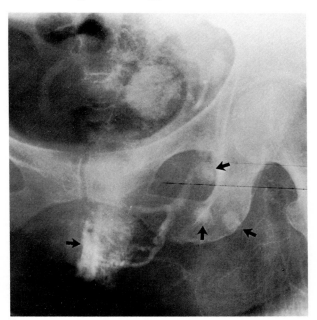

B

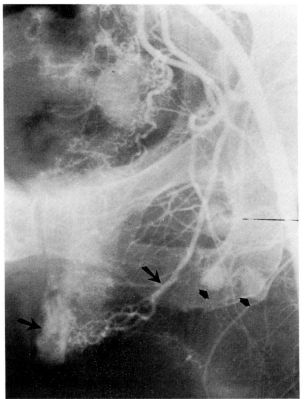

A

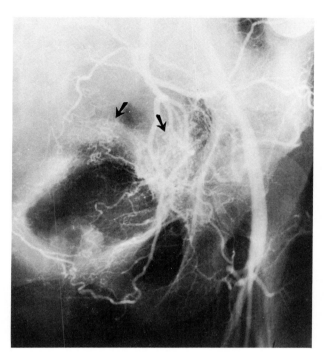

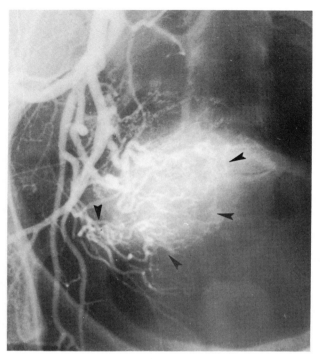

Figure 73-33. Bimanual examination suggested fixation of the right parametrium in this patient treated by surgery and radiation therapy for a stage 2A carcinoma of the cervix. The arteriogram unequivocally demonstrates tumor neovascularity in the region of the left parametrium as well as involving the dome of the bladder and right bladder wall and establishes the diagnosis of recurrence rather than radiation-induced fibrosis (*arrows*).

Figure 73-34. Tumor neovascularity and a tumor stain are seen lateral to the vaginal fornix (*arrowheads*), establishing the diagnosis of carcinoma of the cervix with extension into the parametrium. Physical examination in the patient was handicapped by postsurgical fibrosis attendant on a prior supracervical hysterectomy. (From Lang et al. [75].)

(Fig. 73-33). Similarly, arteriography is the best modality to differentiate extension of a carcinoma of the cervix from postsurgical fibrosis in patients with prior supracervical hysterectomy. The mass attributable to postsurgical fibrosis is avascular, whereas a carcinoma of the cervix will feature characteristic tumor neovascularity [71, 74, 106] (Fig. 73-34).

Arteriography in the Diagnosis of Pelvic Hemorrhage

Massive extraperitoneal hemorrhage is a common and not infrequently fatal complication of pelvic trauma [3, 4, 16, 31, 58, 70, 84, 96, 100, 101, 103–105, 120]. About 65 percent of patients who die as a result of pelvic fractures exsanguinate from related hemorrhage [103]. Postmortem injection studies have demonstrated

multiple lacerations of small and medium-sized arteries and veins [31]. Surgical ligation of the proximal internal iliac artery has only limited effect because of abundant collaterals [18, 27, 31, 97]. However, the risk of incising the retroperitoneum is substantial since loss of this tissue barrier may release the tamponade, which is often the only effective force of hemostasis for venous bleeding [97, 99, 101, 103, 105].

Aortography and selective arteriography of the pelvic vessels permit identification of the bleeding sites and assessment of the magnitude of vascular injury and hematomas and—according to recent publications—can be expanded to control hemorrhage by transcatheter embolization with autologous blood clot or inert embolic material [3, 4, 6, 16, 31, 93, 100, 101, 107, 116].

In addition to external trauma, pelvic hemorrhage may be caused by advanced pelvic neoplasms; childbirth; or iatrogenic injury accompanying transurethral resections of the prostate,

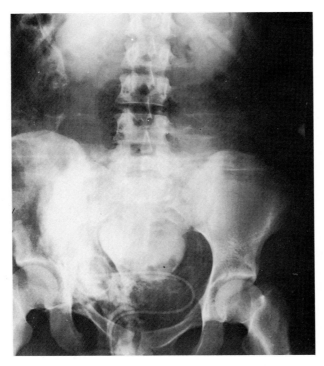

Figure 73-35. Extravasation of contrast medium on a cystogram indicates extraperitoneal and intraperitoneal rupture of the bladder. Moreover, the bladder is displaced from its normal position by an enormous hematoma.

orthopedic surgery such as total hip replacement, or radiation therapy [2, 15, 17, 28, 33, 41, 44–46, 73, 94, 100, 108, 113, 116].

TECHNIQUE

A Seldinger approach via the axillary artery is favored for the examination of patients who have sustained pelvic trauma. A flush aortogram is recommended for initial study. Superselective arteriograms are then obtained for detailed assessment of the vascular injury and in preparation for transcatheter embolization (Figs. 73-35–73-37).

The propensity for injury of the medial circumflex femoral artery attendant on hip replacement surgery calls for study of the common iliac artery to adequately demonstrate this bleeding site [100] (Figs. 73-38, 73-39).

Intractable hemorrhage with advanced pelvic neoplasms or occurring as a complication of transurethral resection of the prostate or following radiation therapy is attributable to diffuse bleeds and hence necessitates study of the anterior divisions of both hypogastric arteries to establish the extent of involvement [2, 28, 44, 71, 73, 113] (Figs. 73-40–73-42).

Figure 73-36. Superselective arteriogram of the right superior vesical artery shows puddling of contrast medium, identifying several of the bleeding sites in this patient, who sustained extensive pelvic injury.

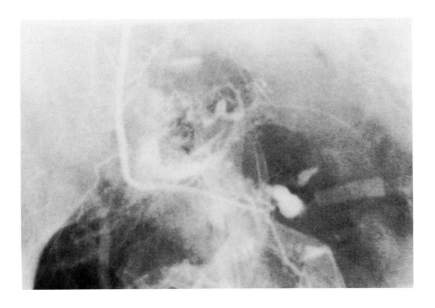

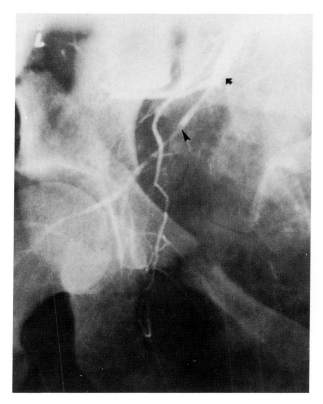

Figure 73-37. After selective transcatheter embolization of the right superior vesical, internal pudendal,
and obturator arteries with Gelfoam particles, a control arteriogram demonstrates appropriate occlusion
of all vessels of the anterior division of the hypogastric artery leading to the bleeding sites (*arrow, arrowhead*).

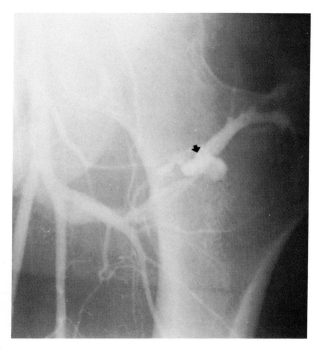

Figure 73-38. An injection of the common femoral
artery demonstrates a pseudoaneurysm (*arrow*) and
active bleeding from the left medial circumflex
femoral artery as a consequence of iatrogenic injury
sustained during surgery on the joint capsule. Note
premature opacification of a draining vein attesting to
the presence of an arteriovenous fistula.

Figure 73-39. Following superselective transcatheter
embolization of the offensive branch of the medial circumflex femoral artery with autologous blood clot
(*arrow*) and placement of a wire coil (*arrowhead*) in the
main segment of the medial circumflex femoral artery,
there is evidence neither of further extravasation of
contrast medium nor of flow through the arteriovenous fistula on the control arteriogram.

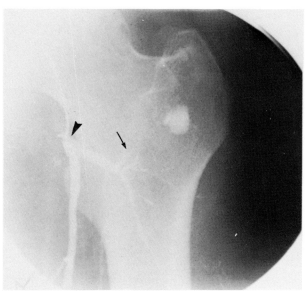

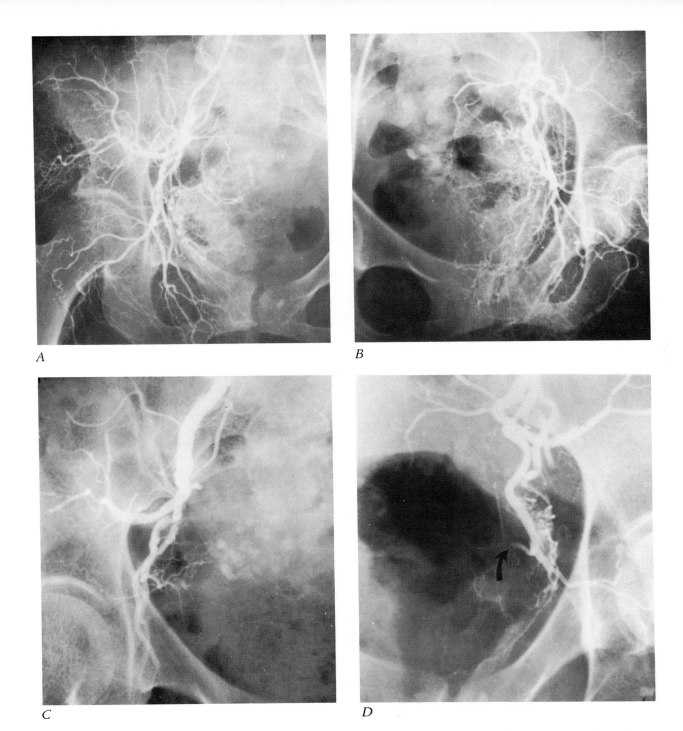

A

B

C

D

Figure 73-40. (A) Selective arteriogram of the anterior division of the right hypogastric artery demonstrates extensive tumor neovascularity involving the entire right half of the bladder. This was attributable to carcinoma of the cervix contiguously extending into the bladder and causing intractable hemorrhage from the bladder. (From Lang et al. [73].) (B) Selective arteriogram of the anterior division of the left hypogastric artery demonstrates identical tumor neovascularity involving the left half of the bladder. (C) Following transcatheter embolization of the branches of the anterior division of the right hypogastric artery with 2 ×

2 × 2-mm Gelfoam particles, the control arteriogram demonstrates occlusion of all tumor vessels and branches of the anterior division but unimpaired flow to the branches of the posterior division of the right hypogastric group. (D) Control arteriogram following a similar transcatheter embolization of the anterior division of the left hypogastric artery shows identical results (*arrow*). The vast collateral network in the pelvis permits embolization of the anterior divisions of both hypogastric arteries without fear of causing necrosis of the bladder.

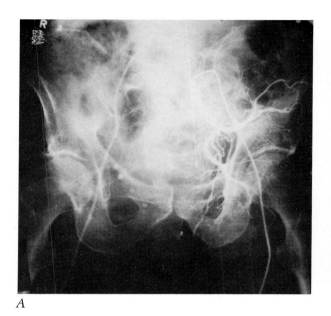

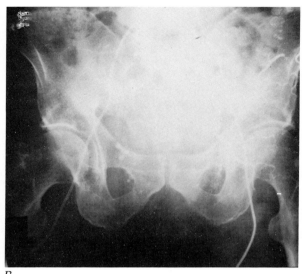

A

B

Figure 73-41. (A) Selective arteriogram of the right hypogastric group demonstrates extravasation of contrast medium in the prostatic fossa. (B) Following transcatheter embolization of both right and left hypogastric arteries, the control arteriogram demonstrates truncation of the feeding arteries and there is no longer evidence of extravasation of contrast medium. The intractable hemorrhage following transurethral resection was controlled by this intervention. (From Faysal [28].)

Figure 73-42. Telangiectatic vessels are seen throughout the bladder (*arrows*). These are felt to be responsible for intractable hemorrhage from innumerable bleeding points, a not uncommon complication of external radiation therapy to bladder neoplasms. (From Lang [67].)

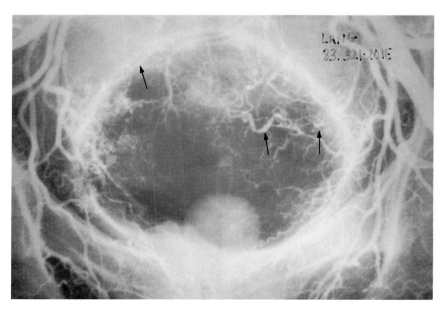

Interventional Arteriography in the Pelvis

The need for selective delivery of highly toxic chemotherapeutic agents first led to the development of superselective catheterization of pelvic vessels [20, 68, 81]. Soon the potential of this technique for selective delivery of embolic material was recognized and its application expanded to the management of pelvic hemorrhage [2–4, 17, 28, 31, 41–43, 46, 72, 73, 84, 87, 88, 93, 94, 100, 101, 107, 108, 113, 114, 116, 120]. Most recently transluminal angioplasty has assumed a prominent role among interventional arteriographic techniques practiced in the pelvic region [33].

Transcatheter Embolization in Management of Patients with Uncontrollable Hemorrhage from Pelvic Organs

The aim of transcatheter embolization in the management of intractable bleeding from pelvic organs is control of hemorrhage and stabilization of the patient without permanent disruption of vascular perfusion and risk of irreversible tissue infarction. To achieve this goal, disruption of blood flow needs to be restricted to the smallest branch vessel effectively curtailing hemorrhage yet not likely to embarrass collateral perfusion. Embolization of vessels at the level of the capillary bed eliminates collateral flow via the precapillary plexus and can result in massive tissue necrosis [15, 49]. To avoid this complication, transcatheter embolization is directed at vessels at the arteriolar level. Appropriate choice of the size and characteristics of the embolic material assures lodging in vessels of the desired size. If later restoration of vascular continuity is desired, embolic material prone to dissolution is chosen [72].

TECHNIQUE

Once the site of hemorrhage is defined on the aortograms, the catheter is advanced under fluoroscopic guidance first into the hypogastric artery and then into its anterior division and/or its branches.

Pharmacologic manipulation of blood flow may be useful to locate bleeding sites and to channel infarct particles into the bleeding vessels. Intraarterial administration of vasoconstrictors such as epinephrine hydrochloride in a dose rate of 5 to 20 μg or vasopressin at a dose rate of 0.05 unit per minute will cause constriction of the normal vascular bed without eliciting a similar response from bleeding vessels. Thus, a preferential flow to bleeding vessels can be created.

Material used for embolization is determined by the size of the vessel to be embolized and whether permanent, semipermanent or short-time occlusion is desired [72, 125]. Autologous blood clot has the advantages of nonantigenicity, ready availability, conformity to the vessel size, and lysis within 8 to 24 hours [3, 17, 31, 41, 44, 58, 72, 100, 105, 116, 120, 125]. The last characteristic makes this the embolic material of choice if later restoration of vascular continuity is desired, as in patients treated for intractable bleeding following orthopedic surgery, transurethral resection of the prostate, puerperal hemorrhage, or hemorrhage secondary to pelvic trauma.

Gelfoam is the most readily available substance suitable for semipermanent occlusion of vessels. In general, Gelfoam is used in the form of small cubes of about 2 × 2 × 2 mm that are suspended in a mixture of saline and contrast medium. Admixed contrast medium facilitates fluoroscopic observation of migration and lodging of Gelfoam particles. Though the cubes of Gelfoam may fragment, collateral flow via the precapillary collaterals is generally maintained [43, 72].

Ivalon (polyvinyl alcohol) is not subject to fragmentation and therefore, if administered in the form of 2 × 2 × 2-mm cubes, tends to lodge in small arteries and virtually assures collateral circulation via the precapillary plexus [125].

Isobutyl 2-cyanoacrylate monomer is a compound favored for occlusion of larger-caliber vessels. The rapid setting of the monomer assures lodging of the embolus in medium-sized arteries and hence unimpaired collateral circulation via the precapillary plexus [32, 39, 125].

If larger vessels such as the main hypogastric artery have to be occluded, detachable balloons, wire coils, or small vascular umbrellas are favored [36, 72, 122, 124].

Clinical Situations Amenable to Management by Transcatheter Embolization

TRAUMATIC HEMORRHAGE

The contraindication to surgical exploration of the retroperitoneal space in patients who have sustained pelvic trauma is attendant loss of tamponading effect, the only force effectively curtailing venous bleeding. This important fact plus the known failure of proximal ligation of the hypogastric artery to control pelvic hemorrhage makes transcatheter embolization with autologous blood clot the method of choice in the management of traumatic pelvic hemorrhage [3, 4, 6, 18, 27, 31, 58, 72, 84, 93, 96, 97, 99, 101, 103–105, 107, 120].

Superselective embolization of the responsible branch with autologous clot is favored to minimize the volume of tissue deprived of its primary vascular supply and to retain some collateral perfusion via the precapillary collateral vessels. Pharmacologic manipulation of flow by intraarterial administration of epinephrine hydrochloride constricts normal arterioles and hence protects normal tissues against embolization while promoting lodging of autologous clots in medium-sized arteries leading to the bleeding sites. This in turn fosters maintenance of some collateral circulation via the precapillary plexus. Maintenance of collateral perfusion and use of embolic material prone to lysis and therefore resulting in later restoration of vascular continuity are important in the prevention of tissue necrosis, which is fostered by the frequently concurrent venous thrombosis [16, 72, 99].

The relationship between specific fracture sites and injury to specific vessels facilitates the task of limiting embolization to a branch artery [100] (see Fig. 73-37). If, however, the bleeding vessel is not identifiable, embolization should be limited to the anterior division of the hypogastric artery on the side of the fracture, which on the basis of probability should give origin to the responsible bleeding branch. Embolization of the posterior division of the hypogastric arteries should be avoided because of intolerance of the gluteal muscle mass to deprivation of vascular supply and infrequency of bleeding from its radicles [72, 73].

Transcatheter embolization with inert embolic material has also been used in the management of intractable puerperal hemorrhage [17, 46].

The technique is equally applicable to the treatment of hemorrhage attendant on transurethral resections and refractory to conventional treatment of this complication [28, 44, 66, 88, 94, 114] (see Fig. 73-41). Contrary to the restricted embolization advocated in the management of traumatic hemorrhage, intractable hemorrhage following transurethral resection calls for embolization of the anterior divisions of both hypogastric arteries, preferably again with autologous blood clot [28, 44, 72, 88, 94].

Intractable hemorrhage occurring as a complication of orthopedic procedures can often be traced to bleeding from a specific branch artery [100] (see Figs. 73-38, 73-39). Superselective engagement and embolization of the branch artery with autologous blood clot is the recommended treatment [72].

In patients with intractable hemorrhage from the bladder attributable to pelvic neoplasms, specific bleeding sites can seldom be identified [71–73, 114]. Generally, arteriograms demonstrate contiguous extension of tumor from or to adjacent organs, creating an extensive parasitic collateral network [41, 49, 71–73, 87, 108, 114] (see Fig. 73-40A). For these reasons, all branches of the anterior division of the hypogastric arteries must be embolized (see Fig. 73-40B, C, D). The abundant parasitic precapillary network safeguards against avascular necrosis of the bladder [15, 49]. Because of the presence of extensive neoplastic neovascularity a more permanent type of occlusion is desirable, and Gelfoam or Ivalon cubes are the embolic material of choice.

Intractable hemorrhage from the bladder following radiation therapy and attributable to telangiectatic vessels diffusely involving the entire bladder is, likewise, best managed by embolization of all branches of the anterior division of both hypogastric arteries [45, 66, 77] (see Fig. 73-42). Once again, one must safeguard against avascular necrosis of the bladder, a protection that is assured by use of 2 × 2 × 2-mm Ivalon cubes guaranteed to lodge in small arteries, hence preserving precapillary collateral flow [15, 49]. In elderly and specifically diabetic and arteriosclerotic patients, the vascular supply of the inferior mesenteric artery must be studied, since necrosis of the colon can result if this organ depends on the collateral supply from the hypogastric arteries slated for embolization [18, 115, 117] (see Fig. 73-5).

The specific bleeding site is usually identifiable

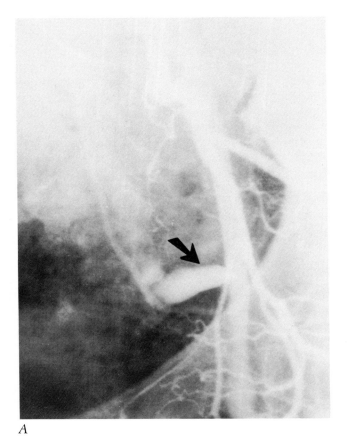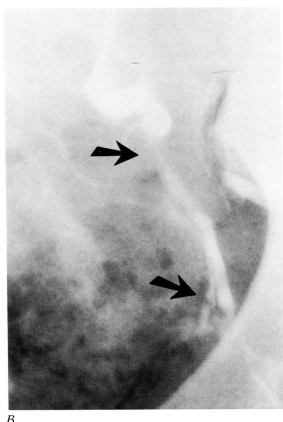

A   B

Figure 73-43. (A) The 1-second arteriogram demon-strates massive extravasation of contrast medium into a huge necrotic carcinoma of the cervix (*arrow*). (B) A control arteriogram after transcatheter embolization with 2 × 2 × 2-mm Gelfoam particles demonstrates satisfactory occlusion of all branches of the anterior division of the left hypogastric artery (*arrows*). Unilat-eral embolization of the offensive branch satisfactorily controlled bleeding. (From Lang [72].)

if hemorrhage occurs from a tumor of the female genital organs [71–73, 113]. Thus embolization can be limited to the offensive vessel or vessel group [2, 87, 113, 114] (Fig. 73-43). Gelfoam or Ivalon cubes are once again the material of choice for the reasons already discussed. In general, the resultant reduction of pressure will cause cessa-tion of hemorrhage. However, in isolated cases embolization of the contralateral anterior division of the hypogastric artery may become necessary to reduce blood flow and pulse pressure further and stop the hemorrhage.

In some instances, transcatheter embolization with radioactive particles may be chosen to treat the neoplasm by high-dose interstitial radiation therapy [69] (Fig. 73-44A, B). Since effective-ness of radiation depends on oxygenation of the tumor tissue, a minimum number of sources must be used to avoid creation of a hypoxic milieu [69].

Transcatheter embolization of arteriovenous malformations involving the bladder yields only limited success. While the initial response to transcatheter embolization with inert embolic material is uniformly favorable, the propensity of such malformations to derive supply from practi-cally all pelvic vessels will generally deny long-term improvement [73] (see Figs. 73-20–73-22). Only total embolization of all small vessels of the arteriovenous malformation itself with Gelfoam powder or isobutyl 2-cyanoacrylate monomer can obliterate this kind of malformation [32]. The technique is fraught with the danger of transmis-sion of the material through the high-flow ar-teriovenous malformation and resultant emboli-zation of the pulmonary vascular bed.

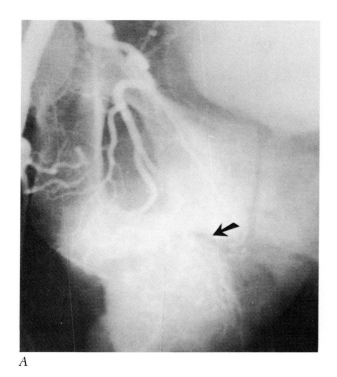

A

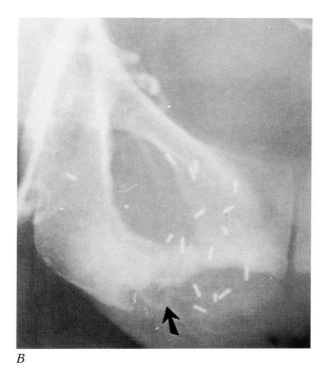

B

Figure 73-44. (A) Intensive tumor neovascularity supplied predominantly from the right internal pudendal and obturator arteries outlines a huge metastasis to the right labium from a carcinoma of the cervix (*arrow*). (B) Transcatheter embolization with radon gold seeds was chosen for treatment of this debilitated octogenarian. The resultant infarct implant delivered a high dose of radiation therapy to the tumor-bearing area (interstitial implant), which caused marked regression in the size of the tumor and reepithelialization of denuded and excoriated areas. On this radiograph obtained 3 months later, there is even evidence of remineralization of a metastatic lesion involving the ischial ramus (*arrow*).

Selective Chemotherapeutic Perfusion

Systemic toxicity of many chemotherapeutic agents has made it necessary to isolate and perfuse selectively the vascular system of a tumor [20, 40, 68, 81, 82]. Surgical isolation of the arterial and venous circulation of pelvic organs or the hind quarter is a difficult and cumbersome task. The availability of chemotherapeutic agents bound to protein to a large extent during their first tissue passage makes possible limitation of both therapeutic and toxic effects to a confined volume of tissue by restriction of the arterial distribution of the chemotherapeutic agent. Superselective catheterization of the vessels supplying the tumor and placement of an indwelling perfusion catheter offer a minimally invasive solution to the problem of isolated organ perfusion (Fig. 73-45). Continued infusion of the chemotherapeutic agents at a constant rate is readily accomplished by use of a one-way valve and slow-flow pump [40]. The effect of chemotherapy can then be monitored by follow-up arteriograms (Fig. 73-45B).

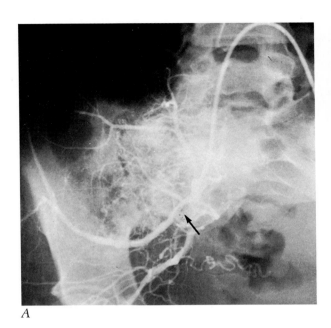

A

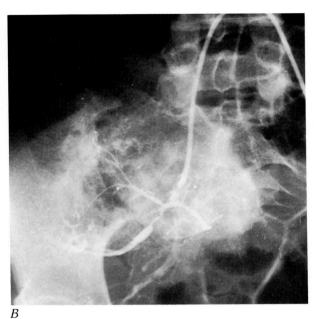

B

Figure 73-45. (A) Superselective arteriogram of the posterior division of the right hypogastric artery demonstrates encasement of the midgluteal artery (*arrow*) and intense tumor neovascularity in a mass involving the right sacroiliac joint and sacrum. (B) Following selective perfusion with bleomycin for 20 days, a control arteriogram demonstrates remarkable changes. The tumor has shrunk considerably and is now hypovascular. The previously noted encasement of the midgluteal artery is more pronounced, perhaps secondary to cicatricial changes; all vessels are much smaller, reflecting the reduced flow.

Pelvic Venography

Pelvic venography is useful for assessment of pelvic vein thrombosis, a common source of pulmonary emboli, for determining traumatic injury of pelvic veins, and for staging of pelvic neoplasms [26, 30, 99].

Transfemoral catheterization of the external and common iliac veins and then retrograde injection into the internal iliac veins usually render adequate demonstration of the pelvic venous system to establish or exclude the diagnosis of pelvic vein thrombosis.

Detailed demonstration of uterine, parametrial, and internal pudendal veins, however, is necessary to stage neoplasms arising from the female genital organs. Transvaginal insertion of a needle into the myometrium and injection of contrast medium constitute the best technique for visualizing uterine and parametrial veins and

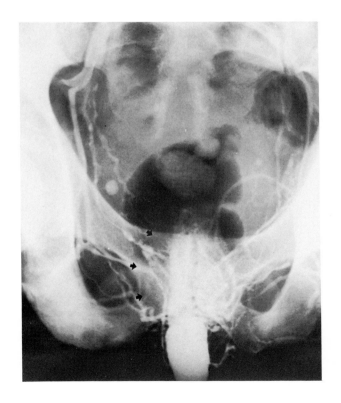

Figure 73-46. Transperineal injection of prostatic veins shows notable absence of filling of the right prostatic and pampiniform plexus. This was proved to be attributable to a carcinoma of the prostate extending through the capsule (*arrows*).

demonstrating direct invasion or encasement of these veins by tumor.

Cannulation of the dorsal vein of the penis or direct injection into the prostatic or pampiniform plexus offers optimal visualization of the perivesical and prostatic venous plexus and internal pudendal vein in the male [26, 30]. Demonstration of filling defects within the veins or frank amputation is a significant indicator of early tumor extension and invasion through the prostatic capsule [26] (Fig. 73-46). Unfortunately, inflammatory disease can cause indistinguishable encasement and amputation of veins, limiting the usefulness of this procedure. Displacement of the internal pudendal vein may reflect the presence of a primary tumor mass or large metastatic nodes.

References

1. Abelson, D.   Diagnostic value of the penile pulse and blood pressure: A Doppler study of impotence in diabetics. *J. Urol.* 113:636, 1975.
2. Athanasoulis, C. A., Waltman, A. C., Barnes, A. B., and Herbst, A. L.   Angiographic control of pelvic bleeding from treated carcinoma of the cervix. *Gynecol. Oncol.* 4:144, 1976.
3. Ayella, R. J., DuPriest, R. W., Jr., Khaneja, S. C., Maekawa, K., Sonderstrom, C. A., Rodriguez, A., and Cowley, R. A.   Transcatheter embolization of autologous clot in the management of bleeding associated with fractures of the pelvis. *Surg. Gynecol. Obstet.* 147:849, 1978.
4. Barlow, B., Rottenberg, R. W., and Santulli, T. V.   Angiographic diagnosis and treatment of bleeding by selective embolization following pelvic fracture in children. *J. Pediatr. Surg.* 10:939, 1975.
5. Batalden, D. J., Wickstrom, P. H., Ruiz, E., and Gustila, R. B.   Value of the G suit in patients with severe pelvic fracture: Controlling hemorrhage shock. *Arch. Surg.* 109:326, 1974.
6. Borell, U., and Fernström, I.   The adnexal branches of the uterine artery: An arteriographic study in human subjects. *Acta Radiol.* (Stockh.) 40:561, 1953.
7. Borell, U., and Fernström, I.   The ovarian artery: An arteriographic study in human subjects. *Acta Radiol.* (Stockh.) 42:253, 1954.
8. Borell, U., and Fernström, I.   Hydatidiform mole diagnosed by pelvic angiography. *Acta Radiol.* (Stockh.) 56:113, 1961.
9. Borell, U., Fernström, I., Lindblom, K., and Westman, A.   The diagnostic value of arteriography of the iliac artery in gynaecology and obstetrics. *Acta Radiol.* (Stockh.) 38:247, 1952.
10. Borell, U., Fernström, I., Moberger, G., and Ohlson, L.   *The Diagnosis of Hydatidiform Mole, Malignant Hydatidiform Mole and Choriocarcinoma with Special Reference to the Diagnostic Value of Pelvic Arteriography.* Springfield, Ill.: Thomas, 1966.
11. Borell, U., Fernström, I., and Ohlson, L.   Diagnostic value of arteriography in cases of placenta previa. *Am. J. Obstet. Gynecol.* 86:535, 1963.
12. Borell, U., Fernström, I., and Westman, A.   The value of pelvic arteriography in the diagnosis of mole and chorionepithelioma. *Acta Radiol.* (Stockh.) 44:378, 1955.
13. Bowie, J. D., Rochester, D., Cadkin, A. V., Cooke, W. T., and Kuuzman, A.   Accuracy of placental localization by ultrasound. *Radiology* 128:177, 1978.
14. Braedel, H. U., and Krauntzun, K.   Die Gefässdarstellung bösartiger Harnblasengeschwülste unter besonderer Berüksichtigung ihrer örtlichen Ausbreitung. *ROEFO* 100:209, 1964.
15. Braf, Z. F., and Koontz, W. W., Jr.   Gangrene of bladder: Complication of hypogastric artery embolization. *Urology* 9:670, 1977.
16. Braunstein, P. W., Skudder, P. A., McCarroll, J. R., Musolino, A., and Wade, P. A.   Concealed hemorrhage due to pelvic fracture. *J. Trauma* 4:832, 1964.
17. Brown, B., Heaston, D. K., Poulson, A. M., Gabert, H. A., Mineau, D. E., and Miller, F. J., Jr.   Uncontrollable postpartum bleeding: A new approach to hemostasis through angiographic arterial embolization. *Obstet. Gynecol.* 54:361, 1979.
18. Burchell, R. C.   Physiology of internal iliac artery ligation. *J. Obstet. Gynaecol. Br. Commonw.* 75:642, 1968.
19. Callen, P. W.   Computed tomographic evaluation of abdominal and pelvic abscesses. *Radiology* 131:171, 1979.
20. Cavanaugh, D., Horadhanakul, P., and Comas, M. R.   Regional chemotherapy—a comparison of pelvic perfusion and intra-arterial infusion in patients with advanced gynecologic cancer. *Am. J. Obstet. Gynecol.* 123:435, 1975.
21. Christenson, R. R., Smith, C. W., and Burko, H.   Arteriographic manifestations of pheochromocytoma. *AJR* 126:567, 1976.
22. Cockshott, W. P., Evans, K. T., and Hendrickse, J. P. DeV.   Arteriography of trophoblastic tumors. *Clin. Radiol.* 15:1, 1964.
23. Conrad, M. R., Davis, G. M., Green, C. E., and Curry, T. S., III.   Real time ultrasound in the diagnosis of acute dissecting aneurysm of the abdominal aorta. *AJR* 132:115, 1979.
24. Cummins, B. H., Hill, S., Path, M. C., and Williams, J. L.   Pheochromocytoma of the urinary bladder. *Br. J. Urol.* 41:71, 1969.

25. Deklerk, D. P., Catalona, W. J., Nime, F. A., and Freeman, C.   Malignant pheochromocytoma of the bladder: Late development of renal cell carcinoma. *J. Urol.* 113:864, 1975.

26. Drosdovskij, B. J., Zyb, A. F., and Duntschik, W. N.   Beckenphlebographie mit Kontrastmittelinjektionen in die Vena dorsalis penis profunda zur Beunteilung der Ausdehnung von Blasen- und Prostata-Carcinomen. *Radiologe* 17: 124, 1977.

27. Fahmy, K.   Internal iliac artery ligation and its efficiency in controlling pelvic hemorrhage. *Int. Surg.* 51:244, 1969.

28. Faysal, M.   Angiographic management of post-prostatectomy bleeding. *J. Urol.* 122:129, 1979.

29. Fernström, I.   Arteriography of the uterine artery. *Acta Radiol.* [*Suppl.*] (Stockh.) 122:1, 1955.

30. Fitzpatrick, T. J.   Venography of the deep dorsal venous and valvular systems. *J. Urol.* 111:518, 1974.

31. Flint, L. M., Jr., Brown, A., Richardson, J. D., and Polk, H. C.   Definitive control of bleeding from severe pelvic fractures. *Ann. Surg.* 189:709, 1979.

32. Freeny, P. C., Bush, W. H., Jr., and Kidd, R.   Transcatheter occlusive therapy of genitourinary abnormalities using isobutyl 2-cyanoacrylate (bucrylate). *AJR* 133:647, 1979.

33. Frieman, D. B., Ring, E. J., Oleaga, J. A., Berkowitz, H., and Roberts, B.   Transluminal angioplasty of the iliac, femoral and popliteal arteries. *Radiology* 132:285, 1979.

34. Fuleihan, F. M., and Cordonnier, J. J.   Hemangioma of the bladder: Report of a case and review of the literature. *J. Urol.* 102:581, 1969.

35. Fuselier, H. A., Jr.   Paraganglioma of the bladder: Report of a case. *J. Urol.* 113:42, 1975.

36. Gianturco, C., Anderson, J. H., and Wallace, S.   Mechanical devices for arterial occlusion. *AJR* 124:428, 1975.

37. Gibod, L. B.   L'impuissance sexuelle organique. Problèmes diagnostiques. Possibilités thérapeutiques (English abstract). *Nouv. Presse Med.* 7:4221, 1978.

38. Ginestié, J., and Romieu, A.   Traitement des impuissances d'origine vasculaire. La revascularisation des corps caverneux (English abstract). *J. Urol. Nephrol.* (Paris) 82:853, 1976.

39. Goldin, A. R., Barnes, D. R., and Jacobsen, I.   Percutaneous infarction of renal tumors: Comparison between gelatin sponge embolization and cyanoacrylate occlusion. *Urology* 11:197, 1978.

40. Goldman, M. L., Bilbao, M. K., Rösch, J., and Dotter, C. T.   Complications of indwelling chemotherapy catheters. *Cancer* 36:1983, 1975.

41. Goldstein, H. M., Meddlin, H., Ben-Manachem, Y., and Wallace, S.   Transcatheter arterial embolization in the management of bleeding in the cancer patient. *Radiology* 115:603, 1975.

42. Grace, D. M., Pitt, D. F., and Gold, R. E.   Vascular embolization and occlusion by angiographic techniques as an aid or alternative to operation. *Surg. Gynecol. Obstet.* 143:469, 1976.

43. Greenfield, A. J., Athanasoulis, C. A., Waltman, A. C., and LeMoure, E. R.   Transcatheter embolization: Prevention of embolic reflux using balloon catheters. *AJR* 131:651, 1978.

44. Hald, T., and Mygind, T.   Control of life-threatening vesical hemorrhage by unilateral hypogastric artery muscle embolization. *J. Urol.* 112:60, 1974.

45. Hassler, O., and Hietala, S. O.   Angiographic abnormalities in the urinary bladder wall after irradiation: I. Animal experiments; II. Clinical investigations. *Acta Radiol.* [*Suppl.*] (Stockh.) 328:1, 1973.

46. Heaston, D. K., Mineau, D. E., Brown, B. J., and Miller, F. J., Jr.   Transcatheter arterial embolization for control of persistent massive puerperal hemorrhage after bilateral surgical hypogastric artery ligation. *AJR* 133:152, 1979.

47. Hendrickse, J. P. deV., Cockshott, W. P., Evans, K. T. E., and Barton, C. J.   Pelvic arteriography in the diagnosis of malignant trophoblastic disease. *N. Engl. J. Med.* 271:859, 1964.

48. Herman, A., Adar, R., and Rubinstein, Z.   Vascular lesions associated with impotence in diabetic and non-diabetic arterial occlusive disease. *Diabetes* 27:975, 1978.

49. Hietala, S. O.   Urinary bladder necrosis following selective embolization of the internal iliac artery. *Acta Radiol.* [*Diagn.*] (Stockh.) 19:316, 1978.

50. Hietala, S. O., and Duchek, M.   Angiography in urinary bladder tuberculosis. *Acta Radiol.* [*Diagn.*] (Stockh.) 16:297, 1975.

51. Hietala, S. O., Ghahremani, G. G., Faunce, H. F., and Yaghmai, I.   Radiologic manifestations of pelvic lipomatosis. *Radiologe* 17:130, 1977.

52. Hietala, S. O., and Hazra, T.   Angiography in vesical and perivesical neoplastic and non-neoplastic lesions. *Acta Radiol.* [*Diagn.*] (Stockh.) 19:447, 1978.

53. Hietala, S. O., Texter, J. H., Jr., and Crane, D. B.   Angiography in pheochromocytoma of the urinary bladder: Report of a case. *Acta Radiol.* [*Diagn.*] (Stockh.) 18:313, 1977.

54. Jaques, P. F., Staab, E., Richey, W., Photopulos, G., and Swanton, M.   CT-assisted pelvic and abdominal aspiration biopsies in gynecological malignancy. *Radiology* 128:651, 1978.

55. Javaheri, P., and Raafat, J.   Malignant phaeochromocytoma of the urinary bladder—report of 2 cases. *Br. J. Urol.* 47:401, 1975.

56. Johnson, D. E., Kaesler, K. E., Kaminsky, S., Jing, B. S., and Wallace, S. Lymphangiography as an aid in staging of bladder cancer. *South. Med. J.* 69:28, 1976.

57. Jones, E. A., and Alexander, M. K. Idiopathic retroperitoneal fibrosis associated with arteritis. *Ann. Rheum. Dis.* 25:356, 1966.

58. Kakish, L. J., Stein, J. M., Kotler, S., Mang, C. I. T., and Barlow, B. Angiographic diagnosis in treatment of bleeding due to pelvic trauma. *J. Trauma* 13:1083, 1973.

59. Kauppila, A., Jouppila, P., Suramo, I., and Vehaskari, A. Pelvic arteriography in the diagnosis of malignant trophoblastic disease. *Ann. Chir. Gynaecol.* 63:130, 1974.

60. Kees, C. J. Angiographic staining and hypervascularity in a case of fibrous retroperitonitis. *Radiology* 113:329, 1974.

61. Kelâmi and Taenzer, B. Fehlinterpretationen, bei der Harnblasenangiographie. *Urol. Int.* 24:349, 1969.

62. Kempezinski, R. F. The role of the vascular diagnostic laboratory in the evaluation of male impotence. *Am. J. Surg.* 138:278, 1979.

63. Klein, T. W., and Kaplan, T. W. Klippel-Trenaunay syndrome associated with urinary tract hemangiomas. *J. Urol.* 114:596, 1975.

64. Kolstad, P., and Liverud, K. Pelvic arteriography in malignant trophoblastic neoplasia. *Am. J. Obstet. Gynecol.* 105:175, 1969.

65. Korobkin, M., Callen, P. W., and Fisch, A. E. Computed tomography of the pelvis and retroperitoneum. *Radiol. Clin. North Am.* 17:301, 1979.

66. Kumar, A. P. M., Wrenn, E. L., Jr., Jayalakshmamma, B., Conrad, L., Quinn, P., and Cox, C. Silver nitrate irrigation to control bladder hemorrhage in children receiving cancer therapy. *J. Urol.* 116:85, 1976.

67. Lang, E. K. Roentgenographic assessment of bladder tumors: A comparison of diagnostic accuracy of roentgenographic techniques. *Cancer* 23:717, 1969.

68. Lang, E. K. Superselective arterial catheterization of tumors of the urogenital tract: A modality used for perfusion of chemotherapeutic agents and infarction with radioactive pellets. *J. Urol.* 104:16, 1970.

69. Lang, E. K. Locoregional treatment of neoplasms by radioactive infarct particles introduced via arterial catheterization. *Panminerva Med.* 17:398, 1975.

70. Lang, E. K. The role of arteriography in trauma. *Radiol. Clin. North Am.* 14:353, 1976.

71. Lang, E. K. Angiography in the diagnosis of pelvic neoplasms. *Radiology* 134:353, 1980.

72. Lang, E. K. Redefinition of goals and techniques of transcatheter embolization of pelvic vessels for control of intractable hemorrhage. *Radiology* 140:331, 1981.

73. Lang, E. K., Deutsch, J. S., Goodman, J. R., Barnett, T. S., LaNasa, J., and Duplessis, G. H. Transcatheter embolization of hypogastric branch arteries in management of intractable bladder hemorrhage. *J. Urol.* 121:30, 1979.

74. Lang, E. K., and Greer, J. L. The value of pelvic arteriography for the staging of carcinoma of the cervix. *Radiology* 92:1027, 1969.

75. Lang, E. K., Simon, K. J., Cummings, D. H., Byrd, E. H., Jr., Moore, H. E., Tannehill, R. H., West, W. C., Jr., Tate, W. B., Brooks, G. G., and Dilworth, E. E. Arteriography, pelvic pneumography and lymphangiography augmenting assessments and staging of carcinoma of the cervix. *South. Med. J.* 63:1249, 1970.

76. Lang, E. K., Wishard, W. N., Jr., Nourse, M., and Mertz, J. H. O. Retrograde arteriography in diagnosis of bladder tumors. *Trans. Am. Assoc. Genitourin. Surg.* 54:15, 1962.

77. Lapides, J. Treatment of delayed intractable hemorrhagic cystitis following radiation or chemotherapy. *J. Urol.* 104:707, 1970.

78. Lee, J. K. T., Stanley, R. J., Sagel, S., and McClenan, B. L. Accuracy of CT in detecting intra-abdominal and pelvic lymph node metastases from pelvic cancers. *AJR* 131:675, 1978.

79. Leestma, J. R., and Price, E. B., Jr. Paraganglioma of the urinary bladder. *Cancer* 28:1063, 1971.

80. Levi, S., and Delval, R. Value of ultrasonic diagnosis of gynecological tumors in 370 surgical cases. *Acta Obstet. Gynecol. Scand.* 55:261, 1976.

81. Lifshitz, S., Railsback, L. D., and Buchsbaum, H. J. Intra-arterial pelvic infusion chemotherapy in advanced gynecologic cancer. *Obstet. Gynecol.* 52:476, 1978.

82. Liukko, P., Gronroos, M., Satokari, K., and Pitkancy, T. Pelvic angiography in the follow-up of chorioadenoma destruens. *Ann Chir. Gynaecol.* 67:147, 1978.

83. Macintosh, P. K., Thomson, K. R., and Barbaric, Z. L. Percutaneous transperitoneal lymphnode biopsy as a means of improving lymphographic diagnosis. *Radiology* 131:647, 1979.

84. Matalon, T. S. A., Athanasoulis, C. A., Margolies, M. N., Waltman, A. C., Novelline, R. A., Greenfield, A. J., and Miller, S. E. Hemorrhage with pelvic fractures: Efficacy of transcatheter embolization. *AJR* 133:859, 1979

85. Merrin, C., Wajsman, Z., Baumgartner, G., and Jennings, E. Clinical value of lymphangiography. Are the nodes surrounding the obturator nerve visualized? *J. Urol.* 117:762, 1977.

86. Michal, V., Kramár, R., and Bartak, V. Femoro-pudendal bypass in the treatment of sexual impotence. *J. Cardiovasc. Surg.* (Torino) 15:356, 1974.

87. Miller, F. J., Jr., Mortel, R., Mann, W. J., and Jahshan, A. E. Selective arterial embolization for control of hemorrhage in pelvic malignancy: Femoral and brachial catheter approach. *AJR* 126:1028, 1976.
88. Mitchell, M. E., Waltman, A. C., Athanasoulis, C. A., Kerr, W. S., and Dretler, S. P. Control of massive prostatic bleeding with angiographic techniques. *J. Urol.* 115:692, 1976.
89. Morton, D. G., Lagasse, L. D., Moore, D. G., Jacobs, M., and Amromin, G. D. Pelvic lymphadenectomy following radiation in cervical carcinoma. *Am. J. Obstet. Gynecol.* 88:932, 1964.
90. Murphy, P. Developments in preoperative staging of bladder tumors. *Urology* 11:109, 1978.
91. Nilsson, J. Angiography in tumors of urinary bladder. *Acta Radiol.* [*Suppl.*] (Stockh.) 263:1, 1967.
92. Park, R. C., Patow, W. E., Rogers, R. E., and Zimmerman, E. A. Treatment of stage I carcinoma of the cervix. *Obstet. Gynecol.* 418:17, 1973.
93. Paster, S. B., Van Houten, F. X., and Adams, D. F. Percutaneous balloon catheterization: A technique for control of arterial hemorrhage caused by pelvic trauma. *J.A.M.A.* 230:573, 1974.
94. Pereiras, R. V., Jr., Meier, W. L., Katz, E. R., and Viamonte, M., Jr. Arteriographic embolization treatment for postprostatectomy hemorrhage. *Urology* 9:705, 1977.
95. Petty, W. M., Teaford, A. K., Park, R. C., and Patow, W. E. Angiographic evaluation of early carcinoma of the cervix. *Gynecol. Oncol.* 1:211, 1973.
96. Quinby, W. C., Jr. Pelvic fractures with hemorrhage. *N. Engl. J. Med.* 284:668, 1971.
97. Ravitch, M. M. Hypogastric artery ligation in acute pelvic trauma. *Surgery* 56:601, 1964.
98. Redman, H. C. Computed tomography of the pelvis. *Radiol. Clin. North Am.* 15:441, 1977.
99. Reynolds, B. M., and Balsano, N. A. Venography in pelvic fractures. A clinical evaluation. *Ann. Surg.* 173:104, 1971.
100. Ring, E. J., Athanasoulis, C., Waltman, A C., Margolies, M. N., and Baum, S. Arteriographic management of hemorrhage following pelvic fracture. *Radiology* 109:65, 1973.
101. Ring., E. J., Waltman, A. C., Athanasoulis, C., Smith, J. C., Jr., and Baum, S. Angiography in pelvic trauma. *Surg. Gynecol. Obstet.* 139:375, 1974.
102. Rodberg, C., and Wickbom, I. Pelvic angiography and pneumoperitoneum in the diagnosis of gynecologic lesions. *Acta Radiol.* [*Diagn.*] (Stockh.) 6:133, 1967.
103. Rothenberger, D. A., Fischer, R. P., and Perry, J. F., Jr. Major vascular injuries secondary to pelvic fractures: An unsolved clinical problem. *Am. J. Surg.* 136:660, 1978.
104. Rothenberger, D. A., Fischer, R. P., Strate, R. G., Velasco, R., and Perry, J. F., Jr. The mortality associated with pelvic fractures. *Surgery* 84:356, 1978.
105. Rothenberger, D. A., Velasco, R., Strate, R. G., Fischer, R. P., and Perry, J. F., Jr. Open pelvic fracture: A lethal injury. *J. Trauma* 18:184, 1978.
106. Scarabelli, C., Schiavino, G., Croce, E., and Fedele, M. Importanza dell angiografia pelvica selettiva en ginecologia. *Minerva Ginecol.* 30:849, 1978.
107. Schroder, J., Terwey, B., Buhr, H. J., and Gerhardt, P. Die Behandlung traumatischer Becken Blutungen durch Embolisation. *Chirurg* 49:286, 1978.
108. Schurhke, T. D., and Barr, J. W. Intractable bladder hemorrhage: Therapeutic angiographic embolization of the hypogastric arteries. *J. Urol.* 116:523, 1976.
109. Seidelmann, F. E., Cohen, W. N., and Bryan, P. J. CT staging of bladder neoplasms. *Radiol. Clin. North Am.* 15:419, 1977.
110. Seidelmann, F. E., Cohen, W. N., Bryan, P. J., Temes, S. P., Kraus, D., and Schoenrock, G. Accuracy of CT staging of bladder neoplasms using the gas-filled method: Report of 21 patients with surgical confirmation. *AJR* 130:735, 1978.
111. Seidelmann, F. E., Reich, N. E., Cohen, W. N., et al. Computed tomography of the seminal vesicles and seminal vesical angle. *J. Comput. Assist. Tomogr.* 1:281, 1977.
112. Seidelmann, F. E., Temes, S. P., Cohen, W. N., Bryan, P. J., Patil, U., and Sherry, R. G. Computed tomography of the gas-filled bladder: Methods of staging bladder neoplasms. *Urology* 9:337, 1977.
113. Smith, D. C., and Wyatt, J. F. Embolization of hypogastric arteries in the control of massive vaginal hemorrhage. *Obstet. Gynecol.* 49:317, 1977.
114. Smith, J. C., Jr., Kerr, W. S., Athanasoulis, C. A., Waltman, A. C., Ring, E. J., and Baum, S. Angiographic management of bleeding secondary to genitourinary tract surgery. *J. Urol.* 113:89, 1975.
115. Smith, R. F., and Szilagyi, D. E. Ischemia of the colon as a complication in surgery of the abdominal aorta. *Arch. Surg.* 80:806, 1960.
116. Tadavarthy, S. M., Knight, L., Ovitt, T. W., Snyder, C., and Amplatz, K. Therapeutic transcatheter arterial embolization. *Radiology* 112:13, 1974.
117. Tajes, R. V. Ligation of the hypogastric arteries and its complications in resection of cancer of the rectum. *Am. J. Gastroenterol.* 26:612, 1956.
118. *TNM Classification of Malignant Tumors* (3rd

ed.).   Geneva: Union Internationale Contre Cancer, 1978.

119. Udoff, E. J., Barth, K. H., Harrington, D. P., Kaufman, S. L., and White, R. I. Hemodynamic significance of iliac artery stenosis: Pressure measurements during arteriography. *Radiology* 132:289, 1979.

120. van Urk, H., Perlberger, R. R., and Muller, H. Selective arterial embolization for control of traumatic pelvic hemorrhage. *Surgery* 83:133, 1978.

121. Wajsman, Z., Baumgartner, G., Murphy, G. P., and Merrin, C. Evaluation of lymphangiography for clinical staging of bladder tumors. *J. Urol.* 114:712, 1975.

122. Wallace, S., Gianturco, C., Anderson, J. H., Goldstein, H. M., Davis, L. J., and Bree, R. L. Therapeutic vascular occlusion utilizing steel coil technique: Clinical applications. *AJR* 127:381, 1976.

123. Walsh, J. W., Rosenfield, A. A., Jaffe, C. C., Shwartz, P. E., Simeone, J., Dembner, A. G., and Taylor, K. J. N. Prospective comparison of ultrasound and computed tomography in the evaluation of gynecologic pelvic masses. *AJR* 131:955, 1978.

124. White, R. I., Jr., Kaufman, S. L., Barth, K. H., DeCaprio, V., and Strandberg, J. V. Embolotherapy with detachable silicone balloons: Technique and clinical results. *Radiology* 131: 619, 1979.

125. White, R. I., Jr., Strandberg, J. V., Gross, G. S., and Barth, K. H. Therapeutic embolization with long-term occluding agents and their effects on embolized tissues. *Radiology* 125:677, 1977.

126. Winterberger, A. R., Jennings, E. C., and Murphy, G. P. Arteriography in metastatic tumors to the bladder. *J. Urol.* 108:577, 1972.

127. Winterberger, A. R., and Murphy, G. P. Correlation of B-scan ultrasonic laminography with bilateral selective hypogastric arteriography and lymphangiography in bladder tumors. *Vasc. Surg.* 8:169, 1974.

128. Winterberger, A. R., Wajsman, Z., Merrin, C., and Murphy, G. P. Eight year experience with arteriographic and lymphangiographic staging of bladder carcinoma. *J. Urol.* 119:208, 1978.

7. Retroperitoneal Arteriography

Retroperitoneal Arteriography in Adults

DAVID C. LEVIN

Retroperitoneal arteriography is performed primarily to evaluate suspected retroperitoneal masses—principally malignant or benign tumors, abscesses and other inflammatory lesions, or hematomas. Retroperitoneal masses are rare. Armstrong and Cohn [1] reviewed 25,647 tumors recorded in the New Orleans Tumor Registry between 1948 and 1962. Only 41 of these tumors (0.16%) arose mainly in the retroperitoneal space. It should be noted that in this discussion and all referenced papers, masses arising in specific organs such as the kidneys, adrenals, duodenum, and pancreas are excluded. The term *retroperitoneal mass* is taken to include only those lesions arising in the amorphous retroperitoneal space in which these organs are contained.

Although retroperitoneal tumors are rare, they provide a distinct challenge from both diagnostic and therapeutic points of view. Because they do not arise in specific organs, symptoms do not occur until relatively late in their course, and the masses are usually rather large at the time of detection. The presenting clinical symptoms and signs can include weight loss, abdominal enlargement or fullness, a palpable mass, nausea, and back pain.

The retroperitoneal space contains a number of different types of tissues: fibrous tissue, muscle, areolar connective tissue, fat, lymph nodes, lymphatics, fascia, sympathetic nervous structures, blood vessels, mesothelial tissues, and remnants of the embryologic urogenital ridge. A wide histologic variety of primary retroperitoneal tumors therefore occur. These can be classified into five major types: (1) Mesenchymal tumors: Liposarcomas, leiomyosarcomas, fibrosarcomas, rhabdomyosarcomas, and spindle cell sarcomas are the most common. Undifferentiated sarcomas and carcinomas, chondrosarcomas, hemangiopericytomas, malignant fibrous histiocytomas, and mesotheliomas occur less commonly. The only benign mesenchymal tumor that appears with any frequency is lipoma. (2) Lymphomas: Between 5 and 10 percent of all lymphomas arise primarily within the abdomen, and approximately half of these occur in the retroperitoneal space [2, 3]. This category does not include the more common cases of lymphoma (which are first detected elsewhere in the body and which occur secondarily in the retroperitoneal space) since these cases are generally not studied arteriographically. (3) Metastatic tumors. (4) Neural tumors: These can be benign or malignant and

1789

include neurofibroma, neurilemoma, extraadrenal neuroblastoma, and ganglioneuroma. (5) Tumors of the urogenital ridge remnant: On rare occasions, a tumor having the histologic appearance of a gonadal tumor develops in the retroperitoneal space when the gonads themselves are normal. Such tumors are thought to arise in the embryonic urogenital ridge remnant.

The most prevalent benign, nonneoplastic causes of retroperitoneal masses are hematomas and inflammatory lesions such as abscesses. Cysts and retroperitoneal fibrosis also occur on rare occasions. Retroperitoneal hematomas may be signaled clinically by the sudden onset of back or flank pain, shock, and a falling hematocrit. They may result from trauma, be caused by rupture of a small metastatic tumor of the adrenal gland or other small retroperitoneal tumor, or occur entirely spontaneously. Retroperitoneal abscesses and other inflammatory masses often present clinically in a manner similar to that of retroperitoneal tumors, except that inflammatory masses are more likely to be accompanied by fever. In some cases of retroperitoneal inflammatory disease, symptoms may be largely or completely absent.

Approximately 80 to 85 percent of retroperitoneal masses are malignant [1]. Their prognosis is generally poor, in part because the lesions are usually rather far advanced before the patient seeks medical attention. Radical surgery is the treatment of choice, except in cases of lymphoma, which are best treated by radiation.

The emergence within the past few years of noninvasive imaging modalities like computed tomography (CT) and ultrasound has greatly altered the diagnostic approach to retroperitoneal lesions. Prior to the advent of CT and ultrasound, the retroperitoneal space was an exceedingly difficult area to visualize, and arteriography was frequently performed as a relatively early screening procedure in cases in which retroperitoneal lesions were suspected. At the present time, CT and ultrasound can both provide excellent visualization of retroperitoneal lesions, so that arteriography need no longer be utilized for screening purposes. However, once CT or ultrasound has suggested the presence of a retroperitoneal mass, arteriography can still provide important information to help in surgical management. This will be discussed in greater detail later in the chapter.

Angiographic Findings in Retroperitoneal Tumors

The arteriographic findings in retroperitoneal tumors have been described in considerable detail by the author and others [4–10]. Although

Figure 74-1. Right retroperitoneal fibrosarcoma. The tumor contains extensive coarse and irregular neovascularity, arising from several right lumbar arteries and both hypogastric arteries. (From Levin et al. [7]. Reproduced with permission from *Radiology*.)

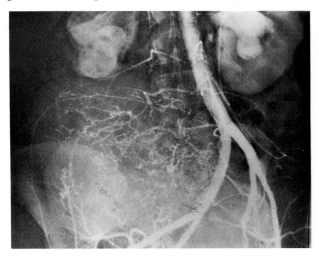

Figure 74-2. Left retroperitoneal leiomyosarcoma. Selective arteriography of a left lumbar artery demonstrates extensive and highly irregular neovascularity with multiple large vascular sinusoids, particularly along the lower and lateral aspects of the tumor. (Courtesy of Iraj Hooshmand, M.D.)

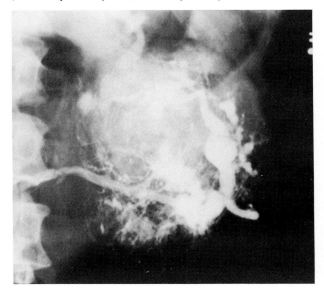

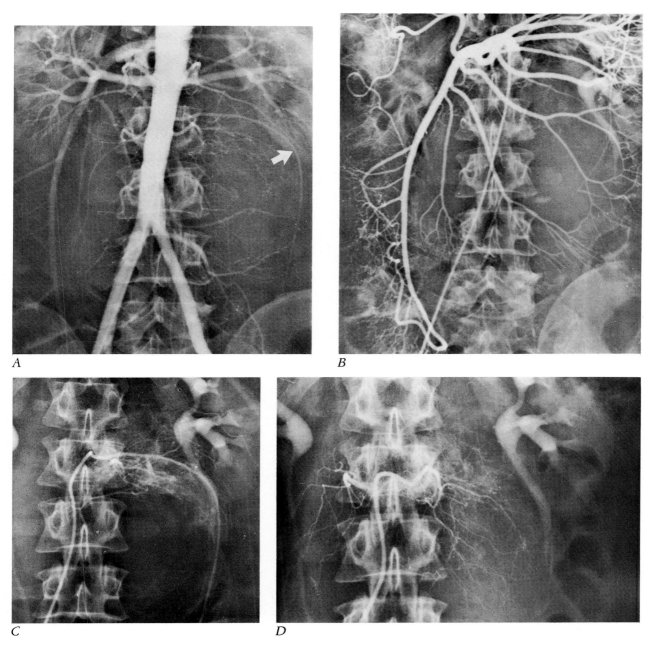

Figure 74-3. Retroperitoneal lymphosarcoma. (A) Initial abdominal aortogram demonstrates displacement of the superior mesenteric artery to the right and displacement of the left testicular artery (*arrow*) around a mass containing fine neovascularity. (B) Superior mesenteric arteriography shows that the artery is draped around the border of the retroperitoneal tumor but does not contribute any neovascularity to it. (C) Selective left testicular ar-teriogram again demonstrates displacement of the artery around the lateral border of the tumor. Some fine neovascularity arises from the proximal portion of the testicular artery as it passes medial to and slightly below the left kidney. (D) Selective left lumbar arteriogram demonstrates fine neovascularity arising from this lumbar branch as well. (A, C, D from Levin et al. [7]. Reproduced with permission from *Radiology*.)

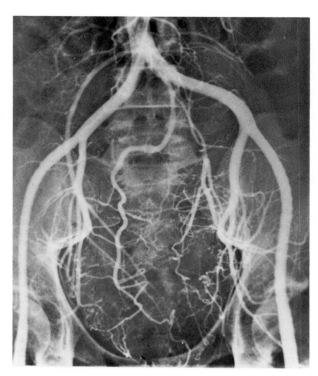

Figure 74-4. Leiomyosarcoma of the pelvic retroperitoneal space. Fine neovascularity is observed throughout the large mass, arising from both hypogastric arteries and the median sacral artery.

often striking, they are nonspecific. These findings can generally be characterized in terms of degree of vascularity and displacement of arteries and/or the kidneys.

Displacement of arteries and/or the kidneys is seen in virtually all but very small retroperitoneal masses. This is not surprising since the abdominal aorta is a retroperitoneal structure and all its major branches pass through the retroperitoneal space for at least part of their course. The kidneys are the largest and most easily visible retroperitoneal organs angiographically, and their displacement also may be one of the first signs, and sometimes the only sign, of a retroperitoneal mass.

The vascularity exhibited by retroperitoneal tumors can be conveniently classified into three major types:

Type I tumors contain vessels that are large, coarse, highly irregular, and ragged and fail to show progressive decrease in caliber as do normal vessels. Sinusoidal pooling of contrast and tumor staining may occur during the capillary phase. In the vast majority of cases exhibiting this type of vascularity, the lesion will prove to be a malig-

nant tumor [9]. However, in rare instances benign neural tumors such as neurofibroma or neurilemoma will produce this same coarse hypervascularity [4, 6]. Figure 74-1 shows a fibrosarcoma in a young woman. Extensive neovascularity is present with supply from multiple lumbar arteries and the iliac arteries on both sides. Figure 74-2 shows a leiomyosarcoma in the left retroperitoneal space. Very large, irregular arteries and vascular sinusoids are present within the tumor. In my experience, among all retroperitoneal neoplasms, leiomyosarcomas and spindle cell sarcomas seem to contain the greatest degree of coarse neovascularity.

Type II tumors also display hypervascularity, but the vessels are of a finer, more reticular character and tend to be distributed in a more homogeneous manner. Diffuse staining is generally seen during the capillary phase, but contrast pooling or vascular sinusoids are usually not seen. As with type I lesions, most type II lesions will prove to be malignant tumors. However, on rare occasions benign neural tumors and lipomas may demonstrate this vascular pattern [8]. Figure 74-3 shows a lymphosarcoma arising primarily in the retroperitoneal space. Fine neovascularity and staining in the area of the tumor can be seen on selective left testicular and lumbar arteriograms. Figure 74-4 shows a leiomyosarcoma of the pelvic retroperitoneal space. The tumor was supplied by multiple arteries. Lymphomas are the most common lesions to exhibit type II hypervascularity.

Type III includes all retroperitoneal tumors that are hypovascular or avascular. Although absence of neovascularity is often considered a sign of a benign lesion, in the retroperitoneal space most hypovascular or avascular masses will nevertheless prove to be malignant tumors. In my experience, slightly fewer than half of all malignant retroperitoneal tumors are hypovascular or totally avascular. Figure 74-5 shows a large liposarcoma that is entirely avascular. Benign retroperitoneal tumors, such as neurofibroma and lipoma, can also have an avascular pattern.

It is apparent from the foregoing discussion that malignant retroperitoneal tumors can be characterized by a broad spectrum of vascularity, ranging from extremely hypervascular to totally avascular. In many instances, lesions of the same histologic type may exhibit widely varying degrees of vascularity in different patients. Any attempt at making a histologic diagnosis based

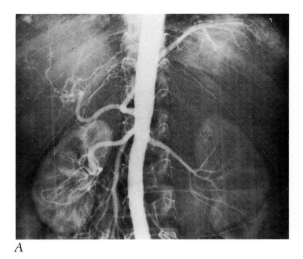

A

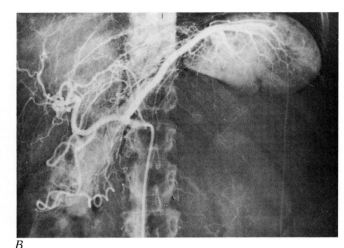

B

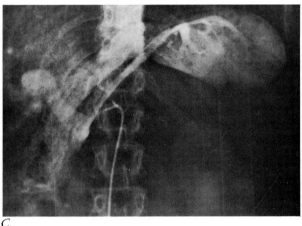

C

Figure 74-5. Left retroperitoneal liposarcoma. (A) Initial abdominal aortogram shows downward displacement of the left renal artery and left kidney, upward displacement of the spleen, and displacement to the right of the lower abdominal aorta. No abnormal vascularity is seen. (B) Celiac axis arteriogram confirms the upward displacement of the spleen. No definite neovascularity is seen. (C) The venous phase of the celiac arteriogram confirms the absence of any tumor staining or pooling. (From Levin et al. [7]. Reproduced with permission from *Radiology*.)

upon the vascular pattern of the tumor should therefore be avoided.

Angiographic Findings in Retroperitoneal Hematomas

Retroperitoneal hemorrhage may result from trauma or rupture of tumors (especially metastatic tumors of the adrenal gland) or may occur spontaneously. Angiography will often fail to reveal the exact source of bleeding but will demonstrate a mass effect with displacement and stretching of major vessels and/or the kidneys. As would be expected, the hematomas are entirely avascular.

Figure 74-6 shows a left retroperitoneal hematoma that was found at surgery to arise from rupture of a metastatic lesion of the left adrenal gland from a primary bronchogenic carcinoma. Figure 74-7 demonstrates an apparently spontaneous left retroperitoneal hemorrhage in a previously healthy 25-year-old woman. No specific cause or source of the hemorrhage was ever found at surgery.

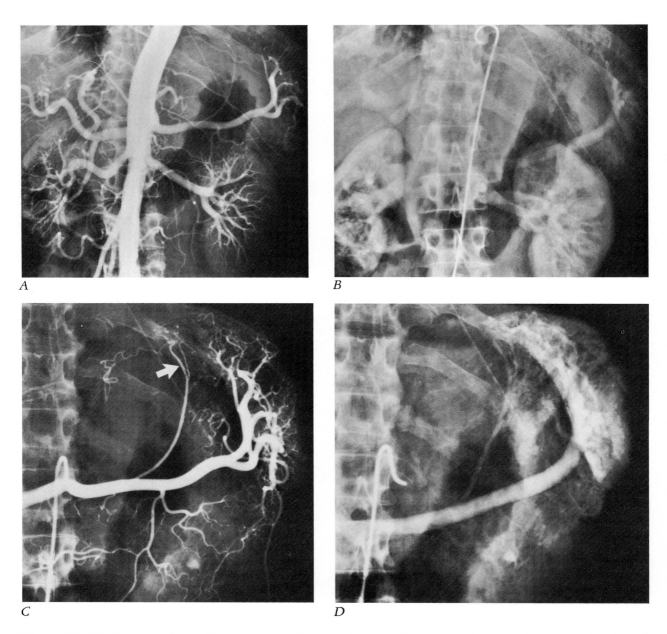

Figure 74-6. Left retroperitoneal hematoma resulting from rupture of the left adrenal gland. The patient had bronchogenic carcinoma, which metastasized to the left adrenal gland. (A and B) Abdominal aortogram, early- and late-phase films. No neovascularity is seen. The left renal artery is slightly straightened, and the left kidney is displaced downward slightly. (C and D) Selective splenic arteriogram, early- and late-phase films. A large avascular mass is present in the left upper quadrant retroperitoneal space. The splenic artery is stretched, particularly a small branch to the upper pole of the spleen (*arrow*). The spleen itself is draped over the lateral border of the mass. The late-phase film shows that there is also displacement and stretching of the splenic vein.

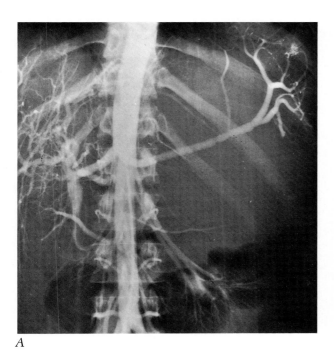

A

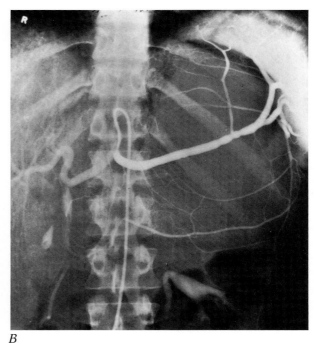

B

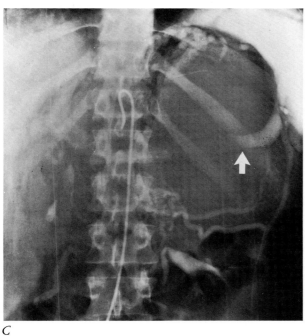

C

Figure 74-7. Spontaneous left retroperitoneal hemorrhage. (A) Initial abdominal aortogram demonstrates a large left upper quadrant avascular mass with marked downward displacement of the left renal arteries and left kidney. (B) Selective splenic arteriogram confirms the avascular nature of the mass. There is stretching of the splenic and pancreatic arteries. Several areas of narrowing are seen in the midportion of the splenic artery, but these were never explained. (C) The late phase of the splenic arteriogram demonstrates the avascular nature of the mass. The central portion of the splenic vein (*arrow*) is not opacified, and some collateral venous pathways are noted in the region of the gastric fundus and the upper pole of the left kidney. This finding suggests splenic vein obstruction, but at operation the splenic vein was noted to be patent. It was simply compressed by the large retroperitoneal hematoma.

Angiographic Findings in Retroperitoneal Inflammatory Disease

The angiographic findings in patients with retroperitoneal abscesses or other types of inflammatory disease are often somewhat more subtle than those in patients who have retroperitoneal tumors. Displacement of vessels by the mass may be present, particularly if the lesion is a relatively large abscess under tension. On the other hand, if the inflammatory process is not encapsulated or confined, displacement of vessels and/or the kidneys may not occur.

The degree of vascularity is also variable. Retroperitoneal inflammatory lesions may be totally avascular or may show a mild degree of fine, somewhat irregular vascularity similar to the type II vascularity described above. If the abscess is vascularized, some staining may occur during the capillary phase, but this is unusual. The degree of vascularity is probably related partly to the proximity of the lesion to well-vascularized ret-

Figure 74-8. Late-phase film of a selective left renal arteriogram in a patient with staphylococcal perinephric abscess. The density just lateral to the catheter tip is caused by overlying barium in the colon. Fine vascularity is seen medial to the upper pole of the left kidney. This case is an example of an inflammatory retroperitoneal lesion exhibiting type II neovascularity similar to that found in many malignant tumors. (Courtesy of Iraj Hooshmand, M.D.)

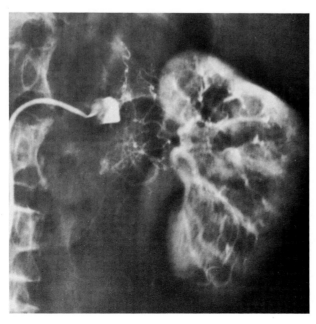

roperitoneal organs such as the kidneys or pancreas. Thus, perinephric or peripancreatic abscesses tend to be somewhat more vascular than psoas abscesses. I have never seen an instance in which an inflammatory retroperitoneal mass contained extremely prominent, coarse type I vascularity. Figure 74-8 illustrates a staphylococcal perinephric abscess. Fine vascularity is seen medial to the kidney, but there was no staining.

Differential Diagnosis

The first sign that should alert the angiographer to the presence of a retroperitoneal mass is displacement of the retroperitoneal segments of major vessels (either arteries or veins) and/or the kidneys. This sign occurs in the vast majority of retroperitoneal mass lesions, although it may be absent in some cases of poorly confined retroperitoneal inflammatory processes.

If the mass, in addition to vascular and/or renal displacement, demonstrates coarse, ragged, highly irregular arteries (type I) with pooling or filling of sinusoids during the late phase, the diagnosis is most likely to be malignant tumor (there is a small possibility that such findings could be caused by a benign neural tumor). If the mass shows fine, somewhat more homogeneous vascularity (type II), the diagnosis is again ordinarily malignant tumor, but the cause could also be benign neural tumors, lipomas, or abscesses. If the mass is hypovascular or completely avascular, the differential diagnosis includes malignant tumors, benign neural tumors or lipomas, hematomas, and abscesses.

The actual cell type of a malignant retroperitoneal tumor cannot be predicted angiographically. As indicated earlier, I have seen numerous examples of a given type of tumor exhibiting widely varying degrees of vascularity and ranging from totally avascular to extremely hypervascular.

Current Role of Angiography in Evaluation of Retroperitoneal Masses

Ultrasound and computed tomography have proved to be reliable in the detection of retroperitoneal masses [10–15]. Therefore, angiography is not necessary as a screening procedure in patients clinically suspected of having such lesions. Once a retroperitoneal mass is detected by ultrasound or CT, however, angiography does have an important role to play prior to surgery [7, 10.] Since the degree of vascularity of these masses is so highly variable, it is important that the surgeon know in advance whether excessive neovascularity is present. If it is, he must be aware of the source from which it arises. If there is significant arterial supply to the mass from renal, celiac, superior mesenteric, or inferior mesenteric arteries, these arteries may have to be sacrificed during the tumor resection, necessitating removal of devascularized organs such as the kidney or portions of bowel. Even if the mass is located posteriorly in the retroperitoneal space and is supplied only by lumbar arteries, it is important to know, prior to ligating them, whether any of these lumbar arteries supply portions of the spinal cord. In rare instances, avascular retroperitoneal masses may invade or encase major arteries or veins [7], thereby necessitating resection of segments of those vessels at the time of resection of the tumor itself. In certain patients with highly vascular retroperitoneal masses, preoperative devascularization by transcatheter embolization might facilitate resection, although there has been very little experience so far with the application of embolization in this area. Finally, Karp et al. [10] have recently pointed out that even with the current availability of sophisticated noninvasive imaging techniques, it may at times be impossible to differentiate intraperitoneal from retroperitoneal lesions if the mass is very large. In such instances the delineation of the source of blood supply by arteriography might indicate whether the mass arises primarily in the retroperitoneal space or is within the peritoneal cavity or one of the intraperitoneal organs.

For all the above reasons, surgeons experienced in treatment of retroperitoneal masses have found angiography to be invaluable in preoperative planning of their approach and have advocated its routine use [15] in dealing with these difficult and dangerous lesions.

References

1. Armstrong, J. R., and Cohn, I., Jr. Primary malignant retroperitoneal tumors. *Am. J. Surg.* 110:937, 1965.
2. Banfi, A., Bonnadonna, G., Carnevali, G., Oldini, C., and Salvini, E. Preferential sites of involvement and spread in malignant lymphoma. *Eur. J. Cancer* 4:319, 1968.
3. Fuller, L. M. Results of large volume irradiation in management of Hodgkin's disease and malignant lymphoma originating in the abdomen. *Radiology* 87:1058, 1966.
4. Bron, K. M., and Sherman, L. Arteriography in evaluating retroperitoneal mass lesions. *N.Y. State J. Med.* 67:1875, 1967.
5. Vinik, M. N., Jr., Neal, M. P., Jr., and Freed, T. A. Retroperitoneal angiography. *South. Med. J.* 61:646, 1968.
6. Lowman, R. M., Grnja, V., Peck, D. R., Osborn, D., and Love, L. The angiographic patterns of the primary retroperitoneal tumors: The role of the lumbar arteries. *Radiology* 104:259, 1972.
7. Levin, D. C., Watson, R. C., and Baltaxe, H. A. Arteriography of retroperitoneal masses. *Radiology* 108:543, 1973.
8. Damascelli, B., Musumeci, R., Botturi, M., Petrillo, R., and Spagnoli, I. Angiography of retroperitoneal tumors. A review. *AJR* 124:565, 1975.
9. Levin, D. C., Gordon, D. H., Kinkhabwala, M., and Becker, J. A. Arteriography of retroperitoneal lymphoma. *AJR* 126:368, 1976.
10. Karp, W., Hafstrom, L. O., Jonsson, P. E. Retroperitoneal sarcoma: Ultrasonographic and angiographic evaluation. *Br. J. Radiol.* 53:525, 1980.
11. Stephens, D. H., Sheedy, P. F., II, Hattery, R. R., and Williamson, B., Jr. Diagnosis and evaluation of retroperitoneal tumors by computed tomography. *AJR* 129:395, 1977.
12. Carter, B. L., and Wechsler, R. J. Computed tomography of the retroperitoneum and abdominal wall. *Semin. Roentgenol.* 13:201, 1978.
13. Bree, R. L., and Green, B. Gray scale sonographic appearance of intraabdominal mesenchymal sarcoma. *Radiology* 128:193, 1978.
14. Korobkin, M., Callen, P. W., and Fisch, A. E. Computed tomography of the pelvis and retroperitoneum. *Radiol. Clin. North Am.* 17:301, 1979.
15. Duncan, R. E., and Evans, A. T. Diagnosis of primary retroperitoneal tumors. *J. Urol.* 117:19, 1977.

Pediatric Angiography in Retroperitoneal Tumors

J. A. GORDON CULHAM

Abdominal angiography in pediatric patients has become an accepted technique in the evaluation of mass lesions of the retroperitoneum. Its acceptance stems from a growing awareness of its contribution to patient care and the increasing safety of pediatric angiographic techniques.

Newer diagnostic modalities, specifically ultrasonography and computed tomography (CT), are contributing greatly to the evaluation of mass lesions, and it is hoped that angiography will not need to be employed to diagnose cystic disease or hydronephrosis. In the diagnosis of solid mass lesions, however, CT is less accurate in young children because of their uncontrolled respiration and poor natural contrast owing to their natural paucity of retroperitoneal fat. Thus we find that once a solid mass lesion is diagnosed, angiography continues to play a significant role in confirming the diagnosis, defining the precise size and location of the lesion, and evaluating the spread of the lesion, as well as the presence of multifocal or bilateral lesions.

Our surgical staff in general feel that valuable knowledge of surgical anatomy and pathology is derived from the angiographic investigations performed and that the rewards in the operating room far outweigh the disadvantage of a delay of a day or two while these investigations are carried out.

Handling the Pediatric Patient

Children range in age from newborn to 16 or 18 years, and in weight from 1 to 80 kg. Thus considerable flexibility is necessary in meeting the needs of such a wide spectrum of patients. The special needs, however, are limited to the younger children and infants.

For babies, safe angiography requires care to prevent heat loss with monitoring of the patient's core temperature during lengthy procedures. The angiography room must be heated for the comfort and safety of the patient, not of the angiographer [45]. Radiant heaters and warming blankets can also be employed. Overhydration or overloading with contrast material happens easily. The volumes of the flushing solution and the contrast material must be carefully monitored.

Most pediatric angiography can be performed without general anesthesia. In children under 3 months we use local anesthesia only and no sedation. In older infants and children we use the following cocktail:

Meperidine (Demerol)	25.00 mg	
Chlorpromazine	6.25 mg	per cc
Promethazine	6.25 mg	

Children are sedated with an intramuscular dose of 0.1 cc per kilogram of body weight, up to a maximum of 2 cc. In about an hour most children will be adequately sedated and will remain so for about 2 hours. Supplemental intravenous sedation may be given during the procedure as required. Older children, who are more cognizant of their fate, may be very anxious. In these patients intravenous diazepam (Valium) is helpful. Rarely, these measures fail, and general anesthesia is required. Our patients are prepared for angiography as they would be for general anesthesia, and so our anesthetists are willing to carry on with general anesthesia without delay.

Younger children are loosely restrained during angiography with clove-hitch bands attached to sandbags. This restraint prevents contamination of the sterile field and is well tolerated.

The above measures, combined with a quiet angiographic suite, a little loving care and consolation, and a favorite toy or blanket nearby, enable most angiographic procedures to be not overly unpleasant for the child or the angiographer.

Equipment

X-ray equipment for pediatric angiography must be of top quality. Small generators are not appropriate for small patients. Indeed, rapid heart rates, rapid circulation, breathing, and other kinds of motion require extremely short exposure times. Small structures in small patients require superb resolution to be adequately displayed. Filming rates of up to six films per second are occasionally required to record rapidly occurring events, but most cases can be studied at maximum filming rates of three films per second. Biplane filming can be useful to limit the contrast dose.

Small is especially appropriate for small children when it comes to needles, guidewires, and catheters. In children who weigh less than 10 kg, femoral puncture is made with a 22-gauge needle inside a Teflon cannula (Deseret R. Angiocath). This cannula allows passage of an 0.018-inch

(0.46-mm) guidewire for subsequent passage of a 3 French catheter (Cook).

	Needle	Guidewire	Catheter
<10 kg	22	0.018 inch (0.46 mm)	3 French
10–20 kg	20	0.025 inch (0.63 mm)	4.1 French
>20 kg	18	0.035 inch (0.89 mm)	5 French

In larger children, larger catheter systems are used, but seldom is a catheter larger than 5 French required. Commercially available aortogram catheters are useful (U.M.I., Cook). When selective injections are required, the appropriate curve depends on the size of the aorta; therefore, each catheter curve is produced after an initial aortogram is viewed. To assure smooth passage of the catheter, each system must be carefully matched so that the tip is precisely tapered to the guidewire [57]. Also, the needle should be no larger than that required to allow passage of the guidewire.

Technique of Percutaneous Puncture in Small Children

The Seldinger technique, which revolutionized angiography, has convincingly come of age in pediatrics [50]. In older children, the techniques of femoral puncture are identical to those used in adults. In very small children, some modification is necessary [18, 53, 56, 57].

First, both sides of the groin are prepared. The course of the femoral artery is carefully palpated. A roll is placed under the baby's buttocks to extend the hips and to improve the ability to palpate the artery. Because the patient is so small, it is often awkward to attempt to place a palpating finger above and below the point of puncture. This difficulty is aggravated by a more shallow angle of puncture used in small children (30–35 degrees). For these reasons, the course of the artery is carefully located and then a skin puncture is made directly over the vessel a centimeter or so distal to the most easily palpated vessel at the inguinal ligament. Local anesthesia is infiltrated in moderation over and about the artery. A small dermatotomy is made at the skin puncture site, with care taken that it remain directly over the artery. Puncture of the artery is then attempted by palpating only above the puncture site with one or two fingers. The angle of entry is such that the artery is encountered where best felt just below the inguinal ligament and below the palpating finger. If palpation of the vessel is very difficult to do with surgical gloves on, we occasionally perform the puncture with an ungloved palpating hand after a 10-minute surgical scrub. We have encountered no problems with wound sepsis with this approach.

No attempt is made to perform single-walled puncture in infants. After transfixing the artery, the needle is removed and the cannula slowly withdrawn. The return of blood is often not forceful, and once any blood returns, gentle passage of the guidewire is attempted. If any resistance is encountered, the guidewire is removed and the cannula position is adjusted. Slight medial, lateral, superior, or inferior position of the hub may facilitate passage of the guidewire. If not, the cannula is withdrawn slightly. If passage is unsuccessful, the vessel is gently compressed for a few minutes to gain hemostasis. Following this, if the vessel remains easily palpable, another attempt can be made. But if the vessel is poorly felt, we move to the other femoral artery.

Once a guidewire has been successfully passed, a catheter is inserted. We prefer not to use the additional exchange necessary to employ a dilator; we find little difficulty in passing a catheter that is well matched to an appropriately sized guidewire. Countertraction on the guidewire will often help in catheter passage.

Femoral venous puncture is performed in essentially the same manner, except that the puncture site is made farther caudal and medial to the site for arterial puncture. Gentle suction on the cannula hub aids the early identification of returning blood. The translucent Teflon cannula also helps in this regard.

Successful femoral puncture is possible in patients of any size; it has been performed in children who weigh just over 1 kg [9].

Complications

The complications of angiography in children are similar to those of angiography in adults. The complications occur at the catheter tip, and they consist of spasm, thromboembolism, intimal dissection or transmural extravasation, and, rarely, catheter knotting or kinking.

Complications also occur at the puncture site and although they are no different in type from those in adults, some occur more frequently in children. Hematoma forms occasionally, but it is rarely a serious problem. Unrecognized retroperitoneal bleeding can occur if the puncture site is too high.

Children's vessels tend to be more reactive, and spasm occurs frequently. Thrombosis also occurs more frequently, particularly in small infants. The incidence of thrombosis varies greatly due to the facts that (1) clinical evaluation alone is likely to underestimate the true incidence, and (2) angiographic techniques vary widely [27]. The Doppler technique, oscillometry, plethysmography, and follow-up arteriographic techniques are more accurate [37]. Many small children will have diminished pulses following angiography, probably due to spasm. If the pulses remain diminished beyond several hours, complicating thrombosis is likely to be present. The high incidence of thrombosis in smaller children may be reduced by the use of smaller catheters for very small patients [2]. A further reduction in the incidence of thrombosis has been achieved by the use of anticoagulation and antiplatelet agents during the procedure [3, 19]. Our experience using the catheter systems described above has been that thrombotic complications are extremely uncommon. When infants in the first week of life are studied, consideration should be given to an umbilical arterial approach. Much useful information can be obtained safely in this way, and, although they are rarely necessary, even selective injections can be done by this route.

Retroperitoneal Tumors

WILMS' TUMOR

Wilms' tumor is the commonest abdominal tumor in children. It and neuroblastoma account for most retroperitoneal tumors (Table 75-1). It is

Table 75-1. Solid Retroperitoneal Tumors Seen at The Hospital For Sick Children in a Recent 5-year Period (1974–1978)

Tumor	Number of Patients
Wilms' tumor	40
Neuroblastoma	33
Rhabdomyosarcoma	5
Adrenal tumors	5
Teratoma	2
Undifferentiated sarcoma	2

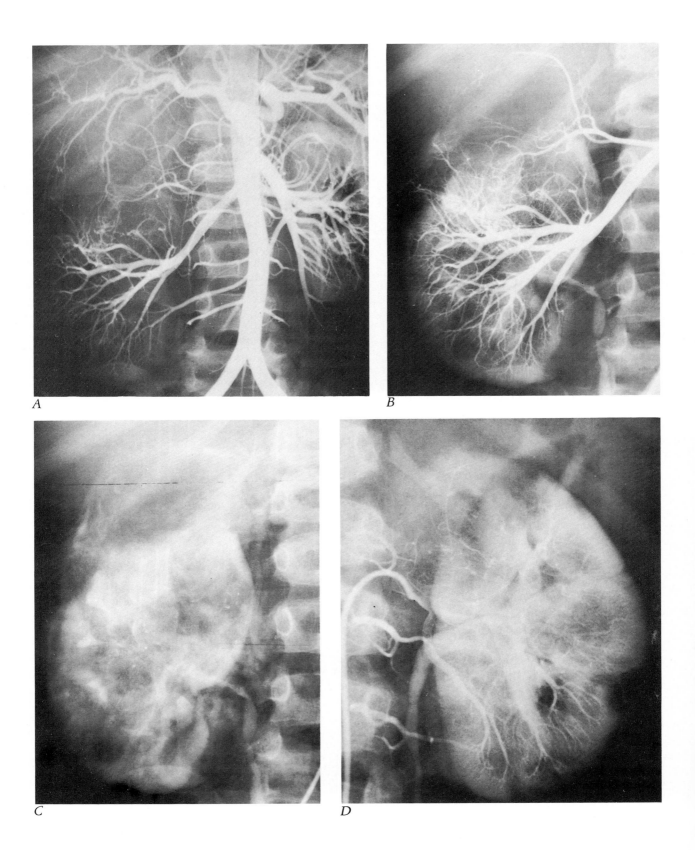

A

B

C

D

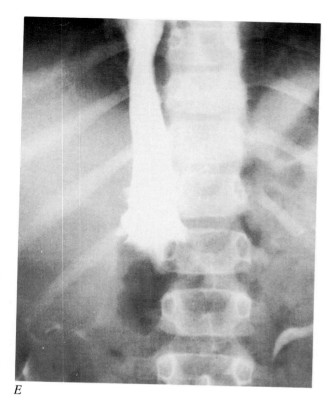

E

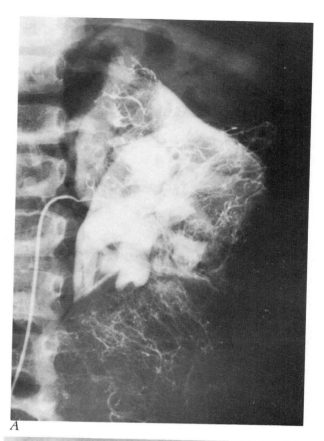

A

◄ **Figure 75-1.** A 5-year-old boy with bilateral Wilms' tumors with extension into the vena cava from the right kidney obstructing the renal vein and cava. (A) Abdominal aortogram showing a tumor of the right kidney. (B and C) Selective renal arteriogram showing a vascular tumor in the upper pole of the right kidney. The later film shows an avascular area in the upper pole and collateral veins. (D) Selective left renal arteriogram shows a small tumor in the medial upper pole. (E) Cavography from above reveals an inferior vena cava obstructed by two tumor nodules.

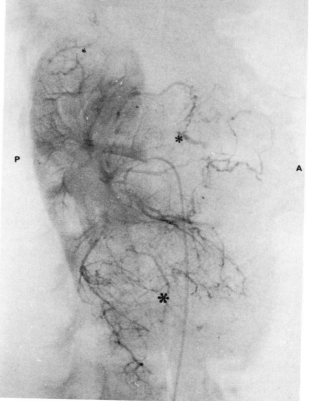

Figure 75-2. A 5-year-old girl with hemihypertrophy has three Wilms' tumors of the left kidney. (A) Selective left renal arteriogram shows three tumors. (B) Lateral view subtracted image shows the three tumors (*stars*). A = anterior; P = posterior.

B

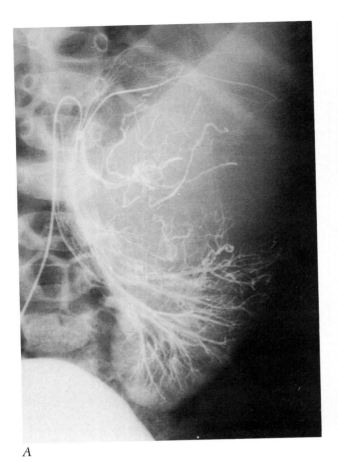

A

B

Figure 75-3. A 3-year-old boy with Wilms' tumor of the left kidney. (A) Selective left renal arteriogram shows a vascular tumor of the upper pole. Curvilinear vessels near the renal hilus supply tumor extending into the renal vein and cava. (B) Inferior vena cavogram shows tumor extending from the renal vein into the vena cava.

the policy at The Hospital For Sick Children in Toronto to study most Wilms' tumors arteriographically. Other institutions do not recommend angiography, or they do so only in suspected cases of bilateral tumor [17, 21]. Recent reports attest to the ability of CT and ultrasonography to demonstrate caval thrombus, but the reliability of these tests is not yet established, particularly in young children [20, 31, 32]. The surgical staff at our hospital feel that the information gleaned at minimal risk is useful in planning the surgical procedure. Angiography consists of an aortogram and bilateral selective renal arteriograms. In addition, a vena cava angiogram and, often, a selective renal venogram are performed. These studies confirm the diagnosis, precisely define the lesions, exclude contralateral disease, and evaluate extension into the surgical margins of the renal veins or into the vena cava. The 10 percent

incidence of bilaterality at presentation and the 16 to 22 percent incidence of spread into renal veins are arguments in favor of routine arteriography [1, 16, 40, 47]. Occasionally, Wilms' tumor extends into the heart [47, 52]. Our surgical staff has had the unfortunate experience of an operative death from a pulmonary embolism due to unrecognized tumor in the cava. Such complications are, I believe, avoidable. The surgical approach has been altered in other children with caval extension.

The arteriographic findings consist of a mass effect with associated tumor vascularity (Fig. 75-1) [13, 14, 16, 23, 26, 34, 39]. The degree of vascularity is variable, but only rarely is the tumor avascular. Focal areas of avascularity are common due to cystic areas, hemorrhage, or necrosis (Fig. 75-1). The tumors are occasionally bilateral or multifocal (Figs. 75-1, 75-2). Extension of tumor

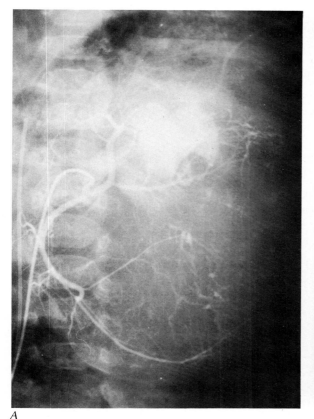

A

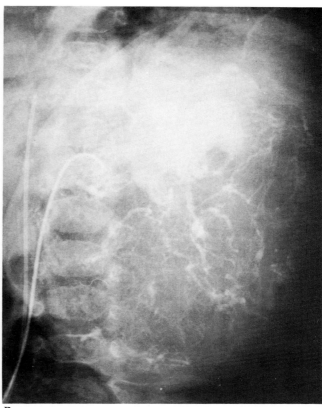

B

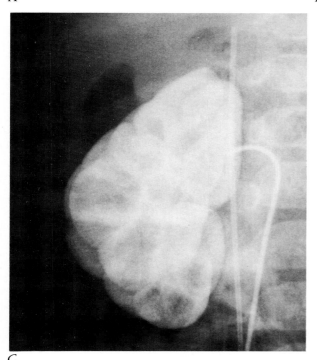

C

Figure 75-4. A 2-month-old child with a large benign hamartoma of the left kidney. Selective left renal arteriogram in early (A) and late (B) arterial phase shows a huge vascular tumor replacing virtually all the left kidney. (C) Nephrogram phase of the right renal arteriogram shows a normal right kidney with prominent fetal lobulation.

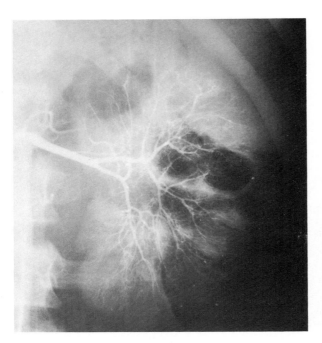

Figure 75-5. A 15-year-old boy with diffuse infiltrating adenocarcinoma of the left kidney. A selective renal arteriogram shows attenuated irregular arteries with fine tumor vessels. The kidney is diffusely enlarged.

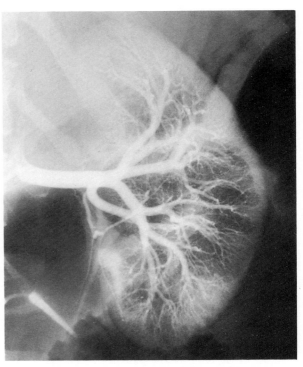

Figure 75-6. A 15-year-old boy developed a painful left flank mass 10 days following an injury. An avascular mass is seen displacing the upper pole laterally and obscuring the renal margin medially. At surgery, a perinephric abscess was drained.

into the veins and the cava can be suspected from the distribution of the tumor arteries and by obstructed venous drainage (Figs. 75-1, 75-3) [31].

Venography confirms caval or renal vein extension (Figs. 75-1, 75-3). Occasionally Wilms' tumors extend out of the kidney and into the retroperitoneum and may be indistinguishable from neuroblastoma. Venography may aid in identifying the organ of origin [1].

In the first 3 months of life, solid renal tumors with identical arteriographic findings are likely to be due to a benign renal tumor: fetal renal hamartoma or mesoblastic nephroma (Fig. 75-4) [4, 6, 29].

Other renal tumors in children include the occasional renal carcinoma and sarcoma (Fig. 75-5). Renal carcinoma accounts for 4 percent of renal tumors and tends to occur in older children; the average age is 13.5 years, approximately 10 years older than the average age in Wilms' tumor [10].

Inflammatory masses may be vascular or avascular, and they may mimic tumor (Fig. 75-6). Redundant renal parenchyma and focal hypertrophy may also cause confusion, on occasion mimicking

a solid mass. Angiography is seldom required to dispel the confusion [41, 42].

Occasionally, a cystic lesion may cause confusion. Occult forms of obstructed duplication, particularly if associated with infection, may simulate tumor [28]. The cystic nature of the lesion should be evident by ultrasonography, but small lesions, particularly in the upper pole of the kidney, may be difficult to assess (Fig. 75-7). Multilocular cyst of the kidney is an uncommon cystic mass lesion that may be related to or associated with Wilms' tumor (Fig. 75-8) [7, 8, 11, 44]. Solitary cystic lesions are uncommon in children. Such a diagnosis should be made only after multilocular cyst, cystic Wilms' tumor, renal cell carcinoma, and polycystic disease have all been excluded.

Children with Beckwith's syndrome, aniridia, and hemihypertrophy (and children of parents with hemihypertrophy) are at risk for Wilms' tumor [22, 30, 35, 36, 38]. The incidence of Wilms' tumor in hemihypertrophy is not known, but 6 percent of children with Wilms' tumor have

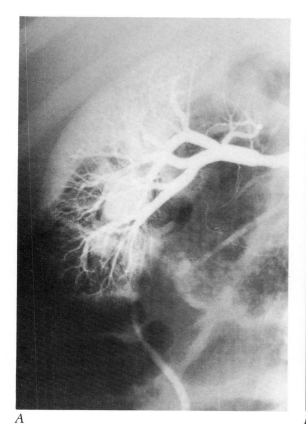

A

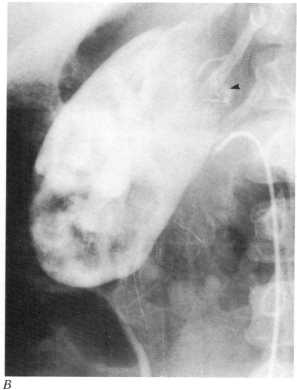

B

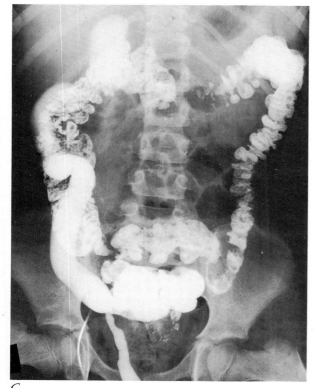

C

Figure 75-7. A 7-year-old girl underwent arteriography to assess a right renal mass. (A) A selective right renal arteriogram shows displaced vessels in the upper pole. (B) In the nephrogram phase, a defect is seen in the upper pole, with slow flow in the neighboring arteries. A fine blush of pathologic vessels is noted (*arrowhead*). (C) Cystoscopy and retrograde pyelography of an ectopic ureter shows a hydronephrotic upper pole collecting system and a dilated ureter. The abnormal arteries are secondary to infection.

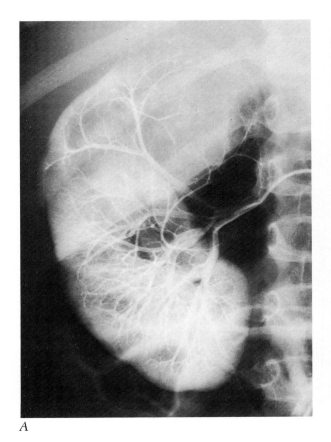

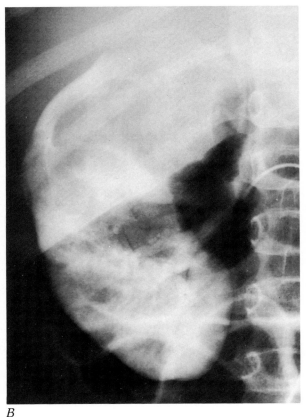

A

B

Figure 75-8. (A and B) Selective right renal arteriography in a 4-year-old girl shows a multiloculated avascular mass that was proved to be due to a multilocular cyst.

hemihypertrophy and 25 percent of children with aniridia develop Wilms' tumor. These children should be followed closely by excretory urography and/or ultrasonography.

NEUROBLASTOMA

Neuroblastoma (and its variants) is the second commonest retroperitoneal tumor in children (see Table 75-1). It occurs twice as often in the sympathetic chain as in the adrenal gland. In very large tumors, it can be difficult to guess the site of origin, and confusion with Wilms' tumor can occur.

Angiography is not routinely employed in neuroblastoma, because often surgery is not indicated [5]. Approximately 70 percent of patients with neuroblastomas have metastatic disease at presentation. Therapy in these patients consists of chemotherapy and radiation. Localized disease in the adrenal gland can be surgically extirpated without angiography. Angiography is indicated when surgery is contemplated for a very large abdominal mass. Severe vessel displacement and encasement can occur, making a preoperative road map extremely useful [33, 34]. The map should include aortography and cavography. Angiography is indicated also when neuroblastoma is suspected on the basis of clinical or laboratory findings but has not been located. Children with a neurologic syndrome characterized by opsoclonus and myoclonus are likely to have neuroblastoma [27, 51].

The laboratory finding of an elevated level of VMA (vanillylmandelic acid) suggests neuroblastoma. These patients should be studied carefully, and it should be remembered that the lesion may be not in the abdomen but in the neck, thorax, or pelvis.

The angiographic findings consist largely of a mass effect that causes major displacement of arteries and veins but that also may encase them (Fig. 75-9) [33, 34]. The surgical implications of tumor around the aorta are obvious. Tumor vascularity is variable but usually present. Tumor

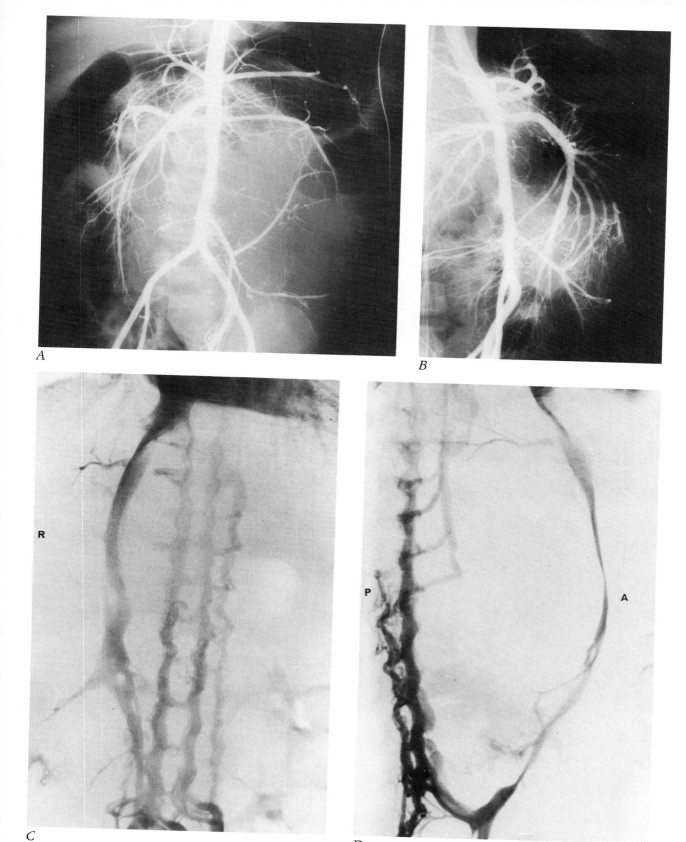

A

B

C

D

Figure 75-9. (A and B) Anteroposterior and lateral views of an abdominal aortogram show anterior displacement and circumferential narrowing of the abdominal aorta. Tumor vessels are present in the left retroperitoneum due to neuroblastoma. (C and D) The inferior vena cava is anteriorly displaced and narrowed but not invaded by the tumor. R = right; A = anterior; P = posterior.

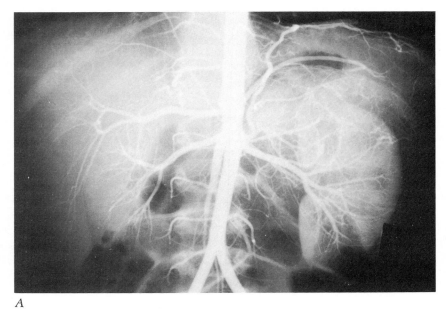

A

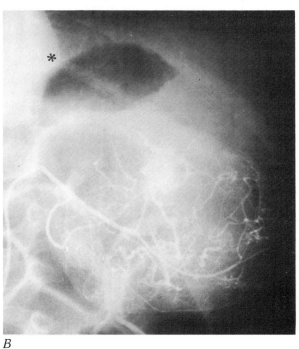

B

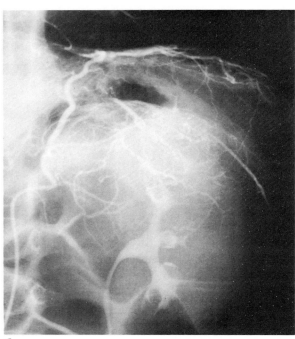

C

Figure 75-10. This 18-month-old boy has a left adrenal neuroblastoma that produces caudal and lateral displacement of the left kidney. (A and B) A selective inferior adrenal arteriogram defines the lower two-thirds of the mass. A paraspinal soft tissue mass is also shown (*star*). (C) A selective inferior phrenic arteriogram shows the remainder of the adrenal tumor, as well as tumor vessels in the paraspinal extension of the tumor.

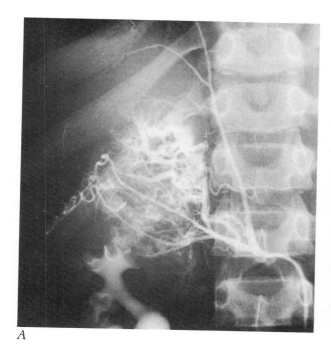

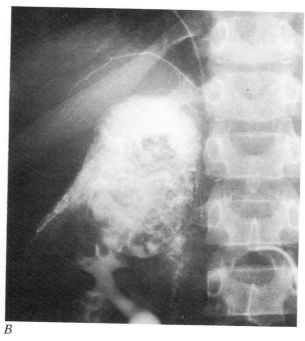

A

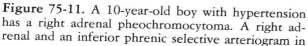

B

Figure 75-11. A 10-year-old boy with hypertension has a right adrenal pheochromocytoma. A right adrenal and an inferior phrenic selective arteriogram in the early (A) and late (B) arterial phase shows a very vascular tumor of the adrenal gland, with tumor vessels, radially oriented circulation, and central necrosis.

may be seen intruding along the paraspinal planes (Fig. 75-10).

Children under 1 year of age have a good prognosis, even those with disseminated disease. Newborns with an adrenal mass may be suspected of having neuroblastoma, but adrenal hemorrhage is more likely and a conservative approach is indicated.

OTHER ADRENAL TUMORS

Pheochromocytoma is the next most common adrenal tumor in children. It is usually diagnosed clinically during an investigation of hypertension. If pheochromocytoma is suspected, arteriography is indicated but should be performed only after adrenergic blockade [58]. Occasional adrenal adenomas and carcinomas occur, usually presenting with characteristic clinical syndromes of hypersecretion: Cushing's syndrome and the adrenogenital syndrome.

The angiographic findings of adrenal tumors are similar and often do not allow differentiation among cortical adenoma, pheochromocytoma, and their malignant counterparts [12, 24]. Central areas of necrosis are common in pheochromocytomas (Fig. 75-11) [55]. If tumor spread is evident, malignancy can be diagnosed (Fig. 75-12) [46, 49].

Extraadrenal and bilateral pheochromocytomas occur commonly in children, particularly in familial cases or in cases associated with medullary carcinoma of the thyroid [15, 48]. Extraadrenal tumors are usually demonstrated by a vascular blush (Fig. 75-13). Renal hilar tumors may produce narrowing of the renal arteries (Fig. 75-13) [54]. The difficulty of locating such lesions at surgery justifies angiography, so that a preoperative diagnosis of the number and the location of the lesions can be made [55].

OTHER RETROPERITONEAL TUMORS

These consist of mostly rhabdomyosarcoma, lymphosarcoma, and undifferentiated sarcoma and teratoma. Angiography is employed to define the precise size, location, and extent of the lesion preparatory to surgical excision. The type of tumor cannot be determined angiographically, nor can the degree of malignancy (Fig. 75-14) [43]. Teratomas tend to be calcified on plain radiography with coarser calcification than is characteristic of neuroblastoma (Fig. 75-15). Mature ossific structures, such as bones and

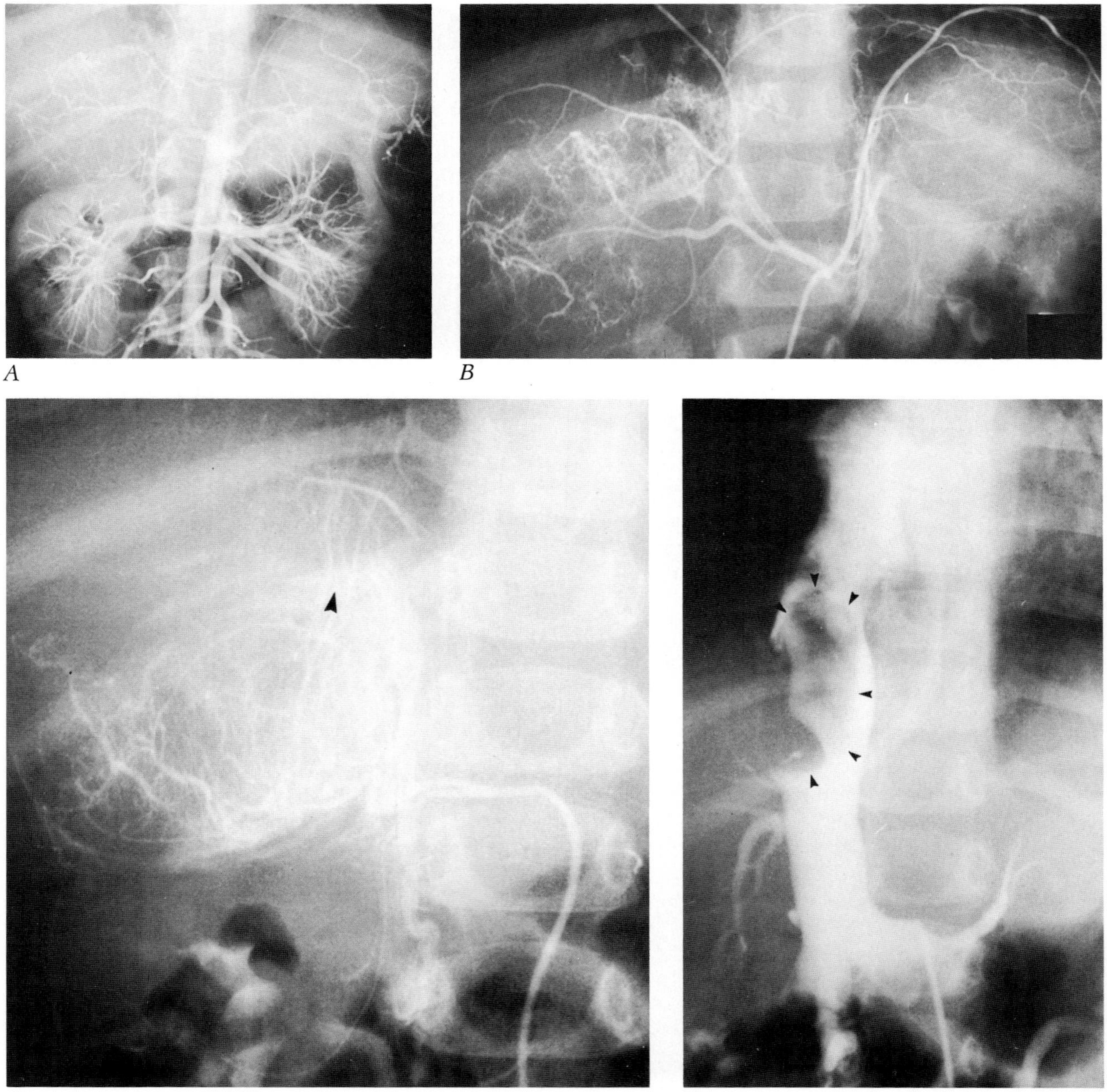

A

B

C

D

Figure 75-12. A 2-year-old girl with virilization has adrenal carcinoma. (A) An abdominal aortogram shows a right suprarenal tumor displacing the kidney inferiorly. (B) A selective inferior phrenic arteriogram shows the tumor vascularity in the adrenal gland. (C) An adrenal arteriogram shows abnormal arteries coursing superomedially (*arrowhead*), supplying (D) an extension of the tumor (*arrowheads*) in the inferior vena cava.

Figure 75-13. An 11-year-old boy undergoing investigation for hypertension has a right renal hilar pheochromocytoma. (A) An abdominal aortogram shows dilated and tortuous arteries with narrowing of two right renal artery branches. (B) A selective right renal arteriogram shows better the two narrowed renal branches. (C) An accessory renal artery supplies the upper pole of the right kidney, the right adrenal gland, and a hilar pheochromocytoma. (D) The capillary phase of the same injection shows the tumor (*star*) intimately related to the two narrowed renal artery branches.

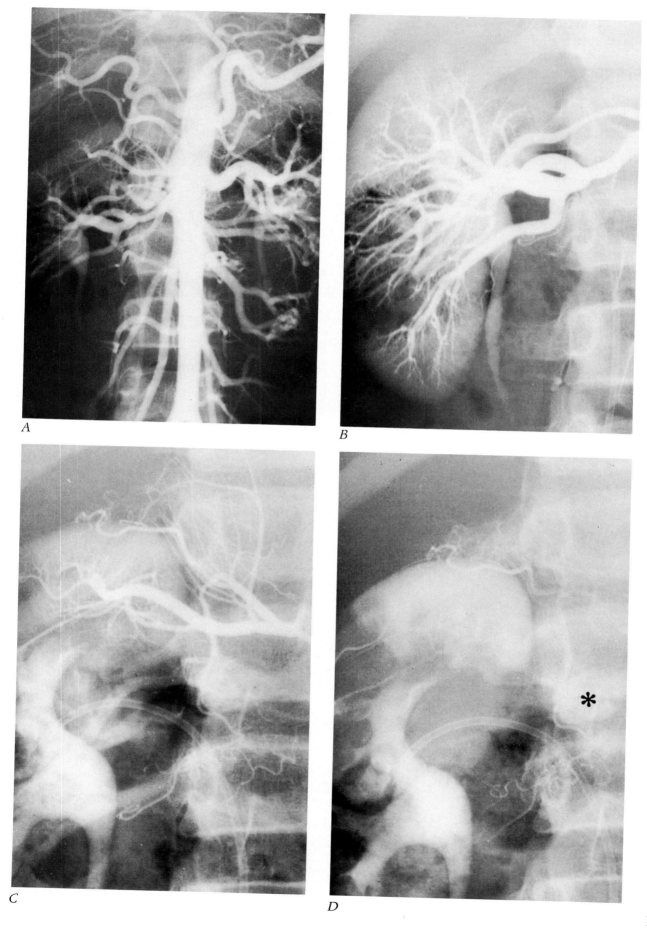

A

B

C

D

*

1813

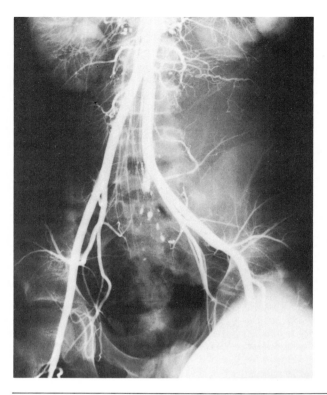

Figure 75-14. A 10-year-old boy with a limp and psoas spasm was found to have a rhabdomyosarcoma in the left lower retroperitoneum. An aortogram shows displacement of the aorta and the left iliac vessels to the right, with sparse tumor vascularity. Residual contrast material from a myelogram is present in the spinal subarachnoid space.

Figure 75-15. A 10-week-old girl presented with congestive heart failure, absent femoral pulses, and an abdominal mass. (A) An aortogram performed from a percutaneous high brachial approach shows an aortic occlusion distal to the renal arteries and an intraluminal thrombus. A large abdominal mass is present, with calcification in the left upper quadrant. (B) A selective left renal arteriogram shows a very stretched renal artery, sparse tumor vascularity, and collateral flow via the ureteric artery. A benign retroperitoneal teratoma was removed surgically.

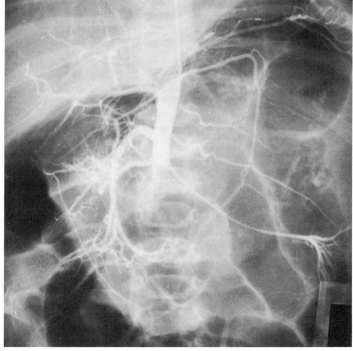

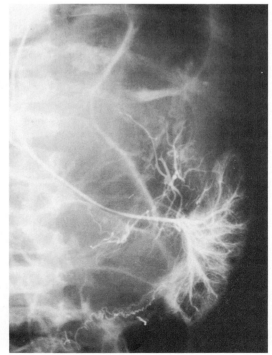

A

B

teeth, can be found in some benign teratomas. Because of the limitations of angiography in determining histology, I believe masses should be biopsied prior to nonsurgical treatment.

References

1. Beckmann, C. F., and Abrams, H. L. Renal venography: Anatomy, technique, applications, analysis of 132 venograms, and a review of the literature. *Cardiovasc. Intervent. Radiol.* 3:45, 1980.
2. Bedford, R. F. Radial artery function following percutaneous cannulation with 18 and 20 gauge catheters. *Anesthesiology* 47:37, 1977.
3. Bedford, R. F., and Ashford, T. P. Aspirin pretreatment prevents post-cannulation radial-artery thrombosis. *Anesthesiology* 51:176, 1979.
4. Berdon, W. E., Wigger, H. J., and Baker, D. H. Fetal renal hamartoma—a benign tumor to be distinguished from Wilms' tumor: Report of 3 cases. *AJR* 118:18, 1973.
5. Berger, P. E., Kuhn, J. P., and Munschauer, R. W. Computed tomography and ultrasound in the diagnosis and management of neuroblastoma. *Radiology* 128:663, 1978.
6. Bolande, R. Congenital and infantile neoplasia of the kidney. *Lancet* 2:1497, 1974.
7. Brown, J. M. Cystic partially differentiated nephroblastoma. *J. Pathol.* 115:175, 1975.
8. Carlson, D. H., Carlson, D., and Simon, H. Benign multilocular cystic nephroma. *AJR* 131:621, 1978.
9. Carter, G. A., Girod, D. A., and Hurwitz, R. A. Percutaneous cardiac catheterization in the neonate. *Pediatrics* 55:662, 1975.
10. Cassady, J. R., Filler, R., Jaffe, N., and Vawter, G. Carcinoma of the kidney in children: Results of an interdisciplinary approach to management. *Radiology* 112:691, 1974.
11. Christ, M. L. Polycystic nephroblastoma. *J. Urol.* 98:570, 1967.
12. Christenson, R., Smith, C. W., and Burko, H. Arteriographic manifestations of pheochromocytoma. *AJR* 126:567, 1976.
13. Clark, R. E., Moss, A. A., deLorimier, A. A., and Palubinskas, A. J. Arteriography of Wilms' tumor. *AJR* 113:476, 1971.
14. Cremin, B. J., and Kaschula, R. O. C. Arteriography in Wilms' tumour—the results of 13 cases and comparison to renal dysplasia. *Br. J. Radiol.* 45:415, 1972.
15. Ekelund, L., and Hoevels, J. Adrenal angiography in Sipple's syndrome. *Acta Radiol. [Diagn.]* (Stockh.) 20:637, 1979.
16. Fay, R., Brosman, S., and Williams, D. I. Bilateral nephroblastoma. *J. Urol.* 110:119, 1973.
17. Fellows, K. E., Jr. The uses and abuses of abdominal and peripheral arteriography in children. *Radiol. Clin. North Am.* 10:349, 1972.
18. Fitz, C. R., and Harwood-Nash, D. C. Special procedure techniques in infants. *Radiol. Clin. North Am.* 13:181, 1975.
19. Freed, M. D., Keane, J. F., and Rosenthal, A. The use of heparinization to prevent arterial thrombosis after percutaneous cardiac catheterization in children. *Circulation* 50:565, 1974.
20. Goldstein, H. M., Green, B., and Weaver, R. M., Jr. Ultrasonic detection of renal tumor extension into the inferior vena cava. *AJR* 130:1083, 1978.
21. Grossman, H., Sullivan, D. C., Kirks, D. R., and Merten, D. F. Integrated imaging for childhood diseases. *Pediatr. Ann.* 9(2):15, 1980.
22. Haicken, B. N., and Miller, D. R. Simultaneous occurrence of congenital aniridia, hamartoma and Wilms' tumor. *J. Pediatr.* 78:497, 1971.
23. Hidai, H., Fukuoka, H., and Murayama, T. Arteriography of Wilms' tumor. *J. Urol.* 110:347, 1973.
24. Hoevels, J., and Ekelund, L. Angiographic findings in adrenal masses. *Acta Radiol. [Diagn.]* (Stockh.) 20:337, 1979.
25. Hohn, A. R., and Craenen, J. Arterial pulses following percutaneous catheterization in children. *Pediatrics* 43:617, 1969.
26. Katzen, B. T., and Markowitz, M. Angiographic manifestations of bilateral Wilms' tumor. *AJR* 126:802, 1976.
27. Keating, J. W., and Cromwell, L. D. Remote effects of neuroblastoma. *AJR* 131:299, 1978.
28. Kittredge, R. D., and Levin, D. C. Unusual aspect of renal angiography in ureteric duplication. *AJR* 119:805, 1973.
29. Larson, D. M. Congenital mesoblastic nephroma. *Am. J. Dis. Child.* 132:318, 1978.
30. Lee, F. A. Radiology of the Beckwith-Wiedemann syndrome. *Radiol. Clin. North Am.* 10:261, 1972.
31. Madayag, M. A., Ambos, M. A., Lefleur, R. S., and Bosniak, M. A. Involvement of the inferior vena cava in patients with renal cell carcinoma. *Radiology* 133:321, 1979.
32. Marks, W. M., Korobkin, M., Callen, P. W., and Kaiser, J. A. C.T. diagnosis of tumor thrombosis of the renal vein and inferior vena cava. *AJR* 131:843, 1978.
33. McDonald, P., and Harwood-Nash, D. C. F. Arterial stenoses in neuroblastoma. *AJR* 112:167, 1971.
34. McDonald, P., and Hiller, H. G. Angiography in abdominal tumours in childhood with particular reference to neuroblastoma and Wilms' tumor. *Clin. Radiol.* 19:1, 1968.
35. Meadows, A. T., Lichenfeld, J. L., and Koop, C. E. Wilms's tumor in three children of a woman with congenital hemihypertrophy. *N. Engl. J. Med.* 291:23, 1974.
36. Miller, R. W., Fraumeni, J. F., Jr., and Manning, M. D. Association of Wilms's tumor with

aniridia, hemihypertrophy and other congenital malformations. *N. Engl. J. Med.* 270:922, 1964.

37. Mortenson, W.   Angiography of the femoral artery following percutaneous catheterization in infants and children. *Acta Radiol. [Diagn.]* (Stockh.) 17:581, 1976.

38. Müller, S., Gadner, H., Weber, B., Vogel, M., and Riehm, H.   Wilms' tumor and adrenocortical carcinoma with hemihypertrophy and hamartomas. *Eur. J. Pediatr.* 127:219, 1978.

39. Pappis, C. H., Moussatos, G. H., Constantinides, C. G., and Kairis, M.   Bilateral nephroblastoma in a horseshoe kidney. *J. Pediatr. Surg.* 14:483, 1979.

40. Perez, C. A. Kaiman, H. A., Keith, J., Mill, W. B., Vietti, T. J., and Powers, W. E.   Treatment of Wilms' tumor and factors affecting prognosis. *Cancer* 32:609, 1973.

41. Pingoud, E. G., and Pais, S. O.   Epinephrine renal venography in pseudotumors consisting of normal renal tissue. *Radiology* 131:65, 1979.

42. Pollack, H. M., Edell, S., and Morales, J. O.   Radionuclide imaging in renal pseudotumors. *Radiology* 111:639, 1974.

43. Polsky, M. S., Shackelford, G. D., Weber, C. H., Jr., and Ball, T. P., Jr.   Retroperitoneal teratoma. *Urology* 8:618, 1976.

44. Redman, J. F., and Harper, D. L.   Nephroblastoma occurring in a multilocular cystic kidney. *J. Urol.* 120:356, 1978.

45. Reilly, B. J., and Harwood-Nash, D. C.   Radiological examination of the newborn. *Radiol. Clin. North Am.* 13:171, 1975.

46. Rote, A. R., Flint, L. D., and Ellis, F. H., Jr.   Intracaval recurrence of pheochromocytoma extending into right atrium: Surgical management using extracorporeal circulation. *N. Engl. J. Med.* 296:1269, 1977.

47. Schullinger, J. N., Santulli, T. V., Casarella, W. J., and MacMillan, R. W.   Wilms' tumor: The role of right heart angiography in the management of selected cases. *Ann. Surg.* 185:451, 1977.

48. Scully, R. E., Galdabini, J. J., and McNeely, B. U. (eds.).   Case records of the Massachusetts General Hospital: Case 45-1975. *N. Engl. J. Med.* 193: 1085, 1975.

49. Scully, R. E., Galdabini, J. J., and McNeely, B. U. (eds.).   Case records of the Massachusetts General Hospital: Case 14-1976. *N. Engl. J. Med.* 295:774, 1976.

50. Seldinger, S. I.   Catheter replacement of needle in percutaneous arteriography: New technique. *Acta Radiol.* (Stockh.) 39:368, 1953.

51. Senelick, R. C., Bray, P. F., Lahey, M. E., Van-Dyk, H. J. L., and Johnson, D. G.   Neuroblastoma and myoclonic encephalopathy: Two cases and a review of the literature. *J. Pediatr. Surg.* 8:623, 1973.

52. Slovis, T. L., Cushing, B., Reilly, B. J., Farooki, Z. Q., Philippart, A. I., Berdon, W. E., Baker, D. H., and Reed, J. O.   Wilms' tumor to the heart: Clinical and radiographic evaluation. *AJR* 131: 263, 1978.

53. Takahashi, M.   Percutaneous Catheterization in Infants and Children. In M. T. Gyepes (ed.), *Angiography in Infants and Children*. New York: Grune & Stratton, 1974.

54. Van Way, C. W., III, Michelakis, A. M., Alper, B. J., Hutcheson, J. K., Rhamy, R. K., and Scott, H. W., Jr.   Renal vein renin studies in a patient with renal hilar pheochromocytoma and renal artery stenosis. *Ann. Surg.* 172:212, 1970.

55. Velasquez, G., Nath, P. H., Zollikofer, C., Valdez-Davila, O., Castaneda-Zuniga, W. R., Formanek, A., and Amplatz, K.   The "ring sign" of necrotic pheochromocytoma. *Radiology* 131: 69, 1979.

56. White, R. I., Jr.   Pediatric Angiography. In R. I. White, Jr. (ed.), *Fundamentals of Vascular Radiology*. Philadelphia: Lea & Febiger, 1976.

57. White, R. I., Jr., Giargiana, F. A., Borushok, M., and Harrington, D. P.   A new system for percutaneous catheterization of the pediatric patient. *Radiology* 107:443, 1973.

58. Zelch, J. V., Meaney, T. F., and Belhobeck, G. H.   Radiologic approach to the patient with suspected pheochromocytoma. *Radiology* 111:279, 1974.

Index

Index

Antibiotic therapy—*Continued*
  in mesenteric ischemia, 1743
  in pyelonephritis, 1178, 1179
  after renal trauma, 1240
Antibodies to contrast media, 27
Anticoagulation therapy
  in abdominal aortography, 1030, 1038
  in mesenteric ischemia, 1743
  in pulmonary embolism, 806, 813
Antidiuretic hormone, 98. *See also* Vaso-
    pressin
Antihistamines, for reactions to contrast
    media, 30, 32, 1983
Antihypertensive medications, 1248,
    1344, 1346
Anxiety of patients
  in abdominal aortography, 1031, 1036
  complications related to, 29–30
  in pediatric angiography, 1800
  in renal angiography, 1091
Aorta
  abdominal, 1018–1088. *See also* Abdom-
    inal aorta
  aneurysms of. *See* Aneurysm(s)
  in aortopulmonary window, 413, 737
  arteriosclerosis of. *See* Arteriosclerosis
  arteritis of, 1060, 1279
  coarctation of. *See* Coarctation, of aorta
  in coronary arteriography, 489–490
  coronary artery bypass grafts attached
    to, 693
  in femoral arteriography, 1840, 1843
  grafts of, 478. *See also* Grafts, aortoiliac
  in lung and mediastinal tumors, 842
  renal arteries from, multiple, 1217–
    1221
  supravalvular ring of, 528
  surgery of, 1819–1831
  thoracic, 338–483. *See also* Thoracic
    aorta
  transluminal angioplasty of, 2120–2123
  trauma of, in angiography, 1047
  in vena cava compression, 960
Aortic arch, 18, 226–227, 345, 475–476,
    480–481
  in aberrant vessels, 475, 481
  in adults, 358, 360–362
  aneurysms of, 429, 430, 431
    pulmonary artery occlusion in, 760
  in coarctation of aorta, 389, 392, 395,
    396, 397, 402
    postoperative evaluation of, 404–405
  double, 475, 481
  in infants, 353, 355
  persistent right, 475
  thoracic aortography in anomalies of,
    345
  in trigeminal artery persistence, 475–
    476
  vascular rings of, 475
Aortic bulb, 528
  in adults, 358, 360
  contrast injections in, 559
  in infants, 353, 355
Aortic lymph nodes, 1990, 1993–1994
  computed tomography of, 2080, 2082
  in lymphomas, 2074
  obstruction of, 2052
  size and shape of, 2051
Aortic root, 528–537, 558
  in adults, 358

Aortic root—*Continued*
  aneurysms of, 431
    dissecting, 443
  in infants, 353
Aortic spindle, compared to ductus diver-
    ticulus, 362–363
Aortic valves, 358–360, 467–472
  catheterization of, 472–475, 480–490
  in coarctation of aorta, 403
  coronary arteriography in assessment of,
    473, 515, 570
  insufficiency of, 472–475
  left coronary cusp of, 528
  noncoronary cusp of, 528, 537
  prosthetic replacement of, 472, 570
    postoperative evaluation of, 478
  reflux of contrast material through, 472–
    474
  right coronary cusp of, 528, 536
  stenosis of, 345, 403, 467–468, 470,
    515, 570
Aortitis
  aneurysms in, 429, 1081
  in syphilis, 429
  Takayasu's, 431
Aortoazygos fistula, posttraumatic, 917
Aortobifemoral bypass grafts, 1853
Aortocoronary bypass grafts, 2094, 2095,
    2096
Aortoenteric fistula, after aortoiliac
    surgery, 1828, 1830–1831
Aortography
  abdominal, 1018–1088. *See also* Abdom-
    inal aortography
  complications of, 25
    fatal, 22–23
    neurologic, 1025
  contrast media for, 17, 19, 31
  after coronary bypass surgery, 699
  global, 845, 846–847
  injection rates for, 196
  lumbar. *See* Abdominal aortography
  in mesenteric ischemia, 1736, 1746,
    1749
  in ovarian tumors, 1769
  in pediatric patients, 339, 340, 341,
    1804, 1808
  in pelvic hemorrhage, 1773, 1774,
    1778
  in pheochromocytoma, 1412
  prior to adrenal arteriography, 1397
  renal, 1092, 1107, 1250, 1252
  in retroperitoneal tumors, 1804, 1808
  thoracic, 338–483. *See also* Thoracic aor-
    tography
Aortoiliac system, 1819–1831
  aneurysms in, 1825, 1828, 1831
  arteriosclerosis of, 1057, 1058, 1827,
    1828, 1853
  barium studies of, 1831
  catheterization of, 1819–1824, 1825,
    1827
  collateral circulation in, 1065, 1069–
    1076
  complications in surgery of, 1827, 1854
  computed tomography of, 1828, 1829,
    1831
  computerized fluoroscopy of, 1825–
    1827
  endarterectomy of, 1853
  endoscopy of, 1831

Aortoiliac system—*Continued*
  filming techniques for, 1824–1825,
    1827, 1828, 1831
  fistula in, 1828, 1830–1831
  grafts in, 1819, 1821, 1823, 1824, 1825,
    1853–1854. *See also* Grafts, aor-
    toiliac
  isotope scan of, 1829
  in Leriche syndrome, 1066
  occlusions of, 1063–1066
    in chronic thrombosis, 1063, 1066
  pseudoaneurysms of, 1825, 1827,
    1828–1830, 1831, 1854
  revascularization of, 1851, 1853–1854
  steal syndrome of, 1749
  transluminal angioplasty in, 2120–2123,
    2130–2131
  ultrasonography of, 1827, 1828, 1829,
    1831
Aortopulmonary window or fenestration,
    413, 737
  pulmonary hypertension in, 764
Aplasia
  of coronary arteries, 531
  of lymphatic systems, 2024
  renal, 1225
Appendiceal arteries, 1024, 1626
Appendix
  blood supply of, 1024, 1026
  carcinoid tumors of, 1651
Aramine, 34
Arch aortography, *See* Thoracic aortog-
    raphy
Arcuate renal arteries, 210, 1109, 1113–
    1115, 1250
Arcuate renal veins, 1332
Arms. *See also* Upper extremity arteriogra-
    phy
  lymphatic system of, 1981–1982, 1994–
    1995
Arrest, cardiopulmonary, as reaction to an-
    giography, 33, 34
  treatment of, 79–87. *See also* Cardiopul-
    monary resuscitation
Arrhythmias
  coronary arteriography in, 571
  as reaction to angiography, 22, 23, 24,
    31–32, 34, 83, 86, 88–90
    in coronary arteriography, 505, 511
    in pulmonary arteriography, 708, 711
    in pulmonary embolism, 812, 813
  treatment of, 34
Arteria
  accessoria, 534
  anastomotica auricularia magna, 639
  magna, 420, 1080
  magna et dolicho, 1080
Arterial sheath, for coronary arteriogra-
    phy, 487–488, 489
Arteriectasis, of upper extremity arteries,
    1928
Arteriomegaly, 1080
Arteriosclerosis, 192
  of abdominal aorta and branches, 1022,
    1029, 1030, 1032, 1038, 1057–
    1076
  aneurysms in, 1063, 1080, 1081,
    1087
  angiographic appearance of, 1058–
    1066
  calcifications in, 1060–1061

Robb needle, in retrograde brachial aortography, 340
Rodriguez-Alvarez catheter, 192
Roentgen, W. C., 3
Roentgen-area-product meter, monitoring patient exposure to radiation, 171
Roentgenographic plain films. *See* Plain films
Roll film
  advantages of, 108, 111
  cameras for, 141
  compared to cut-film, 108, 111
Roll-film changers, 108, 111, 115–120
  Amplatz, 116–119
  CGR, 119–120
  Elema, 115–116
  Franklin, 116
  Ruggles, 105, 106
Rosenthal, basal veins, 257, 259–260, 261
Rotational mounting units, multiangulation, 178–179
Rotational scanography, 123
Ruggles roll-film changer, 105, 106

Saccular aneurysms, of abdominal aorta, 1080, 1084
Sacral arteries
  in aortic occlusion, 1073
  lateral, 1838
  middle, 1025
  supplementary renal arteries from, 1220
Sacral veins, 895, 900
Sacrum, tumors of, embolization therapy for, 2161–2163
Safety
  of angiography, 96
  of equipment
    electrical, 171–172
    quality assurance programs for, 167–169
  of patients, monitoring of, 156–158
Sagittal sinus, superior, 260
Salt, dietary, renin production affected by, 1344
Sanchez-Perez cassette changer, 110, 111
Sandbag use, after angiography, 1046
Saphenous veins, 1880–1881, 1882
  accessory, 1881
  in bypass grafts, 693–695
    in renovascular hypertension, postoperative assessment of, 1291–1293
  incompetence of, 1910–1911, 1915, 1916
  long, 1880–1881
  short, 1880
  varicose, 1908, 1911
  in vertebral venography, 898
Saralasin, in detection of renovascular hypertension, 1253
Sarcoidosis, 929
  hypercalcemia in, 977
  lymphangiography in, 2044
  pulmonary, 749, 750
Sarcomas
  chondrosarcomas, 1869
  embolization of, 1975
  Ewing's, 1954
  fibrosarcomas, 1869
  liposarcomas, 1869
  osteogenic, 1869, 1935, 1947–1952

Sarcomas—*Continued*
  of prostate, 1768
  of pulmonary artery, 842
  renal, 1806
  reticulum cell, 1452, 1558, 1560, 1643, 1653, 1954
  retroperitoneal, 1789, 1792, 1811
  rhabdomyosarcomas, 1789, 1811, 1869, 1969
  of soft tissues, 1969–1970
  synovial, 1968
  of upper extremity, 1935
  of vena cava, 971
Satellite anastomotic circulation, 634
Scalenus anticus syndrome, 1002–1004, 1930
Scanning, radionuclide. *See* Radionuclide studies
Scapular arteries, 393, 395
Schönander film changers, 107, 111
  tubes for use with, 135
  in upper extremity arteriography, 1925
Schoonmaker-King technique, in coronary arteriography, 501
Schwannoma
  renal, 1159
  vascularity of, 301
Scimitar sign and syndrome, in anomalous pulmonary connections, 884, 885, 886, 887–888, 889–890, 891
Scintigraphy, *See* Radionuclide studies
Sclerosing agents, for tissue ablation, 2181–2184
Sclerosing cholangitis, 2369–2373
Sclerosing mediastinitis, vena cava obstruction in, 926
Sclerosis, Mönckeberg's, 574, 582
Screens
  calcium tungstate, 177
  for cine film viewing, 153–154
  in magnification angiography, 207–208
  rare-earth, 137, 176, 177–178
Secobarbital, in arterial portography, 1606
Secondary radiation, affecting radiographic image, 109, 123
Secretion
  in mesenteric angiography, 1631
  in pancreatic angiography, 1438, 1439
Sedatives, in renal angiography, 1091
Segmental pulmonary arteries, 719, 720, 721–722, 739, 792
Segmental renal arteries, 1109–1112
Segmental vertebral veins, 900, 903
Seizure activity, as complication of angiography, 1042
  in spinal arteriography, 320, 333
  in thoracic aortography, 347, 348
  treatment of, 33
Seldinger catheterization technique, 188, 190
  in abscess drainage, modification of, 2340, 2342–2344
  in bone and soft tissue tumors, 1938
  in bronchial arteriography, 853
  in carotid angiography, 219, 221
  in coronary angioplasty, 2088
  in hepatic arterial infusion chemotherapy, 2290
  in jugular venography, 227
  in pediatric angiography, 1800

Seldinger catheterization technique—*Continued*
  in pelvic angiography, 1753, 1774
  in portography, arterial, 1606
  in pulmonary angiography, 818
  in renal angiography, 1091
  in thoracic aortography, 342
  in vena cavography, 941
  in vertebral venography, 897
Selectan, 8, 15
  chemical composition of, 54
  generic name of, 68
Sengstaken-Blakemore tube, 1514
Sensitivity testing, 27, 30, 97, 98
  in abdominal aortography, 1031
  in carotid angiography, 221
  effectiveness of, 30, 1045
  in thoracic aortography, 340
Sensitometric film, in quality control program, 165
Sephadex particles, for embolic material, 2136, 2142
Sepsis, after biliary interventional procedures, 2375, 2376–2377, 2385
Septal defects
  aortic, 413–415
    thoracic aortography in, 344
  atrial. *See* Atrial septal defects
  ventricular, 415. *See also* Ventricles of heart, septal defects of
Septal lines, in anomalous pulmonary vein connections, 876
Septicemia
  after renal biopsy, 2324
  splenic artery aneurysms in, 1550
Sequestration, pulmonary, 476–477, 738
  bronchial arteriography in, 845, 846, 858
  intralobar and extralobar, 858
  thoracic aortography in, 345
Serbinenko balloon catheters, 2225–2226
Serial filming, 105–123. *See also* Rapid filming
Sheath, arterial, in coronary arteriography, 487–488, 489
Sheehan's syndrome, 1419
Shock
  as complication of angiography, 33–34
  in lymphangiography, 1985
  mesenteric ischemia in, 1740
  after renal trauma, 1233, 1234, 1236, 1240
Shunting
  in aortic aneurysm rupture, 434
  in aortic septal defect, 413
  arteriovenous, *See* Arteriovenous fistulas, acquired
  in coronary artery fistulas, 675–677
  in ductus arteriosus patency, 372, 374, 376, 389, 395, 737, 2259, 2260
  hepatic arterial-portal venous, 1482, 1483
  left-to-right, 723
    in anomalous pulmonary vein connections, 873, 875, 886, 890–891
    in aortopulmonary window, 737
    Eisenmenger reaction in, 767
    pulmonary hypertension in, 764, 765, 767, 794
  in lung and mediastinal tumors, 842

Spleen—*Continued*
abscesses of, 1556, 1567, 1568
accessory tissue in, 1545
in anemia, hemolytic, 1531, 1551, 1553
arteriovenous fistula in, 1551
asplenia, 1545–1547
    inferior vena cava in, 949–950
barium studies of, 1545, 1548, 1554,
    1568
computed tomography of, 1531, 1545,
    1568
congenital anomalies of, 1543–1547
cysts of, 1554–1557, 1565
in hypersplenism, 1543, 1551, 1568,
    2135, 2141, 2142, 2176, 2177,
    2199–2201
infarction of, 1151
interventional techniques for, 1567–
    1568, 2135, 2141, 2142, 2176,
    2177–2178, 2198–2201, 2205
nontraumatic rupture of, 1567
normal vascular anatomy of, 1531–
    1539, 1576–1581
polysplenia, 905, 1547
in portal hypertension, 1531, 1551
portography of, arterial, 1606, 1609
radionuclide scanning of, 1543, 1545,
    1547, 1568
in splenomegaly, 1542–1543, 1568
splenoportography of, 1573–1601. *See
    also* Splenoportography
in splenosis, 1545
trauma of, 1531, 1545, 1551, 1560–
    1567, 1568
    conservative management of, 1565
    delayed rupture in, 1565–1567
    diagnostic decision pathway in, 1568
tumors of, 1556, 1558–1560, 1568
    benign, 1558
    malignant, 1558–1560
    metastatic, 1560, 1568
ultrasonography of, 1543, 1545, 1568
in urography. *See* Urography, spleen in
wandering or ectopic, 1543–1545
Splenectomy
medical, 2198–2201
partial, 1565
portography after, arterial, 1606, 1607,
    1615–1616
risks and benefits of, 1568
Splenic arteries, 1531–1568
in abdominal plain films, 1548, 1550
age-related changes in, 1532, 1539
aneurysms of, 1548–1551. *See also* An-
    eurysms, of splenic artery
arteriography of, 1531–1568. *See also*
    Splenic arteriography
arteriosclerosis of, 1023, 1540, 1548
circulation time in, 1539
diameter of, 1538
distribution of, 1532, 1538
    distributed configuration of, 1532,
        1538
    magistral configuration of, 1532,
        1538
gastric, 1535, 1537
gastroepiploic, 1535, 1538
inferior terminal, 1535, 1538
length and width measurements of,
    1532, 1538–1539
in mesenteric angiography, 1630

Splenic arteries—*Continued*
normal anatomy of, 1023–1024, 1427,
    1428, 1531–1539
origin of, 1531–1532, 1537
pancreatic, 1428, 1431–1433, 1532–
    1535, 1537–1538, 1539
in pancreatitis, 1452, 1454, 1455
polar, 1535–1537, 1538
in portography, arterial, 1606, 1607,
    1619
prehilar, 1428, 1532, 1538
prepancreatic, 1428, 1532, 1538, 1539
in renal artery obstruction, 1292
selective catheterization of, 1439
superior terminal, 1535, 1538
suprapancreatic, 1428, 1532, 1537,
    1538–1539
terminal, 1535, 1538
tortuosity of, 1532, 1539
trauma of, 1458
Splenic arteriography, 1531–1568
in abscesses of spleen, 1567
accessory splenic tissue in, 1545
in aneurysms of splenic artery, 1548–
    1551
in arteriosclerosis, 1548
in arteriovenous fistula, splenic, 1551
in arteritis of splenic artery, 1548, 1550
in asplenia, 1545–1547
in cirrhosis, 1551, 1552
compared to other imaging procedures,
    1568
in congenital anomalies, 1543–1547
contrast media in, 18, 21
in cysts of spleen, 1554–1556
in dysplasia of splenic artery, 1548
in gastrointestinal bleeding, 1673, 1677
hepatic arteriography with, 1503
in infarction of spleen, 1551
interventional occlusive techniques in,
    1567–1568, 2141, 2142, 2176,
    2177–2178
    for medical splenectomy, 2198–2201
normal anatomy in, 1531–1539
in pancreatic carcinoma, 1539–1542
in polysplenia, 1547
in portal hypertension, 1551, 1552,
    1619
portal vein in, 1606, 1607, 1619
postoperative, after splenorenal shunts,
    1552
posttraumatic, 1560–1567
spinal cord damage in, 330
in splanchnic vein occlusion, 1552–1554
in splenomegaly, 1542–1543
in thrombosis of splenic artery, 1551
in tumors of spleen, 1556, 1558–1560,
    1568
in wandering spleen, 1543–1545
Splenic lymph nodes, 2074
computed tomography of, 2082
ultrasonography of, 2077
Splenic veins, 1433, 1552–1554, 1613–
    1615
anatomy of, 1467, 1581–1583
arteriovenous fistula of, 1551
catheterization of, 1470–1471
circulation time in, 1539
collateral circulation in obstruction of,
    1590–1591, 1613–1615
dislocation of, 1601

Splenic veins—*Continued*
in pancreatic carcinoma, 1473, 1524
in portal hypertension, 1507, 1509,
    1619
portography of, arterial, 1609, 1613–
    1615, 1619
splenoportography of, 1573–1601. *See
    also* Splenoportography
width of, 1580–1581
Splenomegaly, 1542–1543
diagnostic decision pathway in, 1568
interventional techniques in, 1567–
    1568
portography in, arterial, 1607
splenoportography in, 1575
Splenoportal roentgenography. *See*
    Splenoportography
Splenoportography, 1573–1601
catheters and catheterization techniques
    in, 196, 1574
in cirrhosis, 1587, 1591, 1593–1601
contraindications to, 1576
contrast media in, 18
extrahepatic vessels in, 1601
    anatomy of, 1581–1583
    obstruction of, 1590–1591
hazards of, 1574–1575, 1576
hemodynamics in, 1576–1581
    in vascular obstruction, 1583–1591
in hepatic tumors, 1492, 1601
hepatographic phase of, 1580, 1583,
    1601
historical aspects of, 1573, 1605
indications for, 1575
intrahepatic vessels in
    anatomy of, 1583
    in cirrhosis, 1593–1601
    in malignant tumors, 1601
    obstruction of, 1587–1590, 1591
nonvisualization of splenoportal axis in,
    1617–1619
normal anatomy in, 1581–1583
patient position for, 1520
in portal hypertension, 1587, 1605,
    1609, 1617–1619
in portal vein dislocation, 1601
after portacaval shunt, 1591
in portosystemic collateral flow, 1509
technique of, 1573–1574
Splenorenal surgical shunts, 1616–1617
preoperative and postoperative evalua-
    tion in, 1355–1356
splenic artery changes after, 1552
Splenosis, 1545
Split-function tests, renal, 1253, 1261,
    1266
Spongel, 864
Spot-film techniques, 130
in biliary interventional procedures,
    2386, 2390
cameras for, 141–142, 178
cinefluorography compared to, 141
coning in, 137
costs of, 142
electrical power requirements for, 134
film for, 146, 590
image intensifiers for, 139
in ischemic heart disease, 162
radiographic tubes for, 136, 137
Sprue, mesenteric angiography in, 1643
Squamous cell carcinoma, renal, 1153, 1190

Upper extremity arteriography—*Continued*
  in Raynaud's phenomenon, 1925, 1932, 1933–1934, 1936
  in spasms, arterial, 1934
  in stenoses and thromboses, 1930–1933
  in thoracic outlet syndrome, 1934
  in tumors, 1928–1929, 1936, 1938
Upper extremity lymphatic system, 1994–1995
Urea hydrochloride, as sclerosing agent, 2181
Ureter
  circumcaval, 948
  obstruction of
    after biopsy, 2324, 2325
    hydronephrosis in, 1201–1215. *See also* Hydronephrosis
    oliguria in, 1301, 1316, 1319, 1320, 1322
    nephrostomy in, percutaneous, 2281–2283
    in renal transplantation, 1385–1387
    in renal tumors, 1156
  retrocaval, 948
  retrograde catheterization of, 1301, 1316, 1319
  transcaval, 948
Ureteric artery, 1115
Ureteric veins, 1332, 1334
  in vena cava obstruction, 951–952, 955, 957
Ureteropelvic junction, in hydronephrosis, 1201, 1213, 1215
Urinary tract. *See* Genitourinary tract
Urine
  albumin levels in, after renal angiography, 1100
  blood in. *See* Hematuria
  cytologic examination of, in renal pelvic tumors, 1153
  in oliguria, 1299–1322
Urogenital ridge remnant, tumors of, 1790
Urografin, 19, 70. *See also* Diatrizoate contrast media
  chemical composition of, 43, 46
  generic name of, 70
  in splenoportography, 1574
  in upper extremity arteriography, 1925, 1926
Urography. *See also* Pyelography
  abdominal aortography before, 1035
  in adrenal adenocarcinoma, 1419
  complications of, 1321
    fatal, 26
    respiratory, 25
  contrast media in, 17
  historical aspects of, 4, 7, 15
  lymphangiography with, 1981, 2077
  in renal disorders
    in abscesses, 1181
    in arteriovenous fistulas, 1273
    in carcinoma, 1131
    in cyst(s), 1165–1166
    in cystic disease, 1226
    in fibrolipomatosis, 1356
    in hydronephrosis, 1201, 1202, 1207, 1212, 1213
    in hypertension, 1253
    in pelvic tumors, 1153
    in pseudotumors, 1159

Urography, in renal disorders—*Continued*
    in pyelonephritis, 1178, 1179, 1191, 1197
    in stenosis, 1250
    in thrombosis, 1352
    in trauma, 1232, 1233–1234, 1236, 1237, 1277
    in tuberculosis, 1194, 1195
    in varices, 1353
    in Wilms' tumor, 1125
  in retroperitoneal fibrosis, 2034
  sensitivity testing in, 30
  spleen in, 1568
    in congenital anomalies, 1545
    in cysts, 1556
  thoracic aortography before, 343–344
  in ureteral obstruction in oliguria, 1301, 1316, 1319
Urokinase, in pulmonary embolism, 754, 812, 813
Urokon, 15, 16–17, 1043, 1048. *See also* Acetrizoate sodium
  blood vessel reactions to, 25
  central nervous system reactions to, 20, 22
  chemical composition of, 42
  generic name of, 70
  renal reactions to, 22, 1321
  in thoracic aortography, 346
  toxicity of, 16
Uromiro, 70–71. *See also* Iodamide contrast media
Uroselection, 707. *See also* Neo-Iopax
USCI catheters, 197–200
Uterine arteries, 1027
  in cervical carcinoma, 1769
  in fibromyomas, 1768
  in ovarian tumors, 1769
Uterine veins, 1782–1783
Uterus, 1768, 1769–1773
  carcinoma of
    cervical, 1769–1773, 2052–2053
    in corpus, 2053
    metastatic, 2052–2053
  fibromyomas of, 1768, 1769
  pelvic angiography of, 1768–1773
  radiation-induced fibrosis of, 1770, 1773
  ultrasonography and computed tomography of, 1769, 1770

Vacuum contact system of film cassettes, 110–111
Vagina, carcinoma of, 2053
Valium, 220. *See also* Diazepam (Valium)
Valsalva maneuver, 788, 896
  in adrenal angiography, 1399
  in jugular venography, 227
  in lower extremity venography, 1884, 1885, 1886, 1888, 1911
  in parathyroid venous sampling, 989
  in pulmonary angiography, 817
  in spinal angiography, 321
  in vena cavography, 940, 942, 943, 952, 971
Valsalva sinus, 353, 358, 528
  aneurysms of, 418, 428, 429, 431–434
  aortic narrowing above, 468, 470, 472
  coronary arteries originating from, 678–682, 685
  rupture of, 374, 376

Valves
  aortic. *See* Aortic valves
  in lower extremity veins, 1882, 1883
    normal appearance of, 1888
    in varicose veins, 1908, 1910
  in lymphatic system, 1990, 2003, 2015, 2018
    in fistulas, 2034
    incompetent, 2024, 2025
  mitral. *See* Mitral valves
  pulmonary, stenosis of, 723, 729–731
  in renal veins, 1328, 1338–1339
  in thyroid veins, 989
Vanguard cine viewers, 155
Vanillylmandelic acid levels
  in bladder neoplasms, 1762
  in neuroblastoma, 1808
  in pheochromocytoma, 1411
VariCath films, 147
Varices. *See* Varicosities
Varicocele
  of spermatic vein, angiographic treatment of, 2281
  testicular, balloon occlusion in, 2220–2221
Varicose aneurysm of thoracic aorta, 428
Varicosities
  esophageal. *See* Esophagus, varices of
  gastric, in splenic vein occlusion, 1552–1554
  of lower extremity, 1886, 1891, 1906, 1908–1914, 1916–1917
    centrifugal theory of, 1910
    centripetal theory of, 1910
    primary, 1908, 1910, 1911
    recurrent, 1913–1914
    secondary, 1908, 1910, 1911
  pulmonary artery
    congenital, 738–739
    flow-caliber relationship of vessel in, 791
  sclerosing agents for, 2181
Vasa recta, 1626, 1702
  in colitis, 1722
Vasa vasorum, aortic, 848
  aneurysms in infections of, 428, 429
Vascoray. *See* Iothalamate contrast media, meglumine
Vasoactive drugs, 24–25, 95–102
  availability of, 96
  in bone and soft tissue tumor studies, 1939
  in complications from angiography, 91, 92, 93
  in coronary arteriography, 559
  dose-response curve of, 96
  in femoral arteriography, 1848
  in gastrointestinal bleeding
    for control, 1676–1679
    for studies, 1673
  in hepatic arteriography, 1492–1496
  in mesenteric angiography, 1629, 1631–1635, 1640, 1648, 1651, 1702
  in pancreatic angiography, 1433, 1436–1439, 1440, 1444–1446, 1447
  in pelvic angiography, 1754, 1778, 1779
  in portography, arterial, 1607–1608
  pulmonary hypertension related to, 765
  in renal angiography, 95, 1099. *See also* Renal angiography, vasoactive drugs in

Vasoactive drugs—*Continued*
safety of, 96
tissue ablation with, 2175–2187
vasoconstrictors, 96, 97–98
vasodilators, 96, 98–102
Vasoactive intestinal polypeptide
pancreatic venous sampling for, 1471
tumors producing, 1448, 1473
Vasopressin, 95
antidiuretic properties of, 1676, 1697
in gastrointestinal bleeding, 95, 96,
1676–1679, 1684–1691, 2155–
2156
complications of, 1697
diverticular, 1689–1690, 1724
esophageal, 1677–1679, 1685
in inflammatory disease, 1690–1691
in ischemic colitis, 1724
in tumors, 1695–1697
in hepatic arteriography, 1483, 1492
mesenteric ischemia from therapy with,
1639, 1733, 1740, 1743
in pancreatic angiography, 1436
in pelvic angiography, 1778
in splenic arteriography, posttraumatic,
1562
in splenic hemorrhage, 2176
vasoactive effects of, 96, 98
Vena cava
inferior, 895, 897, 905, 939–973
absence of, 903, 905, 915–916, 949,
950
anomalous pulmonary vein connections with, 872, 873, 883, 884,
885, 887
blood flow velocity in, 970–971
communications of, 900
computed tomography of, 943, 950,
960–962, 971
congenital anomalies of, 947–950,
963–964
drainage into left atrium, 903
embryogenesis of, 945–947
hepatic segment of, 905, 915, 950
interruption of, 905, 916
left-sided, 949
normal anatomy of, 939
obstruction of, 895, 905, 916, 950–
964, 966–968, 971
central collateral channels in, 951, 957
course of communicating vessels in,
950–951
extrinsic, 958–963
infrarenal, 950, 951–955, 964
intermediate collateral channels in,
951–952, 957
intrinsic, 963–964
midcaval, 950, 955–957, 964
portal collateral routes in, 952–953,
954–955, 957, 958
practical and potential collateral
routes in, 950–958
size of communicating stoma in,
951
superficial collateral routes in, 953–
954, 957
upper, 950, 957–958, 963–964
valves in, 951
persistent left, 905, 916
postrenal segment of, 948–949
prerenal segment of, 949

Vena cava, inferior—*Continued*
prophylactic filter in, 941, 968–970
in pulmonary embolism, 916, 966–
970
recanalization of, 968
thrombosis of, 963–964
ultrasonography of, 971
vena cavography of, 940–943. *See also*
Vena cavography, inferior
superior, 895, 903, 923–936
anomalous pulmonary vein connections with, 872, 873, 877, 880,
881, 883, 884–885, 887, 891
bilateral, 905
in coronary artery fistulas, 675, 676
drainage into left atrium, 905
in inferior vena cava obstruction, 957,
958
in lung and mediastinal tumors, 823,
824, 925–926
normal anatomy of, 924
obstruction of
in aneurysms, 929
bypass grafts in, 926
collateral circulation in, 895, 905,
916, 923, 924, 925, 926
in fibrosis, 929
in infectious diseases, 929
in tumors, 925–926, 929
ostium of, 524, 548–549
parathyroid hormone levels in, 990
persistent left, 903, 936
in sclerosing mediastinitis, 926
syndrome of, 923, 924–935
Vena cavography
inferior, 897
in adrenal neoplasms, 959–960
azygos veins in, 915–916
biocclusive, 942
capnocavography technique of, 942
collateral circulation in, 950–958,
966–968, 971
complications of, 972
computed tomography in, 943, 950,
960–962, 971
contrast media in, 18, 940, 941, 942,
953
in extrinsic obstruction, 958–963
femoral approach for, 940–941, 971
filling defects in, 971
historical aspects of, 940–941, 950
in iliac vein spurs, 972–973
indications for, 950
interpretation of, pitfalls in, 971
in intrinsic obstruction, 963–964
limitations of, 962
lymphangiography with, 1981–1985,
2077
in lymphatic tumors, 960, 961–962,
2054
needles used in, 940, 941
in obstruction of vena cava, 950–964
postangiographic procedures in, 941–
942
postoperative, 950, 966–970
in pregnancy, 963
in primary tumors of cava, 971
projections for, 941, 972
in recurrent embolization, 966–970
in renal tumors, 941, 959–960, 964,
1128, 1145, 1339–1342, 1804

Vena cavography, inferior—*Continued*
renal veins in, 1328
in retroperitoneal fibrosis, 2034
^{99m}technetium in, 943
techniques of, 940–943, 971
ultrasonography in, 942–943, 971
superior, 923–936
contrast media in, 18
indications for, 923–924, 936
technique of, 924
in vena cava syndrome, 925–926
Ventilation, artificial, in reactions to angiographic procedures, 81–83, 84,
93–94
Ventricles of brain, tumors of, 303–305
Ventricles of heart, 715, 743–744, 797
akinesis of, 491, 573
aneurysms of, 569
arrhythmias of, 571
asynergy of, 572–573, 620–621
in atrial septal defect, 724
biplane assessment of, 158, 161, 162,
621
in collateral circulation, 636–637, 654,
655
in coronary arteriography, 488–491,
569, 571, 660–661, 697
coronary artery branches to, 525, 538,
540, 542, 545, 558, 559
in coronary artery fistulas, 676, 677
dyskinesis of, 491, 573
hypertrophy of, 743–744
hypokinesis of, 491, 573
in pulmonary circulation, 763
in pulmonary embolism, 751
in pulmonary hypertension, 725, 743–
744, 764, 765, 766, 767–768,
769, 771, 772, 773, 784
radionuclide studies of, 592
reactions to angiography, 88, 89, 90, 91,
93, 160
reflux of contrast media in, 472–474
septal blood supply, 525, 549
septal defects of
in anomalous pulmonary vein connections, 873, 883, 890
bronchial arteriography in, 846, 860–
861
compared to atrial septal defects, 725
pulmonary atresia with, 860–861
pulmonary hypertension in, 725,
743–744, 764, 765
septal perforation, coronary arteriography in, 570
in thoracic aortography, 341
ventriculography of, 158, 491–492. *See
also* Ventriculography
Ventricular cerebral veins, inferior, 260
Ventricularization of pressure, in coronary
arteriography, 492, 494, 495,
661
Ventriculography, 158, 490–491, 568,
592
in anomalous pulmonary vein connections, 881
in aortic stenosis, 468
in asynergy, 572–573, 620–621
biplane technique of, 158, 161, 162
catheter for, 161, 192
complications of, 510
contrast injections for, 161